Y0-BRQ-511

# Acid-Base and Electrolyte Disorders

# Acid-Base and Electrolyte Disorders

## A COMPANION TO *Brenner & Rector's* THE KIDNEY

**Thomas D. DuBose, Jr., MD**
Peter T. Bohan Professor and Chair of Internal Medicine
Professor of Molecular and Integrative Physiology
University of Kansas School of Medicine
Kansas City, Kansas

**L. Lee Hamm, MD**
Professor of Medicine and Physiology
Tulane University School of Medicine
Chief of Nephrology and Hypertension
Vice-Chairman, Department of Medicine
Tulane University Health Sciences Center
New Orleans, Louisiana

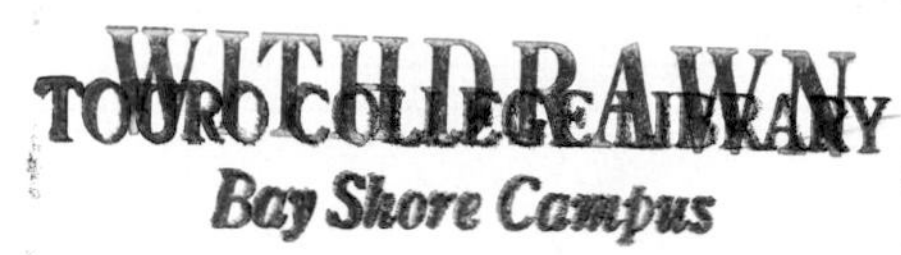


SAUNDERS
An Imprint of Elsevier Science
Philadelphia London New York St. Louis Sydney Toronto

BS

**SAUNDERS**
An Imprint of Elsevier Science

The Curtis Center
Independence Square West
Philadelphia, Pennsylvania 19106

ACID-BASE AND ELECTROLYTE DISORDERS: A COMPANION TO BRENNER & RECTOR'S THE KIDNEY

ISBN 0–7216–8956–6



## Notice

Medicine is an ever-changing field. Standard safety precautions must be followed, but as new research and clinical experience broaden our knowledge, changes in treatment and drug therapy may become necessary or appropriate. Readers are advised to check the most current product information provided by the manufacturer of each drug to be administered to verify the recommended dose, the method and duration of administration, and the contraindications. It is the responsibility of the treating physician, relying on experience and knowledge of the patient, to determine the dosages and the best treatment for each individual patient. Neither the publisher nor the editor assumes any liability for any injury and/or damage to persons or property arising from this publication.

The Publisher

**Library of Congress Cataloging-in-Publication Data**

DuBose, Thomas D.
Acid-base and electrolyte disorders: a companion to Brenner & Rector's the kidney/
Thomas D. DuBose, Jr., L. Lee Hamm.
p. cm.
Includes bibliographical references.
ISBN 0–7216–8956–6
1. Kidneys—Diseases. 2. Kidney. 3. Acid-base imbalances. 4. Water-electrolyte imbalances. I. Hamm, L. Lee. II. Brenner & Rector's the kidney. III. Title.

RC902.K53 2000 Suppl.
616.3′992–dc21 2001032848

*Acquisition Editor:* Sue Hodgson
*Project Manager:* Mary Anne Folcher
*Manuscript Editor:* Marjory Fraser
*Illustration Specialist:* Peg Shaw

Printed in the United States of America

Last digit is the print number: 9 8 7 6 5 4 3 2 1

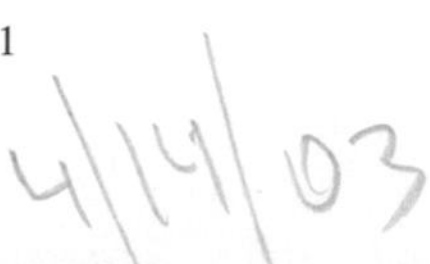

*To our families, trainees, associates, and mentors who have made our work in this fundamental area of nephrology and physiology possible*

*To Donald W. Seldin for his contributions to the field, our personal careers, and most especially his unique ability to correlate pathophysiological concept with clinical medicine in an understandable and inspiring fashion*

# Foreword

The latest edition of *Brenner and Rector's The Kidney,* appeared in the year 2000. Its coverage is comprehensive and thorough, ranging over the entire field of nephrology, probing in depth the pathogenesis, diagnosis, and treatment of renal disease, as well as exploring such basic underlying disciplines as renal physiology, immunonephrology, genetics, and renal endocrinology. This being so, why this additional text, *Acid-Base and Electrolyte Disorders?*

Drs. DuBose and Hamm are fully cognizant of the formidable character of the parent textbook. They have no intention of producing a mere update or precis. Instead, they have designed a novel treatment of a more focused segment of nephrology, which is both fresh and stimulating. This text, unlike its senior companion, is confined to classic renal physiology—an analysis of normal and deranged electrolyte metabolism—not to the entire field of nephrology. This focus allows for a denser treatment of basic principles and their physiologic derangements. There is a deliberate omission of detailed discussions of individual renal diseases. Ketoacidosis, for example, is treated in depth, but the massive and complicated domain of clinical diabetes mellitus is not.

This concentration on normal and deranged renal physiology has great virtues. It affords an understanding of basic processes underlying a whole variety of different disease states. Novel areas, neglected in most textbooks, are treated here in detail. Genetic disorders of epithelial ion transport, renal tubular acidosis, and water transport are given extensive exposition in order to furnish a background for the mechanisms of a broad class of tubular disorders. The treatment of the regulation of specific electrolytes is subdivided into extensive individual chapters, rather than having a chapter or two cover the entire subject matter. Potassium metabolism, for example, is discussed in three individual chapters so as to present a thorough assessment of the entire spectrum of disorders. Similarly, acid-base balance—normal regulation, physiologic disturbances, diagnosis, and treatment—is explored in twelve chapters, thereby providing dense coverage from basic principles to overt disorders.

*Acid-Base and Electrolyte Disorders* also has a practical bent. The physiologic background is carefully interwoven to provide a logical basis for diagnosis and treatment, rather than a simple catalog of diagnostic and therapeutic formulae.

It is a distinct pleasure to welcome this fresh and innovative textbook. Drs. DuBose and Hamm are distinguished investigators who have made significant contributions to the understanding of normal and abnormal electrolyte metabolism. They are both highly competent clinicians, with extensive experience both in nephrology and general internal medicine. Their deep appreciation of basic renal physiology provides the conceptual framework for the diagnosis and treatment of a broad spectrum of renal diseases. The text is a pleasure to read—renal physiology coupled with practical application providing a framework for a rational approach to the patient.

DONALD W. SELDIN, MD
William Buchanan Chair of Internal Medicine
University of Texas Southwestern Medical Center at Dallas, Dallas, Texas

# Preface

*Acid-Base and Electrolyte Disorders: A Companion to Brenner & Rector's The Kidney* is intended for all students who study acid-base and electrolyte disorders. It is particularly useful to medical students, house officers, nephrology fellows, and clinical nephrologists.

We have tried to provide a concise and practical approach by emphasizing pathophysiology. This, in turn, is linked to logical diagnostic approaches and therapy of acid-base and electrolyte abnormalities.

Disorders of acid-base and electrolyte homeostasis have interested nephrologists for many decades. Indeed, this subject represents the very foundation of the subspecialty of nephrology. Accordingly, the challenge of solving difficult acid-base and electrolyte problems has served as an intellectual attraction to the field for many. To appeal to such a diverse audience, the approach in *Acid-Base and Electrolyte Disorders* should be viewed as distinct from the more detailed approach in *Brenner & Rector's The Kidney*. The material in the parent text has served as a springboard from which to launch and amplify discussion of the clinical disorders, avoiding overemphasis on complex physiological and pathophysiological concepts. In this respect, a goal of this text is to provide a practical resource on the subject for students, while serving as a core curriculum for nephrology fellows preparing for their careers.

The text is divided into five sections: acid-base disorders and disorders in metabolism of water, sodium, potassium, and divalent ions. To cover these broad areas, we have selected an internationally distinguished panel of experts as contributors. We have also attempted to separate the subject matter in each section into relatively small self-contained chapters, avoiding repetition and certainly contradiction in subsequent chapters. Diagnostic and treatment algorithms are developed whenever possible. The chapter contributors have provided very specific recommendations for therapy so that the text may serve as a precise guideline, rather than a general review, for therapeutic intervention.

Many of the issues covered in *Acid-Base and Electrolyte Disorders* have not been emphasized in other similar texts. Acid-base disorders in the critical care setting, for example, have not been treated elsewhere comprehensively. Chapters in the areas of renal tubular acidosis; polyuric disorders; renin-angiotensin systems; genetic disorders of renal electrolyte transport; genetic abnormalities associated with hypertension; electrolyte abnormalities in the intensive care patient; and renal calcium receptor and associated abnormalities all represent areas in which late advances in genetics and molecular biology have resulted in an explosion of related knowledge. We have strived that the subject matter be current, and emphasis placed on new developments in the field. We trust that this text will serve as a valuable resource for those in other scientific disciplines who may wish to update their knowledge on the current state of pathophysiology, diagnosis, and therapy of disorders in this rapidly developing field.

Readers are encouraged to refer to the parent text for detailed discussion of the physiology of some of the disorders covered here, as well as a more detailed reference list. We insure that the reference list, while adequate, is highly focused and includes and acknowledges landmark studies.

We thank the contributing authors for their contemporary and scholarly dissertations on these pertinent topics in acid-base and electrolyte homeostasis. Most especially we wish to thank Marla Lampp at the University of Kansas for her skillful organizational and editorial assistance. Finally we wish to thank the staff at Saunders Elsevier Science, especially Richard Zorab and Sabrina Price.

THOMAS D. DUBOSE, JR., MD
L. LEE HAMM, MD

# Contributors

**Horacio J. Adrogué, MD**
Professor of Medicine, Baylor College of Medicine; Chief, Renal Section, Veterans Affairs Medical Center, Houston, Texas
*Respiratory Alkalosis*

**Robert J. Alpern, MD**
Ruth W. and Milton P. Levy, Sr. Chair in Molecular Nephrology; Atticus James Gill, MD, Chair in Medical Science; Dean, Southwestern Medical School, University of Texas Southwestern Medical Center at Dallas, Dallas, Texas
*Urinary Acidification*

**Robert J. Anderson, MD**
Professor of Medicine, Head, Division of General Internal Medicine, University of Colorado Health Sciences Center, Denver, Colorado
*Edematous Disorders*

**Daniel Batlle, MD**
Professor of Medicine and Chief, Division of Nephrology/Hypertension, Northwestern University Medical School, Chicago, Illinois
*Syndromes of Aldosterone Deficiency and Resistance*

**Tomas Berl, MD**
Professor of Medicine, Head, Renal Diseases and Hypertension, University of Colorado Health Sciences Center, Denver, Colorado
*Hyponatremia*

**Daniel G. Bichet, MD**
Professor of Medicine, Career Investigator, le Fonds de la recherche en santé du Québec, Université de Montréal; Director, Clinical Research Unit, Centre de recherche, Hôpital du Sacré-Coeur de Montréal, Montréal, Québec, Canada
*Hypernatremia and the Polyuric Disorders*

**Akhil Bidani, MD, PhD**
Professor of Medicine, Director, Division of Pulmonary and Critical Care Medicine, University of Texas—Houston Health Science Center, Houston, Texas
*Regulation of Whole Body Acid-Base Balance*

**Roland C. Blantz, MD**
Professor of Medicine, University of California, San Diego, School of Medicine, La Jolla; Head, Division of Nephrology-Hypertension, Veterans Administration Hospital, San Diego Healthcare System, San Diego, California
*Renin-Angiotensin-Aldosterone System*

**David Z.I. Cherney, MD**
Medical Resident, University of Toronto Faculty of Medicine, Toronto, Ontario, Canada
*Ketoacidosis*

**Michel Chonchol, MD**
Assistant Professor of Medicine, University of Colorado Health Sciences Center, Denver, Colorado
*Hyponatremia*

**Thomas D. DuBose, Jr., MD**
Peter T. Bohan Professor and Chair of Internal Medicine and Professor of Molecular and Integrative Physiology, University of Kansas School of Medicine; Kansas City, Kansas
*Metabolic Acidosis; Renal Tubular Acidosis*

**David H. Ellison, MD**
Professor of Medicine and Physiology and Pharmacology, Oregon Health Sciences University School of Medicine; Head, Division of Nephrology and Hypertension, Veterans Administration Medical Center, Portland Oregon
*Salt-Wasting Disorders*

**Michael Emmett, MD, MACP**
Chairman, Department of Internal Medicine, Baylor University Medical Center; Clinical Professor of Medicine, University of Texas Southwestern Medical Center at Dallas, Dallas, Texas
*Diagnosis of Simple and Mixed Disorders*

**Kevin W. Finkel, MD**
Associate Professor of Medicine, Division of Renal Diseases and Hypertension, University of Texas—Houston Health Science Center, Houston, Texas
*Metabolic Acidosis, Electrolyte Abnormalities in the Intensive Care Unit*

**Peter A. Friedman, PhD**
Professor of Pharmacology, Departments of Pharmacology and of Medicine, University of Pittsburgh School of Medicine, Pittsburgh, Pennsylvania
*Renal Regulation of Calcium, Phosphate, and Magnesium*

**Francis B. Gabbai, MD**
Associate Professor of Medicine in Residence, University of California, San Diego, School of Medicine, La Jolla; Chief of Nephrology, Veterans Administration Hospital, San Diego Healthcare System, San Diego, California
*Renin-Angiotensin-Aldosterone System*

**John H. Galla, MD**
Emeritus Professor of Medicine, University of Cincinnati College of Medicine, Cincinnati, Ohio
*Metabolic Alkalosis*

**Philippe Gauthier, MD**
Assistant Professor of Medicine, Tulane University School of Medicine, New Orleans, Louisiana
*Acidosis of Chronic Renal Failure*

**Esther A. González, MD**
Assistant Professor of Internal Medicine, Saint Louis University School of Medicine, St. Louis, Missouri
*Abnormal Calcium and Magnesium Metabolism*

**Mitchell L. Halperin, MDCM**
Professor of Medicine, University of Toronto Faculty of Medicine; Attending Staff, St. Michael's Hospital, Toronto, Ontario, Canada
*Ketoacidosis*

**L. Lee Hamm, MD**
Professor of Medicine and Physiology, Tulane University School of Medicine; Chief of Nephrology and Hypertension and Vice Chairman, Department of Medicine, Tulane University Health Sciences Center, New Orleans, Louisiana
*Urinary Acidification*

**Thomas A. Heming, PhD**
Associate Professor of Medicine and of Physiology and Biophysics, University of Texas Medical School at Galveston; Director, Pulmonary Research Laboratories, Division of Pulmonary and Critical Care Medicine, University of Texas Medical Branch, Galveston, Texas
*Regulation of Whole Body Acid-Base Balance*

**Keith A. Hruska, MD**
Professor of Pediatrics, Medicine, and Cell Biology, Washington University School of Medicine; Division Head, Pediatric Nephrology, St. Louis Children's Hospital, St. Louis, Missouri
*Hypophosphatemia and Hyperphosphatemia*

**Kamel S. Kamel, MD**
Associate Professor of Medicine, University of Toronto Faculty of Medicine; Attending Staff, St. Michael's Hospital, Toronto, Ontario, Canada
*Ketoacidosis*

**Bruce C. Kone, MD**
Professor of Internal Medicine and/or Integrative Biology and Pharmacology, Director, Division of Renal Diseases and Hypertension, Vice Chairman, Department of Internal Medicine, University of Texas—Houston Health Science Center, Chief, Section of Nephrology, MD Anderson Cancer Center, Houston, Texas
*Hypokalemia*

**Melvin E. Laski, MD**
Professor, Internal Medicine and Physiology, Texas Tech University Health Sciences Center School of Medicine, Lubbock, Texas
*Lactic Acidosis*

**Jacob Lemann, Jr., MD**
Clinical Professor, Nephrology Section, Department of Medicine, Tulane University School of Medicine, New Orleans, Louisiana
*Acidosis of Chronic Renal Failure*

**Nicolaos E. Madias, MD**
Executive Academic Dean and Professor of Medicine, Tufts University School of Medicine; Staff Physician, Division of Nephrology, New England Medical Center Hospitals, Boston, Massachusetts
*Respiratory Alkalosis*

**Clara E. Magyar, PhD**
Assistant Professor, Department of Pharmacology, University of Pittsburgh School of Medicine, Pittsburgh, Pennsylvania
*Renal Regulation of Calcium, Phosphate, and Magnesium*

**Jean-Pierre Mallié, MD**
Professor of Medicine, Université Henri Poincaré-Nancy, Directeur, Centre hospitalier universitaire de Nancy, Hôpital d'Enfants, Vandoeuvre Cedex, France
*Hypernatremia and the Polyuric Disorders*

**David Marples, MD**
Associate Professor, School of Biomedical Sciences, University of Leeds, Leeds, United Kingdom
*Cell Biology of Vasopressin and Aquaporins*

**Kevin J. Martin, MB, BCh**
Professor of Internal Medicine, Saint Louis University School of Medicine; Director, Division of Nephrology, Saint Louis University Health Science Center, St. Louis, Missouri
*Abnormal Calcium and Magnesium Metabolism*

**Glenn A. McDonald, MD**
Assistant Professor of Internal Medicine, Division of Renal Diseases and Hypertension, University of Texas—Houston Health Science Center, Houston, Texas
*Renal Tubular Acidosis*

**Pierre Meneton, PhD**
Research Investigator, Institut National de la Santé et de la Recherche Médicale, Paris, France
*Genetic Disorders of Renal Apical $Na^+$ Transporters*

**Amit Mitra, MD**
Internal Medicine Resident, Northwestern University Medical School, Chicago, Illinois
*Syndromes of Aldosterone Deficiency and Resistance*

**Søren Nielsen, MD, PhD**
Professor of Cell Biology and Pathophysiology, Department of Cell Biology, Institute of Anatomy, University of Aarhus, Aarhus, Denmark
*Cell Biology of Vasopressin and Aquaporins*

**Young S. Oh, PhD**
Assistant Professor of Medicine and of Neurobiology, University of Alabama at Birmingham School of Medicine, University of Alabama, Birmingham, Alabama
*Genetic Disorders of Renal Apical $Na^+$ Transporters*

**Charles Y.C. Pak, MD**
Distinguished Chair in Mineral Metabolism, Director, Center for Mineral Metabolism and Clinical Research, University of Texas Southwestern Medical Center at Dallas, Dallas, Texas
*Idiopathic Hypercalciuria and Renal Stone Disease*

**Sanford Reikes, MD**
Assistant Professor of Internal Medicine, Saint Louis University School of Medicine; Assistant Medical Director, St. Louis Renal Care, St. Louis, Missouri
*Abnormal Calcium and Magnesium Metabolism*

**Ruth A. Schwalbe, PhD**
Assistant Professor, Research, University of Florida College of Medicine, Gainesville, Florida
*Regulation of Renal Potassium Transport*

**David Sheikh-Hamad, MD**
Associate Professor of Medicine, Division of Nephrology, Baylor College of Medicine, Houston, Texas
*Cell Biology of Vasopressin and Aquaporins*

**Eric E. Simon, MD**
Associate Professor of Medicine, Tulane University School of Medicine; Medical Director, Dialysis Clinics, Inc.; Staff Physician, Tulane University Hospital, VA Medical Center, and Charity Hospital, New Orleans, Louisiana
*Acidosis of Chronic Renal Failure*

**Harold M. Szerlip, MD**
Professor of Medicine and Associate Chairman, Department of Medicine, Nephrology and Pulmonary/Critical Care, Medical College of Georgia School of Medicine, Augusta, Georgia
*Acid-Base Disorders in the Critical Care Setting*

**Galen B. Toews, MD**
Professor of Internal Medicine, University of Michigan Medical School; Chief, Division of Pulmonary and Critical Care Medicine, University of Michigan Health System, Ann Arbor, Michigan
*Respiratory Acidosis*

**Divina M. Tuazon, MD**
Senior Research Fellow, Division of Pulmonary and Critical Care Medicine, University of Texas Medical Branch, Galveston, Texas
*Regulation of Whole Body Acid-Base Balance*

**David G. Warnock, MD**
Professor of Medicine and of Physiology, University of Alabama at Birmingham School of Medicine, University of Alabama; Director, Division of Nephrology, University of Alabama Hospitals, Birmingham, Alabama
*Genetic Disorders of Renal Apical $Na^+$ Transporters*

**I. David Weiner, MD**
Associate Professor of Medicine and Physiology, University of Florida College of Medicine; Attending Physician, Shands at the University of Florida, and Staff Physician, Gainesville, Florida
*Regulation of Renal Potassium Transport, Hyperkalemia*

**Donald E. Wesson, MD**
Professor, Medicine and Physiology, Chair, Department of Internal Medicine, and Chief, Combined Program in Nephrology and Physiology, Texas Tech University Health Sciences Center, Lubbock, Texas
*Lactic Acidosis*

**Gina M. Whitney, MD**
Fellow in Pediatric Critical Care Medicine, Southwestern Medical School, Dallas, Texas
*Acid-Base Disorders in the Critical Care Setting*

**Charles S. Wingo, MD**
Professor of Medicine and Physiology, University of Florida College of Medicine; Chief, Renal Section; Veterans Affairs Medical Center, Gainesville, Florida
*Regulation of Renal Potassium Transport, Hyperkalemia*

# Contents

Section I
## ACID-BASE DISORDERS



Section II
## WATER



Section III
## SODIUM



Section IV
## POTASSIUM

# Section I
# *Acid-Base Disorders*

## CHAPTER 1

# Regulation of Whole Body Acid-Base Balance

Akhil Bidani, MD, PhD ▪ Divina M. Tuazon, MD ▪ Thomas A. Heming, PhD

Whole body acid-base homeostasis involves the integration of a number of physiologic processes, including intra- and extracellular buffering, and the compensatory actions of the kidneys, lungs, and liver[1–3] (Fig. 1–1*A*). The appropriate interpretation of body acid-base status, as revealed by simultaneous measurements of blood electrolytes and arterial blood gases, requires an understanding of these physiologic processes at both cell and organ levels. In healthy humans, arterial blood pH is maintained relatively constant between 7.35 and 7.40 (equivalent to an $H^+$ concentration range of 40 to 45 nM) in the face of wide variations in the daily (and often minute-by-minute) load of acids and bases. Arterial blood pH is vulnerable to significant changes when acid-base regulatory mechanisms are impaired by disease or trauma. Changes in arterial blood pH affect cardiac and central nervous system (CNS) functions, among others. Arterial blood pH values outside the range of 6.7 to 7.7 are incompatible with human life. This pH interval represents an exceedingly narrow range of blood $H^+$ concentration, encompassing only about 140 nM. Viewed in the context of the thousands of millimoles of acid that the body handles daily, the maintenance of normal blood pH attests to the great sensitivity and capacity of the acid-base regulatory systems.

Traditional discussions of acid-base pathophysiology focus primarily on changes that can be measured in blood. However, it is actually the maintenance of normal intracellular pH ($pH_i$) that is vital for cell viability, enzyme functions, and other cellular metabolic processes. Cells are endowed with multiple mechanisms that defend $pH_i$ against intra- and extracellular acid-base challenges. Disruption of $pH_i$ regulation leads to alterations in cell metabolism and function and, ultimately, to tissue and organ failure. Intra- and extracellular pH homeostasis is the result of a balance between those processes that tend to change pH and the body's ability to minimize and compensate for the changes.

## ACID PRODUCTION

The body is continually confronted by a large quantity of endogenously produced acids (Table 1–1),[4, 5] when viewed in the context of a total body buffering capacity of only 1000 mmol. Volatile and nonvolatile (fixed) acids are produced by intermediary metabolism. The largest fraction of daily acid production is the volatile acid $CO_2$. In a normal adult at rest, glucose and fatty acid metabolism produce about 15,000 to 20,000 mmol/day of $CO_2$. An additional 750 to 1500 mmol/day of $CO_2$ are generated by the normal hepatic metabolism of lactate via the Cori cycle. During exercise, $CO_2$ production can increase more than 10-fold. Volatile acid production can also be greatly increased in critically ill patients, due to increased metabolism. Depending on the underlying disease process (e.g., burns, infections, sepsis), the metabolic rate can increase from 30% to 100% with corresponding increases in the rate of $CO_2$ production.

Fixed acid production is approximately 60 to 100 mmol/day in a normal 70-kg adult male. The three primary sources of fixed acid production are diet, metabolism, and base loss in the stool. Each source contributes about 20 to 40 mmol/day of acid. The composition of the resultant acids is highly variable. Sulfuric acid is generated from the oxidation of organic sulfur in methionine and cysteine residues. Organic acids are formed by the incomplete oxidation of carbohydrates, fats, and proteins (as well as nucleic acids). The hydrolysis of phosphate esters in proteins and nucleic acids yields phosphoric acid. Hydrochloric acid is produced when chloride salts of cationic amino acids (e.g., lysine and arginine) are metabolized to neutral products. In addition, the loss of $HCO_3^-$ and base equivalents (e.g., organic anions) in the stool (see Fig. 1–1) acts in effect as an acid-loading process and results in the addition of an equimolar amount of acid to the body. The rate of fixed acid production is greatly enhanced during certain pathologic conditions. For instance, hypoinsulinemia, alcoholism, and starvation lead to increments in ketoacid production. Ingestion of toxins and drugs results in accelerated formation of organic acids such as formic acids from methanol, oxalic acid from ethylene glycol, and salicylic acid from aspirin. Loss of base in the stool is increased in pathologic conditions such as diarrhea. In trauma and sepsis, protein catabolism can increase three- to fourfold with a proportional increase in fixed acid production.

## BUFFER SYSTEMS

Buffer systems are critical to the physiology and pathophysiology of acid-base homeostasis.[6–9] Buffers can be broadly defined as systems that attenuate the

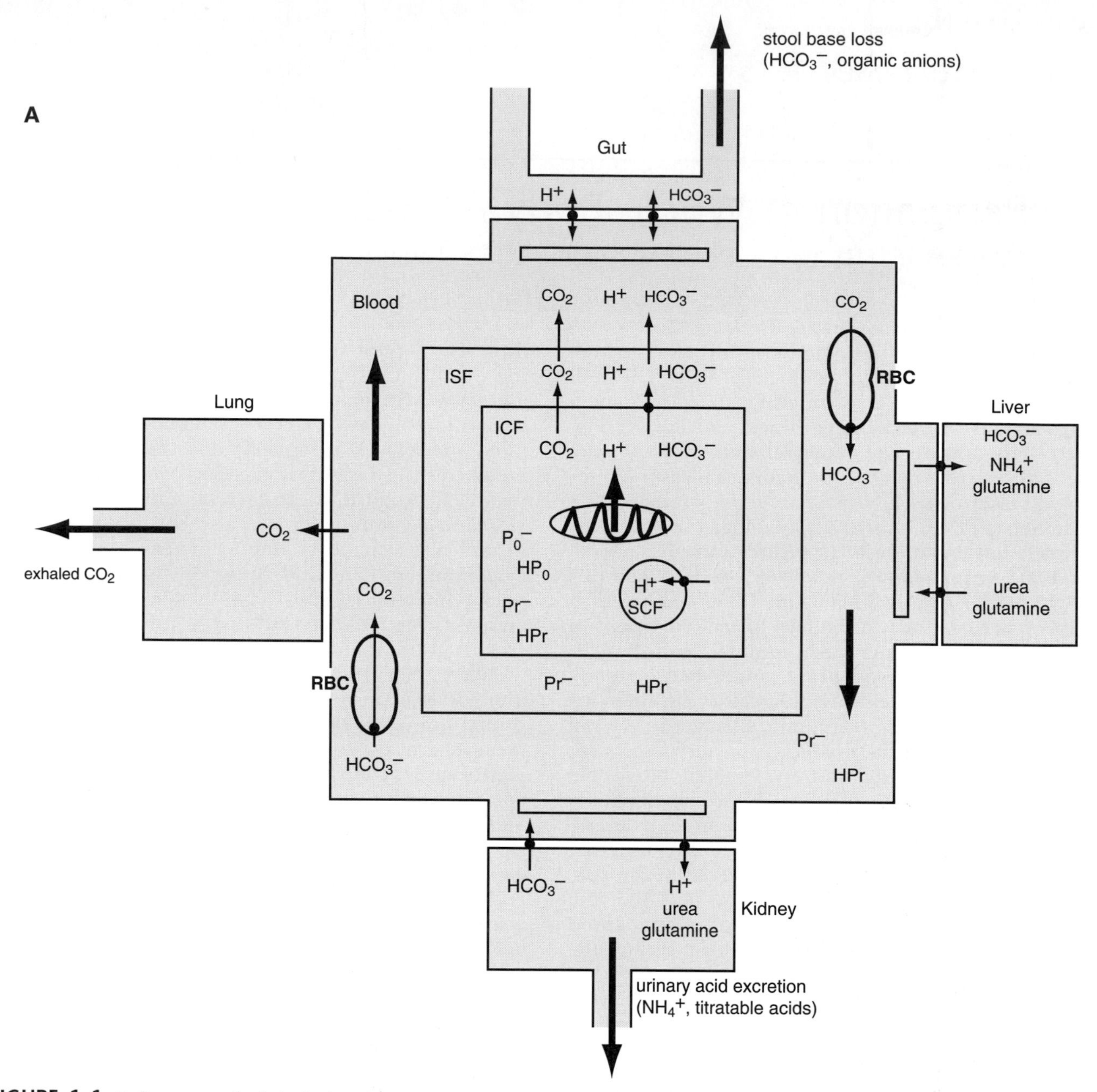


**FIGURE 1–1** ■ Summary of whole body acid-base regulation. *A,* Intra- and extracellular pH homeostasis reflects a balance between processes that produce acids/bases and those that remove acids/bases. *B,* Cell metabolism produces volatile and nonvolatile acids. The resultant acids are buffered by interaction with cell proteins or organic phosphates, by transport across endomembranes into intracellular organelles, or by transport across the plasma membrane. Membrane fluxes of acids/bases are reversible and, thus, the intracellular buffering systems are also available to buffer changes in extracellular pH. *C,* Stomach mucosal cells secrete $H^+$ into the gut lumen and $HCO_3^-$ into the blood. In contrast, most gastrointestinal segments below the pylorus secrete $HCO_3^-$ into the gut lumen and $H^+$ into the blood. Overall, these actions produce a net acid load to the body. *D,* Liver detoxification of $NH_4^+$ can consume blood $HCO_3^-$ via the formation of urea or spare blood $HCO_3^-$ via the formation of glutamine.

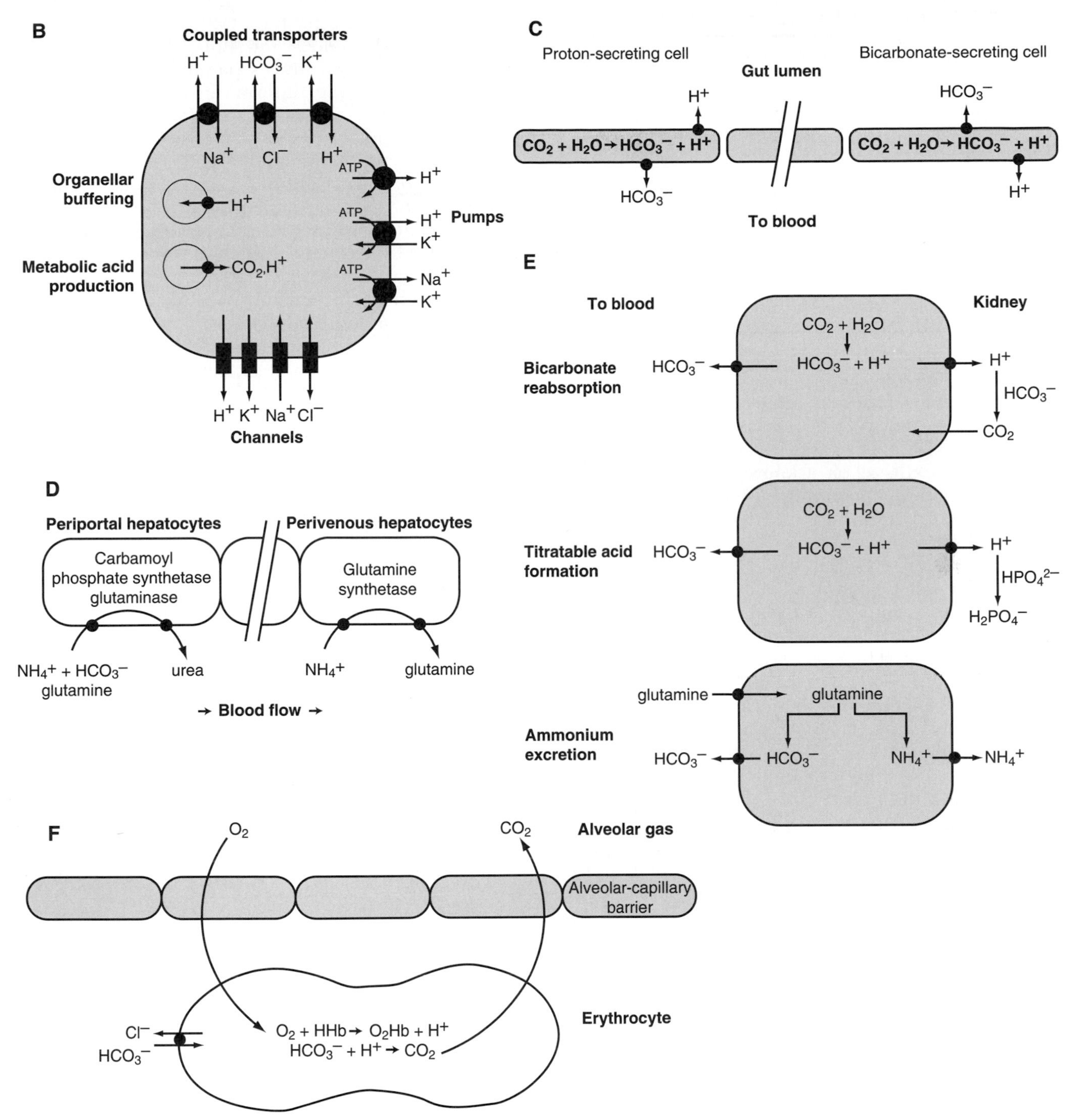


**FIGURE 1–1** *(Continued)* ■ *E,* The kidneys regulate blood $HCO_3^-$ concentration by reabsorbing filtered $HCO_3^-$, forming titratable acids, or by excreting $NH_4^+$. *F,* Blood $HCO_3^-$ is mobilized to $CO_2$ and excreted in the lungs. Consequently, lung function regulates blood $P_{CO_2}$ and, hence, the blood $CO_2$ concentration. ISF, interstitial fluid; ATP, adenosine triphosphate; ICF, intracellular fluid; $P_o^-$ and $HP_o$, organic phosphate buffer pair; $Pr^-$ and HPr, protein buffer pair; RBC, red blood cell; SCF, subcellular (organelle) fluid.

**TABLE 1–1.** Normal Acid-Base Balance

| Acid | Acid Production (mmol/day) | Primary System for Excretion |
|---|---|---|
| | *Volatile Acids* | |
| $CO_2$ | 15,000–20,000 | Pulmonary |
| Lactate (metabolized to $CO_2$) | 750–1500 | Pulmonary |
| | *Fixed Acids* | |
| Sulfuric acid<br>Phosphoric acid<br>Hydrochloric acid<br>Organic acids and others | 60–100 | Renal |

pH change in a solution by removing or releasing free $H^+$. The important role of buffers in attenuating pH changes can be appreciated by comparing the pH change that results when a known amount of acid is added to a solution containing buffers versus a solution lacking buffers. For example, if 10 mmol of strong acid are added to a 1-L solution containing 50 mM of phosphate buffer (e.g., $Na_2HPO_4$-$NaH_2PO_4$) at a pH of 7.0, the pH will decrease to about 6.5. In contrast, when the same amount of acid is added to a 1-L solution at a pH of 7.0 containing no buffer, the pH will fall to about 2.0. Four distinct mechanisms are involved in whole body buffering: (1) physicochemical buffering, (2) biochemical buffering, (3) intracellular organellar buffering, and (4) plasmalemmal flux of acid-base equivalents.

Regardless of the underlying mechanism, the ability of a buffer system to resist changes in pH is quantified via the buffering capacity ($\beta$). $\beta$ is commonly defined as the mM of $H^+$ or $OH^-$ required to cause a given change in pH and is expressed in units of mM/pH or slykes. When the value of $\beta$ is large, a greater concentration of acid or base must be added to the solution to effect a unit change in pH. Conceptually, $\beta$ represents the slope of the pH titration curve at a given pH and, therefore, is itself pH-dependent. An alternative approach to $\beta$ is obtained by considering the general buffer system:

$$Buf\text{-}H^{n+1} \rightleftharpoons Buf\text{-}H^{n} + H^{+} \quad (1)$$

Buf-$H^n$ buffers acid loads by combining with some of the added $H^+$ to form Buf-$H^{n+1}$, whereas Buf-$H^{n+1}$ buffers alkali loads by combining with some of the added $OH^-$ to form Buf-$H^n$ and water. In this generalized scheme, $\beta$ is appropriately calculated as the first derivative *(d)* of the concentration of Buf-$H^n$, with respect to pH:

$$\beta = \frac{d[Buf\text{-}H^{n}]}{dpH} \quad (2)$$

An important determinant of the $\beta$ of any specific buffering mechanism is whether the buffer operates as an open or a closed system. The quantitative behavior of an open-system buffer differs considerably from that of a closed-system buffer (Fig. 1–2). In an open system, the buffer pair (Buf-$H^n$ and Buf-$H^{n+1}$) can be envisioned as occurring in two separate but communicating compartments (i.e., internal and external compartments), such as cytosol and extracellular fluid or pulmonary capillary blood and alveolar gas. At least one component of the buffer pair (usually the uncharged component) diffuses freely between the internal and external compartments, so that the external compartment provides an infinite reservoir for that component. Consequently, when $H^+$ or $OH^-$ is added to the internal compartment, the concentration of the diffusive component remains unchanged. The production or consumption of that component during the buffering process is countered by diffusion across the compartmental interface (e.g., cell plasma membrane or alveolar-capillary barrier). Thus, in an open system, the concentration of the diffusive buffer component can be considered as fixed and unchanged during the addition of either $H^+$ or $OH^-$. The buffering capacity of an open buffer system is:

$$\beta^{open} = 2.303\ [Buf\text{-}H^{n}] \quad (3)$$

$\beta^{open}$ increases steadily with increments in the Buf-$H^n$ concentration or pH. On the other hand, in a closed buffer system, both members of the buffer pair are confined to a single compartment. Consequently, in a closed system, addition of $H^+$ or $OH^-$ alters the concentrations of both buffer components. This limits the ability of the buffer to cope with continued addi-

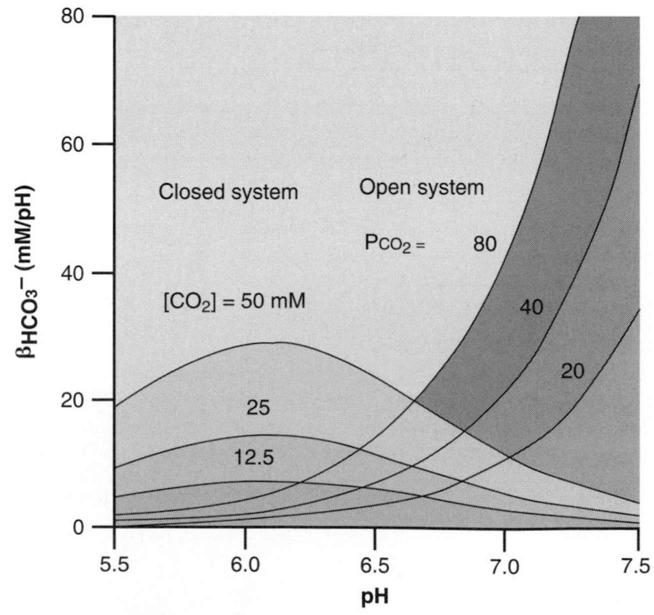


**FIGURE 1–2** ■ Relationship between buffering capacity ($\beta$) and pH for a physicochemical buffer ($CO_2$-$HCO_3^-$) operating as an open system versus a closed system. In a closed system, the total buffer concentration remains constant with changes in pH, albeit the ratio of basic-to-acidic buffer components ($HCO_3^-$:$CO_2$) varies. The $\beta$ of a closed-system buffer peaks at pH = pK′ (6.1 for $CO_2$-$HCO_3^-$). In an open system, the acidic buffer component ($CO_2$) remains constant with changes in pH, whereas concentrations of the basic component ($HCO_3^-$) and total buffer vary directly with pH. The $\beta$ of an open-system buffer increases progressively with increments in pH.

tion of $H^+$ or $OH^-$. The buffering capacity of a closed buffer system is:

$$\beta^{closed} = 2.303 \frac{K'_{buf} \cdot [H^+]}{(K'_{buf} + [H^+])^2} \cdot [TB] \quad (4)$$

where $K'_{buf}$ is the apparent dissociation constant for the buffer pair and [TB] represents the total concentration of buffer (i.e., the sum of $Buf\text{-}H^n$ and $Buf\text{-}H^{n+1}$ concentrations). It is important to note that $\beta^{closed}$ peaks when solution pH = $pK'_{buf}$, at which point,

$$Maximal\ \beta^{closed} = 0.58\ [TB] \quad (5)$$

Body fluids typically contain more than one buffer system. The total β of a solution containing several buffers is the sum of the β of the individual buffers. The Isohydric Principle dictates that the consequences of $H^+$ or $OH^-$ addition are shared among all buffers present in a given solution. In other words, when $H^+$ or $OH^-$ is added to the solution, the $Buf\text{-}H^{n+1}/Buf\text{-}H^n$ ratios of all the buffers in the solution are affected. An important implication of the Isohydric Principle is that quantifying the behavior of any individual buffer system is adequate to predict the quantitative behavior of all other buffers in the solution. This explains why, in the clinical setting, the acid-base status of a patient is most often expressed in terms of the principal extracellular buffer, the $CO_2\text{-}HCO_3^-$ system.

## Physicochemical Buffering

Common physicochemical buffer systems contain two substances—a conjugate acid and its conjugate base. An "acidic" physicochemical buffer contains a weak acid and a salt of the weak acid (i.e., the conjugate base). A "basic" physicochemical buffer contains a weak base and a salt of the weak base (conjugate acid). Together the buffer pair (i.e., the conjugate acid and base) resist changes in solution pH upon the addition of acids or bases by combining partially with the additional $H^+$ or $OH^-$ (see Equation 1). An example of a physicochemical buffer system is a neutral weak acid (HA) together with its conjugate base ($A^-$):

$$HA \leftrightharpoons H^+ + A^- \quad (6)$$

The equilibrium constant for this buffer pair is:

$$K' = \frac{[H^+]\,[A^-]}{[HA]} \quad (7)$$

The prime sign is used to indicate that the true thermodynamic constant (K) is modified by the use of concentrations rather than chemical activities. Accordingly, K′ varies with the temperature and ionic strength of the solution. Taking logarithms of both sides of Equation 7 and defining pK′ as $-\log_{10} K'$, one obtains:

$$pH = pK' + \log_{10}\frac{[A^-]}{[HA]} \quad (8)$$

The value of pK′ provides an estimate of the strength of an acid or base. Strong acids are in essence completely ionized in solution and, thus, have a relatively low pK′ (or a high K′). Conversely, a strong base exists predominantly in the un-ionized form and, therefore, has a high pK′ (or a low K′). Weak acids and bases have intermediate values for pK′ (i.e., close to a value of 7) and, hence, at physiologic pH values, are present in solution as a mixture of conjugate acid and base. From Equation 8, it is easy to see that buffer pairs are half dissociated at pH = pK′. Thus, the pK′ of a buffer pair can also be defined as the pH at which the buffer pair exists 50% as the conjugate acid and 50% as the conjugate base.

**Carbon Dioxide.** Physiologically, the most important physicochemical buffer is the $CO_2\text{-}HCO_3^-$ system. When $CO_2$ is dissolved in water, carbonic acid ($H_2CO_3$) forms and then dissociates to yield $H^+$ and $HCO_3^-$. The overall reaction proceeds slowly in the absence of the enzyme carbonic anhydrase, with an uncatalyzed half-time of about 8 seconds at 37°C. At chemical equilibrium, only about 1 part in 1000 of the total carbon dioxide in solution is $H_2CO_3$. Because the $H_2CO_3$ concentration is low and proportional to that of dissolved $CO_2$, the formation of $H_2CO_3$ is usually ignored and the hydration of $CO_2$ is treated as a single reaction:

$$CO_2 + H_2O \leftrightharpoons H^+ + HCO_3^- \quad (9)$$

It is noteworthy that, in the presence of carbonic anhydrase, the catalyzed reaction proceeds as written in Equation 9 (i.e., without the formation of $H_2CO_3$) and is virtually instantaneous. The Henderson-Hasselbalch equation for $CO_2\text{-}HCO_3^-$ is derived from the equilibrium equation for the simplified reaction (see Equation 9). The most common form of the Henderson-Hasselbalch equation expresses the concentration of dissolved $CO_2$ in terms of the physical solubility coefficient ($\alpha CO_2$) and partial pressure ($P_{CO_2}$) of $CO_2$ (in accordance with Henry's law):

$$pH = pK' + \log_{10}\frac{[HCO_3^-]}{(\alpha_{CO_2}\, P_{CO_2})} \quad (10)$$

The value for pK′ in this case is sensitive to solution temperature, ionic strength, and pH (via the effects on $H_2CO_3$), whereas the value for $\alpha CO_2$ varies with temperature and ionic strength. Using conventional values for the pK′ (6.1) and $\alpha CO_2$ (0.03 mM/mm Hg) of human blood plasma at 37°C and pH 7.4, one obtains the Henderson equation, which is of great use in the clinical interpretation of acid-base data:

$$[H^+]\ (nM) = 24\frac{P_{CO_2}(mm\ Hg)}{[HCO_3^-]\ (nM)} \quad (11)$$

These considerations of the $CO_2\text{-}HCO_3^-$ buffer system are strictly valid only when the buffer system is in a state of chemical equilibrium. In the absence of carbonic anhydrase, the interconversion of $CO_2$ and $HCO_3^-$ (see Equation 9) occurs slowly over many seconds. Under such conditions, reaction limitations can become quite important,[10] and the "apparent" buffering capacity of the $CO_2$-$HCO_3^-$ system becomes time-dependent.

The crucial role of $CO_2$-$HCO_3^-$ as a physiologic buffer system warrants further elaboration.[11] Because buffer efficiency is greatest in the pH range near pK′, it appears at first glance that the $CO_2$-$HCl_3^-$ system (pK′ = 6.1) would not be an effective buffer at physiologic pH values. However, $CO_2$-$HCO_3^-$ is an extremely potent buffer system in vivo and serves as the predominant buffer system for extracellular fluid. The potency and efficacy of the $CO_2$-$HCO_3^-$ system are due mainly to the augmentation of β that accompanies the operation of a buffer in an open system (see Fig. 1–2). Because $CO_2$ diffuses freely across biologic barriers and cell membranes, its concentration in biologic fluids can be modulated rapidly via the ventilatory apparatus. When $H^+$ are added to a body fluid, some of the $H^+$ combine with $HCO_3^-$ and generate molecular $CO_2$. The $CO_2$ diffuses rapidly out of the fluid and is excreted in the lung. Thus, the $CO_2$ concentration of the fluid remains essentially unchanged and $HCO_3^-$ continues to buffer any additional $H^+$. The β of the $CO_2$-$HCO_3^-$ system is increased in hypercapnia and decreased in hypocapnia (see Fig. 1–2). This reflects changes in the concentrations of $HCO_3^-$ and $CO_2$.

**Proteins.** Proteins have prosthetic groups that bind or release $H^+$ and hence are amphoteric; that is, they act as both acids and bases. For example, proteins possess "acidic" free carboxyl groups due to the presence of glutamic and aspartic residues. Carboxyl (-COOH) groups can lose a proton to form $-COO^-$. Proteins also contain "basic" amino groups due to the presence of arginine, lysine, and histidine. Amino ($-NH_2$) groups can accept a proton to become $-NH_3^+$. The β of any given protein reflects the composite contribution of the molecule's complement of dissociable groups. A predominant contribution is provided by the imidazole group of histidine, which has a pK′ of 6.4 to 7.0. Another important contribution is provided by *N*-terminal α-amino groups that have pK′ values in the range of 7.4 to 7.9. Because of the multiplicity of pK′ values within a given protein molecule, the pH titration curve of most proteins is essentially linear. In other words, protein β is relatively constant with changes in pH.

**Phosphates.** Both inorganic and organic phosphates serve as acid-base buffers in body fluids. Inorganic phosphates generate or consume protons via a number of reactions. At physiologic pH, the most important reaction is:

$$H_2PO_4^- \rightleftharpoons H^+ + HPO_4^{2-} \quad (12)$$

with a pK′ of 6.8. Inorganic phosphates contribute little to the buffering capacity of blood, owing to their low concentration in plasma (~2 mM). However, inorganic phosphate is an important buffer in urine, because it is excreted in high concentration (~10-fold higher concentration than in plasma). Urine buffers are important determinants of urinary $H^+$ excretion (see later). Organic phosphates, including 2,3-diphosphoglycerate (2,3-DPG), glucose-1-phosphate, adenosine monophosphate (AMP), adenosine diphosphate (ADP), and adenosine triphosphate (ATP), function as buffers in a manner similar to that of inorganic phosphates. The phosphate moieties in these organic compounds have pK′ values of 6.0 to 7.5. Organic phosphates exist in substantial concentrations within cells and contribute significantly to the intracellular nonbicarbonate β.

**Ammonia.** The ammonia ($NH_3$)-ammonium ($NH_4^+$) buffer system,

$$NH_3 + H^+ \rightleftharpoons NH_4^+ \quad (13)$$

has a relatively high pK′ (~9.5). For this reason, $NH_3$-$NH_4^+$ would be expected to be an inefficient buffer in the physiologic pH range; most of the buffer pair would exist as $NH_4^+$. Nonetheless, the $NH_3$-$NH_4^+$ system plays an important role in urinary $H^+$ excretion and acid-base metabolism (see later).

**Bone as a Buffer.** Bone contains approximately 80% of the total $CO_2$ in the body. About two thirds of this $CO_2$ is in the form of carbonate ($CO_3^-$) complexed with calcium, sodium, and other cations. These carbonates are located in the lattice of the bone crystals. The other third consists of bicarbonate, which appears to be located in the hydration shell of the hydroxyapatite. Swan and Pitts[12] demonstrated that approximately 40% to 60% of administered $H^+$ are buffered outside the extracellular fluid space, specifically by soft tissues and bone. Furthermore, the loss of bone salts during acute and chronic acidoses suggests that bone participates in acid-base buffering in vivo. The mechanism of bone buffering is probably the release of calcium carbonate, which buffers metabolic $H^+$.[13]

## Biochemical Buffering

A number of biochemical reactions generate or consume $H^+$ (e.g., glycolysis, ATP hydrolysis, and phosphorylation of ADP by creatine phosphate).[14–17] Additionally, the hydration of metabolically produced $CO_2$ can result in the net generation of $H^+$. It is reasonable, therefore, to postulate that alterations in biochemical reaction pathways or rates (with consequent changes in cell metabolism) could serve as biochemical buffer systems. The contribution of metabolism to acid-base status appears to be considerably more complicated than was envisioned previously. For example, the amount of $H^+$ released during the metabolism of glucose to lactate depends on the cellular magnesium concentration and $pH_i$. The net generation of $H^+$ can vary from 0 to 2 mol per mol of glucose consumed, the upper limit being realized at high cellular $Mg^{2+}$ concentrations and low $pH_i$ values.[15]

## Intracellular Organellar Buffering

Many intracellular organelles (e.g., mitochondria, lysosomes, sarcoplasmic reticulum, and chromaffin granules) possess acid-base transport systems that are capable of vectorial $H^+$ transport across the organelle endomembrane.[18–20] Changes in $pH_i$ could alter the net flux of acid-base equivalents across organellar membranes by stimulating or inhibiting endomembrane acid-base transporters. Thus, alterations in the extent of $H^+$ sequestration in organelles could represent a mechanism for $H^+$ buffering of the cell cytoplasm.

## Plasmalemmal Flux of Acid-Base Equivalents

The plasma membrane of most cells is endowed with specialized transport mechanisms that play a vital role in both cell and whole body acid-base homeostasis (see Fig. 1–1*B*).[21–26] Plasmalemmal flux of acid-base equivalents represents an important mechanism of $H^+$ buffering of body fluids. Electrolyte transport is an integral part of $pH_i$ regulation. Consequently, plasmalemmal acid-base transporters are important not only in $pH_i$ regulation but also in control of cell volume and plasma membrane potential. Most cells have two or more distinct $pH_i$-regulating transport systems. Baseline $pH_i$ is determined by the relative activity of these transporters (Fig. 1–3). The significance of variations in the distribution and kinetic characteristics of the $pH_i$-regulating transporters is unclear, but redundancy appears to be prevalent.

**$Na^+$-$H^+$ Exchanger.** The $Na^+$-$H^+$ exchanger (NHE) facilitates the one-for-one exchange of extracellular $Na^+$ for intracellular $H^+$, eliciting a rise in $pH_i$.[27–29] The exchange process is secondary active. It is driven by the chemical gradients of $Na^+$ and $H^+$ and, therefore, is dependent on the operation of plasmalemmal $Na^+$-$K^+$-ATPase. The NHE is a nearly ubiquitous feature of the plasma membrane of mammalian cells.[29–33] In epithelial cells, NHE activity has been demonstrated in both basolateral and apical membranes, although not necessarily in the same type of cell. Furthermore, the plasmalemmal density of the transporter (as inferred from rates of $Na^+$ transport) varies greatly among cell types. For example, the rate of $Na^+$-$H^+$ exchange per unit of membrane surface area in lymphocytes is several hundred–fold greater than in erythrocytes. $Na^+$-$H^+$ exchange is very important in the normalization of $pH_i$ after cytosolic acidification.[27–29] In many but not all cell types, the NHE is also important for the maintenance of steady-state $pH_i$. The transporter is regulated by $pH_i$: the NHE is activated by decrements in $pH_i$. Conversely, activity of the transporter is reduced by decrements in extracellular pH, possibly due to competition between $H^+$ and $Na^+$ for the external cation-binding site of the exchanger. The transporter can be activated within minutes by numerous external stimuli, including growth factors, insulin, vasopressin, and other chemical and biologic agents.[27, 28] Typically, rapidly acting agents alter the exchanger's sensitivity to $pH_i$. The NHE also demonstrates slower adaptive changes in activity during states of persistent acidosis or alkalosis. These slow adaptive changes generally reflect changes in the plasmalemmal density of the transporter.

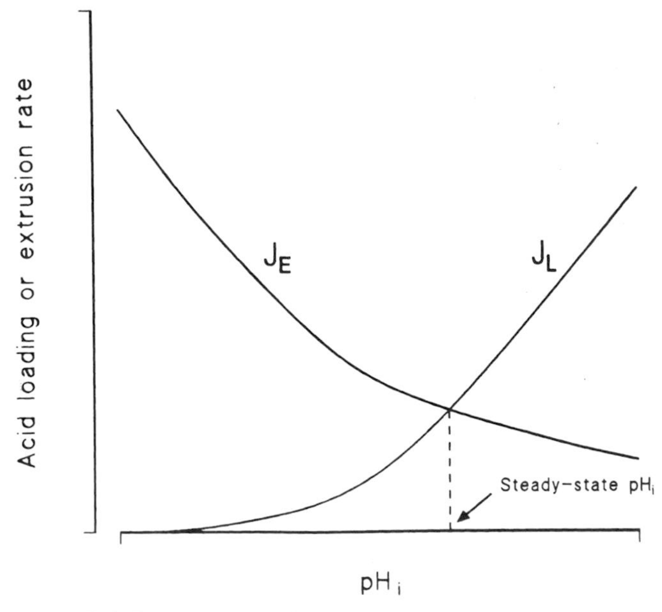


**FIGURE 1–3** ■ Cells express multiple mechanisms for the transport of acid-base equivalents across the plasma membrane. Typically, the rates of acid extrusion ($J_E$) and acid loading ($J_L$; effectively equivalent to base extrusion) are sensitive to intracellular pH ($pH_i$). Steady-state $pH_i$ is determined by the balance of acid loading and extrusion in the cell.

**$HCO_3^-$-Dependent Mechanisms for $pH_i$ Regulation.** Various $HCO_3^-$-dependent mechanisms participate in $pH_i$ regulation, including cation-independent $HCO_3^-$-$Cl^-$ exchange, $Na^+$-dependent $HCO_3^-$-$Cl^-$ exchange, and electrogenic $Na^+$-$HCO_3^-$ cotransport. The cation-independent $HCO_3^-$-$Cl^-$ transporter facilitates the one-for-one exchange of anions across cell membranes. The best studied prototype for this type of transporter is band 3 protein, a major protein in the red blood cell plasmalemma.[30, 31] Cation-independent $HCO_3^-$-$Cl^-$ exchange is reversible. The direction of net transport is determined by the magnitude of the inwardly directed gradient for $Cl^-$ relative to that for $HCO_3^-$. In the red blood cell, the $HCO_3^-$-$Cl^-$ exchanger mediates $HCO_3^-$ flux into the erythrocyte during $CO_2$ excretion in the lung and flux out of the erythrocyte during $CO_2$ loading of blood in peripheral capillaries.[10] In most other cells, the inwardly directed $Cl^-$ gradient is generally larger than the inward $HCO_3^-$ gradient, so that the former dominates and $HCO_3^-$ is transported out of the cell. In these cells, the exchanger plays a crucial role in $pH_i$ recovery from cytosolic alkaline loads. The exchanger is sensitive to $pH_i$: transport increases with increments in $pH_i$. The transporter also is sensitive to physiologic ligands.[32–34]

The $Na^+$-dependent $HCO_3^-$-$Cl^-$ exchanger transports $HCO_3^-$ into the cell and, therefore, functions effectively as an acid extruder.[35, 36] This mechanism is electroneutral and facilitates the exchange of extracellular $Na^+$ and $HCO_3^-$ for intracellular $Cl^-$ (and possibly $H^+$). In some cells, this transporter plays a major role in setting the baseline $pH_i$ and for $pH_i$ recovery following cytosolic acid loads.

The $Na^+$-$HCO_3^-$ cotransporter is electrogenic. It transports $HCO_3^-$ and $Na^+$ out of the cell with a coupling ratio of 3:1, respectively. The cotransporter is energized by the negative membrane potential and the outward gradient for $HCO_3^-$, which together overcome the opposing inward gradient for $Na^+$. This mechanism has been identified in the basolateral (serosal) membrane of proximal tubular cells of the kidneys, where it functions as the main mechanism for $HCO_3^-$ efflux into the blood.[37–39]

**$H^+$-Translocating ATPases.** Proton pumps mediate the active transport of $H^+$ across cell membranes by direct coupling of $H^+$ movement to ATP hydrolysis.[40, 41] The gastric $H^+$-$K^+$ exchanger is an example of an electroneutral $H^+$ pump. This transporter, located in the apical membrane of parietal cells, exchanges external $K^+$ for internal $H^+$.[42] Electrogenic proton pumps are expressed in the endomembranes of all mammalian cells and the plasma membrane of some cells.[43–46] The endomembrane pumps function to acidify the lumens of intracellular organelles (e.g., endosomes, lysosomes, and Golgi apparatus). The plasmalemmal pumps participate in vectorial $H^+$ transport in epithelial cells and in $pH_i$ regulation. It may appear illogical to hydrolyze ATP to extrude $H^+$ inasmuch as hydrolysis of one ATP molecule liberates approximately 0.8 $H^+$-equivalents. However, for the $H^+$-ATPases studied to date, the stoichiometric coupling ratio (2 to 3 $H^+$ transported per ATP molecule hydrolyzed) makes $H^+$ extrusion an energy-efficient process.

**$H^+$-Lactate Cotransport.** Lactic acid is uncharged and can permeate cell membranes by nonionic diffusion. The need for a specific lactic acid transporter is, therefore, not obvious. Nonetheless, an $H^+$-lactate cotransporter has been identified in some cells (e.g., cardiac muscle cells, skeletal muscle cells, and placental cells).[20] Typically, these cells produce a large amount of lactic acid, which is transported rapidly out of the cells. The $H^+$-lactate cotransporter is very effective at increasing $pH_i$ in these cells during a lactic acid load. The driving force is the lactate concentration gradient.

## ROLE OF BUFFERS IN ACID-BASE HOMEOSTASIS

Buffers that are confined to the intracellular space are referred to as intrinsic buffers, whereas buffers that freely communicate with the extracellular space are called extrinsic buffers. Closed-system physicochemical buffers, biochemical buffering, and organellar buffering constitute the intrinsic buffer system. Open-system physicochemical buffers and buffering by plasmalemmal acid-base transport constitute the extrinsic buffer system.

### Intracellular Buffering

The main intracellular buffers are proteins, bicarbonate, and organic phosphates (Table 1–2). The $CO_2$-$HCO_3^-$ system is particularly effective because the components of the system can be independently regulated by the body to maintain acid-base status. The plasma membranes of most (if not all) mammalian cells are highly permeable to $CO_2$ and thus the intracellular $CO_2$ concentration is approximately equal to the extracellular concentration. As a result, the intracellular $CO_2$ concentration is effectively regulated by pulmonary gas exchange. Operation of the $CO_2$-$HCO_3^-$ buffer as an open system greatly augments its effective β (see Fig. 1–2). Furthermore, there are specific plasma membrane transporters for $HCO_3^-$. Thus, the intracellular $HCO_3^-$ concentration can be regulated independently of $CO_2$. Overall, these attributes make the $CO_2$-$HCO_3^-$ system remarkably effective for intracellular buffering. The total intracellular β is approximately doubled in the presence of physiologic concentrations of $HCO_3^-$. In many cells, the baseline $pH_i$ is also elevated in the presence of $HCO_3^-$ due to both the increased β and the activity of the $HCO_3^-$-dependent transport mechanisms. For the same reasons, $pH_i$ recovery from cytosolic acid-base challenges is faster in the presence of $HCO_3^-$ than in its absence.

**TABLE 1–2.** Intracellular Buffer Systems

| Buffer | pK′ | % Contribution to Buffering of Fixed Acid Load |
|---|---|---|
| | *Red Blood Cells* | |
| Proteins (primarily hemoglobin) | 7.0–8.0 | 60 |
| $CO_2$-$HCO_3^-$ | 6.1 | 30 |
| Organic phosphates | 6.0–7.5 | 10 |
| | *Other Cells* | |
| Proteins | 5.5–8.5 | 50 |
| $CO_2$-$HCO_3^-$ | 6.1 | 2 |
| Organic phosphates | 6.0–7.5 | 48 |

### Extracellular Buffering

The main extracellular buffers are bicarbonate, proteins, and inorganic phosphate (Table 1–3). $CO_2$-$HCO_3^-$ is quantitatively the most important extracellular buffer, in part because of its high concentration (~25 mM). The extracellular protein concentration is only 2 to 4 mM, but proteins are efficient buffers due

**TABLE 1–3.** Extracellular Buffer Systems

| Buffer | pK′ | % Contribution to Buffering of Fixed Acid Load |
|---|---|---|
| | *Separated Blood Plasma* | |
| Proteins | 5.5–8.5 | 23 |
| $CO_2$-$HCO_3^-$ | 6.1 | 75 |
| Inorganic phosphates | 6.8 | 2 |
| | *Interstitial Fluid* | |
| Proteins | 5.5–8.5 | 9 |
| $CO_2$-$HCO_3^-$ | 6.1 | 90 |
| Inorganic phosphates | 6.8 | 1 |

**TABLE 1–4.** Whole Blood Buffering Systems

| Buffer | Normal Concentration | pK′ | Base-Acid Ratio at pH of 7.4 | % Contribution to Buffering of Fixed Acid Load |
|---|---|---|---|---|
| ***Bicarbonate Buffers*** | | | | |
| Plasma $CO_2$-$HCO_3^-$ | 18.5 mM | 6.1 | $HCO_3^-$: $CO_2$ = 20 : 1 | 35 |
| Red blood cell $CO_2$-$HCO_3^-$ | 6.5 mM | 6.1 | $HCO_3^-$: $CO_2$ = 20 : 1 | 18 |
| ***Nonbicarbonate Buffers*** | | | | |
| Hemoglobin | 15 g/dL | 7.0–8.0 | $Hb^-$: HHb ~ 4 : 1 | 35 |
| Plasma proteins | 7 g/dL | 5.5–8.5 | $Pr^-$: HPr ~ 4 : 1 | 7 |
| Organic phosphates | 1 mM | 6.0–7.5 | Org-$P^-$: Org-HP ~ 4 : 1 | 3 |
| Inorganic phosphates | 2 mM | 6.8 | $HPO_4^{2-}$: $H_2PO_4^-$ = 4 : 1 | 2 |

to the presence of numerous buffering residues on each molecule. Albumin accounts for most of the nonbicarbonate β of blood plasma. The buffering capacity of albumin is about 0.12 to 0.14 mmol/g/pH. Globulins have a lower buffering capacity (0 to 0.08 mmol/g/pH). The buffering capacity of all plasma proteins cumulatively is 0.08 to 0.10 mmol/g/pH. For a total plasma protein concentration of 7 g/dL, this corresponds to a plasma protein β of 5.8 to 6 mM/pH. The extracellular phosphate concentration is ~2 mM, and this buffer is therefore less important than $HCO_3^-$. Extracellular buffering of fixed acids is very effective. However, because the $CO_2$-$HCO_3^-$ complex is the dominant buffer system, extracellular buffering of changes in $CO_2$ concentration (i.e., $PCO_2$) is rather ineffective. Relatively small variations of blood $PCO_2$ greatly influence the pH of blood plasma. Thus, the main buffering of changes in $CO_2$ concentration takes place in erythrocytes and tissue cells.

## Buffering in Blood and Tissues

The primary buffer systems of whole blood are $CO_2$-$HCO_3^-$ (in red blood cells and plasma), proteins (hemoglobin in red blood cells and plasma proteins in plasma), and organic and inorganic phosphates (in red blood cells and plasma, respectively) (Table 1–4). $CO_2$-$HCO_3^-$ contributes ~50% of the total β of whole blood. The buffering behavior of blood is complicated by the unequal distribution of buffers between red blood cells and plasma and by exchange processes between the two compartments. Buffering in blood is usually examined by the measurement of blood pH after changes of $PCO_2$. Because the resultant changes in free $H^+$ concentration are always small in absolute terms (nM range), they can be ignored against the mM changes in buffer (i.e., Buf-$H^n$ and Buf-$H^{n+1}$) concentrations when considering mass balance. In accordance with the Isohydric Principle, determination of the change in $HCO_3^-$ concentration allows one to assess the effective buffering power of blood nonbicarbonate buffers:

$$\beta_{non\text{-}HCO3} = -\frac{\Delta[HCO_3^-]}{\Delta pH} \quad (14)$$

It is important to note that, in this situation, $HCO_3^-$ serves only as an indicator of the buffering of nonbicarbonate buffers (mainly hemoglobin and plasma proteins) and exerts no buffering action by itself. $\beta_{non\text{-}HCO3}$ is ~25 mM/pH for blood plasma when measured in the presence of red blood cells (true plasma), but only ~5 mM/pH for separated plasma. This difference is due to the fact that, in whole blood, the change in plasma pH is strongly attenuated by $HCO_3^-$ exchange with the red blood cells. Red blood cell hemoglobin is the predominant nonbicarbonate buffer. This reflects the high concentration of hemoglobin in blood and the molecule's high buffering capacity (~2.9 mmol $H^+$/mmol hemoglobin/pH). Significant structural changes occur in hemoglobin during the loading and unloading of oxygen. These changes in turn affect the molecule's buffering properties. The pH titration curves for oxyhemoglobin ($O_2Hb$) and reduced hemoglobin (HHb) are linear over the physiologic pH range, but that for reduced hemoglobin is shifted to the right. In other words, $O_2Hb$ is a stronger acid than HHb. Thus, the binding of oxygen to HHb is associated with a release of $H^+$; the pH of a 1 mM hemoglobin solution decreases by ~0.2 units when the hemoglobin is oxygenated. Preventing this change in pH would require the effective removal of ~0.6 mmol of $H^+$ per mmol of $O_2Hb$ produced.

Experimental measurement of blood and tissue β cannot adequately separate the contributions of physicochemical buffers, biochemical buffering, organellar buffering, and plasmalemmal acid-base fluxes. Tissue buffering power has been defined operationally as the change in "tissue pH" after an imposed disturbance in acid-base status, typically, a change in blood $PCO_2$. An "average intracellular pH" of tissue is obtained using either microelectrodes or the distribution of weak acids. The tissue buffering power is then defined as,[47]

$$\lambda_{tissue} = \frac{\Delta(\log_{10} PCO_2)}{\Delta pH} \quad (15)$$

The relationship between $\lambda_{tissue}$ and total intracellular buffering capacity ($\beta^{tot}_i$) is

$$\lambda_{tissue} = 1 + \frac{\beta^{tot}_i}{2.303\,[HCO_3^-]} \quad (16)$$

Note that to convert $\lambda_{tissue}$ to $\beta^{tot}_i$, it is necessary to specify the intracellular pH, $PCO_2$, and $HCO_3^-$ concentration.

### Whole Body Buffering

Acid- or alkali-loading experiments have demonstrated that the total body buffering capacity is much larger than that predicted from the $HCO_3^-$ content of the extracellular space. For a 70-kg man, the total buffering capacity is estimated at ~1000 mmol, whereas the $HCO_3^-$ content of extracellular fluid is only ~360 mmol.[3] Because $HCO_3^-$ is localized primarily in the extracellular fluid space, about two thirds of the whole body β is dependent on nonbicarbonate intracellular buffering mechanisms. Thus, $H^+$ flux into cells during acid loading and flux out of cells during alkali loading provide rapid buffering that minimizes changes in extracellular pH.

## ROLE OF THE LUNG IN ACID-BASE HOMEOSTASIS

The lung is the primary mechanism for maintaining $CO_2$ homeostasis.[48] $CO_2$ transport and excretion in vivo is an efficient process that accommodates the excretion of ~200 mL/min of $CO_2$ with a $P_{CO_2}$ gradient of only 6 mm Hg between venous blood and alveolar gas. Metabolically produced $CO_2$ diffuses from cellular fluids into tissue capillary blood down a small, but finite, $P_{CO_2}$ gradient. Approximately 10% of the $CO_2$ is transported in blood as dissolved gas (Table 1–5). A small fraction of blood $CO_2$ is also transported bound to proteins as carbamino compounds. The great majority of $CO_2$ entering the blood is hydrated within the red blood cell to $HCO_3^-$, in the presence of carbonic anhydrase.[49] Most of the $H^+$ produced via $CO_2$ hydration is buffered by hemoglobin. The accompanying $HCO_3^-$ exits the red blood cell by electroneutral exchange with $Cl^-$ via band 3 protein. When mixed venous blood arrives at the lung, the sequence of reactions and transport events is reversed and $CO_2$ is excreted rapidly from the body (see Fig. 1–1*F*).

The nonbicarbonate β of blood (due predominantly to hemoglobin) plays a vital role in $CO_2$ transport and excretion in vivo.[49] Nonbicarbonate buffers are crucial to the transport of metabolically produced $CO_2$ in blood predominantly as $HCO_3^-$. If $CO_2$ transport from peripheral tissues were limited to dissolved $CO_2$ in blood, one can estimate that an arteriovenous difference in $P_{CO_2}$ of ~60 mm Hg would be required to transport 200 mL $CO_2$/min with a resting cardiac output of 6 L/min, as opposed to the normal arteriovenous $P_{CO_2}$ gradient of only 6 mm Hg. The presence of nonbicarbonate buffers increases the $CO_2$ transport capacity of blood by buffering the $H^+$ generated during $CO_2$ loading. Pulmonary excretion of $CO_2$ is regulated by the rate of minute ventilation which, along with pulmonary blood flow, determines the value of alveolar $P_{CO_2}$. Patients with limited cardiopulmonary reserve, who are unable to increase either cardiac output or alveolar ventilation, are particularly vulnerable to inhibition of the normal pathways and mechanisms for $CO_2$ transport. Marked increments in tissue and central mixed venous blood $P_{CO_2}$ and decrements in plasma pH have also been described in patients with moderate-to-severe congestive heart failure.[50]

## ROLE OF THE GUT IN ACID-BASE HOMEOSTASIS

The gastrointestinal tract plays a significant role in the control of systemic pH.[2, 3, 51] In many segments of the alimentary canal, $H^+$ or $HCO_3^-$ are secreted into the gut lumen. Although the secretory mechanisms differ, all secreted $H^+$ and $HCO_3^-$ are produced inside gut mucosal cells via the hydration of $CO_2$. $CO_2$ hydration produces $H^+$ and $HCO_3^-$ in equimolar amounts (see Equation 9). Thus, secretion of $H^+$ into the gut lumen effectively leaves behind an excess $HCO_3^-$, and similarly secretion of $HCO_3^-$ leaves behind an excess $H^+$. These "excess" ions exit the gut mucosal cells in the direction opposite to the gut lumen, that is, into the interstitial fluid and blood (see Fig. 1–1*C*). The stomach adds $H^+$ to the gut lumen, thus acidifying its contents, and adds $HCO_3^-$ to the blood, thus alkalinizing it. Almost all the segments below the pylorus have the opposite effect. They add $HCO_3^-$ to the gut lumen and $H^+$ to the blood. Obviously, if the quantities of $HCO_3^-$ and $H^+$ entering the blood from the GI tract were exactly equimolar, the gut would have no net impact on extracellular acid-base balance: the plasma $HCO_3^-$ concentration would not change. However, on balance, more $HCO_3^-$ than $H^+$ is secreted into the gut lumen and, consequently, more $H^+$ than $HCO_3^-$ enter the blood. Overall, the gut liberates ~20 to 40 mmol of net $H^+$ per day into the blood.

The net $HCO_3^-$ secretion (i.e., in excess of $H^+$ secretion) into the gut lumen is in the range of 20 to 40 mmol/day. Given this secretory rate, and the fact that daily stool volume is typically 0.25 L or less, one would expect a stool $HCO_3^-$ concentration of ~80 to 160 mM. However, the fecal $HCO_3^-$ concentration is typically just 15 to 30 mM. In the colon, undigested food is partially metabolized by bacteria to organic acids, especially acetic, propionic, and butyric acids.

**TABLE 1–5.** Pathways for Pulmonary $CO_2$ Excretion

| | Normal (%) | Without Intravascular Lung Carbonic Anhydrase (%) | Without Red Blood Cell $HCO_3^-$-$Cl^-$ Exchange (%) |
|---|---|---|---|
| Dissolved $CO_2$ | 11 | 12 | 16 |
| $HCO_3^-$ dehydration | | | |
| plasma | 7 | <1 | 15 |
| red blood cell | 68 | 74 | 53 |
| Carbamate dissociation | 14 | 14 | 16 |

These acids are neutralized by stool $HCO_3^-$. The anions (i.e., conjugate bases) of the organic acids remain. Their combined stool concentration is often greater than 100 mM. In this way, most secreted $HCO_3^-$ is consumed and replaced with organic anions, resulting in a low stool $HCO_3^-$ concentration and high stool concentration of organic anions.

## ROLE OF THE LIVER IN ACID-BASE HOMEOSTASIS

The balance between metabolic production and consumption of acid-base equivalents can be controlled via the liver and represents a "metabolic" component of whole body acid-base homeostasis.[52, 53] Hepatic detoxification of $NH_4^+$ (an end-product of amino acid metabolism) has been implicated in regulating whole body pH. There are two major pathways for $NH_4^+$ detoxification and excretion (see Fig. 1–1*D*). One pathway involves hepatic synthesis of urea (the urea cycle) and urinary excretion of that compound. Production and excretion of urea via this pathway consume $HCO_3^-$. The second pathway involves hepatic synthesis of glutamine from $NH_4^+$, reconversion of glutamine to $NH_4^+$ in the kidney (renal ammoniagenesis), and urinary excretion of $NH_4^+$. Excretion of $NH_4^+$ via this pathway has no net effect on body $HCO_3^-$. Changes in the hepatic-renal handling of $NH_4^+$ between urea production/excretion (an $HCO_3^-$-consuming pathway) and glutamine production/renal ammoniagenesis (an $HCO_3^-$-neutral pathway) should "metabolically" impact acid-base status. There is a general consensus that normal functioning of the liver is an important determinant of whole body acid-base status. Cirrhosis of the liver is associated with alkalosis in most cases.[54] However, at present, the role of the liver as an important site for "metabolic" control of pH homeostasis is controversial.

At the level of the liver acini, the cellular systems for ureagenesis and glutamine synthesis are anatomically located in series[52, 54] (see Fig. 1–1*D*). Enzymes of the urea cycle are localized in periportal hepatocytes, whereas glutamine synthetase is confined to perivenous hepatocytes. Thus, as blood transits a hepatic sinusoid, it flows first through a urea-synthesizing segment and then through a glutamine-synthesizing segment of the acinus. The rate-controlling enzyme of the urea cycle, carbamoyl phosphate synthetase, has a low affinity for $NH_4^+$ ($K_m$ = 1–2 mM) relative to the physiologic $NH_4^+$ concentration of portal blood (0.2 to 0.3 mM). Urea synthesis is amplified in periportal hepatocytes by mitochondrial co-localization of carbamoyl phosphate synthetase and glutaminase. This arrangement facilitates the degradation of blood glutamine to urea (a net $HCO_3^-$-neutral process). The $NH_4^+$ that spills over from the ureagenic segment of the acinus is scavenged from the sinusoidal blood in the perivenous glutamine-synthesizing segment. Hepatic glutamine synthetase has a relatively high affinity for $NH_4^+$ ($K_m$ = 0.3 mM). Together, the synthesis of glutamine in perivenous hepatocytes (from $NH_4^+$) and degradation of glutamine in periportal hepatocytes (to urea) is referred to as the "intracellular glutamine cycle." In steady-state conditions, the glutamine-synthesizing and -degrading arms of this cycle are balanced.

Nitrogen metabolism is sensitive to pH. Acidosis causes a decrease in urinary excretion of urea and an increase in excretion of $NH_4^+$ (see later). These changes are associated with a decrement in hepatic urea synthesis and increased release of glutamine from the liver. However, it is unclear whether the effects of acidosis on hepatic nitrogen metabolism reflect changes in the conversion of blood $NH_4^+$ to urea or in the intracellular glutamine cycle. Häussinger and coworkers[52, 54] have extensively studied the role of the liver in acid-base regulation. According to their model, acidosis impairs urea synthesis by inhibiting the conversion of blood $NH_4^+$ to urea. Acidosis is proposed to slow the delivery of $NH_4^+$ and $HCO_3^-$ to carbamoyl phosphate synthetase, in part through the effects of pH on mitochondrial carbonic anhydrase. Consequently, there is an increase in the amount of blood $NH_4^+$ that spills over to the perivenous glutamine-synthesizing segment of the acinus. In this model, detoxification of blood $NH_4^+$ is shifted in acidosis from ureagenesis to glutamine synthesis. This is expected to reduce "metabolic" consumption of $HCO_3^-$, in effect sparing $HCO_3^-$, which would then be available to ameliorate the causative acidosis. However, it is possible to explain the pH sensitivity of hepatic ureagenesis and glutamine release without involving changes in the detoxification of blood $NH_4^+$ to urea. Several authors have concluded that acidosis alters hepatic nitrogen metabolism primarily through effects on the intracellular glutamine cycle.[53, 55, 56] Acidosis inhibits amino acid transport across the plasma membrane of hepatocytes.[55, 56] This is expected to decrease the uptake of blood glutamine by periportal hepatocytes and, hence, to increase the availability of glutamine (and other amino acids) to the kidneys. It would also reduce glutaminase-amplification of urea synthesis, without necessarily altering the availability of blood $NH_4^+$ or $HCO_3^-$ to the urea cycle. According to this interpretation of the data, acidosis has little direct effect on the hepatic detoxification of blood $NH_4^+$ to urea and, thus, has little effect on "metabolic" consumption of $HCO_3^-$ by the liver.

## ROLE OF THE KIDNEY IN ACID-BASE HOMEOSTASIS

The kidneys regulate the plasma $HCO_3^-$ concentration through three main processes: reabsorption of filtered $HCO_3^-$; formation of titratable acidity; and excretion of $NH_4^+$ in the urine.[57–61] The first two processes involve $H^+$ secretion, either by $Na^+$-$H^+$ exchange into the proximal tubule or by secretion of $H^+$ in the subsegments of the collecting duct. Whenever $H^+$ is secreted from a renal cell into the tubule fluid, an intracellular $HCO_3^-$ is left behind. Exit of this $HCO_3^-$ from the cell across the basolateral membrane results ultimately in the addition of $HCO_3^-$ to blood. Secreted $H^+$ can combine with intratubular $HCO_3^-$ to form

$CO_2$, catalyzed by extracellular carbonic anhydrase on the apical membrane of proximal tubular cells. Thus, for each secreted $H^+$ combining with an intratubular $HCO_3^-$, there is the consumption of one intratubular $HCO_3^-$ and the addition of one $HCO_3^-$ to the blood (see Fig. 1–1*E*). The net result of this process is reabsorption of almost all filtered $HCO_3^-$ (~80% to 90% in the proximal tubule and remainder in the loop of Henle and collecting duct). Secreted $H^+$, particularly in the distal tubule, can also combine with urinary buffers, primarily inorganic phosphate. For each secreted $H^+$ combining with urinary $HPO_4^{2-}$ to form $H_2PO_4^-$, there is the addition of one $HCO_3^-$ to the peritubular blood (see Fig. 1–1*E*). This additional $HCO_3^-$ is called new or "regenerated" bicarbonate and replaces $HCO_3^-$ consumed in the buffering of metabolically produced $H^+$. Thus, excreted phosphate is replaced in the blood with $HCO_3^-$. The protonation of urinary buffers such as phosphate is referred to as the titratable acidity of the urine. The third process involved in urinary acidification is the excretion of urinary $NH_4^+$. Renal tubular cells synthesize $NH_4^+$ from glutamine. Excretion of $NH_4^+$ leaves behind an intracellular $HCO_3^-$, which is added to peritubular blood. For each $NH_4^+$ excreted in the urine, one new or regenerated $HCO_3^-$ is added to the blood (see Fig. 1–1*E*).

Total renal $H^+$ secretion is the sum of the filtered $HCO_3^-$ that is reabsorbed, the titratable acid in urine, and urinary $NH_4^+$. The net rate of acid excretion, which represents the amount of new or regenerated $HCO_3^-$ added to the blood by the kidney, is equal to the sum of the titratable acid and urinary $NH_4^+$ concentration less any urinary $HCO_3^-$, all multiplied by the rate of urine flow. Both the excretion of $NH_4^+$ and its rate of production are regulated and undergo adaptive changes under conditions of altered acid-base balance. The kidney has a large capacity to increase $NH_4^+$ generation. For this reason, renal $NH_4^+$ generation is the predominant pathway of $HCO_3^-$ generation in chronic acidotic states. Furthermore, an inadequate production of $NH_4^+$ is the main reason why chronic renal failure leads to metabolic acidosis. By regulating urinary excretion of $H^+$ and $HCO_3^-$, the kidneys play an integral role in the acid-base homeostasis of the body. Although it is clear that control of renal production and excretion of $NH_4^+$ plays a central role in the regulation of systemic acid-base balance, control processes in other organs are involved in the overall regulation of $NH_4^+$ excretion. The liver and skeletal muscle play essential roles in the regulation of systemic acid-base balance by influencing the rate of glutamine production, thus controlling glutamine production to match glutamine utilization by the kidney.

## PHYSIOLOGIC COMPENSATORY RESPONSES

Disturbances in acid-base status can originate from changes in metabolism (anaerobic versus aerobic) or diet (including the ingestion of toxins), or from alterations in respiratory, renal, or hepatic function.[62–68] The initial response to an acid-base disturbance includes physicochemical buffering in the extracellular fluid followed by the participation of cellular buffering mechanisms (Fig. 1–4). The latter include both cytosolic physicochemical buffers and transmembrane fluxes of acid and bases. In a metabolic disturbance, physicochemical buffering is shared approximately equally by the intracellular and extracellular buffer systems (Fig. 1–5 and Table 1–6).[67, 68] In a respiratory disturbance, on the other hand, physicochemical buffering occurs predominantly in the intracellular compartment (see Fig. 1–5 and Table 1–6).[65, 66] Extracellular $HCO_3^-$ cannot buffer a change in $CO_2$ because the interconversion of $CO_2$ and $HCO_3^-$ generates or consumes equivalent amounts of $HCO_3^-$ and $H^+$. The relative contribution of the various cellular acid-base transporters to resolution of an acid-base disturbance is dependent on the type of acid-base disturbance (Fig. 1–5). Both $Na^+$-$H^+$ and $K^+$-$H^+$ exchanges make significant contributions in respiratory and metabolic derangements. In respiratory disturbances, $HCO_3^-$-$Cl^-$ exchange assumes a greater role as entry of $CO_2$ into the cell and its subsequent hydration therein produce $H^+$ (which are buffered by intracellular physicochemical buffers) and $HCO_3^-$ (which is exchanged for external $Cl^-$). Although physicochemical buffering occurs

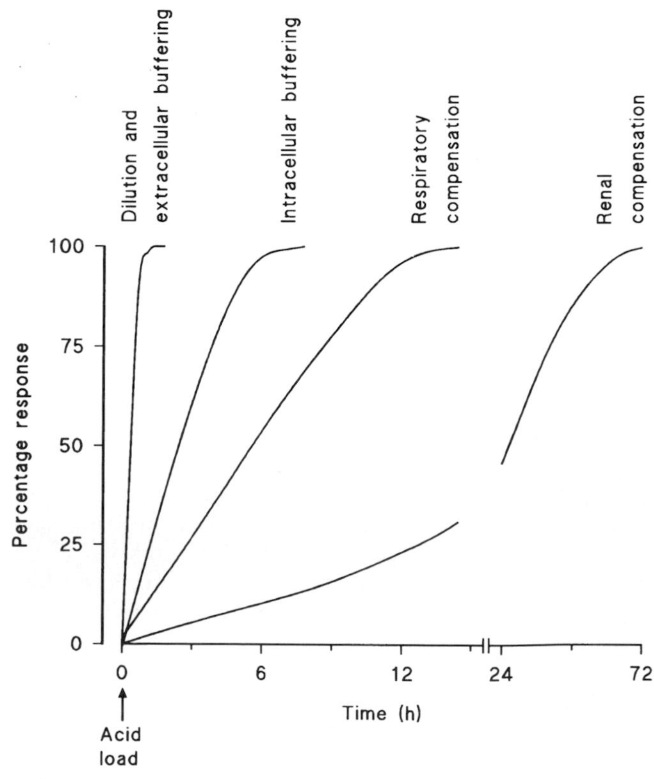


**FIGURE 1–4** ■ Time courses for compensation of extracellular acid-base disturbances. Mixing of added $H^+$ or $OH^-$ with extracellular fluid and buffering in the extracellular space is almost complete within 1 hour. Intracellular buffering involves plasmalemmal fluxes of acid-base equivalents and takes several hours for completion. Respiratory compensation is completed in about 12 to 14 hours, whereas renal compensation is slower and requires about 1 to 2 days for completion.

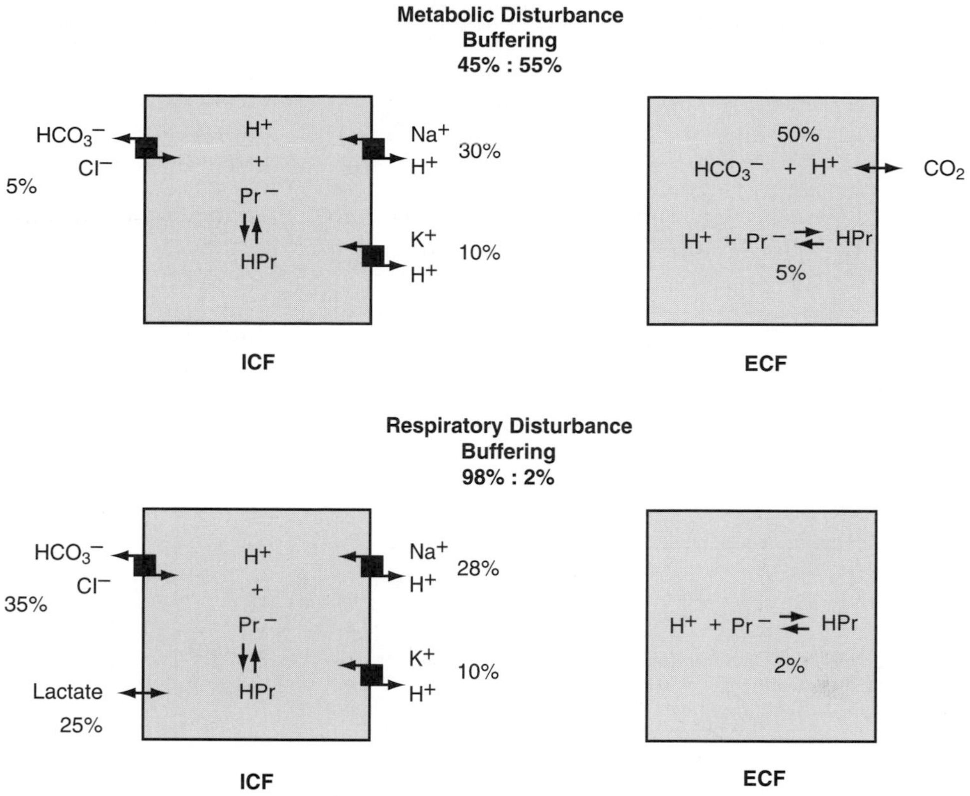

**FIGURE 1–5** ■ Partitioning of buffering of acid-base disturbances between intracellular (ICF) and extracellular (ECF) fluids. ICF and ECF participate almost equally in the buffering of metabolic disturbances, whereas buffering of respiratory disturbances occurs predominantly in the ICF. ECF $HCO_3^-$ plays a major role in the buffering of metabolic disturbances but has no role in the buffering of respiratory disturbances. Buffering in the ICF involves transmembrane flux of acid-base equivalents. $Na^+$-$H^+$ exchange is involved in ICF buffering of both metabolic and respiratory disturbances. The role of $Cl^-$-$HCO_3^-$ exchange is enhanced in respiratory disturbances.

very rapidly over minutes, cellular $H^+$ buffering mediated by alteration in transmembrane acid-base fluxes can require 4 to 6 hours for completion (see Fig. 1–4).

$CO_2$-$HCO_3^-$ buffering and elimination is an efficient system for acid-base regulation as long as the function of the lungs is normal. However, when there is a primary defect in the capacity of the lungs to remove $CO_2$, or when $CO_2$ elimination is inappropriately large, the body experiences a net gain or a net loss of $H^+$. The resultant acid-base disorder is called "respiratory" because it is caused by a primary abnormality in respiratory function. Even though the primary disturbance is in arterial $P_{CO_2}$, it is important to realize that plasma $HCO_3^-$ also changes in acute respiratory acid-base disturbances. This is a consequence of the simultaneous generation of both $H^+$ and $HCO_3^-$ via $CO_2$ hydration in the presence of carbonic anhydrase (see Equation 9). The quantitative relationship between $HCO_3^-$ and $P_{CO_2}$ is described by the $CO_2$ binding curve (Fig. 1–6). When $P_{CO_2}$ first increases, most of the generated $H^+$ are buffered by hemoglobin, leaving $HCO_3^-$ behind and causing an alkaline shift in pH. With continued increases in $P_{CO_2}$, the buffering of $H^+$ becomes less efficient; as a result, the increases in $HCO_3^-$ are less for a given $P_{CO_2}$ change and pH becomes more acid. Note that all along the $CO_2$ binding curve, $HCO_3^-$ and $P_{CO_2}$ change in the same direction, but the ratio between $HCO_3^-$ and $P_{CO_2}$ (and, therefore, pH) declines with increasing $P_{CO_2}$. Hypercapnia is generally well tolerated,[67, 68] except in patients with cardiac arrhythmia, renal insufficiency, or increased intracranial pressure. The corresponding respiratory acidosis is also well tolerated, but sudden changes in arterial pH can have significant adverse effects due to associated changes in cerebral blood flow and ion distributions across cell membranes.

Excessive acid or base loads that consume or produce additional buffer anions (mainly $HCO_3^-$) are the cause of "metabolic" acid-base disorders. The acid load can be the result of altered acid production (e.g., ketoacidosis or lactic acid acidosis), loss of $HCO_3^-$

**TABLE 1–6.** Contributions to Buffering of Acid Loads

| Buffering System | Components | Primary Location | Type of Buffer System | Acids Buffered |
|---|---|---|---|---|
| Bicarbonate | $CO_2$-$HCO_3^-$ | Plasma<br>Interstitial fluid<br>Intracellular fluid | Open | Fixed (50% metabolic $H^+$) |
| Nonbicarbonate | Hemoglobin<br>Other proteins<br>Phosphates | Intracellular fluid<br>Plasma | Closed | Fixed (50% metabolic $H^+$)<br>Volatile (100% respiratory $H^+$) |

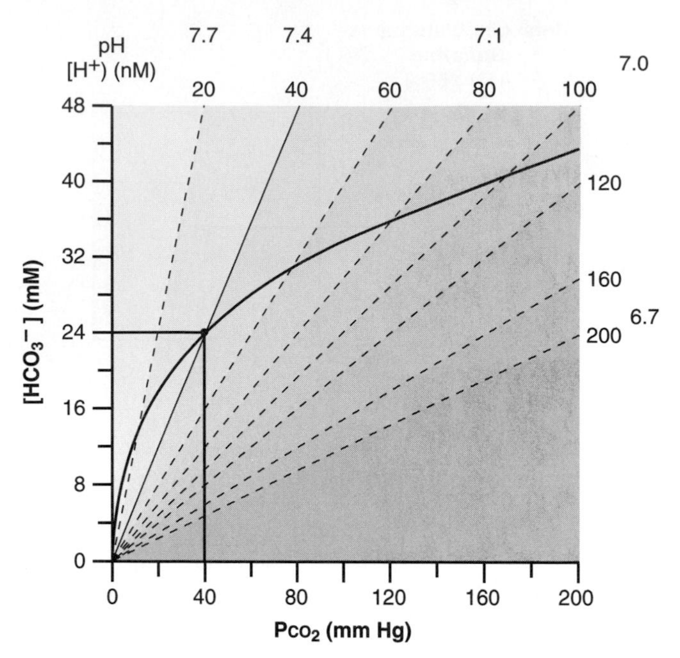


**FIGURE 1–6** ■ $CO_2$ binding curve for whole blood in vitro. Increases in $P_{CO_2}$ from 0 to ~10 mm Hg cause an initial alkalosis, because most of the generated $H^+$ are buffered by hemoglobin. Further increases in $P_{CO_2}$ cause progressive decrements in pH.

(e.g., diarrhea), or inadequate urinary acid excretion (e.g., chronic renal failure). Similarly, a base load can result from increased base production (e.g., consumption of a vegetarian diet), loss of $H^+$ (e.g., vomiting), or inadequate urinary $HCO_3^-$ excretion (e.g., hyperaldosteronism). The primary consequence of all metabolic acid-base disorders is a change in $HCO_3^-$ concentration.

Although cellular and extracellular pH buffering mechanisms are important elements in the defense of acid-base balance, their contributions are limited ultimately by the availability of buffer stores. Thus, pH stability in the face of persistent acid-base abnormalities requires additional homeostatic mechanisms, namely the modulation of renal $HCO_3^-$ reabsorption and pulmonary $CO_2$ excretion. Not all compensations are equally effective. Renal (i.e., metabolic) compensation of respiratory disturbances is generally more efficient than respiratory compensation of metabolic disturbances; that is, the secondary change more closely matches the primary one. It makes sense that renal compensation is more complete; changes in blood $HCO_3^-$ concentration "cost" the body much less than changes in blood $P_{CO_2}$. Altering the blood $HCO_3^-$ concentration requires only a change in renal bicarbonate handling, whereas altering blood $P_{CO_2}$ involves either intense muscular work (i.e., during hyperventilation) or the risk of hypoxemia and hypercapnia (i.e., during hypoventilation). The best-compensated primary disturbance is respiratory alkalosis. In this condition, the secondary fall in blood $HCO_3^-$ concentration so closely matches the primary reduction in blood $P_{CO_2}$ that the pH may actually be in the normal range. Even here, however, the pH does not return to its original set point. In the other primary acid-base disturbances (i.e., respiratory acidosis, metabolic acidosis, and metabolic alkalosis), the pH always remains outside the normal range.

During respiratory disturbances, compensation develops slowly over 2 to 5 days (Fig. 1–7).[63–66] Although the kidney begins to spill $HCO_3^-$ (in respiratory alkalosis) or regenerate $HCO_3^-$ (in respiratory acidosis) within hours, it takes time for these processes to reach peak levels. Additional time is then required for the plasma $HCO_3^-$ concentration to fall or rise to a new steady-state level. When the changes in arterial $P_{CO_2}$ causing a respiratory acid-base disturbance persist, secondary changes in the renal excretion of $H^+$ are initiated. Arterial $P_{CO_2}$ exerts direct control over renal $HCO_3^-$ absorption. In respiratory acidosis, renal ab-

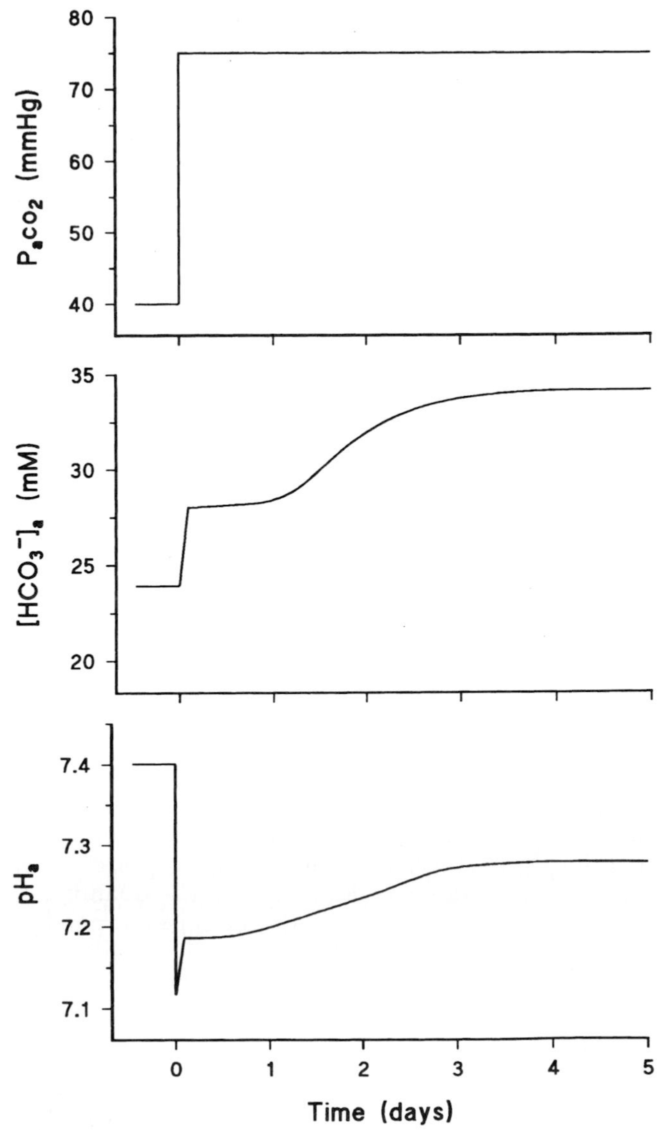


**FIGURE 1–7** ■ Time courses for compensation of respiratory acidosis. Arterial $P_{CO_2}$ is rapidly increased at time zero. This is followed immediately by a rapid increase in plasma $HCO_3^-$ and $H^+$ concentrations. The initial change in $H^+$ concentration (nM versus mM change in $HCO_3^-$) is buffered by hemoglobin and tissue buffers. Plasma $HCO_3^-$ concentration continues to increase slowly over several days as renal compensation takes effect. This returns the plasma $H^+$ concentration toward the normal value.

sorption of $HCO_3^-$ increases, which augments the plasma $HCO_3^-$ concentration. Conversely, the fall in $P_{CO_2}$ in respiratory alkalosis causes an inhibition of renal $H^+$ secretion and $HCO_3^-$ absorption. This loss of $HCO_3^-$ reduces the plasma $HCO_3^-$ concentration. Thus, when a new steady state is reached after several days, the initially large deviations in plasma pH have been substantially (but typically not fully) compensated. The signature of renal compensation is a change in plasma $HCO_3^-$ concentration that is larger than can be accounted for by the law of mass action alone. Compensation develops more slowly in respiratory acidosis than in respiratory alkalosis (3 to 5 days versus 2 to 4 days, respectively) because increased $NH_4^+$ excretion requires changes in proximal tubule enzymes, which occur gradually.

During metabolic disturbances, changes in ventilatory rate develop quickly, and a new steady-state $P_{CO_2}$ is usually reached within about 12 hours (Fig. 1–8).[69, 70] During metabolic acidosis, the kidneys increase net $H^+$ excretion and, hence, $HCO_3^-$ generation. This increase is homeostatic because it adds additional $HCO_3^-$ to the extracellular fluid compartment, thus helping to keep the plasma $HCO_3^-$ concentration from falling as low as it would otherwise. The increase in net $H^+$ excretion is due mainly to a rise in $NH_4^+$ excretion, which can take several days to fully develop but can be quite striking. For example, in metabolic acidosis due to uncontrolled diabetes (i.e., diabetic ketoacidosis), $NH_4^+$ excretion can reach 300 to 500 mmol/day, equivalent to 10 times the normal value. This renal response occurs only during metabolic acidosis of nonrenal origin. For example, in nephrogenic metabolic acidosis, the kidney is itself disabled and is thus unable to greatly augment $H^+$ excretion. Low $pH_i$ appears to act as a signal for increments in $NH_4^+$ excretion. Increments in excretion of titratable acid also serve to increase net $H^+$ excretion, as a compensatory response to metabolic acidosis. The degree to which the excretion of titratable acid can increase is limited in most forms of metabolic acidosis by the availability of phosphate. Nevertheless, metabolic acidosis augments the urinary excretion of phosphate and, therefore, some increase in the formation of titratable acid takes place. For example, titratable acid can increase significantly in diabetic ketoacidosis, where large amounts of β-hydroxybutyrate are generated and excreted. Even though this buffer has a pK′ of 4.8, it can accept at least 150 mmol of $H^+$ per day. In contrast to the formation of titratable acid, renal synthesis of ammonia has a large reserve capacity. The rise in $NH_4^+$ excretion in acidosis reflects both a more effective process of urinary $NH_4^+$ excretion and a higher rate of renal $NH_4^+$ production. These two pathways are sequentially activated. Induction of acidosis is very quickly followed by an increase in $NH_4^+$ excretion. This fast response reflects mainly a boost in the efficiency with which the produced $NH_4^+$ is transferred into the tubular urine and then excreted. With some delay, acidosis stimulates $NH_4^+$ production by upregulating a number of limiting steps in this process, including glutamine release from skeletal muscle, glutamine uptake by renal cells, transport of glutamine into mitochondria, and the activity of enzymes involved in $NH_4^+$ production (e.g., glutaminase, glutamate dehydrogenase). As a consequence of these adjustments, excretion of $NH_4^+$ continues to rise for a number of days. Daily $NH_4^+$ excretion in chronic acidosis can reach 250 to 300 mmol. In most conditions, this increase greatly exceeds the increase in $HCO_3^-$ generation that can be achieved by the excretion of titratable acid.

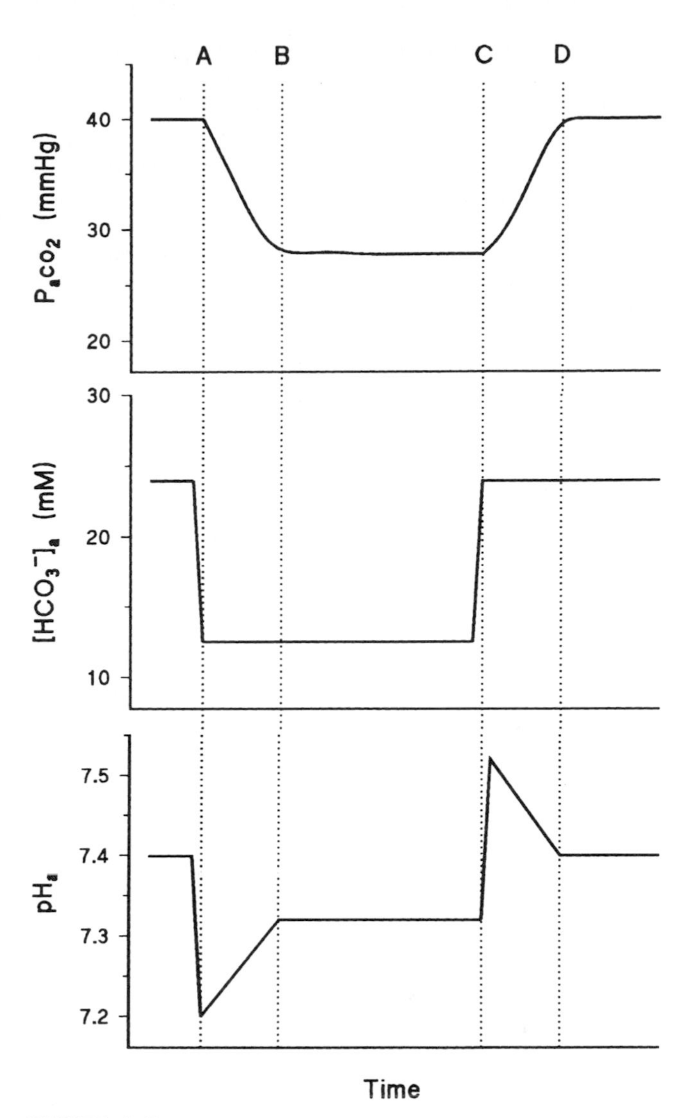


**FIGURE 1–8** ■ Time courses for compensation of a metabolic acidosis. *A,* The initial rapid decline in plasma $HCO_3^-$ concentration causes a rapid increase in plasma $H^+$ concentration, before respiratory compensation occurs. *B,* The plasma $H^+$ concentration returns toward the normal value as respiratory compensation takes effect and $P_{CO_2}$ falls. *C,* The $HCO_3^-$ concentration is normalized faster than the $P_{CO_2}$ and transiently alkalinizes the blood. *D,* Blood pH normalizes as $P_{CO_2}$ returns to normal.

## INDICATORS OF EXTRACELLULAR ACID-BASE STATUS

The quality and extent of acid-base disturbances (acidosis or alkalosis) is indicated by the pH of arterial blood. The respiratory component (primary or compensatory) of the disturbance is indicated by arterial blood $P_{CO_2}$. Unfortunately, various seemingly disparate indices have been used over the past 5 to 6 decades for the quantitative characterization of the nonrespiratory or metabolic component (primary or compensatory). Plasma $HCO_3^-$ concentration is not an ideal index of acid-base disorders. It is not quantitative because it fails to reflect the contribution made by the nonbicarbonate buffers. Moreover, the $HCO_3^-$ concentration varies with $P_{CO_2}$.

Many schemes have been introduced to distinguish between respiratory and metabolic acid-base disturbances.[71–79] On the face of it, these schemes seem at odds with each other. One approach counts weak ions (buffer base), another approach counts strong ions (strong ion difference), and yet another approach counts some strong and some weak ions (anion gap). Some approaches consider plasma parameters ($P_{CO_2}$ versus $HCO_3^-$ concentration), some whole blood (base excess), and other approaches consider all extracellular fluid (standard base excess). The terminology is different and there are important conceptual differences among the different approaches. Nonetheless, these alternative approaches produce quantitatively similar conclusions.

## Total Carbon Dioxide Content of Plasma

The total $CO_2$ content of plasma is the sum of the plasma concentrations of $HCO_3^-$, dissolved $CO_2$, and $H_2CO_3$. The contributions of dissolved $CO_2$ and $H_2CO_3$ are small. For this reason, the total $CO_2$ content of plasma and the plasma $HCO_3^-$ concentrations are often used interchangeably. The particular value of this indicator of acid-base status is that the total $CO_2$ content can be conveniently measured by an automated analyzer. The total $CO_2$ content of venous plasma is often reported routinely along with the electrolytes and urea. Despite the potential loss of $CO_2$ from the venous sample by exposure to air, the measurement offers a useful screening test of acid-base status.

It is traditional to use arterial blood samples for the determination of blood gas parameters ($P_{CO_2}$ and pH) and to use venous blood samples for measurements of serum electrolytes (including total $CO_2$ content). In normal hemodynamically stable adults, the total $CO_2$ content of mixed venous blood is ~2 mM higher than that of arterial blood. Thus, the $HCO_3^-$ concentration calculated from an arterial blood gas sample is generally ~2 mM lower than the total $CO_2$ content measured on a mixed venous blood sample from the same subject. The total $CO_2$ content in a peripheral venous blood sample is variable and depends on the regional blood flow and metabolic rate. However, in all cases it is expected to be higher than the $HCO_3^-$ concentration calculated from an arterial blood gas sample. The seemingly small difference in these values can be significant in patients with severe metabolic acidosis (e.g., diabetic ketoacidosis). Furthermore, calculations of $HCO_3^-$ deficit can be in error because of these intrinsic differences. In patients with impaired cardiac systolic function, such as those with ischemic or hypertensive cardiomyopathies, the discrepancy between arterial and central venous blood gas parameters can be very large when the cardiac output is significantly reduced. Adrogue and associates[50] documented that central venous blood $P_{CO_2}$ can be as high as 65 mm Hg and pH can be as low as 7.25 in patients with severely reduced cardiac output (NYHA class III and IV). Thus, measurements of arterial blood gas values can be misleading in assessing the adequacy of peripheral tissue perfusion and tissue acid-base status.

## Whole Blood Base Excess

The whole blood base excess, usually referred to simply as the base excess (BE), was introduced by Siggaard-Andersen to overcome the limitations of plasma $HCO_3^-$ concentration as an index of acid-base status.[77] It was proposed as an indicator which would not be influenced by changes in the arterial $P_{CO_2}$. Furthermore, it was proposed to provide a quantitative measure of the degree of abnormality in the metabolic component of the acid-base disturbance. BE is derived from the whole blood buffer base, which is defined as the sum of the concentrations of buffer anions (mainly $HCO_3^-$ and hemoglobin) in whole blood. The normal value for whole blood buffer base, determined by titration of whole blood with a strong acid, ranges from 45 to 50 mM. BE is defined as the difference between the observed and normal values for whole blood buffer base. The normal BE value is 0 ± 2.5 mM. Just as $HCO_3^-$ concentration has limitations, so does base excess. First, BE is influenced by arterial $P_{CO_2}$ in vivo. The reason for this is the difference between in vivo and in vitro reactions. In vitro, as the $P_{CO_2}$ changes, the nonbicarbonate buffers accept or donate $H^+$, the $HCO_3^-$ concentration changes in a reciprocal fashion, and the whole blood buffer base (and hence BE) remains unchanged. However, in vivo, as the $P_{CO_2}$ rises, the increase in blood $HCO_3^-$ concentration is attenuated by flux of the anion into the interstitial fluid compartment. Thus, the whole blood buffer base falls and BE assumes a negative value. Changes in BE are related to the whole blood buffering capacity and pH as:

$$\beta_{wholeblood} = \frac{\Delta BE}{\Delta pH} \quad (17)$$

## Standard Base Excess

To overcome the limitation of whole blood base excess, standard base excess (SBE) quantifies the metabolic abnormality of the extracellular fluid. SBE is not the same as the whole blood BE but is the BE of whole blood together with the interstitial fluid. SBE provides an estimate of the change in buffer base needed to restore the metabolic acid-base status to normal in the entire extracellular fluid compartment. SBE is computed from plasma $HCO_3^-$ and plasma:

$$SBE = 0.93\ ([HCO_3^-] - 24.4) + 13.79\ (pH - 7.4) \quad (18)$$

## In Vivo $Pco_2$-$HCO_3^-$ Approach

To circumvent the inaccuracy of BE in vivo, Schwartz and associates[78] determined the differences between the calculated and measured values for blood pH and $Pco_2$ in groups of patients with known acid-base abnormalities in steady states of compensation. The authors described the mean compensatory responses to six primary states of acid-base disorders. Linear equations or maps were used to relate the $H^+$ concentration to $Pco_2$ for primary respiratory disturbances and the $Pco_2$ to $HCO_3^-$ concentration for primary metabolic disorders. Comparison of the measured $HCO_3^-$ concentration with the "expected" concentration provided a quantitative estimate of the metabolic component of the acid-base disturbance. This $Pco_2$-$HCO_3^-$ approach suffers from the same limitations as SBE.

## Weak Anions and Buffer Base

The weak anions consist primarily of $HCO_3^-$ and nonvolatile buffer anions ($A^-$). Weak anions appear or disappear as needed to maintain electroneutrality and chemical equilibrium. The sum of their concentrations was referred to as buffer base (BB)[79]:

$$BB = [HCO_3^-] + [Pr^-] + [HPO_4^-] + [Hb^-] \quad (19)$$

## Nonvolatile Weak Acid Buffer

The nonvolatile weak acid buffers include inorganic phosphate and histidine residues on hemoglobin and albumin. The total concentration of these buffers ($A_{TOT}$) is an independent determinant of acid-base status. $A_{TOT}$ differs from BB in that it includes both the ionized ($A^-$) and un-ionized (HA) species of buffer pairs. $A_{TOT}$ does not include $HCO_3^-$, which is not an independent determinant of acid-base status.

## Strong Ion Difference

The strong ion approach, formalized by Stewart,[73] is based on the principles of electroneutrality (charge balance). In any approach to whole body acid-base status, it is tacitly recognized that acid-base status is controlled via primary regulation of extracellular (i.e., plasma) pH. Whereas cells are endowed with multiple mechanisms for controlling intracellular pH, these in turn are affected by changes in extracellular pH. If one accepts plasma pH to be the regulated parameter, then plasma $H^+$ concentration is the dependent variable and is determined by other independent variables. In classical approaches, the independent variables are blood $Pco_2$ (which in turn is regulated by CNS modulation of ventilatory drive and by metabolism) and plasma $HCO_3^-$ concentration (which is regulated by the kidneys) (Fig. 1–9*A*). Stewart[73] emphasized the distinction between variables capable of acting independently and those whose concentrations are dependent on equilibration among all the systems. He identified the independent variables as the net charge difference between strong ions (the strong ion difference [SID]), the total concentration of weak acid buffers ($A_{TOT}$), and $Pco_2$ (see Fig. 1–9*B*). The dependent variables in the Stewart approach include the concentrations of $H^+$, $HCO_3^-$, and $A^-$ (i.e., the dissociated portion of the weak acid buffers). Changes in water content influence the $H^+$ concentration by changing the independent variables in absolute terms or relative to one another.

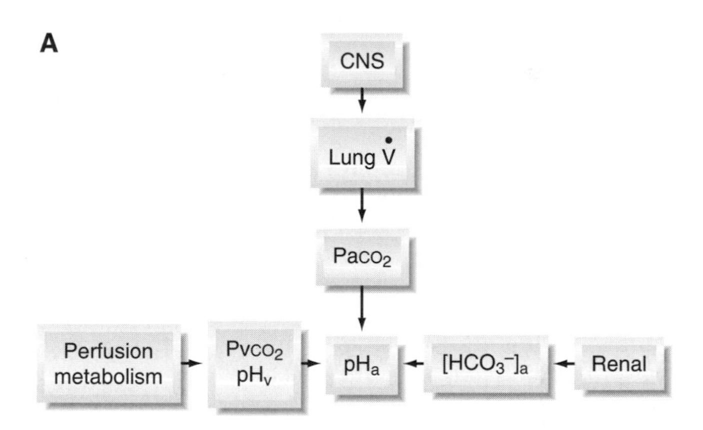


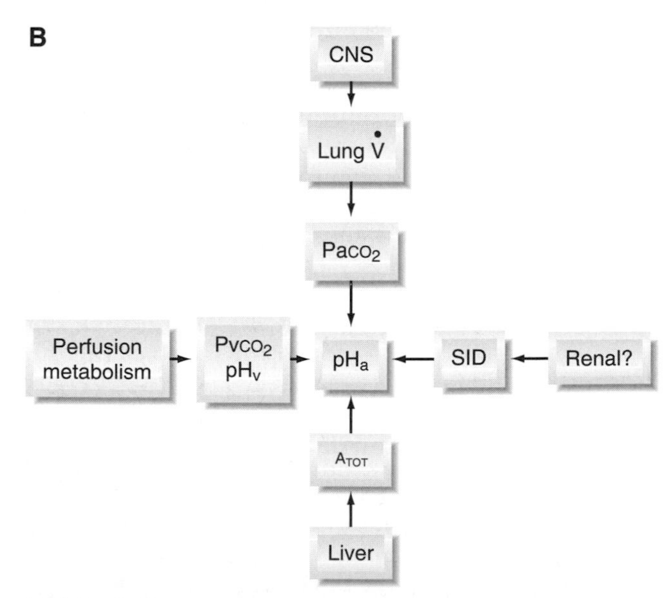


**FIGURE 1–9** ■ Comparison of classical and strong ion difference (SID) approaches to whole body acid-base regulation. In the classical approach *(A)*, the blood $Pco_2$ and $HCO_3^-$ concentration are independent variables that control plasma pH. In the SID approach *(B)*, the independent variables that control the plasma pH are $Pco_2$, the plasma (SID), and total concentration of weak acid buffers ($A_{TOT}$).

By definition of strong cations and anions, electroneutrality dictates:

$$SID = \Sigma\ (strong\ cations) - \Sigma\ (strong\ anions) = [Na^+] + [K^+] - [Cl^-] \quad (20)$$

For practical purposes, no other strong cations in plasma other than $Na^+$ and $K^+$ need to be considered. $Ca^{2+}$ and $Mg^{2+}$ are often considered as strong cations, but they bind reversibly to albumin and other biologic molecules. Additional strong ions, such as β-hydroxybutyrate, acetoacetate, and lactate, can be present in some cases and must then be included in calculating SID. The essence of the Stewart approach is to solve multiple simultaneous equations for electroneutrality and chemical equilibrium for $P_{CO_2}$, SID, and each species contributing to $A_{TOT}$. Typically, SID is estimated in much the same way as Singer and Hastings[79] calculated BB in 1948. However, Stewart's equations describe only plasma, whereas Singer and Hastings' nomogram is for whole blood. Changes in SID are related to the plasma buffer capacity and pH as:

$$\beta_{plasma} = \frac{\Delta SID}{\Delta pH} \quad (21)$$

Stewart's approach implies that the $H^+$ concentration is not controlled by the balance between $P_{CO_2}$ and $HCO_3^-$ concentration. This is consistent with our current understanding that the plasma $HCO_3^-$ concentration is dependent on the interaction of several systems. Furthermore, the approach may have the advantage of linking acid-base changes to other physiologic functions that are influenced by changes in ion concentrations (e.g., membrane potentials, cell volume, and other aspects of fluid and electrolyte regulation). The approach remains a source of controversy, at least in part because of confusion between the concepts involved and the mathematics used to quantify the contributions of independent variables. Conceptually, the approach may call into question some long-held views of the mechanisms that influence the ionic states of different fluid compartments (e.g., $Na^+$-$H^+$ and $Cl^-$-$HCO_3^-$ exchanges). However, the approach cannot identify the mechanisms by which changes are brought about; it can only quantify the effects. The mathematical implications are also controversial. Although $H^+$ concentration can be calculated using the approach, obviously this is not a primary objective; the $H^+$ concentration can be measured. There is generally good concordance between measured and calculated $H^+$ concentrations in plasma, but the accuracy is dependent on the accuracy with which the independent variables are measured. For example, at low SID values, a small error in the determination of SID can have a large effect on the calculated $H^+$ concentration. One of the problems with the SID approach is the large number of measurements of multiple ions that must be made. Another criticism relates to the confidence that can be placed in the equation parameters. The most critical of these are $A_{TOT}$ and the dissociation constants of the various buffer species ($K_A$). In plasma, these values are linked to plasma protein content. The results of classic titration studies established effective $K_A$ values. However, these values for plasma represent the combined effects of many amino acids with widely varying $K_A$, and new mathematical expressions have been derived. Such studies have theoretical importance, but the practical application of the approach has not shown significant advantages.[80–82]

The utility of the SID approach for assessing cellular acid-base regulation has not yet been rigorously evaluated. However, coupled fluxes of acid-base equivalents and counter ions (e.g., $Na^+$ and $Cl^-$) across cell membranes would be expected to impact both the cytosolic SID and $pH_i$. Conversion of SID theory for plasma to whole blood requires computing the hemoglobin buffer strength and its effective dissociation constant and also the exchange of ions between red blood cells and plasma. A theoretical comparison of whole blood SID with BE using Siggaard-Andersen's equations showed no significant difference.[81, 82] The SID approach may be useful when identifying missing ions in plasma. It is, however, difficult to recommend the SID approach in routine clinical practice. Furthermore, the SID approach is only valid for an open system, where $P_{CO_2}$ is an independent variable. In a closed system, such as during cardiac arrest or circulatory insufficiency, $P_{CO_2}$ (particularly venous blood values) becomes perfusion-dependent and the body might behave as a closed system.

## Anion Gap and Strong Ion Gap

Anion gap (AG) was introduced by Emmett and Narins[83] and is based on the electroneutrality principle. It determines the difference between measured and unmeasured ions in plasma:

$$AG = [Na^+] + [K^+] - [Cl^-] - [HCO_3^-] \quad (22)$$

This difference reflects the concentration of buffer anions ($A^-$) and unmeasured strong ions. Normally, $A^-$ is the only unmeasured anion of a significant amount and, hence, AG provides an estimate of the buffer anion concentration. The usual range (when $K^+$ is included) is 3 to 11 mM. When $K^+$ is not included, a normal AG is 8 to 16 mM. The $A^-$ concentration is a function of pH and $A_{TOT}$. In plasma, $A_{TOT}$ seems to be represented solely by albumin and inorganic phosphate. The large normal range of AG limits its ability to detect metabolic acidosis. SBE may be a much better tool for detecting such imbalances. AG is helpful for distinguishing between increased anion gap metabolic acidosis versus normal anion gap metabolic acidosis. The main value of AG may be in identifying a combined chronic respiratory acidosis plus acute metabolic acidosis, in which instance the AG can be elevated despite a normal SBE with elevated $P_{CO_2}$ and normal $P_{CO_2}$-$HCO_3^-$ relationship. A potential improvement on plasma AG is the plasma strong ion gap (SIG):

$$[SIG] = [BB] - [SIG] \quad (23)$$

## GRAPHIC REPRESENTATIONS OF EXTRACELLULAR ACID-BASE STATUS

The acid-base status of body fluids can be graphically represented in numerous ways. Most are based on the Henderson-Hasselbalch equation and the buffer power of blood and, therefore, are equivalent. It is generally assumed for such plots that the nonbicarbonate β is pH independent, which is a reasonable assumption for most extracellular fluids. The traditional technique is the Davenport or pH-$HCO_3^-$ diagram (Fig. 1–10) which results from the analysis of buffering. The iso-$P_{CO_2}$ lines in this diagram rise exponentially with increasing pH. The slope $d(HCO_3^-)/dpH$ at any $CO_2$ isopleth (i.e., at a fixed $P_{CO_2}$) represents the open-system buffering capacity provided by $CO_2$-$HCO_3^-$. In contrast, plots of the change in $HCO_3^-$ concentration versus pH with changes in $P_{CO_2}$ yield the total nonbicarbonate buffering power of the fluid (true plasma β in plots derived from blood data). The ability to analyze abnormalities in acid-base balance using a standard Davenport diagram, although theoretically appealing, is limited by two main factors. First, the number of buffer systems in the body is so large and the distribution of individual buffer systems so complex that it is not possible to define a unique nonbicarbonate buffer line that is applicable to both acute and chronic disturbances. Second, the compensatory physiologic responses of alterations in bicarbonate reabsorption and pulmonary $CO_2$ excretion in the face of primary acid-base abnormalities are complex and variable depending on the type and duration of disturbance. For example, there is a significant difference between the $CO_2$ dissociation curves for whole blood in vitro and for the whole body in vivo. This discrepancy is due to differences in the $HCO_3^-$ distribution space.[11] In vitro, $HCO_3^-$ has access only to plasma, whereas in vivo $HCO_3^-$ can redistribute into the much larger poorly buffered interstitial space. Additionally, mechanisms of $pH_i$ regulation result in a further apparent lowering of the buffer capacity of the extracellular space. The net effect of these two processes is to reduce the slope of the in vivo $CO_2$ dissociation curve by 30% to 50%, depending on the size of the extra- and intracellular fluid compartments. Furthermore, the in vivo mechanisms of biochemical and organellar buffering are difficult to separate quantitatively. To obviate these theoretical and practical difficulties, it is customary to use empirically determined relationships between pH and $P_{CO_2}$ (or $HCO_3^-$) for various idealized simple acid-base relationships. Several points of caution are worth reiterating in the use of such acid-base maps or nomograms. It is assumed that sufficient time has elapsed for the full compensatory response (e.g., 6 to 12 hours for ventilatory compensation in primary metabolic disturbances and as much as 2 to 4 days for the metabolic response to primary respiratory disturbances). Furthermore, finding acid-base values within a shaded area does not necessarily imply the existence of a simple acid-base disorder.

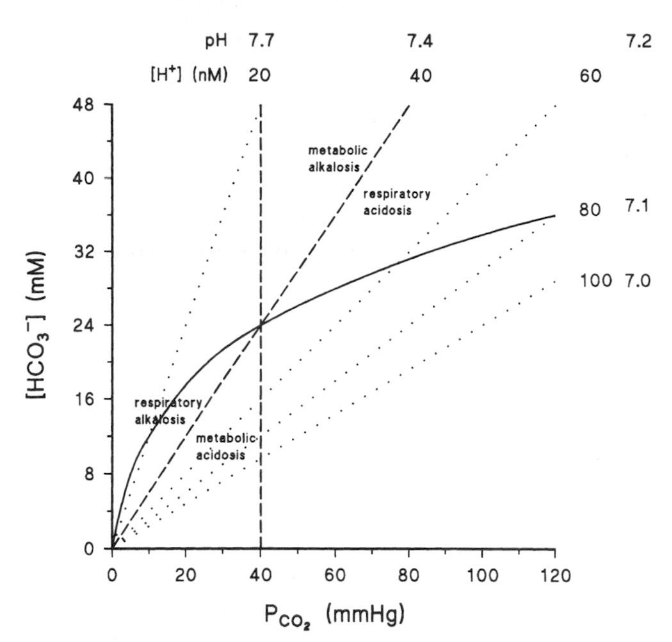


FIGURE 1–11 ■ Plot of blood $P_{CO_2}$ versus $HCO_3^-$ concentration, indicating regions corresponding with the particular acid-base disorders. The isopleths are blood pH.

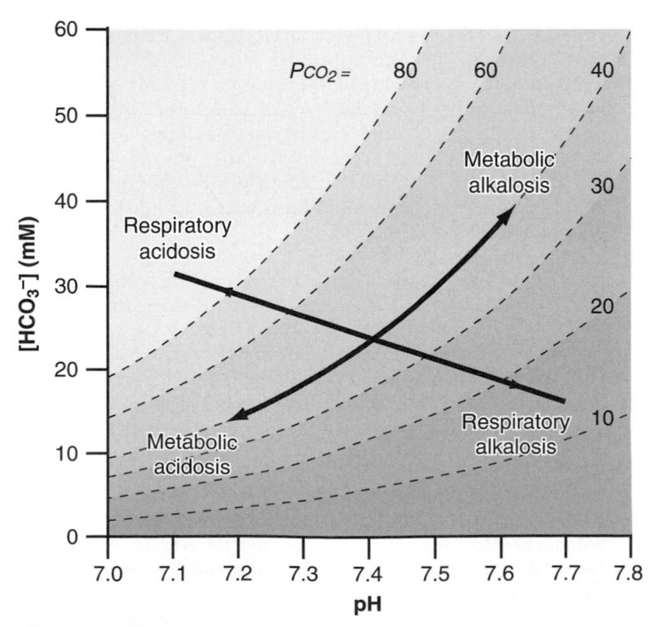


FIGURE 1–10 ■ Davenport diagram of blood pH versus $HCO_3^-$ concentration, indicating the effects of particular acid-base disorders. Isopleths are blood $P_{CO_2}$. The slope of the *straight solid line* represents the nonbicarbonate buffering capacity.

The $P_{CO_2}$-$HCO_3^-$ diagram (Fig. 1–11) follows from the blood $CO_2$ dissociation curve. The $(HCO_3^-)/(CO_2)$ ratio is shown by the slope of the iso-pH lines.

The pH-log $P_{CO_2}$ diagram (Fig. 1–12) offers the advantage of plotting the directly measured variables $P_{CO_2}$ and pH against each other. It is widely used today.[8] The nonbicarbonate buffering power of true plasma is represented by the difference in negative slope of the (slightly curved) lines and lines of constant $HCO_3^-$ concentration. The latter have a slope of −1. Metabolic disturbances are represented by displacements parallel to the abscissa.

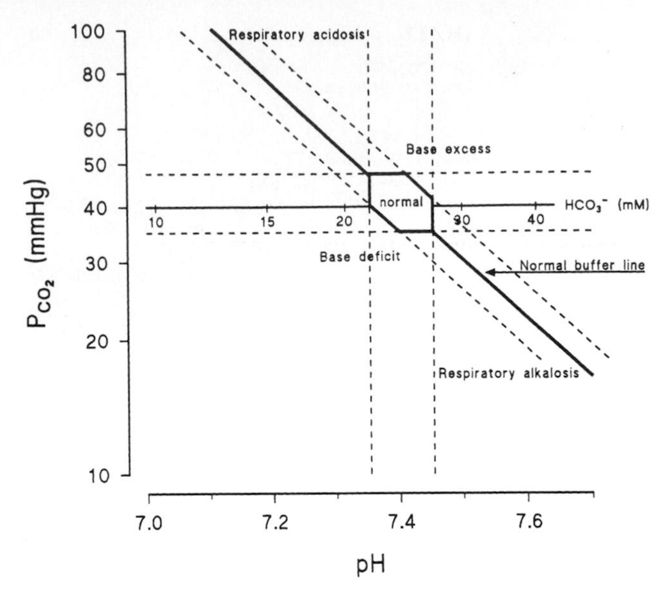


**FIGURE 1–12** ■ Plot of blood pH versus the logarithm of $P_{CO_2}$, indicating regions corresponding to particular acid-base disorders.


## ACKNOWLEDGMENTS

Supported by NIH HL51421 and Constance Marsili Schafer Research Fund.


## REFERENCES


1. Thompson WST, Adams JF, Cowan RA: Clinical Acid-Base Balance. New York, Oxford University Press, 1997.
2. Valtin H, Gennari FJ: Acid Base Disorders: Basic Concepts and Clinical Management. Boston, Little, Brown, 1987.
3. Bidani A, DuBose TD: Acid-base regulation: Cellular and whole body. In Arieff AI, DeFronzo RA (eds): Fluid, Electrolyte, and Acid Base Disorders. New York, Churchill Livingstone, 1995, pp 69–104.
4. Kleinman JG, Lemann J: Acid production. In Maxwell MH, Kleeman CR, Narins RG (eds): Clinical Disorders of Fluid and Electrolyte Metabolism. New York, McGraw-Hill, 1987, pp 159–174.
5. Abelow B: Understanding Acid-Base. Baltimore, Williams & Wilkins, 1998.
6. Madias NE, Cohen JJ: Acid base chemistry and buffering. In Cohen JJ, Kassirer JP (eds): Acid-Base. Boston, Little, Brown, 1982, pp 3–12.
7. Gennari FJ, Cohen JJ: Intracellular acid, base physiology. In Cohen JJ, Kassirer JP (eds): Acid-Base. Boston, Little, Brown, 1982, pp 25–40.
8. Davenport HW: The ABC of Acid-Base Chemistry. Chicago, University of Chicago Press, 1983.
9. Boron WF: Chemistry of buffer equilibria in blood plasma. In Seldin DW, Giebisch G (eds): The Regulation of Acid Base Balance. New York, Raven Press, 1989, pp 3–32.
10. Bidani A, Crandall ED: Quantitative aspects of capillary $CO_2$ exchange. In Chang HK, Paiva M (eds): Respiratory Physiology: An Analytical Approach. New York, Marcel Dekker, 1989, pp 371–419.
11. Fernandez PC, Cohen RM, Feldman GM: The concept of bicarbonate distribution space: The crucial role of bicarbonate buffers. Kidney Int 36:747–752, 1989.
12. Swan RG, Pitts RF: Neutralization of infused acid by nephrectomized dogs. J Clin Invest 34:205–212, 1955.
13. Bushinsky DA: Internal exchanges of hydrogen ions: Bone. In Seldin DW, Giebisch G (eds): The Regulation of Acid Base Balance. New York, Raven Press, 1989, pp 69–88.
14. Gevers W: Generation of protons by metabolic processes in heart cells. J Mol Cell Cardiol 9:867–874, 1977.
15. Hochachka PW, Mommsen TP: Protons and anaerobiosis. Science 219:1391–1397, 1983.
16. Gevers W, Dowdle E: The effect of pH on glycolysis in vitro. Clin Sci 25:343–349, 1963.
17. Relman AS: Metabolic consequences of acid-base disorders. Kidney Int 1:347–359, 1972.
18. Mellman I, Fuchs R, Helenius A: Acidification of the endocytic and exocytic pathways. Annu Rev Biochem 55:663–700, 1986.
19. Ohkuma S, Poole B: Fluorescence probe measurement of the intralysosomal pH in living cells and the perturbation of pH by various agents. Proc Natl Acad Sci U S A 75:3327–3331, 1978.
20. Nomura K, Nakamura Y: Determination of the intravesicular pH of fragmented sarcoplasmic reticulum with 5,5-dimethyl-2,4-oxazolidinedione. J Biochem 80:1393–1399, 1976.
21. Putnam RW, Roos A: Intracellular pH. In Hoffman JF, Jamieson JD (eds): Handbook of Physiology. Section 14: Cell Physiology. New York, Oxford University Press, 1997, pp 389–440.
22. Tennessen TI: Intracellular pH and electrolyte regulation. In Grenvik A, Ayres SM, Holbrook PR, Shoemaker WC (eds): Textbook of Critical Care. Philadelphia, WB Saunders, 2000, pp 507–522.
23. Boron WF: Cellular buffering and intracellular pH. In Seldin DW, Giebisch G (eds): The Regulation of Acid Base Balance. New York, Raven Press, 1989, pp 33–56.
24. Boron WF: Control of intracellular pH. In Seldin DW, Giebisch G (eds): The Kidney: Physiology and Pathophysiology. New York, Raven Press, 1992, pp 219–263.
25. Madshus IH: Regulation of intracellular pH in eukaryotic cells. Biochem J 250:1–8, 1988.
26. Hoffman EK, Simonsen LO: Membrane mechanisms in volume and pH regulation in vertebrate cells. Physiol Rev 69:315–382, 1989.
27. Mahnesmith RL, Aronson PS: The plasma membrane sodium-hydrogen exchanger and its role in physiologic and pathophysiologic processes. Circ Res 56:774–782, 1985.
28. Grinstein S, Rothstein A: Mechanisms of regulation of the $Na^+/H^+$ exchanger. J Membr Biol 90:1–12, 1986.
29. Benos DJ: Amiloride: Chemistry, kinetics, and structure-activity relationships. In Grinstein S (ed): $Na^+/H^+$ Exchange. CRC Press, Boca Raton, FL, pp 121–136, 1988.
30. Lowe AG, Lambert A: Chloride bicarbonate exchange and related transport processes. Biochem Biophys Acta 694:353–374, 1983.
31. Gunn RB: Transport of anions across red cell membranes. In Giebisch G, Tosteson DC, Ussing HH (eds): Membrane Transport in Biology. New York, Springer-Verlag, 1979, pp 59–80.
32. Reinertsen KV, Tennessen TI, Jacobsen J, et al: Role of chloride/bicarbonate antiport in the control of cytosolic pH: Cell-line differences in activity and regulation of antiport. J Biol Chem 263:11117–11125, 1988.
33. Lin P, Ahluwalia M, Grinstein E: An alkaline pH-activated $Cl^-$ anion exchanger regulates pH homeostasis in fibroblasts. Am J Physiol 258:C132–C139, 1990.
34. Ludt J, Tennessen TI, Sandvig K, Olsnes S: Evidence for involvement of protein kinase C in regulation of intracellular pH by $Cl^-/HCO_3^-$ antiport. J Membr Biol 119:179–186, 1991.
35. Alpern RJ, Chambers M: Basolateral membrane $Cl^-/HCO_3^-$ exchange in the rat proximal convoluted tubule: Na-dependent and -independent modes. J Gen Physiol 89:581–598, 1987.
36. Boyarsky G, Ganz MB, Sterzel RB, Boron WF: pH regulation in single glomerular mesangial cells. II: $Na^+$-dependent and -independent $Cl^-$-$HCO_3^-$ exchangers. Am J Physiol 255:C857–C869, 1988.
37. Aronson PS, Soleimani M, Grassl SM: Properties of the renal $Na^+$-$HCO_3^-$ cotransporter. Semin Nephrol 11:28–36, 1991.
38. Soleimani M, Aronson PS: Ionic mechanism of $Na^+$-$HCO_3^-$ cotransport in rabbit renal basolateral membrane vesicles. J Biol Chem 264:18302–18308, 1989.
39. Alpern RJ: Mechanism of basolateral membrane $H^+/OH^-/HCO_3^-$ transport in the rat proximal convoluted tubule: A sodium-coupled electrogenic process. J Gen Physiol 86:613–636, 1985.
40. Schuurmans-Stekhoven F, Bonting SL: Transport adenosine tri-

phosphatases: Properties and functions. Physiol Rev 61:1–76, 1981.
41. Stone DK, Xie XS: Proton translocating ATPases: Issues in structure and function. Kidney Int 33:767–774, 1988.
42. Sachs G, Wallmark B, Saccomani G, et al: The ATP-dependent component of gastric acid secretion. In Slayman CL (ed): Current Topics in Membranes and Transport, vol 16. New York, Academic Press, pp 135–151, 1982.
43. Bowman BJ, Bowman EJ: $H^+$-ATPases from mitochondria, plasma membranes, and vacuoles of fungal cells. J Membr Biol 94:83–97, 1986.
44. Kinne-Saffran E, Beauwens R, Kinne R: An ATP-driven proton pump in brush-border membranes from rat renal cortex. J Membr Biol 64:67–76, 1982.
45. Bidani A, Brown SES, Heming TA, et al: Cytoplasmic pH in pulmonary macrophages: Recovery from acid load is $Na^+$ independent and NEM sensitive. Am J Physiol 257:C65–C76, 1989.
46. Swallow CJ, Grinstein S, Rotstein O: A vacuolar type $H^+$-ATPase regulates cytoplasmic pH in murine macrophages. J Biol Chem 265:7645–7654, 1990.
47. Roos A: Intracellular pH and buffering power of the rat brain. Am J Physiol 221:176–181, 1971.
48. Roughton FJW: Transport of oxygen and carbon dioxide. In Fenn WO, Rahn H (eds): Handbook of Physiology. Section 3: Respiration, vol I. Washington, DC, American Physiological Society, 1964, pp 767–825.
49. Bidani A: Analysis of abnormalities of capillary $CO_2$ exchange in vivo. J Appl Physiol 70:1686–1699, 1991.
50. Adrogue HJ, Rashad MN, Gorin AB, et al: Assessing acid-base status in circulatory failure: Differences between arterial and central venous blood. N Engl J Med 320:1312–1316, 1989.
51. Knauf H, Sachs G: $H^+/HCO_3^-$ transport by the gastrointestinal tract. In Häussinger D (ed): pH Homeostasis: Mechanisms and Control. New York, Academic Press, 1988, pp 427–445.
52. Häussinger D: Liver regulation of acid-base balance. Miner Electrolyte Metab 23:249–252, 1997.
53. Schoolwerth AC, O'Donovan DJ: Effects of acid-base alterations and protein deletion on hepatic nitrogen metabolism. Adv Exp Med Biol 420:217–227, 1997.
54. Häussinger DA, Meijer AJ, Gerok W, Sies H: Hepatic nitrogen metabolism and acid-base homeostasis. In Häussinger D (ed): pH Homeostasis: Mechanisms and Control. New York, Academic Press, 1988, pp 337–377.
55. Boon L, Blommaart JE, Meijer AJ, et al: Acute acidosis inhibits liver amino acid transport: No primary role for the urea cycle in acid-base balance. Am J Physiol 267:F1015–F1020, 1994.
56. Boon L, Blommaart JE, Meijer AJ, et al: Response of hepatic amino acid consumption to chronic metabolic acidosis. Am J Physiol 271:F198–F202, 1996.
57. DuBose TD Jr, Good DW, Hamm LL, Wall SM: Ammonium transport in the kidney: New physiological concepts and their clinical implications. J Am Soc Nephrol 1:1193–1203, 1991.
58. Good DW: New concepts in renal ammonia excretion. In Seldin DW, Giebisch G (eds): The Regulation of Acid Base Balance. New York, Raven Press, 1989, pp 169–184.
59. Knepper MA: Renal transport of ammonia in systemic pH regulation. In Häussinger D (ed): pH Homeostasis: Mechanisms and Control. New York, Academic Press, 1988, pp 305–322.
60. Alpern RJ, Rector FC: Renal regulation of acid-base metabolism. In Maxwell MH, Kleeman CR, Narins RG (eds): Clinical Disorders of Fluid and Electrolyte Metabolism. New York, McGraw-Hill, 1987, pp 175–206.
61. Schnermann JB, Sayegh SI: Kidney Physiology. Philadelphia, JB Lippincott, 1997.
62. Woodbury JW: Body acid-base state and its regulation. In Patton HD, Fuchs AF, Hille B, et al (eds): Textbook of Physiology. Philadelphia, WB Saunders, 1989, pp 1114–1138.
63. Madias NE, Cohen JJ: Respiratory acidosis. In Cohen JJ, Kassirer JP (eds): Acid-Base. Boston, Little, Brown, 1982, pp 307–348.
64. Molony RD, Scheiss MC, Dosekun AK: Respiratory acid-base disorders. In Kokko JP, Tannen RL (eds): Fluid and Electrolytes. Philadelphia, WB Saunders, 1996, pp 267–342.
65. Gennari FJ: Respiratory acidosis and alkalosis. In Maxwell MH, Kleeman CR, Narins RG (eds): Clinical Disorders of Fluid and Electrolyte Metabolism. New York, McGraw-Hill, 1987, pp 713–742.
66. Madias NE, Cohen JJ: Respiratory alkalosis and acidosis. In Seldin DW, Giebisch G (eds): The Kidney: Physiology and Pathophysiology. New York, Raven Press, 1992, pp 2837–2872.
67. Bidani A, Tzouanakis AE, Cardenas V, Zwischenberger J: Permissive hypercapnia in acute respiratory failure. JAMA 272:957–962, 1994.
68. Bidani A, Cardenas V, Tzouanakis AE, Zwischenberger J: Permissive hypercapnia. In Bone RC (ed): Pulmonary and Critical Care Medicine, vol 3. Chicago, Mosby-Year Book, 1995, pp 1–17.
69. Alpern RJ, Emmett M, Seldin DW: Metabolic alkalosis. In Seldin DW, Giebisch G (eds): The Kidney: Physiology and Pathophysiology. New York, Raven Press, 1992, pp 2733–2758.
70. Emmett M, Alpern RJ, Seldin DW: Metabolic acidosis. In Seldin DW, Giebisch G (eds): The Kidney: Physiology and Pathophysiology. New York, Raven Press, 1992, pp 2759–2836.
71. Gattinoni L, Lissoni A: Pathophysiology and diagnosis of respiratory acid-base disturbances in patients with critical illness. In Ronco C, Bellmomo R (eds): Critical Care Nephrology. Boston, Kluwer Academic, 1998, pp 297–311.
72. Holmes O: Human Acid-Base Physiology. New York, Chapman & Hall, 1993.
73. Stewart PA: How to Understand Acid-Base: A Quantitative Acid-Base Primer for Biology and Medicine. New York, Elsevier, 1981.
74. Jones NL: A quantitative physicochemical approach to acid-base physiology. Clin Biochem 23:189–195, 1990.
75. Jones NL: Acid-base physiology. In Crystal RG, West JB, Barnes PJ, Weibel ER (eds): The Lung—Scientific Foundations. Philadelphia, Lippincott-Raven, 1997, pp 1657–1672.
76. Schlichtig R, Grogono AW, Severinghaus JW: Current status of acid-base quantitation in physiology and medicine. Anesthesiol Clin North Am 16:211–233, 1998.
77. Severinghaus JW: Acid-base balance controversy. J Clin Monitor 7:274–277, 1991.
78. Schwartz WB, Brackett NC, Cohen JJ: The response of extracellular hydrogen ion concentration to graded degrees of hypercapnia: The physiological limits of defense of pH. J Clin Invest 44: 291–301, 1965.
79. Singer RB, Hastings AB: Improved clinical method for estimation of disturbances of acid-base balance of human blood. Medicine 27:223–242, 1948.
80. Schlichtig R: Base excess and strong ion difference during $O_2$-$CO_2$ exchange. Adv Exp Med Biol 411:97–102, 1997.
81. Schlichtig R: Base excess vs strong ion difference. Which is more helpful? Adv Exp Med Biol 411:91–95, 1997.
82. Siggaard-Andersen O, Fogh-Andersen N: Base excess or buffer base (strong ion difference) as measure of a non-respiratory acid-base disturbance. Acta Anaesthesiol Scand Suppl 107:123–128, 1995.
83. Emmett M, Narins RG: Clinical use of the anion gap. Medicine 56:38–54, 1977.

CHAPTER 2

# Urinary Acidification

Robert J. Alpern, MD ▪ L. Lee Hamm, MD

The kidneys are the predominant organs responsible for maintenance of the nonrespiratory components of acid-base balance, the so-called metabolic component. This chapter summarizes renal acid-base transport; references are selective. More extensive details are provided in other recent reviews.[1, 2]

The acid-base functions of the kidney involve maintenance of body buffers (principally via maintenance of a normal plasma bicarbonate [$HCO_3^-$] concentration) and excretion of nonvolatile acids (essentially all acids except carbon dioxide [$CO_2$]). Under most conditions, the kidneys accomplish this by two main processes: reabsorption of all bicarbonate filtered at the glomerulus, and excretion of acid in the form of titratable acid and ammonium ($NH_4^+$), to produce new bicarbonate. With alkali loads, the kidneys can also restore acid-base balance by the urinary excretion of alkali into the urine. Quantitatively, the absolute amount of bicarbonate filtered and reabsorbed on a daily basis is some 4000 mEq/day (glomerular filtration rate [GFR] × plasma bicarbonate), much greater than urinary acid excretion.

Net acid excretion (NAE) by the kidneys is expressed by the equation:

$$NAE = TA + NH_4^+ - HCO_3^-$$

where TA is titratable acid, and bicarbonate is urinary bicarbonate, which, under most conditions, is negligible. Because urinary $NH_4^+$ is not an acid in a chemical sense, as discussed later, this equation in essence represents not the rate of acid excretion by the kidneys but the rate of "new" bicarbonate production by the kidneys during excretion of titratable acid and ammonium. Ordinarily, NAE is approximately 50 to 100 mEq/day, depending on diet. Ammonium excretion usually represents approximately two thirds of NAE under usual conditions but can adapt upward to an even larger proportion under conditions of acid loads. *Titratable acid* is a term used to express the amount of acid that has been added to urine. Because urine contains a mixture of many buffers in variable amounts, the urine pH alone poorly reflects the amount of acid the kidneys are excreting. To determine titratable acid, urine is titrated from its collected pH up to plasma pH with the strong alkali sodium hydroxide (NaOH). The amount of alkali used to bring the urine pH up to plasma pH is quantitatively titratable acid. The principal urinary buffer is phosphate, which has a $pK_a$ of approximately 6.8. Other urinary buffers are present in much lower concentrations and include such substances as creatinine and citrate.[3] Ammonia/ammonium ($NH_3/NH_4^+$) is a rather poor buffer in the physiologic pH range, because the $pK_a$ of $NH_4^+$ is 9, well above both plasma and particularly urine pH.

The kidneys accomplish acid-base homeostasis by means of an elegant and complex system of transport processes along the nephron. Both bicarbonate reabsorption and titratable acid excretion are accomplished by hydrogen ion ($H^+$) secretion into the tubule lumen, via a variety of transport proteins in the apical membranes of various cell types in different nephron segments. Ammonium excretion depends on both the biochemical production of ammonium, principally in the proximal tubule, and the transport of ammonium into the final urine, which occurs through a complex process that is linked to $H^+$ transport in various ways (discussed later).

The proximal tubule is responsible for the majority of bicarbonate reabsorption, the production of ammonium, and the initiation of titratable acid excretion. The more distal parts of the nephron are conceptually the site of final regulation of titratable acid excretion, ammonium excretion, and final lowering of urine pH. The processes of bicarbonate reabsorption and $H^+$ secretion are discussed in sequential order from proximal tubule to thick ascending limb to collecting duct. Ammonium excretion is considered separately because of its unique aspects. Carbonic anhydrase is important in most aspects of acid-base transport and is therefore discussed first.

## CARBONIC ANHYDRASE

Carbonic anhydrase (CA) facilitates acid-base transport all along the nephron. CA catalyzes the reversible reaction:

$$CO_2 + OH^- \leftrightarrow HCO_3^-$$

This equation, when considered with the reaction $H_2O \leftrightarrow H^+ + OH_3^-$, is equivalent to the more commonly written equation:

$$CO_2 + H_2O \leftrightarrow HCO_3^- + H^+$$

Although carbonic acid ($H_2CO_3$) was previously considered an intermediate, this is not the case at the molecular level.[4] By greatly accelerating the interconversion of $CO_2$ and $HCO_3^-$, CA effectively increases the buffering ability of the $CO_2/HCO_3^-$ buffer system. In tissues or organs with $H^+$ and/or $HCO_3^-$ transport, the absence or inhibition of CA allows the local accumulation of $H^+$ (or $HCO_3^-$), which impedes further transport.

Two isoforms of CA are predominant in the kidney: cytosolic type II and membrane-bound type IV.[1] Type II CA is widely distributed in cells along the nephron involved in acid-base transport. Membrane-bound type IV CA also appears to be important in several nephron segments. CA type IV on the apical or luminal membrane of most of the proximal tubule facilitates $HCO_3^-$ reabsorption resulting from $H^+$ secretion.[5, 6] Also, CA type IV resides in the basolateral membrane of the proximal tubule, probably facilitating $HCO_3^-$ efflux from tubule cell to interstitium and, ultimately, venous blood.[7] Similarly, CA type IV is present on both apical and basolateral membranes of the thick ascending limb.[6] Some cells of the distal tubule and collecting duct also have at least luminal CA type IV.[8–10] However, most segments of the collecting duct and the final portion of the proximal tubule, the $S_3$ segment, do *not* have luminal membrane CA type IV.[6, 11] (The exact locations vary with the techniques used to examine localization and with the experimental species.[1]) Those nephron segments with no luminal CA type IV absorb luminal $HCO_3^-$ at slower rates, but luminal pH will be lower. The lower luminal pH may serve several physiologic functions but clearly aids in trapping $NH_4^+$ in the luminal fluid (see later). Recent studies demonstrated that both CA types II and IV increase with metabolic acidosis in experimental animals, presumably facilitating increased rates of acid-base transport.[12–14] Despite the importance of CA, significant rates of $HCO_3^-$ reabsorption persist at the whole kidney level (but not in most isolated nephron segments in vitro) during complete inhibition of CA activity. The mechanisms of the compensatory CA-independent $HCO_3^-$ reabsorptive processes have not been fully delineated.[1]

## PROXIMAL TUBULE

The proximal tubule reabsorbs the majority of filtered $HCO_3^-$, lowering luminal $HCO_3^-$ concentration from approximately 25 mEq/L to 5 to 8 mEq/L. This is accompanied by luminal acidification from a pH of 7.25 to 7.35 at the beginning of the tubule to a pH of 6.7 at the end. Classically, the proximal tubule was divided into the proximal convoluted tubule and the proximal straight tubule, based on its shape. More recently, it has been divided into $S_1$, $S_2$, and $S_3$ segments. The $S_1$ segment comprises the first portion of the proximal convoluted tubule and is very short, the $S_2$ segment encompasses the remaining portion of the proximal convoluted tubule and the beginning of the proximal straight tubule, and the $S_3$ segment is the terminal portion of the proximal straight tubule. Rates of acidification are greatest in $S_1$ and least in $S_3$.

### Transcellular Acidification

Acidification of the proximal tubular fluid involves the active addition of acid to the luminal fluid. As such, it is a transcellular process. Because the proximal tubule cell has a voltage of approximately −70 mV, acid extrusion, or equivalently base entry, is an active process that requires the input of energy. Base efflux across the basolateral membrane can occur passively, driven by the cell's negative voltage.

#### APICAL MEMBRANE $H^+$ SECRETION

Active acid extrusion across the apical membrane is mediated by active $H^+$ secretion from cell to lumen. This was first proved by the demonstration of an acid disequilibrium pH.[15, 16] When luminal fluid was exposed to a cell-impermeable CA inhibitor, luminal pH decreased. Because secreted $H^+$ ions could no longer be buffered by $OH^-$ ions generated from $HCO_3^-$ through the CA reaction (see later), the concentration of free $H^+$ ions increased (acid disequilibrium pH). These classic studies proved that $H^+$ ions were added to the luminal fluid and thus were secreted into the lumen; equally important, they proved that the luminal fluid is exposed to CA activity.

Further support for the concept of $H^+$ transport on the apical membrane derives from the use of isolated membrane vesicles where $CO_2/HCO_3^-$ can be removed, and transport can be studied in its absence. These studies consistently showed that $CO_2/HCO_3^-$ is not required for $H^+$ transport. More recently, these $H^+$-secreting transport proteins have been cloned and their expression demonstrated on the apical membrane.

**Acidification and Carbonic Anhydrase.** The proximal tubule contains CA intracellularly and on both the apical and the basolateral cell membranes. Based on the finding of an acid disequilibrium pH described earlier, it has been concluded that the luminal fluid is exposed to CA. Figure 2–1 shows how CA facilitates $HCO_3^-$ absorption in the proximal tubule. $H^+$ ions secreted into the luminal fluid react with $OH^-$ ions, causing pH to decrease. The associated decrease in $OH^-$ ions causes $HCO_3^-$ to dissociate to $CO_2$ and $OH^-$, catalyzed by CA. This causes the disappearance of luminal $HCO_3^-$ and alkalinizes the luminal fluid, allowing $H^+$ secretion to proceed.

In the cell, $H_2O$ dissociates into $H^+$ and $OH^-$. The $H^+$ is secreted across the luminal membrane. $CO_2$ formed in the lumen diffuses into the cell, where it reacts with $OH^-$ to form $HCO_3^-$, again catalyzed by CA. The $HCO_3^-$ then exits across the basolateral membrane. The net result is the loss of $HCO_3^-$ from the lumen and the appearance of an equivalent amount of $HCO_3^-$ in the renal interstitium, which is returned to the systemic circulation via the renal vein.

**Na-H Exchanger.** $H^+$ transport across the apical membrane is mediated by two transporters. The first one identified was an Na-H exchanger or antiporter.[17, 18] This protein exchanges one $Na^+$ for one $H^+$ ion. The Na,K ATPase on the basolateral membrane maintains cell $Na^+$ concentration at a low level, which provides a driving force for $Na^+$ entry into the cell. The approximately 10-fold $Na^+$ gradient (lumen >

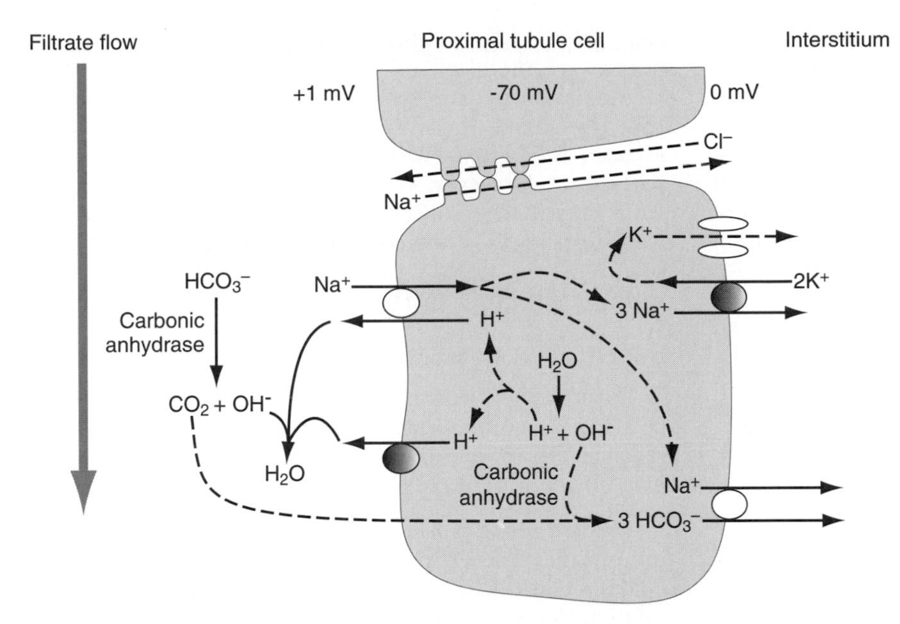


**FIGURE 2–1** ■ Cell model for proximal tubule acidification. $H^+$ secretion into the proximal tubule lumen is mediated by an Na-H exchanger and a vacuolar $H^+$ pump. In the lumen, $H^+$ reacts with $OH^-$, which causes $HCO_3^-$ to dissociate to $OH^-$ and $CO_2$. This latter reaction is catalyzed by carbonic anhydrase. In the cell, $H_2O$ dissociates into $H^+$ and $OH^-$. The $H^+$ is secreted into the lumen, while $OH^-$ reacts with $CO_2$ in the cell to form $HCO_3^-$, again catalyzed by carbonic anhydrase. $HCO_3^-$ then exits the cell on an electrogenic $Na^+$-$HCO_3^-$ cotransporter. (Courtesy of University of Texas Southwestern Web Curriculum.)

cell) provides a driving force that allows the transporter to establish a 10-fold $H^+$ gradient. Given that proximal tubular cell pH is approximately 7.3, the Na-H exchange can establish a luminal pH of 6.3. This thermodynamic capacity is more than sufficient for the proximal tubule, given that the luminal fluid is acidified only to a pH of 6.7 in vivo.

The Na-H exchangers are inhibited by amiloride.[19] Amiloride analogues with hydrophobic substitutions in the 5-amino nitrogen demonstrate increased potency against Na-H exchangers.[20] An example is the now commonly used ethylisopropyl amiloride. Na-H exchangers are also inhibited by a series of Hoechst compounds, including HOE694.[21]

A family of genes, referred to as NHE, have been cloned that encode Na-H exchangers.[22] Five of these encode mammalian plasma membrane proteins (NHE-1 to NHE-5), and four of these are expressed in the kidney (NHE-1 to NHE-4). NHE-1 and NHE-4 are expressed in nonpolar cells or on the basolateral membrane of epithelial cells, and their roles appear to be more related to cellular housekeeping functions, such as the maintenance of intracellular homeostasis. NHE-2 and NHE-3 are expressed on the apical membrane of epithelia and mediate transepithelial transport.

Current evidence strongly supports the fact that the proximal tubule Na-H antiporter is encoded by NHE-3. NHE-3 is unusual among the Na-H exchangers in that although it is inhibited by the same inhibitors that act on other Na-H exchangers, it is significantly more resistant, requiring higher concentrations of inhibitors such as amiloride and its analogues and HOE694.[21, 23] This characteristic had previously been described for the proximal tubule apical membrane Na-H antiporter. Immunohistochemical studies have localized NHE-3 to the proximal tubule apical membrane, and no other isoforms have been localized there (Fig. 2–2).[24, 25] In addition, NHE-3 is regulated in a manner that is identical to the regulation of the apical membrane Na-H exchanger (see later). Last, in mice in which the NHE-3 gene has been genetically disrupted, 61% of proximal tubule acidification is inhibited, approximating the percentage of acidification attributable to the Na-H exchanger (see later).[26]

All the NHE genes include an N-terminal domain that includes 10 to 12 transmembrane domains and mediates transport. The C-terminal domain is cytoplasmic and appears to play an important role in regulation.

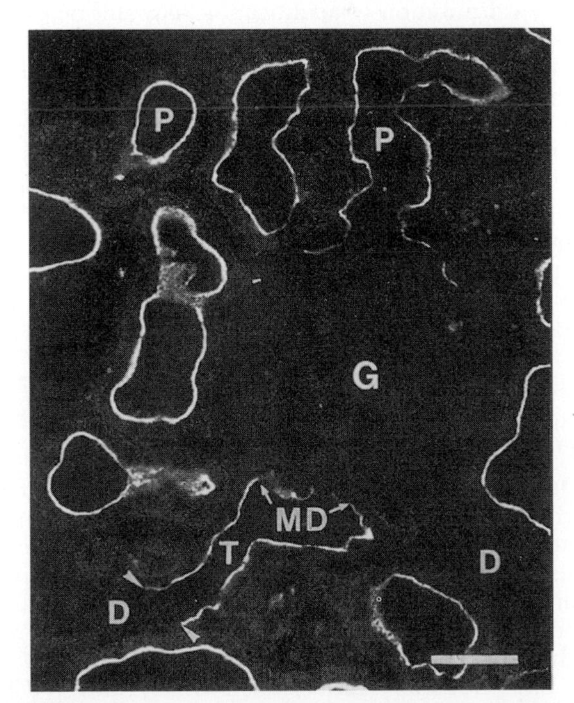


**FIGURE 2–2** ■ Immunohistochemical localization of NHE-3 on the apical membrane of the proximal tubule and thick ascending limb. D, distal convoluted tubule; G, glomerulus; MD, macula densa; P, proximal tubule; T, thick ascending limb. (From Amemiya M, Lotting J, Lötscher M, et al: Expression of NHE-3 in the apical membrane of rat renal proximal tubule and thick ascending limb. Kidney Int 48:1206–1215, 1995.)

**Vacuolar $H^+$ Pump.** The proximal tubule apical membrane also possesses an electrogenic vacuolar $H^+$ pump. This pump is a member of a family of proton pumps composed of multiple subunits and is present in many intracellular organelles, such as endosomes, the endoplasmic reticulum, the Golgi apparatus, and lysosomes.[27] Antibodies against subunits of this vacuolar pump label the apical membrane of the proximal tubule.[28] In addition, this transporter mediates electrogenic transport in the proximal tubule. If all organic solutes are removed from the luminal fluid of the microperfused proximal tubule, the tubule develops a transepithelial lumen positive voltage that is related to acidification and is due to the vacuolar $H^+$ pump.[29] Vacuolar $H^+$ pumps are inhibited by N,N′-dicyclohexylcarbodiimide (DCCD) and by the more specific inhibitor bafilomycin A1.[30]

**Roles of NHE-3 and the Vacuolar $H^+$ Pump in Proximal Tubule Acidification.** The roles of these two transporters in proximal tubule acidification have been studied extensively. When $Na^+$ is removed from the luminal and peritubular fluid, all bicarbonate absorption is inhibited.[31–33] This was interpreted as indicating that all acidification is mediated by the Na-H antiporter, but these results are complicated by the fact that the mechanism of basolateral base exit is Na-coupled (see later). A second approach demonstrated that peritubular potassium (K) removal, which inhibits Na,K ATPase, inhibits all acidification.[31, 34] Inhibition of Na,K ATPase increases cell Na concentration, which would be expected to inhibit Na-H exchange but stimulate the basolateral membrane Na-coupled transporter. However, inhibition of acidification may still be due to the slowing of base exit, because inhibition of Na,K ATPase causes cell depolarization, which would inhibit the basolateral membrane electrogenic Na-coupled base exit step (see later). The most useful approach has been to use inhibitors of the Na-H antiporter, such as amiloride and amiloride analogues.[35, 36] These studies have shown that approximately two thirds of acidification is mediated by the Na-H antiporter, with one third mediated by an Na-independent mechanism. This result was confirmed by the finding that two-thirds of bicarbonate absorption is inhibited in NHE-3 null mice.[26] Also consistent with these results is the finding that DCCD, an inhibitor of the vacuolar $H^+$ pump, inhibits approximately 21% of bicarbonate absorption.[37]

**Other Transporters.** In addition to the transporters described earlier, the proximal tubule apical membrane expresses other transporters that are relevant to acidification but quantitatively less important. Apical membrane chloride-base exchangers mediate sodium chloride (NaCl) absorption by functioning in parallel to the Na-H antiporter. The net result is that $H^+$ and base transport cancel each other, and NaCl is transported. The Cl-base exchangers expressed on the apical membrane include Cl-formate, Cl-oxalate, and Cl-OH. In theory, Cl-base exchange should cause luminal alkalinization or slow luminal acidification, but quantitatively, the effect is small.

Absorption of citrate and other organic anions is also relevant to acidification, in that these organic anions are metabolized to $HCO_3^-$. Citrate absorption is mediated by an Na-coupled transporter, NaDC-1, that transports three $Na^+$ for each citrate.[38] It is increased in acidosis, which serves to increase alkali absorption.[39] However, this effect is quantitatively small with regard to acidification. It is, however, important with respect to stone disease. Accelerated citrate absorption leads to low urinary citrate (hypocitraturia), which predisposes to stone disease.

## BASOLATERAL MEMBRANE BASE EFFLUX

As described earlier, because the proximal tubule cell has an interior negative voltage, base can exit passively. In theory, this could be mediated by a simple $H^+$, $OH^-$, or $HCO_3^-$ channel.

**Electrogenic Na-$HCO_3$ Cotransport.** Basolateral membrane base efflux is mediated by an electrogenic Na-$HCO_3$ cotransporter. This was first identified in the salamander proximal tubule and then later shown in the rat and rabbit.[40–42] Base efflux is coupled to $Na^+$, with $Na^+$ transport in the same direction as base transport. Transport is electrogenic, in that it generates a negative voltage; it is voltage sensitive, in that the transporter runs faster in response to a more negative cell voltage and slower in response to a less negative cell voltage. This implies that the transporter carries a negative charge, and thus that the stoichiometry is base charge greater than $Na.^+$ If one calculates the required stoichiometry for the transporter to run in the efflux mode, 3 base:1 Na is required. Indeed, this is the stoichiometry that has been found.[43, 44] The transporter has been found to be dependent on $CO_2$-$HCO_3^-$, suggesting that $HCO_3^-$ is at least one of the base moieties transported.[7] Studies have suggested that the transporter functions as an Na-$HCO_3$-$CO_3$ cotransporter.[45] $CO_3^{2-}$ is equivalent to two $HCO_3^-$ ions, in that two $HCO_3^-$ ions react to form one $CO_3$ and one $CO_2$. The Na-$HCO_3$ cotransporter is inhibited by disulfonic stilbenes such as SITS (4′-acetamido-4′-isothiocyanostilbene-2,2′-disulfonic acid) and DIDS (4,4′-dithiocyanostilbene-2,2′-disulfonic acid). These inhibitors, however, inhibit many anion transporters and should not be considered specific.

The Na-$HCO_3$ transporter has now been cloned by expression cloning.[46, 47] It is encoded by NBC-1 (*N*a *b*icarbonate *c*otransporter). This cDNA encodes a protein that is 25% to 40% identical to the AE (*a*nion *e*xchanger) family of Cl-$HCO_3^-$ exchangers. They possess an N-terminal cytoplasmic domain that interacts with the cytoskeleton, and a C-terminal portion that contains 10 transmembrane domains. Antibodies to NBC-1 have confirmed its localization to the basolateral membrane of the proximal tubule (Fig. 2–3).[48] Subsequently, two other related cDNAs have been cloned, NBC-2 and NBC-3.

**Other Transporters.** The basolateral membrane also possesses an Na-H exchanger encoded by NHE-1.[49] This transporter likely participates in housekeeping roles such as regulation of cell pH, cell volume, the cytoskeleton, and cell growth.

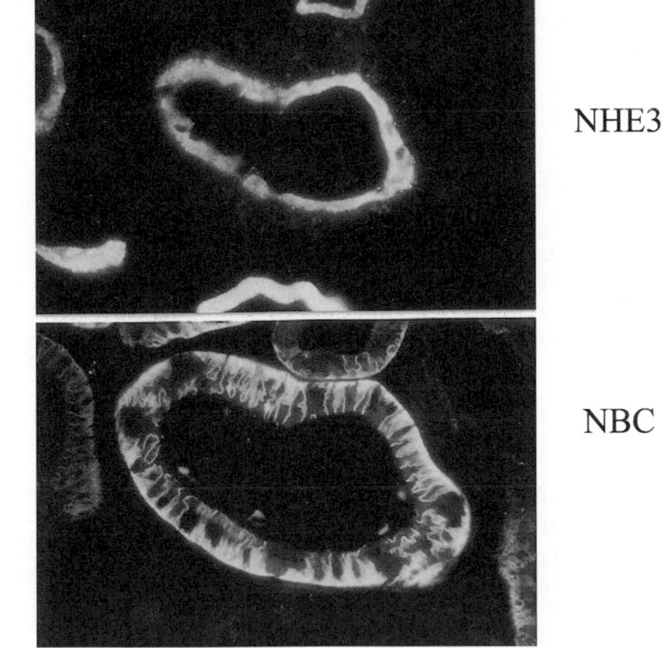


**FIGURE 2–3** ■ Immunohistochemical localization of NHE-3 and NBC-1 on the apical and basolateral membranes, respectively, of the proximal tubule. (Courtesy of Bernhard Schmitt, Walter Boron, and Daniel Biemesdorfer.)

Also on the basolateral membrane is an Na-coupled Cl-$HCO_3$ exchanger, likely an $Na(HCO_3)_2$-Cl exchanger.[50] This transporter may play a role in basolateral membrane $Cl^-$ exit, but it does not appear to play a significant role in base efflux.

**Role of NBC-1 in Basolateral Base Efflux.** Evidence strongly suggests that NBC-1 mediates all basolateral membrane base efflux. First, bicarbonate absorption is Na-dependent and Cl-independent.[31] Second, the majority of basolateral membrane H-$HCO_3^-$ permeability is Na-dependent and Cl-independent.[41, 50] Third, disulfonic stilbenes inhibit acidification in the proximal tubule.[51, 52] Fourth, cell depolarization with barium inhibits $HCO_3^-$ absorption.[53]

### LEAK PATHWAYS

As fluid proceeds along the proximal tubule, its pH and $HCO_3^-$ concentration decrease. This creates a driving force for passive backleak of alkali into the lumen or acid from the lumen. Although $H^+$ permeability is great, the concentrations of $H^+$ are small, and passive transepithelial fluxes are therefore small.[54] Because of the cell's negative voltage, passive $H^+$ diffusion may occur from lumen to cell. A more significant passive flux is mediated by $HCO_3^-$ diffusion across the paracellular pathway.[55]

All these passive fluxes are minor when considering total fluxes of H-$HCO_3^-$ across the tubule. However, these fluxes can become significant when considering net fluxes in the late proximal tubule (Fig. 2–4). Although the rates of $HCO_3^-$ absorption are low in this part of the tubule, they are very important because they determine the end proximal $HCO_3^-$ concentration and pH and thus determine the amount of $HCO_3^-$ delivered distally. Thus, changes in net $H^+$-$HCO_3^-$ transport in the late proximal tubule do not significantly affect total proximal tubule transport but do significantly affect distal delivery of $HCO_3^-$, which can be physiologically important.

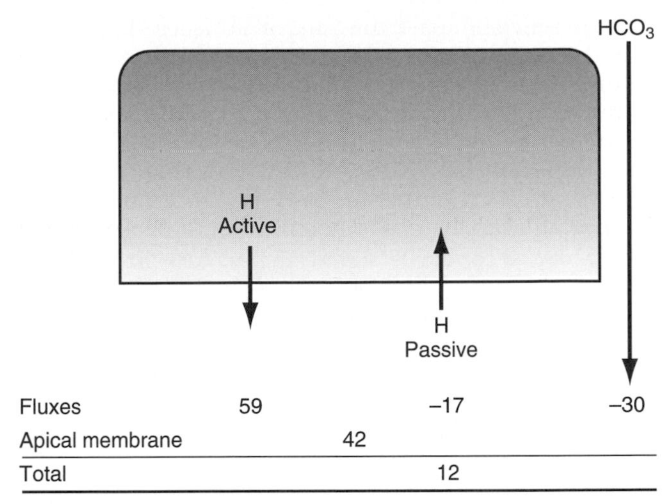


**FIGURE 2–4** ■ Passive fluxes in the late proximal tubule. (From Alpern RJ: Cell mechanisms of proximal tubule acidification. Physiol Rev 70: 79–114, 1990.)

## Regulation of Acidification

### GLOMERULOTUBULAR BALANCE: LUMINAL AND FLOW DEPENDENCE

One of the major obstacles the kidney faces in renal acidification is that of reabsorbing filtered $HCO_3^-$. The human kidney filters about 4000 mEq of $HCO_3^-$ each day and must reabsorb this $HCO_3^-$ before dealing with challenges imposed by extrarenal acid accumulation. Because filtered $HCO_3^-$ can vary, rates of $H^+$ secretion must vary in parallel. This is referred to as glomerulotubular balance.

A number of mechanisms contribute to glomerulotubular balance. First is the effect of luminal pH and $HCO_3^-$ concentration on rates of acidification. As luminal $HCO_3^-$ concentration and pH decrease along the nephron, rates of $H^+$ secretion slow. This relationship between luminal $HCO_3^-$ concentration and net $H^+$ secretion is linear in luminal $HCO_3^-$ concentrations up to 45 mEq/L.[55, 56] This is due to the fact that transcellular $H^+$ secretion is stimulated by luminal alkalinization, and to the effect of luminal $HCO_3^-$ concentration on paracellular $HCO_3^-$ diffusion.

If GFR increases, the filtered load of $HCO_3^-$ increases. If the rate of $HCO_3^-$ absorption does not change, luminal $HCO_3^-$ concentration will fall at a slower rate, leading to a higher luminal concentration, which then stimulates net $H^+$ secretion. However, this can explain only a small proportion of the effect of flow rate.[52, 57] In addition, increases in luminal flow rate directly stimulate the rate of $H^+$ secretion.[58] This may be due to a flow-dependent diffusion barrier, wherein the pH in the vicinity of the transporters is lower than that in the bulk luminal fluid. Increases in flow rate, by decreasing the size of the diffusion barrier, would alkalinize the fluid adjacent to the transporter and secondarily increase its rate. Conversely, it is possible that changes in flow rate modify cell shape, which can secondarily signal an increase in acidification rate.

In addition to these effects of flow rate, which occur instantaneously, there are chronic effects of changes in GFR. These chronic increases in GFR increase the apical Na-H antiporter and basolateral Na-$HCO_3$ transporter activity and increase the capacity of the tubule for transepithelial $HCO_3^-$ absorption.[59]

### PERITUBULAR pH

The kidney regulates the rate of $H^+$ secretion in response to disorders of blood pH, so as to return blood pH to normal values. In acidosis, the proximal tubule increases the rate of $H^+$ secretion, whereas in alkalosis, it decreases $H^+$ secretion. A number of mechanisms contribute. Changes in peritubular pH do not affect paracellular permeability, but they do regulate the gradients across the paracellular pathway.[60] However, the most significant regulation occurs with regard to transcellular transport.

Acidosis causes a decrease in cell pH; metabolic acidosis does so by causing a driving force for enhanced $HCO_3^-$ exit, and respiratory acidosis does so by $CO_2$ diffusion into the cell. Decreases in cell pH then stimulate apical membrane transport in a number of ways. Decreases in cell pH stimulate the $H^+$ efflux on NHE-3 by altering the driving force across the transporter. In addition, increases in intracellular $H^+$ concentration increase the rate of NHE-3 to a greater extent than can be explained by a change in driving force. This direct activation of NHE-3 by decreases in cell pH is a type of allosteric regulation of NHE-3.[61] Allosteric regulation is instantaneous.

In addition to these forms of regulation, NHE-3 is regulated by more chronic mechanisms. Chronic metabolic acidosis increases the rate of bicarbonate absorption to a greater extent than is seen with acute pH changes of similar magnitude.[62] This is due to chronic increases in apical membrane NHE-3 and basolateral membrane NBC-1 activities.[63, 64] Chronic metabolic acidosis causes an increase in apical membrane NHE-3 abundance.[65, 66] At this time, it appears that this effect is due mostly to exocytic insertion of NHE-3 from a pool of intracellular vesicles into the apical membrane.[67] As will be discussed later, endothelin-1 (ET-1) increases apical NHE-3 activity by causing exocytic insertion of NHE-3 into the apical membrane. Chronic acidosis causes an increase in renal cortical ET-1 production, which is then responsible for exocytic insertion of NHE-3.[68] Acidosis also causes increased cortisol secretion, which contributes to the increase in NHE-3 activity.[69]

Respiratory acidosis causes adaptations that stimulate $HCO_3^-$ absorption.[70] These adaptations are associated with increases in NHE-3 and NBC-1 activities.[71] Acidosis has also been shown to cause exocytic insertion of vacuolar $H^+$ pumps.[72]

### POTASSIUM DEPLETION

Potassium depletion causes intracellular acidification that is due to cell hyperpolarization.[73] The effect on the proximal tubule is similar to that of metabolic acidosis—increased $HCO_3^-$ absorption and increased activities of NHE-3 and NBC-1.[74, 75] This contributes to the clinical observation that potassium deficiency causes metabolic alkalosis.

### EXTRACELLULAR FLUID VOLUME

Extracellular volume contraction is the most important cause of maintenance of metabolic alkalosis. This is due in part to increased proximal tubule $HCO_3^-$ absorption. One mechanism for this is that volume contraction decreases paracellular $HCO_3^-$ permeability.[60] This decreases $HCO_3^-$ backleak and allows increased net $HCO_3^-$ absorption. In addition, volume contraction causes an increase in NHE-3 activity.[76] This may be due to increased angiotensin II or catecholamine levels in volume contraction (see later).

### HORMONAL REGULATION

Proximal tubule acidification is regulated by a number of hormones and autocrine and paracrine factors. Dopamine and parathyroid hormone (PTH) serve as inhibitors of acidification. PTH-induced inhibition has been extensively studied and is due at least in part to activation of adenylyl cyclase and increased levels of cyclic adenosine monophosphate (cAMP). Increased cAMP activates protein kinase A (PKA), which then phosphorylates NHE-3, leading to inhibition.[77] NHE-3 inhibition also requires the presence of a protein, NHERF (*NHE regulatory factor*), which serves as a scaffolding protein to bring PKA and NHE-3 together.[78]

Angiotensin II, catecholamines, and ET-1 stimulate $HCO_3^-$ absorption and NHE-3 activity. Angiotensin II and ET-1 cause trafficking of NHE-3 to the apical membrane.[79, 80] Catecholamine-induced NHE-3 stimulation is mediated by $\alpha_2$-adrenergic receptors and by $\beta_2$-adrenergic receptors. $\beta_2$-Adrenergic receptors have been demonstrated to activate NHE-3 by sequestering NHERF.[81] Angiotensin II and ET-1 both inhibit adenylyl cyclase and stimulate tyrosine kinase pathways, contributing to NHE-3 activation.[82–85] ET-1 has also been demonstrated to increase cell calcium and activate CaM kinase, contributing to NHE-3 activation.[83]

## LOOP OF HENLE AND THICK ASCENDING LIMB

Water abstraction in the thin descending limb concentrates luminal bicarbonate, thereby alkalinizing lu-

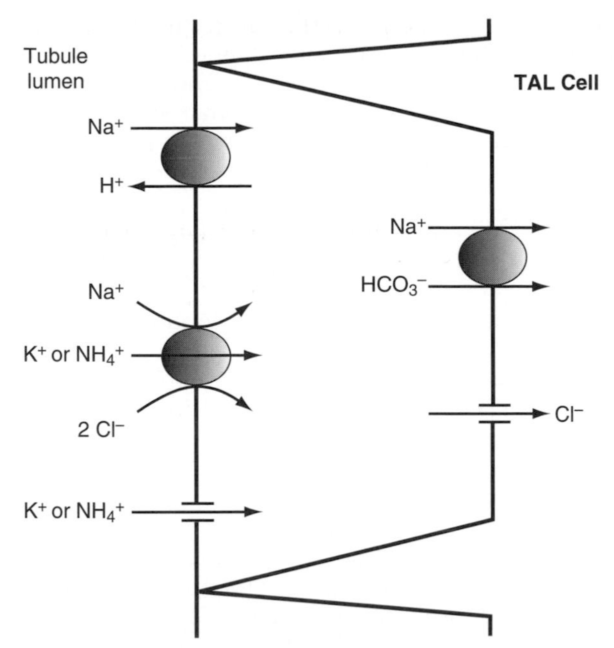


**FIGURE 2–5** ■ Model of acid-base transport in the thick ascending limb (TAL). The predominant transporters responsible for transepithelial transport are an apical Na-H exchanger and a basolateral Na-$HCO_3^-$ cotransporter. Also shown are some pathways for $NH_4^+$ transport on the apical membrane: $NH_4^+$ transport via the Na-K-2Cl cotransporter and via $K^+$ channels. Other probable pathways for $NH_3$ and $NH_4^+$ transport (such as basolateral mechanisms) are not shown.

minal fluid.[86, 87] This alkalinization is important in $NH_3$ diffusion out of the ascending limb of the loop of Henle into the papillary interstitium and ultimately into the medullary collecting ducts. The elevation of luminal bicarbonate is also thought to be important in bicarbonate absorption during inhibition of CA.[1]

Subsequent to this concentration of luminal bicarbonate, the thick ascending limb reabsorbs 50% to 70% of the bicarbonate delivered out of the proximal tubule lumen.[88, 89] The mechanisms of this bicarbonate reabsorption are depicted in Figure 2–5. The apical Na-H exchanger accounts for most of the bicarbonate reabsorption, although an apical $H^+$ ATPase may also be present.[29, 90] The apical Na-H exchanger has been identified as NHE-3, but NHE-2 may also be present.[91, 92] A basolateral Na-H exchanger, NHE-1, has been identified both in functional studies and by immunocytochemical studies.[93–95] Basolateral Na-H exchange probably functions in cell volume and cell pH regulation, but not in transepithelial bicarbonate transport. To accomplish net transepithelial bicarbonate reabsorption in series with the apical Na-H exchange, bicarbonate transport out of the cell into the interstitium probably occurs via an Na-$HCO_3^-$ cotransporter that is related to, but distinct from, that found in the proximal tubule.[94, 96]

Bicarbonate reabsorption in the thick ascending limb is regulated by a variety of factors. Acute and chronic metabolic acidosis stimulates bicarbonate reabsorption, and metabolic alkalosis inhibits bicarbonate reabsorption.[97, 98] Glucocorticoids, mineralocorticoids, and sodium delivery appear to have counteracting effects on bicarbonate reabsorption in the thick ascending limb. For instance, NaCl restriction, which decreases sodium delivery to the thick ascending limb, decreases bicarbonate reabsorption in the thick ascending limb, but high doses of mineralocorticoids increase bicarbonate reabsorption.[98, 99] A variety of peptide hormones have also been found to regulate thick ascending limb bicarbonate reabsorption, probably via changes in cAMP, but the overall physiologic significance of these effects is not clear. For instance, arginine vasopressin (AVP) inhibits bicarbonate reabsorption in the thick ascending limb by the stimulation of adenyl cyclase.[100, 101] Increasing osmolality also inhibits bicarbonate reabsorption. Furosemide stimulates thick ascending limb bicarbonate reabsorption.[90]

In sum, the thick ascending limb contributes substantially to bicarbonate reabsorption along the nephron and is regulated by acid-base status and a variety of hormones. However, unique roles of the thick ascending limb in pathophysiologic circumstances are still poorly understood because of the larger upstream reabsorption of bicarbonate in the proximal tubule and the downstream regulation of urine acidification by more distal segments.

## DISTAL NEPHRON

The distal nephron past the thick ascending limb and macula densa is composed of several distinct segments. They are discussed together because of many similar characteristics; each segment has unique features that are also noted. The distal nephron is responsible for the reabsorption of any remaining filtered bicarbonate (approximately 5% to 10% of the filtered load) that has not been reabsorbed upstream, the generation of additional titratable acid by the secretion of protons, and the "trapping" of $NH_4^+$ in the collecting duct for excretion into the final urine. Therefore, the distal nephron, despite a limited capacity for $H^+$ secretion, is responsible for the final regulation of urinary acid excretion. Despite this importance, these segments have not been studied as extensively as the proximal tubule, in part because of limited absolute tissue mass for each segment, and in part because of their inaccessibility.

The initial parts of the distal nephron, comprising the connecting segment and the distal convoluted tubule, have been studied predominantly with micropuncture of the superficial distal tubule. The cortical collecting duct and the outer medullary collecting duct have been studied almost exclusively with in vitro microperfusion techniques and, to a much lesser extent, with cell culture techniques. The inner medullary collecting duct has been studied by a variety of techniques, including some in vitro microperfusion studies, microcatheterization studies, micropuncture studies, acute isolation of enriched cell preparations, and cell culture. In addition to these techniques for studying these nephron segments, the turtle urinary bladder proved to be an invaluable model for understanding

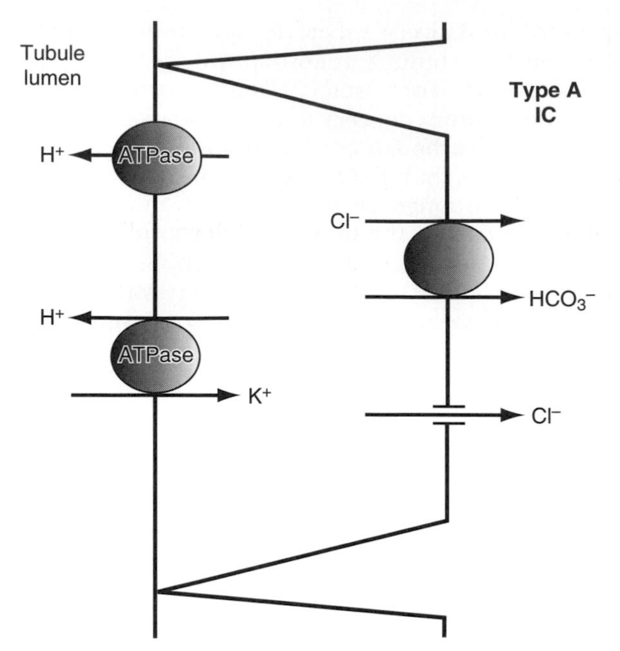


**FIGURE 2–6** ■ Model of acid-base transport in type A intercalated cells (and related cell types) in collecting duct segments. The exact contribution of $H^+$ ATPase versus $H^+$, $K^+$ ATPase in various conditions differs.

the basic mechanisms of distal nephron acid secretion, particularly before the development of in vitro microperfusion studies.

The general model for acid secretion in the distal nephron is depicted in Figure 2–6. Proton secretion into the luminal fluid occurs across the apical membrane via a vacuolar-type $H^+$ ATPase. In the distal convoluted tubule and the connecting segment, there is also an apical Na-H exchanger (probably NHE-2) present that is responsible for some of the proton secretion.[102, 103] Also along the collecting duct in many segments, one of at least two types of $H^+$,$K^+$ ATPase is present. The roles and details of this $H^+$,$K^+$ ATPase are discussed later. On the basolateral membrane of many acid-secreting distal tubule cells, a Cl-$HCO_3^-$ exchanger is present, mediating bicarbonate extrusion across the basolateral membrane into the interstitium and peritubular blood. The luminal proton secretion, coupled with the basolateral bicarbonate extrusion, results in reabsorption of any luminal bicarbonate and the production of "new" bicarbonate in the absence of luminal bicarbonate. Most, if not all, cell types secreting $H^+$ in the distal nephron have cytosolic CA type II. Only a minority of cells along the distal nephron have luminal membrane CA type IV. Although this general model pertains to many cells along the distal nephron that secrete acid, there are differences among the various segments, and the particular details of each segment vary in some cases with the experimental species.

The cell model depicted in Figure 2–6 most closely approximates the type A or α intercalated cell in the cortical collecting duct. Intercalated cells in the distal nephron are the prototypical acid-secreting cells that are dispersed among the more numerous principal cells, which are responsible for sodium absorption, potassium secretion, and AVP-dependent water transport. In the cortical collecting duct and in the connecting tubule, there are also bicarbonate-secreting intercalated cells, usually referred to as B or β intercalated cells. All intercalated cells have cytoplasmic CA.

## Bicarbonate Secretion

Bicarbonate secretion has been found in the superficial distal nephron and in the cortical collecting duct of both rats and rabbits.[104–106] (Bicarbonate secretion has also been found in the model epithelia, the turtle urinary bladder.) The transport process is electroneutral, sodium independent, and coupled to chloride reabsorption.[1] The bicarbonate secretion occurs via type B intercalated cells, as modeled in Figure 2–7. As discussed in other sections later, basolateral $H^+$ ATPase probably mediates the active component of bicarbonate secretion, with transepithelial bicarbonate transport mediated specifically by an apical Cl-$HCO_3^-$ exchanger. Bicarbonate secretion is stimulated by metabolic alkalosis, mineralocorticoids (possibly via metabolic alkalosis), and isoproterenol.[107–109] Bicarbonate secretion is inhibited by acid loads.[110]

## Segmental Characteristics

The distal convoluted tubule and connecting segment have been studied best using micropuncture of the superficial distal tubule. Some studies have differentiated the early and late regions of the superficial distal nephron and, therefore, have studied predominantly the connecting segment versus the distal convo-

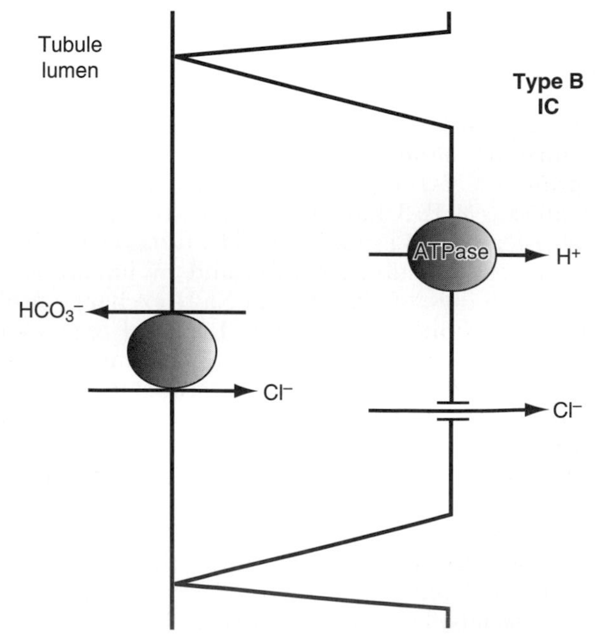


**FIGURE 2–7** ■ Model of acid-base transport in type B intercalated cells of the cortical collecting duct.

luted tubule and initial collecting duct. In the early superficial distal nephron, both an apical Na-H exchanger and an $H^+$ ATPase (distinguished by amiloride analogue and bafilomycin sensitivity, respectively) have been found to account for luminal acidification.[102] In the later aspects of the superficial distal tubule, an $H^+$ ATPase, and probably an $H^+,K^+$ ATPase, accounts for most of the luminal acidification.[111] The superficial distal tubule has also been found to secrete bicarbonate under some circumstances, such as alkali loading of animals.[106] The more distal aspects of the superficial distal nephron (connecting tubule) clearly have intercalated cells, whereas the earlier aspects do not.

The cortical collecting duct has both type A and type B intercalated cells and can both reabsorb and secrete bicarbonate.[1] Type B intercalated cells predominate in the initial cortical collecting duct, and type A intercalated cells predominate in the inner cortical collecting duct. This segment has probably been the most studied of the distal nephron segments, predominantly by in vitro microperfusion of rabbit (and rat) cortical collecting duct. With significant sodium reabsorption in this segment, transepithelial voltage significantly modulates acid secretion. With acid loading, tubules reabsorb bicarbonate; with alkali loading or chloride deficiency, bicarbonate secretion predominates. Transepithelial transport of bicarbonate can also be clearly influenced in this segment by transepithelial chloride gradients based on the apical $Cl\text{-}HCO_3^-$ exchanger in type B cells and the basolateral $Cl\text{-}HCO_3^-$ exchanger present in type A cells.[112] Interconversion of type A and type B intercalated cells has been supported by some studies of the cortical collecting duct, a concept countered by other investigations. However, a variety of studies using different techniques have suggested that intermediate cell types may function to modulate the magnitude and direction of bicarbonate transport, depending on overall acid-base homeostasis.[113] For instance, intercalated cells with both apical and basolateral $Cl\text{-}HCO_3^-$ exchangers have been demonstrated in both rabbits and rats, the two predominant experimental species for these types of studies.[114]

The outer medullary collecting duct has distinct subsegments, the outer and the inner stripe, differing in morphology and function. The outer stripe has both sodium-reabsorbing principal cells and type A or acid-secreting intercalated cells. In contrast, the inner stripe appears to have no sodium transport and, as in the outer stripe, only type A intercalated cells. In fact, some studies have suggested that all cells in the inner stripe, particularly the innermost aspect, have only a single cell type that secretes acid, but with some cells having more baseline activity.[115, 116] The inner stripe differs from the preceding outer stripe, in that the luminal voltage is positive due to $H^+$ secretion with no sodium absorption. Interestingly, the inner stripe also has luminal CA, facilitating a higher rate of bicarbonate reabsorption.[117] This contrasts with most segments of the distal tubule, which have no luminal CA. In nephron segments with luminal delivery of bicarbonate, CA eliminates the acid disequilibrium pH, which slows $H^+$ secretion. Variations in luminal pH influence the rate of not only bicarbonate reabsorption but also ammonium secretion, with a lower luminal pH facilitating $NH_4^+$ trapping.

The inner medullary collecting duct has been subdivided morphologically into three subsegments, but for acid-base transport, few distinctions can be made. The outermost part of the inner medullary collecting duct has distinct intercalated cells—at least in several species—whereas the inner part of the inner medullary collecting duct has no distinct intercalated cells.[118] In fact, the cell type and cellular mechanisms of acid secretion and bicarbonate reabsorption in the inner medullary collecting duct have not been definitely established. Particularly in the innermost part of the inner medullary collecting duct and in cultured inner medullary collecting duct cells, all cells appear similar, and all appear to have proton secretion. However, distinct cellular localization of several key acid-base transport proteins has been difficult, such as for $H^+$ ATPase, anion exchanger 1 (AE1), and CA. Activities for each of these proteins can be found in cell preparations, but immunocytochemical studies have been negative in many instances.

## $H^+$ ATPase

An apical membrane $H^+$ ATPase has been thought to be responsible for most of the acid secretion along the distal nephron,[1, 119, 120] although an important role for $H^+,K^+$ ATPase has been found in certain circumstances in recent years (see later). The $H^+$ ATPase in the distal nephron is a multi-subunit, "vacuolar-type" ATPase. Several of the subunits have been cloned and characterized. The $H^+$ ATPase is the same as or similar to that found in many intracellular organelles, such as lysosomes and clathrin-coated vesicles. This $H^+$ ATPase also shares most subunits with the proximal tubule $H^+$ ATPase; however, there is a distinct 56-kilodalton subunit present in the proximal tubule (B2-subunit, or "brain isoform"), which is different from that expressed in the distal nephron (B1, or "kidney isoform").[121] Other subunits may differ as well.[122] By transporting a single positive charge, the $H^+$ ATPase is electrogenic and hence influenced by membrane voltage. In intracellular organelles, a chloride channel shunts the current and hence allows acidification of the organelle. However, most studies of $H^+$-secreting cells of the distal nephron have failed to identify a luminal or apical chloride channel. Rather, the current is thought to be shunted paracellularly; that is, chloride enters the lumen via a paracellular pathway. The vacuolar-type $H^+$ ATPase is sensitive to *N*-ethylmaleimide (NEM) and bafilomycin A, the latter a distinguishing feature among ATPases.

Regulation of $H^+$ ATPase in the distal nephron is thought to occur predominantly by insertion (and retrieval) of $H^+$ ATPase into the apical membrane via fusion of subapical vesicles with the apical membrane.[1, 119] The stimulus for this involves intracellular acidification or increased $P_{CO_2}$ and probably increased intracellular calcium.[123, 124] In addition, stimulatory and inhibitory proteins have been identified in the cytosol, but their role remains uncertain.[125, 126] $H^+$ ATPase appears to be regulated to a lesser extent, if at all, by transcriptional and translational mechanisms.[113]

Basolateral $H^+$ ATPase probably mediates $HCO_3^-$ secretion from type B intercalated cells.[1] But basolateral $H^+,K^+$ ATPase may also contribute to this function in some circumstances.[107]

## $H^+,K^+$ ATPase

In recent years, an important role for $H^+,K^+$ ATPase in distal nephron acid secretion has been demonstrated in several studies, but the role during baseline conditions remains controversial.[1, 127, 128] In fact, animals with knockouts for either gastric $H^+,K^+$ ATPase or colonic $H^+,K^+$ ATPase have normal acid-base status.[129, 130] This does not negate an important role for $H^+,K^+$ ATPase however, because compensatory mechanisms may exist. $H^+,K^+$ ATPase exchanges two cations ($H^+$ and $K^+$) and therefore is electroneutral and not influenced by membrane voltage. The $H^+,K^+$ ATPase in the distal nephron appears to involve at least two isoforms—gastric $H^+,K^+$ ATPase (also called HK-α 1 or HKg), identical to that in gastric parietal cells, and colonic $H^+,K^+$ ATPase (also called HK-α 2 or HKc), identical to that originally isolated from the colon.[127, 128] The latter has at least two mRNA isoforms.[128] In addition, there may be at least one additonal type of $H^+,K^+$ ATPase present in the distal nephron. Gastric $H^+,K^+$ ATPase is a heterodimer composed of α- and β-subunits analogous to Na,K ATPase, which is in the same family of ATPases. The colonic $H^+,K^+$ ATPase α-subunit, in contrast, associates with Na,K ATPase β-subunits, particularly $\beta_1$.[131–133] Colonic $H^+,K^+$ ATPase may also substitute $Na^+$ for $H^+$ and function as $Na^+$,K ATPase[134] or substitute $NH_4^+$ for $K^+$ and secrete $NH_4^+$.[135, 136]

The role of $H^+,K^+$ ATPase is most dramatic in states of potassium depletion, where there is an upregulation of omeprazole and SCH28080-sensitive $HCO_3^-$ absorption and colonic $H^+,K^+$ ATPase mRNA, particularly in the medullary collecting duct.[137–142] There is also an adaptation during potassium depletion of $H^+,K^+$ ATPase in the cortical collecting duct, but this may involve gastric $H^+,K^+$ ATPase. Metabolic acidosis may also stimulate $H^+,K^+$ ATPase.[137] The mechanisms of cellular regulation of $H^+,K^+$ ATPase have not been completely delineated but involve upregulation of mRNA and protein levels of the colonic $H^+,K^+$ ATPase α isoform. There has also been some suggestion that $H^+,K^+$ ATPase plays a role in bicarbonate secretion, but this has not been completely characterized.[107] Although $H^+,K^+$ ATPase is present in type B intercalated cells, it is probably localized at the apical membrane, rendering the function unclear.[143, 144] A role for $H^+,K^+$ ATPase in sodium absorption has also been proposed; consistent with this role, studies have demonstrated that sodium can substitute for potassium to accomplish sodium absorption.[134, 145]

Confusion regarding the roles of gastric versus colonic $H^+,K^+$ ATPase (and versus another isoform) derives from differences between functional studies in collecting ducts and proteins expressed in heterologous systems such as *Xenopus* oocytes.[127] For instance, in expression studies, gastric $H^+,K^+$ ATPase is invariably inhibited by low concentrations of SCH28080, whereas colonic $H^+,K^+$ ATPase is sensitive to high concentrations of ouabain but not to SCH28080; however, in the distal tubule, some studies have identified acid secretion sensitive to SCH28080 simultaneous with upregulation of colonic $H^+,K^+$ ATPase and downregulation of gastric $H^+,K^+$ ATPase.[127] Three distinct types of $H^+,K^+$ ATPase activity have been determined in enzyme activity studies.[127] Therefore, it appears that another nongastric $H^+,K^+$ ATPase exists in kidney that is upregulated by chronic hypokalemia. A number of laboratories are currently working to define the molecular equivalent of so-called type III $H^+,K^+$ ATPase.[127]

## Basolateral Chloride-Bicarbonate Exchange

In the distal nephron, basolateral bicarbonate extrusion occurs predominantly via a truncated form of AE1, also known as band 3 protein, the red cell exchanger involved in $CO_2$ transport from tissues to lung.[146, 147] AE1 is the first of a family of $Cl\text{-}HCO_3^-$ exchangers in a larger family of bicarbonate-transporting proteins. The kidney form of AE1 has an alternative start site and therefore differs from the erythrocyte protein in lacking a C-terminal portion that is involved in binding to the cytoskeleton in red cells.[148, 149] However, both proteins—the erythrocyte and kidney form of AE1—exchange one chloride for one bicarbonate ion in an electroneutral fashion. Cell chloride is much lower than plasma or interstitial chloride, and therefore the out-to-in chloride gradient partially drives the exchange process. AE1 is clearly present in the basolateral membrane of type A intercalated cells but is probably also located in the inner medullary collecting duct cells in lower density.

## Other Transporters

In addition to the transporters discussed earlier that have clearly established roles in acid-base transport, several other transporters are known to be present in the distal nephron and to potentially contribute to acid-base transport. First, a basolateral Na-H exchanger is present in virtually all cells along the distal nephron.[150, 151] Probably this basolateral transporter contributes to intracellular pH and intracellular volume regulation, but not to transepithelial acid-base transport.

Basolateral chloride channels are also present in the collecting duct.[152, 153] Basolateral chloride channels may recycle the chloride that enters the cell via the basolateral $Cl\text{-}HCO_3^-$ exchanger. In this fashion, these chloride channels may regulate transepithelial acid-base transport, but this has not been clearly established; however, several cloned chloride channels (CLC) have been localized to collecting duct cells. The molecular function of particular chloride channels has not been established with certainty, but ClC-5 (the mutated gene in Dent disease) and ClC-3 have been localized to type A and type B intercalated cells, respectively, but their functions there are unknown.[154, 155] CFTR is also located in the collecting duct, but its function is uncertain.[156]

The molecular identity of the $Cl\text{-}HCO_3^-$ exchanger in the apical membrane of bicarbonate-secreting type B intercalated cells has not been established with certainty. Although some studies of cultured collecting duct cells suggested that kidney AE1 accounts for bicarbonate secretion,[157, 158] recent studies strongly suggest that pendrin may be the apical $Cl\text{-}HCO_3^-$ exchanger.[159] Pendrin was previously cloned as the gene responsible for Pendred syndrome, an autosomal recessive disease causing deafness and goiter. Pendrin was previously identified as an iodine transporter.

Also, at least one member of the NBC family has been localized to the apical membrane of type A intercalated cells and the basolateral membrane of type B intercalated cells.[160–162] How these contribute to transepithelial acid-base transport has not been established.

## Regulation of Distal Nephron Acidification

### pH

Both acute and chronic acidosis stimulate distal nephron acid-base transport. This has been shown by both in vivo and in vitro studies.[1, 2] Acutely, in vitro, either lowering peritubular bicarbonate or raising $P_{CO_2}$ increases collecting duct luminal acidification or bicarbonate reabsorption.[163, 164] The acute effect is likely secondary to decreases in intracellular pH, which stimulates exocytic insertion of $H^+$ ATPase into the apical membrane from subapical vesicles.[123] This process is likely calcium and microtubule or microfilament dependent and similar to mechanisms of neurosecretory exocytosis.[164–166] In addition to the exocytic insertion of $H^+$ pumps, reductions in peritubular bicarbonate also kinetically stimulate basolateral $Cl\text{-}HCO_3^-$ exchange.

Chronic changes in acid-base balance also dramatically alter acid-base transport in the distal nephron. In vitro studies of tissues obtained from chronically acid- or alkali-loaded animals demonstrate that the chronic changes persist, implying chronic adaptations. Several studies demonstrate morphologic changes in the intercalated cells of the collecting duct. With acid loading, the bicarbonate-secreting B cells undergo both functional and morphologic changes.[167, 168] Some investigators have suggested that there is an interconversion of type B cells to type A intercalated cells, but this remains controversial.[167] Immunocytochemical studies have clearly shown changes in staining patterns of intercalated cells for $H^+$ ATPase with acid or alkali loads.[113] Chronically, there does not seem to be an increase of mRNA for $H^+$ ATPase,[113] but there is an increase in mRNA and protein of AE1 with acidosis.[169, 170] The mediators of the changes associated with chronic acidosis are not known with certainty; the initiator may be changes in systemic pH, bicarbonate, or $P_{CO_2}$, and hormones such as endothelin (discussed later) may be involved.

Luminal pH probably also affects acid secretion. This has been shown most clearly in the turtle bladder model, where a decreasing mucosal pH (equivalent to luminal pH) decreased the rate of $H^+$ ATPase pumping.[171] The distal nephron represents a tight epithelium, so a low luminal pH (high $H^+$ concentration) can be maintained without significant effects on either intracellular pH or paracellular fluxes of $H^+$.

### SODIUM DELIVERY VOLTAGE IN MINERALOCORTICOIDS

In contrast to the proximal tubule, the effects of volume status on distal nephron acid-base homeostasis are probably secondary to changes in NaCl delivery and mineralocorticoid status, rather than a direct effect of volume status on acid-base transport. Many studies, ranging from in vitro studies to clinical studies, have demonstrated that distal delivery of sodium and the characteristics of the accompanying ion and mineralocorticoid status influence distal tubule acidification.[1, 2, 172–174] Most, if not all, of the effect of sodium delivery and the accompanying ion is accounted for by the transepithelial voltage influencing the rate of $H^+$ ATPase. Because $H^+$ ATPase is an electrogenic pump, a more negative lumen voltage stimulates $H^+$ secretion. With increasing sodium delivery, poorly reabsorbable anions (anions other than chloride) and mineralocorticoids increase the magnitude of the lumen negative voltage.[174–176] Chloride delivery also influences the apical $Cl\text{-}HCO_3^-$ exchanger in type B intercalated cells; limited chloride delivery inhibits bicarbonate secretion in the collecting duct.[177]

In addition to their effects on sodium reabsorption and transepithelial voltage, mineralocorticoids directly stimulate $H^+$ ATPase.[173, 178, 179] Mineralocorticoids also stimulate bicarbonate secretion by type B cells, but this may be secondary to the associated metabolic alkalosis.[109]

### POTASSIUM

Potassium depletion has been associated with increased distal nephron acidification of the urine; however, usually this results when an excess mineralocorticoid state stimulates both urine acidification and urinary potassium loss. Pure potassium depletion suppresses aldosterone secretion and thus may indirectly decrease urine acidification. However, potassium depletion (in addition to its well-known effects of increasing proximal bicarbonate reabsorption and ammonium production and excretion) probably can increase distal nephron acidification.[180, 181]

Recent work has demonstrated that potassium

depletion increases $H^+,K^+$ ATPase activity and function in the collecting duct.[127] This allows both potassium reabsorption in the collecting duct and $H^+$ secretion. Most studies are consistent with potassium depletion increasing the colonic isoform of $H^+,K^+$ ATPase, in contrast to a higher activity of gastric $H^+,K^+$ ATPase under normal conditions.[127]

**OTHER HORMONES**

A variety of hormones have been found to regulate distal nephron acid-base transport, but the clinical implications of many of these have not been established. Recent studies with endothelin are particularly important.[182] ET-1 levels have been found to be increased in the renal interstitium of acidotic rats, and this increase in ET-1 levels appears to stimulate superficial distal tubule $H^+$ secretion via the $ET_B$ receptor, as in the proximal tubule.[183, 184] This ET-1 may be released from the microvascular endothelial cells in response to acidosis.[184]

AVP, isoproterenol, vasoactive intestinal polypeptide, angiotensin II, PTH, prostaglandins $E_2$ and $I_2$, and glucagon have all been found to alter distal nephron acid-base transport, but their physiologic and pathophysiologic roles in acid-base balance have not been determined.[1, 2]

## AMMONIUM EXCRETION

Renal excretion of ammonium is critical for normal acid-base homeostasis, normally accounting for at least two thirds of net acid excretion. Ammonium is a weak acid with a $pK_a$ of approximately 9.0:

$$NH_4^+ \rightarrow NH_3 + H^+$$

Therefore, at pH 7, the ratio of $NH_4^+$ to $NH_3$ is approximately 100:1; at pH 7.4, the ratio is 40:1. Hence, little $NH_3$ is available to buffer $H^+$, and $NH_4^+/NH_3$ is not an effective urinary or physiologic buffer; the excretion of $NH_4^+$ does not represent the direct elimination of acid. However, physiologically, the excretion of ammonium represents the production of new bicarbonate when ammonium production and excretion are considered as a whole. Ammonium is produced predominantly from glutamine.[1, 185, 186] The metabolism of the carbon skeleton of glutamine (resulting from the deamidation of glutamine) produces bicarbonate.

Most of the ammonium from the metabolism of glutamine is excreted into urine, and bicarbonate is returned to the blood. Without the urinary excretion of ammonium, it would be consumed with bicarbonate to produce urea in the liver and would result in no new bicarbonate formation. Hence, the excretion of ammonium in the urine from the metabolism of glutamine represents the production of new bicarbonate by the kidney, the equivalent of acid excretion.

Ammonium excretion usually represents approximately two thirds of net acid production per day. This excretion can undergo significant upregulation during chronic acid loads and appears to be regulated at several steps, as discussed later.

### Ammoniagenesis

Ammonium can be produced via several metabolic pathways; the most important appears to be mitochondrial glutaminase I (also called phosphate-dependent glutaminase) in the proximal tubule.[185, 186] Glutaminase is present in other nephron segments, but in these other locations it is quantitatively not as important and is not significantly upregulated by chronic acidosis, as in the proximal tubule. Glutaminase deamidation of glutamine yields glutamate, which is deamidated by glutamate dehydrogenase to form ammonia and α-ketoglutarate. Glutaminase and glutamate dehydrogenase are upregulated by chronic metabolic acidosis, predominantly via an increase in mRNA stability.[187–190] These mitochondrial pathways, coupled with the Krebs cycle enzymes, ultimately produce malate, which is transported to the cytoplasm, where it is converted to oxaloacetate and finally to phosphoenolpyruvate by the key enzyme phosphoenolpyruvate carboxykinase. This enzyme is also important because of its critical regulation by acid-base homeostasis. The phosphoenolpyruvate can subsequently be metabolized either to glucose via gluconeogenesis or to bicarbonate.

Ammonia synthesis is upregulated by both acute and chronic acidosis.[185] Chronic potassium deficiency also stimulates ammoniagenesis, possibly by a reduction in cell pH. In contrast, hyperkalemia reduces ammoniagenesis and transport of ammonium into the collecting duct.[191] A variety of hormones increase ammoniagenesis. Importantly, angiotensin II increases both ammonia synthesis and proximal tubule secretion of ammonia.[192, 193] Other hormones reported to increase ammoniagenesis include insulin, PTH, dopamine, and α-adrenergic agonists.[185, 194] In contrast, prostaglandins appear to inhibit ammoniagenesis.[195]

### $NH_4^+$ and $NH_3$ Transport

Traditionally, virtually all of total ammonia transport was thought to occur by $NH_3$ diffusion through the lipid membranes. $NH_4^+$ was considered to be impermeable across cell membranes and tubules. This resulted in $NH_4^+$ trapping, as $NH_3$ would diffuse across membranes, and total ammonia (the sum of $NH_3$ and $NH_4^+$) would accumulate substantially in the most acid environment, where the concentration of $NH_3$ would be kept low. This traditional concept has been found to be overly simplistic. Studies in the last 2 decades have shown that $NH_3$ is not freely permeable across some cell membranes, and $NH_4^+$ is transported by a variety of membrane transporters.[196, 197]

Ammonium produced in the proximal tubule is secreted predominantly into the luminal fluid. This occurs both by $NH_3$ diffusion into the more acid luminal fluid and by $NH_4^+$ transport in exchange for sodium on the Na-H exchanger.[198, 199] In this manner, regulation of apical Na-H exchange regulates ammonium secretion into the lumen of the proximal tubule. In addition to these steps of regulation, increasing luminal flow rate and angiotensin II may have other more direct mechanisms of stimulating ammonium secretion into the lumen.[193, 200] Despite these mechanisms for proximal tubule secretion of ammonium, a significant amount of synthesized ammonia (>20%) is released across the basolateral membrane of the proximal tubule or escapes from the lumen of the proximal tubule into the basolateral interstitial compartment and ultimately reaches renal venous blood.[186, 201]

Ammonium secreted into the lumen of the proximal tubule does not simply continue into the urine. In the loop of Henle and thick ascending limb, total ammonia appears to undergo a recycling and a countercurrent concentration.[196, 202] Total ammonia may be secreted into the descending limb of the loop of Henle but is then reabsorbed in the thick ascending limb.[203] Ammonia lost in the loop of Henle is transported into the collecting duct. Interstitial total ammonia concentrations rise from the outer medullary region to the highest concentration in the deep papilla, as illustrated in Figure 2–8. The principal driving force for this medullary concentration of ammonia appears to be reabsorption of total ammonia in the thick ascending limb. The thick ascending limb has been found to have unique $NH_3/NH_4^+$ transport characteristics. First, the apical membrane of the thick ascending limb has a very low permeability to $NH_3$.[204] In contrast, $NH_4^+$ is reabsorbed from the lumen into the cell via substitution for potassium on both the Na-K-2Cl cotransporter and the apical membrane potassium channel (see Fig. 2–5).[205, 206] In addition, $NH_4^+$ reabsorption may be driven passively by the lumen's positive voltage in the thick ascending limb. Not only is $NH_4^+$ transported in the thick ascending limb, but this transport appears to be regulated, in that increasing potassium concentrations inhibit $NH_4^+$ transport.[205] Factors that alter the rate of the Na-K-2Cl cotransporter are also likely to alter $NH_4^+$ transport in the thick ascending limb.

With ammonium removal in the loop of Henle and thick ascending limb, total ammonia delivery to the lumen of the distal convoluted tubule is lower than that to the end of the proximal tubule.[202] But total ammonia is secreted along the length of the collecting duct. Most, if not all, of this secretion appears to occur by nonionic diffusion of $NH_3$ along the length of the collecting duct from the progressively increasing concentrations of ammonia in the interstitium.[207] Acid secretion along the length of the collecting duct (including the acid disequilibrium pH in most segments of the collecting duct) keeps luminal concentrations of $NH_3$ low, maintaining an $NH_3$ gradient from interstitium to lumen for $NH_3$.[207] Although nonionic diffusion of $NH_3$ across the apical membrane of collecting duct cells appears to be the rate-limiting step, $NH_4^+$ may be transported by other transporters in the collecting duct.[208] $NH_4^+$ can be transported into inner medullary collecting duct cells on $Na^+$, $K^+$ ATPase in substitution for $K^+$.[208] Also, $NH_4^+$ may be transported on the $H^+$,$K^+$ ATPase present along the collecting duct (see earlier).

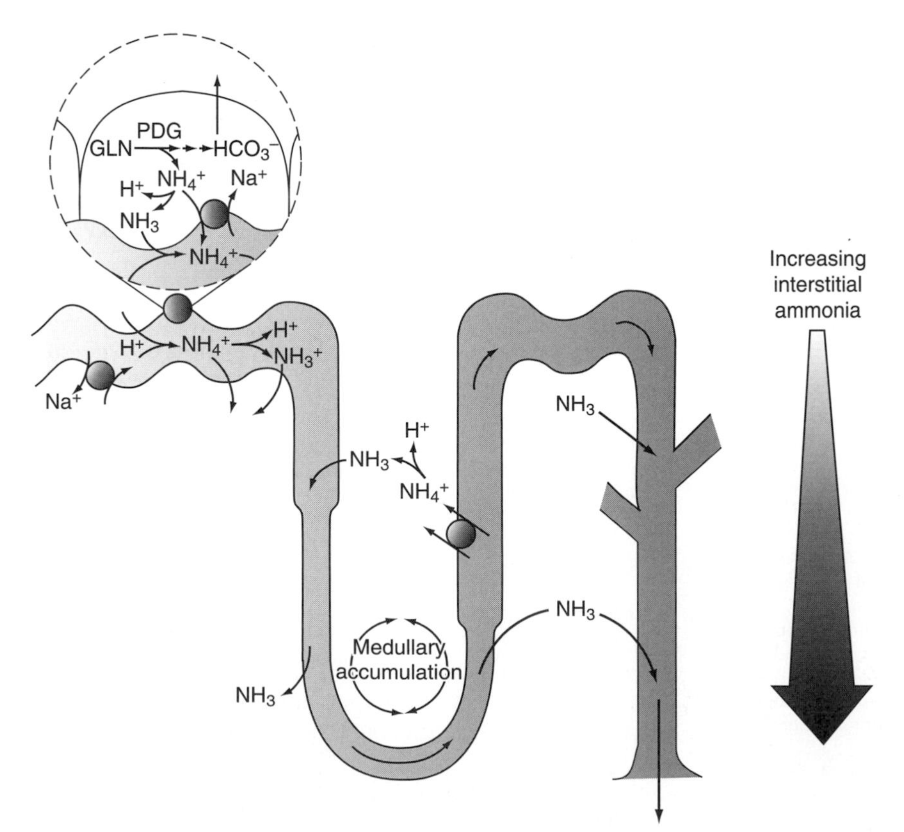


**FIGURE 2–8** ■ Model of ammonia-ammonium transport along the nephron. Ammonium is made predominantly in the proximal tubule from glutamine (GLN). Both $NH_3$ and $NH_4^+$ are likely secreted into the lumen of the proximal tubule. $NH_3$ and $NH_4^+$ are concentrated in the renal medulla; this process is accomplished in large part via $NH_4^+$ reabsorption in the thick ascending limb. $NH_3$ diffuses from the medullary interstitium into the medullary collecting duct. Other potential pathways are not illustrated.

The multiple and complex steps of total ammonia transport in the kidney allow for regulation of total ammonia transport, in addition to regulation of ammoniagenesis (discussed earlier).[3, 197] Clearly, acidosis stimulates not only ammoniagenesis but also ammonium excretion into the urine. Some portion of this is likely secondary to enhanced $H^+$ secretion along the collecting duct. However, the other transport mechanisms for ammonium may allow independent regulation, particularly based on factors such as potassium.

## REFERENCES


1. Alpern RJ: Renal acidification mechanisms. In Brenner BM (ed): The Kidney, 6th ed. Philadelphia, WB Saunders, 2000, pp 455–519.
2. Hamm LL, Alpern RJ: Cellular mechanisms of renal tubular acidification. In Seldin D, Giebisch G (eds): The Kidney: Physiology and Pathophysiology, 3rd ed. Philadelphia, Lippincott Williams & Wilkins, 2000, pp 1935–1979.
3. Hamm LL, Simon EE: Roles and mechanisms of urinary buffer excretion. Am J Physiol 253:F595–F605, 1987.
4. Silverman DN, Vincent SH: Proton transfer in the catalytic mechanism of carbonic anhydrase. Crit Rev Biochem 14:207–255, 1983.
5. Lucci MS, Tinker JP, Weiner IM, DuBose TD Jr: Function of proximal tubule carbonic anhydrase defined by selective inhibition. Am J Physiol 245:F443–F449, 1983.
6. Brown D, Zhu XL, Sly WS: Localization of membrane-associated carbonic anhydrase type IV in kidney epithelial cells. Proc Natl Acad Sci U S A 87:7457–7461, 1990.
7. Krapf R, Alpern RJ, Rector FC Jr, Berry CA: Basolateral membrane Na/base cotransport is dependent on $CO_2/HCO_3$ in the proximal convoluted tubule. J Gen Physiol 90:833–853, 1987.
8. Dobyan DC, Magill LS, Friedman PA, et al: Carbonic anhydrase histochemistry in rabbit and mouse kidneys. Anat Rec 204: 185–197, 1982.
9. Star RA, Burg MB, Knepper MA: Luminal disequilibrium pH and ammonia transport in outer medullary collecting duct. Am J Physiol 252:F1148–F1157, 1987.
10. Wall SM, Flessner MF, Knepper MA: Distribution of luminal carbonic anhydrase activity along rat inner medullary collecting duct. Am J Physiol 260:F738–F748, 1991.
11. Kurtz I, Star R, Balaban RS, et al: Spontaneous luminal disequilibrium pH in $S_3$ proximal tubules. J Clin Invest 78:989–996, 1986.
12. Tsuruoka S, Kittelberger A, Schwartz GJ: Carbonic anhydrase II and IV mRNA in rabbit nephron segments: Stimulation during metabolic acidosis. Am J Physiol 274:F259–F267, 1998.
13. Brion LP, Zavilowitz BJ, Rosen O, Schwartz GJ: Changes in soluble carbonic anhydrase activity in response to maturation and $NH_4Cl$ loading in the rabbit. Am J Physiol 261:R1204–R1213, 1991.
14. Brion LP, Zavilowitz BJ, Suarez C, Schwartz GJ: Metabolic acidosis stimulates carbonic anhydrase activity in rabbit proximal tubule and medullary collecting duct. Am J Physiol 266:F185–F195, 1994.
15. Vieira FL, Malnic B: Hydrogen ion secretion by rat renal cortical tubules as studied by an antimony microelectrode. Am J Physiol 214:710–718, 1968.
16. Rector FC Jr, Carter NW, Seldin DW: The mechanism of bicarbonate reabsorption in the proximal and distal tubules of the kidney. J Clin Invest 44:278–290, 1965.
17. Murer H, Hopfer U, Kinne R: Sodium/proton antiport in brush-border membrane vesicles isolated from rat small intestine and kidney. Biochem J 154:597–604, 1976.
18. Kinsella JL, Aronson PS: Properties of the Na-H exchanger in renal microvillus membrane vesicles. Am J Physiol 238:F467–F469, 1980.
19. Kinsella JL, Aronson PS: Amiloride inhibition of the Na-H exchanger in renal microvillus membrane vesicles. Am J Physiol 241:F374–F379, 1981.
20. Kleyman TR, Cragoe EJ Jr: Amiloride and its analogs as tools in the study of ion transport. J Membr Biol 105:1–21, 1988.
21. Kelly MP, Quinn PA, Davies JE, Ng LL: Activity and expression of $Na^+$-$H^+$ exchanger isoforms 1 and 3 in kidney proximal tubules of hypertensive rats. Circ Res 80:853–860, 1997.
22. Counillon L, Pouyssegur J: The expanding family of eucharyotic Na/H exchangers. J Biol Chem 275:1–4, 2000.
23. Haggerty JG, Agarwal N, Reilly RF, et al: Pharmacologically different Na/H antiporters on the apical and basolateral surfaces of cultured porcine kidney cells ($LLC-PK_1$). Proc Natl Acad Sci U S A 85:6797–6801, 1988.
24. Amemiya M, Loffing J, Lotscher M, et al: Expression of NHE-3 in the apical membrane of rat renal proximal tubule and thick ascending limb. Kidney Int 48:1206–1215, 1995.
25. Biemesderfer D, Pizzonia J, Exner M, et al: NHE3: A Na/H exchanger isoform of the renal brush border. Am J Physiol 265:F736–F742, 1993.
26. Schultheis PJ, Clarke LL, Meneton P, et al: Renal and intestinal absorptive defects in mice lacking the NHE3 $Na^+/H^+$ exchanger. Nat Genet 19:282–285, 1998.
27. Stone DK, Xie XS: Proton translocating ATPases: Issues in structure and function. Kidney Int 33:767–774, 1988.
28. Brown D, Hirsch S, Gluck S: Localization of a proton-pumping ATPase in rat kidney. J Clin Invest 82:2114–2126, 1988.
29. Fromter E, Gessner K: Active transport potentials, membrane diffusion potentials, and streaming potentials across rat kidney proximal tubule. Pflugers Arch 351:85–98, 1974.
30. Bowman EJ, Siebens A, Altendorf K: Bafilomycins: A class of inhibitors of membrane ATPases from microorganisms, animal cells, and plant cells. Proc Natl Acad Sci U S A 85:7972–7976, 1988.
31. Burg MB, Green N: Bicarbonate transport by isolated perfused rabbit proximal convoluted tubules. Am J Physiol 233:F307–F314, 1977.
32. Chantrelle B, Cogan MG, Rector FC Jr: Evidence for coupled sodium/hydrogen exchange in the rat superficial proximal convoluted tubule. Pflugers Arch 395:186–189, 1982.
33. Ullrich KJ, Rumrich G, Baumann K: Renal proximal tubular buffer-(glycodiazine) transport. Pflugers Arch 357:149–163, 1975.
34. Sasaki S, Shiigai T, Takeuchi J: Intracellular pH in the isolated perfused rabbit proximal tubule. Am J Physiol 249:F417–F423, 1985.
35. Preisig PA, Ives HE, Cragoe EJ, et al: Role of the Na/H antiporter in rat proximal tubule bicarbonate absorption. J Clin Invest 80:970–978, 1987.
36. Chan YL, Giebisch G: Relationship between sodium and bicarbonate transport in the rat proximal convoluted tubule. Am J Physiol 240:F222–F230, 1981.
37. Bank N, Aynedjian HS, Mutz BF: Evidence for a DCCD-sensitive component of proximal bicarbonate reabsorption. Am J Physiol 249:F636–F644, 1985.
38. Pajor AM: Sequence and functional characterization of a renal sodium/dicarboxylate cotransporter. J Biol Chem 270:5779–5785, 1995.
39. Aruga S, Wehrli, S, Kaissling B, et al: Chronic metabolic acidosis increases NaDC-1 mRNA and protein abundance in rat kidney. Kidney Int 58:206–215, 2000.
40. Boron WF, Boulpaep EL: Intracellular pH regulation in the renal proximal tubule of the salamander: Basolateral $HCO_3$ transport. J Gen Physiol 81:53–94, 1983.
41. Alpern RJ: Mechanism of basolateral membrane $H/OH/HCO_3$ transport in the rat proximal convoluted tubule. J Gen Physiol 86:613–636, 1985.
42. Akiba T, Alpern RJ, Eveloff J, et al: Electrogenic sodium/bicarbonate cotransport in rabbit renal cortical basolateral membrane vesicles. J Clin Invest 78:1472–1478, 1986.
43. Yoshitomi K, Fromter E: Cell pH of rat renal proximal tubule in vivo and the conductive nature of peritubular $HCO_3(OH^-)$ exit. Pflugers Arch 402:300–305, 1984.
44. Soleimani M, Grassl SM, Aronson PS: Stoichiometry of $Na$-$HCO_3$ cotransport in basolateral membrane vesicles isolated from rabbit renal cortex. J Clin Invest 79:1276–1280, 1987.
45. Soleimani M, Aronson PS: Ionic mechanism of $Na:HCO_3$ cotransport in renal basolateral membrane vesicles (BLMV). J Biol Chem 264:18302–18308, 1989.

46. Romero MF, Fong P, Berger UV, et al: Cloning and functional expression of rNBC, an electrogenic $Na^+$-$HCO_3^-$ cotransporter from rat kidney. Am J Physiol 274:F425–F432, 1998.
47. Romero MF, Hediger MA, Boulpaep EL, Boron WF: Expression cloning and characterization of a renal electrogenic $Na^+$/$HCO_3^-$ cotransporter. Nature 387:409–413, 1997.
48. Schmitt BM, Biemesderfer D, Boulpaep E, et al: Immunolocalization of the electrogenic Na/$HCO_3$ cotransporter (NBC) in mammalian and amphibian kidney [abstract]. J Am Soc Nephrol 8:10A, 1997.
49. Biemesderfer D, Reilly RF, Exner M, et al: Immunocytochemical characterization of Na-H exchanger isoform NHE-1 in rabbit kidney. Am J Physiol 263:F833–F840, 1992.
50. Alpern RJ, Chambers M: Basolateral membrane Cl/$HCO_3$ exchange in the rat proximal convoluted tubule. J Gen Physiol 89:581–598, 1987.
51. Ullrich KJ, Capasso G, Rumrich G, et al: Coupling between proximal tubular transport processes: Studies with ouabain, SITS and $HCO_3$-free solutions. Pflugers Arch 368:245–252, 1977.
52. Chan YL, Biagi B, Giebisch G: Control mechanisms of bicarbonate transport across the rat proximal convoluted tubule. Am J Physiol 242:F532–F543, 1982.
53. Sasaki S, Berry CA, Rector FC Jr: Effect of potassium concentration on bicarbonate reabsorption in the rabbit proximal convoluted tubule. Am J Physiol 224:F122–F128, 1983.
54. Preisig PA, Alpern RJ: Contributions of cellular leak pathways to net $NaHCO_3$ and NaCl absorption. J Clin Invest 83:1859–1867, 1989.
55. Alpern RJ, Cogan MG, Rector FC Jr: Effect of luminal bicarbonate concentration on proximal acidification in the rat. Am J Physiol 243:F53–F59, 1982.
56. Malnic G, deMello-Aires M: Kinetic study of bicarbonate reabsorption in proximal tubule of the rat. Am J Physiol 220: 1759 1767, 1971.
57. Alpern RJ, Cogan MG, Rector FC Jr: Flow dependence of proximal tubular bicarbonate absorption. Am J Physiol 245: F478–F484, 1983.
58. Preisig PA: Luminal flow rate regulates proximal tubule H-$HCO_3$ transporters. Am J Physiol 262:F47–F54, 1992.
59. Preisig PA, Alpern RJ: Increased Na/H antiporter and Na/3$HCO_3$ symporter activities in chronic hyperfiltration. J Gen Physiol 97:195–217, 1991.
60. Alpern RJ, Cogan MG, Rector FC Jr: Effects of extracellular fluid volume and plasma bicarbonate concentration on proximal acidification in the rat. J Clin Invest 71:736–746, 1983.
61. Aronson PS, Nee J, Suhm MA: Modifier role of internal H in activating the Na-H exchanger in renal microvillus membrane vesicles. Nature 299:161–163, 1982.
62. Kunau RT Jr, Hart JI, Walker KA: Effect of metabolic acidosis on proximal tubular total $CO_2$ absorption. Am J Physiol 249: F62–F68, 1985.
63. Akiba T, Rocco VK, Warnock DG: Parallel adaptation of the rabbit renal cortical sodium/proton antiporter and sodium/bicarbonate cotransporter in metabolic acidosis and alkalosis. J Clin Invest 80:308–315, 1987.
64. Preisig PA, Alpern RJ: Chronic metabolic acidosis causes an adaptation in the apical membrane Na/H antiporter and basolateral membrane $Na(HCO_3)_3$ symporter in the rat proximal convoluted tubule. J Clin Invest 82:1445–1453, 1988.
65. Ambühl PM, Amemiya M, Danczkay M, et al: Chronic metabolic acidosis increases NHE3 protein abundance in rat kidney. Am J Physiol 271:F917–F925, 1996.
66. Wu MS, Biemesderfer D, Giebisch G, Aronson P: Role of NHE3 in mediating renal brush border $Na^+$-$H^+$ exchange: Adaptation to metabolic acidosis. J Biol Chem 271:32749–32752, 1996.
67. Yang X, Amemiya M, Peng Y, et al: Acid incubation causes exocytic insertion of NHE3 in OKP cells. Am J Physiol 279: C410–C419, 2000.
68. Laghmani K, Ohuchi T, Preisig PA, et al: $ET_B$ receptor contributes to acidosis induced activation of the renal cortical apical mebrane Na/H antiporter [abstract]. J Am Soc Nephrol 9: 7A, 1998.
69. Ambühl PM, Yang X, Peng Y, et al: Glucocorticoids enhance acid activation of $Na^+/H^+$ exchanger 3 (NHE3). J Clin Invest 103:429–435, 1999.
70. Cogan MG: Chronic hypercapnia stimulates proximal bicarbonate reabsorption in the rat. J Clin Invest 74:1942–1947, 1984.
71. Ruiz OS, Arruda JAL, Talor Z: Na-$HCO_3$ cotransport and Na-H antiporter in chronic respiratory acidosis and alkalosis. Am J Physiol 256:F414–F420, 1989.
72. Schwartz GJ, Al-Awqati Q: Carbon dioxide causes exocytosis of vesicles containing H pumps in isolated perfused proximal and collecting tubules. J Clin Invest 75:1638–1644, 1985.
73. Amemiya M, Tabei K, Kusano E, et al: Incubation of OKP cells in low-$K^+$ media increases NHE3 activity after early decrease in intracellular pH. Am J Physiol 276:C711–C716, 1999.
74. Capasso G, Kinne R, Malnic G, Giebisch G: Renal bicarbonate reabsorption in the rat. I. Effects of hypokalemia and carbonic anhydrase. J Clin Invest 78:1558–1567, 1986.
75. Soleimani M, Bergman JA, Hosford MA, McKinney TD: Potassium depletion increases luminal Na/H exchange and basolateral Na:$CO_3$:$HCO_3$ cotransport in rat renal cortex. J Clin Invest 86:1076–1083, 1990.
76. Moe O, Tejedor A, Levi M, et al: Dietary NaCl modulates Na-H antiporter activity in renal cortical apical membrane vesicles. Am J Physiol 260:F130–F137, 1991.
77. Moe OW, Amemiya M, Yamaji Y: Activation of protein kinase A acutely inhibits and phosphorylates Na/H exchanger NHE-3. J Clin Invest 96:2187–2194, 1995.
78. Weinman EJ, Steplock D, Tate K, et al: Structure-function of recombinant Na/H exchange regulatory factor (NHE-RF). J Clin Invest 101:2199–2206, 1998.
79. Peng Y, Amemiya M, Yang X, et al: $ET_B$ receptor activation causes exocytic insertion of NHE3 in OKP cells. Am J Physiol 280:F34–42, 2001.
80. Bloch RD, Zikos D, Fisher KA, et al: Activation of proximal tubular Na-H exchange by angiotensin II. Am J Physiol 263: F135–F143, 1992.
81. Hall RA, Premont RT, Chow CW, et al: The $B_2$-adrenergic receptor interacts with the $Na^+/H^+$-exchanger regulatory factor to control $Na^+/H^+$ exchange. Nature 392:626–630, 1998.
82. Liu FY, Cogan MG: Angiotensin II (AII) stimulates early proximal bicarbonate absorption in the rat by decreasing cyclic adenosine monophosphate. J Clin Invest 84:83–91, 1989.
83. Chu TS, Peng Y, Cano A, et al: $Endothelin_B$ receptor activates NHE-3 by a $Ca^{2+}$-dependent pathway in OKP cells. J Clin Invest 97:1454–1462, 1996.
84. Chu TS, Tsuganezawa H, Peng Y, et al: Role of tyrosine kinase pathways in $ET_B$ receptor activation of NHE3. Am J Physiol 271:C763–C771, 1996.
85. Tsuganezawa H, Preisig PA, Alpern RJ: Dominant negative c-Src inhibits angiotensin II induced activation of NHE3 in OKP cells. Kidney Int 54:394–398, 1998.
86. DuBose TD Jr, Lucci MS, Hogg RW, et al: Comparison of acidification parameters in superficial and deep nephrons of the rat. Am J Physiol 244:F497–F503, 1983.
87. Buerkert J, Martin D, Trigg D: Segmental analysis of the renal tubule in buffer production and net acid formation. Am J Physiol 244:F442–F454, 1983.
88. DuBose TD Jr, Pucacco LR, Lucci MS, Carter NW: Micropuncture determination of pH, $P_{CO_2}$, and total $CO_2$ concentration in accessible structures of the rat renal cortex. J Clin Invest 64: 476–482, 1979.
89. Buerkert J, Martin D, Trigg D: Segmental analysis of the renal tubule in buffer production and net acid formation. Am J Physiol 244:F442–F454, 1983.
90. Good DW: Sodium-dependent bicarbonate absorption by cortical thick ascending limb of rat kidney. Am J Physiol 248: F821–F829, 1985.
91. Amemiya M, Loffing J, Lotscher M, et al: Expression of NHE-3 in the apical membrane of rat renal proximal tubule and thick ascending limb. Kidney Int 48:1206–1215, 1995.
92. Sun AM, Liu Y, Tse CM, et al: $Na^+/H^+$ exchanger isoform (NHE2) is expressed in the apical membrane of the medullary thick ascending limb. J Membr Biol 160:85–90, 1997.
93. Biemesderfer D, Reilly RF, Exner M, et al: Immunocytochemical characterization of Na-H exchanger isoform NHE-1 in rabbit kidney. Am J Physiol 263:F833–F840, 1992.
94. Krapf R: Basolateral membrane H/OH/$HCO_3$ transport in the rat cortical thick ascending limb. J Clin Invest 82:234–241, 1988.

95. Hebert SC: Hypertonic cell volume regulation in mouse thick limbs. II. Na-H and Cl-$HCO_3$ exchange in basolateral membranes. Am J Physiol 250:C920–C931, 1986.
96. Vorum H, Kwon TH, Fulton C, et al: Immunolocalization of electroneutral Na-HCO(3)(−) cotransporter in rat kidney. Am J Physiol Renal Fluid Electrolyte Physiol 279:F901–909, 2000.
97. Capasso G, Unwin R, Ciani F, et al: Bicarbonate transport along the loop of Henle. II. Effects of acid-base, dietary, and neurohormonal determinants. J Clin Invest 94:830–838, 1994.
98. Good DW: Adaptation of $HCO_3^-$ and $NH_4^+$ transport in rat MTAL: Effects of chronic metabolic acidosis $Na^+$ intake. Am J Physiol 258:F1345–F1353, 1990.
99. Unwin R, Capasso G, Giebisch G: Bicarbonate transport along the loop of Henle: Effects of adrenal steroids. Am J Physiol 268:F234–F239, 1995.
100. Good DW: Inhibition of bicarbonate absorption by peptide hormones and cyclic adenosine monophosphate in rat medullary thick ascending limb. J Clin Invest 85:1006–1013, 1990.
101. Bichara M, Mercier O, Houillier P, et al: Effects of antidiuretic hormone on urinary acidification and on tubular handling of bicarbonate in the rat. J Clin Invest 80:621–630, 1987.
102. Wang T, Malnic G, Giebisch G, Chan YL: Renal bicarbonate reabsorption in the rat. IV. Bicarbonate transport mechanisms in the early and late distal tubule. J Clin Invest 91:2776–2784, 1993.
103. Chambrey R, Warnock DG, Podevin R-A, et al: Immunolocalization of the $Na^+/H^+$ exchanger isoform NHE2 in rat kidney. Am J Physiol 275:F379–F386, 1998.
104. McKinney TD, Burg MB: Bicarbonate transport by rabbit cortical collecting tubules: Effect of acid and alkali loads in vivo on transport in vitro. J Clin Invest 60:766–768, 1977.
105. Knepper MA, Good DW, Burg MB: Ammonia and bicarbonate transport by rat cortical collecting ducts perfused in vitro. Am J Physiol 249:F870–F877, 1985.
106. Levine DZ, Iacovitti M, Nash L, Vandorpe D: Secretion of bicarbonate by rat distal tubules in vivo. J Clin Invest 81: 1873–1878, 1988.
107. Gifford JD, Rome L, Galla JH: H-K-ATPase activity in rat collecting duct segments: Am J Physiol 262:F692–F695, 1992.
108. Hayashi M, Yamaji Y, Iyori M, et al: Effect of isoproterenol on intracellular pH of the intercalated cells in the rabbit cortical collecting ducts. J Clin Invest 87:1153–1157, 1991.
109. Garcia-Austt J, Good DW, Burg MB, Knepper MA: Deoxycorticosterone-stimulated bicarbonate secretion in rabbit cortical collecting ducts: Effects of luminal chloride removal and in vivo acid loading. Am J Physiol 249:F205–F212, 1985.
110. Hamm L, Vehaskari VM, Hering-Smith K: Control of bicarbonate transport in collecting tubules from normal and remnant kidneys. Am J Physiol 256:F680–F687, 1989.
111. Wesson DE: Na/H exchange and H-K-ATPase increase distal tubule acidification in chronic alkalosis. Kidney Int 53:945–951, 1998.
112. Laski ME, Warnock DG, Rector FC Jr: Effects of chloride gradients on total $CO_2$ flux in the rabbit CCT. Am J Physiol 244: F112–F121, 1983.
113. Bastani B, Purcell H, Hemken P, et al: Expression and distribution of renal vacuolar proton-translocating adenosine triphosphatase in response to chronic acid and alkali loads in the rat. J Clin Invest 88:126–136, 1991.
114. Emmons C, Kurtz I: Functional characterization of three intercalated cell subtypes in the rabbit outer cortical collecting duct. J Clin Invest 93:417–423, 1994.
115. Ridderstrale Y, Kashgarian M, Koeppen B, et al: Morphological heterogeneity of the rabbit collecting duct. Kidney Int 34: 655–670, 1988.
116. Weiner ID, Wingo CS, Hamm LL: Regulation of intracellular pH in two cell populations of inner stripe of rabbit outer medullary collecting duct. Am J Physiol 265:F406–F415, 1993.
117. Star RA, Burg MB, Knepper MA: Luminal disequilibrium pH and ammonia transport in outer medullary collecting duct. Am J Physiol 252:F1148–F1157, 1987.
118. Madsen KM, Clapp WL, Verlander JW: Structure and function of the inner medullary collecting duct. Kidney Int 34:441–454, 1988.
119. Brown D, Breton S: Structure, function, and cellular distribution of the vacuolar $H^+$ ATPase ($H^+$ V-ATPase) proton pump. In Seldin D, Giebisch G (eds): The Kidney: Physiology and Pathophysiology. Philadelphia, Lippincott Williams & Wilkins, 2000, pp 171–191.
120. Gluck S, Nelson R: The role of the V-ATPase in renal epithelial $H^+$ transport. J Exp Biol 172:205–218, 1992.
121. Nelson RD, Guo XL, Masood K, et al: Selectively amplified expression of an isoform of the vacuolar H-ATPase 56-kilodalton subunit in renal intercalated cells. Proc Natl Acad Sci U S A 89:3541–3545, 1992.
122. Hemken P, Guo XL, Wang ZQ, et al: Immunologic evidence that vacuolar H ATPases with heterogeneous forms of $M_r$ = 31,000 subunit have different membrane distributions in mammalian kidney. J Biol Chem 267:9948–9957, 1992.
123. Gluck S, Cannon C, Al-Awqati Q: Exocytosis regulates urinary acidification in turtle bladder by rapid insertion of H pumps into the luminal membrane. Proc Natl Acad Sci U S A 79: 4327–4331, 1982.
124. Schwartz GJ, Al-Awqati Q: Regulation of transepithelial $H^+$ transport by exocytosis and endocytosis. Annu Rev Physiol 48: 153–161, 1986.
125. Zhang K, Wang ZQ, Gluck S: Identification and partial purification of a cytosolic activator of vacuolar H-ATPases from mammalian kidney. J Biol Chem 267:9701–9705, 1992.
126. Zhang K, Wang ZQ, Gluck S: A cytosolic inhibitor of vacuolar H-ATPases from mammalian kidney. J Biol Chem 267:14539–14542, 1992.
127. Doucet A, Horisberger J: Renal ion-translocating ATPases: The P-type family. In Seldin D, Giebisch G (eds): The Kidney: Physiology and Pathophysiology. Philadelphia, Lippincott Williams & Wilkins, 2000, pp 140–170.
128. Caviston TL, Campbell WG, Wingo CS, Cain BD: Molecular identification of the renal $H^+$, $K^+$-ATPases. Semin Nephrol 19: 431–437, 1999.
129. Spicer Z, Miller ML, Andringa A, et al: Stomachs of mice lacking the gastric H,K-ATPase alpha-subunit have achlorhydria, abnormal parietal cells, and ciliated metaplasia. J Biol Chem 275:21555–21565, 2000.
130. Meneton P, Schultheis PJ, Greeb J, et al: Increased sensitivity to $K^+$ deprivation in colonic H,K-ATPase–deficient mice. J Clin Invest 101:536–542, 1998.
131. Kraut JA, Hiura J, Shin JM, et al: The $Na^+$-$K^+$-ATPase $\beta_1$ subunit is associated with the HK$\alpha$2 protein in the rat kidney. Kidney Int 53:958–962, 1998.
132. Codina J, Delmas-Mata JT, DuBose TD Jr: The $\alpha$ subunit of the colonic $H^+$-$K^+$-ATPase assembles with $\beta_1$-$Na^+$-$K^+$-ATPase in kidney and distal colon. J Biol Chem 273:7894–7899, 1998.
133. Sangan P, Kolla SS, Rajendran VM, et al: Colonic H-K-ATPase beta-subunit: Identification in apical membranes and regulation by dietary K depletion. Am J Physiol 276:C350–C360, 1999.
134. Cougnon M, Bouyer P, Planelles G, Jaisser F: Does the colonic H,K-ATPase also act as an Na,K-ATPase? Proc Natl Acad Sci U S A 95:6516–6520, 1998.
135. Cougnon M, Bouyer P, Jaisser F, et al: Ammonium transport by the colonic $H^+$-$K^+$-ATPase expressed in *Xenopus* oocytes. Am J Physiol 277:280C–287, 1999.
136. Nakamura S, Amlal H, Galla JH, Soleimani M: $NH_4^+$ secretion in inner medullary collecting duct in potassium deprivation: Role of colonic $H^+$,$K^+$ ATPase. Kidney Int 56:2160–2167, 1999.
137. Silver RB, Mennitt PA, Satlin LM: Stimulation of apical H-K-ATPase in intercalated cells of cortical collecting duct with chronic metabolic acidosis. Am J Physiol 270:F539–F547, 1996.
138. Guntupalli J, Onuigbo M, Wall S, et al: Adaptation to low-$K^+$ media increases $H^+$-$K^+$-ATPase but not $H^+$-ATPase-mediated pH (i) recovery in OMCD1 cells. Am J Physiol 42:C558–C571, 1997.
139. Ahn KY, Park KY, Kim KK, Kone B: Chronic hypokalemia enhances exprssion of the $H^+$-$K^+$-ATPase$_2$-subunit gene in renal medulla. Am J Physiol 271:F314–F321, 1996.
140. Marsy S, Elalouf JM, Doucet A: Quantitative RT-PCR analysis of mRNAs encoding a colonic putative H,K-ATPase alpha subunit along the rat nephron: Effect of $K^+$ depletion. Pflugers Arch 432:494–500, 1996.
141. Wang T, Malnic G, Giebisch G, Chan YL: Renal bicarbonate reabsorption in the rat. IV. Bicarbonate transport mechanisms

in the early and late distal tubule. J Clin Invest 91:2776–2784, 1993.

142. Nakamura S, Wang Z, Galla JH, Soleimani M: $K^+$ depletion increases $HCO_3^-$ reabsorption in OMCD by activation of colonic $H^+$-$K^+$-ATPase. Am J Physiol 274:F687–F692, 1998.
143. Weiner ID, Milton AE: $H^+$-$K^+$-ATPase in rabbit cortical collecting duct B-type intercalated cell. Am J Physiol 270:F518–F530, 1996.
144. Silver RB, Frindt G: Functional identification of H-K-ATPase in intercalated cells of cortical collecting tubule. Am J Physiol 264:F259–F266, 1993.
145. Zhou X, Wingo CS: H-K-ATPase enhancement of Rb efflux by cortical collecting duct. Am J Physiol 263:F43–F48, 1992.
146. Schuster VL, Bonsib SM, Jennings ML: Two types of collecting duct mitochondria-rich (intercalated) cells: Lectin and band 3 cytochemistry. Am J Physiol 251:C347–C355, 1986.
147. Drenckhahn D, Schluter K, Allen DP, Bennett V: Colocalization of band 3 with ankyrin and spectrin at the basal membrane of intercalated cells in the rat kidney. Science 230:1287–1289, 1985.
148. Kudrycki KE, Shull GE: Primary structure of the rat kidney band 3 anion exchange protein deduced from a cDNA. J Biol Chem 264:8185–8192, 1989.
149. Brosius FC III, Alper SL, Garcia AM, Lodish HF: The major kidney band 3 gene transcript predicts an aminoterminal truncated band 3 polypeptide. J Biol Chem 264:7784–7787, 1989.
150. Weiner ID, Hamm LL: Regulation of intracellular pH in the rabbit cortical collecting tubule. J Clin Invest 85:274–281, 1990.
151. Hays SR, Alpern RJ: Apical and basolateral membrane H extrusion mechanisms in inner stripe of rabbit outer medullary collecting duct. Am J Physiol 259:F628–F635, 1990.
152. Koeppen BM: Conductive properties of the rabbit outer medullary collecting duct: Inner stripe. Am J Physiol 248:F500–F506, 1985.
153. Pappas CA, Koeppen BM: Electrophysiological properties of cultured outer medullary collecting duct cells. Am J Physiol 263:F1004–F1010, 1992.
154. Gunther W, Luchow A, Cluzeaud F, et al: ClC-5, the chloride channel mutated in Dent's disease, colocalizes with the proton pump in endocytotically active kidney cells. Proc Natl Acad Aci U S A 95:8075–8080, 1998.
155. Obermuller N, Gretz N, Kriz W, et al: The swelling-activated chloride channel C1C-2, the chloride channel C1C-3, and C1C-5, a chloride channel mutated in kidney stone disease, are expressed in distinct subpopulations of renal epithelial cells. J Clin Invest 101:635–642, 1998.
156. Todd-Turla KM, Rusvai E, Naray-Fejes-Toth A, Fejes-Toth G: CFTR expression in cortical collecting duct cells. Am J Physiol 270:F237–F244, 1996.
157. Al-Awqati Q, Vijayakumar S, Hikita C, et al: Phenotypic plasticity in the intercalated cell: The hensin pathway. Am J Physiol 275:F183–F190, 1998.
158. van Adelsberg JS, Edwards JC, Al-Awqati Q: The apical Cl/$HCO_3$ exchanger of β intercalated cells. J Biol Chem 268: 11283–11289, 1993.
159. Soleimani M, Greeley T, Petrovic S, et al: Pendrin: An apical $Cl^-$/$OH^-$$HCO_3^-$ exchanger in the kidney cortex. Am J Physiol Renal Physiol 280:F356–F364, 2001.
160. Kwon TH, Pushkin A, Abuladze N, et al: Immunoelectron microscopic localization of NBC3 sodium-bicarbonate cotransporter in rat kidney. Am J Physiol Renal Fluid Electrolyte Physiol 278:F327–F336, 2000.
161. Pushkin A, Yip KP, Clark I, et al: NBC3 expression in rabbit collecting duct: Colocalization with vacuolar $H^+$-ATPase. Am J Physiol 277:F974–F781, 1999.
162. Pushkin A, Abuladze N, Lee I, et al: Cloning, tissue distribution, genomic organization, and functional characterization of NBC3, a new member of the sodium bicarbonate cotransporter family. J Biol Chem 274:16569–16575, 1999.
163. Breyer MD, Kokko JP, Jacobson HR: Regulation of net bicarbonate transport in rabbit cortical collecting tubule by peritubular pH, carbon dioxide tension, and bicarbonate concentration. J Clin Invest 77:1650–1660, 1986.
164. McKinney TD, Davidson KK: Effects of respiratory acidosis on $HCO_3$ transport by rabbit collecting tubules. Am J Physiol 255: F656–F665, 1988.
165. Banerjee A, Li G, Alexander EA, Schwartz JH: Role of SNAP-23 in trafficking of $H^+$-ATPase in cultured inner medullary collecting duct cells. Am J Physiol Cell Physiol 280:C775–C781, 2001.
166. Banerjee A, Shih T, Alexander EA, Schwartz JH: SNARE proteins $H^+$-ATPase redistribution to the apical membrane in rat renal inner medullary collecting duct cells. J Biol Chem 274: 26518–26522, 1999.
167. Schwartz GJ, Barasch J, Al-Awqati Q: Plasticity of functional epithelial polarity. Nature 318:368–371, 1985.
168. Satlin LM, Schwartz GJ: Cellular remodeling of $HCO_3$-secreting cells in rabbit renal collecting duct in response to an acidic environment. J Cell Biol 109:1279–1288, 1989.
169. Teixeira da Silva JC Jr, Perrone RD, Johns CA, Madias NE: Rat kidney band 3 mRNA modulation in chronic respiratory acidosis. Am J Physiol 260:F204–F209, 1991.
170. Sabolic I, Brown D, Gluck S, Alper S: Regulation of AE1 anion exchanger and $H^+$-ATPase in rat cortex by acute metabolic acidosis and alkalosis. Kidney Int 51:125–137, 1997.
171. Steinmetz PR, Lawson LR: Effect of luminal pH on ion permeability and flows of Na and H in turtle bladder. Am J Physiol 220:1573–1580, 1971.
172. Schwartz WB, Jenson RL, Relman AS: Acidification of the urine and increased ammonium excretion without change in acid-base equilibrium: Sodium reabsorption as a stimulus to the acidifying process. J Clin Invest 34:673–680, 1955.
173. Stone DK, Seldin DW, Kokko JP, Jacobson HR: Mineralocorticoid modulation of rabbit medullary collecting duct acidification: A sodium independent effect. J Clin Invest 72:77–83, 1983.
174. Laski ME, Kurtzman NA: Characterization of acidification in the cortical and medullary collecting tubule of the rabbit. J Clin Invest 72:2050–2059, 1983.
175. Tam SC, Goldstein MB, Stinebaugh BJ, et al: Studies on the regulation of hydrogen ion secretion in the collecting duct in vivo: Evaluation of factors that influence the urine minus blood $P_{CO_2}$ difference. Kidney Int 20:636–642, 1981.
176. Al-Awqati Q, Muller A, Steinmetz PR: Transport of H against electrochemical gradients in turtle urinary bladder. Am J Physiol 233:F502–F508, 1977.
177. Star RA, Burg MB, Knepper MA: Bicarbonate secretion and chloride absorption by rabbit cortical collecting ducts. J Clin Invest 76:1123–1130, 1985.
178. Al-Awqati Q, Norby LH, Mueller A, Steinmetz PR: Characteristics of stimulation of H transport by aldosterone in turtle urinary bladder. J Clin Invest 58:351–358, 1976.
179. Hulter HN, Ilnicki LP, Harbottle JA, Sebastian A: Impaired renal H secretion and $NH_3$ production in mineralocorticoid-deficient glucocorticoid-replete dogs. Am J Physiol 232:F136–F146, 1977.
180. Hays SR, Seldin DW, Kokko JP, Jacobson HR: Effect of K depletion on $HCO_3$ transport across rabbit collecting duct segments [abstract]. Kidney Int 29:368A, 1986.
181. Capasso G, Jaeger P, Giebisch G, et al: Renal bicarbonate reabsorption in the rat. J Clin Invest 80:409–414, 1987.
182. Wesson DE: Physiologic and pathophysiologic renal consequences of H(+)-stimulated endothelin secretion. Am J Kidney Dis. 35:LII–LV, 2000.
183. Wesson DE: Endogenous endothelins mediate increased distal tubule acidification induced by dietary acid in rats. J Clin Invest 99:2203–2211, 1997.
184. Wesson DE, Dolson GM: Endothelin-1 increases rat distal tubule acidification in vivo. Am J Physiol 273:F586–F594, 1997.
185. Nagami GT: Renal ammonia production and excretion. In SeldinD, Giebisch G (eds): The Kidney: Physiology and Pathophysiology, (3rd ed.). Philadelphia, Lippincott Williams & Wilkins, 2000, pp 1996–2013.
186. Tanner RL: Renal ammonia production and excretion. In Windhager EE (ed): Handbook of Physiology: Renal Physiology. New York, Oxford University Press, 1992, pp 1017–1059.
187. Laterza OF, Curthoys NP: Effect of acidosis on the properties of the glutaminase mRNA pH-response element binding protein. J Am Soc Nephrol 11:1583–1588, 2000.
188. Laterza OF, Hansen WR, Taylor L, Curthoys NP: Identification of an mRNA-binding protein and the specific elements that

may mediate the pH-responsive induction of renal glutaminase mRNA. J Biol Chem 272:22481–22488, 1997.
189. Wright PA, Packer RK, Garcia-Perez A, Knepper MA: Time course of renal glutamate dehydrogenase induction during $NH_4$ Cl loading in rats. Am J Physiol 262:F999–F1006, 1992.
190. Kaiser S, Hwang JJ, Smith H, et al: Effect of altered acid-base balance and of various agonists on levels of renal glutamate dehydrogenase mRNA. Am J Physiol 262:F507–F512, 1992.
191. DuBose TD Jr, Good DW: Chronic hyperkalemia impairs ammonium transport and accumulation in the inner medulla of the rat. J Clin Invest 90:1443–1449, 1992.
192. Nagami GT: Effect of angiotensin II on ammonia production and secretion by mouse proximal tubules perfused in vitro. J Clin Invest 89:925–931, 1992.
193. Nagami GT: Effect of luminal angiotensin II on ammonia production and secretion by mouse proximal tubules. Am J Physiol 269:F86–F92, 1995.
194. Schoolwerth AC: Regulation of renal ammoniagenesis in metabolic acidosis (nephrology forum). Kidney Int 40:961–973, 1991.
195. Jones ER, Beck TR, Kapoor S, et al: Prostaglandins inhibit renal ammoniagenesis in the rat. J Clin Invest 74:992–1002, 1984.
196. Knepper MA, Packer R, Good DW: Ammonium transport in the kidney. Physiol Rev 69:179–249, 1989.
197. DuBose TD Jr, Good DW, Hamm LL, Wall SM: Ammonium transport in the kidney: New physiological concepts and their clinical implications. J Am Soc Nephrol 1:1193–1203, 1991.
198. Kinsella JL, Aronson PS: Interaction of $NH_4$ and Li with the renal microvillus membrane Na-H exchanger. Am J Physiol 241:C220–C226, 1981.
199. Nagami GT: Luminal secretion of ammonia in the mouse proximal tubule perfused in vitro. J Clin Invest 81:159–164, 1988.
200. Nagami GT, Kurokawa K: Regulation of ammonia production by mouse proximal tubules perfused in vitro. J Clin Invest 75: 844–849, 1985.
201. Good DW, DuBose TD Jr: Ammonia transport by early and late proximal convoluted tubule of the rat. J Clin Invest 79: 684–691, 1987.
202. Buerkert J, Martin D, Trigg D: Ammonium handling by superficial and juxtamedullary nephrons in the rat: Evidence for an ammonia shunt between the loop of Henle and the collecting duct. J Clin Invest 70:1–12, 1978.
203. Good DW, Knepper MA, Burg MA: Ammonia and bicarbonate transport by thick ascending limb of rat kidney. Am J Physiol 247:F35–F44, 1984.
204. Kikeri D, Sun A, Zeidel ML, Hebert SC: Cell membranes impermeable to $NH_3$ Nature 339:478–480, 1989.
205. Good DW: Active absorption of $NH_4$ by rat medullary thick ascending limb: Inhibition by potassium. Am J Physiol 255: F78–F87, 1988.
206. Kikeri D, Sun A, Zeidel ML, Hebert SC: Cellular $NH_4^+/K^+$ transport pathways in mouse medullary thick limb of Henle: Regulation by intracellular pH. J Gen Physiol 99:435–461, 1992.
207. Good DW, Caflisch CR, DuBose TD Jr: Transepithelial ammonia concentration gradients in inner medulla of the rat. Am J Physiol 252:F491–F500, 1987.
208. Wall SM, Trinh HN, Woodward KE: Heterogeneity of NH + 4 transport in mouse inner medullary collecting duct cells. Am J Physiol 269:F536–F544, 1995.

CHAPTER 3

# Diagnosis of Simple and Mixed Disorders

Michael Emmett, MD, MACP

The Henderson-Hasselbalch equation describes the relationship between the pH, $P_{CO_2}$, and $HCO_3$ concentrations:

$$pH = 6.1 + \log \frac{[HCO_3]}{(0.03)\ \alpha P_{CO_2}} \quad \text{Equation 1}$$

A primary elevation of the $P_{CO_2}$ (respiratory acidosis), or fall in plasma $[HCO_3]$ (metabolic acidosis), reduces the pH, producing acidemia. A primary reduction in $P_{CO_2}$ (respiratory alkalosis), or elevation of plasma $[HCO_3]$ (metabolic alkalosis), increases the pH and produces alkalemia. Whenever one of these primary disorders increases, or reduces, the $P_{CO_2}$ or $HCO_3$, a compensatory response should develop. Compensation drives the opposite parameter (i.e., the $HCO_3$ or $P_{CO_2}$) in the same direction as the initial disturbance. As can be seen in Equation 1, if the numerator and denominator both move in the same direction—both increase or decrease—the pH tends to normalize. The magnitude of the compensatory response for each simple acid-base disorder can be predicted. Figure 3–1 shows one of many acid-base nomograms that define the 95% confidence ranges for the compensatory response produced by each primary disorder.[1] These ranges represent the compensatory responses exhibited by 95% of otherwise normal individuals who have developed a single acid-base derangement (or in whom an acid-base derangement has been experimentally produced). Table 3–1 shows several mathematical equations and other arithmetical relationships that also predict these compensatory responses. When a simple acid-base disorder is identified, determine whether the appropriate compensatory response exists. If an appropriate level of compensation is not present, then a mixed or complex acid-base disorder may exist.

Although compensation drives the pH toward normal, the pH generally remains slightly acid or alkaline (chronic respiratory alkalosis is an exception to this rule—see later). By convention, compensatory responses are expected physiologic consequences of each primary disorder and should not be called secondary acid-base disorders. For example, when hyperventilation reduces the $P_{CO_2}$ to compensate for metabolic acidosis, this low $P_{CO_2}$ should not be considered to be a "compensatory respiratory alkalosis." Furthermore, because a patient with metabolic acidosis should have an appropriately reduced $P_{CO_2}$, a "normal," or frankly elevated $P_{CO_2}$, indicates absence, or failure, of compensation. This does define a second acid-base disorder; in this example, respiratory acidosis also exists (i.e., the $P_{CO_2}$ is too high). Alternatively, if respiratory alkalosis complicates metabolic acidosis, then the $P_{CO_2}$ is reduced below the level expected for compensation for metabolic acidosis. Such mixed metabolic-respiratory acid-base disorders can be identified only if the $P_{CO_2}$ level that should exist for a given degree of metabolic acidosis is known.

The following sections review each of the four simple disorders and define the expected levels of compensation and the time frame within which they develop.

## SIMPLE ACID-BASE DISORDERS

### Metabolic Acidosis

Metabolic acidosis is a pathologic process that causes the plasma $[HCO_3]$ to fall. One or more of following mechanisms is usually responsible for the development of this disorder:

1. Accelerated alkali loss into the stool or urine
2. Increased rates of endogenous acid generation, the ingestion or infusion of acid loads that exceed either the normal acid excretory capacity or the rate of metabolic conversion of acids to neutral compounds or $CO_2$ and $H_2O$
3. Decreased renal capacity to excrete normal acid loads

It is helpful to separate the metabolic acidoses into two groups on the basis of the anion gap (AG).[2] All metabolic acidoses have either an increased AG or an increased chloride concentration [Cl]. (Hyperchloremia is defined as a [Cl] that is increased relative to the [Na] (i.e., the [Cl]:[Na] ratio is greater than the normal 1:1.4). Figure 3–2 shows how the anion gap is calculated, and Figure 3–3 demonstrates why the [AG] or [Cl], or both, must increase when the $[HCO_3]$ falls. It is important to note that the quantitative increase in [AG] or [Cl] should approximate the quantitative reduction in $[HCO_3]$.[3] A disruption of this relationship is a helpful clue to the presence of certain types of mixed acid-base disorders (see the subsequent section on the anion gap for a more complete discussion of the AG and the $HCO_3$–AG relationship).

#### HYPERCHLOREMIC METABOLIC ACIDOSIS

Hyperchloremic metabolic acidosis reduces the $[HCO_3]$ and increases the [Cl]; the [AG] remains normal. Hyperchloremic acidosis generally develops as a result of one the following abnormalities: (1) fluids containing a high concentration of $NaHCO_3$, or poten-

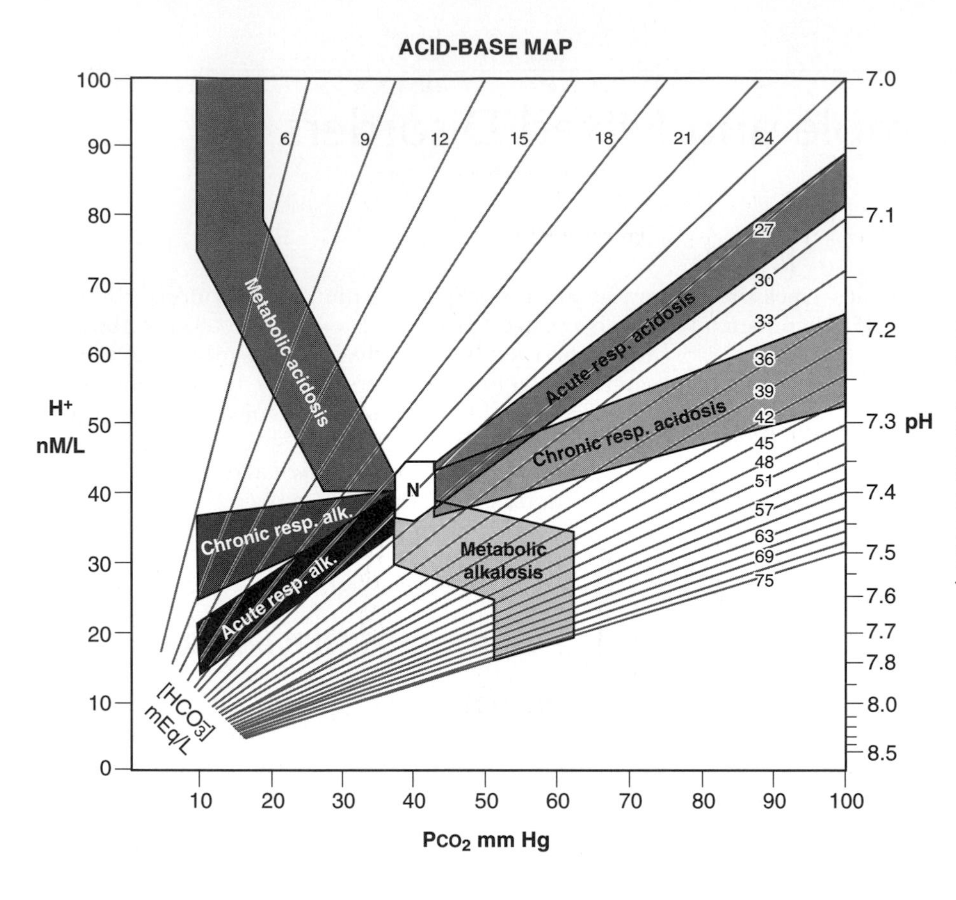


FIGURE 3–1 ■ Acid-base nomogram showing the 95% compensation confidence bands for each simple acid-base disorder. The $P_{CO_2}$ is shown on the X axis and the pH or hydrogen ion concentration on the Y axis. The diagonal lines represent isopleths of the blood bicarbonate concentration. (From Goldberg M, et al: Computer-based instruction and diagnosis of acid-base disorders: A systematic approach. JAMA 223:266–275, 1973.)

tial $NaHCO_3$, are lost from the extracellular fluid (ECF); and (2) HCl, or potential HCl, is added to the ECF.

Any organic sodium salt that can be metabolized to $NaHCO_3$ represents potential $NaHCO_3$. For example, Na lactate, Na citrate, Na acetate, and Na butyrate all generate $NaHCO_3$ when the organic anion (and a proton) is metabolized to glucose or to $CO_2$ and $H_2O$. The addition of such salts to the ECF is equivalent to the addition of $NaHCO_3$, and the loss of such salts is equivalent to the loss of $NaHCO_3$. In contrast, organic chloride salts that can be metabolized to neutral substances represent potential HCl. Examples include $NH_4Cl$, lysine Cl, histidine Cl, and arginine Cl. The hyperchloremic metabolic acidosis of diarrhea develops because of the loss of $NaHCO_3$ and potential $NaHCO_3$ salts, such as Na acetate and Na butyrate, into the stool. The ingestion or infusion of $NH_4Cl$ also generates hyperchloremic acidosis. The common causes of hyperchloremic acidosis are shown in Table 3–2.

The various types of renal tubular acidosis (RTA) all produce hyperchloremic acidosis. Proximal RTA results from a reduced renal $NaHCO_3$ reabsorptive capacity. If the serum [$HCO_3$] increases above the abnormally low renal tubule threshold, $NaHCO_3$ is excreted into the urine. When the serum [$HCO_3$] falls below this threshold level, $NaHCO_3$ excretion ceases and the distal tubule can appropriately acidify the urine because the distal tubule acidification mechanisms remain normal in this disorder. Distal RTA results from an inability of the distal renal tubules to

**TABLE 3–1.** Acid-Base Disorders and Compensatory Responses

| Disorder | $H^+$ | pH | $HCO_3$ | $Pa_{CO_2}$ | Adaptive Response | Time for Adaptation |
|---|---|---|---|---|---|---|
| Metabolic acidosis | ↑ | ↓ | ↓↓ | ↓ | $\Delta P_{CO_2} = (1.5)HCO_3 + 8$<br>$\Delta P_{CO_2} = HCO_3 + 15$ | 12–24 hr |
| Metabolic alkalosis | ↓ | ↑ | ↑↑ | ↑ | $\Delta P_{CO_2} = (0.4–0.6)HCO_3$ | 24–36 hr |
| Respiratory acidosis | | | | | | |
| Acute | ↑ | ↓ | ↑ | ↑↑ | $\Delta HCO_3 = 0.1\ \Delta P_{CO_2}$ | Minutes–Hours |
| Chronic | ↑ | ↓ | ↓ | ↑↑ | $\Delta HCO_3 = 0.3\ \Delta P_{CO_2}$ | Days |
| Respiratory alkalosis | | | | | | |
| Acute | ↑ | ↓ | ↑ | ↓↓ | $\Delta HCO_3 = 0.2\ \Delta P_{CO_2}$ | Minutes–Hours |
| Chronic | ↓ | ↑ | ↑ | ↓↓ | $\Delta HCO_3 = 0.4\ \Delta P_{CO_2}$ | Days |

Double arrows indicate the primary disturbance.

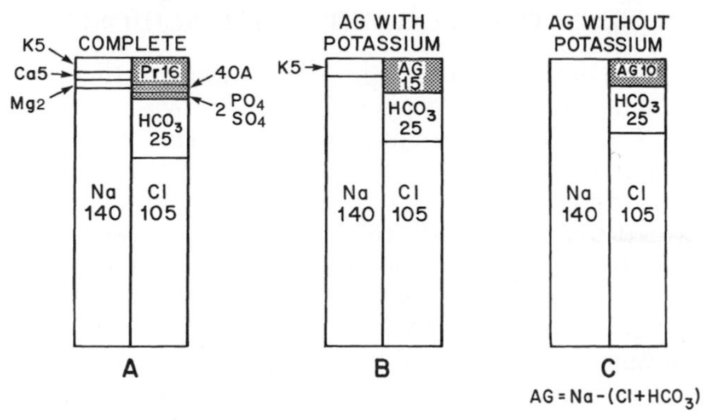


**FIGURE 3–2** ■ The ionic anatomy of serum is shown. *A,* The entire cation and anion composition is displayed. The total anion concentration must equal the total cation concentration. *B,* Measurement restricted to the four major electrolytes K, Na, Cl, and $HCO_3$. Under normal conditions, concentration of the sum of (Na + K) exceeds the sum of (Cl + $HCO_3$). This results in an anion gap, which is shown here to be 15 mEq/L. *C,* The anion gap calculation excluding K. The potential K variation is small compared with the other three variables; therefore, it may be disregarded for the purposes of this calculation. The anion gap, which is calculated as [Na − Cl + $HCO_3$], is shown to be 10 mEq/L.

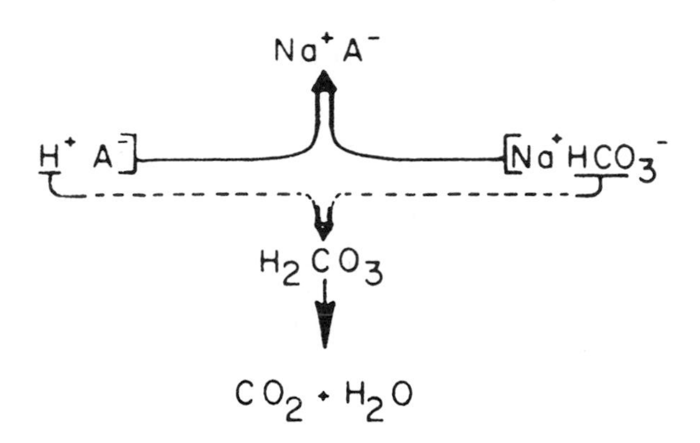


**FIGURE 3–3** ■ Metabolic acidosis and the anion gap. The addition of a relatively strong acid such as $H^+A^-$ to the extracellular fluid (ECF) alters the electrolyte profile as shown. If the acid is HCl, the reduction in [$HCO_3$] is matched by a reciprocal increase in [Cl]. If a non-HCl acid, such as lactic acid, is added to the ECF, the reduction in [$HCO_3$] is matched by a reciprocal increase in the anion gap, while [Cl] remains relatively stable. (The loss of $NaHCO_3$ from the body also produces a hyperchloremic acidosis.)

**TABLE 3–2.** Causes of Metabolic Acidosis

**Hyperchloremic (Normal Anion Gap) Metabolic Acidosis**

GI Loss of $HCO_3$

Diarrhea
Ureterosigmoidostomy

Renal $HCO_3$ Loss

- Proximal RTA
  - Isolated—sporadic, familial
  - Fanconi's syndrome with phosphaturia, glucosuria, uricosuria, aminoaciduria
    - Familial, cystinosis, tyrosinemia, multiple myeloma, Wilson's disease, ifosfamide, osteopetrosis
- Carbonic anhydrase inhibitors
- Ileal bladder

Reduced Renal $H^+$ Secretion

- Distal RTA
  - Familial, hypercalcemic/hypercalciuric states, Sjögren's syndrome, autoimmune diseases, amphotericin, renal transplant
- Type 4 RTA
  - Hyporeninemic-hypoaldosteronism—diabetes mellitus, tubulointerstitial disease, NSAIDs
  - Defective MC synthesis or secretion—Addison's disease, chronic heparin therapy, congenital adrenal defects
  - Inadequate renal response to MC–sickle cell disease, SLE, K-sparing diuretics, "chloride shunts"
- Early uremia

HCl/HCl precursor ingestion/infusion

HCl
$NH_4Cl$
Arginine HCl

Other

Post chronic hyperventilation
Recovery from diabetic ketoacidosis
Toluene inhalation

**High Anion Gap Metabolic Acidosis**

1. Lactic acidosis
   a. D-Lactic Acidosis
2. Ketoacidosis
3. Uremia
4. Methanol ingestion
5. Ethylene glycol ingestion
6. Salicylate poisoning

GI, gastrointestinal; MC, mineralocorticoid; NSAIDs, nonsteroidal anti-inflammatory drugs; RTA, renal tubular acidosis; SLE, systemic lupus erythematosus.

generate or maintain a normal pH gradient (the normal minimal urine pH is <5.5). Therefore, these patients always excrete inappropriately alkaline urine despite systemic acidemia. Distal RTA is also often associated with renal medullary calcifications and development of calcium renal stones, which develop as a result of hypercalciuria and reduced urine citrate excretion. Distal RTA also generally causes hypokalemia as a result of renal potassium losses. Alkaline urine in a patient with hyperchloremic metabolic acidosis and hypokalemia suggests the diagnosis of distal RTA. However, several other conditions must be excluded. Some bacteria metabolize urine urea to generate ammonium and $CO_2$. This alkalizes the urine in the bladder after the kidney has formed it. Therefore, a urinary tract infection must be ruled out. Patients with severe diarrhea may also develop laboratory findings that suggest distal RTA. The hyperchloremic acidosis of diarrhea is caused by the loss of alkali in stool (see earlier).

Normal kidneys should maximally acidify the urine in response to this acid stress, and they do. However, marked hypokalemia also generally develops as a result of stool potassium loss, and this stimulates renal ammoniagenesis and ammonia excretion. Very high urine ammonium levels increase the urine pH. This does not represent a renal acidification defect (in fact, net renal acid excretion in these patients is very high).[4] In contrast, patients with distal RTA have low ammonium excretion rates. Type 4 RTA is a hyperkalemic, hyperchloremic acidosis that is usually caused by hypoaldosteronism or an inadequate renal tubule response to aldosterone. Reduced potassium excretion produces hyperkalemia, which inhibits renal $NH_4$ synthesis and excretion. (Hypokalemia stimulates and hyperkalemia inhibits renal ammonium synthesis and excretion.) The reduction in $NH_4$ excretion reduces renal net acid excretion and contributes to the development of metabolic acidosis.

If a segment of intestine is exposed to urine, the intestinal epithelium absorbs chloride and secretes $HCO_3$. Potassium is also secreted into the urine. Excretion of $NaHCO_3$ and potassium-rich urine results in hypokalemic, hyperchloremic metabolic acidosis. Ureterosigmoidostomy, ileal loop bladders, and bowel segment interposition into the urinary stream are clinical examples of this pathophysiology.

## METABOLIC ACIDOSIS WITH AN INCREASED ANION GAP

AG metabolic acidosis develops when organic acids or non-Cl inorganic acids such as $H_2SO_4$ or $NaH_2PO_4$ accumulate at rates that exceed the rates of their removal via renal excretion or metabolism. The common causes of AG acidosis are listed in Table 3–2. Lactic acidosis is most often caused by ischemia resulting from local or systemic underperfusion or overt shock. Drugs and toxins that impair oxidative metabolism can also produce lactic acidosis. For example, metformin generates profound lactic acidosis when toxic levels accumulate in patients with renal insufficiency. Cyanide and carbon monoxide poisoning also produce lactic acidosis. Lactic acidosis can also develop as a result of a number of inherited and acquired enzyme disorders, especially those affecting the glycolytic or mitochondrial metabolic pathways.

Ketoacidosis may develop in diabetic patients with poor glucose control. It is often precipitated by the metabolic stress of intercurrent medical or surgical complications. Ketoacidosis can also complicate chronic alcohol abuse.

Methanol ingestion causes formic acidosis, whereas ingested ethylene glycol is metabolized to glyoxalate acid and oxalic acid. Oxalic acid precipitates with calcium and deposits in the brain, lungs, peripheral nerves, and kidneys. Severe renal failure often occurs.

## COMPENSATION FOR METABOLIC ACIDOSIS

The compensatory hyperventilation produced by metabolic acidosis is triggered primarily by a fall in the blood and brain interstitial fluid pH. This stimulates chemoreceptors located in the respiratory centers of the medulla.[5] Activation of peripheral chemoreceptors, located in the carotid arteries and aorta, also contributes to hyperventilation, but they play a secondary role. The maximal respiratory response to a rapid change in serum [$HCO_3$] develops over 12 to 24 hours. Conversely, when metabolic acidosis has existed for days or more and is then rapidly corrected, the hyperventilation may persist for many hours. This can result in a period of respiratory alkalosis following correction of metabolic acidosis. The delay in the development of compensatory hyperventilation and its relatively slow reversal are probably due to slow pH equilibration among the central nervous system (CNS), interstitial fluid, and the blood following rapid changes in blood $HCO_3$ concentration.[5]

The magnitude of the hyperventilatory response and the $P_{CO_2}$ level that develops in metabolic acidosis are proportional to the reduction in blood $HCO_3$ concentration. Albert and associates[6] determined this relationship in 60 patients with established, untreated metabolic acidosis (Fig. 3–4). They showed that through most of the pathophysiologic range, the relationship was linear and derived the following equation (often called Winters' equation):

$$\text{Expected } P_{CO_2} = 1.5\ (\text{measured } HCO_3) + 8 \pm 2 \qquad \text{Equation 2}$$

This relationship generally holds regardless of the specific etiology of the metabolic acidosis. For example, assume that a patient with renal failure develops renal

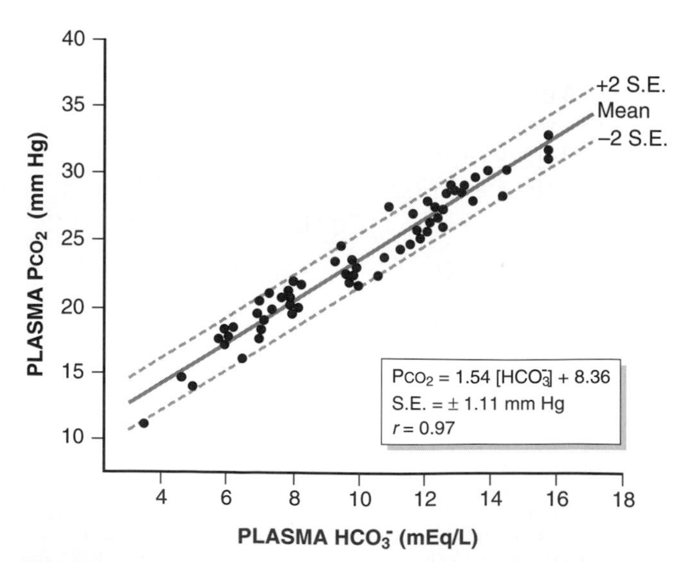


**FIGURE 3–4** ■ The relationship between the plasma [$HCO_3$] and the plasma $P_{CO_2}$ in patients with metabolic acidosis. (From Albert MD, et al: Quantitative displacement of acid-base equilibrium in metabolic acidosis. Ann Intern Med 66:312, 1967.)

acidosis and has a serum $HCO_3$ of 10 mEq/L and a $Pco_2$ of 22 mm Hg. How do we know whether the magnitude of the hypocapnia is appropriate for the degree of acidosis or whether an additional independent respiratory disorder exists? The formula indicates that when metabolic acidosis reduces the serum $HCO_3$ to 10 mEq/L, the $Pco_2$ should be about 23 mm Hg (range, 21–25). If the patient's $Pco_2$ had been $<21$ or $>25$ mm Hg, then the respiratory response would be inappropriate (either inadequate or excessive) for the degree of metabolic acidosis, and a superimposed respiratory alkalosis or acidosis should be considered. This can also be determined from the acid-base nomogram (Fig. 3–1).

In addition to the graphic relationships shown in Figure 3–1 and the relatively cumbersome Winters' equation, several other, simpler formulas and relationships have been described that predict the compensatory response to metabolic acidosis. An equation almost as accurate as Equation 2 follows:

$$Pco_2 = HCO_3 + 15 \qquad \text{Equation 3}$$

This equation predicts a $Pco_2$ of 25 mm Hg in the uremic patient whose metabolic acidosis has reduced the $HCO_3$ to 10 mEq/L. Yet another helpful relationship is that the $Pco_2$ should decrease by approximately 1 to 1.3 mm Hg for each 1 mEq/L fall in serum $HCO_3$. This formula predicts that the $Pco_2$ in our uremic patient should be 20 to 25 mm Hg. Finally, it has been observed that in steady-state metabolic acidosis, the $Pco_2$ should approximate the last two digits of the measured arterial pH.[7] The uremic patient had a serum $HCO_3$ of 10 mEq/L, a $Pco_2$ of 22 mm Hg, and a pH of 7.23. Because the $Pco_2$ is near 23, this also indicates that appropriate compensation exists.

As noted, the compensatory respiratory response to metabolic acidosis is generally independent of the cause of the metabolic acidosis. Thus, the acidosis produced by severe diarrhea, diabetic ketoacidosis, and renal tubular dysfunction all generate a similar degree of hyperventilation for any given $HCO_3$ reduction. (Lactic acidosis may generate slightly greater respiratory responses than other metabolic acidoses, but the differences are subtle and have no clinical importance.[8])

These compensatory rules have several caveats. First, the metabolic acidosis must have been present for at least 12 to 24 hours. Metabolic acidosis of brief duration may not reduce the $Pco_2$ to these predicted levels. Therefore, use of predictive formulas or nomograms in that setting could incorrectly indicate that the $Pco_2$ is inappropriately high (i.e., that respiratory acidosis complicates the metabolic acidosis). Second, maximal hyperventilation in response to severe acidosis rarely reduces the $Pco_2$ below a minimal value of about 10 to 12 mm Hg.

Madias and associates[9] described a potentially harmful effect of the hyperventilatory response in patients with severe chronic metabolic acidosis. Hyperventilation and hypocarbia cause transient bicarbonaturia and decrease net renal acid excretion. These effects reduce the $HCO_3$ concentration. This is most apparent in patients with chronic respiratory alkalosis, where it is recognized as appropriate metabolic compensation (see later). However, these renal effects of hypocapnia also occur when patients with metabolic acidosis hyperventilate. The compensatory decrease in $Pco_2$ triggered by a low $HCO_3$ concentration can therefore further reduce the $HCO_3$ concentration. The impact of this additional reduction in $HCO_3$ concentration on the arterial pH varies with the severity of the metabolic acidosis. Patients with severe metabolic acidosis may develop worse acidemia as a result of this "maladaptive" hyperventilatory response to metabolic acidosis.

## Metabolic Alkalosis

Metabolic alkalosis is a disorder that generates a primary increase in $[HCO_3]$. Normal kidneys can rapidly excrete large quantities of $NaHCO_3$. Therefore, the administration or generation of $HCO_3$ does not greatly increase the $HCO_3$ concentration unless conditions exist that reduce renal $NaHCO_3$ excretion. Renal maintenance of metabolic alkalosis may be caused by a global reduction in renal function or stimulation of renal tubule $HCO_3$ reabsorption. Whenever metabolic alkalosis develops, both the process responsible for increasing the $[HCO_3]$ and the reason why the kidneys are not efficiently excreting the additional $HCO_3$ must be determined.[10] Decreased $HCO_3$ filtration reflects a reduced glomerular filtration rate (GFR), whereas increased renal tubule reabsorption is generally caused by ECF volume contraction, hypokalemia, or elevated mineralocorticoid activity. The increased $HCO_3$ concentration of metabolic alkalosis is associated with a proportionate reduction in the Cl concentration and almost invariable hypokalemia.

Gastric fluid contains HCl, NaCl, a small amount of KCl, and water. Its loss from the body via vomiting or nasogastric (NG) suction generates a metabolic alkalosis and simultaneously contracts the ECF volume and triggers renal potassium losses that produce hypokalemia. The later effects reduce the GFR and simultaneously stimulate renal $NaHCO_3$ reabsorption. Another common cause of metabolic alkalosis is the administration of thiazide or loop diuretics. Diuretics increase renal NaCl and water excretion, which contracts the ECF and stimulates the renin-angiotensin-aldosterone axis. Persistent distal NaCl delivery (owing to the diuretic), combines with volume and chloride depletion and increased aldosterone activity to accelerate distal tubule Na reabsorption, potassium secretion, and proton secretion. This generates hypokalemia and metabolic alkalosis. The hypokalemia, ECF contraction, and continued distal tubule reabsorption of Na and secretion of protons maintain the alkalosis. Thus, the kidney is the site of $HCO_3$ generation and the site of alkalosis maintenance in diuretic-induced metabolic alkalosis. Gastric fluid loss and diuretic use probably account for approximately 90% of all cases of metabolic alkalosis.

The metabolic alkaloses can be separated into two groups based on the patient's "effective arterial volume." If the kidneys perceive a reduced "effective arterial volume," then they avidly reabsorb filtered Na, $HCO_3$, and Cl. The urine chloride concentration is generally a good indirect indicator of the kidney's perception of the effective arterial volume. Table 3–3 divides the metabolic alkaloses on the basis of a spot urine Cl concentration. A urine [Cl] <20 mEq/L generally indicates that effective arterial volume is reduced, and this contributes to the maintenance of the metabolic alkalosis. The metabolic alkaloses in the low urine [Cl] group are also called "chloride- or saline-sensitive," because administration of chloride-containing fluids such as NaCl will expand the ECF, restore effective arterial volume, and thus cause an $NaHCO_3$ diuresis that corrects the alkalosis. However, conditions such as congestive heart failure, cirrhosis, and nephrotic syndrome have low effective arterial volume that does not improve with saline expansion. Expansion of the effective arterial volume in such patients requires treatment of the underlying pathology. The metabolic alkaloses with high urine [Cl] (>20 mEq/L) have either an expanded effective arterial volume or a renal tubule defect that causes inappropriate renal NaCl excretion. Many patients with metabolic alkalosis and a high urine chloride concentration have $HCO_3$ generation and maintenance mechanisms related to persistent mineralocorticoid stimulation and hypokalemia. This group includes the metabolic alkalosis of primary hyperaldosteronism, renin-secreting tumors, Cushing's disease, and the ingestion of exogenous mineralocorticoids. These disorders are associated with ECF expansion and hypertension. Liddle's syndrome is due to a genetic defect that causes mineralocorticoid independent acceleration of distal tubule $Na^+$ reabsorption. This leads to clinical and electrolyte abnormalities similar to primary hyperaldosteronism. Generally, NaCl infusion does not correct metabolic alkaloses in the high urine [Cl] group. Consequently, these disorders are also called the chloride-, or saline-, unresponsive, or resistant, metabolic alkaloses.

Diuretic-induced metabolic alkalosis is a special case that straddles these urine [Cl] categories. Soon after ingestion or infusion of a diuretic, the urine [Cl] increases above 20 mEq/L owing to the diuretic effect. Later, as the diuretic effect wanes, the urine [Cl] falls below 20 mEq/L, which reflects ECF contraction. The maintenance phase of diuretic alkalosis is linked to effective arterial volume contraction. Volume expansion should correct the alkalosis but may not be possible if the diuretics are indicated. Therefore, diuretic alkalosis behaves as "volume-sensitive" or low urine [Cl] metabolic alkalosis, although the urine [Cl] may be low (remote from the diuretic) or high (recent diuretic). Bartter's and Gitelman's syndromes are also high urine [Cl] metabolic alkaloses. Most of these disorders are caused by an inherited defect in the thick limb of Henle or distal tubule NaCl transporters. These are the same transporters that can be inhibited by loop and thiazide diuretics. Consequently, these patients behave as though exposed to a constant infusion of a loop (Bartter's syndrome) or thiazide (Gitelman's syndrome) diuretic. ECF contraction, low blood pressure, high renin and aldosterone levels, and persistently high urine [Cl] are characteristic features.

**TABLE 3–3.** Differential Diagnosis of Metabolic Alkalosis

| Low urine [Cl] (<20 mEq/L) chloride-responsive | High urine [Cl] (>20 mEq/L) chloride-unresponsive |
|---|---|
| Diuretics (remote) ⟷ | Diuretics (recent) |
| Vomiting/NG suction | High blood pressure |
| S/P chronic hypercarbia | Primary hyperaldosteronism |
| Chloridorrhea | Cushing disease |
| | Ectopic ACTH |
| | Exogenous mineralocorticoids |
| | Mineralocorticoid-like substances |
| | Liddle syndrome |
| | Low blood pressure |
| | Bartter syndrome |
| | Gitelman syndrome |
| | Severe K depletion |

ACTH, adrenocorticotropic hormone; NG, nasogastric; S/P, status post.

### COMPENSATION FOR METABOLIC ALKALOSIS

When metabolic alkalosis increases the plasma $HCO_3$ concentration and the arterial pH, these changes are detected by central and peripheral chemosensory receptors that direct the respiratory center to decrease minute ventilation. The $P_{CO_2}$ increases. This reduces the $HCO_3/P_{CO_2}$ ratio and drives the pH toward normal. It is generally agreed that the respiratory response to metabolic alkalosis is less predictable than the response to metabolic acidosis. This variation among patients has been attributed to complicating respiratory disorders, hypoxia, differing degrees of intracellular alkalosis, and the effects of potassium depletion. However, more recent studies have found less variation.[11]

Patients with metabolic alkalosis should have an elevated $P_{CO_2}$ (>40 mm Hg). Therefore, the patient with an elevated $HCO_3$ and a reduced $P_{CO_2}$ clearly has mixed metabolic alkalosis and respiratory alkalosis. A normal or only slightly increased $P_{CO_2}$ in a patient with a major $HCO_3$ elevation also indicates inadequate compensation or "relative hyperventilation." The $P_{CO_2}$ should increase by about 0.4 to 0.6 mm Hg for each 1 mEq/L $HCO_3$ increment.[11] At the other extreme, maximal respiratory compensation for metabolic alkalosis rarely increases the $P_{CO_2}$ above 60 mm Hg. A $P_{CO_2}$ tension above this level usually indicates that respiratory acidosis coexists.

## Respiratory Acidosis

About 15,000 to 20,000 mm of $CO_2$ is produced and excreted each day, and respiration normally maintains the arterial $P_{CO_2}$ at about 40 mm Hg. Disorders that compromise ventilation may create transient imbalances between the rates of $CO_2$ production and excretion that result in hypercapnia. A higher $P_{CO_2}$ level permits a greater quantity of $CO_2$ to be excreted at any

**TABLE 3–4.** Causes of Respiratory Acidosis

| |
|---|
| 1. CNS depression<br>Sedatives/CNS lesions |
| 2. Neuromuscular disorders<br>Myopathies/neuropathies |
| 3. Thoracic cage restriction<br>Kyphoscoliosis/scleroderma |
| 4. Impaired lung motion<br>Pleural effusion/pneumothorax |
| 5. Acute obstructive lung disease<br>Aspiration/tumor/bronchospasm |
| 6. Chronic obstructive lung disease |
| 7. Miscellaneous<br>Ventilator malfunction/CPR |

CNS, central nervous system; CPR, cardiopulmonary resuscitation.

given minute ventilation. Consequently, at the onset of hypoventilation, the $P_{CO_2}$ increases until it once more matches $CO_2$ production and excretion. Thus, with steady-state hypercapnia, the lungs excrete the generated $CO_2$ at the expense of a sustained elevation of arterial $P_{CO_2}$. (The patient only "retains" $CO_2$ transiently. After the higher $P_{CO_2}$ has stabilized, acid balance is restored.) The causes of respiratory acidosis are shown in Table 3–4.

### COMPENSATION FOR RESPIRATORY ACIDOSIS

Respiratory acidosis is characterized by an increased $P_{CO_2}$ and carbonic acid concentration ($0.03 \times P_{CO_2}$). The $HCO_3/P_{CO_2}$ ratio falls and reduces the pH. Compensation for respiratory acidosis increases the $HCO_3$ concentration, thus raising the $HCO_3/P_{CO_2}$ ratio and driving the pH back toward the normal range. The magnitude of the compensatory response and the source of the additional $HCO_3$ vary with the duration of the respiratory acidosis. Consequently, it is important to distinguish between acute and chronic respiratory acidosis. Compensation for acute respiratory acidosis is caused by tissue buffering of some of the carbonic acid. The increased $P_{CO_2}$ and carbonic acid concentration drives the reaction in Equation 4 toward the right:

$$\uparrow P_{CO_2} \rightarrow \overrightarrow{\uparrow H_2CO_3 \rightleftharpoons HCO_3 + H^+} \qquad \text{Equation 4}$$

This shift increases the $H^+$ concentration and reduces the pH. Simultaneously, extracellular and intracellular nonbicarbonate buffers take up most of the "excess" $H^+$ (about one third of these protons are taken up by hemoglobin). To the extent that such buffering occurs, $HCO_3$ is formed. When the pH decreases from 7.4 to 7.1, the free $H^+$ concentration increases by only 0.04 mEq/L. However, this acute metabolic compensatory mechanism is very limited. Brackett and associates carefully analyzed the metabolic response to acute hypercapnia and derived 95% confidence bands and an equation describing the relationship between $P_{CO_2}$ and $HCO_3$ in these patients.[12] The plasma $HCO_3$ concentration increased by about 1 mEq/L for each 10–mm Hg increase in $P_{CO_2}$. Thus, an acute rise in $P_{CO_2}$ from 40 to 70 mm Hg should increase the $HCO_3$ concentration from 24 to 27 mEq/L. Consequently, even severe acute respiratory acidosis cannot increase the $HCO_3$ concentration by more than 4 to 5 mEq/L.

Respiratory acidosis and hypercarbia also stimulate the kidney to increase acid excretion and $HCO_3$ reabsorption. Although this response begins rapidly, it takes several days to develop fully. Acidemia, hypercarbia, and high carbonic acid levels stimulate renal ammonia synthesis and accelerate renal acid excretion. If renal acid excretion exceeds the patient's requirement to excrete the normal "fixed" acid load, new $HCO_3$ is being synthesized. Excretion of $NH_4Cl$, and to lesser degrees NaCl and KCl, also generates hypochloremia, which is characteristic of chronic respiratory acidosis. Hypercapnia also stimulates renal tubule $HCO_3$ reclamation, mainly in the proximal renal tubule. In this manner, increased $HCO_3$ synthesis and tubular reabsorption are coordinated to stabilize the plasma $HCO_3$ at a higher concentration. Once the plasma $HCO_3$ concentration stabilizes at a higher steady-state level, renal acid excretion falls to again match the "fixed" acid load (steady-state conditions are restored).

Brackett and associates[13] also studied the compensatory response to chronic respiratory acidosis in humans and identified the relationship between the $P_{CO_2}$ and plasma $HCO_3$ concentration. This relationship is shown in Figure 3–1. The $HCO_3$ should increase by about 3.5 mEq/L for each 10–mm Hg increase in $P_{CO_2}$ in patients with chronic respiratory acidosis. This increase in $HCO_3$ is not usually enough to restore the pH to the mid-normal range. Patients with mild chronic respiratory acidosis generally have a low normal pH, whereas patients whose $P_{CO_2}$ is chronically elevated above 50 mm Hg almost always remain acidemic despite full metabolic compensation.[14]

## Respiratory Alkalosis

Increased alveolar ventilation, or hyperventilation, results in a transient imbalance between $CO_2$ production and excretion. As described earlier, a lower alveolar $CO_2$ tension, or $P_{CO_2}$, will cause less $CO_2$ to be excreted at any given level of minute ventilation. Therefore, when hyperventilation persists, and a lower $P_{CO_2}$ stabilizes, $CO_2$ balance is restored despite hypocapnia. A low $P_{CO_2}$ and carbonic acid concentration ($0.03 \times P_{CO_2}$), together with alkalemia, define respiratory alkalosis. The causes of respiratory alkalosis are shown in Table 3–5.

### COMPENSATION FOR RESPIRATORY ALKALOSIS

Compensation for respiratory alkalosis reduces the $HCO_3$ concentration (and elevates the chloride concentration), and this drives the $HCO_3/P_{CO_2}$ ratio and pH back toward the normal range. The compensatory responses generated by acute and chronic respiratory

**TABLE 3–5.** Causes of Respiratory Alkalosis

1. Anxiety
2. CNS disorders
   CVA/tumor/infection
3. Hormones
   Progesterone/catecholamines
4. Drugs
   Salicylates/analeptics
5. Sepsis/endotoxemia
6. Hyperthyroidism
7. Hypoxia
8. Pregnancy
9. Cirrhosis
10. Pulmonary edema
11. Lung diseases
    Restriction/pulmonary emboli/pneumonia
12. Ventilator induced

CNS, central nervous system; CVA, cerebrovascular accident.

alkalosis mirror those described in response to acute and chronic respiratory acidosis.

$$\downarrow P_{CO_2} \leftarrow \downarrow H_2CO_3 \rightleftharpoons HCO_3 + H^+ \qquad \text{Equation 5}$$

Acute respiratory alkalosis reduces the $P_{CO_2}$ and $H_2CO_3$ concentration that drives Equation 5 toward the left. The reduction in $H^+$ concentration (alkalemia) causes the release of $H^+$ from extracellular and intracellular buffers. This $H^+$ combines with ECF $HCO_3$ to generate $H_2CO_3$, which reduces the $HCO_3$ concentration. This acute fall in the $HCO_3$ concentration occurs within minutes and is of a relatively small magnitude. Arbus and associates[15] studied this acute response and found that the $HCO_3$ concentration falls by about 2 mEq/L for each 10–mm Hg decrement in $P_{CO_2}$. If respiratory alkalosis persists, the kidneys generate a much greater compensatory $HCO_3$ reduction. Although these renal mechanisms are engaged rapidly, their effects are not clinically important for 12 to 24 hours. Early bicarbonaturia is followed by reduced renal $NH_4Cl$ and titratable acid excretion. This produces positive acid balance and reduces the $HCO_3$ concentration. After a stable lower $HCO_3$ concentration has been achieved, renal acid excretion again increases to match acid production, and acid balance is restored.

The expected compensatory response to chronic respiratory alkalosis has been determined by studying normal subjects who either travel to, or live at, high altitude.[16] These studies show that compensation for chronic respiratory alkalosis reduces the plasma $HCO_3$ concentration by about 5 mEq/L for each 10–mm Hg reduction in $Pa_{CO_2}$. Chronic respiratory alkalosis is unique among the simple acid-base disturbances. It is the only disorder for which compensation returns the pH to the mid-normal range. Thus, this disorder is the exception to the rule that compensation returns the pH *toward* normal but does not restore a normal pH. This $P_{CO_2}/HCO_3$ relationship indicates that when chronic respiratory alkalosis produces a sustained $P_{CO_2}$ of 20 mm Hg, the serum $HCO_3$ should fall from 24 to 14 mEq/L; this results in a pH of 7.46.

# MIXED ACID-BASE DISORDERS

As discussed, compensation for each primary disorder is to be expected and does not represent an independent, or second, acid-base disorder. However, the absence of compensation does indicate that a mixed acid-base disorder may exist. The mixed disorders resulting from a lack of compensation have a synergistic effect on the pH. They cause a more severe degree of acidemia, or alkalemia, than would occur with a primary compensated disorder. They include mixed metabolic acidosis and respiratory acidosis and mixed metabolic alkalosis and respiratory alkalosis. When severe, these mixed acid-base disorders cause the $P_{CO_2}$ and $HCO_3$ to move in opposite directions from their normal ranges (i.e., one is increased and the other is decreased). The other mixed disorders, which include mixed respiratory alkalosis and metabolic acidosis, mixed respiratory acidosis and metabolic alkalosis, and mixed metabolic acidosis and metabolic alkalosis, have opposing effects on the pH, which may be low, normal, or high, depending on the relative severity of each disorder. Triple acid-base disorders are usually caused by the combination of metabolic acidosis, metabolic alkalosis, and a respiratory acid-base abnormality.

## Anion Gap

The ion profile of normal serum is shown in Figure 3–2. The law of electroneutrality mandates that the number of positive charges (cations) in any solution must equal the number of negative charges (anions). Consequently, if the charge concentration (expressed as mEq/L) of every serum, or plasma, ion is determined, then the concentration of positive and negative charges must be the same. If one focuses only on the three ions that exist in the largest concentration (Na, Cl, and $HCO_3$), then the Na concentration normally exceeds the sum of the Cl and $HCO_3$ concentrations. The difference $[Na] - ([Cl] + [HCO_3])$ is called the anion gap (AG). The normal anion gap, calculated in this manner, is $12 \pm 4$ mEq/L ($\pm$ 2 SD). Each laboratory must determine the normal range of the AG, because the normal range of each analyte is laboratory- and instrument-dependent. Potassium is not included in the calculation because of its relatively small quantitative contribution. The AG is a virtual measurement. It does not actually represent the concentration of any specific ion or group of ions. It consists of the anionic contributions of albumin, inorganic phosphate, sulfate, and multiple organic anions that balance a component of the Na concentration.

The AG is used to separate the metabolic acidoses into two groups: (1) the high anion gap metabolic acidoses and (2) the normal anion gap, or hyperchloremic, metabolic acidoses. The causes of the metabolic acidoses are listed in Table 3–2. The AG is also an important clue to the existence of certain mixed acid-base disorders.

When protons accumulate in the ECF, they are buffered by the following reaction:

$$H^+ + HCO_3 \rightarrow H_2CO_3 \rightarrow CO_2 + H_2O$$

Therefore, as is shown in Figure 3–3, when X mm/L of the acid HA accumulates in the ECF, the $HCO_3$ concentration falls by X mm/L and "A" concentration increases by X mm/L. If HA is any non-HCl acid (e.g., lactic, keto, or formic acid), $HCO_3$ falls and Cl and Na concentrations do not change. Consequently, the $HCO_3$ reduction is associated with a reciprocal increase in the AG ([Na] − ([Cl] + [$HCO_3$])). If the accumulating acid is HCl, then the reduction in $HCO_3$ is accompanied by a similar increase in Cl and the AG does not change. In addition, whenever $NaHCO_3$ is lost from the body, hyperchloremic acidosis also develops. This occurs because the loss of $NaHCO_3$ contracts the ECF, which shrinks the Cl space and increases the Cl concentration. Dietary chloride may also be retained. Note that the magnitude of increase in the AG, or the chloride concentration, is similar to the decrease in the $HCO_3$ concentration.

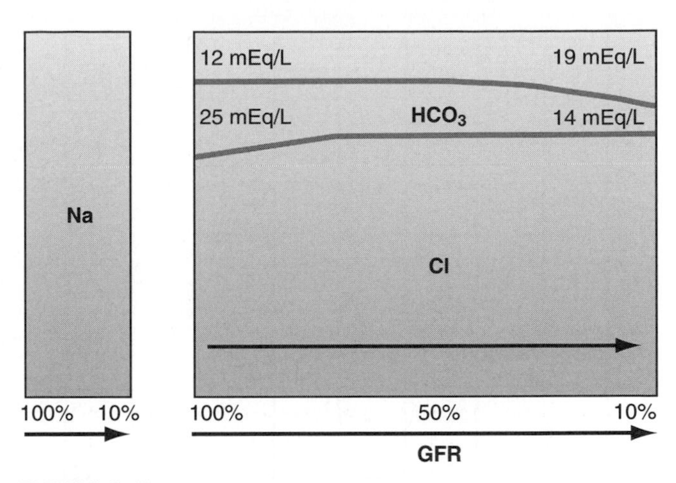


**FIGURE 3–5** ■ The progressive decline in [$HCO_3$] and changes in the Cl and anion gap concentrations over time in patients with progressive renal insufficiency. (Adapted from Widmer B, et al: Serum electrolyte and acid base composition: The influence of graded degrees of chronic renal failure. Arch Intern Med 139: 1099–1102, 1979.)

## Mixed Metabolic Acidoses

Sometimes anion gap and hyperchloremic acidosis develop together. This is technically a "mixed" acid-base disorder, although that designation usually refers to combinations of respiratory and metabolic disorders or to mixed metabolic acidosis and alkalosis. When anion gap and hyperchloremic acidosis coexist, the reduction in $HCO_3$ is partially balanced by an AG increase and partially by hyperchloremia. Mixed hyperchloremic and anion gap metabolic acidosis may occur during the evolution of chronic renal failure. Hyperchloremic acidosis is more common during the early phase of this disease and is the result of reduced renal $NH_4Cl$ excretion. Late in the course of renal failure, more typical uremic anion gap acidosis evolves (Fig. 3–5).[17] Patients with severe diarrhea can also develop this type of mixed metabolic acidosis. The alkali lost in the stool generates a hyperchloremic acidosis. The associated volume depletion sometimes adds a component of lactic acidosis,[18] and starvation may produce ketoacidosis. A third clinical setting in which mixed hyperchloremic/AG acidosis develops is one in which the high AG acidosis is caused by acids containing an anion that the kidney can efficiently excrete as a sodium salt. If an organic acid is added to the ECF and the anion is then excreted as a sodium salt, hyperchloremic acidosis develops.[19] Clinical examples include the acidosis produced by glue sniffing. The inhaled toluene is metabolized to benzoic acid and hippuric acid, and the kidney then excretes Na and K benzoate and hippurate.[20] The treatment phase of ketoacidosis also often transforms an AG acidosis into a hyperchloremic acidosis. The major cause is volume re-expansion, which increases renal excretion of Na acetoacetate and Naβ-OH-butyrate.[21] Technically, combinations of various AG acidoses can also be classified as mixed disorders. For example, ketoacidosis and lactic acidosis may coexist. Several toxins also generate mixed organic metabolic acidosis.

## Mixed Metabolic Acidosis and Metabolic Alkalosis

The AG-$HCO_3$ relationship is an essential clue to the existence of mixed anion gap metabolic acidosis and metabolic alkalosis. Always compare the magnitude of the AG increase with the decrement in the $HCO_3$ concentration. If the anion gap increases significantly more than the reduction in $HCO_3$, this mixed disorder may exist. Figure 3–6 shows the development of this mixed disturbance in a patient who initially had uremic, high AG, acidosis. First, the development of classic late-phase uremic acidosis is shown—the magnitude of the AG increase is similar to the magnitude of the $HCO_3$ reduction. The patient then develops nausea and vomiting. The loss of gastric HCl increases the $HCO_3$ and reduces the Cl concentrations. The AG remains large despite normalization of the $HCO_3$ (because the Cl concentration falls). The resultant discrepancy between the AG increase and $HCO_3$ decrease indicates that metabolic alkalosis preceded, coincided with, or followed the development of the anion gap metabolic acidosis. The relationship between the changes in the anion gap and $HCO_3$ concentrations are sometimes referred to as the Δ/Δ (delta/delta). Table 3–6 shows another example of this mixed disorder. Note that if metabolic alkalosis complicates hyperchloremic acidosis, there is no residual clue of a large AG to indicate the existence of this mixed disorder. In this case, the hyperchloremic metabolic acidosis increases the Cl concentration and reduces the $HCO_3$ concentration, whereas the metabolic alkalosis moves each of these parameters in the opposite directions. Recognition of this disorder re-

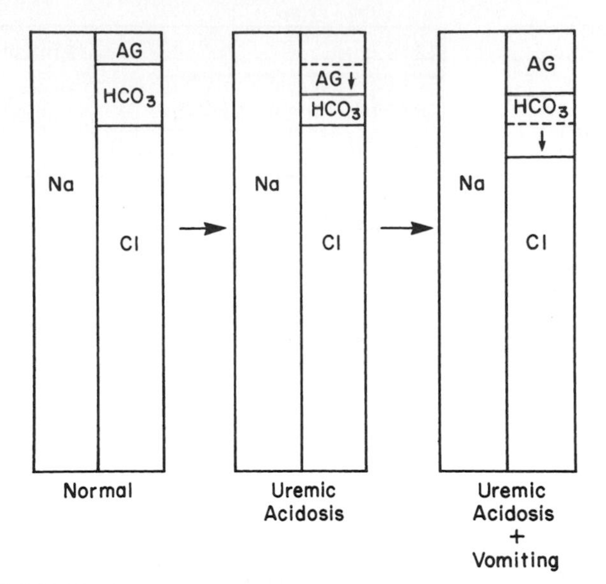


**FIGURE 3–6** ■ A patient develops uremic metabolic acidosis. The [$HCO_3$] falls, and the anion gap increases reciprocally. The patient then begins to vomit, which increases the [$HCO_3$] while reducing [Cl]. In the example, the [$HCO_3$] has been restored to normal. Mixed metabolic acidosis and metabolic alkalosis are now present. The correct diagnosis is suggested by the large anion gap and a coexisting normal [$HCO_3$] (resulting from the low [Cl]).

quires knowledge of sequential chemistries and other historical and clinical clues.

The two components of this mixed disorder have opposing effects on the pH and may, therefore, be acidic, normal, or alkaline.

## Mixed Metabolic Acidosis and Respiratory Acidosis

When metabolic acidosis reduces the $HCO_3$ concentration but the $P_{CO_2}$ is inadequately reduced, then mixed metabolic and respiratory acidosis may coexist. Table 3–7 shows some examples of this mixed disorder. Absence of compensation for metabolic acidosis indicates a milder form of this mixed disorder, whereas overt hypercarbia combined with metabolic acidosis indicates a more severe disorder. Mixed acute metabolic and respiratory acidosis occurs commonly in patients who have suffered cardiopulmonary arrest and also occurs in patients with severe pulmonary edema. If metabolic acidosis is complicated by severe hypokalemia or severe hypophosphatemia, these patients may develop respiratory acidosis as a result of respiratory muscle weakness. A number of drug overdoses and poisons can generate metabolic acidosis and simultaneously depress respiration, which causes coexisting respiratory acidosis. Finally, patients with obstructive lung disease and chronic respiratory acidosis should manifest an appropriate increase in $HCO_3$ concentration (see the section on respiratory acidosis). If they develop a complicating metabolic acidosis, then their $HCO_3$ concentration falls and indicates the presence of this mixed disorder.

## Mixed Metabolic Alkalosis and Respiratory Acidosis

Chronic respiratory acidosis should produce a compensatory increase in $HCO_3$ as described earlier. If the $HCO_3$ increase is greater than the level expected for compensation, this indicates that mixed metabolic alkalosis and respiratory acidosis exists. The expected $HCO_3$ compensatory increase in patients with chronic respiratory acidosis should not restore the pH to the mid-normal range. Table 3–8 shows several examples of this mixed disorder. Metabolic alkalosis often complicates respiratory acidosis as a result of diuretic use and low-salt diets. The resultant "normal" pH can reduce respiratory drive and thus worsen the respiratory acidosis. The pulmonary status of such patients improves if the diuretic is switched to an acidifying agent, such as acetazolamide, so that the $HCO_3$ is reduced to the appropriate level.[22] Respiratory acidosis can also be superimposed on an underlying metabolic alkalosis. Severe hypokalemia may develop with metabolic alkalosis and can depress muscle strength, thus generating respiratory acidosis.

**TABLE 3–6.** Mixed Metabolic Acidosis and Metabolic Alkalosis

| | | | | Mixed Metabolic Alkalosis and Metabolic Acidosis | |
|---|---|---|---|---|---|
| | Normal | High AG Metabolic Acidosis | Normal AG Metabolic Acidosis | *High AG Metabolic Acidosis* | *Normal AG Metabolic Acidosis* |
| Na (mEq/L) | 140 | 140 | 140 | 140 | 140 |
| K (mEq/L) | 4.0 | 5.0 | 5.0 | 3.5 | 3.5 |
| Cl (mEq/L) | 105 | 105 | 115 | 95 | 105 |
| $HCO_3$ (mEq/L) | 25 | 15 | 15 | 25 | 25 |
| Anion gap | 10 | 20 | 10 | 20 | 10 |
| $P_{CO_2}$ (mm Hg) | 40 | 31 | 31 | 40 | 40 |
| pH | 7.42 | 7.31 | 7.31 | 7.42 | 7.42 |

AG, anion gap.

**TABLE 3–7.** Mixed Metabolic Acidosis and Respiratory Acidosis

| | Normal | Metabolic Acidosis | Mixed Metabolic Acidosis and Respiratory Acidosis | |
|---|---|---|---|---|
| | | | *Mild* | *Severe* |
| Na (mEq/L) | 140 | 140 | 140 | 140 |
| K (mEq/L) | 4.0 | 4.5 | 5.0 | 5.0 |
| Cl (mEq/L) | 105 | 104 | 102 | 102 |
| $HCO_3$ (mEq/L) | 25 | 16 | 18 | 18 |
| Anion gap | 10 | 20 | 20 | 20 |
| $PCO_2$ (mm Hg) | 40 | 30 | 38 | 50 |
| pH | 7.42 | 7.35 | 7.30 | 7.18 |

**TABLE 3–8.** Mixed Metabolic Alkalosis and Respiratory Acidosis

| | Normal | Chronic Respiratory Acidosis | Metabolic Alkalosis | Chronic Respiratory Acidosis and Metabolic Alkalosis |
|---|---|---|---|---|
| Na (mEq/L) | 140 | 140 | 140 | 140 |
| K (mEq/L) | 4.0 | 4.0 | 3.0 | 3.5 |
| Cl (mEq/L) | 105 | 97 | 92 | 88 |
| $HCO_3$ (mEq/L) | 25 | 33 | 36 | 42 |
| Anion gap | 10 | 10 | 12 | 10 |
| $PCO_2$ (mm Hg) | 40 | 60 | 46 | 67 |
| pH | 7.42 | 7.36 | 7.52 | 7.42 |

**TABLE 3–9.** Mixed Metabolic Acidosis and Respiratory Alkalosis

| | Normal | Metabolic Acidosis | Metabolic Acidosis and Respiratory Alkalosis | |
|---|---|---|---|---|
| | | | *Mild* | *Severe* |
| Na (mEq/L) | 140 | 140 | 140 | 140 |
| K (mEq/L) | 4.0 | 3.5 | 4.0 | 3.5 |
| Cl (mEq/L) | 105 | 106 | 106 | 106 |
| $HCO_3$ (mEq/L) | 25 | 14 | 14 | 13 |
| Anion gap | 10 | 20 | 20 | 21 |
| $PCO_2$ (mm Hg) | 40 | 29 | 24 | 15 |
| pH | 7.42 | 7.31 | 7.39 | 7.56 |

**TABLE 3–10.** Simple and Mixed Alkaloses

| | | Simple Alkalosis | | Mixed Alkalosis | |
|---|---|---|---|---|---|
| | Normal | *Metabolic* | *Chronic Respiratory* | *Mild* | *Severe* |
| Na (mEq/L) | 140 | 140 | 140 | 140 | 140 |
| K (mEq/L) | 4 | 3 | 3.5 | 3.0 | 2.8 |
| Cl (mEq/L) | 105 | 92 | 109 | 92 | 92 |
| $HCO_3$ (mEq/L) | 25 | 35 | 17 | 32 | 32 |
| Anion gap | 10 | 13 | 14 | 16 | 16 |
| $PCO_2$ (mm Hg) | 40 | 47 | 25 | 38 | 30 |
| pH | 7.42 | 7.49 | 7.46 | 7.55 | 7.65 |

## Mixed Metabolic Acidosis and Respiratory Alkalosis

When metabolic acidosis is associated with a $P_{CO_2}$ that is lower than the predicted compensatory level, mixed metabolic acidosis and respiratory alkalosis may exist. From the other perspective, if respiratory alkalosis develops first it should appropriately reduce the $HCO_3$ concentration. If the $HCO_3$ concentration is lower than predicted for a given level of respiratory alkalosis, this also indicates a mixed metabolic acidosis and respiratory alkalosis. Table 3–9 shows several examples of this mixed disorder.

This mixed disorder often occurs in patients with salicylate poisoning. Toxic levels of salicylate directly stimulate the CNS respiratory center, thus causing hyperventilation and respiratory alkalosis. Simultaneously, salicylate intoxication uncouples mitochondrial oxidative phosphorylation and this causes multiple organic acids (including ketoacids and lactic acid) to accumulate. Salicylic acid itself is a relatively strong acid that contributes to the AG metabolic acidosis. Although both respiratory alkalosis and metabolic acidosis coexist in both infants and adults, the former usually have more severe AG metabolic acidosis and profound acidemia, whereas respiratory alkalosis, and an alkaline or normal pH, is more often the dominant abnormality in older children and adults.[23] Patients with chronic liver disease are also at risk for this mixed disorder. The respiratory alkalosis in these patients is caused by stimulation of the respiratory center by a combination of factors, including high levels of ammonia and other biogenic amines, hypoxia, and elevated progesterone levels.[24] These patients may also develop metabolic acidosis as a result of RTA (e.g., autoimmune hepatitis, Wilson's disease, primary biliary acidosis), and the late stages of liver failure may be complicated by hepatorenal syndrome (uremic acidosis) and lactic acidosis.[25,26]

This mixed acid-based disorder also occurs commonly in the intensive care unit (ICU). Respiratory alkalosis occurs in patients due to mechanical overventilation, pain, hypoxia, sepsis, stress (high catecholamine levels), neurologic dysfunction, and hypotension.[27] Many of these critically ill patients also develop lactic acidosis, uremic acidosis, or diarrheal acidosis.

## Mixed Metabolic Alkalosis and Respiratory Alkalosis

The combination of a low $P_{CO_2}$ and high $HCO_3$ concentration is diagnostic of metabolic alkalosis and respiratory alkalosis. Table 3–10 shows several examples of this mixed disorder. Mixed metabolic and respiratory alkalosis has a synergistic elevating effect on the pH, leading to extreme alkalemia. Marked alkalemia produces multiple adverse pathophysiologic effects, including cerebral vasoconstriction, increased hemoglobin affinity for oxygen (reducing tissue oxygen unloading), hypokalemia, and cardiac arrhythmias.[28,29] This spectrum of adverse effects contributes to the high mortality rate associated with extreme alkalemia. Metabolic and respiratory alkalosis occurs relatively frequently in the surgical ICU. The causes of the respiratory component were listed earlier (see Mixed Metabolic Acidosis and Respiratory Alkalosis). The metabolic alkalosis in these surgical patients may result from NG suction, the alkali load contained in blood products, and the frequent use of diuretics. Development of mixed metabolic and respiratory alkalosis in the ICU has an ominous prognosis. If the pH exceeds 7.64, the mortality rate is 80%.[28] This mixed disorder may also occur in the pregnant woman. High progesterone levels, arteriovenous shunting, and diaphragm elevation associated with pregnancy cause hyperventilation.[30] This is a normal physiologic manifestation of pregnancy and results in a $P_{CO_2}$ of about 30 mm Hg and a $HCO_3$ of about 20 mEq/L (compensatory decrease) during the third trimester. Metabolic alkalosis may develop as a result of vomiting or the use of diuretics. The $HCO_3$ concentration increases, and metabolic and respiratory alkalosis ensues.

## Triple Acid-Base Disorders

Triple acid-base disorders exist when metabolic acidosis and metabolic alkalosis combine with either respiratory acidosis or respiratory alkalosis. Coexistent metabolic acidosis and alkalosis results in a low, normal or elevated $HCO_3$ concentration. Whatever the $HCO_3$ concentration, it should be associated with an appropriate $P_{CO_2}$. Therefore, if the final $HCO_3$ concentra-

**TABLE 3–11.** Metabolic Acidosis, Metabolic Alkalosis, Metabolic Acidosis and Alkalosis, and Triple Acid-Base Disturbance

| | Normal | Metabolic Alkalosis | Metabolic Acidosis (Anion Gap) | Metabolic Acidosis and Metabolic Alkalosis | Respiratory Alkalosis with Metabolic Acidosis and Metabolic Alkalosis (Triple Disturbance) |
|---|---|---|---|---|---|
| Na (mEq/L) | 140 | 140 | 140 | 140 | 140 |
| K (mEq/L) | 4.0 | 3.0 | 4.5 | 4.0 | 3.3 |
| Cl (mEq/L) | 105 | 92 | 105 | 90 | 88 |
| $HCO_3$ (mEq/L) | 25 | 35 | 10 | 25 | 25 |
| Anion gap | 10 | 13 | 25 | 25 | 27 |
| $P_{CO_2}$ (mm Hg) | 40 | 47 | 24 | 40 | 30 |
| pH | 7.42 | 7.49 | 7.24 | 7.42 | 7.54 |

tion is reduced, then the $Pco_2$ should be reduced to the levels described for metabolic acidosis; if the $HCO_3$ concentration is normal, then the $Pco_2$ should be normal; if the $HCO_3$ concentration is elevated, then the $Pco_2$ should increase to the level described with metabolic alkalosis. If the $Pco_2$ falls outside the expected range, a coexisting respiratory disorder may exist. Patients with severe liver disease often develop triple acid-base disorders.[24] Metabolic acidosis may be caused by uremia, lactic acidosis, RTA, or diarrhea. Metabolic alkalosis may develop as a result of vomiting, use of diuretics, or NG suction. When the metabolic acidosis is of the high anion gap variety, the anion gap increase exceeds the reduction of the $HCO_3$ concentration (see Mixed Metabolic Acidosis and Alkalosis). Finally, patients with liver failure often develop chronic hyperventilation and respiratory alkalosis as a result of stimulation of the CNS respiratory center by ammonia and other accumulating toxic compounds, high progesterone levels, and hypoxia produced by elevation of the diaphragm (from ascites) and arteriovenous shunting. Table 3–11 shows an example of this mixed disorder.

## REFERENCES


1. Goldberg M, Green SB, Moss ML, et al: Computer-based instruction and diagnosis of acid-base disorders: A systematic approach. JAMA 223:266–275, 1973.
2. Emmett M, Narins RG: Clinical use of the anion gap. Medicine (Baltimore) 56:38–54, 1977.
3. Narins RG, Emmett M: Simple and mixed acid-base disorders: A practical approach. Medicine (Baltimore) 59:161–187, 1980.
4. Schloeder FX, Griffith DP, Stinebaugh BJ: Evaluation of renal acidification in patients with urea-splitting organisms. Investig Urol 15:299–302, 1978.
5. Pappenheimer JR: The ionic composition of cerebral extracellular fluid and its relation to control of breathing. Harv Lect 61: 71–94, 1967.
6. Albert MD, Dell RB, Winters RW: Quantitative displacement of acid-base equilibrium in metabolic acidosis. Ann Intern Med 66: 312, 1967.
7. Fulop M: A guide for predicting arterial $CO_2$ tension in metabolic acidosis. Am J Nephrol 17:421–424, 1997.
8. Relman AS: Lactic acidosis. Trans Am Clin Climatol Assoc 82: 70–76, 1970.
9. Madias NE, Adrogue HG, Cohen JJ: Maladaptive renal response to secondary hypercapnia in chronic metabolic alkalosis. Am J Physiol 238:F283–F289, 1980.
10. Seldin DW, Rector FC Jr: The generation and maintenance of metabolic alkalosis. Kidney Int 1:306–321, 1972.
11. Javaheri S, Kazemi H: Metabolic alkalosis and hypoventilation in humans. Am Rev Respir Dis 136:1101–1116, 1987.
12. Brackett NC Jr, Cohen JJ, Schwartz WB: Carbon dioxide titration curve of normal man: Effect of increasing degrees of acute hypercapnia on acid-base equilibrium. N Engl J Med 272:6, 1965.
13. Brackett NC Jr, Wingo CF, Muren O, et al: Acid-base response to chronic hypercapnia in man. N Engl J Med 280:124, 1969.
14. van Ypersele de Strihou C, Brasseur CL, De Connick J: The "carbon dioxide response curve" for chronic hypercapnia in man. N Engl J Med 275:117, 1966.
15. Arbus GS, Hebert LA, Levesque PR, et al: Characterization and clinical application of the "significance band" for acute respiratory alkalosis. N Engl J Med 280:117, 1969.
16. Weil JV: Ventilatory control at high altitude. In Fishman AP (ed): Handbook of Physiology. Section 3: The Respiratory System. Bethesda, Md, American Physiological Society, 1986, pp 703–727.
17. Widmer B, Gerhardt RE, Harrington JT, et al: Serum electrolyte and acid-base composition: The influence of graded degrees of chronic renal failure. Arch Intern Med 139:1099–1102, 1979.
18. Wang F, Butler T, Rabbani GH, et al: The acidosis of cholera: Contributions of hyperproteinemia, lactic acidemia, and hyperphosphatemia to an increased serum anion gap. N Engl J Med 315:1591–1595, 1986.
19. Emmett M, Seldin DW: Evaluation of acid-base disorders from plasma composition. In Seldin DW, Giebisch G (eds): The Regulation of Acid-Base Balance. New York, Raven Press, 1989, pp 213–263.
20. Carlisle EJ, Donnelly SM, Vasuvattakul S, et al: Glue-sniffing and distal renal tubular acidosis: Sticking to the facts. J Am Soc Nephrol 1:1019–1027, 1991.
21. Adrogue HJ, Wilson H, Boyd AE III, et al: Plasma acid-base patterns in diabetic ketoacidosis. N Engl J Med 307:1603–1610, 1982.
22. Bear R, Goldstein M, Phillipson E, et al: Effect of metabolic alkalosis on respiratory function in patients with chronic obstructive lung disease. Can Med Assoc J 117:900–903, 1977.
23. Gabow PA, Anderson RJ, Potts DE, et al: Acid-base disturbances in the salicylate-intoxicated adult. Arch Intern Med 138:1481–1484, 1978.
24. Mulhausen R, Eichenholz A, Blumentals A: Acid-base disturbances in patients with cirrhosis of the liver. Medicine 46:185–189, 1967.
25. Pares A, Rimola A, Bruguera M, et al: Renal tubular acidosis in primary biliary cirrhosis. Gastroenterology 80:681–686, 1981.
26. Heinig RE, Clarke EF, Waterhouse C: Lactic acidosis and liver disease. Arch Intern Med 139:1229–1232, 1979.
27. Steer ML, Cloeren SE, Bushnell LS, et al: Metabolic alkalosis and respiratory failure in critically ill patients. Surgery 72:408–413, 1972.
28. Wilson RF, Gibson D, Percinel AK, et al: Severe alkalosis in critically ill surgical patients. Arch Surg 105:197–203, 1972.
29. Anderson LE, Heinrich WL: Alkalemia-associated morbidity and mortality in medical and surgical patients. South Med J 80: 729–733, 1987.
30. Machida H: Influence of progesterone on arterial blood and CSH acid-base balance in women. J Appl Physiol 51:1433–1436, 1981.

CHAPTER 4

# Metabolic Acidosis

Kevin W. Finkel, MD ▪ Thomas D. DuBose, Jr., MD

Metabolic acidosis may be asymptomatic or associated with numerous life-threatening illnesses. If left untreated, it leads to several adverse hemodynamic and metabolic consequences. Therefore, physicians often intervene aggressively by increasing an intubated patient's minute ventilation and administering intravenous alkali. However, correction of abnormal pH values without consideration of the underlying pathophysiologic process resulting in the acidosis is often ineffective and can be associated with significant deleterious effects. Therefore, the treatment of metabolic acidosis should be directed at the underlying disease process while minimizing excessive ventilation and alkali administration.

**Cardiovascular Effects.** Systemic acidosis, with the subsequent fall in intracellular pH, can result in decreased cardiac contractility, central venous vasoconstriction, and decreased arterial blood pressure.[1,2] Conversely, correction of acidosis has been shown to reverse these adverse hemodynamic effects.[3] The degree to which acidosis suppresses cardiac contractility is controversial. It has been argued that the methods utilized to produce metabolic acidosis in older animal studies, such as the administration of phenformin or surgical hepatectomy, may have effects on cardiac performance that are independent of acidosis. In fact, more recent animal studies have demonstrated that myocardial function is well preserved until extracellular pH falls below 7.0.[4] One mechanism by which intracellular acidosis appears to impair contractility is interference with calcium binding to troponin.[2] Metabolic acidosis also results in an increase in sympathetic tone.[5] This increased activity may partially compensate for acidosis-induced cardiac depression by augmenting contractility, venous blood return, and heart rate. At the same time, however, acidosis decreases responsiveness to catecholamines.[6] Therefore, the net effect of acidosis on cardiovascular stability is determined by the interaction of these two competing mechanisms. Finally, metabolic acidosis is associated with an increase in the incidence of cardiac dysrhythmias.[7]

**Respiratory Effects.** Metabolic acidosis induces a compensatory increase in minute ventilation in an attempt to lower the $Pa_{CO_2}$. This increased work of breathing can be deleterious for patients who have underlying lung disease or for patients who are being weaned from mechanical ventilation by producing respiratory muscle fatigue and failure. Similar to hypoxemia, metabolic acidosis causes pulmonary vasoconstriction, which leads to right ventricular failure and low cardiac output.

**Skeletal Effects.** Excess circulating protons are titrated by the skeleton, the largest buffering system in the body. This leads to an osteopenic form of metabolic bone disease, hypercalciuria, and possible nephrolithiasis and nephrocalcinosis. During acute metabolic acidosis, serum calcium levels rise rapidly, representing mineral dissolution.[8] This proton-mediated release of bone calcium appears to be the result of alterations in the physiochemical factors that govern the deposition and dissolution of bone mineral.[9] On the other hand, during chronic metabolic acidosis, the release of bone calcium is induced by an increase in cell-mediated bone reabsorption, in addition to the alteration in the physiochemical properties of bone.[10]

**Nutritional Effects.** Metabolic acidosis also contributes to negative nitrogen balance, particularly in critically ill patients who already are hypercatabolic. Metabolic acidosis increases protein degradation.[11] This effect is partially explained by an increase in renal ammoniagenesis, which requires extrarenal glutamine generation.[12] In addition, metabolic acidosis also accelerates amino acid oxidation and muscle branched-chain ketoacid dehydrogenase activity.[13] These changes lead to increased net protein degradation and the generation of a catabolic state during metabolic acidosis. Alkali treatment reverses the process.

## DEFINITION AND FUNDAMENTAL CONCEPTS

Metabolic acidosis occurs as a result of a marked increase in endogenous production of acid (e.g., lactic and ketoacids), loss of bicarbonate stores (e.g., diarrhea or renal tubular acidosis), or progressive accumulation of endogenous acids in the setting of renal insufficiency. Metabolic acidosis is recognized by the presence of acidemia (pH $<7.35$), a low serum bicarbonate concentration, and a compensatory decrease in the $Pa_{CO_2}$. It can also be detected by an elevation of the anion gap, even when the pH and serum bicarbonate values are normal. The anion gap serves a useful role in the initial evaluation of metabolic acidosis. A metabolic acidosis with a *normal anion gap* (hyperchloremic) suggests that bicarbonate has been effectively replaced by chloride. This occurs when bicarbonate is lost from the kidneys or the gastrointestinal tract, there is defective urinary acidification by the renal tubules, or renal failure impairs the excretion of metabolically produced acid. In contrast, metabolic acidosis with a *high anion gap* indicates addition of an acid other than hydrochloric acid or its equivalent to the extracellular fluid (ECF). If the accompanying nonchloride anion cannot be excreted in relation to the rate of production and is retained following bicarbonate titration, the anion replaces titrated bicarbonate without disturbing the chloride concentration. Thus, the acidosis is normochloremic and the anion gap increases.

## ANION GAP

All evaluations of acid-base disorders should include a determination of the anion gap. The anion gap (AG) is calculated as follows: $AG = Na^+ - (Cl^- + HCO_3^-) = 10$ mEq/L. The anion gap represents unmeasured anions that are normally present in serum, including anionic proteins (mainly albumin), phosphate, sulfate, and organic anions. When excess anions are produced in clinical settings such as diabetic ketoacidosis or lactic acidosis, the anion gap increases above the normal value. Changes in electrolyte balance can also affect the anion gap without necessarily altering a patient's acid-base status. This nuance is best understood by rearranging the formula for calculating the anion gap as follows:

$$\text{Unmeasured cations (UC)} + Na^+ = \text{unmeasured anions (UA)} + (Cl^- + HCO_3^-).$$

$$\text{Therefore, } AG = Na^+ - (Cl^- + HCO_3^-) = UA - UC, \text{ or } AG = UA - UC.$$

Based on this formula, an increase in the anion gap would be expected by a decrease in unmeasured cations or an increase in unmeasured anions. For example, the anion gap may increase secondary to an increase in anionic albumin as a consequence of either an increased albumin concentration or alkalemia. The modest rise of the anion gap that is seen during alkalosis is partially explained by an increased net negative charge of albumin. A fall in the anion gap is generated by either an increase in unmeasured cations or a decrease in unmeasured anions. A decrease in the anion gap can result from: (1) an increase in unmeasured cations (i.e., calcium, magnesium, and potassium), or (2) the addition to the blood of abnormal cations, such as lithium (lithium intoxication) or cationic immunoglobulins (IgG) in plasma cell dyscrasias. This effect explains why a narrowed anion gap is a clue to the diagnosis of multiple myeloma. The anion gap also decreases if the quantity of the major plasma anionic substituent albumin is low, such as in nephrotic syndrome or cirrhosis of the liver. As a general rule, the anion gap falls by 2.5 mEq/L for every 1 g/dL decrease in albumin concentration.[14] Finally, laboratory errors can create a false low anion gap. Hyperviscosity and hyperlipidemia lead to an underestimation of the true sodium concentration, and bromide intoxication causes an overestimation of the true chloride concentration.

In the face of a normal serum albumin, elevation of the anion gap is usually due to the addition to the blood of non–chloride-containing acids. The anions accompanying such acids include inorganic (e.g., phosphate, sulfate), organic (e.g., ketoacids, lactate, uremic organic anions), exogenous (e.g., salicylate or ingested toxins with organic acid production), or unidentified anions. The chloride concentration is not altered when the new acid anion is added to the blood, thus the "gap" increases. If the anion is not excreted by the kidney, the magnitude of the decrement in bicarbonate concentration will equal the increase in the unmeasured anion concentration and the anion gap. If the retained anion can be metabolized back to bicarbonate (e.g., ketones or lactate, after successful treatment), normal acid-base balance will be restored as the anion gap returns toward the normal value of 10 mEq/L.

Another calculation that is useful in properly evaluating metabolic acidosis is the delta $HCO_3^-$ to delta AG ratio: ($\Delta HCO_3^-/\Delta AG$). In a pure anion gap metabolic acidosis, the fall in bicarbonate concentration should roughly equal the increase in the anion gap ($\Delta HCO_3^-/\Delta AG = 1$). If the fall in bicarbonate concentration is much greater than the rise in the anion gap ($\Delta HCO_3^-/\Delta AG = 2$), then there exists both an anion gap and non-anion gap metabolic acidosis. Conversely, if the $\Delta HCO_3^-/\Delta AG = 0.5$, both an anion gap metabolic acidosis and a metabolic alkalosis are present. In this case, the fall in bicarbonate does not match the addition of anions as determined by the change in the AG.

Calculation of the anion gap is the first step in the diagnostic approach to metabolic acidosis (Fig. 4–1).

## RESPIRATORY COMPENSATION FOR METABOLIC ACIDOSIS

When a primary decrease occurs in the plasma bicarbonate concentration, a compensatory increase in minute ventilation to lower $Pa_{CO_2}$ is expected from stimulation of medullary chemoreceptors in the brain by acidemia. As a result, the pH returns toward, but not to, normal. The hypocapnic response to metabolic acidosis is predictable in simple acid-base disorders and blunts the magnitude of the decline in pH that would otherwise occur. The degree of respiratory compensation expected in a simple form of metabolic acidosis can be predicted from the relationship:

$$Pa_{CO_2} = (1.5 \times HCO_3^-) + 8$$

Thus, in a patient with metabolic acidosis and a plasma bicarbonate concentration of 12 mEq/L, a $Pa_{CO_2}$ between 24 and 28 mm Hg would be anticipated. Values for $Pa_{CO_2}$ below 24 or greater than 28 mm Hg illustrate a mixed disturbance (i.e., metabolic acidosis and respiratory alkalosis, or metabolic acidosis and respiratory acidosis, respectively). Whereas this relationship is accurate within ±2 mm Hg, the $Pa_{CO_2}$ can also be estimated more conveniently by adding 15 to the patient's serum $HCO_3^-$ concentration. Another

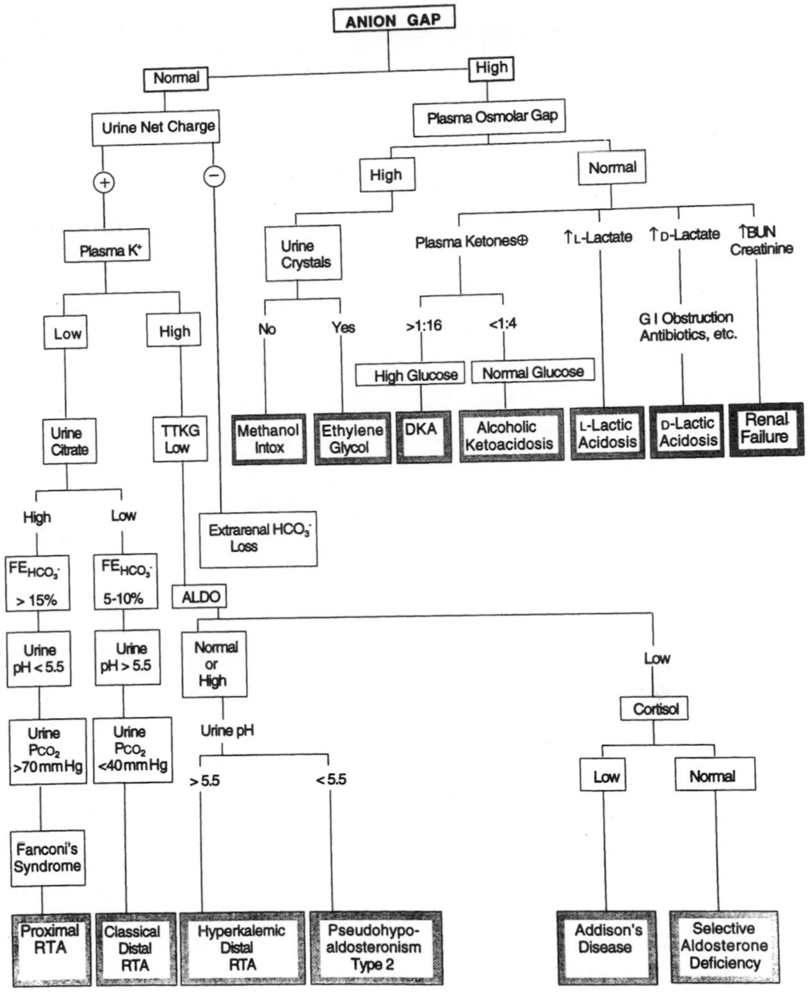

**FIGURE 4–1** ■ Flow diagram of the approach to metabolic acidosis. The anion gap is the entry point and divides the types of metabolic acidoses into the high anion gap and normal anion gap categories. Final diagnoses are displayed in *hatched boxes*. ALDO, aldosterone; BUN, blood urea nitrogen; DKA, diabetic ketoacidosis; GI, gastrointestinal; RTA, renal tubular acidosis; TTKG, transtubular potassium gradient.

commonly used formula to calculate the expected decline in the $PaCO_2$ level is:

$$\Delta PaCO_2 = 1.25 \times \Delta HCO_3^-$$

Deviations from anticipated values imply a coexisting disturbance such as respiratory acidosis or alkalosis.

## RENAL RESPONSE TO ACIDOSIS

The kidneys regulate plasma bicarbonate through three processes: (1) reabsorption of filtered $HCO_3^-$, (2) excretion of titratable acidity, and (3) synthesis and excretion of $NH_4^+$. Net acid excretion is defined as the sum of titratable acidity and ammonium excretion, less any bicarbonate that appears in the urine. Approximately 80% to 90% of the filtered bicarbonate is reabsorbed in the proximal tubule. Under normal conditions, the distal nephron reabsorbs the remainder (~5% to 10%). In addition to the amount of $H^+$ secreted to absorb the filtered bicarbonate, the collecting duct must secrete an additional quantity of protons equal to that generated from metabolism and digestion of dietary protein. The quantity of acids produced on a daily basis is approximately 1 mEq/kg/day. Thus, an equal amount of acid must be secreted to prevent the development of chronic positive hydrogen ion balance and metabolic acidosis. Ammonium excretion is the major component of net acid excretion and is regulated by both ammoniagenesis and by ammonium transport.

## ESTIMATING URINARY $NH_4^+$ EXCRETION: THE URINE NET CHARGE AND OSMOLAL GAP

When renal function is normal, the kidney responds to chronic metabolic acidosis by increasing ammonium production and excretion. Ammonium production and excretion by the kidney are impaired in chronic renal failure, hyperkalemia, and renal tubular acidosis (RTA). Because diarrhea or RTA can cause a hyperchloremic metabolic acidosis, it is important to delineate whether the kidney is responding to systemic acidosis appropriately by increasing ammonium excretion. Ammonium excretion can be estimated with a spot urine sample by determining the urine net charge (UNC) or urinary osmolol gap. The UNC is

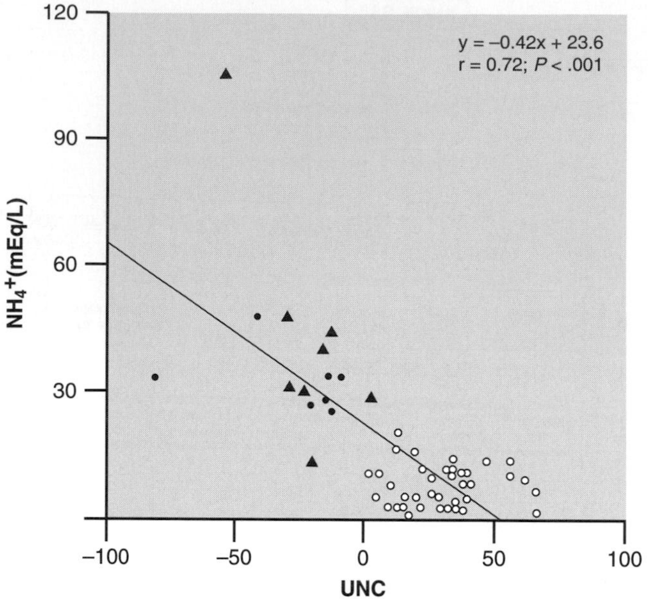

**FIGURE 4–2** ■ Urinary ammonium ($NH_4^+$) in relation to the urinary net charge (UNC). The 38 patients with altered distal urinary acidification are represented by *open circles*; the 7 normal subjects receiving ammonium chloride, by *closed circles*; and the 8 patients with hyperchloremic metabolic acidosis associated with diarrhea, by *triangles*. (Modified from Batlle DC, Hizon M, Cohen E, et al: The use of the urinary anion gap in the diagnosis of hyperchloremic metabolic acidosis. N Engl J Med 318:594, 1988.)

defined as the difference in the concentration of urinary chloride ($Cl^-$) and the sum of the urinary cations $Na^+$ and $K^+$: UNC = $[Na^+ + K^+]_u - [Cl^-]_u$. In chronic metabolic acidosis of nonrenal origin (e.g., diarrhea), the expected response by the kidney is to increase ammonium production and excretion. The increase in $NH_4^+$ concentration in the urine in this condition will manifest as an increase in the negative UNC ($Cl^-$ concentration will exceed the sum of $Na^+$ and $K^+$, and the UNC will be a negative value). In contrast, in hyperchloremic metabolic acidosis from RTA, the UNC will be zero or positive, denoting little or no increase in $NH_4^+$ excretion.[15] This inappropriate renal response to the metabolic acidosis is due to impaired ammoniagenesis or a tubular defect in $H^+$ secretion (Fig. 4–2). The utility of the UNC in estimating urinary ammonium has been verified, but caution is urged if $NH_4^+$ is excreted with an anion other than $Cl^-$. For example, the presence in the urine of ketones, drug anions, and toxins such as toluene metabolites all invalidate this method. Furthermore, the acidification of the urine is dependent on adequate distal delivery of sodium, thus the utility of this test is also questionable when urinary sodium concentration is less than 20 mEq/L.

The urinary ammonium ($U_{NH_4}{}^+$) can also be estimated from the measured urine osmolality (UOsm), urine $[Na^+ + K^+]$, and urine urea and glucose (all expressed in mmol/L):

$$U_{NH_4}{}^+ = 0.5(\text{UOsm} - [2(Na^+ + K^+) + \text{urea} + \text{glucose}]$$

# CLINICAL EXAMPLES OF METABOLIC ACIDOSIS

## Hyperchloremic Metabolic Acidosis (Normal Anion Gap Acidosis)

### PATHOGENESIS AND DIFFERENTIAL DIAGNOSIS

The diverse clinical disorders that may result in a hyperchloremic metabolic acidosis are outlined in Table 4–1. Hyperchloremic metabolic acidosis occurs most often as a result of loss of bicarbonate from the gastrointestinal tract or as a result of a renal acidification defect. In these disorders, a normal anion gap results from reciprocal changes in chloride and bicarbonate concentrations. Therefore, in a simple hyperchloremic acidosis, the rise in chloride level is matched by a decline in the bicarbonate concentration. A mixed disorder is suggested by an absence of this relationship. Diarrhea causes metabolic acidosis because of the loss of large quantities of bicarbonate and bicarbonate decomposed by reaction with organic acids. Because diarrheal stools contain a higher concentration of bicarbonate and decomposed bicarbonate than plasma, volume depletion and metabolic acidosis develop. Hypokalemia is often encountered because large quantities of potassium are lost from stool and because volume depletion causes synthesis of renin and aldosterone, enhancing renal potassium excretion. Instead of an acid urine pH, which is often anticipated with diarrhea, a pH higher than 6.0 is occasionally observed. The alkaline urinary pH occurs because metabolic acidosis and hypokalemia both increase renal

**TABLE 4–1.** Causes Of Hyperchloremic Metabolic Acidosis*

I. Gastrointestinal bicarbonate loss
  A. Diarrhea
  B. External pancreatic or small bowel drainage
  C. Ureterosigmoidostomy, jejunal loop
  D. Drugs
    1. Calcium chloride (acidifying agent)
    2. Magnesium sulfate (diarrhea)
    3. Cholestyramine (bile acid diarrhea)
II. Renal tubular acidification defects
  A. Hypokalemia
    1. Proximal renal tubular acidosis (RTA) (type 2 RTA)
    2. Classical distal RTA (type 1 RTA)
  B. Hyperkalemia
    1. Generalized distal nephron dysfunction (type 4 RTA)
    2. Mineralocorticoid deficiency
    3. Mineralocorticoid resistance
    4. Decreased delivery of $Na^+$ to the distal nephron
      a. Liver disease
  C. Normokalemia or hyperkalemia
    1. Early renal failure
III. Other
  A. Acid loads (ammonium chloride, hyperalimentation with insufficient alkali infusion)
  B. Loss of potential bicarbonate: ketosis with ketone excretion
  C. Expansion acidosis (rapid saline administration)
  D. Posthypocapnic state
  E. Glue sniffing

*Must rule out hypoalbuminemia, pseudohyponatremia, pseudohyperchloremia, and paraproteinemia.

**TABLE 4–2.** Distinguishing Features of Hyperchloremic Acidoses

| | Proximal RTA (Type 2 RTA) | Classical Distal RTA (Type 1 RTA) | Generalized Distal Defect (Type 4 RTA) | Extrarenal $HCO_3^-$ Loss |
|---|---|---|---|---|
| Anion gap | Normal | Normal | Normal | Normal |
| Plasma $[K^+]$ | Low (with $R_x$) | Low | High | Low |
| Urine anion gap or urine osmolal gap | Low | Low | Very low | High |
| Urine pH | Low | High | Low or high | Low or high |
| Urine $P_{CO_2}$ | >70 | <40 | <40 | >70 |
| $FE_{HCO_3^-}$ | >15% (with $R_x$) | 5–10% | 10–15% | <5% |
| Urine citrate | High | Low | Low | Normal |
| TTKG | High | High | Low (not high) | Low |

RTA, renal tubular acidosis; TTKG, transtubular potassium gradient.

ammonium synthesis and excretion, thus providing more urinary buffer, which allows urine pH to increase above 6.0.

Metabolic acidosis due to gastrointestinal losses with a high urine pH must be differentiated from RTA. Urinary $NH_4^+$ excretion is typically low in RTA, whereas $NH_4^+$ excretion is high in patients with diarrhea. The adequacy of urinary ammonium excretion in metabolic acidosis can be estimated by calculating the UNC or osmolal gap as previously discussed. Because $NH_4^+$ is assumed to be present if the sum of the major cations ($Na^+ + K^+$) is less than the $Cl^-$ concentration in urine, a negative UNC is taken as evidence of increased ammonium in the urine in the face of diarrhea. Conversely, urine that contains little or no $NH_4^+$ will have more $Na^+ + K^+$ than $Cl^-$ and the UNC is positive. This finding suggests a renal mechanism for the hyperchloremic acidosis, such as RTA. Distinguishing features of hyperchloremic acidoses are outlined in Table 4–2.

**Urinary Intestinal Diversions.** Numerous metabolic disorders, including hyperchloremic metabolic acidosis, may develop in patients who have surgically created urinary diversions (ureterosigmoidostomy or ileal loop conduit), usually after treatment of urogenital malignancies. It has been shown that these gastrointestinal segments secrete sodium and bicarbonate and reabsorb ammonia, hydrogen ions, and chloride when exposed to urine.[16] Perfusion studies have demonstrated that sodium is secreted in exchange for hydrogen ion and bicarbonate is secreted in exchange for chloride. It has also been documented that ammonium transport plays a major role in generating the metabolic acidosis of urinary diversions.[17] Ammonium is absorbed primarily in its ionized form, and the rate of absorption is directly proportional to the luminal ammonium concentration. Hyperchloremic metabolic acidosis develops in 30% to 80% of patients with a ureterosigmoidostomy, and most require long-term treatment with alkali therapy.[18] The acidosis can be acutely exacerbated by pyelonephritis and worsening renal function. The development of a hyperchloremic acidosis is encountered less frequently in patients with an ileal loop, because of decreased contact time between the urine and this type of urinary diversion. However, if the loop is exceptionally long, or becomes obstructed, then acidosis can occur.

Dilutional acidosis, acidosis due to exogenous acid loads, and the post-hypocapnic state are less recognized causes of hyperchloremic acidosis; these causes can usually be excluded with history. When large volumes of isotonic saline are infused rapidly, particularly into patients with renal insufficiency, the plasma bicarbonate declines reciprocally in relation to chloride. By the addition of acid or acid equivalents to blood, infusion of arginine or lysine HCl during parenteral hyperalimentation can lead to hyperchloremic metabolic acidosis.

## Hyperchloremic Acidosis of Chronic Renal Failure

**Pathophysiology.** Loss of functioning renal parenchyma by progressive renal disease is commonly associated with metabolic acidosis. Typically, the acidosis is hyperchloremic when the glomerular filtration rate is between 20 and 50 mL/min but may convert to the typical high anion gap acidosis of uremia with more advanced renal failure. Although it is assumed that this pattern is observed more commonly in patients with renal failure from tubulointerstitial diseases, hyperchloremic metabolic acidosis is just as frequent in advanced glomerular diseases. In fact, when patients are first initiated on hemodialysis, the prevalence of hyperchloremic acidosis and anion gap acidosis is roughly equivalent.[19] The major defect in acidification in renal failure is reduced ammoniagenesis proportional to decreased renal mass. Also, medullary ammonium accumulation and trapping in the collecting duct are impaired. Typically, patients have normal serum potassium levels because of adaptive increases in potassium secretion by the colon and distal nephron. If hyperkalemia does develop, a further reduction occurs in ammonium production and excretion because hyperkalemia directly suppresses ammonium synthesis. In addition, potassium ion competes with ammonium for transport in the proximal tubule, loop of Henle, and the collecting duct—all of which reduce ammonium excretion, and thus net acid excretion.

## Renal Tubular Acidosis

### PROXIMAL RENAL TUBULAR ACIDOSIS

**Diagnostic Points.** Although proximal RTA can result from an isolated defect in bicarbonate reclama-

**TABLE 4–3.** Disorders Associated with Proximal RTA

| Disorders |
|---|
| **Isolated Defect** |
| Primary |
| Decreased carbonic anhydrase activity |
| Acetazolamide |
| **Generalized Defect (Fanconi Syndrome)** |
| Primary |
| Genetic or sporadic |
| Secondary |
| Cystinosis |
| Wilson disease |
| Lowe syndrome |
| Tyrosinemia |
| Dysproteinemias |
| Multiple myeloma |
| Light chain disease |
| Monoclonal gammopathy |
| Drugs or toxins |
| Ifosfamide |
| Tubulointerstitial disease |
| Sjögren syndrome |
| Medullary cystic disease |

tion, in most cases it occurs in association with generalized proximal tubular dysfunction manifested by glycosuria, generalized aminoaciduria, hypercitraturia, and phosphaturia. This generalized failure of proximal tubular function is referred to as *Fanconi syndrome.* The clinical disorders associated with proximal RTA are outlined in Table 4–3. Patients with proximal RTA generally present in the steady state with a chronic hyperchloremic metabolic acidosis, an acid urine pH, hypokalemia, and a small amount of bicarbonate excretion. An initial bicarbonaturia causes renal potassium wasting and mild volume depletion. The ensuing rise in renin and aldosterone levels further aggravates the renal potassium losses. Upon infusion of $NaHCO_3$, bicarbonaturia predictably ensues because of an abnormally low renal bicarbonate absorption threshold. Therefore, the urine becomes alkaline. The diagnosis is confirmed by demonstrating an inappropriately high rate of bicarbonate excretion ($FE_{HCO_3^-} > 10\%$ to 15%) in the face of a near-normal serum bicarbonate concentration (>21 mEq/L). Nephrolithiasis and nephrocalcinosis are not usually seen in patients with proximal RTA, because the acidic tubular pH keeps calcium and phosphate in solution. However, most patients do develop skeletal abnormalities, which are manifested as rickets in children and osteopenia in adults.

**Treatment.** The magnitude of the bicarbonaturia (>10% of the filtered load) requires that large amounts of bicarbonate be administered to correct the bicarbonate concentration. For example, 10 to 30 mEq/kg/day of bicarbonate or its metabolic equivalent (citrate) is required to maintain the plasma bicarbonate concentration at normal levels. Supplementation with potassium is also often necessary because of the kaliuresis induced by high distal bicarbonate delivery when the plasma bicarbonate concentration is normalized. Therefore, large alkali loads are not advised; rather, smaller amounts of alkali therapy can be provided as either sodium citrate solutions or $NaHCO_3$ tablets. If there is a compelling reason to correct the plasma bicarbonate concentration back to normal (growing children), the addition of hydrochlorothiazide may diminish requirements for bicarbonate supplementation by causing volume contraction and enhanced proximal bicarbonate reabsorption. It is usually necessary in children to provide vitamin D and phosphate supplementation orally.

## CLASSICAL DISTAL RENAL TUBULAR ACIDOSIS

**Pathophysiology and Diagnostic Points.** The typical findings in classical distal RTA include hypokalemia, hyperchloremic acidosis, low urinary ammonium excretion (positive UNC or low osmolal gap), and an inability to acidify the urine appropriately during spontaneous or chemically induced metabolic acidosis. Under several different circumstances, including acute acid infusion, patients with classical hypokalemic RTA are unable to lower their urine pH below 5.5 and uniformly display a lower urinary $Pa_{CO_2}$ than do normal subjects. These abnormalities suggest that one or both of the active proton pumps present in the collecting duct—the $H^+$-ATPase or the $H^+/K^+$-ATPase—are defective. Patients with classical hypokalemic RTA also excrete lower amounts of urinary ammonium for the degree of systemic acidosis. This occurs because of a failure to trap ammonium in the medullary collecting duct as a result of higher than normal tubular pH and a loss of a functional $H^+$ pump. The pathophysiologic basis of most forms of classical distal RTA is an abnormality of one of the acid-base transporters in the cortical or medullary collecting duct. Those pumps shown to be involved in the development of distal RTA to date include the apical electrogenic $H^+$-ATPase (in both an autosomal recessive genetic defect and in acquired forms of the disease) and the basolateral $HCO_3^-/Cl^-$ exchanger (described in families with an autosomal dominant variety). The autosomal recessive form is associated with hereditary nerve deafness and has been shown to be a result of an abnormality in the gene that encodes one of the subunits of the apical $H^+$-ATPase. It is associated with a marked reduction in the urinary $P_{CO_2}$ during bicarbonate diuresis. The autosomal dominant disorder results from a missense mutation of the *AE1* gene causing insertion of the $HCO_3^-/Cl^-$ exchanger into the apical rather than the basolateral membrane of the collecting duct. If this assessment is correct, patients with this inherited form of distal RTA would manifest an abnormally high urinary $P_{CO_2}$. Recent studies in these patients have suggested that this is indeed the case. In contrast, the only example of a "gradient" or "back-leak" lesion is that caused by amphotericin B nephrotoxicity. In this disorder, the urinary $P_{CO_2}$ is normal, denoting preservation of pump integrity. A defect in the apical $H^+/K^+$-ATPase has not yet been described.

Hypokalemia and hypercalciuria often accompany this disorder, but proximal tubule reabsorptive function is preserved. The dissolution of bone is the result of chronic positive acid balance, which causes calcium, magnesium, and phosphate wasting. Because chronic metabolic acidosis also decreases renal production of citrate, the resultant hypocitraturia in combination with hypercalciuria and high intratubular pH creates an environment that is favorable for urinary stone formation and nephrocalcinosis. Nephrocalcinosis is a reliable marker of classical distal RTA, because this disorder does not occur in proximal RTA or the generalized dysfunction of the nephron associated with hyperkalemia. Nephrocalcinosis further aggravates the reduction in net acid excretion by impairing the transfer of ammonia from the loop of Henle to the collecting duct. The disorders associated with classical distal RTA are displayed in Table 4–4.

**Treatment.** In either inherited or acquired forms of distal RTA, correction of chronic metabolic acidosis can usually be achieved by administration of alkali in an amount sufficient to neutralize the production of metabolic acids derived from the diet. In adult patients with distal RTA, this is usually equal to no more than 1 to 3 mEq/kg/day. Larger amounts of bicarbonate must be administered to correct the acidosis and maintain normal growth in children. In patients with distal RTA, potassium deficits may be severe, and the provision of bicarbonate may drive potassium into cells, worsening the hypokalemia. Thus, substantial deficits should be corrected before initiating alkali therapy. Once hypokalemia is resolved, correction of acidosis with alkali therapy will restore ECF volume and decrease the stimulus for potassium excretion. A major benefit from correction of the acidosis is prevention of progressive renal failure, particularly in the presence of nephrocalcinosis. Also, the frequency of nephrolithiasis is usually greatly reduced by alkali therapy.

**TABLE 4–4.** Causes of Distal Renal Tubular Acidosis

|  |
|---|
| **Classical Distal Renal Tubular Acidosis (Type 1 RTA)** |
| I. Primary inherited forms (usually with nephrocalcinosis, hypercalciuria, and urolithiasis) |
| II. Secondary acquired forms |
| A. Associated with nephrocalcinosis |
| 1. Primary hyperparathyroidism |
| 2. Medullary sponge kidney |
| B. Associated with hyperglobulinemia |
| 1. Hyperglobulinemic purpura |
| 2. Sjögren syndrome |
| 3. Cryoglobulinemia |
| 4. Polyarteritis nodosa |
| C. Drugs and toxins |
| 1. Amphotericin B |
| 2. Analgesic abuse |
| 3. Ifosfamide |
| D. Tubulointerstitial diseases |
| 1. Chronic pyelonephritis |
| 2. Renal transplant rejection |
| E. In association with genetically transmitted diseases |
| 1. Sickle cell anemia |
| 2. Medullary cystic disease |
| **Generalized Distal Tubule Dysfunction (Type 4 RTA)** |
| I. Primary mineralocorticoid deficiency |
| A. Addison disease |
| B. Isolated mineralocorticoid deficiency |
| 1. Chronic idiopathic hypoaldosteronism |
| 2. Heparin administration in the critically ill patient |
| II. Hyporeninemic hypoaldosteronism |
| A. Diabetic nephropathy |
| B. AIDS nephropathy |
| C. Tubulointerstitial disease |
| D. Obstructive uropathy |
| E. Systemic lupus erythematosus |
| III. Angiotensin II–impaired production or reduced sensitivity |
| A. Angiotensin-converting enzyme inhibitors |
| B. Angiotensin II receptor antagonists |
| IV. Aldosterone resistance |
| A. Pseudohypoaldosteronism types I and II |
| B. Sickle cell nephropathy |
| C. Salt-wasting nephropathy |
| D. Drugs |
| 1. Amiloride |
| 2. Trimethoprim |
| 3. Triamterene |
| 4. Pentamidine |
| 5. Cyclosporin A |
| 6. Spironolactone |

## GENERALIZED DISTAL NEPHRON DYSFUNCTION (TYPE 4 RENAL TUBULAR ACIDOSIS)

**Pathophysiology and Diagnostic Points.** Although hyperchloremic, hyperkalemic metabolic acidosis is common in advanced renal failure, in patients with type 4 RTA the hyperkalemia is disproportionate to the fall in glomerular filtration rate. In such patients, a unique dysfunction of potassium and acid secretion by the collecting tubule coexists. Urinary ammonium excretion is decreased, and renal function is usually compromised. The causes of type 4 RTA are listed in Table 4–4.

Hyperkalemia, by direct effects in the kidney and by stimulation of aldosterone release, usually induces a brisk kaluresis. In type 4 RTA, an inappropriate renal response to hyperkalemia can be demonstrated by measuring the osmolality and potassium of both urine and serum and calculating the transtubular $K^+$ gradient (TTKG):

$$\text{TTKG} = (U_{K}^{+}/P_{K}^{+}) \div (\text{UOsm}/\text{POsm})$$

In patients with impaired renal excretion of potassium in the face of hyperkalemia, the TTKG is inappropriately low (<6). Conversely, when hyperkalemia arises from nonrenal sources (e.g., rhabdomyolysis or tumor lysis syndrome), the TTKG will be high (>6 to 10), signifying intact tubular function. Impaired ammonium production and excretion, in part due to hyperkalemia, lead to decreased net acid excretion and systemic acidosis.

Type 4 RTA can be attributed in many cases to *hyporeninemic hypoaldosteronism.* This disorder is a frequent cause of hyperkalemic, hyperchloremic metabolic acidosis and is typically seen in older adults with diabetes mellitus or tubulointerstitial disease and renal insufficiency. Patients usually have mild-to-moderate renal insufficiency, metabolic acidosis, modest hyperkalemia (5.5 to 6 mEq/L), and concurrent hypertension and congestive heart failure. Hyporeninemic hypoaldosteronism is also seen with some regularity in patients with sickle cell disease, HIV-associated nephropathy, systemic lupus erythematosus, and transplant rejection.

Medications such as trimethoprim, pentamidine, and potassium-sparing diuretics are important and common causes of hyperkalemia. Although these agents do not cause hyperchloremic metabolic acidosis directly, they are often associated with this acid-base disorder in patients with moderate-to-severe renal insufficiency. Metabolic acidosis is the result of the suppression by hyperkalemia of renal ammonium production and, thus, a decrease in net acid excretion. The mechanism common to these agents is impairment of sodium reabsorption in the collecting duct. Decreased sodium transport in this nephron segment dissipates the electronegative potential, which normally favors potassium secretion. This "voltage defect" may cause hyperkalemia and decreased ammonium excretion.

Angiotensin-converting enzyme inhibitors (ACEIs) and *angiotensin II receptor blockers* (ARBs), by interfering with angiotensin II–mediated aldosterone release, can lead to hyperkalemia and subsequent metabolic acidosis, particularly in patients with diabetes mellitus, renal insufficiency, or congestive heart failure. Because ACEIs and ARBs have been shown to decrease progression of numerous renal diseases and prolong survival in patients with congestive heart failure, treatment of hyperchloremic, hyperkalemic metabolic acidosis is usually undertaken to allow for continued use of these agents. The combination of spironolactone and ACEIs or ARBs can result in severe hyperkalemia in susceptible patients. Nevertheless, this combination will become more commonplace with the publication of a study showing improved survival rates in patients with congestive heart failure treated with both ACEIs and spironolactone.[20]

The presence of hyperchloremic metabolic acidosis with hyperkalemia can also be a sign of *urinary tract obstruction.* Three mechanisms have been found to explain this finding: (1) aldosterone deficiency secondary to decreased renal production of renin, (2) a defect in distal nephron sodium reabsorption that decreases the intraluminal negative potential difference, impairing potassium and hydrogen ion secretion (voltage defect), and (3) a combination of these two defects.[21] Obstructive uropathy should be considered in any patient with unexplained renal failure and hyperchloremic metabolic acidosis with hyperkalemia.

Several patients without glomerular or tubulointerstitial disease have been described who have hyperchloremic, hyperkalemic metabolic acidosis with undetectable renin and aldosterone levels (pseudohypoaldosteronism type 2 [PHA2]). The defect, which appears to be the result of enhanced distal chloride reabsorption, decreases ("shunts") the electronegative potential in the collecting duct that promotes potassium secretion. Such patients respond to therapy with thiazide diuretics, which has suggested to some that the molecular defect is a gain-in-function mutation of the $Na^+$-$Cl^-$ exchanger in the distal tubule. Nevertheless, genetic studies in patients with PHA2 have not demonstrated co-segregation of this clinical syndrome with the gene that encodes for the $Na^+$-$Cl^-$ exchanger. The acidosis is usually mild, and renal potassium excretion is resistant to mineralocorticoid administration. Renin and aldosterone levels normalize if volume expansion is corrected with salt restriction or diuretic therapy.

An autosomal recessive form of pseudohypoaldosteronism type 1 (PHA1) occurs because of an inherited loss-of-function mutation in the gene that encodes the epithelial $Na^+$ channel (ENaC) protein of the cortical collecting duct principal cell. This defect impairs sodium absorption and potassium secretion and causes salt wasting, hyperkalemia, and acidosis that is resistant to correction by aldosterone. These children respond to generous administration of NaCl supplements. This defect is more severe and persists throughout life. An autosomal dominant form of PHA1 that exists is less severe and often resolves by puberty. Studies have revealed that autosomal dominant PHA1 is caused by a mutation of the mineralocorticoid receptor (MLR) gene.

**Treatment.** Reduction in serum potassium levels enhances renal ammoniagenesis and ammonium excretion, thus improving or correcting the metabolic acidosis. Patients with combined deficits in glucocorticoids and mineralocorticoids should receive supplements of both adrenal hormones. Patients with hyporeninemic hypoaldosteronism respond to a cation exchange resin (sodium polystyrene sulfonate) and alkali therapy. Treatment with a loop diuretic to induce renal potassium and salt excretion as well as dietary potassium restriction are useful. The correction of the hyperkalemia is often associated with restoration of renal ammonium excretion and, thus, correction of the acidosis. Volume depletion should be avoided unless the patient is volume overexpanded or hypertensive. Supraphysiologic doses of mineralocorticoids may be necessary but should be administered cautiously and only in combination with a loop diuretic to avoid volume overload or aggravation of hypertension. PHA1 in children should be treated with avid sodium chloride intake. PHA2 in adults responds to thiazide diuretics and dietary salt restriction. In patients who continue to receive ACEIs or spironolactone, administration of a loop diuretic and a cation exchange resin may be required.

## High Anion Gap Acidoses (Anion Gap >10 mEq/L)

Identification of the underlying cause of a high anion gap metabolic acidosis is facilitated by consideration of the clinical setting and associated laboratory values. Five disorders cause a high anion gap acidosis, as outlined in Table 4–5: (1) L-lactic acidosis, (2) ketoacidosis, (3) toxin-induced acidoses, (4) uremic acidosis, and (5) D-lactic acidosis from gastrointestinal overproduction. Initial screening to differentiate the high anion gap acidoses should include: (1) a history or other evidence for drug and toxin ingestion, (2) historical evidence of diabetes (e.g., diabetic ketoacidosis), (3) evidence of alcoholism or increased levels of β-hydroxybutyrate (alcoholic ketoacidosis), (4) observation for clinical signs of uremia and determination of

**TABLE 4–5.** Causes of High Anion Gap Acidosis

| | |
|---|---|
| Ketoacidosis | Renal failure |
| Diabetic ketoacidosis | Acute |
| Alcoholic ketoacidosis | Chronic |
| Starvation ketoacidosis | Toxins |
| Lactic acidosis | Ethylene glycol |
| L-Lactic acidosis | Methyl alcohol |
| Type A | Salicylates |
| Type B | |
| D-Lactic acidosis | |

the blood urea nitrogen (BUN) and creatinine (uremic acidosis), (5) determination of the serum osmolal gap and inspection of the urine for oxalate crystals (ethylene glycol), (6) recognition of the numerous settings in which lactate levels may be increased (e.g., hypotension, cardiac failure, leukemia, drugs, and cancer), (7) arterial blood gas analysis to detect concurrent respiratory alkalosis (salicylate intoxication), and (8) determination of D-lactate levels in the presence of gastrointestinal ileus, obstruction or pouches, bacterial overgrowth, or antibiotic therapy.

## L-LACTIC ACIDOSIS

**Pathophysiology.** L-Lactic acidosis occurs in a diverse group of disorders and is a marker of decreased survival rates. Although lactate metabolism bears a close relationship to that of pyruvate, lactate is a metabolic dead-end pathway with pyruvate as its only outlet. Lactate is produced predominantly by the brain, gastrointestinal tract, muscle, skin, and red blood cells. Lactate synthesis is altered by changes in systemic pH that control the rate of glycolysis by acting on the rate-limiting enzyme phosphofructokinase (PFK). Acidosis decreases while alkalosis increases lactate production. The other major determinants of L-lactate levels are the concentrations of pyruvate and the NADH to $NAD^+$ ratio. The principal organs that remove lactate are the liver, kidneys, and muscle. Hepatic utilization of lactate can be impeded by several factors: poor blood flow to the liver, primary liver disease, and tissue anoxia or ischemia. Clinically significant lactic acidosis (lactate >4 mmol/L) is most often the result of tissue hypoxia, so-called *type A lactic acidosis.* It is seen commonly in scenarios such as cardiac arrest, ischemic limbs or gut, cardiogenic shock, hemorrhage, sepsis, and multiple organ dysfunction syndrome (MODS). Lactic acidosis also develops in patients with malignancies or enzymatic defects or in patients receiving certain drugs or toxins, such as phenformin or nucleoside analogues for HIV infection. This form of acidosis, where tissue hypoxia is not operative, is called *type B lactic acidosis.* It is important to note that although lactic acidosis is typically listed as a cause of anion gap acidosis, studies have shown that in up to 50% of patients with lactic acidosis, the acidosis is either wholly or, in part, hyperchloremic in origin.[22, 23]

**Treatment.** The basic principle of therapy for L-lactic acidosis is that the underlying condition initiating the disruption in normal lactate metabolism must first be corrected. Every attempt should be made to restore tissue perfusion when it is inadequate. Vasoconstricting agents should be used cautiously, because they can potentiate the hypoperfused state. Alkali therapy has been generally recommended for acute, severe acidosis (pH <7.1) to improve cardiac performance, response to vasoconstrictors, and lactate utilization. However, the use of bicarbonate in lactic acidosis remains controversial. Animal studies have shown that bicarbonate administration increases lactate production by increasing PFK activity, enhances $CO_2$ production, and impairs cardiac performance. Most of these animal models, however, do not accurately mimic the clinical scenario of lactic acidosis and often employ fixed ventilation. Bicarbonate infusion in such circumstances would be expected to fail, because the underlying pathophysiology is never treated. The use of bicarbonate in lactic acidosis has also been indicted in human studies because of its inability to improve outcome. However, any therapy in lactic acidosis is futile if the underlying cause of tissue hypoxia cannot be corrected. Fluid overload may also occur with bicarbonate therapy because the amount required is often massive, necessitating diuretics, ultrafiltration, or dialysis with a bicarbonate buffer. This volume administration is poorly tolerated because of central venoconstriction and decreased cardiac output. In order to avoid the potential deleterious effects of bicarbonate administration, several other buffering agents have been suggested for the treatment of lactic acidosis. *Dichloroacetate* (DCA) decreases lactate levels by stimulating the enzyme pyruvate dehydrogenase and improves pH, acidosis, and survival in animal studies. However, in a large clinical trial, although DCA improved several laboratory parameters in patients with sepsis and lactic acidosis, it had no beneficial effect on the outcome.[24] *Carbicarb,* an equimolar solution of sodium bicarbonate and sodium carbonate, may offer equivalent buffering capacity to bicarbonate without increasing the $Paco_2$. However, no head-to-head comparisons in patients with lactic acidosis have been performed. *THAM* is a proton and $CO_2$ scavenger that can correct both metabolic and respiratory acidosis. Its use has been limited by side effects such as hypoglycemia, hyperkalemia, respiratory failure, and skin necrosis. As is the case with Carbicarb, THAM has not been proved to be clinically more efficacious than bicarbonate. In patients with severe metabolic acidosis and marked hypercapnia from acute lung injury, THAM may be a useful therapeutic agent. However, such patients have a very high mortality rate, so that THAM may ultimately prove to be ineffective in this setting. If the underlying cause of the lactic acidosis can be remedied, blood lactate will be reconverted to bicarbonate. Bicarbonate derived from lactate conversion, in addition to any new bicarbonate generated by renal mechanisms during acidosis and from exogenous alkali therapy, is additive and may result in an overshoot alkalosis. When bicarbonate is administered, the goal should be to raise the pH to no more than 7.2 to 7.25. Reports suggest that continuous venovenous hemodialysis (CVVHD) may offer some advantages to patients who have lactic acidosis. However, controversy surrounds the alkali source used in this procedure. Some studies have found that use of lactate-based dialysis is deleterious in patients with lactic acidosis. This disadvantage can be overcome in CVVHD by regional anticoagulation with sodium citrate. Here, citrate is converted into bicarbonate by the liver. However, we have previously reported impaired citrate utilization in some patients with liver failure.[25] Several groups have developed bicarbonate-based continuous therapies that offer physiologic dialysate and improved hemodynamic stability.

## D-LACTIC ACIDOSIS

**Pathophysiology.** D-Lactate is produced by bacteria that may overgrow in the gastrointestinal tract in association with jejunoileal bypass, intestinal obstruction, antibiotic therapy, or ileus.[26] The diagnosis requires specifically measuring D-lactate, because it is not detected by the measurement of L-lactate levels.

**Treatment.** The potential danger in D-lactic acidosis is from an accumulation of toxic products rather than from the acidosis itself. Initial therapy includes: (1) cessation of feeding, (2) eradication of bacterial overgrowth, and (3) enhanced gastrointestinal motility. Long-term treatment may necessitate removal of the intestinal bypass if stasis and bacterial overgrowth persist or are recurrent.

## KETOACIDOSIS

### *Diabetic Ketoacidosis*

**Pathophysiology.** Diabetic ketoacidosis (DKA) results from increased fatty acid metabolism and accumulation of acetoacetate and β-hydroxybutyrate due to insulin deficiency and relative excess of glucagon. The absence of insulin promotes lipolysis and fatty acid release, whereas glucagon stimulates the hepatic metabolism of fatty acids to keto acids.

**Diagnostic Points.** DKA typically develops in association with intercurrent illness, particularly infection, that temporarily increases insulin requirements. The diagnosis is established by the concurrence of metabolic acidosis, strongly positive plasma ketones in undiluted serum, hyperglycemia, ECF volume depletion, and Kussmaul respiration. If patients are able to avoid volume depletion, the urinary loss of potential bicarbonate in the form of keto acids will lead to a hyperchloremic metabolic acidosis. However, most patients will be volume-depleted, leading to retention of ketones and an anion gap acidosis.

**Treatment.** The mainstay of therapy is the administration of insulin to inhibit keto acid production and also intravenous fluids for ECF volume restoration and correction of electrolyte abnormalities. Most, if not all, patients with DKA require correction of the volume depletion that almost invariably accompanies the osmotic diuresis and ketoacidosis. Initial therapy with isotonic saline may require rates in excess of 1000 mL/hr intravenously. When the pulse and blood pressure have stabilized and the corrected serum sodium concentration is in the range of 130 to 135 mEq/L, switch to 0.45% NaCl. Ringer lactate should be avoided. If the blood sugar declines below 250 to 300 mg/dL, 0.45% NaCl with 5% dextrose should be administered. Low-dose intravenous insulin therapy (0.1 U/kg/hr) smoothly corrects the biochemical abnormalities and minimizes hypoglycemia and hypokalemia. Although regular insulin may also be administered intramuscularly (0.2 mg/kg initially, then 6 U every hour), this method may not be effective in volume-depleted patients, which is often the case in ketoacidosis.

Total body potassium depletion is universally present in patients with DKA because of increased urinary loss from osmotic diuresis, ketonuria, high aldosterone levels, and vomiting. However, the potassium level on admission is typically elevated. This paradoxical hyperkalemia is caused by: (1) insulin deficiency that allows transcellular shifting of potassium out of cells, (2) hypertonicity, which osmotically drags potassium out of cells, and (3) decreased distal sodium delivery to the kidneys because of ECF volume depletion, which impairs renal potassium secretion. A normal or reduced potassium level on admission signals severe depletion. Administration of fluid, insulin, and alkali may cause the potassium level to decline further. Because therapy must be individualized, frequent monitoring of plasma potassium concentration is mandatory. When the urine output has been established, and the serum potassium falls below 5 mEq/L, 20 mEq KCl can be administered in each liter of fluid. Care should be taken in the presence of hyperkalemia, especially if the patient has renal insufficiency, because the usual therapy may not correct the hyperkalemia.

The routine administration of phosphate (usually as potassium phosphate) is not advised because of the potential for hyperphosphatemia and hypocalcemia. A significant number of patients with DKA will have significant hyperphosphatemia before the initiation of therapy. In the volume-depleted, malnourished patient, however, a normal or elevated phosphate concentration on admission may be followed by a rapid fall in plasma phosphate levels within 2 to 6 hours after the initiation of therapy. Bicarbonate therapy is usually unnecessary. In general, the increased anion gap represents the "potential" bicarbonate present in the circulation, which can be realized when the ketoacids are metabolized to bicarbonate with insulin treatment. If bicarbonate is administered, there is a risk of developing an "overshoot alkalosis" once ketones are converted back to bicarbonate.

## ALCOHOLIC ACIDOSIS

**Pathophysiology and Diagnostic Points.** Chronic alcoholics may develop ketoacidosis when alcohol consumption is abruptly curtailed, usually as a result of vomiting, abdominal pain, starvation, and volume depletion. This disorder, which is more common in women who are binge drinkers, is often underdiagnosed and should be suspected in alcoholics presenting with an anion gap acidosis. The glucose concentration is frequently low or normal, and the acidosis may be severe, particularly in the face of ECF volume depletion. The anion gap is expanded because of elevated ketones, which are predominantly β-hydroxybutyrate. Mild lactic acidosis may coexist because of an alteration in the redox state by ethanol in the liver or tissue hypoxia because of severe volume depletion. The nitroprusside reaction (Acetest) detects acetoacetic acid preferential to β-hydroxybutyrate, hence early on ketones may be weakly positive or negative. Typically, insulin levels are low, and levels of cortisol, glucagon, and growth hormone are high, leading to ketoacidosis.

**Treatment.** The mainstay of treatment consists of intravenous volume repletion and glucose administration (5% dextrose in 0.9% NaCl, not saline alone). Glucose increases the insulin-to-glucagon ratio, which suppresses keto acid production. Hypophosphatemia, hypokalemia, and hypomagnesemia often occur. Hypophosphatemia usually emerges 12 to 24 hours after the patient is admitted to the hospital, thus the need for therapy can be overlooked, especially if the serum phosphorus concentration on the patient's admission is normal. Such patients are at risk of developing "refeeding syndrome," in which administration of carbohydrate enhances insulin release and severe hypophosphatemia, hypokalemia, hypomagnesemia, and vitamin deficiency ensue.[27] Severe hypophosphatemia can result in rhabdomyolysis, hemolysis, platelet dysfunction, and respiratory failure.

## RENAL FAILURE

**Pathophysiology.** Progressive renal failure will eventually convert the hyperchloremic acidosis of early renal insufficiency to a high anion gap acidosis. The elevated anion gap is the result of retention of acid anions (e.g., phosphates and sulfates) as the glomerular filtration rate declines. Classical uremic acidosis is also characterized by a reduced rate of ammonium production and excretion, primarily due to decreased renal mass. The bicarbonate concentration decreases but rarely falls below 15 mEq/L, and the anion gap rarely exceeds 20 mEq/L. The retained acid in patients with chronic renal failure is partly buffered by alkaline salts contained in the skeleton. As a consequence, patients develop a form of metabolic bone disease due to acid-induced demineralization. Thus, an additional "trade-off" in chronic renal failure is a decrease in bone mineral content and negative calcium balance.

**Treatment.** Uremic acidosis requires oral alkali therapy to maintain the bicarbonate concentration above 22 mEq/L. This can be accomplished with relatively modest amounts of alkali (1 to 1.5 mEq/kg/day). Sodium citrate solution or sodium bicarbonate tablets are equally effective. Sodium citrate solution should never be given to patients receiving aluminum-containing antacids, because it greatly increases gastrointestinal absorption of aluminum and precipitates aluminum intoxication.

## TOXIN INGESTION

**Pathophysiology.** Under most physiologic conditions, sodium, urea, and glucose generate the osmotic pressure of plasma. Plasma osmolality (mOsm/kg) is calculated according to the following expression: $P_{Osm} = 2Na^+ + Glu/18 + BUN/2.8$. The calculated and measured osmolality should agree within 10 to 15 mOsm/kg. When the measured osmolality exceeds the calculated osmolality by more than 15 to 20 mOsm/kg, one of two circumstances prevails. First, the serum sodium may be spuriously low, which occurs with hyperlipidemia or hyperproteinemia (pseudohyponatremia), or second, osmolytes other than sodium salts, glucose, or urea have accumulated in plasma. Examples include mannitol infusion, radiocontrast media, or the accumulation of other solutes including the alcohols, ethylene glycol, or acetone. In these examples, the difference between calculated and measured osmolality is proportional to the concentration of unmeasured solutes and is referred to as the *osmolal gap*. With an appropriate clinical history and index of suspicion, the osmolal gap becomes a helpful screening tool in poison-associated anion gap acidosis.

### *Ethylene Glycol Intoxication*

**Diagnostic Points.** Ingestion of ethylene glycol leads to a metabolic acidosis in addition to severe central nervous system, cardiopulmonary, and renal damage. Early, patients appear intoxicated and can rapidly develop seizures and coma. In the next 12 to 24 hours, signs of cardiopulmonary dysfunction such as heart failure, pulmonary edema, or respiratory failure may be seen. If left untreated, renal failure eventually ensues from intratubular obstruction with oxalate and myoglobinuria. The increased anion and osmolal gaps can be attributed to ethylene glycol metabolites, especially oxalic acid, glycolic acid, and other incompletely identified organic acids. Lactic acid production also increases owing to a toxic depression in the reaction rates of the citric acid cycle and altered intracellular redox state. Diagnosis is facilitated by recognizing oxalate crystals in the urine.

**Treatment.** Treatment includes the prompt institution of a saline or osmotic diuresis, thiamine and pyridoxine supplements, fomepizole or ethanol, and hemodialysis. The intravenous administration of the new alcohol dehydrogenase inhibitor fomepizole (4-methylpyrazole) (7 mg/kg as a loading dose) or ethanol intravenously to achieve a level of 22 mmol/L (100 mg/dL), serves to lessen toxicity, because they compete with ethylene glycol for metabolism by alcohol dehydrogenase. Fomepizole, although expensive, offers the advantages of a predictable decline in ethylene glycol levels without the adverse effects, such as excessive obtundation, associated with ethyl alcohol infusion.[28]

### *Methanol Intoxication*

**Diagnostic Points.** Methanol ingestion causes metabolic acidosis in addition to severe optic nerve and central nervous system manifestations due to its metabolism to formic acid from formaldehyde. Nausea, vomiting, and abdominal pain are usually present. Lactic acids and ketoacids as well as other unidentified organic acids may contribute to the acidosis. Due to its low molecular weight, an osmolal gap is usually present.

**Treatment.** Therapy is generally similar to that for ethylene glycol intoxication, including general supportive measures, volume expansion, ethanol or fomepizole administration, and hemodialysis. Initiation of a saline diuresis is unnecessary, because renal toxicity is not a direct effect of methanol or its metabolites.

### *Salicylate Intoxication*

**Diagnostic Points.** The most common form of salicylate is aspirin. Other sources include methyl salicylate (oil of wintergreen), sodium salicylate, and many over-the-counter products. Acetosalicylic acid is rapidly converted after ingestion to salicylic acid, and this metabolite exerts the drug's toxic effects. Early symptoms of toxicity include tinnitus, vertigo, nausea, vomiting, and diarrhea. Severe intoxication can result in altered mental status, coma, noncardiogenic pulmonary edema, and death. Salicylate intoxication can cause several acid-base abnormalities: respiratory alkalosis, metabolic acidosis, or mixed metabolic acidosis-respiratory alkalosis. Salicylates directly stimulate the respiratory center resulting in a rapid fall in $Pa_{CO_2}$. Respiratory alkalosis promotes lactic acid production, and this augments the development of metabolic acidosis. The high anion gap results primarily from accumulation of organic acids such as lactate and ketones. Salicylic acid itself contributes little to the increased anion gap.

**Treatment.** The initial step in therapy should include gastric lavage and activated charcoal administration. To facilitate removal of salicylate, intravenous sodium bicarbonate administration in amounts adequate to alkalinize the urine and to maintain urine output may be required (urine pH $>7.5$). Although this form of therapy is straightforward in acidotic patients, alkalemia from a respiratory alkalosis may make this approach hazardous. Hypokalemia may occur as a result of an alkaline diuresis from sodium bicarbonate or acetazolamide and should be treated promptly. Glucose-containing fluids should be administered because of the danger of hypoglycemia. If renal failure prevents rapid clearance of salicylate, hemodialysis is very effective. Dialysis is also indicated in the setting of salicylate intoxication with volume overload, coma, or progressive clinical deterioration.

## REFERENCES


1. Madias NE: Lactic acidosis. Kidney Int 29:752, 1986.
2. Orchard CH, Kentish JC: Effects of changes of pH on the contractile function of cardiac muscle. Am J Physiol 258:C967, 1990.
3. Wildenthal K, Mierzwiak D, Meyers R, Mitchell J: Effects of acute lactic acidosis on left ventricular performance. Am J Appl Physiol 214:1352, 1968.
4. Cooper D, Herbertson M, Werner H, Walley K: Bicarbonate does not increase left ventricular contractility during L-lactic acidemia in pigs. Am Rev Respir Dis 148:317, 1993.
5. Rocomora J, Downing S: Preservation of ventricular function by adrenergic influences during metabolic acidosis in the cat. Circ Res 24:373, 1969.
6. Bygdeman S: Vascular reactivity in cats during induced changes in acid-base balance of the blood. Acta Physiol Scand 61 (suppl 2):1, 1963.
7. Orchard CH, Cingolani HE: Acidosis and arrhythmias in cardiac muscle. Cardiovasc Res 28:1312, 1994.
8. Kraut JA, Mishler DR, Kurkawa K: Effect of colchicine and calcitonin on calcemic response to metabolic acidosis. Kidney Int 25:608, 1984.
9. Bushinsky D: The contribution of acidosis to renal osteodystrophy. Kidney Int 47:1816, 1995.
10. Kraut JA, Mishler DR, Singer FR, Goodman WG: The effects of metabolic acidosis on bone formation and bone resorption in the rat. Kidney Int 30:694, 1986.
11. Alpern RJ: Trade-offs in the adaptation to acidosis. Kidney Int 47:1205, 1995.
12. Price S, Mitch W: Metabolic acidosis and uremic toxicity: Protein and amino acid metabolism. Semin Nephrol 14:232, 1994.
13. Mitch WE: Influence of metabolic acidosis on nutrition. Am J Kidney Dis 29:xlvii, 1997.
14. Gabow P: Disorders associated with an altered anion gap. Kidney Int 27:472, 1985.
15. Batlle D, Hizon M, Cohen E, et al: The use of the urinary anion gap in the diagnosis of hyperchloremic metabolic acidosis. N Engl J Med 318:594, 1988.
16. McDougal W: Metabolic complications of urinary intestinal diversion. J Urol 147:1199, 1992.
17. Hal MC, Koch MO, McDougal WS: Metabolic consequences of urinary diversion through intestinal segments. Urol Clin North Am 18:725, 1991.
18. Cruz DN, Huot SJ: Metabolic complications of urinary diversions: An overview. Am J Med 102:477, 1997.
19. Wallia R, Greensberg A, Piraino B, et al: Serum electrolyte patterns in end-stage renal disease. Am J Kidney Dis 8:98, 1986.
20. Pitt B, Zannad F, Remme W, et al: The effect of spironolactone on morbidity and mortality in patients with severe heart failure. N Engl J Med 341:709, 1999.
21. Batlle D, Arruda J, Kurtzman N: Hyperkalemic distal renal tubular acidosis associated with obstructive uropathy. N Engl J Med 304:373, 1981.
22. Iberti T, Leibowitz A, Papadakos P, Fischer E: Low sensitivity of the anion gap as a screen to detect hyperlactatemia in critically ill patients. Crit Care Med 18:275, 1990.
23. Levraut J, Bounatirou T, Ichai C, et al: Reliability of anion gap as an indicator of blood lactate in critically ill patients. Intensive Care Med 23:417, 1997.
24. Stacpoole P, Wright E, Baumgartner T, et al: A controlled clinical trial of dichloroacetate for treatment of lactic acidosis in adults. N Engl J Med 327:1564, 1992.
25. Meier-Kriesche H-U, Finkel KW, Gitomer J, DuBose TD Jr: Unexpected severe hypocalcemia during continuous venovenous hemodialysis with regional citrate anticoagulation. Am J Kidney Dis 33:E8, 1999.
26. Halperin M, Kamel K: D-Lactic acidosis: Turning sugar into acids in the gastrointestinal tract. Kidney Int 49:1, 1996.
27. Solomon S, Kirby D: The refeeding syndrome: A review. JPEN 14:90, 1990.
28. Brent J, McMartin K, Phillips S, et al: Fomepizole for the treatment of ethylene glycol poisoning. N Engl J Med 340:832,1999.
29. DuBose TD Jr: Metabolic acidosis. In Brady H, Wilcox C (eds): Therapy in Nephrology and Hypertension: A Companion to Brenner & Rector's The Kidney. Philadelphia, WB Saunders, 1999, pp 279–286.
30. DuBose TD Jr: Acidosis and alkalosis. In Fauci A, Braunwald E, Isselbacher K, et al (eds): Harrison's Principles of Internal Medicine, 14th ed. New York, McGraw-Hill, 1998, pp 277–286.
31. DuBose TD Jr: Acid-base disorders. In Brenner B (ed): Brenner & Rector's The Kidney, 6th ed. Philadelphia, WB Saunders, 2000, pp 925–997.
32. Bushinsky D: Metabolic acidosis. In Jacobson H, Striker G, Klahr S (eds): The Principles and Practice of Nephrology, 2nd ed. St. Louis, CV Mosby, 1995, pp 924–931.

CHAPTER 5

# Ketoacidosis

Mitchell L. Halperin, MD ▪ David Z.I. Cherney, MD ▪ Kamel S. Kamel, MD

Ketoacids are water-soluble, four-carbon, energy-rich circulating fuels that are formed during the partial oxidation of fatty acids in liver mitochondria. The control mechanisms that underlie the formation and set limits on the rate of production of ketoacids probably originated evolutionarily in Paleolithic times to permit survival during prolonged fasting.[1,2] The chapter is divided into six sections. In the first section, the role of ketoacids in fasting is examined. The next two sections include a quantitative analysis of both ketoacid production and removal, including renal excretion (Fig. 5–1). The fourth section considers acid-base aspects of ketoacidosis. In the fifth section, biochemical aspects of hyperglycemia are considered. In the final section, the emphasis is on diabetic ketoacidosis (DKA) and the ketoacidosis that may occur when ethanol is ingested (i.e., alcoholic ketoacidosis [AKA]). Although the ketoacidosis of starvation may have little clinical significance, this setting can still provide insights into the biochemical and quantitative aspects of ketoacid production and removal (for a more detailed discussion, see reference 3).

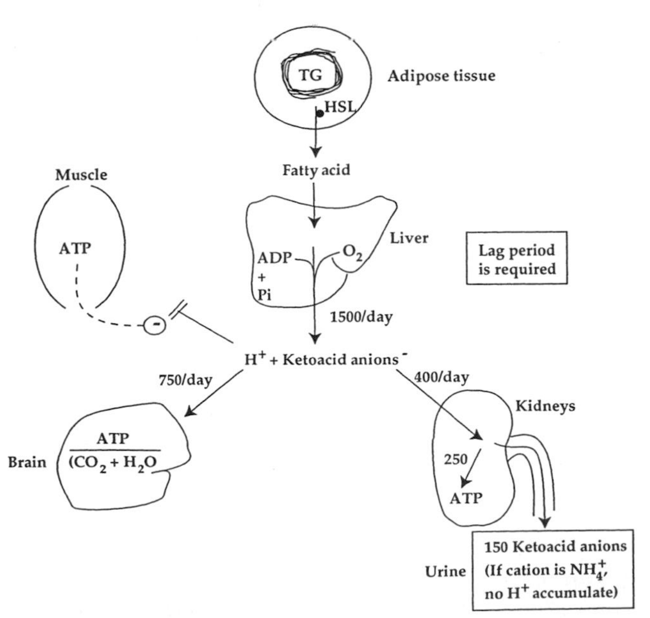


**FIGURE 5–1** ▪ The metabolic process involved in ketoacid metabolism. The metabolic process begins with activation of hormone-sensitive lipase (HSL) in adipose tissue. After a lack of insulin and a rise in glucagon for several days, the production of ketoacids in the liver rises progressively to 1500 mmol/day. The main sites of removal of ketoacids are the brain (750 mmol/day) and the kidneys (400 mmol/day).

## KETOACIDS AND THE STRATEGY FOR SURVIVAL DURING FASTING

The prerequisites for ketoacid accumulation in plasma and the possible impact of their formation follow.

### Settings Where Ketoacids Are Important in Intermediary Metabolism

The important function of energy fuels is to regenerate enough useful energy in the form of adenosine triphosphate (ATP) to carry out biologic work (i.e., mechanical work, ion pumping, and biosynthesis).[4] When there is no intake of food, all the fuels oxidized must come from endogenous sources. The answers to the following four questions are central to understand metabolic regulation during caloric deprivation. Which organ should be dominant? Which fuel type will that critical organ oxidize (i.e., carbohydrate, protein, or fat)? How much fuel will that organ need to oxidize? What is the "price to pay" for this new metabolic pattern? Succinct responses to these questions follow. The most important organ necessary for survival is the brain. The dominant fuel consumed by the brain during starvation must be water-soluble and derived from storage fat. The quantity of fuels synthesized should match the anticipated metabolic needs of the brain. The "price to pay" when a fat-derived fuel becomes the principal substrate for the brain is an excess of hydrogen ions ($H^+$). Each of these points is now considered in more detail.

#### METABOLIC ISSUES IN THE BRAIN

The first issue to consider is which fuel should be oxidized in the brain. During the fed state (or an overnight fast), glucose is its major fuel because when measurements are made, glucose is virtually the only fuel extracted from the arterial blood supply.[2] Moreover, in quantitative terms, the amount of glucose extracted by the brain is sufficient to account for all its oxygen consumption. In contrast, in states with prolonged caloric deprivation, ketoacids (not glucose) appear to be the main fuel oxidized by the brain.[5]

The fact that the brain burns ketoacids during prolonged fasting has several important metabolic implications. First, there is a hierarchy of fuel oxidation with fatty acids being the fuel of first choice if they are able to enter cells at a sufficiently rapid rate. If fatty acids

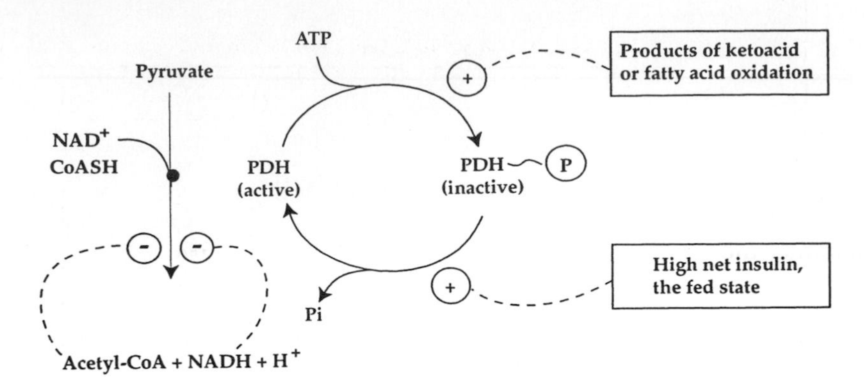


**FIGURE 5–2** ■ Central role of pyruvate dehydrogenase. Pyruvate dehydrogenase (PDH) catalyzes an irreversible reaction essential for the complete oxidation of glucose. When ketoacids or fatty acids are oxidized, PDH is phosphorylated and becomes inactive. The end-products of their oxidation, acetyl-coenzyme A (CoA) and NADH, inhibit the residual active PDH enzymatic activity.

cannot gain access to cells (e.g., brain cells, because of the blood-brain barrier [BBB]), ketoacids are the fuel selected if their concentration is high enough in plasma and a transport system is present in the BBB. Data in humans suggest that ketoacids are oxidized in preference to glucose in the brain when both fuels are provided in millimolar amounts.[6] The biochemical basis for this hierarchy of fuel oxidation is that the products of fatty acid or ketoacid oxidation inhibit pyruvate dehydrogenase (PDH), the key enzyme-catalyzed reaction that is mandatory for the complete oxidation of carbohydrates (Fig. 5–2).[4, 6, 7] Another example of this "fuel selection" is presented in the section on renal metabolism, where ketoacids displace glutamine as the preferred fuel to regenerate ATP in cells of the proximal convoluted tubule (PCT).

The second issue to consider is how many ketoacids the brain can oxidize. As a general rule, the rate of turnover of ATP in cells sets an upper limit on the rate of oxidation of fuels.[4, 5] This aspect is critical not only to determine how many ketoacids are oxidized daily in the brain but also how this rate can be altered in vivo (Fig. 5–3). ATP and adenosine diphosphate (ADP) are present in catalytic amounts; therefore, one can only regenerate as much ATP as was used to perform biologic work.[4, 5]

**Quantitative Issues.** The brain consumes approximately 4000 mmol of oxygen and regenerates 24,000 mmol of ATP per day in an adult. This quantity is relatively constant unless coma or drugs decrease biologic work performed by the brain. Therefore, to regenerate most of this ATP during prolonged fasting, the brain oxidizes 750 mmol of the principal ketoacid in the circulation, β-hydroxybutyric acid (H·β-HB) per day (Equation 1).

$$\text{H·β-HB} + 4.5\ O_2 \rightarrow 4\ CO_2 + 4\ H_2O + 27\ \text{ATP} \quad \text{(Equation 1)}$$

## METABOLIC DEMANDS OF THE KIDNEY DURING KETOACIDOSIS

Renal issues must also be integrated into the setting of ketoacidosis caused by prolonged fasting.[6] The kidney removes approximately 400 mmol of ketoacids—250 mmol/day by oxidation and 150 mmol by excretion as their ammonium ($NH_4^+$) salts.[7] Although this ketonuria may be thought of simply as a "waste of energy," it has biologic advantages. These ketoacid anions are excreted mainly with $NH_4^+$. During prolonged fasting, the excretion of the usual osmoles—urea, sodium ($Na^+$), potassium ($K^+$), and chloride ($Cl^-$)—is very low.[8] Therefore, the excretion of 300 mOsm of these solutes ($NH_4^+$ and ketoacid anions) daily will achieve a small, but sufficient volume of urine to minimize the risk of kidney stone formation (Equation 2).[8] Although the source of glutamine used for ammoniagenesis was derived from endogenous protein, the loss of lean body mass is significantly lower than if this osmolar excretion rate was in the form of urea.[6]

$$\text{Urine volume} = \text{number of osmoles excreted/[Osm] urine} \quad \text{(Equation 2)}$$

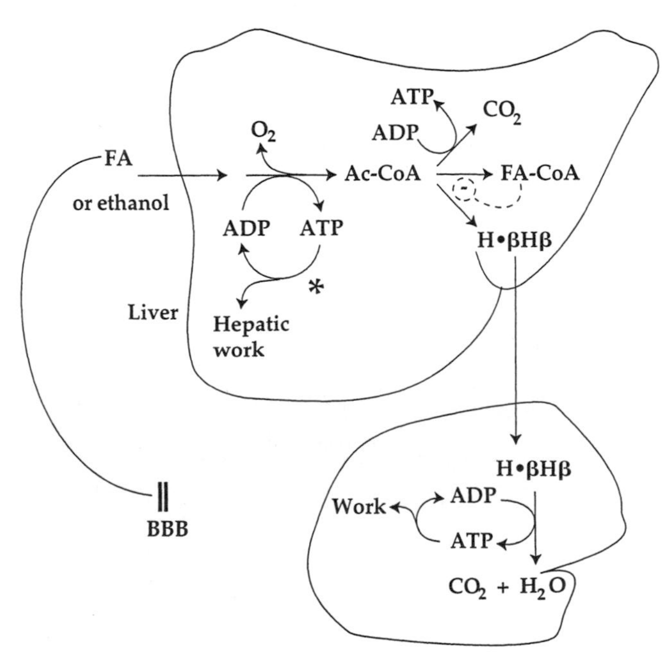


**FIGURE 5–3** ■ Requirement for a source of adenosine diphosphate (ADP) in the control of a metabolic process. The upper structure is the liver; the lower structure is the brain. When fatty acids (FA) or ethanol are oxidized in the liver to yield adenosine triphosphate (ATP) and acetyl-coenzyme A (CoA) a source of ADP is needed. This ADP availability is dependent on the hydrolysis of ATP to perform work in hepatocytes. Availability of ADP sets the upper limit on hepatic ketogenesis and on the rate of oxidation of ketoacids in the brain.

Three renal factors permit the appropriate rate of excretion of $NH_4^+$ in prolonged fasting. First, glutamine is the fuel oxidized to regenerate ATP in cells of the PCT during metabolic acidosis.[9] Second, the upper limit for the rate of ATP regeneration in the PCT is set by the rate of reabsorption of filtered $Na^+$, the major process that converts ATP to ADP in these cells.[5,10] Third, complete oxidation of glutamine, the renal precursor of $NH_4^+$ and bicarbonate ions ($HCO_3^-$), is reduced when ketoacids are reabsorbed and oxidized in these cells (the fuel selection issue discussed in the hierarchy of fuels[11]). In fact, the oxidation of glutamine or H·β-HB in the cells of the PCT produces an equivalent amount of ATP (27 mmol of ATP per mmol of fuel).[12]

#### METABOLIC DEMANDS OF OTHER ORGANS

In general, other than the intestinal tract,[13] little oxidation of ketoacids occurs in the remaining organs, probably because they oxidize fatty acids.[11] Because intestinal work (absorption/secretion) is quite low during prolonged fasting, the ketoacids formed in the liver are fuels that are oxidized primarily in the brain and kidneys. A summary of the quantitative issues concerning the capacity to produce and utilize ketoacids is provided in Table 5–1. These aspects are considered in more detail later in this chapter.

### Unanswered Questions

The following questions still do not have clear answers. First, what are the control mechanisms that permit muscles to oxidize ketoacids if ketoacids are available very early in fasting, but prevent them from oxidizing appreciable quantities of ketoacids later in fasting? Second, why is there a lag period in ketoacid oxidation by the brain when ketoacids are produced very quickly?[14] This is important primarily to understand the clinical syndrome of AKA and is considered in more detail later in this chapter.

## METABOLIC PRODUCTION OF KETOACIDS

With prolonged fasting, the production of ketoacids is matched by their rate of removal in the steady state, avoiding the development of progressive metabolic acidosis.[12] Two factors are needed to develop severe degrees of ketoacidosis in DKA and AKA. First, there must be the "usual" stimulated rate of ketoacid formation (i.e., that observed in prolonged fasting). Second, and of greater importance, there must be a reduced rate of ketoacid oxidation because of a reduced rate of metabolic work in the brain and the kidneys—the two major organs that oxidize ketoacids (see Fig. 5–1).

**TABLE 5–1.** Ketoacid Turnover During Prolonged Fasting*

| Organ | Metabolism (mmol/day) |
|---|---|
| Liver | +1500 |
| Brain | −750 |
| Kidney | |
| Metabolism | −250 |
| Excretion | −150 |
| Other organs | −200 |
| Conversion to acetone | −150 |

*The rate of production is denoted by a + sign and the rate of removal is denoted by a − sign.

### Lag Period Before Ketoacids Accumulate

It is well documented that the concentration of ketoacids in plasma rises appreciably, but only after several days of fasting.[7] This lag period is also observed during the development of DKA.[15] Although the biochemical basis of this lag period is unclear, it may be related to the time required for the induction of components of the transport system for entry of fatty acyl groups into the mitochondria.

### Control of Ketogenesis

The metabolic process involved in the formation of ketoacids can be viewed as having two levels of regulation. First, one must ensure that there is enough substrate for ketogenesis (i.e., to supply fatty acids to the liver). Second, controls must be present within the liver to prevent excessive production of ketoacids (constraints due to the availability of ADP).

**Supply of Fatty Acids.** Because the function of ketogenesis is to provide a water-soluble fat-derived fuel for the brain (i.e., ketoacids) when the availability of the alternate fuel (glucose) is in short supply in the circulation, the signal to initiate the formation of ketoacids is a reduction in glycemia. The sensor to initiate this metabolic process is in the β cells in the islets of Langerhans. A fall in the level of insulin causes the activation of hormone-sensitive lipase[16] in adipocytes and leads to a rise in the level of free fatty acids in plasma (Fig. 5–4). The observed level of fatty acids in plasma during DKA and prolonged fasting is approximately 1 mmol/L. Because each liter of blood has 0.6 L of plasma and hepatic blood flow is close to 1 L/min,[17] the liver receives 0.6 mmol/min of fatty acids. If the liver extracted 50% of these fatty acids in a single pass, the maximum possible rate of ketogenesis would be 1.2 mmol/min (4 mmol of ketoacids per mmol of palmitate, see Equation 3). The aforementioned implies no other hepatic fate for acetyl coenzyme A (CoA) derived from fatty acids; that is, oxidation in the tricarboxylic acid (TCA) cycle (Equation 4).

$$\text{Palmitate} + 6\ O_2 + 27\ (\text{ADP} + \text{Pi}) \rightarrow 4\ \text{ketoacids} + 27\ \text{ATP} \qquad \text{(Equation 3)}$$

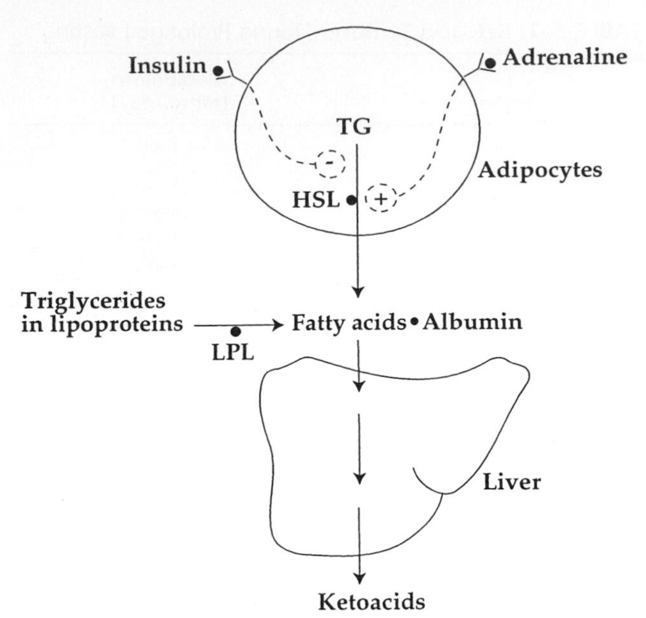


**FIGURE 5–4** ■ Supply of fatty acids to the liver. There are two possible sources of fatty acids for the liver. The major source is from adipose tissue triglycerides. This requires activation of hormone-sensitive lipase (HSL) by hormones whose actions oppose those of insulin. The second potential source of fatty acids is the hydrolysis of circulating triglycerides by hepatic lipoprotein lipase (LPL).

$$\text{Palmitate} + 23\ O_2 \rightarrow 8 \text{ acetyl CoA} + 35 \text{ ATP, or } 16\ (CO_2 + H_2O) + 129 \text{ ATP} \quad \text{(Equation 4)}$$

**Controls in the Liver.** The next step in the production of ketoacids occurs in hepatocytes (see Fig. 5–3). Here, under the hormonal influence primarily of high levels of glucagon, the entry of fatty acyl groups into the mitochondria is stimulated. Key regulators in this entry step are carnitine, which acts as a catalyst,[18] and low levels of malonyl CoA, which acts as a stimulator.[19] Under conditions involving a lack of insulin and high levels of glucagon, the activity of the enzyme that leads to the synthesis of malonyl CoA, acetyl-CoA carboxylase, is inhibited (Fig. 5–5). Therefore, the level of malonyl CoA should decline; this allows for a rapid entry of fatty acyl CoA groups into hepatic mitochondria.[19] Once inside mitochondria, β-oxidation of fatty acids occurs, yielding acetyl CoA, nicotinamide adenine dinucleotide [reduced form] (NADH), and flavin adenine dinucleotide [reduced form] ($FADH_2$); reoxidation of these latter cofactors in the presence of ADP ultimately regenerates ATP. Within the hepatic mitochondria, the precursor for the synthesis of ketoacids is acetyl CoA. Whereas this metabolic intermediate can be derived from three main sources (i.e., pyruvate, β-oxidation of free fatty acids, and ethanol), only the latter two substrates are precursors for ketogenesis, because the oxidation of fatty acids or ethanol leads to inhibition of PDH (see Fig. 5–2).

The next site of regulation within hepatocytes is at the acetyl CoA crossroads (see Fig. 5–3). Regulation here involves controls exerted by the provision of ADP as a result of the rate of turnover of ATP in hepatocytes to perform biologic work. Because there is little room to vary the rate of hepatic work, ketoacid production is ultimately limited by the availability of ADP in hepatocytes (see Table 5–1).[4, 5] If another pathway regenerates ATP, the rate of ketoacid formation is even lower than the limit set by the rate of hepatic work (i.e., the availability of ADP).

**Quantitative Aspects.** The rate of consumption of oxygen by the liver is approximately 3000 mmol/24 hr. In addition, based on nitrogen balance data during prolonged fasting, 600 mmol of oxygen are consumed in the conversion of protein to glucose[20]; therefore, only the remaining 2400 mmol of oxygen can be used

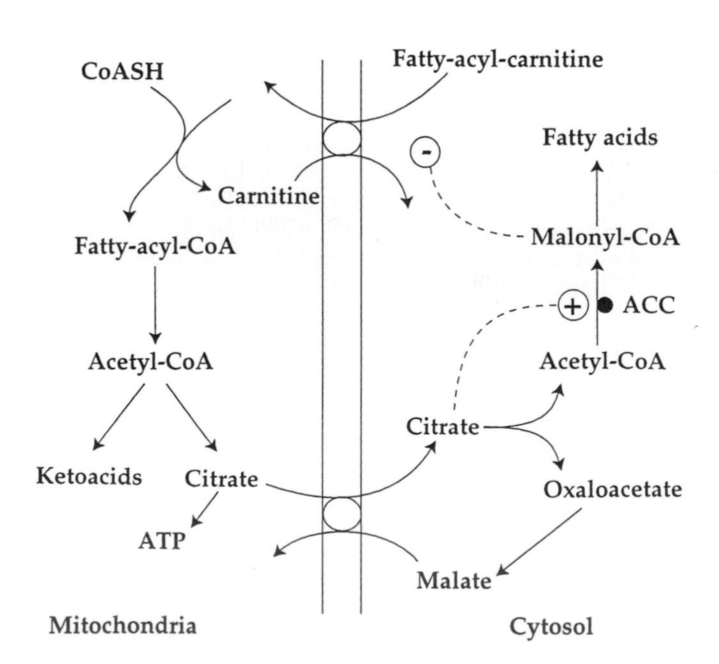


ACC is activated by insulin and inhibited by glucagon

**FIGURE 5–5** ■ Control of fatty acid oxidation in the liver. The parallel vertical lines represent the hepatic inner mitochondrial membrane. The rate-limiting step for the β-oxidation of fatty acids is their entry into mitochondria as a carnitine ester. This step is inhibited by cytosolic malonyl-coenzyme A (CoA), the product of the regulated cystosolic enzyme, acetyl-CoA carboxylase (ACC). ACC is inhibited in insulin deficiency states where fatty acid oxidation occurs at a rapid rate.

in ketogenesis. Because the oxidation of 1 mmol of palmitate to equal proportions of H·β-HB and acetoacetic acid (H·AcAc) consumes 6 mmol of oxygen and produces 4 mmol of ketoacids (see Equation 4), one can deduce that the maximal rate of ketogenesis is close to 1600 mmol/day (see Table 5–1).

### Ketoacids Formed During the Oxidation of Ethanol

The ingestion of ethanol may lead to a severe degree of ketoacidosis in the absence of diabetes mellitus.[21] The following components are required for the development of AKA. First, one needs a deficiency of insulin and high levels of hormones whose actions oppose those of insulin. This usually comes about because of protracted vomiting and extracellular fluid (ECF) volume contraction, a result of excessive ethanol intake. The secretion of insulin is inhibited by the α-adrenergic actions of catecholamines released in response to the low ECF volume despite the presence of a mild degree of hyperglycemia.[22, 23] Second, at the hepatic level, the metabolism of ethanol is rapid because ethanol levels are considerably higher than the concentration of ethanol required for half-maximal activity (Km) of alcohol dehydrogenase (<1 mmol/L).[24] This can lead to high levels of acetyl CoA over a relatively short time.[21] If alternate fates for this acetyl CoA are blocked (e.g., fatty acid synthesis because of low levels of insulin, see Fig. 5–3), acetyl CoA levels rise and lead to higher rates of ketogenesis. Of note, by using ethanol as the substrate for ketogenesis, the slow step of fatty acid entry into hepatic mitochondria is bypassed. Therefore, almost no lag period may occur before a maximum rate of ketogenesis could be achieved. Third, there is the issue of turnover of ATP to provide ADP in hepatocytes. The major point to emphasize in this regard is that the generation of acetyl CoA from ethanol and fatty acids yields almost the same amount of ATP per acetyl CoA formed (Equation 5; see also Equation 4).

$$\text{Ethanol} + 4\ \text{ADP} + 4\ \text{Pi} + \text{CoASH} \rightarrow \text{acetyl CoA} + 4\ \text{ATP} \quad \text{(Equation 5)}$$

Hence, the maximum rate of ketogenesis should be similar with ethanol or fatty acids as the substrate. Fourth, there is an important and unique feature with regard to the oxidation of ketoacids. The rate of removal of ketoacids is limited by the same constraints related to the rate of turnover of ATP in the brain and the kidneys (see Fig. 5–3). The "sedative effect" of alcohol and the possible presence of brain atrophy in the chronic alcoholic may diminish the metabolic work performed in the brain. Furthermore, there appears to be a time lag before the brain is fully adapted to the use of ketoacids for oxidation.[14] Therefore, in the setting of "rapid ketogenesis" from ethanol, ketoacids may accumulate more quickly because the brain may not be fully prepared for their rapid utilization. Also, with a low glomerular filtration rate (GFR) due to a contracted ECF volume, the rate of consumption of oxygen and thus the oxidation of fuels (ketoacids in this example) in the kidney is reduced.

## REMOVAL OF KETOACIDS

Three possible routes by which ketoacids are removed from the body are: (1) oxidation to $CO_2$ and water, (2) conversion to acetone (and its subsequent elimination via pulmonary exhalation), and (3) urinary excretion of ketoacid anions together with $NH_4^+$ or $H^+$.

### Oxidation of Ketoacids

The main organs that are able to oxidize ketoacids are the brain and the kidney.[7] Therefore, a reduced rate of biologic work in one or both of these organs can lead to a reduced availability of ADP followed by a lower rate of oxidation of ketoacid anions and also a more severe degree of acidosis. In the brain during severe DKA and AKA, cerebral metabolism is reduced, possibly because of hyperosmolarity or acidosis in DKA and also because of the sedative effects of ethanol in AKA.[14] Renal metabolic rate is diminished in these conditions because the contracted ECF volume leads to a fall in the GFR. As a result, less $Na^+$ is filtered and thus reabsorbed.[5] Reabsorption of $Na^+$ is the major reason for increasing the turnover of ATP and, as a result, fuel consumption by the kidney.

### Elimination of Acetone

When H·AcAc is converted to acetone, and the acetone is subsequently eliminated via the lungs, $H^+$ are consumed (Equation 6). An enzyme does not catalyze this process; thus it is directly proportional to the concentration of H·AcAc. During ketoacidosis of fasting, this process is responsible for the removal of approximately 150 mmol of ketoacid anions plus $H^+$ per day.[25] In the presence of a high NADH-to-$NAD^+$ ratio (e.g., while ethanol is being metabolized or in the setting of L-lactic acidosis), the equilibrium between H·AcAc and H·β-HB is shifted toward H·β-HB (Equation 7). As a result, the steady-state concentration of H·AcAc declines and, therefore, less acetone is produced (see Equation 6). This means that yet another route for the elimination of ketoacids is compromised.

$$\text{AcAc}^- + H^+ \rightarrow \text{acetone} + CO_2 \quad \text{(Equation 6)}$$

$$\text{AcAc}^- + \text{NADH} + H^+ \leftrightarrow \beta\text{-HB}^- + \text{NAD}^+ \quad \text{(Equation 7)}$$

### Urinary Loss of Ketoacid Anions

During the ketoacidosis of fasting, approximately 150 mmol of ketoacid anions are excreted daily in the urine.[7] Excretion of ketoacid anions represents the loss of "potential bicarbonate" in the urine. If this rate is matched by the rate of excretion of $NH_4^+$, acid-base balance is maintained. If a significant quantity of ketoacid anions is lost in the urine during the early course of ketoacidosis with a cation other than $NH_4^+$ or $H^+$ ($Na^+$ or $K^+$), a more severe degree of acidosis will develop. Such a large urinary loss of ketoacid anions without $NH_4^+$ occurs most commonly in the setting of salicylate ingestion or concomitant L-lactic acidosis.[12]

## KETOACIDOSIS: ACID-BASE BALANCE

### Production of H+

One can determine if $H^+$ were produced or consumed in any metabolic process by simply counting the net valence of all the substrates and products except those of adenine nucleotides and catalysts[26]; $H^+$ accumulate if the net anionic charge of products exceeds that of the substrates.

### Removal of H+ by Metabolism

In the metabolic process of ketoacid formation in the liver and its oxidation in the brain or kidneys, there is no net production or removal of $H^+$ (see Fig. 5–1). Rather, $H^+$ accumulate when ketoacid anions accumulate in the body or when these anions are excreted as their $Na^+$ or $K^+$ salts rather than as their $NH_4^+$ salts. A quantitative analysis is helpful to illustrate this point about accumulation of ketoacids. First, the total content of $HCO_3^-$ in the ECF compartment of a 70-kg adult is 375 mmol (15 L × 25 mmol/L). If the oxidation of ketoacids in the brain were reduced by 50% in the brain, the quantity of $H^+$ retained in a day would be equivalent to the total amount of $HCO_3^-$ in the ECF compartment in a normal subject. A similar 50% reduction in renal removal of ketoacids would add another 200 mmol of $H^+$ to the body per day. Hence, these daily additions of $H^+$ are close to 50% of the capacity of the body buffer systems to remove them safely.

### Buffering of H+

Although it is customary to rely on measurements in the ECF (i.e., pH, $P_{CO_2}$, $HCO_3^-$) to assess an acid-base disturbance, it is important to recognize that events in the ECF, and especially in arterial blood, may not reflect the acid-base status in the intracellular fluid (ICF).[27] Furthermore, the severity of ICF acidosis, and more specifically the degree of binding of $H^+$ to intracellular proteins, is probably detrimental to cellular function.[28] Two aspects of the clinical presentation in patients with DKA or AKA could be important in this regard.

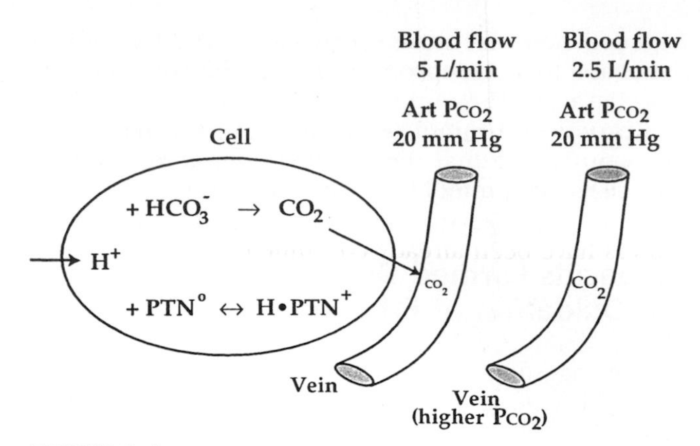


**FIGURE 5–6** ■ Role of tissue $P_{CO_2}$ in the selection of intracellular buffer systems. When the tissue $P_{CO_2}$ rises, the $[H^+]$ in the cells should also rise and require buffering on intracellular proteins (H·APTN+) rather than by bicarbonate buffers. There is a larger rise in tissue and venous $P_{CO_2}$ when the blood flow rate is slower (2.5 L/min in this example) secondary to the extracellular fluid (ECF) volume contraction as shown on the right. When the ECF volume is re-expanded and the blood flow rate is raised to normal (5 L/min in this example), the tissue and venous $P_{CO_2}$ fall. As a result, $H^+$ are displaced from proteins in the intracellular fluid.

**Tissue $P_{CO_2}$.** For more buffering by intracellular proteins, one needs either a very large $H^+$ load or a smaller proportion of buffering of $H^+$ by bicarbonate buffers. A major factor that influences this distribution of buffering is a change in the tissue $P_{CO_2}$.[28] In more detail (Fig. 5–6), a rise in tissue $P_{CO_2}$ causes the intracellular $[H^+]$ and $[HCO_3^-]$ to rise. This rise in intracellular $[H^+]$ will force $H^+$ to bind to proteins in the ICF, shifting them toward a more positively charged form. Patients with DKA and AKA who have a marked degree of ECF volume contraction would have a decreased cardiac output. Even with no change in $CO_2$ production, each liter of blood in the capillaries must now carry more $CO_2$ and have a higher $P_{CO_2}$. The higher tissue $P_{CO_2}$ will lead to more $H^+$ binding to ICF proteins, with potentially harmful consequences. Although the brain is protected early on by autoregulation of its blood flow rate, this system will fail with a marked reduction in cardiac output. Perhaps this is the stage that precipitates coma and an accelerated ketoacid accumulation due to a low rate of ketoacid oxidation in the brain.

**$CO_2$ Production.** For the same rate of alveolar ventilation, a lower arterial $P_{CO_2}$ will be found when there is a smaller rate of production of $CO_2$. Several factors may lead to a lower rate of metabolic production of $CO_2$ in patients with DKA or AKA.[29] In addition to hypothermia, there are factors that are specific to certain organs. For example, alcohol or coma can suppress metabolism in the brain. Metabolism in the kidney can be suppressed because hypovolemia leads to a low GFR. Muscle metabolism can be low because of inactivity, cachexia, or muscle wasting. There will be no production of $CO_2$ by the liver if it regenerates ATP from the conversion of ethanol or fatty acids to ketoacids. Furthermore, a higher NADH-to-$NAD^+$ ratio in the liver could shift H·AcAc to H·β-HB and hence reduce the formation of $CO_2$ by diminishing the amount of H·AcAc available to generate acetone plus $CO_2$.

$CO_2$ is produced when $H^+$ ions are titrated by the bicarbonate buffer system. This production of $CO_2$ diminishes in magnitude when the degree of metabolic acidosis becomes more severe because bicarbonate buffers have been already consumed.

# HYPERGLYCEMIA

In general, an increase in the concentration of a metabolite in plasma is due to an excessive rate of input or a decrease in the rate of output of that metabolite from the plasma compartment. With respect to glucose, there are three major sources of input: (1) diet, (2) glycogen in the liver, and (3) gluconeogenesis. The disposal of glucose occurs via oxidation to regenerate ATP, the conversion of glucose into storage forms of energy such as glycogen in the liver or triglycerides, or the excretion of glucose in the urine. A marked degree of hyperglycemia almost always requires a significant reduction in the rate of excretion of glucose in the urine; this low glucosuria implies that the GFR is very low. This point becomes evident when the quantitative aspects of glucose input and removal are considered later.

## Input of Glucose

**Diet.** The input of glucose from the diet varies. In an adult on a typical Western diet, the consumption of carbohydrates is approximately 250 g/day. Most patients with DKA, however, have a limited intake of carbohydrates unless fruit juice or sugar-containing soft drinks are consumed in large quantities in response to thirst. For example, 1 L of apple juice contains approximately 120 g of glucose.[3]

**Glycogen in the Liver.** The quantity of glycogen in the liver of a 70-kg adult is approximately 100 g; this can supply about 110 g (617 mmol) of glucose. Nevertheless, by the time that patients with DKA arrive in the emergency room, hepatic glycogen breakdown is likely to have occurred several days ago.

**Gluconeogenesis.** New glucose is formed when amino acids (but not L-lactate when the L-lactate was derived from muscle glycogen) are converted to glucose.[11] The rate of gluconeogenesis from amino acids can be estimated from the rate of appearance of urea. For each millimole of glucose made in this process, 1.8 mmol of urea is formed.[11] Given a daily excretion of urea in these patients of 400 to 500 mmol/day, the input of glucose via gluconeogenesis from amino acids is approximately 40 to 50 g (250 mmol) per day. Notwithstanding, this rate could be higher if there is excessive catabolism (e.g., infections) or other sources of protein breakdown (e.g., digestion of blood in the gastrointestinal tract).

## Output of Glucose

Glucose can be removed via its two major metabolic processes, oxidation to regenerate ATP and conversion into storage forms of energy (glycogen and triglycerides), or it can be excreted in the urine during hyperglycemia. During states of lack of insulin, flux through storage pathways is small in magnitude. With regard to the rate of oxidation of glucose, this is determined by the rate of turnover of ATP and also by the presence of other fuels that compete with glucose for oxidation. The oxidation of other fuels (e.g., fatty acids in muscles, ketoacids in the brain) to regenerate ATP will inhibit flux through PDH (see Fig. 5–2) and thus decrease the complete oxidation of glucose. As pointed out by Halperin and associates[3] from their analysis of the data of Atchley and colleagues[15] in a patient with insulin-dependent diabetes mellitus who had his insulin held for 4 days, only 40 g of glucose was oxidized on day 3 of insulin deprivation. Thus, it seems that when ketoacids are present, they are oxidized in preference to glucose by the brain even during states where hyperglycemia is present.

Glucosuria represents the major route for removal of glucose in patients with hyperglycemia.[3] If the filtered load of glucose exceeds its maximum rate of reabsorption of about 325 g/day (1800 mmol/day), glucosuria should be present. With a normal GFR of 180 L/day, glucosuria occurs when the concentration of glucose in plasma exceeds its renal threshold (180 mg/dL, 10 mmol/L).[30] Reducing the GFR will have a considerable quantitative impact on the degree of hyperglycemia. For example, consider a subject who has a blood glucose level of 500 mg/dL (27.8 mmol/L) and a GFR of 150 L/day and who stays in balance with a daily input and excretion of glucose of 425 g. If the input of glucose remains constant but the GFR declines to 100 and then 50 L/day, glycemia would increase to 750 mg/dL (40 mmol/L) and 1500 mg/dL (82.5 mmol/L), respectively. Similarly, during therapy in a patient with a significant contraction of the ECF volume, which is the usual clinical setting in a patient with DKA, a significant reduction in glycemia would occur with the re-expansion of the ECF volume and the expected increase in GFR even without any metabolic effects of insulin.[3]

# CLINICAL CONDITIONS WHERE KETOACIDS ACCUMULATE

DKA is the metabolic consequence of a lack of insulin and a rise in hormone levels with actions that oppose those of insulin (e.g., glucagon, adrenaline, cortisol, adrenocorticotropic hormone, growth hormone, thyroid hormone). It is characterized by the accumulation of a large quantity of glucose and ketoacids in the body. Due to hyperglycemia, there is an excessive renal excretion of glucose, water, and electrolytes. The metabolic acidosis is usually accompanied by strongly positive clinical tests for ketones and the appearance of new anions in the plasma or urine. DKA is the mode of presentation of some previously undiagnosed diabetics, but more often it occurs in patients with known insulin-dependent diabetes mellitus. The precipitating causes include failure to take insulin, an intercurrent illness, or other situations where counter-regulatory hormones may be present in excess (e.g., thyrotoxicosis, hyperadrenocorticism, acromegaly, pregnancy, and surgery). In addition, emotional and psychological upheaval may precipitate episodes of DKA, especially in children. More rarely, DKA can occur in the older patient with non–insulin-dependent diabetes mellitus, especially if drugs such as phenytoin (Dilantin) or thiazide diuretics lead to inhibited release of insulin. There is also often a decreased metabolism of ketoacids due to impaired level of consciousness and a greatly decreased GFR.

Most of the clinical manifestations of DKA are readily explained as the expected consequences of major biochemical changes. Thus, because of hyperglycemia and the resultant osmotic diuresis, the patient presents with a variable duration of thirst, polydipsia, polyuria, weakness, lethargy, and malaise. The blood pressure may be low and postural hypotension, tachycardia, and reduced jugular venous pressure are often found. The metabolic acidosis results in an increased rate and depth of breathing (Kussmaul respiration). The conversion of H·AcAc to acetone imparts the characteristic fruity odor to the breath. The severe acidemia may also have a negative inotropic effect on the heart and has been implicated as a cause of peripheral vasodilatation, both of which can aggravate the hypotension from ECF volume contraction.

Not all the clinical findings, however, are completely explained in terms of the biochemical aberrations. Anorexia, nausea, vomiting, and abdominal pain are frequent, whereas nonspecific gastrointestinal complaints are more common in children. These symptoms together with abdominal tenderness, decreased bowel sounds, guarding, and leukocytosis may be so severe as to mimic an acute abdominal emergency. Rebound tenderness is usually (but not universally) absent, and the presence of glycosuria and ketonemia should signal the correct diagnosis. The cause for the abdominal pain is not entirely clear, but in some cases it may be related to hypertriglyceridemia. Some degree of drowsiness is common, but coma is seen in fewer than 10% of patients with DKA. The state of consciousness does not correlate well with the concentration of ketoacids in plasma. A much better correlation has been found between the level of stupor and coma and the serum osmolality.[31] Focal neurologic signs or seizures should not be attributed to ketoacidosis. Another feature of DKA that remains unexplained is hypothermia, even in the presence of infection. Therefore, the absence of fever and the usual presence of leukocytosis lead to difficulty in diagnosing infection. The signs and symptoms of any precipitating disorder should be appreciated; in fact, these may dominate the clinical picture. Life-threatening issues include hyperkalemia, hemodynamic collapse, the precipitating illness, and rarely, the accumulation of $H^+$.

**Factors Unique to AKA.** AKA is also the metabolic consequence of a lack of insulin, but its basis is that the α-adrenergic action inhibits the release of insulin.[32] It is not essential for ethanol to be present at the time of diagnosis of AKA. AKA is characterized by the accumulation of large quantities of ketoacids, but hyperglycemia is not a prominent feature; in fact, it might not even be present as long as ethanol metabolism inhibits hepatic glucose production. Therefore, polyuria is not a usual presenting feature. One unique feature of AKA is the prominence of multiple episodes of vomiting. The usual reason for this is alcoholic gastritis. As the vomiting becomes protracted, the ECF volume becomes even more contracted than in DKA. Because of the absence of severe acidemia (a combination of metabolic acidosis and metabolic alkalosis due to vomiting), Kussmaul respiration may not be seen. Acetone is not detected on the breath because of the low concentration of H·AcAc (most of the ketoacids are in the form of H·β-HB). The major threats to life are hemodynamic collapse, a much larger deficiency of $K^+$ causing a severe degree of hypokalemia, and specific problems related to ethanol such as central nervous system depression, aspiration pneumonitis, alcohol withdrawal, or a deficiency of thiamine.

## Laboratory Evaluation

**Glucose.** The degree of hyperglycemia varies markedly in patients with DKA and usually exceeds 250 mg/dL (14 mmol/L). Higher values can be seen if there is a marked reduction in the GFR or if the patient has consumed a large quantity of carbohydrate.[3] If the ECF volume is very contracted, not only will there be an exaggerated degree of hyperglycemia, but also glycosuria may be reduced considerably because the filtered load of glucose may not exceed the tubular capacity to reabsorb it.

***Factors Unique to AKA.*** There is often a much less severe degree of hyperglycemia. This is usually attributed to inhibition of gluconeogenesis by the products of ethanol metabolism.

**Ketosis.** In DKA, serum ketones are usually strongly positive up to a dilution of 1 in 8. However, only H·AcAc and acetone yield a positive reaction with the clinical screening test for ketoacids (e.g., nitroprusside test). If there is an increase in the NADH-to-$NAD^+$ ratio as occurs with hypoxia, ketoacids will be almost exclusively in the form of H·β-HB, which is not detected by these clinical tests; a specific enzymatic analysis will be necessary to confirm the presence of H·β-HB.[33] Rarely, ketonemia can be less evident in patients with DKA if the ketoacid anions are being excreted in the urine.[34] In this case, a hyperchloremic type of metabolic acidosis will be present and excessive excretion of ketoacid anions can be detected by finding new anions in the urine (the rate of excretion of major urine cations [$Na^+$ + $K^+$ + $NH_4^+$] is significantly higher than that of $Cl^-$). Conversely, screening tests for ketoacids in the urine may reveal low or undetectable levels in patients with DKA and a very contracted ECF volume, because the filtered load of ketoacid anions may be very low when the GFR falls. The poor delivery of oxygen will result in the conversion of H·AcAc to H·β-HB. Therefore, if serum ketones are only weakly positive, one should perform a direct assay for H·β-HB and, if there is no significant increase in the anion gap in plasma, examine the urine for ketoacid anions by calculating the urine anion[35] and osmolar gaps.[36–38]

***Factors Unique to AKA.*** The very low ECF volume causes insulin deficiency because of the high levels of α-adrenergics. The latter leads to ketoacidosis (i.e., a rise in the plasma anion gap and a fall in plasma bicarbonate). Ketoacids accumulate for two major reasons—an increase in their production (low insulin) and a decrease in their removal rate (sedative effect of ethanol and the low GFR). Because of the oxidation of ethanol and the high NADH-to-$NAD^+$ ratio, the predominant form of acid released is H·β-HB; this accounts for the weakly positive clinical test result for these ketoacids (i.e., a low acetoacetate level). Typically, the concentration of $HCO_3^-$ in plasma may not be very different from normal, reflecting a process that elevates it (metabolic alkalosis due to vomiting) and another process that lowers it (metabolic acidosis).

**Plasma [$Na^+$].** In adults, it is common to observe a low plasma [$Na^+$] due to hyperglycemia. In children, hyperglycemia tends to be less severe and the plasma [$Na^+$] may not be low despite the presence of hyperglycemia.[39] The two major causes of hyponatremia are: (1) the movement of water primarily from muscle cells into the ECF compartment due to hyperglycemia, and (2) the reduced ability to excrete ingested water because vasopressin is released in response to a contracted ECF volume. In quantitative terms, the plasma [$Na^+$] should fall 1 mmol/L for every 72-mg/dL (4-mmol/L) rise in glucose in blood above normal providing that glucose was added without water.[40] If hyponatremia does not accompany hyperglycemia, the intake of water was probably low due to impaired thirst, a decreased ability to obtain or ingest water (e.g., coma), a shift of water into cells due to the development of mild rhabdomyolysis, or the presence of nephrogenic diabetes insipidus.

***Factors Unique to AKA.*** Because hyperglycemia is not as important in AKA, there is less hyponatremia for this reason. Hyponatremia now reflects the large intake of water with ethanol in the face of vasopressin release due to the low ECF volume, stress, and nausea and/or vomiting.

**Plasma [$K^+$].** Even though the plasma [$K^+$] is usually in the 5.5 mmol/L range because $K^+$ has shifted from the ICF to the ECF compartment due to the lack of insulin, there is almost always a decrease in the total body content of $K^+$. The principal reason for this loss of $K^+$ is the glucose-induced osmotic diuresis. Typically, the urine [$K^+$] is close to 30 mmol/L on admission.[3] Additional loss of $K^+$ can occur because of vomiting, diarrhea, or if an ileus was present.

***Factors Unique to AKA.*** In AKA, the deficit of $K^+$ is large and the plasma [$K^+$] might be in the hypokalemic range due to renal loss of $K^+$ or a shift of $K^+$ into cells if metabolic alkalosis predominates. The presence of normal or elevated plasma [$K^+$] may alert the clinician to the presence of rhabdomyolysis.

**Acid-Base.** The plasma [$HCO_3^-$] is reduced because H·β-HB and H·AcAc were added to the ECF compartment. The data in Table 5–2 depict a fall in the plasma [$HCO_3^-$] that is equal to the rise in anion gap in patients with DKA. Nevertheless, there was a component of "indirect" loss of $NaHCO_3$ that is not revealed by the 1:1 ratio of the rise in the plasma anion gap and the decline in the plasma [$HCO_3^-$] because of the contraction in the ECF volume. An indirect loss of $NaHCO_3$ occurs when $H^+$ of H·β-HB convert $HCO_3^-$ to $CO_2 + H_2O$ and the β-$HB^-$ anions are excreted in the urine as their $Na^+$ salts (Fig. 5–7). Accordingly, after 12 hours of successful therapy with a re-expanded ECF volume, hyperchloremic metabolic acidosis will usually be evident (plasma $HCO_3^-$ 16 to 18 mmol/L and a normal value for the anion gap).

**TABLE 5–2.** Extracellular Fluid Bicarbonate and Organic Anion Data in Diabetic Ketoacidosis*

| | | Value (mEq/L) | | |
|---|---|---|---|---|
| | | *Time (hr) after Therapy Started* | | |
| **Parameter** | **Normal Values** | *0* | *12–24* | *48+* |
| ECF volume | 14 | 11 | 14 | 14 |
| [$HCO_3^-$] | 24 | 6 | 16 | 24 |
| [Organic anion] | 1 | 19 | 1 | 1 |
| ECF $HCO_3^-$ content | 336 | 66 | 224 | 336 |
| ECF OA content | 14 | 209 | 14 | 14 |
| ECF $HCO_3^-$ + OA contents | 350 | 275 | 238 | 350 |

*All units are expressed in mEq/L, except for extracellular fluid (ECF), which is in liters. The ECF content of $HCO_3^-$ is the product of the concentration of $HCO_3^-$ and the ECF volume. The ECF organic anion content is the product of the sum of β-HB, AcAc, and L-lactate concentrations multiplied by the ECF volume. Despite the fact that the fall in $HCO_3^-$ concentration was equal to the rise in organic anion concentration, their contents were very different due to the change in ECF volume. The sum of ECF $HCO_3^-$ plus organic anion contents represents the total $HCO_3^-$ in the ECF after therapy. The fact that this content decreased after 12 to 24 hours probably reflects $H^+$ movement into the ECF from the ICF as the ECF pH rises.

OA, organic anions.

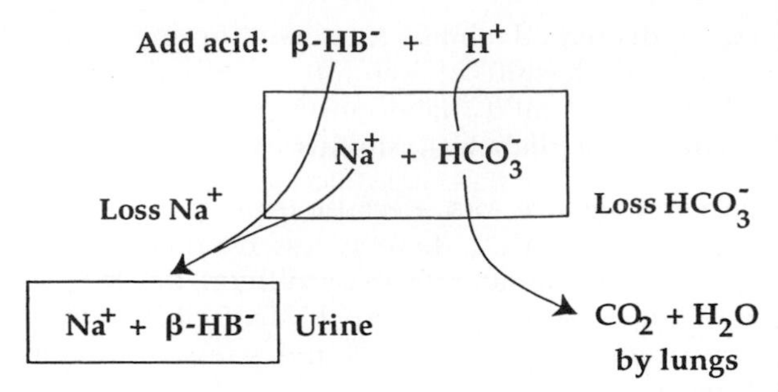


**FIGURE 5–7** ■ Indirect loss of $NaHCO_3$. The *rectangle* depicts the body, and it contains $Na^+ + HCO_3^-$ ions. When H·AβHB is added, its $H^+$ are removed by reacting with $HCO_3^-$. The lungs exhale the resultant $CO_2$. The anion βHB is excreted along with $Na^+$ for electroneutrality. This excretion occurs when the urine contains more βHB than $NH_4^+$; thus it is more prominent when $NH_4^+$ excretion is low.

There is a predictable degree of hypocapnia depending on the degree of metabolic acidosis. Because hypothermia may occur in patients with DKA, one should take this into consideration when interpreting the values reported by the laboratory, because the measurements are made at 37°C.

The arterial $Po_2$ should be elevated owing to the low arterial $Pco_2$. A large increase in the alveolar-arterial $Po_2$ difference may indicate that intrinsic lung disease is present, but it often represents the usual or increased admixture of venous blood that has a very low $Po_2$.[27] The lower the oxygen content of admixed blood, the greater is the decline in the arterial $Po_2$ if it is close to 100 mm Hg because of the shape of the oxyhemoglobin dissociation curve.[27]

***Factors Unique to AKA.*** In AKA, the concentration of $HCO_3^-$ in plasma is often much higher because of the high prevalence of vomiting. In these patients, the anion gap may be increased greatly.[41]

**Blood Urea Nitrogen (BUN) and Creatinine Level in Plasma.** Patients with DKA and AKA have a contracted ECF volume and thus a significant reduction in their GFR. Therefore, the concentrations of urea and creatinine in plasma are elevated. The BUN or urea is also influenced by other factors, such as protein intake, tissue catabolism, rate of gluconeogenesis, and the urine flow rate; thus it is less reliable as an index of the GFR. There are problems with the creatinine assay in DKA depending on the method used. Higher values are reported with the picric acid method if the level of H·AcAc is elevated,[42] whereas lower values are reported with severe hyperglycemia if the enzymatic assay for creatinine is performed on the Kodak analyzer.[43]

**Serum Phosphorus.** The presence of a deficiency of phosphorus in DKA has been known for several decades.[44] Like $K^+$, the concentration of phosphate in the plasma is usually in the normal range on presentation with DKA despite the marked total body deficit. This deficit becomes evident as very severe hypophosphatemia develops once insulin acts.

## Treatment

DKA and AKA are medical emergencies that demand urgent treatment. A general approach to treatment could be made on the basis of threats to the patient's life as they appear during the course of treatment of DKA (Table 5–3). Treatment is divided into considerations of fluid and electrolytes, insulin, $NaHCO_3$, the predisposing factors, and the avoidance of complications.

### Sodium

***Principle.*** The number of particles restricted to the ECF compartment determines its volume. These ECF solutes are usually $Na^+$ and its matching anions, $Cl^-$, $HCO_3^-$, and in these cases ketoacid and possibly L-lactate anions. In DKA and to a lesser extent in AKA, hyperglycemia contributes to defense of the ECF volume.

***Quantities.*** Two points are emphasized.

1. *Units:* Because DKA is most common and a potentially devastating illness in children, we shall discuss quantities in mmol $Na^+$ per kg body weight terms so that values will be similar to those in adults. A simple example of a 50-kg non-obese person with 60% body water helps to illustrate this point. The total body water is 30 L (60% of weight) and 1/3 or 10 L of this volume are in the ECF compartment. With plasma $[Na^+]$ of 140 mmol/L, the total content of $Na^+$ in the ECF is 1400 mmol. Therefore, the normal value is approximately 30 mmol $Na^+$ per kg body weight. Accordingly, a 10% reduction in the ECF volume will be a deficit of 3 mmol $Na^+$/kg body weight. To replace this with isotonic saline,

**TABLE 5–3.** Potential Causes of Death During Diabetic Ketoacidosis

| Cause | Time | Treatment |
|---|---|---|
| • Hyperkalemia-induced cardiac arrhythmia | • Admission | • Insulin |
| • Aspiration | • While CNS depressed<br>• Dilated stomach | • Intubation, NG suction, position, antibiotics |
| • Hypokalemia | • 2 hr or more after insulin is given | • KCl to yield $[K^+]$ of 4 mmol/L |
| • Relative hypoglycemia | • 6–8 hr later | • Give IV $D_5W$ once glucose falls to 250 mg/dL (14 mmol/L) |
| • Underlying lesion and complications | • All times | • Specific measures |

CNS, central nervous system; IV, intravenous; NE, nasogastric.

**TABLE 5–4.** Typical Deficits in a Patient with Diabetic Ketoacidosis

| | Quantity | Comment | Danger |
|---|---|---|---|
| • $Na^+$<br>• $K^+$ | • 3–9 mmol/kg<br>• 4–6 mmol/kg | • Restore $Na^+$ deficit, but not too quickly<br>• Must await insulin action to shift $K^+$ into cells<br>• Examine plasma [$K^+$] | • Cerebral edema if early and too rapid<br>• Initial hyperkalemia<br>• >1.5 hr, hypokalemia |
| • Water<br>• Bicarbonate | • Usually many liters<br>• Can be >500 mmol of $H^+$ buffered | • Half ICF, half ECF<br>• If increased anion gap, need not give bicarbonate unless *very* severe acidosis | • Do not repair water deficit too early<br>• Strong opinions held, but not backed up with clean data |

one simply calculates how many milliliters of 150 mmol $Na^+$ per liter contains 3 mmol of $Na^+$ (1/50 of 1 L or 20 mL) and multiply by body weight. Therefore, the patient should receive 20 mL isotonic saline per kg body weight when one wants to replace a deficit of 3 mmol of $Na^+$ per kg body weight.

2. *The deficit of "effective particles" in the ECF compartment:* Hyperglycemia minimizes the degree of ECF volume contraction that would have resulted from the deficit of $Na^+$. This must be taken into consideration when glycemia falls with therapy.

***Target for Therapy.*** The target for therapy is to replace the deficit of $Na^+$. In most patients with DKA, this is reported to be 3 to 9 mmol $Na^+$/kg body weight (10% to 30% of the ECF $Na^+$ content) (Table 5–4). Nevertheless, two additional facts are important. First, the deficit of $Na^+$ in the ECF compartment early on is made less serious because of the degree of hyperglycemia as discussed earlier. Second, because approximately 50% of the deficit of $K^+$ is due to a gain of cations (mainly $Na^+$) in the ICF compartment,[44] the deficit of $Na^+$ in the body is less severe than the actual deficit in the ECF compartment. With a deficit of $K^+$ of 4 to 6 mmol/kg in DKA, the $Na^+$ deficit in the body is likely to be overestimated by an analysis restricted to the ECF compartment. Accordingly, the target for replacement of $Na^+$ in the ECF compartment should be met in part by giving KCl, with $K^+$ entering and $Na^+$ exiting the ICF compartment *after* insulin acts.

***Rate of Replacement of the Deficit of $Na^+$.*** The issue here is the need to restore systemic hemodynamics bearing in mind the risk of development of cerebral edema; this complication is predominantly seen in children treated for DKA (see later). Our advice is to use clinical judgment. Very aggressive therapy is indicated only if the patient is hemodynamically compromised. In the face of frank hypotension, we would give 3 mmol $Na^+$ (20 mL isotonic saline) per kg body weight over 30 to 60 minutes depending on the degree of hypotension. This aggressive therapy would be continued only as long as the hemodynamic threat was present. When the evidence for a significant hemodynamic compromise is not present, the rate of administration of $Na^+$ should be much slower. The upper limit for $Na^+$ administration should be the expected deficit of $Na^+$ (3 to 9 mmol/kg, see Table 5–4) together with the replacement of ongoing losses (glucosuria-induced loss of close to 2 mmol $Na^+$/kg body weight). This replacement should occur in the first 12 hours. Moreover, most of the $K^+$ that is retained will reduce the need for $Na^+$ from an ECF volume and $Na^+$ content point of view.

***Dangers of Giving $Na^+$ Rapidly.*** This is a major clinical concern in the young child with DKA because of the danger of inducing cerebral edema. The issue is that a rapid bolus of saline distributes initially in the blood volume. The plasma volume is 60% of the blood volume and is close to 25 mL/kg. It is easy to imagine that giving "albumin-free saline" at a very rapid rate can lower the colloid osmotic pressure and raise the hydrostatic pressure in blood delivered to the brain on first pass. Moreover, with a BBB that may not be intact,[45, 46] there is a distinct danger of raising the ECF volume of the brain acutely by this treatment (Fig. 5–8). Therefore, timing of saline administration, the volume infused, and the cardiac output at that moment all contribute to this potential danger in the first 30 to 60 minutes of therapy.

***Clinical Practice.*** It may seem surprising, but there is little excretion of $Na^+$ when the ECF volume is reexpanded in the first 24 hours. Hence if more $Na^+$ is given than needed, an expanded ECF volume is likely

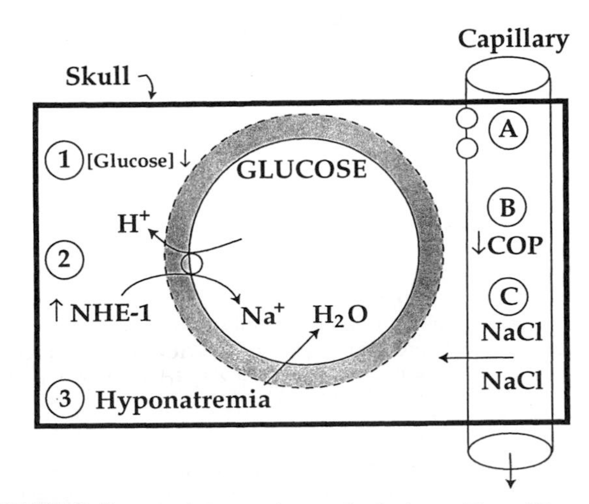


**FIGURE 5–8** ■ Risk factors for cerebral edema. The *solid rectangle* represents the skull. The three risk factors for swelling of brain cells are shown on the left and include a higher concentration of glucose or its metabolites in the brain due to rapid lowering of the blood glucose level (site 1), activation of the $Na^+$:$H^+$ exchanger-1 (NHE-1) by insulin (site 2), and the development of hyponatremia (site 3). The factors causing expansion of the extracellular fluid volume are shown on the right and could be the result of a less restrictive blood-brain barrier (site A), a fall in the colloid osmotic pressure (COP) in plasma (site B), or the excessive administration of saline (site C).

to develop. For example, in a recent chart review of patients who had a serious degree of DKA, the total amount of $Na^+$ given was 25 mmol $Na^+$ per kg body weight.[47] Surely these patients had not lost 80% of their ECF volume prior to therapy. Therefore, if this experience mirrors that in the community, far too much saline is being given to treat patients with DKA.

***Unique Aspects for AKA.*** The patients with AKA often need more aggressive therapy with saline to defend their hemodynamics.

**Water**

***Principle.*** To avoid swelling of cells in the first 12 hours of therapy, the aim of therapy should be to prevent a fall in the "effective osmolality" of plasma ($2 \times [Na^+]$ + glucose [mmol/L]).

***Quantities.*** The usual deficit of water in a patient with a relatively severe degree of DKA is 100 mL/kg body weight. Approximately half of this deficit is in the ECF compartment. Two factors help explain this redistribution. First, the deficit of isotonic saline is entirely from the ECF compartment. Second, there was a shift of water from the ICF to the ECF compartment due both to hyperglycemia and the loss of osmoles from the ICF compartment ($K^+$ + phosphate[44]).

***Target for Therapy.*** To keep the "effective osmolality" of the ECF compartment constant, the target for the plasma $[Na^+]$ is the current plasma $[Na^+]$ plus one half of the expected fall in glycemia. The plasma glucose concentration should fall close to 5.5 mmol/L (100 mg/dL) per hour until it reaches 15 mmol/L (270 mg/dL) (Table 5–5) at which time glucose is usually infused to prevent a further fall in glycemia.

***Implications for Therapy.*** There is not usually a problem with this strategy in adults with DKA because hyponatremia is the usual consequence of hyperglycemia. In children with a severe degree of hyperglycemia (900 mg/dL, 50 mmol/L), the plasma $[Na^+]$ is higher—approximately 140 mmol/L[39, 47] compared with that of adults (126 mmol/L).[40] Therefore, the target for the plasma $[Na^+]$ is to raise it by one half of the fall in glycemia (50 to 15 mmol/L) or by 17 mmol/L in this example. Thus, in adults the target value is 143 mmol/L, whereas it is 157 mmol/L in the child with this blood glucose level. Although nephrologists may be uncomfortable about this degree of hypernatremia, it is the necessary "price to pay" to avoid a fall in the "effective" osmolality of plasma.

**TABLE 5–5.** Anticipated Results of Therapy for Diabetic Ketoacidosis

| | |
|---|---|
| Glucose: | • Will fall 5.5 mmol/L (100 mg/dL) over each of the first 6 hours; reasons for fall are dilution (early), glucosuria (mid-time), and metabolism (late) |
| Sodium: | • Rise in the plasma $[Na^+]$ of 1.4 mmol/L per 100 mg/dL (5.5 mmol/L) decline in glycemia owing to a shift of water into the ECF |
| Potassium: | • Sudden fall over 1–2 hours owing to shift of $K^+$ into cells when insulin acts<br>• The best early indicator of the biologic actions of insulin |
| Bicarbonate: | • Will not rise for several hours<br>• Concentration of bicarbonate close to 16–18 mmol/L once ketoacidosis largely disappears (6 to 8 hours later) |
| Ketoacids: | • Slow, steady decline over 8 hours to 1 mmol/L range<br>• The quick test may actually become more positive, despite less ketoacidosis owing to conversion of H·β-HB to H·AcAc. |
| Anion gap: | • Fall in parallel with ketoacids; returns to normal in 8–12 hours |
| Complications: | • See Table 5–6 |

ECF, extracellular fluid.

***Clinical Practice.*** Although many think that it is advisable to use half-isotonic saline early in therapy because of the hyperosmolar state, we think that it is more important to defend the "effective osmolality" in plasma with isotonic saline initially. Part of our reasoning is that the contribution of glucose to the high osmolality will be reversed by metabolism of glucose. Restoration of the ICF volume must await the synthesis of organic phosphate and the administration of a sufficient amount of $K^+$ so that the need for electrolyte-free water occurs after the emergency therapy. We use half-isotonic saline when the plasma $[Na^+]$ rises above our target value for the plasma $[Na^+]$. It is appropriate to replace large losses of urine with hypotonic saline[3] and to accommodate KCl (or $NaHCO_3$) administration (add KCl or $NaHCO_3$ to hypotonic saline to keep solutions close to isotonic body fluids). This caution against hypotonic saline is particularly important in children to avoid a fall in the effective plasma osmolality (see the section on cerebral edema).

**Potassium**

***Principle.*** $K^+$ is the principle cation in the ICF compartment. It is retained in cells by an electrical-negative voltage created ultimately by the $Na^+$, $K^+$, and ATPase. This voltage is diminished in an insulin-deficient state so that there is a redistribution of $K^+$ from the ICF to the ECF compartment in DKA. Nevertheless, there is a total body deficit of $K^+$ due to enhanced renal loss of $K^+$ in the osmotic diuresis.

***Quantities.*** There is a deficit of $K^+$ in the ICF in DKA of 4 to 6 mmol/kg body weight (see Table 5–4). Approximately half of this deficit of $K^+$ is due to catabolism (largely a decrease in organic phosphate (+ $K^+$) in RNA).[44] The other half of the deficit of $K^+$ is accompanied by a gain of $Na^+$ and $H^+$ in the ICF compartment.

***Target for Therapy.*** The objective is to keep the plasma $[K^+]$ in the 4 to 5 mmol/L range. That portion of the deficit of $K^+$ that was due to catabolism of RNA cannot be replaced until anabolism has occurred. Therefore, in the first day of therapy, the expectation is to replace only half of the deficit of $K^+$.

***Rate of Therapy.*** The actual rate of administration of KCl is dictated by subsequent plasma $[K^+]$. $K^+$ should not be given until the plasma [$K^+$] falls below 5 mmol/L. We do not place much value on the urine flow rate for this decision because the urine $K^+$ loss/min is tiny. Even with a urine output of 100 mL/hr, because the urine [$K^+$] is approximately 30 mmol/L, the loss of $K^+$ is only 3 mmol/hr. Compare this value with the $K^+$ deficit of approximately 300 mmol or a rate of infusion of $K^+$ that might be 30 mmol/hr between 2 and 6 hours of therapy. The highest KCl concentration that is usually infused is 40 mmol/L of intravenous (IV) fluid in a peripheral vein. Add KCl to half-isotonic saline if the "effective osmolality" of plasma is higher than you want it to be.

***Dangers of Therapy.*** The main danger is the development of hypokalemia once insulin acts (1 to 2 hours after giving insulin) and when anabolism occurs (several days later). At all times, there is a danger of hyperkalemia. This is the earliest sign that insulin is no longer acting if an excessive amount of $K^+$ was not given. More caution is needed if there is renal failure.

***Unique Aspects for AKA.*** Hypokalemia is a common finding in patients with alcohol intoxication.[21] When $K^+$ shifted from in the ICF into the ECF compartment, electroneutrality was maintained. This could be achieved if the $K^+$ were lost from the ICF along with intracellular anions (phosphate), or if $K^+$ are exchanged for extracellular cations ($Na^+$ or $H^+$). To the extent that there is a net shift of $K^+$ for $H^+$, the degree of intracellular acidosis will become more severe.[28]

**Insulin**

***Principles.*** The lack of insulin and rise in hormones with counter-insulin actions led to the hyperglycemia and ketoacidosis. This was also the cause of the hyperkalemia. The major acute effect that reflects insulin action during therapy is a fall in the plasma [$K^+$]. The initial fall in glycemia is due to dilution (saline infusion) and possibly glucosuria.[48] Correction of acidosis and a fall in serum ketones does not occur promptly. Low-dose short-acting insulin regimens are now used most commonly. Given the uncertainty of complete and rapid absorption with other routes, we recommend the IV route of administration. The typical dose is 0.1 U/kg as an IV bolus, followed by a constant infusion of 0.1 U/kg/hr. We do *not* give a bolus of insulin in children (see section on Cerebral Edema).

Insulin therapy has potentially detrimental effects that should be anticipated and monitored, including hypokalemia, hypophosphatemia and eventually hypoglycemia. Given that hypokalemia is also a significant risk with bicarbonate therapy, if a patient presents with a low plasma [$K^+$] and acidemia severe enough to require $NaHCO_3$, one could make a case for withholding insulin therapy for an hour or so until sufficient bicarbonate and $K^+$ has been administered. On the surface this may seem inadvisable. Nevertheless, because the rate of ketoacid production minus its removal by oxidation in the brain and kidneys is less than 1 mmol/minute, withholding insulin will not have a major acid-base impact because more $NaHCO_3$ than this is given to treat life-threatening acidemia.

When the concentration of glucose in plasma falls below 250 mg/dL (14 mmol/L), glucose should be added to the infusate either as 5% dextrose in water or in 0.45% saline (depending on the status of the ECF and ICF volumes). Further fluid therapy is determined by the clinical assessment, biochemical measurements, and calculated losses.

***Unique Aspects for AKA.*** We would not give insulin at the outset to patients with AKA.[21] Our reasoning is that hypokalemia is a major danger, hyperglycemia is not an acute medical emergency, and there is not usually an acid-base emergency. Later, hypoglycemia may become a problem. Finally, those patients with normal β cells will release insulin once the ECF volume is re-expanded and the α-adrenergic inhibition of insulin release is removed.

**Acid-Base.** If a patient has inadequate respiratory compensation, they should be treated first with ventilatory support. Therapy with $NaHCO_3$ is only indicated if acidosis is life threatening (plasma $HCO_3^-$ <4 mmol/L). There is no need to raise the plasma [$HCO_3^-$] more than twofold because this will raise the pH 0.3 U if the $P_{CO_2}$ does not rise. Once the plasma [$HCO_3^-$] rises twofold or approaches 8 mmol/L the infusion of $NaHCO_3$ should stop. Severe hyperkalemia is a possible indication for the use of $NaHCO_3$. At least in theory, consideration should be given to use $NaHCO_3$ initially in patients with less severe acidosis who have a decreased ability to oxidize ketoacids, such as those who are comatose and have a low GFR. After ketoacidosis has been successfully treated, patients with a persistent hyperchloremic metabolic acidosis owing to a low rate of excretion of $NH_4^+$ may require $NaHCO_3$.

***Unique Aspects for AKA.*** By considering buffering in the ICF compartment (see Fig. 5–6), it becomes evident that the aggressive administration of isotonic saline and the replacement of part of the $K^+$ deficit would go a long way toward restoring the appropriate charge on intracellular proteins.

Thiamine deficiency merits emphasis; this nutritional deficit is more commonly seen in the chronic alcoholic, and it will compromise PDH activity. In more detail, when the ECF volume is re-expanded, insulin levels rise, and now brain cells become dependent on glucose (instead of ketoacid) oxidation to regenerate their requisite ATP. These effects of thiamine deficiency will be most felt in cells with the highest rate of turnover of ATP or those most easily depleted of thiamine. Thus, there is a danger to these cells due to $H^+$ accumulation or a lack of ATP when ketoacids are no longer available. In therapy, the only extra additional aspect is to add thiamine to the first IV bottle if there is a suspicion of thiamine deficiency.

**Cerebral Edema.** Cerebral edema is a dreaded complication of DKA, because it is responsible for at least 50% of the mortality in children who present with DKA.[49, 50] In addition, children with cerebral edema who survive may be left with significant dysfunction. Even those who seem to be intact may have subtle cognitive and behavioral deficits.

Cerebral edema is the result of a rise in brain ICF and ECF volumes and intracranial pressure because of the fixed volume of the skull.[50] Cerebral edema occurs most commonly 5 to 15 hours after initiating treatment for DKA. Cerebral edema is suspected when there is an unanticipated decline in brain function with signs of drowsiness, irritability, decreased level of consciousness, or focal neurologic deficits. Computed tomography (CT) or magnetic resonance imaging confirms the diagnosis. The pathophysiology of cerebral edema is considered under the following two headings (see Fig. 5–8).

***Factors Related to an Expansion of the ECF Compartment of the Brain.*** These factors include a less restrictive BBB, volume and timing of the saline infusion, and a decline in the colloid osmotic pressure of plasma. There is evidence of subclinical cerebral edema before therapy is instituted when CT scans of the brain are taken.[51] This is likely to be the result of a less restrictive BBB that permits the intracranial ECF volume to increase, effectively bypassing the protective mechanisms that normally exist to prevent this type of fluctuation in intracranial pressure. The second factor is the infusion of IV saline. Two aspects are important to consider in this regard. First, if a bolus is given initially, it will be distributed on first pass in the blood volume and cause a sudden rise in hydrostatic pressure and a fall in the colloid osmotic pressure. Hence, Starling forces and a less restrictive BBB could act in concert to expand the volume of the intracerebral ECF compartment further. A large bolus of saline has been associated with an increased risk of developing cerebral edema.[49] To minimize this risk, a bolus of saline should NOT be given unless there is frank hemodynamic collapse in children with DKA. A third possible factor is a fall in colloid osmotic pressure due to a decrease in the Donnan force in plasma. This could be the result of a less anionic charge on albumin due to rapid reexpansion of the ECF volume.[41, 47]

***Factors Associated with a Rise in Brain Cell Volume.*** There are three factors to consider, a fall in the effective osmolality of plasma ($P_{Osm}$), a rise in intracellular osmoles (insulin bolus), and the development of hyponatremia (see Fig. 5–8). Treatment regimens that have been associated with cerebral edema usually cause important changes in "effective" $P_{Osm}$ (Equation 8).

$$\text{Effective } P_{Osm} = 2 \times [Na^+]_{plasma} + \text{glucose (mmol/L)} \quad \text{(glucose mg/dL/18)} \qquad \text{(Equation 8)}$$

A rapid fall in glycemia may predispose to cerebral edema by allowing the shift of electrolyte-free water from the intravascular space (a compartment with a decreasing osmolality) into brain cells (a compartment with an osmolality that decreases less rapidly). There is evidence to suggest that maintaining a constant "effective" $P_{Osm}$ at the expense of hypernatremia may protect against cerebral edema.[47] This can be accomplished by permitting the plasma [$Na^+$] to rise by half the fall in glycemia in mmol/L terms (see Equation 8), thus keeping the "effective" $P_{Osm}$ constant. For example, when the plasma glucose concentration falls by 30 mmol/L (540 mg/dL), the plasma [$Na^+$] would have to rise to 155 mmol/L (an increase of 15 mmol/L) to keep the "effective" $P_{Osm}$ constant. To achieve this aim, the IV solutions must be isotonic and NOT hypotonic saline.

Second, one should avoid an initial bolus of insulin, because it may cause an increase in the number of intracellular particles in the brain.[51] In more detail, insulin activates the $Na^+$-$H^+$ exchanger in the cell membrane. By causing an increase in the entry of $Na^+$ into brain cells along with the exit of $H^+$ that were bound to intracellular proteins (see Fig. 5–8), there will be a net increase in intraneuronal osmolality, favoring water movement into cells of the brain. As a partial compensation for the hypertonic plasma of a patient with DKA, the brain accumulated osmoles such as sorbitol, fructose, taurine, and glutamine that minimize the degree of shift of water across brain cells. Once the intravascular osmolality falls, however, these osmoles cannot be removed rapidly from the brain and attract electrolyte-free water and thus contribute to cerebral edema.[52]

## Issues for Therapy

The initial saline infusion should be targeted to avoid circulatory collapse. We would not otherwise give a bolus of saline. An example of the rate of saline administration is 3 mmol of NaCl/kg (20 mL isotonic saline per kg) over 90 minutes. Once the patient is hemodynamically stable, the $Na^+$ deficit should be replaced slowly, with an upper limit of 6 to 9 mmol/kg depending on the initial clinical impression of the degree of ECF volume contraction (a crude guess). In children, we would only use isotonic saline to avoid a fall in the "effective" $P_{Osm}$. The target value for the plasma [$Na^+$] in the first 5 to 15 hours is that which keeps a constant "effective" $P_{Osm}$. We would *not* give a bolus of insulin to treat DKA in children.

If signs of cerebral edema did develop, hypertonic saline or mannitol should be infused rapidly to reverse cerebral edema by drawing water out of the brain. Our aim would be to increase the "effective" $P_{Osm}$ by 10 mOsm/kg $H_2O$ (administer 10 mmol of mannitol or 5

**TABLE 5–6.** Complications to Avoid During Therapy

| |
|---|
| On admission |
| Peripheral hypoperfusion |
| Aspiration pneumonitis |
| Thrombotic episodes |
| Hyperkalemia with cardiac arrhythmias |
| From 1.5 hr onward |
| Hypokalemia with cardiac arrhythmias |
| From 6 hr onward |
| Neuroglucopenia, especially at 6 hr time onward |
| From 5–15 hr |
| Brain lesions secondary to cerebral edema |
| Any time |
| Complications of the underlying illness |
| Lack of insulin actions at any time |

mmol of hypertonic NaCl/kg leter of total body water over 5 hours, giving half in the first hour). We speculate that if the BBB were less permeable to mannitol than $Na^+$, one might obtain more therapeutic leverage with mannitol.

**Phosphate.** The usual deficit of phosphate is 1.4 to 2.6 mmol/kg body weight and, whereas only about 11% of patients have hypophosphatemia at diagnosis, once therapy is instituted almost all patients become profoundly hypophosphatemic.[44] There are no controlled studies documenting the absolute benefits of replacement of phosphate. If given, the maximum rate of infusion of phosphate is 50 mmol/8 hr. Because much more $K^+$ than this is required in this time, most of the $K^+$ must be given as KCl.

**Precipitating Event.** Concurrent with the treatment of DKA, it is necessary to treat any precipitating event or accompanying illness.

**Complications Observed During Therapy.** Problems that complicate therapy include hypokalemia, hypoglycemia, and relapse into ketoacidosis (Table 5–6). Alterations in central nervous system function suggest that cerebral edema might be developing. Although clinical rhabdomyolysis is uncommon, enzymes of muscle origin (creatine phosphokinase, aspartate transaminase, and lactate dehydrogenase) are often elevated in plasma. Thrombotic events in veins due to a slow blood flow rate should also be recognized.

## REFERENCES


1. McGarry JD: Disordered metabolism in diabetes: Have we underemphasized the fat component? J Cell Biochem 55:S29–S38, 1994.
2. Kety SS, Polis BD, Nadler CS, et al: The blood flow and oxygen consumption of the human brain in diabetic acidosis and coma. J Clin Invest 27:500–510, 1948.
3. Kamel KS, Stinebaugh BJ, Schloeder FX, et al: Kidney in starvation. In Seldin DW, Giebisch G (eds): The Kidney, Physiology and Pathophysiology. New York, Raven Press, Vol 3, 1992, pp 3457–3470.
4. Flatt JP: On the maximal possible rate of ketogenesis. Diabetes 21:50–53, 1972.
5. Halperin ML, Jungas RL, Pichette C, et al: A quantitative analysis of renal ammoniagenesis and energy balance: A theoretical approach. Can J Physiol Pharmacol 60:1431–1435, 1982.
6. Kamel KS, Lin S-H, Cheema-Dhadli S, et al: Prolonged total fasting: A feast for the integrative physiologist. Kidney Int 53: 531–539, 1998.
7. Cahill GFJ: Starvation in man. N Engl J Med 282:668–675, 1970.
8. Soroka SD, Chayaraks S, Honrath U, et al: Minimum urine flow rate during water deprivation: Importance of the urea and nonurea osmole concentration and excretion rate. J Am Soc Nephrol 8:880–886, 1997.
9. Halperin ML, Kamel KS, Ethier JH, et al: Biochemistry and physiology of ammonium excretion. In Seldin DW, Giebisch G (eds): The Kidney, Physiology and Pathophysiology, Vol 2, 2nd ed. New York, Raven Press, 1992, pp 2645–2679.
10. Lemieux G, Vinay P, Robitaille P, et al: The effect of ketone bodies on renal ammoniagenesis. J Clin Invest 50:1781–1791, 1971.
11. Halperin ML, Rolleston FS: Clinical Detective Stories: A Problem-Based Approach to Clinical Cases in Energy and Acid-Base Metabolism. London, England, Portland Press, 1993, p 1.
12. Schreiber M, Kamel KS, Cheema-Dhadli S, et al: Ketoacidosis, emphasis on acid-base aspects. Diabetes Rev 2:98–114, 1994.
13. Windmueller HG: Glutamine utilization by the small intestine. Adv Enzymol 53:201–237, 1982.
14. Schreiber M, Steele A, Cheema-Dhadli S, et al: Can ketoacidosis develop overnight? J Am Soc Nephrol 7:191–197, 1996.
15. Atchley DW, Loeb RF, Richards DW Jr, et al: On diabetic acidosis: A detailed study of electrolyte balances following withdrawal and reestablishment of insulin therapy. J Clin Invest 12:297–326, 1933.
16. Jungas RL, Ball EG: Studies on the metabolism of adipose tissue. XII: The effects of insulin and epinephrine on free fatty acid and glycerol production in the presence and absence of glucose. Biochemistry 2:283–388, 1963.
17. Brauer RW: Liver circulation and function. Physiol Rev 43:115–213, 1965.
18. Fritz IB: An hypothesis concerning the role of carnitine in the control of interrelations between fatty acid and carbohydrate metabolism. Perspect Biol Med 10:643–677, 1967.
19. McGarry JD, Woeltje KF, Kuwajima M, et al: Regulation of ketogenesis and the renaissance of carnitine palmitoyl transferase. Diabetes Metab Rev 5:271–284, 1989.
20. Jungas RL, Halperin ML, Brosnan JT: Lessons learned from a quantitative analysis of amino acid oxidation and related gluconeogenesis in man. Physiol Rev 72:419–448, 1992.
21. Halperin ML, Hammeke M, Josse RG, et al: Metabolic acidosis in the alcoholic: A pathophysiologic approach. Metabolism 32: 308–315, 1983.
22. Denton RM: Early events in insulin action. Adv Cyclic Nucl Prot Phos Res 20:293–341, 1986.
23. Rosen OM: After insulin binds. Science 237:1452–1458, 1988.
24. Khanna JM, Israel Y: Ethanol metabolism. Int Rev Physiol 21: 275–315, 1980.
25. Reichard GA, Owen OE, Haff AC, et al: Ketone body production and oxidation in fasting obese humans. J Clin Invest 53:508–515, 1974.
26. Halperin ML, Kamel KS, Cheema-Dhadli S: Lactic acidosis, ketoacidosis, and energy turnover: "Figure" you made the correct diagnosis only when you have "counted" on it—Quantitative analysis based on principles of metabolism. Mt Sinai J Med 59: 1–12, 1992.
27. Halperin ML, Goldstein MB: Fluid, Electrolyte and Acid-Base Physiology: A Problem-Based Approach. Philadelphia, WB Saunders, 1998.
28. Vasuvattakul S, Warner LC, Halperin ML: Quantitative role of the intracellular bicarbonate buffer system in response to an acute acid load. Am J Physiol 262:R305–R309, 1992.
29. Kamel KS, Richardson RMA, Goguen JM, et al: Rate of production of carbon dioxide in patients with a severe degree of metabolic acidosis. Nephron 64:514–517, 1993.
30. Deetjen P, Baeyer HV, Drexel H: Renal glucose transport. In Seldin D, Giebisch G (eds): The Kidney: Physiology and Pathophysiology, Vol 2, 2nd ed. New York, Raven Press, 1992, pp 2873–2888.
31. Fulop M, Rosenblatt A, Kreitzer SM, et al: Hyperosmolar nature of diabetic coma. Diabetes 24:594–599, 1975.
32. Porte D Jr: Sympathetic regulation of insulin secretion. Arch Intern Med 123:252–260, 1969.
33. Marliss EB, Ohman JL, Aoki TT: Altered redox state obscuring ketoacidosis in diabetic patients with lactic acidosis. N Engl J Med 283:978, 1970.
34. Adrogue HH, Eiknoyan G, Suki WN: Diabetic ketoacidosis: Role of the kidney in the acid-base homeostasis re-evaluated. Kidney Int 25:591–598, 1984.
35. Goldstein MB, Bear R, Richardson RMA, et al: The urine anion gap: A clinically useful index of ammonium excretion. Am J Med Sci 29:198–202, 1986.
36. Dyck R, Asthana S, Kalra J, et al: A modification of the urine osmolal gap: An improved method for estimating urine ammonium. Am J Nephrol 10:359–362, 1990.
37. Halperin ML, Margolis BL, Robinson LA, et al: The urine osmolal gap: a clue to estimate urine ammonium in "hybrid" types of metabolic acidosis. Clin Invest Med 11:198–202, 1988.
38. Kamel K, Ethier J, Richardson R, et al: Urine electrolytes and osmolality: When and how to use them. Am J Nephrol 10: 89–102, 1990.

39. Mahoney CP, Vlcek BW, DelAguila M: Risk factors for developing brain herniation during diabetic ketoacidosis. Pediatr Neurol 21:721–727, 1999.
40. Roscoe JM, Halperin ML, Rolleston FS, et al: Hyperglycemia-induced hyponatremia: Metabolic considerations in calculation of serum sodium depression. CMAJ 112:452–453, 1975.
41. Kamel KS, Cheema-Dhadli S, Halperin FA, et al: Anion gap: Do the anions restricted to the intravascular space have modifications in their valence? Nephron 73:382–389, 1996.
42. Nanji A, Campbell D: Falsely-elevated serum creatinine values in diabetic ketoacidosis: Clinical implications. Biochemistry 14: 91–93, 1981.
43. Gerrard S, Khayam-Bashi H: Negative interference with the Ektachem (Kodak) enzymic assay for creatinine by high serum glucose [Letter]. Clin Chem 30:1884, 1984.
44. Butler AM, Talbot NB, Burnett CH, et al: Metabolic studies in diabetic coma. Trans Assoc Am Phys 60:102–109, 1947.
45. Hoffman WH, Steinhart CM, Gammal TE, et al: Cranial CT in children and adolescents with diabetic ketoacidosis. Am J Neuroradiol 9:733–739, 1988.
46. Krane EJ, Rockoff MA, Wallman LK, et al: Subclinical brain swelling in children during the treatment of diabetic ketoacidosis. N Engl J Med 312:1147–1151, 1985.
47. Carlotti APCP, Bohn D, Halperin ML: Factors predisposing to cerebral edema (CE) in children presenting with a severe degree of diabetic ketoacidosis (DKA). J Am Soc Nephrol 10:121A, 1999.
48. West ML, Marsden PA, Singer GG, et al: A quantitative analysis of glucose loss during acute therapy for the hyperglycemia hyperosmolar syndrome. Diabetes Care 9:465–471, 1986.
49. Duck SC, Wyatt DT: Factors associated with brain herniation in the treatment of diabetic ketoacidosis. J Pediatr 113:10–14, 1988.
50. Glasser N, Barnett P, McCaslin I, et al: Risk factors for cerebral edema in children with diabetic ketoacidosis. N Engl J Med 344: 264–269, 2001.
51. Van der Meulen JA, Klip A, Grinstein S: Possible mechanism for cerebral oedema in diabetic ketoacidosis. Lancet ii:306–308, 1987.
52. Silver SM, Clark EC, Schroeder BM, et al: Pathogenesis of cerebral edema after treatment of diabetic ketoacidosis. Kidney Int 51:1237–1244, 1997.

CHAPTER 6

# Lactic Acidosis

Melvin E. Laski, MD ▪ Donald E. Wesson, MD

Claussen first described acidosis associated with an increased concentration of lactic acid in the blood in 1925.[1, 2] The currently accepted definition and classification of lactic acidosis are derived from the studies of Huckabee[3, 4] and the multitude of clinical reviews based on this definition and classification that followed.[5–16] Two levels of lactic acidosis were initially described: type I, characterized by a proportional increase in lactate and pyruvate, and type II, characterized by a greater increase in lactate than pyruvate.[3–5] As currently understood, the term *lactic acidosis* generally indicates the latter state (type II lactic acidosis).

Lactate production increases out of proportion to pyruvate production when metabolically active tissues become hypoxic or when carbohydrate metabolism is disrupted for other reasons.[2–16] The production of both pyruvate and lactate rises whenever the rate of glycolysis accelerates. The highest lactate concentrations develop when hypoxia or metabolic abnormalities coincide with high rates of glycolysis. Alternatively, the serum lactate concentration can increase due to decreased lactate use if there is serious disease of lactate-consuming organs. Type A lactic acidosis indicates that the acidosis resulted from generalized or regional tissue hypoxia. Type B lactic acidosis indicates that the acidosis developed due to biochemical abnormalities resulting from malignancy, liver disease, inborn errors of metabolism, or ingestion of metabolic toxins.[2–16]

Type A and type B lactic acidosis share a fundamentally similar pathophysiology. The increased lactic acid production that characterizes both syndromes results from defective aerobic metabolism. Aerobic energy production fails due to a lack of oxygen in type A lactic acidosis; it fails due to its inhibition by a drug, toxin, or inborn error of metabolism in type B lactic acidosis. The intermediate cellular events that follow are similar, though. Because mitochondrial metabolism is impaired, intracellular adenosine triphosphate (ATP) levels fall, and the amount of the reduced form of nicotinamide adenine dinucleotide (NADH) relative to nicotinamide adenine dinucleotide (NAD) increases. Because lactate produced by anaerobic processes cannot be oxidized back to pyruvate, the ratio of the lactate concentration relative to the pyruvate concentration rises. Inadequate ATP production stimulates glycolysis, yet more lactate and pyruvate are produced. A brief description of the biochemical reactions that underlie these processes follows.

## CARBOHYDRATE METABOLISM

Carbohydrate catabolism involves two distinct processes: glycolysis, an anaerobic series of reactions that occurs in the cytosol, and oxidative phosphorylation, an aerobic process that proceeds within mitochondria. Glycolysis converts 1 mol of glucose to 2 mol of pyruvate, with a net energy yield of 2 mol of ATP and the reduction of 2 mol of NAD to NADH. The glycolytic pathway involves 11 reaction steps that can be subdivided into two fairly distinct parts. The initial reactions consume ATP and produce a pair of phosphorylated 3-carbon intermediates; the later steps generate energy through the conversion of these intermediates to pyruvate and lactate. Figure 6–1 outlines the steps of glycolysis.

Glycolysis begins with the phosphorylation of glucose to glucose 6-phosphate by either hexokinase or glucokinase. This consumes a single ATP. Phosphoglucoisomerase then reversibly converts the glucose 6-phosphate to fructose 6-phosphate. In the next step, the enzyme phosphofructokinase catalyzes a second phosphorylation reaction to form fructose-1,6-bisphosphate. The activity of phosphofructokinase is enhanced by hypoxia and by depleted states of high-energy intermediates (the Pasteur effect).[17] Phosphofructokinase activity is also stimulated by elevation of intracellular pH.[18–21] The overall rate of glycolysis is regulated at this reaction, which consumes the second ATP molecule used by the pathway. The fructose-1,6-diphosphate so generated is next split by the enzyme aldolase into two phosphorylated 3-carbon compounds—glyceraldehyde 3-phosphate and dihydroxyacetone phosphate. These two intermediates are freely interconverted by triose phosphate isomerase.

The second part of glycolysis starts as glyceraldehyde-3-phosphate is converted to 1,3-diphosphoglycerate, with the concurrent production of ATP and NADH. Glyceraldehyde-3-phosphate is oxidized and phosphorylated by glyceraldehyde-3-phosphate dehydrogenase. Two hydrogen ions are removed from the initial compound, NAD is reduced to NADH, a proton is released, and an inorganic phosphate molecule is added to the glyceraldehyde-3-phosphate to form 1,3-diphosphoglycerate, a so-called high-energy intermediate. 1,3-Diphosphoglycerate is rapidly dephosphorylated by phosphoglycerate kinase, forming 3-phosphoglycerate and producing ATP. Phosphoglycerate mutase rearranges the 3-phosphoglycerate to generate 2-phosphoglycerate, which is subsequently converted to phosphoenolpyruvate by the enzyme enolase. Phosphoenolpyruvate contains a high-energy phosphate bond. The dephosphorylation of phosphoenolpyruvate by pyruvate kinase consumes adenosine diphosphate (ADP), generating pyruvate and another ATP.

The two pyruvate molecules that result from glycolysis undergo one of several metabolic fates. Pyruvate

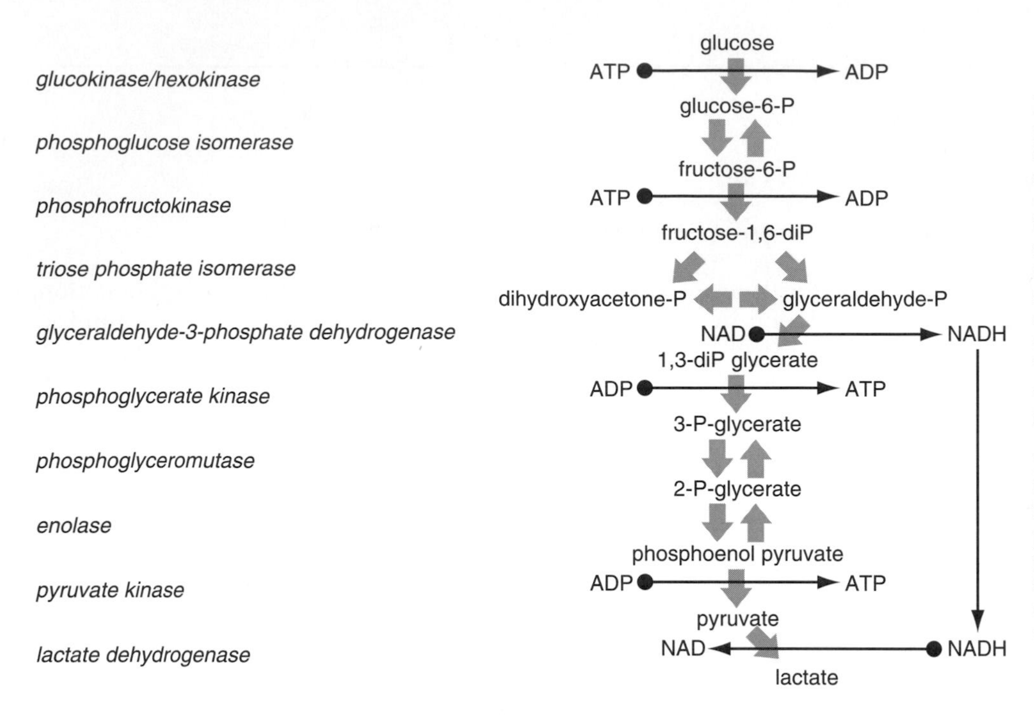


**FIGURE 6–1** ■ The glycolytic pathway diagram illustrates the reactions involved in glycolysis. The enzymes that characterize each step are given at left in italics. "P" indicates phosphate. The initial reactions consume ATP; reactions after the formation of the three carbon intermediates—dihydroxyacetone, phosphate, and glyceraldehyde-3-phosphate—produce ATP. Two ATP molecules are used in the priming reactions; four are produced after the fructose is split (two from each of the three carbon intermediates that result). If lactate is produced, no net NADH is produced. ADP, adenosine diphosphate; ATP, adenosine triphosphate; NAD, nicotinamide adenine dinucleotide; NADH, the reduced form of nicotinamide adenine dinucleotide.

may be reduced to lactate or undergo amination to form alanine in the cytoplasm, and it may be carboxylated to form oxaloacetate or dehydrogenated to produce acetyl coenzyme A (CoA) and carbon dioxide ($CO_2$) within the mitochondria by pyruvate dehydrogenase. The reduction of pyruvate to lactate oxidizes the cofactor NADH to NAD. The reaction may proceed in either direction, depending on the availability of the substrates. The overall reaction is generally written as:

$$\text{Pyruvate} + \text{NADH} \leftrightarrow \text{lactate} + \text{NAD} + \text{H}^+$$

As pointed out by many, these equations can be rearranged to yield:

$$\text{Lactate/pyruvate} = \text{NADH/NAD}$$

The lactate-pyruvate ratio is thereby regulated by the ratio of reduced to oxidized NAD and thus the oxidation reduction (redox) potential of the cell. If the rate of glycolysis is increased but the intracellular redox potential is normal, the lactate concentration increases in proportion to the increase in pyruvate. Conversely, if the redox potential tilts away from oxidation to reduction (more NADH is available than NAD), the lactate concentration increases with respect to the pyruvate concentration. The normal lactate-to-pyruvate ratio is less than 10:1. Any significant elevation of the ratio indicates that there is a change in the redox potential due to disordered aerobic mitochondrial metabolism, whether from lack of oxygen or another cause.

Most of the pyruvate produced by glycolysis is normally consumed within the confines of the mitochondrial membranes by the tricarboxylic acid cycle. The tricarboxylic acid cycle, or Krebs cycle, is more efficient than glycolysis. It is obligatorily aerobic. The glycolysis of 1 mol of glucose to two pyruvate molecules generates 2 mol (net) of ATP and 2 mol of NADH. The production of lactate from pyruvate consumes the NADH. The aerobic metabolism of pyruvate yields much more energy than glycolysis does, when both the tricarboxylic acid cycle and subsequent oxidative phosphorylation are considered. Glycolysis reduces NAD to NADH and shifts the redox potential toward a more reduced state, driving the conversion of pyruvate to lactate. In contrast, NADH is oxidized to NAD in the tricarboxylic acid cycle and the associated electron transport chain, which shifts the redox potential toward the oxidized state. When glycolysis is the predominant form of carbohydrate metabolism, the tissue redox potential is thus shifted to the reduced state, and the ratio of NADH/NAD rises. The Krebs cycle yields oxidized end-products and lowers the NADH/NAD ratio.

A general outline of carbohydrate metabolism is shown in Figure 6–2. The first step of aerobic carbohydrate metabolism, which occurs within mitochondria, is the conversion of pyruvate to acetyl CoA and $CO_2$ in a reaction catalyzed by pyruvate dehydrogenase (PDH; or pyruvate dehydrogenase complex [PDC]). Acetyl CoA derived from pyruvate may then combine with oxaloacetate to form citrate and initiate the tricarboxylic acid cycle. A complex cycle of coordinated reactions that involves eight major intermediates then proceeds. The cycle eventually regenerates the oxaloacetate after production of 1 mol of guanosine triphosphate (GTP), the reduction of 5 mol of NAD to NADH, and the reduction of 1 mol of flavin adenine dinucleotide (FAD) to its reduced form ($FADH_2$) per each mole of acetyl CoA. The carbon in the acetyl CoA is oxidized to $CO_2$. In series of concurrent and tightly

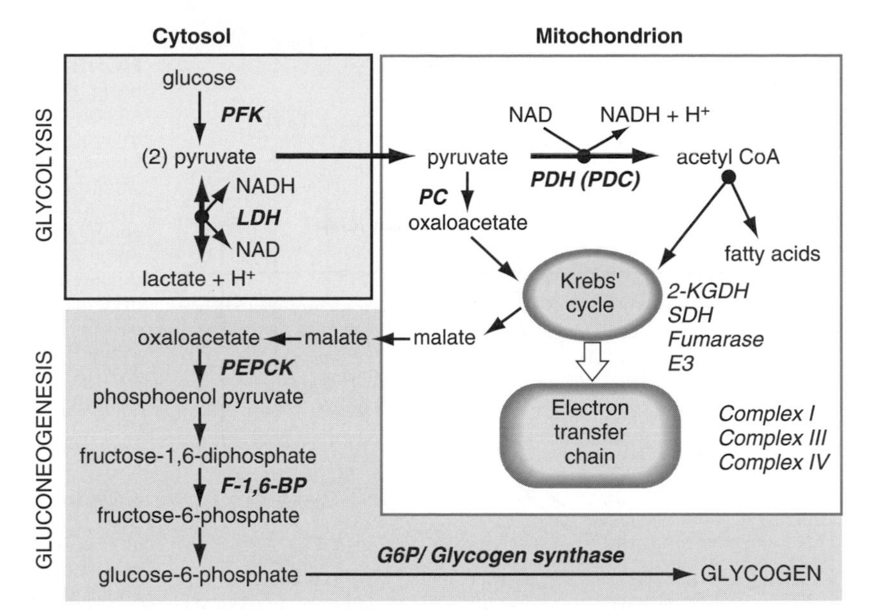


**FIGURE 6–2** ■ This diagram illustrates the major processes involved in carbohydrate metabolism and the key regulatory enzymes for each process. Enzymes are indicated in italics. Glycolysis (*upper left*) is principally regulated by the activity of phosphofructokinase (PFK). PFK is regulated by cell pH, insulin, catecholamines, and cellular adenosine triphosphate (ATP) production. The rate of glycolysis determines the total concentration of pyruvate plus lactate. The ratio of pyruvate to lactate is dictated by the ratio of the reduced form of nicotinamide adenine dinucleotide (NADH) to nicotinamide adenine dinucleotide (NAD); the reaction is otherwise freely reversible and catalyzed by lactate dehydrogenase (LDH). Within the mitochondrion, two enzymes control pyruvate metabolism. Pyruvate dehydrogenase complex (PDH/PDC) catalyzes the formation of acetyl coenzyme A, which then can enter the Krebs cycle or contribute to fatty acid synthesis. PDC deficiency is the most common cause of congenital lactic acidosis. PDC activity is stimulated by dichloroacetate. Pyruvate carboxykinase (PC) adds a carbon to pyruvate to produce oxaloacetate, which replenishes the stores of four carbon intermediates for the Krebs cycle and is also critical for gluconeogenesis (*lower left*). Rare cases of PC deficiency are known. Oxaloacetate produced from pyruvate may be transformed to malate and leave the mitochondrion. In the cytosol, malate is converted back to oxaloacetate, which is a substrate for phosphoenolpyruvate carboxykinase (PEPCK). PEPCK is also critical to the process of gluconeogenesis. Fructose-1,6-bisphosphatase (F-1,6-BP) controls the formation of fructose-1-phosphate. Deficiency of F-1,6-BP leads to glycogen storage disease type II. Glucose-6-phosphatase (G6P) is critical for normal glycogen formation. Abnormal G6P activity is responsible for von Gierke disease. Glycogen synthase deficiency causes a rarer form of glycogen storage disease. 2-Ketoglutarate dehydrogenase (2-KGDH), succinate dehydrogenase (SDH), lipoamide oxidoreductase (E3), and fumarase catalyze steps in the Krebs cycle. Deficiency of any of these enzymes causes congenital lactic acidosis associated with severe clinical syndromes and limited survival. Complexes I, III, and IV are critical to the electron transfer chain. Defects of these complexes are responsible for congenital or acquired lactic acidosis with a complex set of potential clinical presentations.

coordinated reactions, the NADH and $FADH_2$ donate electrons to ubiquinone and the electron transport chain (Fig. 6–3). Eventually the mitochondrial proton ATPase pump transports protons back across the inner membrane, generating ATP in the process. The oxidation of each mole of NADH to NAD thereby results in the production of 3 mol of ATP, the oxidation of $FADH_2$ yields a further mole of ATP, and the previously generated GTP represents another ATP equivalent. Thus, 38 mol of ATP is produced by the metabolism of a single mole of glucose—2 mol by glycolysis, and 36 mol by oxidative phosphorylation.

The complexity of oxidative carbohydrate metabolism cannot be overstated. The electron transport chain involves the action of five large protein complexes derived from two distinct genomes. Complex I (NADH ubiquinone oxidoreductase) pumps protons from the inner membrane to the outer membrane, oxidizes NADH to NAD, and reduces ubiquinone (Q), to $QH_2$. Complex I contains more than 40 subunits; 7 of these are encoded by mitochondrial DNA rather than by nuclear DNA. Complex II is smaller (four peptides) and is completely encoded by nuclear DNA. Complex III, also called succinate ubiquinone oxidoreductase, catalyzes the oxidation of succinate to fumarate and transfers electrons to ubiquinone. Ubiquinol cytochrome *c* cytoreductase, or complex III, has 11 protein subunits, 10 of which are coded by the nucleus, and one of which is mitochondrial in origin. Complex III transfers protons across the mitochondrial membrane as electrons move from ubiquinol to cytochrome *c*. Cytochrome *c* carries electrons from complex III to complex IV. Complex IV, or cytochrome *c* oxidase, transfers electrons from cytochrome *c* and generates water from protons and oxygen. This complex has 13 proteins in 8 subunits. Three of its subunits are of mitochondrial derivation. The final complex, complex V, comprises the $F_0$-$F_1$ proton pumping ATPase. Fourteen of its 16 subunits are encoded on nuclear DNA; the remaining 2 are products of the mitochondrial genome.

PDH (PDC), which generates acetyl CoA from pyruvate, initiates the Krebs cycle and thus is a critical enzyme in lactate-pyruvate metabolism. PDH (PDC) is activated by insulin, which has clinical relevance in type I diabetes.[22, 23] PDH (PDC) activity is also stimulated by ADP and adenosine monophosphate (AMP) and is inhibited by elevated ATP concentrations. Con-

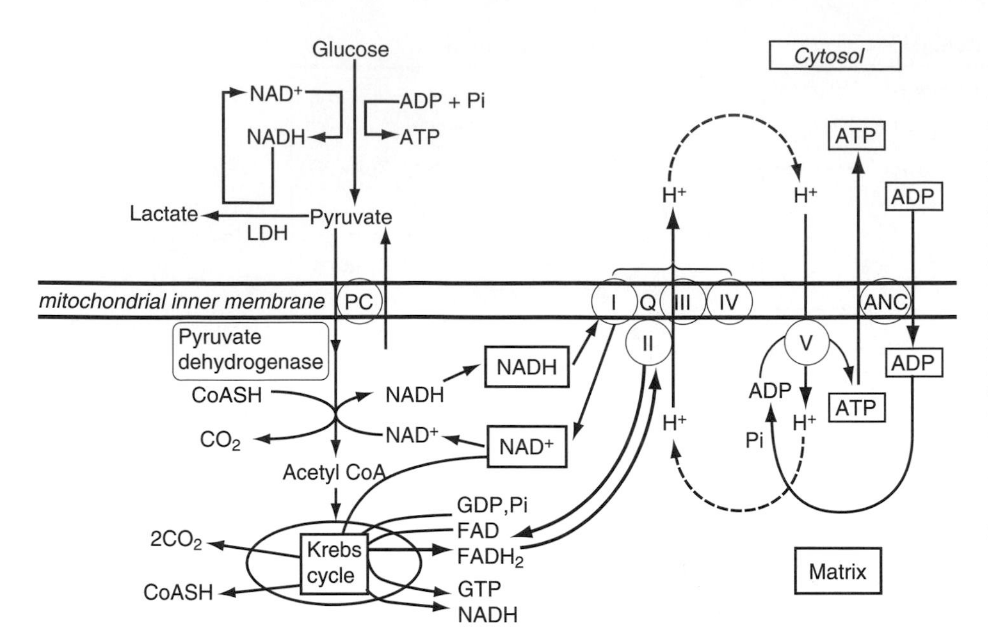


**FIGURE 6–3** ■ The diagram illustrates the major relationships of mitochondrial redox reactions with the totality of carbohydrate metabolism. Reduced cofactors (NADH and $FADH_2$) produced in the Krebs cycle or pyruvate dehydrogenation interact with complexes I, II, III, and IV as well as ubiquinone (Q) and release protons that are transported into the mitochondrial matrix by the ATPase pump (complex V). The ATP generated by the pump is exchanged for ADP, returning ATP to the cytosol. ANC indicates an adenine nucleotide carrier. ATP, adenosine triphosphate; $FADH_2$, flavin adenine dinucleotide (reduced form); NADH, the reduced form of nicotinamide adenine dinucleotide. (Redrawn from Ventura FV, Ruiter JPN, IJlst L, et al: Lactic acidosis in long-chain fatty acid beta-oxidation disorders. J Inherit Metab Dis 21:652, 1998.)

versely, low levels of intracellular ATP stimulate phosphofructokinase and glycolysis, which helps restore ATP levels.

Lactate dehydrogenase catalyzes the oxidation of lactate to pyruvate. There is no other metabolic use for lactic acid. Lactate oxidation proceeds readily when the NADH/NAD ratio favors oxidation; otherwise, lactate persists as a "dead-end" waste product. When tissue oxygenation and redox potential are normal, lactate can be oxidized to pyruvate, and pyruvate can move into the tricarboxylic acid cycle or contribute to gluconeogenesis. If the tissue redox potential is inadequate to permit the regeneration of pyruvate from lactate, the tissue lactate concentration rises. Lactate generated by skeletal muscle or the splanchnic bed under conditions of relative local tissue hypoxia may be released in the circulation and travel to a distant site, usually the liver or the kidney, where the redox potential supports the regeneration of pyruvate and gluconeogenesis (the Cori cycle).

Tissues are divisible into those that normally produce and release lactate to the circulation and those that consume circulating lactate.[24–32] Lactate-producing tissues include skeletal muscle, skin, red blood cells (which are incapable of aerobic metabolism due to the absence of mitochondria), intestine, brain, and renal medulla. The liver consumes lactate by generating pyruvate and then using pyruvate in gluconeogenesis. The renal cortex also consumes significant amounts of lactate and is another significant site of gluconeogenesis. Skeletal muscle is also capable of using lactate to form glycogen under specific conditions.[27, 31]

Lactate production and consumption are balanced in the normal resting state. Approximately 15 to 20 mg lactate/kg body weight/day is generated and used under basal conditions.[24] Although the rate of lactate generation is immense relative to the mass of available circulating buffer, the serum lactate concentration is normally maintained at 1 to 2 mmol/L.[11] The blood and tissue lactate concentration may vary widely on a minute-to-minute basis, however. Lactate production rises rapidly during any intense exercise.[33–35] The local accumulation of lactate in skeletal muscles results in pain and fatigue. The degree to which lactate accumulation is tolerated depends on the muscular conditioning of the individual.

Lactic acidosis is a major concern for students of exercise physiology. Because lactate production during exercise is not pathologic, the degree of acidosis that develops during exercise is ill appreciated in medicine. Better conditioning produces a greater tolerance of anaerobic metabolism. Trained athletes develop lactate levels up to 22 mmol/L with as little as 12 minutes of activity, indicating both the effect of training to enhance anaerobic capacity and the relative nontoxicity of lactic acidosis per se.[34, 35] In contrast, poorly conditioned individuals fail to tolerate lactate accumulation in exercise and develop fatigue after only limited effort at much lower lactate concentrations.[36] The speed of clearance of lactate so generated varies, taking up to 12 hours if the individual rests after the activity, or minutes with a "cool down."[33–35]

As a final note, because lactate is generated at varying rates in different tissue pools, peripheral venous lactate measurement is not always accurate. Arterial lactate concentration should be measured when possible. Peripheral venous lactate concentration correlates with, but is not equivalent to, arterial lactate concentration.[37] Similarly, arterial lactate levels do not always predict the mixed venous lactate levels.[38, 39]

# TYPE A LACTIC ACIDOSIS

## Pathophysiology

The pathophysiology of type A lactic acidosis is not overly complex. Type A lactic acidosis can develop

**TABLE 6–1.** Conditions Associated with Type A Lactic Acidosis

| |
|---|
| Shock |
| Hypovolemic shock |
| Cholera |
| Septic shock |
| Cardiogenic shock |
| Low-output heart failure |
| High-output heart failure |
| Regional hypoperfusion |
| Severe hypoxia |
| Severe asthma |
| Carbon monoxide poisoning |
| Severe anemia |

whenever tissue oxygenation is insufficient to permit aerobic metabolism to continue.[2–16] Conditions associated with type A lactic acidosis are shown in Table 6–1. Oxidative phosphorylation simply cannot proceed during severe tissue hypoxia, because oxygen serves as the ultimate electron acceptor as protons are generated and pumped across the mitochondrial membranes. Glycolysis, in contrast, is not directly affected by tissue oxygen tension. Glycolysis does slow in the presence of the higher ATP availability when oxidation proceeds normally, and it is accelerated when metabolic production of high-energy phosphate intermediates lessens. Glycolysis is also stimulated by catecholamines, and circulating catecholamines are usually increased in patients with shock due to both endogenous release and exogenous administration. Systemic or regional hypoxemia results in generalized or localized tissue hypoxia, which inhibits oxidative phosphorylation and secondarily stimulates glycolysis in the affected tissue beds. In these conditions, pyruvate is produced from glycolysis at increased rates at the precise time it cannot be oxidatively metabolized. As long as glucose remains available, glycolysis continues. The products of glycolysis accumulate, but the metabolism of pyruvate through acetyl CoA and the Krebs cycle cannot proceed. The oxidation of NADH in the mitochondria fails because oxygen is not available to accept electrons, and the local ratio of NADH to NAD rises. The ratio of lactate to pyruvate follows the NADH/NAD ratio, and as further glycolysis proceeds and pyruvate is continually produced, lactate concentration rises sharply. If tissue hypoxia is not generalized, the excess lactate may be shuttled to a site where tissue perfusion and oxygenation allow its oxidation to pyruvate, generally the liver. If the hypoxia is systemic or if liver and kidney function are impaired, there is no respite provided by a lactate shuttle.

## Causes

### SHOCK

Circulatory shock is the most common cause of lactic acidosis, and the presence of lactic acidosis in shock indicates a grim prognosis.[3–16, 40–45] Shock is defined, in part, by properties that lead to lactate generation: inadequate cardiac output and oxygen delivery to some or all tissues and organs. The total cardiac output in shock may be low due to ventricular failure, hemorrhage, or volume depletion, or it may be high due to sepsis or burn, but the tissue oxygen delivery and oxygen extraction are subnormal in either instance. Both high- and low-output cardiac failure can produce lactic acidosis.[40–47] Hypoperfusion and tissue hypoxia invariably increase lactate production by any tissue that depends on oxidative metabolism. Hypoxia inhibits oxidative mitochondrial metabolism, which alters the intracellular NAD/NADH ratio and favors lactate generation. Hypoxia also renders tissue totally dependent on glycolysis for energy. The low ATP levels that develop secondary to inhibition of aerobic metabolism stimulate glycolysis (the Pasteur effect); lactate and pyruvate production rises.

An additional factor affecting lactic acidosis in shock is the inhibition of hepatic lactate extraction.[48, 49] This may occur for the same reason that peripheral lactate generation increases. Splanchnic hypoxia impedes hepatic lactate use; lactate cannot be oxidized to pyruvate, and lactate accumulation is enhanced.[48, 49] Acidosis itself also appears to inhibit lactate use by the liver.[50–53]

In clinical practice, the situation is more complex than the basic scenario. Most patients with shock and low peripheral vascular resistance are given pressor agents in an attempt to reverse the state of low peripheral vascular resistance and thereby the shock state.[54–56] The sepsis syndrome plays a significant role in some instances.[57] Norepinephrine or epinephrine is commonly administered to hypotensive patients. Investigators reviewing the incidence of lactic acidosis following cardiac bypass procedures found that lactic acidosis occurs more frequently when norepinephrine is used to increase systemic resistance than when epinephrine is given, all other aspects of care being similar.[54, 55] Mixed venous oxygen tension and arterial oxygen saturation do not correlate well with lactate production in these cases. One interpretation is that norepinephrine stimulation of glycolysis is responsible for excessive lactate production. Thus, these individuals may have a mix of type A and type B lactic acidosis. Notably, the post–cardiac surgery lactic acidosis described in these articles cleared with time, and mortality was not increased. Other reports described the impact of vasoconstrictor agents on the development of lactic acidosis in septic patients.[56]

Septic shock is a complex state, and the standard argument that lactic acidosis in septic shock occurs primarily because of impaired tissue oxygen delivery has been questioned. When dichloroacetate—which diverts pyruvate metabolism away from lactate but does not alter the overall rate of pyruvate production by glycolysis—is given to patients with septic shock and lactic acidosis, the net rate of pyruvate production falls. This indicates that accelerated pyruvate production also plays a significant role in the generation of increased lactate levels.[58] Epinephrine administration might increase the risk of lactic acidosis in sepsis as well.[56] Nonsteroidal anti-inflammatory drugs also affect pyruvate and lactate generation in sepsis. Hypothesizing that arachidonic acid products play an important role in the sepsis syndrome, Bernard and coworkers administered ibuprofen to a series of patients with sepsis.[59] Ibuprofen lowered oxygen use and lactate production as it decreased prostacyclin and thromboxane levels, but unfortunately, the rate at which overt shock developed and the overall survival of the patients were unaffected.

In addition to septic shock and severe cardiovascular failure, other notable shock states associated with lactic acidosis include lactic acidosis with severe volume depletion in Asiatic cholera.[60] Extreme volume depletion of any cause may carry a similar risk. When volume depletion results in shock and lactic acidosis, the treatment must include aggressive rehydration. Care is required, however, because acidemia renders these individuals at risk for pulmonary edema by its effects on pulmonary and systemic resistance and cardiac performance.[60] It is recommended that pH be partially corrected (to approximately 7.1 to 7.2) by alkali administration as volume is restored. Finally, acute hemorrhage with shock is a well-appreciated cause of lactic acidosis.

## REGIONAL HYPOPERFUSION

Regional hypoperfusion affects localized tissue beds in the same way that systemic shock affects the general circulation. Whereas shock represents a severe decline in cardiac output or massive shunting of the cardiac output from oxygen-dependent organs, regional development of lactic acidosis requires only that a single limb or organ be underperfused. The predominant clinical cause of regional hypoperfusion is arterial compromise, but local tissue lactate concentrations rise whenever oxygen demand exceeds oxygen delivery. Usually the local lactate increase is diluted in the general circulation, and the excess lactate is delivered to the liver or kidney, where it is taken up and metabolized. The usual cost of accelerated regional lactate production is localized muscle pain and cramping, and the individual stops the exercise, depending on whether the anticipated gain is felt to be worth the current pain. It is only when lactate production continues, and the rate of production exceeds the capacity of other sites to consume the product, that a generalized elevation of the serum lactate may persist and cause clinical disease. Clinical examples include peripheral vascular disease affecting a limb and mesenteric arterial disease with a resultant ischemic bowel. When these tissues become hypoxic, lactate production increases, and local lactic acidosis develops. In the case of mesenteric ischemia and ischemic bowel, unexplained lactic acidosis may be the only clue to the diagnosis.[61] Visceral hypoxia with subsequent lactate production has been described during laparoscopic surgery at high intraperitoneal pressure.[62]

An important variation on the theme of localized lactic acidosis is delayed release of lactate to the circulation ("wash-out"). Lactic acidosis may develop only after reperfusion of the previously ischemic region.[63] In this scenario, the lactate generated in the hypoperfused region remains in that tissue bed until the circulation of the region is restored. When the initial circulatory lesion is repaired, the lactate is "washed out" to the body as a whole. Although the load can usually be handled effectively in the absence of liver or kidney disease, a temporary state of systemic lactic acidosis may be observed and may have significant clinical consequences on hemodynamics. Such patients should typically recover with proper support.

## SEVERE HYPOXIA

In theory, arterial hypoxemia should cause tissue hypoxia, as do shock and regional hypoperfusion, and produce lactic acidosis.[64] In fact, chronic arterial hypoxia caused by pulmonary disease usually does not lead to lactic acidosis.[65] In many patients with chronic lung disease, hypoxemia is accompanied by $CO_2$ retention and respiratory acidosis. The acidemia inhibits glycolysis and slows the production of pyruvate and lactate. In acidemia, tissue oxygen delivery is enhanced by a decrease in the avidity of hemoglobin for oxygen at low pH (the Bohr effect). Chronic respiratory acidosis stimulates the generation of 2,3-diphosphoglycerol, which further decreases the affinity of hemoglobin for oxygen, again favoring oxygen delivery to tissue. The combination of these effects shifts the oxygen dissociation curve farther "to the right." The role of this "rightward shift" in extreme acidemia is limited. When acidemia is severe, little additional effect is found as pH falls.[66] Finally, chronic hypoxia is a powerful stimulus to erythropoiesis, and erythrocytosis supports oxygen delivery even as it makes cyanosis more evident. The net result of all these factors is that lactic acidosis does not develop until hypoxia is extreme.

In contrast to the situation in chronic hypoxia, acute hypoxia is not countered by the chronic adaptive mechanisms that serve to increase oxygen delivery, and tissue oxygenation may be markedly compromised. Lactic acidosis may develop in acute respiratory failure at lesser degrees of hypoxia.[64] In the adult respiratory distress syndrome, the lungs may even contribute to lactate production.[67]

## SEVERE ASTHMA

Asthma is associated with two respiratory abnormalities that increase the likelihood that lactic acidosis will occur. First, during the evolution of a severe attack of asthma, the respiratory rate rises and the $PCO_2$ falls. Alkalosis stimulates glycolysis. The respiratory alkalosis that occurs in asthma thus increases the production of lactate and pyruvate. Second, as a severe asthma attack continues, the patient becomes progressively more hypoxic. Now the larger mass of pyruvate and lactate that is present because of the earlier effect of respiratory alkalosis cannot be effectively consumed by oxidative metabolism. Lactate levels increase, and lactic acidosis ensues.[68] β-Adrenergic stimulation, a cornerstone of asthma therapy, increases lactate production by accelerating glycolysis.[69, 70]

### CARBON MONOXIDE POISONING

Carbon monoxide is a more effective ligand for hemoglobin than for oxygen; it binds more avidly to hemoglobin than does oxygen, and it is not as easily displaced. In the presence of carbon monoxide, less oxygen is carried on circulating hemoglobin, and far less is released to the peripheral tissues. This sharply decreases tissue oxygenation, and lactic acidosis develops.[71] The impact of tissue hypoxia on aerobic metabolism in carbon monoxide poisoning is enhanced by the inhibition of cytochromes *a* and $a_3$ by carbon monoxide. Both effects alter the tissue redox potential, and the ratio of pyruvate to lactate is tipped toward lactate generation.

Carbon monoxide poisoning is often massive and acute; in such instances, victims arrive unconscious to the emergency room with classic cherry red mucosal membranes and papilledema on funduscopic examination. Carbon monoxide poisoning can also present in a subacute form. Patients may complain of headache and malaise without classic findings on examination when malfunctioning heating units cause chronic, low-level elevations of carbon monoxide. Treatment includes general support measures, oxygen at high partial pressure, and avoidance of further exposure to carbon monoxide.

### SEVERE ANEMIA

Because the vast majority of oxygen carried by the circulation is bound to hemoglobin, the mass of hemoglobin per liter of blood is a critical issue for oxygen delivery. When anemia becomes critical, the extreme tissue hypoxia that follows induces lactic acidosis.[72–75] This occurs when the blood hemoglobin concentration falls below 4 g/dL. Several reports describe the occurrence of lactic acidosis in patients with severe malaria.[73, 74] Dietary thiamine deficiency exacerbated by rapid use of the vitamin due to rapid red cell turnover may play a role in these cases. The acuity of the anemia may be critical; the patients in case reports tend to have acute hemolytic crises due to malaria. Lactic acidosis has also been described in a patient with paroxysmal nocturnal hemoglobinemia and a sudden fall in hematocrit.[75] A final issue related to anemia is the state of iron stores. Patients with severe iron deficiency and anemia may become iron depleted to the extent that the iron-dependent enzymes of the electron transport chain are affected.[76]

## Treatment

The diagnosis of lactic acidosis is made in about 1% of hospital admissions.[7, 77] The overall mortality in lactic acidosis is 60% to 70%; mortality is virtually 100% when hypotension is also present.[5, 7, 77–81] As pointed out eloquently by Stacpoole, these data indicate that present therapy, which has not advanced significantly since the date of his article (1986), is inadequate at best.[77] Theoretically, the most appropriate treatment of type A lactic acidosis is to reverse the underlying metabolic abnormality that generated it.[2–16] In addition, severe acidosis has deleterious effects on cardiac output and blood pressure, and a response to the acidemia may be indicated. Thus, the therapy for lactic acidosis has two distinct aims. The first is to curtail the excess production of lactic acid by restoring normal oxidative metabolism. The second goal is to raise the acidic pH toward normal. If the underlying metabolic abnormality is not addressed effectively, the chances for a good outcome sharply decrease. Conversely, if the excess lactate production responsible for the acidosis can be halted, the pH may correct without direct intervention.

The only treatment of known efficacy for lactic acidosis in shock remains the reversal of shock. The tissue that generates excess lactate is usually not diseased. If the circulation to the tissue or organ is restored, lactate generation will cease, the accumulated lactate will be metabolized, and acidosis will reverse. If the underlying failure of tissue oxygenation is not corrected, a fatal outcome is almost inevitable.

The root cause of type A lactic acidosis is the tissue hypoxia that develops as a result of shock, severe anemia, or respiratory failure in asthma. Tissue hypoxia is readily reversed in anemic patients by transfusion. Improving oxygenation by mechanical ventilation reverses lactic acidosis when respiratory failure is the cause. The shock state presents a more complex problem, but the basic principles remain true. Shock physiology is characterized by tissue hypoperfusion with subsequent tissue hypoxia. If lactic acidosis is to be successfully treated, the shock state must be reversed. How this is accomplished depends on the type and cause of shock. Septic shock requires control of the underlying infection, improvement of cardiac performance is required in cardiogenic shock, and volume resuscitation is beneficial in hypovolemic shock. In each instance the fundamental concern is to improve the cardiac output and general hemodynamics to restore adequate tissue oxygen delivery. Vasocontrictors are commonly given when the systemic vascular resistance is low, but these must be used with care because some catecholamines increase the rate of glycolysis and lactate generation.[55, 56] Volume support is provided in septic shock up to, and sometimes beyond, the point at which edema is clinically problematic. Hypothetically, interruption of the cytokine cascade in the sepsis syndrome represents a rational approach to limit the damage, but therapy directed against tumor necrosis factor and several of the interleukins has yet to be proved clinically useful in shock. The cardiovascular findings of the ibuprofen trial are promising, but patient survival was not altered.[59] Further study is clearly necessary.

When direct treatment of the cause of shock fails to reverse lactic acidosis, attention is directed at the arterial pH because of the effects of acidemia on the cardiovascular system. Acidemia causes vasodilatation and reduces the sensitivity of the vasculature to catecholamine stimulation (when the pH falls below 7.1).[80, 81] The direct cardiovascular effects of critically low pH also include reduced left ventricular function and an increased tendency to develop ventricular fibrillation.[82–84] Although vasodilatation is commonly viewed as a major clinical problem because it results in hypotension, vasodilatation may initially be a useful response to cardiac dysfunction that allows output to remain elevated in the presence of a low-output state. Conversely, in high-output shock there is no physiologic advantage to vasodilatation. Certainly the reduction of ventricular pump function in severe acidemia is a significant problem. It is largely because of these effects that attempts are made to improve the clinical state by raising serum pH.

Although the use of bicarbonate in the treatment of lactic acidosis has been debated and has recently been somewhat discouraged, bicarbonate remains the most commonly administered agent for the treatment of lactic acidosis. Bicarbonate administration addresses the second of the two major therapeutic aims in lactic acidosis: correction of serum and tissue pH. Two major factors support the continued use of bicarbonate: first, bicarbonate is readily available to a physician who feels pressured to intervene in acidosis, and, second, it is not unusual for the pH to rise after bicarbonate is administered, a response that is commonly viewed as an overall treatment success. However, the use of bicarbonate has numerous negative effects that have convinced some to limit its use in lactic acidosis.[77]

The most significant arguments against the use of sodium bicarbonate in the treatment of lactic acidosis are as follows. First, sodium bicarbonate is most commonly provided in prepackaged 50-mL ampules containing 44 mEq of the salt, a highly hypertonic solution. Whenever a significant number of ampules of sodium bicarbonate are administered, critical hypernatremia and hyperosmolarity may follow.[85] Second, a significant quantity of sodium is given whenever sodium bicarbonate is administered. In those patients with problems related to volume expansion (e.g., pulmonary edema) in addition to lactic acidosis, the additional volume is often deleterious. Third, bicarbonate buffers protons by first reacting to form carbonic acid, which further decomposes to $CO_2$ and water. In an "open" buffer system (one in which the $CO_2$ is lost to the environment) the loss of $CO_2$ greatly extends the buffering power of bicarbonate. If the ability to dispose of $CO_2$ is limited, as is the case for a paralyzed patient whose ventilation is mechanically controlled, the arterial $P_{CO_2}$ will rapidly rise, and acidosis and acidemia may paradoxically worsen. Even a small increase in the $CO_2$ tension paradoxically lowers the intracellular pH. Paradoxical acidosis also develops in the cerebrospinal fluid after bicarbonate administration because the $CO_2$ generated in the buffering process freely crosses the blood-brain barrier, whereas bicarbonate does not, due to its limited permeability across that structure.[86] The resultant fall in cerebrospinal fluid pH may depress consciousness and extend or exacerbate a coma state. Fourth, when the administration of bicarbonate effectively raises both the extracellular and the intracellular pH, lactate production may be accelerated.[17, 18, 87] Elevation of the intracellular pH increases the velocity of the reaction catalyzed by phosphofructokinase. Phosphofructokinase effectively controls the rate of glycolysis and, thus, the rate at which pyruvate is produced. Acceleration of pyruvate production increases the production of lactate if circumstances limit further aerobic metabolism. Therefore, if the intracellular pH is raised, but the factors that prevent oxidative metabolism from proceeding normally are still in place, the result of the rise in pH will be acceleration of lactic acid production. Whether this is necessarily deleterious is a point of some contention. One of the most severe problems in lactic acidosis is that energy production is limited and cellular ATP levels fall. Although the acceleration of glycolysis by pH elevation results in greater lactate levels, it also provides ATP. Fifth, to the extent that the Bohr effect increases oxygen delivery to the tissues, any correction of the pH tends to reduce oxygen delivery, an untoward effect if cardiac output or tissue oxygen delivery is impaired.[88] Finally, if the patient improves during the course of therapy, the circulating lactate will eventually be converted to bicarbonate by the liver and kidneys. If a substantial amount of bicarbonate has already been given in an attempt to raise pH, the combined load of administered and metabolically generated bicarbonate may far exceed the amount needed to restore pH to normal, resulting in "overshoot" alkalemia, with all its attendant problems.[89, 90]

Separate from these effects of bicarbonate administration, but an equally serious issue, is the question of the effectiveness of bicarbonate in terms of survival.[91–93] It remains fair to state that there are no controlled studies based on final outcome (patient survival rather than pH increase or cardiovascular improvement) that provide clear evidence that bicarbonate administration is an effective treatment of lactic acidosis. Bicarbonate treatment arms in studies of alternative buffering agents yield low survival rates.[94–96] However, because the causes of lactic acidosis are many, and because the overall clinical condition of patients with the disorder varies so widely, it is understandable that there are no survival data that illustrate any effectiveness of bicarbonate, or any other agent, in lactic acidosis.

Several animal models of lactic acidosis have been used in studies evaluating therapy. Graf and colleagues rendered dogs severely hypoxic and compared the response of the animals to maintenance intravenous fluids, saline expansion, and bicarbonate infusion.[97] The bicarbonate-infused animals exhibited greater rates of lactate generation and had lower blood pressure and lower cardiac indices than the dogs that were saline supported or merely given maintenance fluids. Arieff and coworkers also compared saline and bicarbonate infusion in diabetic dogs with phenformin-induced lactic acidosis.[98] In this model, bicarbonate-treated dogs developed a greater degree of intracellular acidosis, greater lactate production rates, and lower cardiac output. Survival was not altered by any therapy. An older study reported that bicarbonate infusion increased mortality in phenformin-induced lactic acidosis in dogs.[99] In contrast, a more recent study performed in rats reported a favorable result in bicarbonate-treated animals, at least with regard to the maintenance of cardiac output.[100]

Given the preceding information, one is left to make a decision whether to give bicarbonate to a patient, generally in shock, with ongoing lactic acidosis and significant acidemia. Despite the attendant problems, and in the face of a paucity of supportive data, the standard of care is to administer bicarbonate if the arterial pH is significantly low, usually interpreted as below 7.1 to 7.2.[101] It is at or about this pH that severe cardiac complications are more likely to be an issue. To withhold bicarbonate at these pH levels is difficult to defend in lactic acidosis, although some studies of ketoacidosis suggest that that condition can be successfully treated without the use of bicarbonate despite an extremely low pH.[102]

If bicarbonate is to be administered, what is the proper dose? The volume of distribution of bicarbonate in individuals of normal body habitus has been estimated to be slightly less than the total body water, or about 50% of the body weight (BW) in kilograms.[103, 104] The amount of bicarbonate required to correct the plasma bicarbonate ($[HCO_3]p$) is thus estimated as:

$$\text{Dose of bicarbonate} = (0.5 \times \text{BW}) \times (\text{desired } [HCO_3]p - \text{current } [HCO_3]p)$$

This must be viewed as a very rough estimate, however. Lactate production will continue, and its rate may be accelerated if the pH rises. Any change in the blood pH will alter the respiratory component of acid-base balance if the patient is breathing spontaneously. Severe acidosis may expand the volume of distribution of bicarbonate and cause underestimation of the required bicarbonate dose. Conversely, the estimated bicarbonate dose may be excessive in the very obese, because fat increases weight but not total body water. What is required is careful monitoring of the response to bicarbonate and timely reassessment of the bicarbonate concentration and arterial pH. The target of therapy should be some normalization of pH, usually aiming at an arterial pH above 7.2 and a plasma bicarbonate about 15 mEq/L. Above this pH value, the effects of acidemia are not life threatening, and the risks of therapy remain.

Overt shock with lactic acidosis is often accompanied by acute renal insufficiency or frank renal failure. Bicarbonate is more difficult to administer in this situation owing to the increased risk of volume overload and pulmonary edema. Hemodialysis, which is performed using bicarbonate-based dialysate solutions in most institutions, provides bicarbonate and clears lactate while controlling volume.[105] The limitations of acute hemodialysis include its short duration, which is followed by reaccumulation of lactate and worsening lactic acidosis after treatment, and the fact that many patients with lactic acidosis secondary to shock are simply too ill and too hypotensive to tolerate acute hemodialysis. Peritoneal dialysis is a more gentle therapy, but it rarely provides adequate dialysis in a patient with acute renal failure.[106] Furthermore, most peritoneal dialysis solutions are lactate based, limiting the utility of technique to clear lactate.

Continuous dialysis therapies such as continuous arteriovenous or venovenous hemodialysis (CAVHD, CVVHD, respectively) are better tolerated by severely ill patients than is acute hemodialysis. Unfortunately, these continuous therapies are often performed using peritoneal dialysis solutions as dialysate and Ringer lactate solution as replacement fluid, which limits their ability to remove lactate and may even cause lactate levels to increase. A better option is to perform the procedure using bicarbonate-based solutions for dialysate and replacement.[107–111] Unfortunately, bicarbonate-based dialysis solutions appropriate for CAVHD and CVVHD are not universally available, and it may be necessary to formulate solutions for the treatment on site, which is an expensive proposition open to error. Although the continuous dialysis treatments in lactic acidosis show promise, there are few, if any, current data that demonstrate an improvement in survival when such therapy is provided, a finding likely influenced by the dire prognosis of the patient population before therapy.

Other treatments for severe lactic acidosis have been considered. Carbicarb is a specifically compounded mixture of sodium bicarbonate and sodium carbonate.[112] The mix offers a buffering capacity equal to sodium bicarbonate with somewhat less risk of hyperosmolarity and no elevation of $CO_2$ tension. Data do not indicate that its use improves patient survival, and the mixture is not commercially available. Carbicarb is patented, and it may not be compounded without permission.

Dichloroacetate stimulates PDH and therefore pyruvate consumption. It does so by inhibiting a kinase that downregulates the enzyme.[113–117] The stimulation of pyruvate consumption diverts metabolism away from lactate generation and reduces lactate and pyruvate levels if oxygenation is adequate. The clinical efficacy of dichloroacetate has been evaluated in several clinical trials.[94–96] The data from these trials show that dichloroacetate often elevates the serum bicarbonate and pH, and serum lactate levels decline. Unfortunately, these presumably beneficial effects are not accompanied by an increase in patient survival. As a result, the use of dichloroacetate for the treatment of lactic acidosis in patients with shock and lactic acidosis has not been adopted by most centers. In contrast, dichloroacetate appears to have clinical utility in hereditary forms of type B lactic acidosis, as discussed later in this chapter.

Tromethamine (THAM) is a non-sodium-containing buffer with a pK nearer to physiologic pH than bicarbonate or other commonly used bases.[118] It buffers carbonic acid by accepting a proton and also generates bicarbonate. THAM does not raise the $CO_2$ tension directly, and therefore the intracellular pH and cerebrospinal fluid pH do not fall when it is used. However, THAM has not been shown to be any more clinically effective than bicarbonate. In addition, THAM has significant side effects, including hypoglycemia, hyperkalemia, ventilatory depression, and, in children, hepatic injury.

Tribonat is a proprietary mixture of THAM, acetate, sodium bicarbonate, and phosphate that has undergone clinical trials. Although it appears to be an effective buffer, no survival advantage has yet been noted.[119]

Additional therapeutic options have been tried. Because of the poor tissue perfusion in shock, nitroprusside has been recommended for the treatment of shock with lactic acidosis. No significant benefit has been demonstrated, and nitroprusside may contribute to lactate generation.[120, 121] Methylene blue has also been administered without success.[122]

# TYPE B LACTIC ACIDOSIS

## Pathophysiology

Type B lactic acidosis occurs in a diffuse group of conditions that disrupt aerobic metabolism or accelerate glycolysis and increase lactate production despite the presence of adequate cardiac output and tissue oxygenation (Table 6–2). Its causes include hepatic failure, endocrinopathy, vitamin deficiency, exposure to metabolic toxins, and inherited and acquired disorders of mitochondrial metabolism. Although the presence of lactic acidosis indicates serious disease, type B lactic acidosis is often more chronic in nature and may have a considerably better prognosis than type A. Finally, as opposed to the absence of effective therapy for type A lactic acidosis, specific treatment is sometimes available for type B.

**TABLE 6–2.** Conditions Associated with Type B Lactic Acidosis

Endocrine disease and organ failure
- Liver disease
- Diabetes mellitus
- Catecholamine excess
  - Endogenous
  - Exogenous

Thiamine deficiency

Intracellular inorganic phosphate depletion
- Intravenous fructose
- Intravenous xylose
- Intravenous sorbitol

Alcohols and other ingested compounds metabolized by alcohol dehydrogenase
- Ethanol
- Methanol ingestion
- Ethylene glycol ingestion
- Propylene glycol ingestion

Mitochondrial toxins
- Salicylate intoxication
- Cyanide poisoning
- 2,4-dinitrophenol ingestion
- Non-nucleoside anti–reverse transcriptase drugs

Other drugs

Malignancy

Seizure

Inborn errors of metabolism

## Causes

### LIVER DISEASE

The liver is the primary site of gluconeogenesis. It consumes more lactate than any other organ.[123–125] In severe liver disease, whether acute or chronic, the consumption of lactate could theoretically fall so low as to permit serum levels of lactate to accumulate when peripheral production of lactate is not increased. This degree of hepatic failure is typically associated with hypoglycemia and hyperalaninemia, which result from impaired gluconeogenesis and the subsequent excess alanine production.[126–128] Still, lactic acidosis is not especially common in hepatic disease.[129] Lactic acidosis has been noted to develop after large-volume partial hepatectomy, but such instances are rare.[130] More important is that hepatic insufficiency may increase the possibility that lactic acidosis will develop during sepsis or shock.

### DIABETES MELLITUS

Diabetic patients are at increased risk for lactic acidosis, which may complicate ketoacidosis (up to 10% of cases) or nonketotic hyperglycemic coma (up to 40% to 60% of cases).[6, 7, 131–135] Several factors drive the tendency to develop lactic acidosis. First, almost all patients with diabetic coma, whether ketotic or nonketotic, are volume depleted owing to the solute diuresis that results from uncontrolled hyperglycemia. The effect of volume depletion and hormonal responses to this state impact the delivery of cardiac output to a variety of tissue beds and increase the likelihood that tissue hypoxia will develop. Second, in the absence of insulin, PDH (PDC) is relatively inhibited, and less pyruvate is metabolized to acetyl CoA. Pyruvate and lactate concentrations rise as a result. PDH (PDC) inhibition slows oxidative metabolism in mitochondria and decreases the production of NAD and ATP. Because the ratio of lactate to pyruvate reflects the ratio of NAD to NADH, the relative amount of lactate will rise. A second effect of the altered NADH/NAD ratio is that β-hydroxybutyrate becomes the predominant ketone product rather than acetoacetate.[134] If an altered redox state is suspected, specific testing for β-hydroxybutyrate should be done. The decrease in ATP stimulates glycolysis and thus drives the system to produce more lactate as well. In opposition to the forces that increase lactate production, lactate uptake and use in hepatic gluconeogenesis are increased in diabetes.[132, 133] Patients with diabetes have accelerated cardiovascular disease, increased incidence of peripheral vascular disease, and greater rates of infection than do patients without diabetes, and they are exposed to a greater risk of lactic acidosis as a result. Finally, diabetic patients may be treated with the biguanide drugs phenformin and metformin, which may induce lactic acidosis (see later). Some data show that the incidence of lactic acidosis in diabetic patients is similarly increased in the presence or the absence of metformin therapy, although it seems likely that this drug significantly increases the probability that lactic acidosis will develop.[131, 132]

**Phenformin.** Once used for the treatment of diabetes, phenformin was removed from clinical use in the United States owing to the occurrence of lactic acidosis. Its precise mechanism of action has yet to be adequately explained, but it is known to stimulate glycolysis and inhibit gluconeogenesis.[132, 136–138] It also inhibits PDH (PDC) and lactate uptake by the liver.[139] The incidence of lactic acidosis in phenformin users was in the range of 40 to 64 cases per 100,000 patient-years of drug use.[93, 136–140] Although phenformin was removed from the U.S. market many years ago, sporadic cases of phenformin-related lactic acidosis still occur due to illegal importation of the agent.[141–143] Phenformin remains in use outside the United States, and recent case reports highlight the need for awareness that the drug may be brought in by visitors to Mexico or purchased on the Internet. In Europe, phenformin remains available in Italy and elsewhere.[144]

**Metformin.** Metformin is a dimethylbiguanide related to phenformin. As is true for phenformin, its mechanism of action remains unknown but is unrelated to the alteration of insulin release.[132] Metformin was first used in obese diabetic patients in the 1950s in Europe and achieved popularity in the 1980s. The risk for lactic acidosis with metformin use is roughly one twentieth that seen with phenformin use.[145–148] Recent estimates of the risk for lactic acidosis range from 3 to 25 cases per 100,000 patient-years, but in all surveys, lactic acidosis occurred in patients who were given the drug despite the presence of recognized contraindications (Table 6–3). Rare cases without underlying disease are occasionally reported.[149] The mortality rate reported in a series of individuals with metformin-induced lactic acidosis was 45%. The best recent estimate of the fatality rate due to metformin is only 0.015 fatality per 1000 patient-years. Current recommendations are that the drug not be used in patients with congestive heart failure, chronic pulmonary disease, cirrhosis, or significant renal insufficiency (creatinine >1.6 mg/dL).[150–153] Further recommendations include that metformin be discontinued when patients are admitted to the hospital with significant medical disease or for serious surgery, and that metformin treatment be stopped at least 3 days before the performance of radiologic procedures that involve the use of iodine-containing intravenous contrast material.[154–158] The latter recommendation is made largely because of the risk for acute renal dysfunction following dye use.

**TABLE 6–3.** Contraindications to Metformin Use

| |
|---|
| Liver disease |
| Renal insufficiency (creatinine >1.5 mg/dL) |
| Congestive heart failure |
| Significant acute medical disease |
| Perioperative period, significant surgical procedure |
| Impending exposure to intravenous radiocontrast material |

## CATECHOLAMINE EXCESS

Catecholamines stimulate glycolysis.[64] Epinephrine prepares the organism for fight or flight, both of which demand increased energy production and may require that activity continue even if anaerobic exercise is necessary. This causes the concentration of both lactate and pyruvate, the end-products of glycolysis, to increase significantly. Stimulating glycolysis does not necessarily cause acidosis in and of itself. If oxidative metabolism is functioning normally, the newly produced pyruvate can be oxidized effectively by mitochondria. Local lactate excess can be returned to the liver and used in gluconeogenesis. If catecholamines are present in markedly increased concentrations, however, the peripheral vasoconstriction engendered will reduce the mitochondrial metabolism of pyruvate, lower the redox potential, and force lactate concentrations to rise, resulting in lactic acidosis.

Excessive catecholamine administration has been indicted as a cause of lactic acidosis following cardiovascular surgery and in sepsis.[54–56] β-Blockade, in contrast, may reduce the incidence of lactic acidosis in hemorrhage.[159] Lactic acidosis due to excessive circulating catecholamines is a known complication of pheochromocytoma.[160, 161]

## THIAMINE DEFICIENCY

The PDC, which catalyzes the formation of acetyl CoA from pyruvate before the initiation of aerobic metabolism, is thiamine sensitive. If thiamine deficiency is severe, PDH (PDC) is inhibited, and carbohydrate metabolism is limited to glycolysis. Overt thiamine deficiency is rare in the First and Second Worlds, except in alcoholics. However, thiamine deficiency is a known complication of chemotherapy.[162] Thiamine deficiency also may be partially causal in the lactic acidosis of patients with falciparum malaria.[163] The most clinically relevant reports of lactic acidosis occurring because of thiamine deficiency have been related to shortages of injectable multivitamins for patients receiving total parenteral nutrition.[164–167] In these instances, the patients, most of whom had significant chronic bowel disease, developed lactic acidosis when total parenteral nutrition was continued in the absence of appropriate vitamin support. Thiamine supplementation reverses the condition. Thiamine deficiency has also been noted in patients with increased thiamine requirements secondary to pregnancy or inborn errors of metabolism.[168, 169]

## PHOSPHATE DEPLETION

Severe depletion of intracellular phosphate stores inhibits aerobic metabolism because ATP generation requires adequate availability of inorganic phosphate and ADP. Intracellular phosphate depletion of this degree is far more likely a result of "trapping" (see "Glycogen Storage Diseases" and "Hereditary Fructose Intolerance") than of total body phosphate depletion.[170] Phosphate trapping may develop in otherwise normal individuals given intravenous fructose (which bypasses the slow normal absorption, phosphorylation, and release of fructose by the intestinal mucosa), sorbitol, or xylitol.[171–175] Systemic phosphate depletion increases the susceptibility to trapping, but otherwise it is not known to cause lactic acidosis.[174]

## ETHANOL

The ability of ethanol intake to provoke lactic acidosis results from its hepatic metabolism.[176–179] The incidence of alcoholic lactic acidosis may be considerably greater than appreciated.[179] Alcohols are dehydrogenated by alcohol dehydrogenase. The reaction also reduces NAD to NADH. Given the large quantities of alcohol imbibed during a serious drinking binge, the detoxification of alcohol may generate large quantities of NADH and consume large amounts of NAD. The liver is the primary site for lactate use in the Cori cycle. If the redox potential of the liver is reset to a highly reduced state by ethanol metabolism, pyruvate regeneration from lactate will be inhibited, and lactic acidosis and hypoglycemia will ensue.

Two other aspects of alcohol intake also impact the development of lactic acidosis. First, acetaldehyde, a metabolic product of ethanol metabolism, inhibits PDH ($K_i$ = 50 μmol).[180] Second, individuals with chronic alcoholism are at increased risk of developing thiamine deficiency. As discussed earlier, PDH is thiamine dependent; its activity is depressed by thiamine deficiency.

## METHANOL

Like ethanol, methanol is metabolized by alcohol dehydrogenase. The molecular weight of methanol is only 33, and the amount of methanol in even small volumes is significant; fatalities have been reported after ingestion of 30 mL of methanol. Methanol poisoning is typically accompanied by a large increase in serum osmolarity and an osmolar gap.[181]

Lactic acidosis is not the primary acid-base disorder associated with methanol intoxication. Methanol poisoning is more associated with toxicity due to formic acid and formaldehyde, which cause pruritus (formication) and central nervous system and optic symptoms. However, lactic acid is detectable in many cases of methanol ingestion.[182, 183] Because of the high risk of fatality in methanol ingestion, treatment should be initiated as soon as the diagnosis is suspected. The metabolites of methanol are more toxic than methanol itself. Ethanol infusion has been used because ethanol competes with methanol at alcohol dehydrogenase. Alternatively, fomepizole is a nonintoxicating inhibitor of alcohol dehydrogenase that has recently been released for clinical use.[184] If the amount of methanol ingestion is significant, dialysis should be considered.[182, 183]

## ETHYLENE GLYCOL POISONING

Lactic acidosis may develop as one of several organic acidoses during ethylene glycol poisoning.[185] An osmolal gap is generally present.[181, 185] The metabolism of ethylene glycol rests on the action of alcohol dehydrogenase, and the redox potential is affected, as it is in other forms of alcohol toxicity. When ethylene glycol ingestion is suspected, the urine should be examined for oxalate crystals. Therapy involves supportive care, ethanol or fomepizole infusion to block metabolism, and in severe cases, dialysis.[184]

## SALICYLATES

As is the case in methanol and ethylene glycol poisoning, lactic acidosis in salicylate intoxication is a secondary issue in a complex condition. Two other acid-base abnormalities are considerably more prominent. First, low levels of salicylate intoxication are associated with respiratory alkalosis due to salicylate stimulation of the respiratory center. The respiratory alkalosis leads to increased lactate production. Second, salicylate is an organic acid that may accumulate in quantities high enough to explain metabolic acidosis. However, salicylate intoxication is also associated with lactic acidosis and ketoacidosis. In high concentrations, salicylate is an inhibitor of oxidative phosphorylation, with consequences similar to 2,4-dinitrophenol (2,4-DNP; see later), including dependence on glycolysis for energy metabolism and acceleration of lactate and pyruvate production.[186] Stimulation of glycolysis combined with inhibition of oxidative phosphorylation results in increased lactate production.

## CYANIDE POISONING

Cyanide is a highly effective inhibitor of cytochrome $a$ and cytochrome $a_3$, key participants in oxidative phosphorylation.[187] Cellular ATP levels fall as ATP generation fails. In addition, oxidation of NADH to NAD is blocked. The redox potential of the cell shifts to the reduced state at the same time that metabolism becomes increasingly dependent on glycolysis. Lactate concentration increases to a greater extent than does pyruvate. Cyanide poisoning may result from industrial accidents or deliberate ingestion or poisoning. As mentioned earlier, excessive and prolonged exposure to nitroprusside may also lead to cyanide toxicity. Treatment is not often successful, but if the patient can be supported, cyanide is a small molecule that is readily dialyzed, although its volume of distribution is very large. Survival after dialysis has been reported despite severe poisoning.[188]

## 2,4-DINITROPHENOL

2,4-DNP uncouples the mitochondrial reactions that generate ATP from the reactions that oxidize NADH.[189] NAD is produced, but ATP is not generated. Redox potential is less affected than is the case in cyanide poisoning, but the failure of the respiratory chain means that glycolysis is the only source of cellular energy. Lactate and pyruvate concentrations rise. Though a less severe poisoning than that seen with cyanide ingestion, 2,4-DNP ingestion is associated with fatalities. Ingestion is occasionally reported owing to the inclusion of the inhibitor in unapproved weight-loss formulations.

## NUCLEOSIDE ANTI–REVERSE TRANSCRIPTASE DRUGS

Antiretroviral drugs used in the treatment of human immunodeficiency virus (HIV) infection include anti-protease agents, nucleoside anti–reverse transcriptase drugs, and non-nucleoside anti–reverse transcriptase drugs. The most common treatment regimens include multiple agents from at least two categories, generally a combination referred to as highly active antiretroviral therapy (HAART). Because of the complexity of the drug regimens, and because of the coexistence of disease states that may contribute to acid-base abnormalities, it is somewhat difficult to clearly establish whether any single agent is responsible for the occurrence of lactic acidosis. Nonetheless, enough reports have accumulated to indicate that the nucleoside anti–reverse transcriptase class of agents appears to produce lactic acidosis in a subgroup of patients with acquired immunodeficiency syndrome (AIDS). Zidovudine (ZDV), didanosine (ddI), zalcitabine (ddC), fialuridine (experimental agent), and stavudine (D4T) have all been reported to cause lactic acidosis.[190–197] In addition to lactic acidosis, these patients have been noted to develop hepatic steatosis without inflammation.[191, 192, 194] Biopsies of skeletal muscle have shown abnormal mitochondrial structure and intramitochondrial crystalline inclusions. The agents in question have been found to inhibit mitochondrial DNA polymerase, which disrupts mitochondrial DNA synthesis. Mitochondrial dysfunction follows, and cellular energy metabolism becomes disrupted, with loss of aerobic metabolism and dependence on glycolysis. Further effects of zidovudine on mitochondrial respiration have also been reported in laboratory studies, but these require higher drug concentrations than needed to disrupt DNA synthesis. Lactic acidosis appears to be associated with chronic rather than acute use of the agents in question, so the DNA hypothesis appears to be a better fit. If the syndrome is suspected, the offending drugs must be discontinued, although this may not result in the resolution of lactic acidosis or liver disease. It has been suggested that the administration of riboflavin, a precursor of FAD, may be of some benefit, but the data are limited.[198] Whether other underlying processes must be present for lactic acidosis to develop is not known. Vigilance is required.

## OTHER DRUGS

Lactic acidosis due to other drugs has been reported in limited numbers of cases (Table 6–4). Propofol is a sedative used in the management of patients receiving mechanical ventilation and in induction of anesthesia. Metabolic acidosis and lactic acidosis have been noted in children given the drug.[199] Propofol uncouples oxidative phosphorylation in vitro, and this may be the mechanism of lactic acidosis in these cases, although most of the children also had clinically significant bradycardia or other dysrhythmia which could impair circulation. Continuous venovenous hemofiltration and plasmapheresis have been used with good results, and the suggestion has been made that a water-soluble metabolite of propofol may be responsible for the acidosis.

**TABLE 6–4.** Drugs Associated with Type B Lactic Acidosis

| |
|---|
| **Biguanide Oral Hypoglycemic Agents** |
| Phenformin |
| Metformin |
| **Non-nucleoside Anti–reverse Transcriptase Drugs** |
| Zidovudine(ZDV) |
| Didanosine (ddI) |
| Zalcitabine (ddC) |
| Fialuridine |
| Stavudine (D4T) |
| **Miscellaneous Drugs** |
| Propofol |
| Almitrine besmesylate |
| Clozapine |
| Niacin |
| Germanium |
| Streptozotocin |
| Kombucha tea |
| Ritodrine |
| Terbutaline |
| Metaproterenol |
| Propylene glycol |

Almitrine besmesylate is an orally administered vasoconstrictor that has been used in Europe for the management of chronic obstructive pulmonary disease. In theory, increased pulmonary vasoconstriction enhances the redistribution of flow and is thought to improve gas exchange. Intravenous administration of almitrine has been used in acute pulmonary failure as well. A study of 25 patients given the agent intravenously while suffering respiratory failure found that 8 of the 25 developed hepatic dysfunction and lactic acidosis.[200] Both problems resolved after the drug was discontinued, and 6 of the 8 patients survived.

Another drug recently associated with a case of lactic acidosis is clozapine.[201] Several other drugs have been associated with lactic acidosis, including niacin,[202] germanium,[203] propylene glycol,[204] and streptozocin.[205] Lactic acidosis or metabolic acidosis has been noted after the consumption of a folk remedy called Kombucha tea, which is made by growing a Japanese mushroom in strong tea and ingesting the tea.[206] The mechanism is unknown, but the beverage should be avoided. Finally, prior reports have indicated that lactic acidosis may be observed after the use of ritodrine, terbutaline, and inhaled metaproterenol.[2]

## MALIGNANCY

An increased incidence of lactic acidosis has long been noted in patients with solid tumors and hematologic malignancies.[87, 207–217] Several hypotheses have been advanced to explain this occurrence. First of all, large and especially fast-growing tumor masses may outgrow their blood supply, creating areas of localized tissue hypoxia within the tumor. If the rate of lactate production in these regions exceeds ongoing clearance of lactate by the liver, systemic lactic acidosis will develop. Second, a given tumor may be characterized by abnormal oxidative phosphorylation or pyruvate metabolism due to mutation of one or more enzymes. All tumor cells so affected produce lactate, and production may exceed hepatic clearance. Third, some malignancies exhibit accelerated rates of glycolysis. Fourth, tumor lysis syndrome may develop in response to therapy (and, rarely, spontaneously); lactic acidosis may be seen in this circumstance. Fifth, lactate production may be a result of elevated tumor necrosis factor-α or other cytokines produced by the tumor or in response to the malignancy.[215] Finally, there is an increased risk for factitious lactic acidosis in the presence of severe leukocytosis due to in vitro glycolysis after blood samples are collected.

### SEIZURE

Grand mal seizures represent extreme levels of muscular exertion, and hence lactate production.[218, 219] Further, because the muscle activity is involuntary in seizure, it may continue long after pain or fatigue would cause a conscious individual to stop. In prolonged seizure, there may also be compromise of arterial flow to limb beds by continuous muscular contraction. Lactate levels can be extreme, and average arterial lactic acid concentrations exceed 12 mmol/L in the period immediately following a grand mal seizure.[218] Fortunately, recovery is rapid, and lactate levels return to normal within 90 minutes of the seizure in the absence of any specific intervention. Although technically not seizures per se, strychnine poisoning and heatstroke also represent states of extreme muscular stress and may be associated with lactic acidosis.[220, 221]

## INBORN ERRORS OF METABOLISM

The inherited metabolic disorders associated with the occurrence of lactic acidosis are highly complex. These disorders are seen primarily by pediatricians, predominantly in the neonatal period, but in some instances, the defects are relatively mild and permit survival to adulthood and thus may be seen in adult medicine. Further, owing to the unique inheritance of several of these conditions, it is possible that there are undiagnosed and unsuspected cases of inherited metabolic disease underlying some "typical" cases of lactic acidosis.

The first distinction to be made among the inherited causes of lactic acidosis is between those conditions in which lactic acidosis is a secondary, or indirect, consequence of the abnormality and those in which lactic acidosis is a direct result of the metabolic defect in question (Table 6–5 and Fig. 6–4).[180] "Secondary"

**TABLE 6–5.** Inborn Errors of Metabolism Associated with Lactic Acidosis

| Inborn Errors Associated with "Primary" Lactic Acidosis |
|---|
| Glycogen storage diseases |
| von Gierke disease |
| Fructose-1,6-bisphosphatase deficiency |
| Glycogen synthase deficiency |
| Glycogenosis III |
| Hereditary fructose intolerance |
| Pyruvate dehydrogenase complex deficiency |
| Pyruvate carboxylase deficiency |
| Phosphoenol pyruvate carboxykinase deficiency |
| Disorders of tricarboxylic acid (Krebs) cycle enzymes |
| 2-Ketoglutarate dehydrogenase deficiency |
| Succinate dehydrogenase deficiency |
| Lipoamide oxidoreductase (E3) deficiency |
| Fumarase deficiency |
| Disorders of the electron transport chain |
| Complex I deficiency |
| Complex I, III, and IV deficiency |
| Complex I and IV deficiency |
| **Inborn Errors Associated with "Secondary" Lactic Acidosis** |
| Organic acidurias |
| Propionic acidemia |
| Methylmalonic acidemia |
| Hydroxymethylglutaric aciduria |
| Isovaleric aciduria |
| Fatty acid oxidation disorders |
| Multiple acyl-CoA dehydrogenase deficiency (glutaric aciduria type III) |
| Long-chain fatty acid oxidation defects |
| Urea cycle defects |
| Carbamyl phosphate synthetase deficiency |
| Citrullinemia |
| Ornithine carbamyltransferase deficiency |

lactic acidosis thus occurs in several of the hereditary organic acidurias, in disorders of the urea cycle, and in the presence of enzyme defects affecting fatty acid synthesis. In contrast, "primary" hereditary lactic acidosis occurs in the presence of abnormal hepatic glycogen metabolism, gluconeogenesis, lactate-pyruvate oxidation, Krebs cycle metabolism, or electron transfer–respiratory chain activity. Those conditions associated with "primary" lactic acidosis are considered in some detail.

### Glycogen Storage Diseases

The disorders of gluconeogenesis and glycogen storage that are most associated with lactic acidosis are type 1 glycogen storage disease (von Gierke disease) and fructose-1,6-bisphosphatase deficiency.[222–228] The former condition is subdivided into four subtypes: type 1a, caused by an abnormality of either the catalytic subunit of glucose 6-phosphatase, or the glucose 6-phosphatase regulatory protein in the liver; type 1b, caused by deficient hepatic microsomal glucose 6-phosphate transport; type 1c, caused by deficiency of hepatic microsomal phosphate transport; and, in one instance, type 1d, caused by deficiency of the GLUT 7 transporter in the liver.[222] Hepatic gluconeogenesis effectively stops after the formation of glucose 6-phosphate. Glucose cannot be released to the circulation,

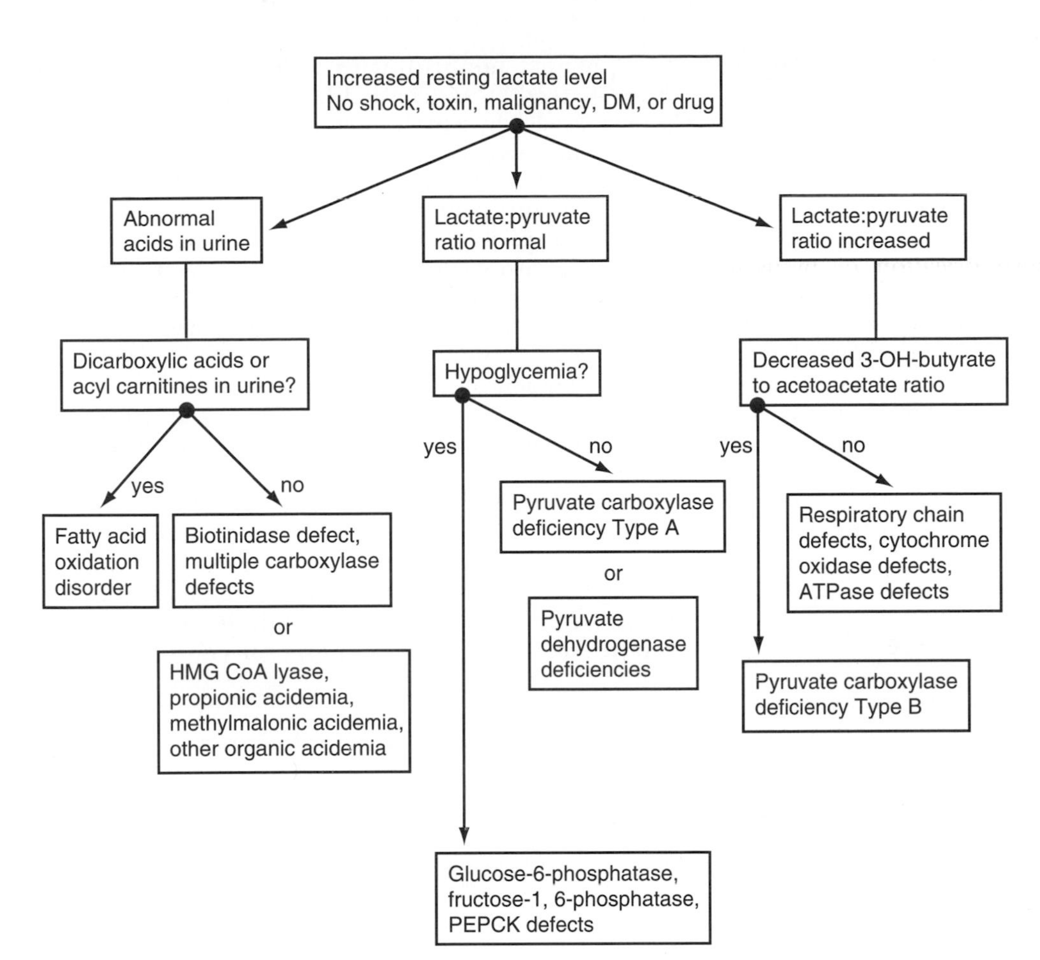


**FIGURE 6–4** ■ Algorithm for evaluation of inherited or acquired lactic acidosis. This simplified flow chart uses clinical biochemistry results to indicate the most likely enzyme defects present in patients with lactic acidosis secondary to inherited or acquired metabolic disorders. The presence of shock, toxins, diabetes (DM), malignancy, or any drug known to induce lactic acidosis excludes the use of this schema. Key issues are the presence or absence of abnormal urinary organic acids and the presence or absence of a lactate: pyruvate ratio significantly over 10:1. Definitive diagnosis of respiratory chain defects, cytochrome oxidase defects, or ATPase defects requires specific measurements of enzyme (complex) activity in affected tissues. Negative studies on circulating blood cells do not rule out the diagnosis. Muscle or liver biopsy may be necessary. ATPase, adenosine triphosphatase; PEPCK, phosphoenol pyruvate carboxykinase.

and hypoglycemia develops after short periods of fasting.[222–226] Glycogen can be made but not consumed, and the liver and kidneys are enlarged due to increased tissue glycogen. When these patients are fasted, hypoglycemia develops, insulin levels fall, and glucagon, growth hormone, and catecholamine concentrations rise. Hepatic glycogenolysis accelerates and increases hepatic glucose 6-phosphate levels, but glucose cannot be formed or released to the circulation. Glycolysis is accelerated, and the intracellular concentration of triose phosphates and pyruvate increases. Some of these intermediates are metabolized via the pentose pathway, but this system has limited capacity. The excess pyruvate is metabolized to acetyl CoA, which drives increased fatty acid synthesis (and hypertriglyceridemia), and the rate of oxidative phosphorylation is increased. Mitochondrial metabolism eventually saturates owing to the excess load and is further limited by the trapping of inorganic phosphate in glucose 6-phosphate and other phosphorylated intermediates. Both pyruvate and lactate concentrations increase, but the ratio shifts to lactate production when mitochondrial oxidation slows. As oxidation fails, intracellular pyruvate levels rise, and pyruvate use in alanine production increases, resulting in hyperalaninemia. Uric acid concentrations rise due to the catabolism of excess AMP and ADP.[225]

Fructose-1,6-bisphosphatase deficiency also leads to failure of gluconeogenesis, but there is less hypoglycemia because stored glycogen can be effectively used to make glucose. Hypoglycemia develops only after a prolonged fast.[222, 227, 228] Again, hypoglycemia stimulates counterregulatory hormone release, which stimulates the glycolytic pathway, but glucose cannot be released to the circulation. Phosphate is trapped in metabolic intermediates, and increased pyruvate production results in increased lactate and fatty acid production. The consequences are similar to those of von Gierke disease. In addition, patients with fructose-1,6-bisphosphatase deficiency develop ketoacidosis during fasting.

Both von Gierke disease and fructose-1,6-bisphosphatase deficiency respond to dietary manipulations designed to avoid hypoglycemia, and patients survive into adulthood if properly treated.[222] The hypoglycemia improves with time in the case of type 1 glycogen storage disease. Acute lactic acidosis and hypoglycemia in either disease may be reversed by the administration of intravenous glucose. Chronic treatment for type 1 glycogen storage disease includes nasogastric administration of glucose solution during sleep and repetitive feeding with uncooked corn starch.[222] Diazoxide has been added in some cases to avoid hypoglycemia and promote growth in growth-retarded children as well.[226] The primary treatment of chronic fructose-1,6-bisphosphatase deficiency is the avoidance of fasting. It is also recommended that fructose and sorbitol be avoided because of the increased risk for phosphate trapping in these patients.

Glycogen synthase deficiency and glycogenosis type III are two other hepatic glycogen storage diseases associated with increased serum lactate concentrations.[222] Glycogen synthase deficiency is characterized by the inability of the liver to synthesize glycogen. If glucose is consumed in excess, the liver responds to the load by preferentially accelerating glycolysis and lactate production. Treatment of the disorder involves frequent feeding to address the tendency toward hypoglycemia caused by the absence of glycogen stores and use of a higher-protein, lower-carbohydrate diet. Glycogenosis type III results from a defect in the enzymes responsible for glycogen branching. Glycogen production and consumption are abnormal, and fasting hypoglycemia and postprandial lactic acidosis are noted.

## Hereditary Fructose Intolerance

The biochemical abnormality present in patients with hereditary fructose intolerance is depression of the activity of fructose 1-phosphate aldolase.[229, 230] This enzyme catalyzes the breakdown of fructose 1-phosphate to D-glyceraldehyde and dihydroxyacetone phosphate. Fructose ingestion by these individuals leads to accumulation of fructose 1-phosphate and depletion of intracellular inorganic phosphate stores. Low phosphate availability limits the ability of the tricarboxylic acid cycle to generate ATP and leads to the accumulation of ADP and AMP. Decreased ATP stimulates PDH (PDC) and thereby accelerates glycolysis and increases extra mitochondrial energy generation. This, however, leads to increased production of lactate and pyruvate at a time when further pyruvate metabolism is limited and NAD levels fall. The ratio of lactate concentration to pyruvate concentration rises, and acidosis follows.

Notable to nephrology is that hereditary fructose intolerance is associated with a form of proximal renal tubular acidosis that resembles Fanconi syndrome.[231, 232] In patients who present with Fanconi syndrome, the work-up should consider the possibility of fructose intolerance.

## Pyruvate Dehydrogenase Complex Deficiency

The most common inherited disorders that cause lactic acidosis are those associated with PDC deficiency.[180, 233] PDC deficiencies are relatively rare but account for the majority of cases of congenital lactic acidosis. Any of the five major components (E1, E2, E3, X-lipoate, and pyruvate dehydrogenase phosphatase) of the PDC may be affected. Both isolated (primary) PDC deficiency and secondary PDC deficiency due to abnormal biotinidase and holoenzyme synthetase activity have been described. E1 complex disorders are associated with an X-linked mutation but behave as if they are autosomal dominant due to an X inactivation phenomenon.[233] Infants with the French phenotype (marked by an elevated lactate-pyruvate ratio and a decreased 3-hydroxybutyric acid–acetoacetate ratio) die within months of delivery; a North American phenotype with a different biochemical profile presents later in infancy and permits survival for a longer period. Some patients present only with ataxic episodes and mild, carbohydrate-intake-sensitive lactic acidosis. Degenerative lesions of the white matter are found on magnetic resonance imaging or brain autopsy and are related to the absence of the enzyme in astrocytic cells, which metabolically support the neurons. The severity of the lesions varies from cystic lesions and cerebral and basal ganglia involvement and cerebral atrophy to absence of neuropathology in the mildest cases.

In patients with milder forms of PDC deficiency, episodes of ataxia may be induced by carbohydrate ingestion. In these instances, a ketogenic diet may be useful.[180, 234] The administration of thiamine has also been recommended, although only some cases have shown evidence of thiamine responsiveness.[235]

## Pyruvate Carboxylase Deficiency

Pyruvate carboxylase (PC) is an intramitochondrial enzyme that regulates the first step of gluconeogenesis. The highest levels of PC are found in liver and kidney. PC deficiency is a rare autosomal recessive disorder.[180, 236] The few individuals found to be lacking in enzyme activity have presented with lactic acidosis, some with an elevated lactate-pyruvate ratio and others with a normal ratio. α-Ketoglutarate is found in excess in the urine. The severity of these disorders falls in three categories, from a devastating disease of infants who have elevated serum ammonium, citrulline, and lysine and severe lactic acidosis and extremely limited survival; to others with lactic acidosis, delayed development, and severe mental retardation if surviving past infancy; and one patient with lactic acidosis but no neurologic consequences. The neurologic consequences of the disorder may be related to the role of PC in astrocyte glutamine-glutamate-GABA metabolism. Some patients present with Leigh disease (see later). Liver and kidney abnormalities may also be present.

## Phosphoenolpyruvate Carboxykinase Deficiency

Phosphoenolpyruvate carboxykinase (PEPCK) deficiency has been described on several occasions and is associated with lactic acidosis, hypoglycemia, hypotonia, hepatomegaly, and failure to thrive.[180] PEPCK catalyzes the decarboxylation of oxaloacetate to phosphoenolpyruvate and is a regulatory step in gluconeogenesis. Deficiency of the enzyme limits gluconeogenesis. The catecholamine response to hypoglycemia accelerates glycolysis and pyruvate and lactate production.

## Mitochondrial Disease

Several disorders of the Krebs cycle enzymes have been described. These include 2-ketoglutarate dehydrogenase deficiency (psychomotor retardation, pyramidal and extrapyramidal dysfunction in early childhood), succinate dehydrogenase deficiency, lipoamide oxidoreductase deficiency (E3), and fumarase deficiency (early onset, progressive encephalopathy, hypotonia, failure to thrive, severe retardation, and early death).[180] There is also a considerable literature regarding inherited and acquired disorders of oxidative phosphorylation and the electron transport chain. Because they induce failure of oxidative phosphorylation and the electron transport chain, these abnormalities result in chronic lactic acidosis.

The heredity of electron transport chain or oxidative phosphorylation disease is complex.[180, 237–241] The system may be disrupted by genetic errors in the mitochondrial genome or the nuclear genome (Fig. 6–5). Mitochondrial inheritance is totally maternal but is not sex linked. Further, spontaneous mutations are known to occur and are the most common cause of some of these syndromes.

Each mitochondrion within a cell carries its own DNA, and cells may contain both affected and normal mitochondria. Complicating matters further is that a given mitochondrion may have multiple copies of DNA—some normal, some abnormal. Because of these factors, some tissues in an affected individual may be normal, others abnormal. The greater the dependence of the organ or tissue in question on oxidative metabolism, the more likely that a mitochondrial defect will be expressed as an organ dysfunction. Another consideration is the effect of mitochondrial lesions on the population dynamics of cells with rapid turnover. In this circumstance, the inheritance of abnormal mitochondria has a survival disadvantage for the clones of affected cells, and, if the individual survives long enough, there is a tendency to outgrow some of the original clinical defects. Stem cells with defects fail to survive, and a healthy population eventually predominates. Some patients with mitochondrial lesions may initially have anemia, leukopenia, and thrombocytopenia, but they recover normal function with time. In contrast, cells with slow turnover and less active metabolism may exhibit symptoms later in life as the proportion of abnormal mitochondria tends to increase. In short, the complex inheritance and the variable expression of mitochondrial defects severely complicate diagnosis. Many of the defects are best described in syndromic terms, but these syndromes have variable expression, and diagnosis is difficult even at this level (Table 6–6). Lactic acidosis occurs in many of the mitochondrial disease syndromes, and investigation of the acidosis is a common starting point toward diagnosis. It is possible that some instances of lactic acidosis in adults are due to unsuspected, partially expressed mitochondrial disorders.[237]

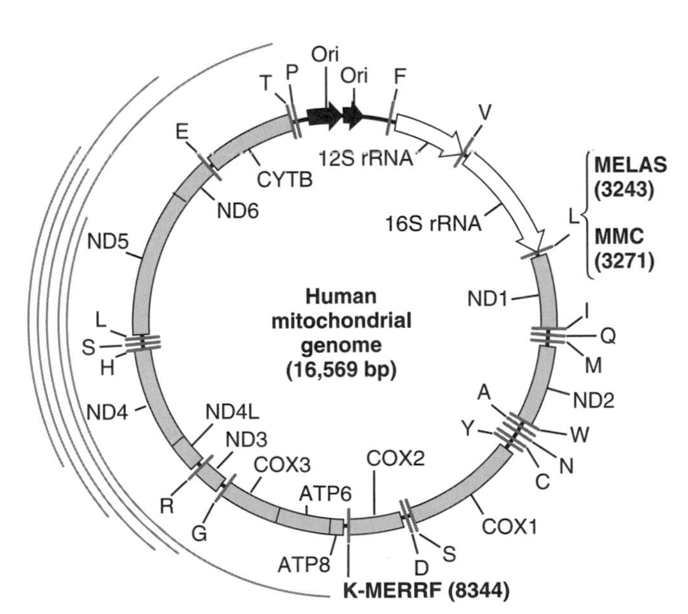


**FIGURE 6–5** ■ The human mitochondrial genome. The variously shaded areas indicate the location of specific rRNA and protein genes. Bars indicate tRNA genes, and the letters at these sites indicate the cognate amino acid for the tRNA. The MELAS and MERRF mutation sites are shown. The 8993 mutation mentioned in the text is not illustrated. The large arcs outside the circular DNA construct indicate recognized large gene deletions associated with the Kearns-Sayre syndrome or the Pearson marrow pancreas syndrome. ATP, hydrogen adenosine triphosphatase; COX, cytochrome oxidase; ND, NADH dehydrogenase. The genome is available in detail from the NIH databank. (Redrawn from NIH databank, accession number NC_001807.)

**TABLE 6–6.** Clinical Syndromes in Disorders of Mitochondrial Metabolism

| |
|---|
| MELAS |
| MERRF |
| Leigh syndrome |
| Pearson marrow pancreas syndrome |
| Kearns-Sayre syndrome |
| Progressive external ophthalmoplegia |

### MELAS

MELAS is the acronym for a clinical syndrome characterized by mitochondrial encephalomyopathy, lactic acidosis, and strokelike episodes.[180, 238–240, 242–249] Most cases (approximately 80%) appear to be due to a mutation of the mitochondrial genome for mitochondrial tRNA-Leu at nucleotide 3243 (see Fig. 6–5). The results of this mutation include the impairment of complex I, complex III, and complex IV function and, thereby, severe defects of mitochondrial energy metabolism. The full extent of the syndrome varies, but it may include hearing loss, hypertrophic cardiomyopathy, ataxia, basal ganglia calcifications, ophthalmoplegia, and diabetes mellitus.[180, 242–249] The disorder is generally considered to be a pediatric condition, but patients survive into adolescence or later. Strokelike episodes are universal by the fifth decade. A survey of adults in a northern district of Finland suggested that the prevalence of the mutation among adults in that region may be as high as 16%.[242] Lactic acidosis was not mentioned among the active clinical problems in these adults, but it is typically found in pediatric cases.

### COMPLEX I DEFICIENCY

Patients with the MELAS syndrome have defects of complex I, but not all patients with complex I disorders are said to have the MELAS syndrome. The cases of complex I deficiency described in the literature had a variety of clinical presentations.[250–253] The cause of the complex I lesion has been localized to a defective synthesis of mitochondrial tRNA (site 3243, 3271, 8344, or 8993 in Fig. 6–5). The lesion is defined by specialized analysis of muscle biopsy material. In a few cases, the lesion is due to a nuclear mutation and is not due to mtRNA, and the disorder does not follow maternal inheritance.[254, 255] Alternative presentations include neonatal fatal lactic acidosis and Leigh disease (subacute necrotizing encephalomyelopathy).

### MERRF

The MERRF (myoclonic epilepsy with ragged red fibers) syndrome presents with myoclonus, ataxia, muscular weakness, and seizure activity.[180, 238–241, 249, 256] The onset of symptoms is in childhood or early adulthood. Cerebral and cerebellar atrophy is found on computed tomography scans, and calcifications of the basal ganglia are suggestive of the disorder. Muscle biopsy reveals ragged red muscle fibers and abnormal mitochondria. Most cases are associated with a heteroplasmic point mutation of residue 8344 of the mitochondrial tRNA gene (lysine). Synthesis of complexes I and IV is affected. The severity of the syndrome varies, depending on the extent to which the total amount of mitochondrial DNA is affected.

### PEARSON MARROW PANCREAS SYNDROME AND KEARNS-SAYRE SYNDROME

The Pearson marrow pancreas syndrome is a complex condition of early life marked by refractory sideroblastic anemia, thrombocytopenia, neutropenia, and defects of pancreatic exocrine function.[180, 238–241, 249, 257, 258] In addition, renal disease, liver failure, hyperparathyroidism, and diabetes may be present. Diarrhea develops due to the pancreatic insufficiency, and lactic acidosis is part of the syndrome. The disorder develops as a consequence of deletions in the mitochondrial genome in the affected tissues. The size of the deletion is noted to vary significantly among affected individuals. Affected enzymes include NADH dehydrogenase subunits, and abnormalities of two mitochondrial tRNAs have also been noted. Most cases are due to spontaneous mutation and are not inherited. The severity of the lesion varies from tissue to tissue in affected individuals. Those patients who survive the initial onset of the condition may go on to exhibit the Kearns-Sayre syndrome.[257] The explanation offered for this transformation is that the mitochondrial gene disorder may be present in only a subpopulation of the cells of the affected tissue. Owing to the rapid turnover of the hematopoietic stem cells and the poor survival of those cells that bear the mutation, there is strong pressure favoring the expansion of the normal population and the eventual total suppression of the affected clones. Thus the anemia and thrombocytopenia disappear as the normal clones expand over time. If neuromuscular cells are also affected, the expression of this portion of the disorder develops as the proportion of affected mitochondria in the nerve and muscle tissue increases. As a result, some individuals survive the Pearson syndrome to develop the Kearns-Sayre syndrome.

The Kearns-Sayre syndrome and progressive external ophthalmoplegia develop before age 20 and are variably marked by ophthalmoplegia, retinal degeneration, heart block, and elevated cerebrospinal fluid protein levels.[180, 249, 257] Enzyme abnormalities found in patients with the syndromes include succinyl dehydrogenase and cytochrome *c* reductase deficiency in the affected tissue. The genetic basis is usually a large-scale mitochondrial DNA deletion, although other mitochondrial genetic duplications have also been found. Lactic acid develops due to the abnormalities of mitochondrial oxidative metabolism.

### LEIGH SYNDROME

Leigh syndrome is characterized by progressive, subacute, necrotizing encephalopathy and is caused by any of a number of mitochondrial enzyme abnormalities. It is seen early in infancy and childhood.[180, 249, 258–260] The syndrome is expressed in patients with PDC deficiency and deficiencies of complex I, complex IV, PC, and mitochondrial ATPase. Lactic acidosis occurs due to the effects on oxidative metabolism.

## Treatment of Lactic Acidosis in Disorders of Mitochondrial Metabolism

The clinical syndromes associated with defective mitochondrial metabolism are often marked by devastating neuromuscular symptoms, but symptoms may be significantly milder in given individuals. The lactic acidosis seen in these syndromes also varies considerably in severity. Typically, it is chronic in nature, and, unlike type A lactic acidosis, lactic acidosis in these diseases does not indicate imminent death. Therapy therefore is aimed at the enhancement of lactate or pyruvate use by other metabolic routes.

Dichloroacetate inhibits a kinase that inactivates PDC and thus stimulates PDC activity.[261–263] This shifts some pyruvate catabolism away from the formation of more lactic acid. The available literature indicates that the efficacy of dichloroacetate in these syndromes varies. Clinical trials are very limited owing to both the rarity of the conditions and the variability of their actual genetic defects and the expression of those defects. Significant toxicity has not been reported, and in those cases in which lactate levels fall, the response can often be maintained.[264]

Other suggested therapy includes the administration of coenzyme Q10, which serves as an antioxidant and potentially affects mitochondrial membrane fluidity.[262] Riboflavin has been reported to improve metabolism in some patients with complex I deficiency.[263] Lipoamide dehydrogenase (E3) deficiency may respond to lipoic acid administration. Menadione (vitamin $K_3$) is a synthetic naphthoquinone derivative that can accept electrons at a potential that could permit the transfer of electrons between ubiquinone and cytochrome *c* in the absence of complex III.[262] Administration of menadione and ascorbic acid has been reported to improve muscle metabolic function in patients with complex III deficiency, but treatment did not alter the circulating lactate level.

## D-LACTIC ACIDOSIS

D-Lactic acidosis differs from typical lactic acidosis in several highly significant ways.[265–273] First, the compound in question is the D stereoisomer of lactate, which is a bacterial product and not a result of mammalian metabolism. Second, D-lactic acidosis is essentially due to the unintentional ingestion of D-lactic acid, not metabolic overproduction. Finally, the symptom complex associated with D-lactic acidosis is far more reflective of intoxication than of acidosis.

The source of D-lactate reported in the clinical literature is its production by colonic bacteria. In most instances there is a history of previous bowel surgery and the presence of a blind loop of gut in which bacterial overgrowth is supported.[265–273] Overproduction of D-lactate occurs when an excess of metabolizable carbohydrates is introduced into this waiting pool of bacteria. The syndrome is rare, because under normal circumstances, human gastrointestinal anatomy and physiology do not allow the prerequisite bacterial overgrowth to occur. A review published in 1998 gleaned only 20 cases from the literature, but many cases doubtless go unreported.[269] In contrast, D-lactic acidosis is well recognized as a disorder of ruminants in the veterinary literature. In these species, the rumen always has a vast population of carbohydrate-metabolizing bacteria that digest otherwise poorly digestible cellulose. If an animal attains access to a food source too rich in easily digestible carbohydrates, however, accelerated bacterial metabolism generates large amounts of D-lactate. The observed signs in the animal include gait disturbances, blindness, and death.

A review of the data pertaining to D-lactate metabolism reveals that humans can clear the compound at rates approaching 100 mmol/h.[267] Some clearance occurs by conversion to pyruvate by the enzyme D-α-hydroxy acid dehydrogenase. This enzyme appears to be inhibited by oxalate, which is present in high concentrations in patients with short bowel syndrome. An additional element of D-lactate clearance is provided by renal excretion of the compound; renal insufficiency probably heightens susceptibility to the syndrome.

The presentation of D-lactic acidosis in humans includes symptoms that echo the observations made in the veterinary disorder. Patients develop confusion, slurred speech, ataxia, and loss of memory.[274] Alcohol ingestion may be suspected. It is currently believed that the apparent intoxication is related to a number of other products of bacterial fermentation with effects on the central nervous system other than D-lactate, but significant amounts of ethanol are not produced.

D-Lactate is not detected by the standard clinical assay for lactate. The standard reagents react only with the L-isomer. It can be detected by nuclear magnetic resonance spectroscopy.[273] D-Lactate can be measured by a relatively simple adaptation of the standard assay. The commercially available assay uses a kit that measures NADH generation by L-lactic dehydrogenase. Substitution of D-lactic dehydrogenase for the L enzyme permits the measurement of D-lactate concentration. Although D-lactic acidosis is considered an anion gap acidosis, in some cases of D-lactic acidosis, only a minimal concentration of D-lactate is present. If D-lactate is present in quantity, a significant anion gap will be present. However, because D-lactate may be effectively cleared by the kidney, some confirmed cases of D-lactic acidosis have presented with a normal anion gap.

The acidemia of D-lactic acidosis can be severe. Serum bicarbonate falls as the lactate (pK = 3.8) is buffered. Arterial pH may fall to as low as 7.1, but more commonly it is somewhat higher. Because the lactate is not produced by the patient but is, in a sense, ingested, administration of bicarbonate is useful if the pH becomes a serious issue.

Treatment of the intoxication syndrome requires supportive measures. Three D-lactate–specific measures should be considered. First, the diet should be adjusted to reduce the delivery of simple carbohydrate to the bacteria-rich colon. In some instances, all oral intake has been stopped and the patient supported with parenteral nutrition. Second, metronidazole or neomycin can be given to alter the bowel flora (vancomycin use should be avoided because of the possible development of vancomycin-resistant enterococci). Finally, if these measures fail and the particular circumstances of the patient permit, surgery to eliminate the blind loop should be considered to avoid recurrence of the disease.

## FACTITIOUS LACTIC ACIDOSIS

When assessing the potential occurrence of lactic acidosis, one must consider the possibility that both the low bicarbonate and the elevated lactate levels detected on a venous blood sample may be artifactual. A single blood sample may provide erroneous data due to two distinct errors of collection and handling. First, excessive and prolonged constriction of blood flow, especially if combined with energetic fist clenching to increase the prominence of forearm veins, may result in temporary and irrelevant local lactate production in the arm from which blood is drawn. Second, improper handling of the collected blood sample may result in lactate production in vitro. Red blood cells lack mitochondria and are incapable of aerobic metabolism. When vials of blood are maintained at room temperature for excessive lengths of time in the absence of a metabolic inhibitor, the red cells continue to metabolize the ambient glucose, generating lactate as a metabolic end-product. This process is more evident when large numbers of white blood cells are present in the sample, as is the case in leukemia. Large amounts of lactate may be produced, with secondary consumption of bicarbonate buffer. The first abnormality noticed is low serum bicarbonate. If this is carefully assessed by performance of an arterial blood gas measurement, the error will be noted. If, however, it is assumed that acidosis is present, subsequent measurement of lactate levels may compound the error unless care is taken to keep the sample chilled or to use a vial containing an inhibitor.[275]

### ACKNOWLEDGMENT

The authors would like to thank Professor Elmus Beale, Ph.D., Department of Cell Biology and Biochemistry, Texas Tech University Health Sciences Center, Lubbock, Texas, for his careful review of the manuscript and his invaluable assistance in generating Figure 6–5.

## REFERENCES

1. Claussen SW: Anhydremic acidosis due to lactic acid. Am J Dis Child 29:761, 1925.
2. Mizock BA: Lactic acidosis. Dis Mon 35:233, 1989.
3. Huckabee WE: Abnormal resting blood lactate. I. The significance of hyperlactatemia in hospitalized patients. Am J Med 30:833, 1961.
4. Huckabee WE: Abnormal resting blood lactate. II. Lactic acidosis. Am J Med 30:840, 1961.
5. Oliva PB: Lactic acidosis. Am J Med 48:209, 1970.
6. Cohen RD, Woods HF: Clinical and Biochemical Aspects of Lactic Acidosis. Oxford, Blackwell Scientific, 1976.
7. Cohen RD, Woods HF: Lactic acidosis revisited. Diabetes 32: 181, 1983.
8. Kreisberg RA: Lactate homeostasis and lactic acidosis. Ann Intern Med 92:227, 1980.
9. Park R, Arieff AI: Lactic acidosis: Current concepts. Clin Endocrinol Metab 12:339, 1983.
10. Frommer JP: Lactic acidosis. Med Clin North Am 67:815, 1983.
11. Narins RG, Jones ER, Townsend R, et al: Metabolic acid-base disorders: Pathophysiology, classification, and treatment. In Arieff AI, DeFronzo RA (eds): Fluid Electrolyte and Acid-Base Disorders. New York, Churchill Livingstone, 1985, p 269.
12. Relman AS: Lactic acidosis. In Brenner BM, Stein JH (eds): Contemporary Issues in Nephrology. Acid-Base and Potassium Homeostasis, vol 2. New York, Churchill Livingstone, 1978, p 65.
13. Park R, Arieff AI: Lactic acidosis. Adv Intern Med 25:33, 1980.
14. Madias NE: Lactic acidosis. Kidney Int 29:752, 1986.
15. Halperin ML, Fields ALA: Review: Lactic acidosis: Emphasis on the carbon precursors and buffering of the acid load. Am J Med Sci 289:154, 1985.
16. DuBose TD: Acid-base disorders. In Brenner BM (ed): Brenner and Rector's The Kidney, 7th ed. Philadelphia, WB Saunders, 2000, pp 925–997.
17. Gevers W, Dowdle E: The effect of pH on glycolysis in vivo. Clin Sci 25:343, 1963.
18. Hood VL, Schubert C, Keller V, Muller S: Effect of system pH on pHi and lactic acid generation in exhaustive forearm exercise. Am J Physiol 255:F479, 1988.
19. Davies SF, Iber C, Keene SA, et al: Effect of respiratory alkalosis during exercise on blood lactate. J Appl Physiol 61:948, 1986.
20. Bersin RM, Arieff AI: Primary lactic alkalosis. Am J Med 85: 867, 1988.
21. Halperin ML, Connors HP, Relman AS, Kamovsky ML: Factors that control the effect of pH on glycolysis in leukocytes. J Biol Chem 244:384, 1969.
22. Moorehouse JA: Pyruvate tolerance tests in healthy and diabetic subjects. Lancet 1:689, 1964.
23. Taylor WM, Halperin ML: Regulation of pyruvate dehydrogenase in muscle: Inhibition by citrate. J Biol Chem 248:6080, 1973.
24. Kriesberg RA: Glucose-lactate interrelations in man. N Engl J Med 287:132, 1972.
25. Cohen RD, Iles RA: Lactic acidosis: Some physiological and clinical considerations. Clin Sci Mol Med 53:405, 1977.
26. Owen OE, Felig P, Morgan AP, et al: Liver and kidney metabolism during prolonged starvation. J Clin Invest 48:1589, 1967.
27. Wahren J, Felig P, Ahlborg T, Jorfeldt L: Glucose metabolism during leg exercise in man. J Clin Invest 50:2715, 1971.
28. Yudkin J, Cohen RD: The contribution of the kidney to the removal of a lactic acid load under normal and acidotic conditions in the conscious rat. Clin Sci Mol Med 48:121, 1975.
29. Berry MN: The liver and lactic acidosis. Proc R Soc Med 60: 1260, 1967.
30. Sestoft L, Trap-Jensen J, Lyngsoe J, et al: Regulation of gluconeogenesis and ketogenesis during rest and exercise in diabetic subjects and normal men. Clin Sci Mol Med 53:411, 1977.
31. McLane JA, Holloszy JO: Glycogen synthesis from lactate in the three types of skeletal muscle. J Biol Chem 254:6548, 1979.
32. Arieff AI, Park R, Leach WJ, Lazarowitz VC: Pathophysiology of experimental lactic acidosis. Am J Physiol 239:F135, 1980.
33. Bruce RA, Jones JW, Strait GB: Anaerobic metabolic responses to acute maximal exercise in male athletes. Am Heart J 67: 643, 1964.
34. Hermansen L, Machlum S, Pruett EDR, et al: Lactate removal at rest and during exercise. In Howald H, Portman JR (eds): Metabolic Adaptation to Prolonged Physical Exercise. Basel, Birkhauser Verlag, 1975, p 101.
35. Osnes JB, Hermansen L: Acid-base balance after maximal exercise of short duration. J Appl Physiol 32:59, 1972.
36. Lundin AP, Stein RA, Brown CD, et al: Fatigue, acid-base and electrolyte changes with exhaustive treadmill exercise in hemodialysis patients. Nephron 46:57, 1987.
37. Gallagher EJ, Rodriguez K, Touger M: Agreement between peripheral venous and arterial lactate levels. Ann Emerg Med 29:479, 1997.
38. Weil MH, Rackow EC, Trevino R, et al: Difference in acid-base state between venous and arterial blood during cardiopulmonary resuscitation. N Engl J Med 315:153, 1986.
39. Adrogué HJ, Rashad MN, Gorin AB, et al: Assessing acid-base status in circulatory failure: Differences between arterial and central venous blood. N Engl J Med 320:1312, 1989.
40. Schumer W: Lactic acid as a factor in the production of irreversibility in oligaemic shock. Nature 212:1210, 1966.
41. Arieff AI, Gertz EW, Park R, et al: Lactic acidosis and the cardiovascular system in the dog. Clin Sci 64:573, 1983.
42. Peretz DL, Scott HM, Duff J, et al: The significance of lactic acidemia in the shock syndrome. Ann N Y Acad Sci 119: 1133, 1965.
43. MacLean LD, Mulligan WG, McLean APH, Duff JH: Patterns of septic shock in man—a detailed study of 56 patients. Ann Surg 166:543, 1967.
44. Vincent JL, Dufaye D, Berre J, et al: Serial lactate determinations during circulatory shock. Crit Care Med 11:449, 1983.
45. Cloutier CT, Lowery BD, Carey LC: Acid-base disturbances in hemorrhagic shock. Arch Surg 98:551, 1969.
46. Aberman A, Fulop M: The metabolic and respiratory acidosis of acute pulmonary edema. Ann Intern Med 76:173, 1972.
47. Fulop M, Horowitz M, Aberman A, Jaffe ER: Lactic acidosis in pulmonary edema due to left ventricular failure. Ann Intern Med 79:180, 1973.
48. Tashkin DP, Goldstein PJ, Simmon DH: Hepatic lactate uptake

during decreased liver perfusion and hypoxemia. Am J Physiol 223:968, 1972.
49. Berry MN, Scheuer J: Splanchnic lactic acid metabolism in hyperventilation, metabolic alkalosis and shock. Metabolism 16:537, 1967.
50. Lloyd MH, Iles RA, Simpson BR, et al: The effect of simulated metabolic acidosis on intracellular pH and lactate metabolism in the isolated perfused rat liver. Clin Sci Mol Med 45:543, 1973.
51. Iles RA, Cohen RD, Rist AH, Baron PG: The mechanism of inhibition by acidosis of gluconeogenesis from lactate in rat liver. Biochem J 164:185, 1977.
52. Baron PG, Iles RA, Cohen RD: Effect of varying $Pco_2$ on intracellular pH and lactate consumption in the isolated perfused rat liver. Clin Sci Mol Med 55:175, 1978.
53. Iles RA, Baron PG, Cohen RD: Mechanism of the effect of varying $Pco_2$ on gluconeogenesis from lactate in the perfused rat liver. Clin Sci Mol Med 55:183, 1978.
54. Raper RF, Cameron G, Walker D, Bowey CJ: Type B lactic acidosis following cardiopulmonary bypass. Crit Care Med 25: 46, 1997.
55. Totaro RJ, Raper RF: Epinephrine-induced lactic acidosis following cardiopulmonary bypass. Crit Care Med 25:1693, 1997.
56. Day NP, Phu NH, Bethell DP, et al: The effects of dopamine and adrenaline infusions on acid-base balance and systemic haemodynamics in severe infection. Lancet 348:219, 1996.
57. Cremer J, Martin M, Redl H, et al: Systemic inflammatory response syndrome after cardiac operations. Ann Thorac Surg 61:1714, 1996.
58. Gore DC, Jahoor F, Hibbert JM, DeMaria EJ: Lactic acidosis during sepsis is related to increased pyruvate production, not deficits in tissue oxygen availability. Ann Surg 224:97, 1996.
59. Bernard GR, Wheeler AP, Russell JA, et al: The effects of ibuprofen on the physiology and survival of patients with sepsis. The Ibuprofen in Sepsis Study Group. N Engl J Med 336: 912, 1997.
60. Harvey RM, Enson Y, Lewis ML, et al: Hemodynamic effects of dehydration and metabolic acidosis in Asiatic cholera. Trans Assoc Am Physicians 79:177, 1966.
61. Bondeu EB, Boley SJ: Early diagnosis of acute mesenteric ischemia. J Crit Illness 1:17, 1986.
62. Taura P, Lopez A, Lacy AM, et al: Prolonged pneumoperitoneum at 15 mmHg causes lactic acidosis. Surg Endosc 12: 198, 1998.
63. Krahenbuhl N: Blood lactate measurement in peripheral arterial disease. In Moret PR, Weber J (eds): Lactate: Physiologic, Methodologic, and Pathologic Approach. New York, Springer-Verlag, 1980, p 174.
64. Huckabee WE: Relationships of pyruvate and lactate during anaerobic metabolism. III. Effect of breathing low-oxygen gases. J Clin Invest 37:264, 1958.
65. Eldridge F: Blood lactate and pyruvate in pulmonary insufficiency. N Engl J Med 274:878, 1966.
66. Refsum HE, Opdahl H, Leraand S: Effect of extreme metabolic acidosis on oxygen delivery capacity of the blood—an in vitro investigation of changes in the oxyhemoglobin dissociation curve in blood with pH values of approximately 6.30. Crit Care Med 25:1497, 1997.
67. Brown SD, Clark C, Gutierrez G: Pulmonary lactate release in patients with sepsis and the adult respiratory distress syndrome. J Crit Care 11:2, 1996.
68. Rabbat A, Laaban JP, Boussairi A, Rochemaure J: Hyperlactatemia during acute severe asthma. Intensive Care Med 24: 304, 1998.
69. Cori CF, Cori GT: Mechanism of epinephrine action. IV: The influence of epinephrine on lactic acid production and sugar utilization. J Biol Chem 84:683, 1929.
70. Maury E, Ioos V, Lepecq B, et al: A paradoxical effect of bronchodilators. Chest 111:1766, 1997.
71. Buehler JH, Berns AS, Webster JR Jr, et al: Lactic acidosis from carboxyhemoglobinemia after smoke inhalation. Ann Intern Med 82:803, 1975.
72. Siebert DJ, Ebaugh FG Jr: Assessment of tissue anoxemia in chronic anemia by the arterial lactate/pyruvate ratio and excess lactate formation. J Lab Clin Med 69:177, 1967.
73. Krishna S, Supanaranond W, Pukrittayakamee S, et al: The disposition and effects of two doses of dichloroacetate in adults with severe falciparum malaria. Br J Clin Pharmacol 41:29, 1996.
74. English M, Muambi B, Mithwani S, Marsh K: Lactic acidosis and oxygen debt in African children with severe anaemia. QJM 90:563, 1997.
75. Essex DW, Jin DK, Bradley TP: Lactic acidosis secondary to severe anemia in a patient with paroxysmal nocturnal hemoglobinuria. Am J Hematol 55:110, 1997.
76. Finch CA, Gollnick PD, Hlastala MP, et al: Lactic acidosis as a result of iron deficiency. J Clin Invest 64:129, 1979.
77. Stacpoole PW: Lactic acidosis: The case against bicarbonate therapy. Ann Intern Med 105:276, 1986.
78. Luft D, Deichsel G, Schmulling RM, et al: Definition of clinically relevant lactic acidosis in patients with internal diseases. Am J Clin Pathol 80:484, 1983.
79. Peretz DI, McGregor M, Dossetor JB: Lactic acidosis: A clinically significant aspect of shock. Can Med Assoc J 90:673, 1964.
80. Blair E, Cowley RA, Tait MK: Refractory septic shock in man: Role of lactate and pyruvate metabolism and acid-base balance in prognosis. Am Surg 31:537, 1965.
81. MacLean LD, Mulligan WG, McLean AP, Duff JH: Patterns of septic shock in man—a detailed study of 56 patients. Ann Surg 166:543, 1967.
82. Medgett IC, Hicks PE, Lasger SZ: Effect of acidosis on 1- and 2-adrenoceptor-mediated vasoconstrictor responses in isolated arteries. Eur J Pharmacol 135:443, 1987.
83. Wildenthal K, Mierzwiak DS, Myers RW, Mitchell JH: Effects of acute lactic acidosis on left ventricular performance. Am J Physiol 214:1352, 1968.
84. Orchard CA, Houser SR, Kort AA, et al: Acidosis facilitates spontaneous sarcoplasmic reticulum Ca release in rat myocardium. J Gen Physiol 253:145, 1987.
85. Mattar JA: Cardiac arrest in the critically ill: Hyperosmolar states following cardiac arrest. Am J Med 56:162, 1974.
86. Posner J, Plum F: Spinal fluid pH and neurologic symptoms in systemic acidosis. N Engl J Med 277:605, 1967.
87. Fraley DS, Adler S, Bruns FJ, Zett B: Stimulation of lactate production by administration of bicarbonate in a patient with a solid neoplasm and lactic acidosis. N Engl J Med 303:1100, 1980.
88. Bellingham AJ, Detter JC, Lenfant C: Regulatory mechanisms of hemoglobin affinity in acidosis and alkalosis. J Clin Invest 50: 700, 1971.
89. Robin ED: Dynamic aspects of metabolic acid-base disturbances: Phenformin lactic acidosis with alkaline overshoot. Trans Am Assoc Physicians 85:317, 1972.
90. Whang R: Bicarbonate overshoot: An indication for acetazolamide therapy. South Med J 68:733, 1972.
91. Mathieu D, Neviere P, Beilard D, et al: Effects of bicarbonate therapy on hemodynamics and tissue oxygenation in patients with lactic acidosis: A prospective, controlled clinical study. Crit Care Med 19:1352, 1991.
92. Cooper DJ, Walley KR, Wiggs BR, et al: Bicarbonate does not improve hemodynamics in critically ill patients who have lactic acidosis. Ann Intern Med 112:492, 1990.
93. Luft D, Schmulling RM, Eggstein M: Lactic acidosis in biguanide treated diabetics: A review of 330 cases. Diabetologia 14: 75, 1978.
94. Stacpoole PW, Harman EM, Curry SH, et al: Treatment of lactic acidosis with dichloroacetate. N Engl J Med 309:390, 1983.
95. Stacpoole PW, Lorenz AC, Thomas RG, Harman EM: Dichloroacetate in the treatment of lactic acidosis. Ann Intern Med 108:58, 1988.
96. Stacpoole PW, Wright EC, Baumgartner TG, et al: A controlled clinical trial of dichloroacetate for treatment of lactic acidosis in adults. The Dichloroacetate–Lactic Acidosis Study Group. N Engl J Med 327:1564, 1992.
97. Graf H, Leach W, Arieff AI: Metabolic effects of sodium bicarbonate in hypoxic lactic acidosis in dogs. Am J Physiol 249: F630, 1985.
98. Arieff AI, Leach W, Park R, Lazarowitz VC: Systemic effects of $NaHCO_3$ in experimental lactic acidosis in dogs. Am J Physiol 242:F586, 1982.

99. Minot AS, Dadd K, Saunders JM: The acidosis of guanidine intoxication. J Clin Invest 13:781, 1934.
100. Halperin FA, Cheema-Dhadli S, Chen CB, Halperin ML: Alkali therapy extends the period of survival during hypoxia: Studies in rats. Am J Physiol 271:R381, 1996.
101. Narins RG, Cohen JJ: Bicarbonate therapy for organic acidosis: The case for its continued use. Ann Intern Med 106:615, 1987.
102. Morris LR, Murphy MB, Kitabchi AE: Bicarbonate therapy in severe diabetic ketoacidosis. Ann Intern Med 105:836, 1986.
103. Garella S, Dana CL, Chazan JA: Severity of metabolic acidosis as a determinant of bicarbonate requirements. N Engl J Med 289:121, 1973.
104. Hazzard PB, Griffin JP: Calculation of sodium bicarbonate requirement in metabolic acidosis. Am J Med Sci 283:18, 1982.
105. Gudis SM, Mangi S, Feinroth M, et al: Rapid correction of severe lactic acidosis with massive isotonic bicarbonate infusion and simultaneous ultrafiltration. Nephron 33:65, 1983.
106. Vaziri ND, Ness R, Wellikson L, et al: Bicarbonate buffered peritoneal dialysis: An effective adjunct in the treatment of lactic acidosis. Am J Med 67:392, 1979.
107. Morgera S, Heering P, Szentandrasi T, et al: Comparison of a lactate versus acetate-based hemofiltration replacement fluid in patients with acute renal failure. Ren Fail 19:155, 1997.
108. Levraut J, Ciebiera JP, Jambou P, et al: Effect of continuous venovenous hemofiltration with dialysis on lactate clearance in critically ill patients. Crit Care Med 25:58, 1997.
109. Roy D, Hogg RJ, Wilby PA, et al: Continuous veno-venous hemodiafiltration using bicarbonate dialysate. Pediatr Nephrol 11:680, 1997.
110. Mariano F, Benzi L, Cecchetti P, et al: Efficacy of continuous venovenous haemofiltration (CVVH) in the treatment of severe phenformin-induced lactic acidosis. Nephrol Dial Transplant 13:1012, 1998.
111. Hilton PJ, Taylor J, Forni LG, Treacher DF: Bicarbonate-based haemofiltration in the management of acute renal failure with lactic acidosis. QJM 91:279, 1998.
112. Sun JH, Filley GF, Hord K, et al: Carbicarb: An effective substitute for $NaHCO_3$ for the treatment of acidosis. Surgery 102: 835, 1987.
113. Whitehouse S, Cooper RH, Randle PJ: Mechanism of activation of pyruvate dehydrogenase by dichloroacetate and other halogenated carboxylic acids. Biochem J 141:761, 1974.
114. Crabb DW, Yount EA, Harris RA: The metabolic effects of dichloroacetate. Metabolism 30:1024, 1981.
115. Blackshear PJ, Holloway PAH, Alberti GMM: The metabolic effects of sodium dichloroacetate in the starved rat. Biochem J 142:279, 1974.
116. Stacpoole PW, Moore GW, Kornhauser DM: Metabolic effects of dichloroacetate in patients with diabetes mellitus and hyperlipoproteinemia. N Engl J Med 298:526, 1978.
117. Graf H, Leach W, Arieff AI: Effects of dichloroacetate in the treatment of hypoxic lactic acidosis in dogs. J Clin Invest 96: 919, 1985.
118. Brasch H, Thies E, Iven H: Pharmacokinetics of TRIS (hydroxymethyl-) aminomethane in healthy subjects and in patients with metabolic acidosis. Eur J Clin Pharmacol 22:257, 1982.
119. Bjemeroth G: Alkaline buffers for correction of metabolic acidosis during cardiopulmonary resuscitation with focus on Tribonat. Resuscitation 37:161, 1998.
120. Taradash MR, Jacobson LB: Vasodilator therapy of idiopathic lactic acidosis. N Engl J Med 293:468, 1975.
121. Humphrey SH, Nash DA Jr: Lactic acidosis complicating sodium nitroprusside therapy. Ann Intern Med 88:58, 1978.
122. Tranquada RE, Bernstein S, Grant WJ: Intravenous methylene blue in the therapy of lactic acidosis. Arch Intern Med 114: 13, 1964.
123. Woll PJ, Record CO: Lactate elimination in man: Effects of lactate concentration and hepatic dysfunction. Eur J Clin Invest 9:397, 1979.
124. Connor H, Woods HF, Murray JD, Ledingham JGG: Utilization of L(+) lactate in patients with liver disease. Ann Nutr Metab 26:308, 1982.
125. Heinig RE, Clarke EF, Waterhouse C: Lactic acidosis and liver disease. Arch Intern Med 139:1229, 1979.
126. Maguire LC, Sherman BM, Whalen JE: Glucose therapy of recurrent lactic acidosis. Am J Med Sci 276:305, 1978.
127. Medalle R, Webb R, Waterhouse C: Lactic acidosis and associated hypoglycemia. Arch Intern Med 128:273, 1971.
128. Marliss EB, Aoki TT, Toews CJ, et al: Amino acid metabolism in lactic acidosis. Am J Med 52:474, 1972.
129. Record CO, Iles RA, Cohen RD, Williams R: Acid-base and metabolic disturbances in fulminant hepatic failure. Gut 16: 144, 1975.
130. Davidson BR, Rai R: Prolonged lactic acidosis after extended hepatectomy under in situ hypothermic perfusion. Liver Transpl Surg 5:151, 1999.
131. Fulop M, Hoberman HD, Rascoff JH, et al: Lactic acidosis in diabetic patients. Arch Intern Med 136:987, 1976.
132. Felig P, Bergman M: The endocrine pancreas: Diabetes mellitus. In Felig P, Baxter JD, Frohman LA (eds): Endocrinology and Metabolism, 3rd ed. New York, McGraw-Hill, 1995, p 1107.
133. Wahren J, Felig P, Cerasi E, Luft R: Splanchnic and peripheral glucose and amino acid metabolism in diabetes mellitus. J Clin Invest 51:1870, 1972.
134. Marliss EB, Ohman JL Jr, Aoki TT, Kozak GP: Altered redox state obscuring ketoacidosis in diabetic patients with lactic acidosis. N Engl J Med 283:978, 1973.
135. Brown JB, Pedula K, Barzilay J, et al: Lactic acidosis rates in type 2 diabetes. Diabetes Care 21:1659, 1998.
136. Conlay LA, Loewenstein JE: Phenformin and lactic acidosis. JAMA 235:1575, 1976.
137. Misbin RI: Phenformin-associated lactic acidosis: Pathogenesis and treatment. Ann Intern Med 87:591, 1977.
138. Davidoff F: Guanidine derivatives in medicine. N Engl J Med 289:141, 1973.
139. Assan R, Heuclin C, Girard JR, et al: Phenformin-induced lactic acidosis in diabetic patients. Diabetes 24:791, 1975.
140. Johnson HK, Waterhouse C: Relationship of alcohol and hyperlactatemia in diabetic subjects treated with phenformin. Am J Med 45:98, 1968.
141. Gan SC, Barr J, Arieff AI, Pearl RG: Biguanide-associated lactic acidosis: Case report and review of the literature. Arch Intern Med 152:2333, 1992.
142. Kwong SC, Brubacher J: Phenformin and lactic acidosis: A case report and review. J Emerg Med 16:881, 1998.
143. Rosand J, Friedberg JW, Yang JM: Fatal phenformin-associated lactic acidosis. Ann Intern Med 127:170, 1997.
144. Enia G, Garozzo M, Zoccali C: Lactic acidosis induced by phenformin is still a public health problem in Italy. BMJ 315: 1466, 1997.
145. Stang M, Wysowski DK, Butler-Jones D: Incidence of lactic acidosis in metformin users. Diabetes Care 22:925, 1999.
146. Chan NN, Brain HP, Feher MD: Metformin-associated lactic acidosis: A rare or very rare clinical entity? Diabet Med 16: 273, 1999.
147. Howlett HC, Bailey CJ: A risk-benefit assessment of metformin in type 2 diabetes mellitus. Drug Saf 20:489, 1999.
148. Stacpoole PW: Metformin and lactic acidosis: Guilt by association? Diabetes Care 21:1587, 1998.
149. Pepper GM, Schwartz M: Lactic acidosis associated with Glucophage use in a man with normal renal and hepatic function. Diabetes Care 20:232, 1997.
150. Safadi R, Dranitzki-Elhalel M, Popovtzer M, Ben-Yehuda A: Metformin-induced lactic acidosis associated with acute renal failure. Am J Nephrol 16:520, 1996.
151. Jurovich MR, Wooldridge JD, Force RW: Metformin-associated nonketotic metabolic acidosis. Ann Pharmacother 31:53, 1997.
152. Sulkin TV, Bosman D, Krentz AJ: Contraindications to metformin therapy in patients with NIDDM. Diabetes Care 20:925, 1997.
153. Schmidt R, Horn E, Richards J, Stamatakis M: Survival after metformin-associated lactic acidosis in peritoneal dialysis–dependent renal failure. Am J Med 102:486, 1997.
154. Nawaz S, Cleveland T, Gaines PA, Chan P: Clinical risk associated with contrast angiography in metformin treated patients: A clinical review. Clin Radiol 53:342, 1998.
155. McCartney MM, Gilbert FJ, Murchison LE, et al: Metformin and contrast media—a dangerous combination? Clin Radiol 54:29, 1999.
156. Heupler FA Jr: Guidelines for performing angiography in patients taking metformin. Members of the Laboratory Perfor-

mance Standards Committee of the Society for Cardiac Angiography and Interventions. Cathet Cardiovasc Diagn 43:121, 1998.
157. Thomsen HS, Morcos SK: Contrast media and metformin: Guidelines to diminish the risk of lactic acidosis in non-insulin-dependent diabetics after administration of contrast media. ESUR Contrast Media Safety Committee. Eur Radiol 9:738, 1999.
158. Rasuli P, Hammond DI: Metformin and contrast media: Where is the conflict? Can Assoc Radiol J 49:161, 1998.
159. Luchette FA, Robinson BR, Friend LA, et al: Adrenergic antagonists reduce lactic acidosis in response to hemorrhagic shock. J Trauma 46:873, 1999.
160. Bornemann M, Hill SC, Kidd GS: Lactic acidosis in pheochromocytoma. Ann Intern Med 105:880, 1986.
161. Bischof T, Gunthard H, Straumann E, Bertel O: [Splenic infarct, lactate acidosis, and pulmonary edema as manifestations of a pheochromocytoma]. Schweiz Med Wochenschr J Suisse Med 127:261, 1997.
162. Romanski SA, McMahon MM: Metabolic acidosis and thiamine deficiency. Mayo Clin Proc 74:259, 1999.
163. Krishna S, Taylor AM, Supanaranond W, et al: Thiamine deficiency and malaria in adults from Southeast Asia. Lancet 353: 546, 1999.
164. Anonymous: From the Centers for Disease Control and Prevention. Lactic acidosis traced to thiamine deficiency related to nationwide shortage of multivitamins for total parenteral nutrition—United States, 1997. JAMA 278:109, 1997.
165. Nakasaki H, Ohta M, Soeda J, et al: Clinical and biochemical aspects of thiamine treatment for metabolic acidosis during total parenteral nutrition. Nutrition 13:110, 1997.
166. Anonymous: Lactic acidosis traced to thiamine deficiency related to nationwide shortage of multivitamins for total parenteral nutrition—United States, 1997. MMWR Morb Mortal Wkly Rep 46:523, 1997.
167. Remond C, Viard L, Paut O, et al: Severe lactic acidosis and thiamine deficiency during parenteral nutrition in a child. Ann Fr Anesth Reanim 18:445, 1999.
168. Mukunda BN: Lactic acidosis caused by thiamine deficiency in a pregnant alcoholic patient. Am J Med Sci 317:261, 1999.
169. Mayatepek E, Schulze A: Metabolic decompensation and lactic acidosis in propionic acidaemia complicated by thiamine deficiency. J Inherit Metab Dis 22:189, 1999.
170. Emmett M, Seldin DW: Disturbances in acid-base balance during hypophosphatemia and phosphate depletion. In Massry SG, Ritz E, Rapado A (eds): Homeostasis of Phosphate and Other Minerals. New York, Plenum, 1978, p. 313.
171. Craig GM, Crane CW: Lactic acidosis complicating liver failure after intravenous fructose. BMJ 4:211, 1971.
172. Hessov I: Effects of fructose and glucose infusions on blood acid-base equilibrium in the postoperative period. Acta Chir Scand 140:347, 1974.
173. Woods HF, Alberti KGMM: Dangers of intravenous fructose. Lancet 2:1354, 1972.
174. Morris RC Jr, Nigon K, Reed EG: Evidence that the severity of depletion of inorganic phosphate determines the severity of the disturbance of adenine nucleotide metabolism in the liver and renal cortex of the fructose-loaded rat. J Clin Invest 61: 209, 1978.
175. Buijs EJ, van Zuylen HJ: Metabolic consequences of a sorbitol overdose during neurosurgery. J Neurosurg Anesthesiol 9:17, 1997.
176. Kreisberg RA, Owen WC, Siegal AM: Ethanol-induced hyperlactic acidemia: Inhibition of lactate utilization. J Clin Invest 50: 166, 1971.
177. Lieber CS, Teschke R, Hasumura Y, Decarli LM: Differences in hepatic and metabolic changes after acute and chronic alcohol consumption. Fed Proc 34:2060, 1975.
178. Ishii K, Kumashiro R, Koga Y, et al: Two survival cases of alcoholic lactic acidosis complicated with diabetes mellitus and alcoholic liver disease. Alcohol Clin Exp Res 20:387A, 1996.
179. Brinkmann B, Fechner G, Karger B, DuChesne A: Ketoacidosis and lactic acidosis—frequent causes of death in chronic alcoholics? Int J Legal Med 111:115, 1998.
180. Robinson BH: Lactic acidemia (disorders of pyruvate carboxylase, pyruvate dehydrogenase). In Scriver CR, Beaudet AL, Sly WS, Valle D (eds): The Metabolic Basis of Inherited Disease, 7th ed. New York, McGraw-Hill, 1995, p. 1479.
181. Jacobsen D, Bredesen JE, Ostborg J: Anion and osmolal gaps in the diagnosis of methanol and ethylene glycol poisoning. Acta Med Scand 212:17, 1982.
182. Bennett IL Jr, Cary FH, Mitchell GL Jr, Cooper MN: Acute methyl alcohol poisoning: A review based on experiences in an outbreak of 323 cases. Medicine (Baltimore) 32:431, 1953.
183. Kreisberg RA, Wood BC: Drug and chemical induced metabolic acidosis. Clin Endocrinol Metab 12:391, 1983.
184. Galliot M, Astier A, VuBien D, et al: Treatment of ethylene glycol poisoning with intravenous 4-methylpyrazone. N Engl J Med 319:97, 1988.
185. Gabow PA, Clay K, Sullivan JB, Lepoff R: Organic acids in ethylene glycol intoxication. Ann Intern Med 105:16, 1986.
186. Smith MJH, Jeffrey SW: The effects of salicylate on oxygen consumption and carbohydrate metabolism in the isolated rat diaphragm. Biochem J 63:524, 1956.
187. Graham DL, Laman D, Theodore J, Robin ED: Acute cyanide poisoning complicated by lactic acidosis and pulmonary edema. Arch Intern Med 137:1051, 1977.
188. Wesson DE, Foley R, Wharton J, et al: Treatment of acute cyanide intoxication with hemodialysis. Am J Nephrol 5:121, 1985.
189. Leverve X, Sibille B, Devin A, et al: Oxidative phosphorylation in intact hepatocytes: Quantitative characterization of the mechanisms of change in efficiency and cellular consequences. Mol Cell Biochem 184:53, 1998.
190. Roy PM, Gouello JP, Pennison-Besnier I, Chennebault JM: Severe lactic acidosis induced by nucleoside analogues in an HIV-infected man. Ann Emerg Med 34:282, 1999.
191. Lenzo NP, Garas BA, French MA: Hepatic steatosis and lactic acidosis associated with stavudine treatment in an HIV patient: A case report. AIDS 11:1294, 1997.
192. Chariot P, Drogou I, de Lacroix-Szmania I, et al: Zidovudine-induced mitochondrial disorder with massive liver steatosis, myopathy, lactic acidosis, and mitochondrial DNA depletion. J Hepatol 30:156, 1999.
193. Aggarwal A, al-Talib K, Alabrash M: Type B lactic acidosis in an AIDS patient treated with zidovudine. Md Med J 45: 929, 1996.
194. Acosta BS, Grimsley EW: Zidovudine-associated type B lactic acidosis and hepatic steatosis in an HIV-infected patient. South Med J 92:421, 1999.
195. Scalfaro P, Chesaux JJ, Buchwalder PA, et al: Severe transient neonatal lactic acidosis during prophylactic zidovudine treatment. Intensive Care Med 24:247, 1998.
196. Sundar K, Suarez M, Banogon PE, Shapiro JM: Zidovudine-induced fatal lactic acidosis and hepatic failure in patients with acquired immunodeficiency syndrome: Report of two patients and review of the literature. Crit Care Med 25:1425, 1997.
197. Charton-Bain MC, Flamant M, Aubertin JM, et al: [Lactic acidosis and hepatic mitochondrial changes during treatment with zidovudine]. Gastroenterol Clin Biol 21:979, 1997.
198. Fouty B, Frerman F, Reves R: Riboflavin to treat nucleoside analogue-induced lactic acidosis. Lancet 352:291, 1998.
199. Cray SH, Robinson BH, Cox PN: Lactic acidemia and bradyarrhythmia in a child sedated with propofol. Crit Care Med 26: 2087, 1998.
200. B'chir A, Mebazaa A, Losser MR, et al: Intravenous almitrine bismesylate reversibly induces lactic acidosis and hepatic dysfunction in patients with acute lung injury. Anesthesiology 89: 823, 1998.
201. Koren W, Kreis Y, Duchowiczny K, et al: Lactic acidosis and fatal myocardial failure due to clozapine. Ann Pharmacother 31:168, 1997.
202. Earthman TP, Odom L, Mullins CA: Lactic acidosis associated with high-dose niacin therapy. South Med J 84:496, 1994.
203. Krapf R, Schaffner T, Iten PX: Abuse of germanium associated with fatal lactic acidosis. Nephron 62:351, 1992.
204. Cate JC, Hedrick R: Propylene glycol intoxication and lactic acidosis. N Engl J Med 303:1237, 1980.
205. Narins RG, Blumenthal SA, Fraser WD, et al: Streptozotocin induced lactic acidosis. Am J Med Sci 265:455, 1973.

206. Anonymous: Unexplained severe illness possibly associated with consumption of Kombucha tea—Iowa, 1995. From the Centers for Disease Control and Prevention. JAMA 275:96, 1996.
207. Stacpoole PW, Lichenstein MJ, Polk JR, Greco FA: Lactic acidosis associated with metastatic osteogenic sarcoma. South Med J 74:868, 1981.
208. Spechler SJ, Esposito AL, Koff RS, Hong WK: Lactic acidosis in oat cell carcinoma with extensive hepatic metastasis. Arch Intern Med 138:1663, 1978.
209. Rice K, Schwartz SH: Lactic acidosis with small cell carcinoma. Am J Med 79:501, 1985.
210. Raju RN, Kardinal CG: Lactic acidosis in lung cancer. South Med J 76:397, 1983.
211. Fields ALA, Wolman SL, Halperin ML: Chronic lactic acidosis in a patient with cancer: Therapy and metabolic consequences. Cancer 47:2026, 1981.
212. Arseneau JC, Canellos GP, Banks PN, et al: American Burkitt's lymphoma: A clinicopathologic study of 30 cases. Am J Med 58:314, 1975.
213. Field M, Block JB, Levin R, Rall DP: Significance of blood lactate elevations among patients with acute leukemia and other neoplastic proliferative disorders. Am J Med 40:528, 1966.
214. Wainer RA, Wiernik PH, Thompson WL: Metabolic and therapeutic studies of a patient with acute leukemia and severe lactic acidosis of prolonged duration. Am J Med 55:255, 1973.
215. Durig J, Fiedler W, de Wit M, et al: Lactic acidosis and hypoglycemia in a patient with high-grade non-Hodgkin's lymphoma and elevated circulating TNF-alpha. Ann Hematol 72:97, 1996.
216. Block JB, Bronson WR, Bell W: Metabolic abnormalities of lactic acid in Burkitt type lymphoma with malignant effusions. Ann Intern Med 65:101, 1966.
217. Roth GJ, Porte D: Chronic lactic acidosis and acute leukemia. Arch Intern Med 125:317, 1970.
218. Orringer CE, Eustace JC, Wunsch CD, Gardener LB: Natural history of lactic acidosis after grand-mal seizures: A model for the study of an anion-gap acidosis not associated with hyperkalemia. N Engl J Med 297:796, 1977.
219. Johnson S, O'Meara M, Young JB: Acute cocaine poisoning: Importance of treating seizures and acidosis. Am J Med 75: 1061, 1983.
220. Boyd RE, Brennan PT, Deng J-F, et al: Strychnine poisoning: Recovery from profound lactic acidosis, hyperthermia, and rhabdomyolysis. Am J Med 74:507, 1983.
221. Hart GR, Anderson RJ, Crumpler CP, et al: Epidemic classical heat stroke: Clinical characteristics and course of 28 patients. Medicine 61:189, 1982.
222. Chen YT, Burchell A: Glycogen storage diseases. In Scriver CR, Beaudet AL, Sly WS, Valle D (eds): The Metabolic Basis of Inherited Disease, 7th ed. New York, McGraw-Hill, 1995, pp 935–966.
223. Sokal JE, Lowe CH, Sarcione EJ, et al: Studies of glycogen metabolism in liver glycogen disease (von Gierke's disease): Six cases with similar metabolic abnormalities and responses to glucagon. J Clin Invest 40:364, 1961.
224. Zuppinger K, Rossi E: Metabolic studies in liver glycogen disease with specific reference to lactate metabolism. Helv Med Acta 35:406, 1969.
225. Greene HL, Wilson FA, Herreran P, et al: ATP depletion, a possible role in the pathogenesis of hyperuricemia in glycogen storage disease type I. J Clin Invest 62:321, 1978.
226. Nuoffer JM, Mullis PE, Wiesmann UN: Treatment with low-dose diazoxide in two growth-retarded prepubertal girls with glycogen storage disease type Ia resulted in catch-up growth. J Inherit Metab Dis 20:790, 1997.
227. Baker L, Winegard AI: Fasting hypoglycemia and metabolic acidosis associated with deficiency of hepatic fructose-1,6-diphosphatase. Lancet 2:13, 1970.
228. Pagliara AS, Karl IE, Keating JP, et al: Hepatic fructose-1,6-diphosphatase deficiency: A cause of lactic acidosis and hypoglycemia in infancy. J Clin Invest 51:2115, 1972.
229. Lamiere N, Mussche M, Baele M, et al: Hereditary fructose intolerance: A difficult diagnosis in the adult. Am J Med 65: 416, 1978.
230. Richardson RMA, Little JA, Patten RA, et al: Pathogenesis of acidosis in hereditary fructose intolerance. Metabolism 28: 1133, 1978.
231. Morris RC Jr: An experimental renal acidification defect in patients with hereditary fructose intolerance. I. Its resemblance to renal tubular acidosis. J Clin Invest 47:1389, 1968.
232. Morris RC Jr: An experimental renal acidification defect in patients with hereditary fructose intolerance. II. Its distinction from classic renal tubular acidosis: Its resemblance to the renal acidification defect associated with the Fanconi syndrome of children with cystinosis. J Clin Invest 47:1648, 1968.
233. Geoffroy V, Fouque F, Benelli C, et al: Defect in the X-lipoyl-containing component of the pyruvate dehydrogenase complex in a patient with neonatal lactic acidemia. Pediatrics 97:267, 1996.
234. Falk RE, Cederbaum SD, Blass JP, et al: Ketotic diet in the management of pyruvate dehydrogenase deficiency. Pediatrics 58:713, 1976.
235. Naito E, Ito M, Yokota I, et al: Thiamine-responsive lactic acidaemia: Role of pyruvate dehydrogenase complex. Eur J Pediatr 157:648, 1998.
236. Wallace JC, Jitrapakdee S, Chapman-Smith A: Pyruvate carboxylase. Int J Biochem Cell Biol 30:1, 1998.
237. Sussman KE, Alfrey A, Kirsch WM, et al: Chronic lactic acidosis in an adult. Am J Med 48:104, 1970.
238. Greene CL, Goodman SI: Catastrophic metabolic encephalopathies in the newborn period: Evaluation and management. Clin Perinatol 24:773, 1997.
239. Adams PL, Turnbull DM: Disorders of the electron transport chain. J Inherit Metab Dis 19:463, 1996.
240. Stacpoole PW: Lactic acidosis and other mitochondrial disorders. Metabolism 46:306, 1997.
241. Wallace DC: Mitochondrial genetics: A paradigm for aging and degenerative diseases? Science 256:628, 1992.
242. Majamaa K, Moilanen JS, Uimonen S, et al: Epidemiology of A3243G, the mutation for mitochondrial encephalomyopathy, lactic acidosis, and strokelike episodes: Prevalence of the mutation in an adult population. Am J Hum Genet 63:447, 1998.
243. Hsieh F, Gohh R, Dworkin L: Acute renal failure and the MELAS syndrome, a mitochondrial encephalomyopathy. J Am Soc Nephrol 7:647, 1996.
244. Terauchi A, Tamagawa K, Morimatsu Y, et al: An autopsy case of mitochondrial encephalomyopathy, lactic acidosis and stroke-like episodes (MELAS) with a point mutation of mitochondrial DNA. Brain Dev 18:224, 1996.
245. Vilarinho L, Santorelli FM, Rosas MJ, et al: The mitochondrial A3243G mutation presenting as severe cardiomyopathy. J Med Genet 34:607, 1997.
246. Suzuki Y, Goto Y, Taniyama M, et al: Muscle histopathology in diabetes mellitus associated with mitochondrial tRNA(Leu(-UUR)) mutation at position 3243. J Neurol Sci 145:49, 1997.
247. Melberg A, Akerlund P, Raininko R, et al: Monozygotic twins with MELAS-like syndrome lacking ragged red fibers and lactacidaemia. Acta Neurol Scand 94:233, 1996.
248. Kishnani PS, Van Hove JL, Shoffner JS, et al: Acute pancreatitis in an infant with lactic acidosis and a mutation at nucleotide 3243 in the mitochondrial DNA tRNALeu(UUR) gene. Eur J Pediatr 155:898, 1996.
249. Saudubray J-M, Carpentier C: Clinical phenotypes: Diagnosis/algorithms. In Scriver CR, Beaudet AL, Sly WS, Valle D (eds): The Metabolic Basis of Inherited Disease, 7th ed. New York, McGraw-Hill, 1995, pp 327–400.
250. Pitkanen S, Feigenbaum A, Laframboise R, Robinson BH: NADH-coenzyme Q reductase (complex I) deficiency: Heterogeneity in phenotype and biochemical findings. J Inherit Metab Dis 19:675, 1996.
251. Mazzella M, Cerone R, Bonacci W, et al: Severe complex I deficiency in a case of neonatal-onset lactic acidosis and fatal liver failure. Acta Paediatr 86:326, 1997.
252. Houshmand M, Larsson NG, Oldfors A, et al: Fatal mitochondrial myopathy, lactic acidosis, and complex I deficiency associated with a heteroplasmic A — G mutation at position 3251 in the mitochondrial tRNALeu(UUR) gene. Hum Genet 97: 269, 1996.
253. Ellaway C, North K, Arbuckle S, Christodoulou J: Complex I deficiency in association with structural abnormalities of the diaphragm and brain. J Inherit Metab Dis 21:72, 1998.

254. Procaccio V, Mousson B, Beugnot R, et al: Nuclear DNA origin of mitochondrial complex I deficiency in fatal infantile lactic acidosis evidenced by transnuclear complementation of cultured fibroblasts. J Clin Invest 104:83, 1999.
255. Frerman FE, Goodman SI: Nuclear-encoded defects of the mitochondrial respiratory chain, including glutaric acidemia type II. In Scriver CR, Beaudet AL, Sly WS, Valle D (eds): The Metabolic Basis of Inherited Disease, 7th ed. New York, McGraw-Hill, 1995, pp 1611–1630.
256. Sanger TD, Jain KD: MERRF syndrome with overwhelming lactic acidosis. Pediatr Neurol 14:57, 1996.
257. Muraki K, Goto Y, Nishino I, et al: Severe lactic acidosis and neonatal death in Pearson syndrome. J Inherit Metab Dis 20: 43, 1997.
258. Seneca S, De Meirleir L, De Schepper J, et al: Pearson marrow pancreas syndrome: A molecular study and clinical management. Clin Genet 51:338, 1997.
259. Elia M, Musumeci SA, Ferri R, et al: Leigh syndrome and partial deficit of cytochrome *c* oxidase associated with epilepsia partialis continua. Brain Dev 18:207, 1996.
260. van der Knaap MS, Jakobs C, Valk J: Magnetic resonance imaging in lactic acidosis. J Inherit Metab Dis 19:535, 1996.
261. Stacpoole PW, Barnes CL, Hurbanis MD, et al: Treatment of congenital lactic acidosis with dichloroacetate. Arch Dis Child 77:535, 1997.
262. Morris AA, Leonard JV: The treatment of congenital lactic acidoses. J Inherit Metab Dis 19:573, 1996.
263. Kuroda Y, Ito M, Naito E, et al: Concomitant administration of sodium dichloroacetate and vitamin $B_1$ for lactic acidemia in children with MELAS syndrome. J Pediatr 131:450, 1997.
264. Stacpoole PW, Moore GW, Kornhauser DM: Toxicity of chronic dichloroacetate. N Engl J Med 300:372, 1979.
265. Dahlquist NR, Perrault JA, Callaway CW, Jones JD: D-Lactic acidosis and encephalopathy after jejunoileostomy: Response to overfeeding and to fasting in humans. Mayo Clin Proc 59: 141, 1984.
266. Day AS, Abbott GD: D-Lactic acidosis in short bowel syndrome. N Z Med J 112:277, 1999.
267. Halperin ML, Kamel KS: D-Lactic acidosis: Turning sugar into acids in the gastrointestinal tract. Kidney Int 49:1, 1996.
268. Bongaerts GP, Tolboom JJ, Naber AH, et al: Role of bacteria in the pathogenesis of short bowel syndrome–associated D-lactic acidemia. Microb Pathog 22:285, 1997.
269. Uribarri J, Oh MS, Carroll HJ: D-Lactic acidosis: A review of clinical presentation, biochemical features, and pathophysiologic mechanisms. Medicine 77:73, 1998.
270. Ramakrishnan T, Stokes P: Beneficial effects of fasting and low carbohydrate diet in D-lactic acidosis associated with short-bowel syndrome. J Parenter Enteral Nutr 9:361, 1985.
271. Oh MS, Phelps K-R, Traube M, et al: D-Lactic acidosis in a man with the short-bowel syndrome. N Engl J Med 301:249, 1979.
272. Stolberg L, Rolfe R, Gitlin N, et al: D-Lactic acidosis due to abnormal gut flora. N Engl J Med 306:1344, 1982.
273. Traube M, Bock JL, Boyer JL: D-Lactic acidosis after jejunoileal bypass: Identification of organic anions by nuclear magnetic resonance spectroscopy. Ann Intern Med 98:161, 1983.
274. Thurn JR, Pierpont GL, Ludvigsen CW, Eckfeldt JH: D-Lactate encephalopathy. Am J Med 79:717, 1985.
275. Savoy J, Kaplan A: A gas chromatographic method for determination of lactic acid in blood. Clin Chem 12:559, 1966.

CHAPTER 7

# Metabolic Alkalosis

John H. Galla, MD

Metabolic alkalosis is an acid-base disorder in which a primary disease process leads to the net accumulation of base within, or the net loss of acid from, the extracellular fluid (ECF). Although in strict terms of acid-base chemistry this occurs because of a decrease in the strong ion difference,[1] metabolic alkalosis is more commonly recognized as an increase in plasma bicarbonate concentration and a consequent decrease in arterial $H^+$ concentration, which is reported again more commonly as an elevation in arterial blood pH or alkalemia.

Unopposed by other primary acid-base disorders, this increase in arterial blood pH promptly, normally, and predictably depresses ventilation and results in increased $Pa_{CO_2}$ and buffering at the magnitude of the alkalemia. The confidence bands for the compensatory respiratory response are the widest and most deformed of the acid-base disorders; these are probably related to the patient populations or the model used to study the response.[2] The most authoritative studies predict an increase in $Pa_{CO_2}$ of 0.6 to 0.7 mm Hg for every 1 mM increase in plasma bicarbonate concentration.[2] Although a $Pa_{CO_2}$ greater than 55 mm Hg is uncommonly encountered, compensatory increases in $Pa_{CO_2}$ to 60 mm Hg have been documented in cases of severe metabolic alkalosis. Experimental evidence now favors a degree of physiologic compensation that is related directly to the extent of the alkalosis and to the degree of elevation of the plasma bicarbonate, irrespective of its etiology and of whether or not there is an intracellular acidosis.[3] Hypokalemia, hypoxemia, and azotemia do not appear to alter the hypoventilatory response. Based on this predictive formula, an insufficient compensatory increase in $Pa_{CO_2}$ should be interpreted as a mixed acid-base disturbance in which a primary stimulus to hyperventilation—respiratory alkalosis—is also present with the metabolic alkalosis; similarly, an excessive compensatory increase in $Pa_{CO_2}$ (higher than predicted) also means a mixed disorder with respiratory acidosis and metabolic alkalosis.

## PREVALENCE AND OUTCOME

Data on the prevalence and outcome of metabolic alkalosis are sparse. In a study at one medical center,[4] metabolic alkalosis was common—half of all acid-base disorders. Because vomiting, nasogastric suction, and the use of chloruretic diuretics are also common among hospitalized patients, this should not be surprising. The mortality rate associated with severe metabolic alkalosis is substantial: Wilson and associates[5] determined a mortality rate of 45% in patients with alkalemia of 7.55 and of 80% when the pH was greater than 7.65; a high mortality (48.5%) for alkalemia greater than 7.60 has been confirmed.[6] Although this relationship between alkalemia and mortality is not necessarily causal, severe alkalosis should be viewed with concern and treatment should be undertaken promptly when the arterial blood pH exceeds 7.55.

## CLASSIFICATION AND DEFINITIONS

The major clinically and pathophysiologically relevant classification is based on whether or not the metabolic alkalosis is dependent on chloride depletion. The chloride-depletion forms, also called the chloride-responsive alkaloses, are more common. The other major grouping, which is not related to chloride depletion, is that of the chloride-resistant alkaloses, most of which are due to potassium depletion with mineralocorticoid excess. Chloride-depletion metabolic alkalosis (CDA), by definition, can be corrected without potassium repletion, although a modest degree of potassium depletion (or at least hypokalemia) is common in CDA because in these circumstances the kidney tends to be "potassium-wasting" and potassium shifts into cells in exchange for protons.[7] Although experimental studies have shown that potassium repletion is not essential to correct CDA,[8] mixed potassium and chloride-depletion metabolic alkalosis also occurs in humans[9, 10] and has been studied experimentally in animals.[11] Several other relatively uncommon causes constitute the balance of etiologies of metabolic alkalosis (Table 7–1).

Disequilibrium metabolic alkalosis occurs in acute or acute-on-chronic metabolic alkalosis, when generation of bicarbonate and resultant elevation of plasma bicarbonate exceeds the capacity of the renal tubule to reabsorb bicarbonate.[12] Transient bicarbonaturia with resultant sodium loss ensues until a new steady state of chronic metabolic alkalosis is achieved and bicarbonate excretion ceases.

The course of metabolic alkalosis can be divided into generation, maintenance, and recovery phases[12]; these phases are examined generally and specifically for each etiology as appropriate. Generation occurs by loss of protons from the ECF into the external environment or into the cells, by gain of base by the oral or intravenous route, or from the base stored in bone apatite. Important maintenance mechanisms are chloride depletion, mineralocorticoid excess and potassium depletion, and states of low or absent glomerular filtration rate (GFR) associated with base excess. In some cases, mechanisms generating and maintaining alkalosis may be occurring simultaneously.

**TABLE 7–1.** Etiologies of Metabolic Alkalosis

**Chloride Depletion**

Gastric losses—vomiting, mechanical drainage, bulimia
Chloruretic diuretics—bumetanide, chlorothiazide, metolazone, etc.
Diarrheal states—villous adenoma, congenital chloridorrhea
Posthypercapneic state
Dietary chloride deprivation with base loading—chloride-deficient infant formulas
Gastrocystoplasty
Cystic fibrosis (high sweat chloride)

**Potassium Depletion–Mineralocorticoid Excess**

Primary aldosteronism—adenoma, idiopathic hyperplasia, renin-responsive, glucocorticoid-suppressible carcinoma
Apparent mineralocorticoid excess
Primary deoxycorticosterone excess—11β- and 17α-hydroxylase deficiencies
Drugs—licorice (glycyrrhizic acid) as a confection or flavoring, carbenoxolone
Liddle syndrome
Secondary aldosteronism
Adrenal corticosteroid excess—primary, secondary, or exogenous
Severe hypertension—malignant, accelerated, renovascular
Hemangiopericytoma, nephroblastoma, renal cell carcinoma
Laxative abuse, clay ingestion[202]
Bartter and Gitelman syndromes and their variants

**Hypercalcemic States**

Hypercalcemia of malignancy
Acute or chronic milk-alkali syndrome

**Other**

Carbenicillin, ampicillin, penicillin
Bicarbonate ingestion—massive or with renal insufficiency
Recovery from starvation
Hypoalbuminemia

# PATHOPHYSIOLOGY OF CHLORIDE-DEPLETION ALKALOSES

## Generation

**Loss of Gastric Acid.** The parietal cell of the gastric epithelium secretes gastric fluid with a proton concentration of 160 to 170 mM (pH ~ 1), sodium 2 to 4 mM, potassium about 10 mM, and chloride about 180 mM in a volume of 2 to 3 L/day; the daily output in pyloric stenosis or Zollinger-Ellison syndrome can be massive. The basal rate of gastric acid is not influenced by the state of acid-base balance but is stimulated by histamine, cholinergic agents, and gastrin and inhibited by somatostatin, β-adrenergic agonists, and enteroglucagon.[13] This transport of HCl is effected by the gastric isoform of $H^+,K^+$ATPase[14] at the luminal membrane, which is inhibitable by omeprazole but not by digitalis glycosides or by an anion antiporter at the basolateral membrane that transports chloride into the cell in a 1:1 exchange for bicarbonate into the extracellular compartment. The loss of gastric fluid by vomiting or iatrogenic removal results in alkalosis, because the bicarbonate generated during the production of gastric acid is not subsequently balanced by the absorption of acid in the more distal segments of the gut.

Although sodium and potassium loss by the gastric route varies in amount and may rise with protracted vomiting, the deficits of these cations occur predominantly by urinary losses and are obligated by bicarbonaturia, which is particularly intense during the generation of alkalosis (i.e., the disequilibrium phase).

Gastrocystoplasty has been introduced for bladder augmentation. The favorable acid environment is protective against infection. However, excessive HCl production may result in urinary losses sufficient to produce alkalosis.[15]

**Chloruretic Diuretics.** This class of diuretics commonly causes metabolic alkalosis, which is more likely to occur when diuretics are used to treat edema rather than hypertension.[16] Chloruretic agents all directly produce initial losses of chloride, sodium, potassium, and fluid in the urine. Chlorothiazide and its congeners inhibit the NaCl symporter in the luminal membrane of the distal convolution.[17] Furosemide and its congeners and ethacrynic acid inhibit the $Na^+$-$2Cl^-$-$K^+$, cotransporter in the ascending thick limb of the loop of Henle; they also increase urinary ammonium, titratable acid, and net acid excretion.[18, 19] In normal humans, furosemide treatment for 2 days induced chloride depletion and alkalosis even when potassium depletion was prevented[20]; potassium balance remained positive until the third day of the maintenance period with stable alkalosis throughout (Fig. 7–1). Generation was, thus, clearly related to chloride depletion.

To counteract these diuretic-induced losses, several renal compensatory mechanisms are evoked and may further generate or maintain alkalosis. The resultant ECF volume contraction accelerates isotonic fluid reabsorption by the proximal tubule, which returns a fluid that is relatively rich in bicarbonate to the plasma. Volume contraction also stimulates renin and aldosterone secretion. Increased aldosterone can accelerate proton secretion and bicarbonate reabsorption by a sodium-independent mechanism in the medullary collecting duct[21] and perhaps in other collecting duct segments.

Potassium excretion is accelerated by several mechanisms and may contribute to the generation and maintenance of alkalosis. Loop diuretics directly decrease potassium uptake in the ascending limb of the loop of Henle.[18] Diuretic-induced increases in sodium and fluid delivery to the late distal convolution and collecting duct accelerate potassium secretion, and increased aldosterone further augments potassium secretion in the collecting duct. Potassium depletion per se effects a shift of protons into the intracellular fluid, thus enhancing alkalosis in the ECF. The resultant intracellular acidosis in renal epithelial cells would enhance proton secretion with resultant bicarbonate reabsorption.

In the proximal tubule, potassium depletion,[22] chloride depletion, and hypercarbia, which occur as a compensatory response to metabolic alkalosis, all may further augment bicarbonate reabsorption. Which of the aforementioned mechanisms primarily engenders renal proton loss and generates alkalosis or participates in maintenance has not yet been established for any of these diuretics.

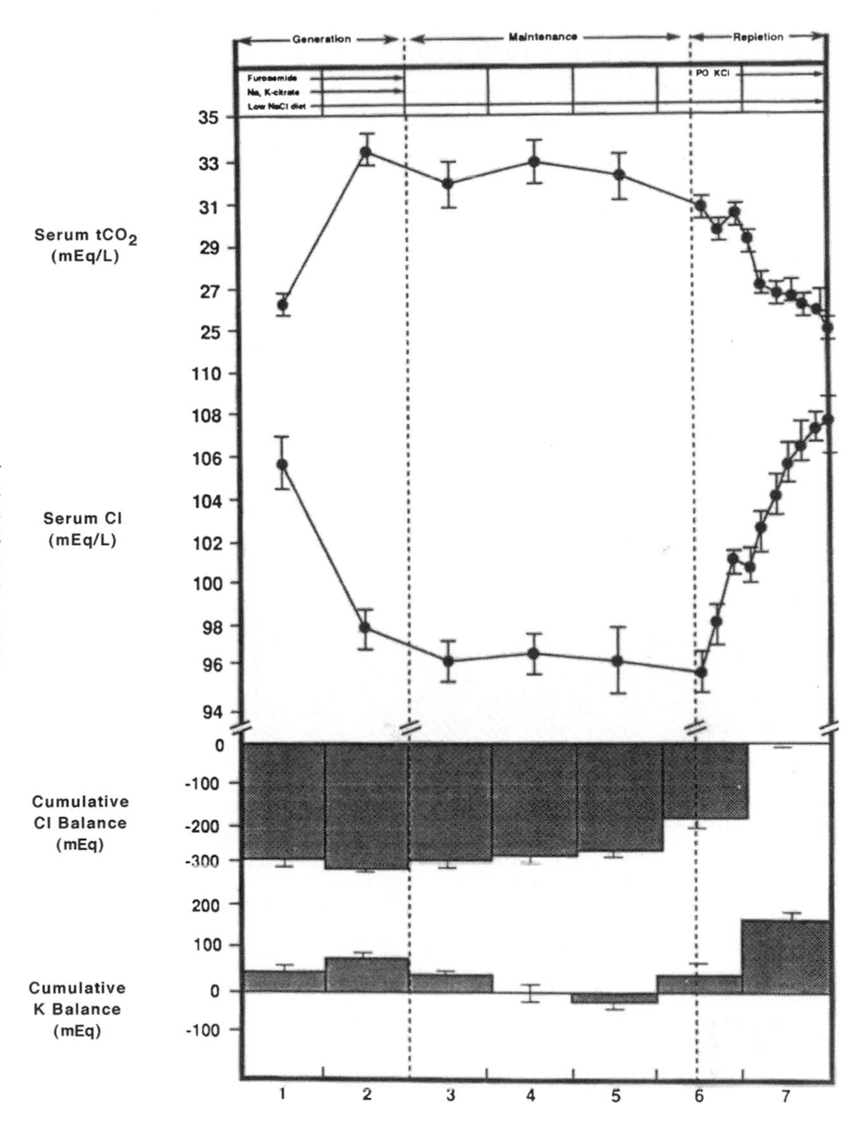


**FIGURE 7–1** ■ Diuretic-induced alkalosis in humans. Furosemide induced chloride depletion and alkalosis, whereas sodium and potassium depletions were prevented by supplementation. Alkalosis was maintained along with neutral potassium balance until day 5 and was then corrected with quantitative chloride repletion. (From Rosen RA, Julian BA, Dubovsky EA, et al: On the mechanism by which chloride corrects metabolic alkalosis in man. Am J Med 84:449, 1988.)

**Posthypercapnea.** Respiratory acidosis is compensated by accelerated renal bicarbonate reabsorption and urinary net acid and chloride excretion, leading to a state of chloride depletion but with intra- and extracellular acidosis.[23, 24] Chloruresis begins within a few hours after the induction of respiratory acidosis and is complete usually within 24 to 48 hours. The responses of the individual nephron segments are incompletely understood, but bicarbonate reabsorption in the proximal tubule of the rat is enhanced[25] and chloride reabsorption in the ascending limb of loop of Henle in the rabbit is diminished.[26] The collecting duct may also participate in generation: type A intercalated cells (ICs) in the cortical collecting duct (CCD) and outer medullary collecting duct (OMCD) are stimulated,[27, 28] bicarbonate absorption is augmented,[29] and mRNA for the basolateral anion exchanger of the type A IC is increased.[30] When respiratory acidosis is corrected, accelerated bicarbonate reabsorption, which is no longer appropriate, will persist if insufficient chloride is available (Fig. 7–2). The patient with respiratory failure and congestive heart failure managed with NaCl restriction epitomizes this presentation.

**Villous Adenoma.** Although villous adenomas of the colon usually produce a hyperchloremic metabolic acidosis because of the loss of large volumes of colonic fluid rich in potassium and bicarbonate, a few (10% to 15%) of these tumors secrete considerable chloride, which results in metabolic alkalosis.[31] With continued growth of the tumor, the volume of the secretion may become massive.[32]

**Chloridorrhea.** Defective apical chloride/bicarbonate exchange in the colon and perhaps the ileum is the primary defect[33] that results in congenital diarrhea with alkalosis, Gastric and jejunal functions are normal. Although fecal sodium and potassium concentrations are normal, the unremitting copious watery stool results also in sodium, potassium, and volume losses. This autosomal recessive disease[34] is caused by a mutation of the downregulated in adenoma (DRA) gene,[35] leading to chloride losses and bicarbonate retention.[34] The renal response mediated by aldosterone is intense sodium and water reabsorption at the expense of proton and potassium secretion, thus further promoting alkalosis.

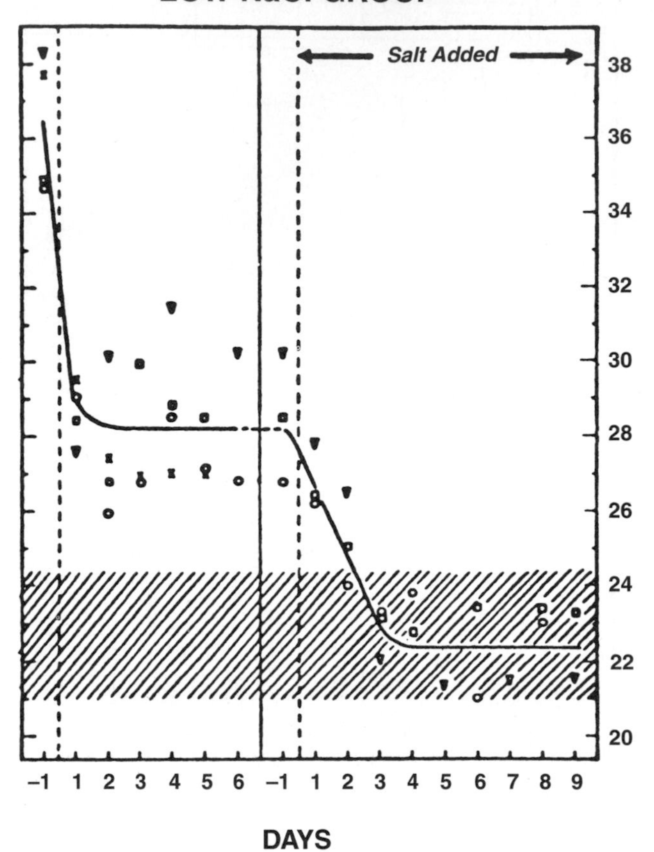


**FIGURE 7–2** ■ Posthypercapneic metabolic alkalosis in dogs; serum ($HCO_3$) is shown on the ordinate. When NaCl is restricted during respiratory acidosis, a residual metabolic alkalosis persists after exposure to high $CO_2$ ceases on day 1. The alkalosis is corrected when NaCl is added to the diet. (From Schwartz WB, Hays RM, Polak A, Haynie GD: Effects of chronic hypercapnia on electrolyte and acid-base equilibrium, II: Recovery with special reference to the influence of chloride intake. J Clin Invest 40:1238, 1961.)

**Cystic Fibrosis.** Skin losses of chloride can generate alkalosis in cystic fibrosis. Alkalosis may even be the presenting feature in adolescence with a few of the several hundred mutations in the cystic fibrosis transmembrane regulator (CFTR) gene.[36]

## Maintenance

The cessation of events that generate alkalosis, such as the discontinuance of diuretics or nasogastric suction, is not necessarily accompanied by resolution of the alkalosis, unlike the usual course in metabolic acidosis. To account for the maintenance of metabolic alkalosis in these instances, the kidney must, a priori, retain bicarbonate by either a decrease in filtered bicarbonate load, an increase in bicarbonate reabsorption, or both.

Concurrent deficits of sodium, potassium, and fluid as well as chloride usually occur in CDA and give rise to controversy as to which of these deficits is responsible for maintenance. In dogs rendered alkalotic by $NaNO_3$ infusion,[37] gastric drainage,[38] or prior hypercapnea[39–41] and maintained on chloride-deficient diets, the resultant alkalosis has been corrected completely by either NaCl or KCl despite persistent deficits of either sodium or potassium; volume contraction also occurred in some models.[38] Furthermore, in men given chloruretic diuretics, infused with $NaNO_3$,[42] or selectively depleted of gastric HCl,[43] alkalosis occurred despite replacement of sodium and potassium losses and was corrected completely with either NaCl or KCl.[43] These studies show that complete correction of CDA can be effected by chloride without repletion of either potassium or sodium per se; thus, deficits of those cations—but not necessarily plasma or ECF volume depletion—cannot be specific causes of maintained alkalosis induced by chloride depletion.[44]

To separate the correction of volume depletion from that of chloride depletion, Cohen[45, 46] maintained alkalosis for 5 days in dogs treated with ethacrynic acid and a NaCl-deficient diet. Cohen then expanded the ECF volume with a fluid that contained chloride and bicarbonate in concentrations identical to that in the alkalemic plasma, thus excluding the possibility that the plasma anion composition was altered by the anion composition of the infused fluid. These infusions completely corrected alkalosis in 24 hours without an increase in GFR. Despite increasing potassium depletion, chloride repletion also occurred. These studies led to the "volume" hypothesis in which the intranephronal redistribution of fluid reabsorption plays the central role: ECF volume depletion accompanying alkalosis augments fluid reabsorption in the proximal tubule where bicarbonate is preferentially reabsorbed compared with chloride; the increased bicarbonate reabsorption in this segment maintains the alkalosis.[47] During correction, volume expansion decreases proximal tubule fluid reabsorption, thus delivering more bicarbonate to the distal nephron, which has a limited capacity to reabsorb bicarbonate. Bicarbonaturia ensues, and the alkalosis is corrected. In this hypothesis, chloride administration has only a permissive role; volume expansion is regarded as the extrarenal impetus to the kidney for correction.

This volume hypothesis has been reexamined in studies of both acute and chronic CDA produced in humans by diuretics and in rats by peritoneal dialysis that produces selective chloride depletion. In rats with CDA given 70 mM chloride ad libitum to drink as either sodium or choline salts, acute CDA was completely corrected within 24 hours despite negative sodium and potassium balances, decreased body weight, and, by experimental design, obligatory bicarbonate loading.[48] After acute bilateral nephrectomy in this model, chloride infusion did not correct CDA, which shows that correction was dependent on a renal response.[49] To exclude a role for volume in the maintenance or correction in this model in a more rigorous manner, alkalotic rats were infused with 5% dextrose solutions that contained either 6% albumin at 2.5 mL/hr/100 g body weight or 80 mM chloride at only 0.6 mL/hr/100 g.[50] In the rats infused with the albumin-containing solution, alkalosis was maintained despite plasma volume expansion by 15% and a normal GFR, whereas in the rats infused with 80 mM chloride, alkalosis was corrected progressively with increased bicarbonate excretion despite persistent volume contraction and a decreased GFR.

In normal men with alkalosis induced by furosemide and maintained by chloride restriction for 5 days,[20] alkalosis was completely corrected as chloride was quantitatively repleted with KCl similar to the experience of Kassirer and Schwartz[8] (see Fig. 7–1). Plasma volumes estimated serially by $^{131}$I-albumin space as well as GFR and estimated renal plasma flow decreased after generation and persisted throughout both maintenance and correction.[20]

Thus, in contradiction to the volume hypothesis, studies in rats and humans that have rigorously separated repletion of volume from that of chloride show that CDA can be corrected by chloride administration without repair of ECF volume contraction and by a renal mechanism in either the acute or chronic CDA model. This extends the earlier conclusion of Schwartz and coworkers: chloride is necessary and *sufficient* for the correction of CDA.

Others have proposed a "cation-depletion" hypothesis[51, 52]; in support of this concept, they cite data in which serum potassium concentration rises with the correction of alkalosis.[20, 50] Although potassium metabolism (but not repletion) may have an important role in correction and alkalosis may promote potassium wasting, the studies cited show persistent or increasing potassium deficits in the face of the correction of CDA, which is clear evidence against a causative role for potassium depletion in alkalosis generated in this manner. In humans,[20] KCl corrected CDA whereas equimolar KCl loading in subjects that were sodium-depleted but not chloride-depleted and alkalotic produced no change in systemic acid-base balance or in urinary net acid excretion. Much earlier, potassium depletion had been shown not to be a causative factor in the pathogenesis of CDA.[43] Suffice it to say that chloride with any of several different cations under various conditions has been reported to correct CDA, whereas no cation administered without chloride has been shown to do so under any condition.

The concept that chloride is necessary and sufficient for the correction of CDA should not be construed to indicate that volume and alkalosis are unrelated; they may be associated events. Garella and coworkers produced CDA in dogs by isovolemic hemofiltration in which the replacement solution contained bicarbonate as the only anion.[53] Cumulative sodium balance decreased minimally compared with the decrease in ECF volume. Because the reduction in ECF volume cannot be explained by urinary losses, it must be linked to the movement of solute and fluid from the ECF into the intracellular space in the setting of chloride depletion or alkalosis in the ECF.

Although the cellular mechanism(s) by which chloride depletion or alkalosis may be associated with fluid shifts between body compartments is unclear, both cell volume and intracellular pH may be regulated by some of the same transport systems.[54–57] Furthermore, the maintenance of intracellular volume has been associated with transport of both chloride and bicarbonate across the cell membrane. For example, when chloride is partially replaced in the medium by an anion with a different reflection coefficient, a different steady-state cell volume may be attained.[57] The result may be cell shrinkage when the substitute is nonpermeant (e.g., gluconate) or cell swelling when it is more permeant (e.g., acetate). Whereas extrapolation from in vitro studies such as this to systemic in vivo events is problematic, it is plausible that alterations in volume detected in both the intracellular and extracellular compartments may occur as a consequence of changes in extracellular anion composition and without an alteration in total body water rather than vice versa. Rather than "contraction alkalosis," this association may be more aptly called "alkalotic contraction."

The foregoing data reinforce the conclusion that chloride depletion is necessary and sufficient to maintain CDA by a renal mechanism. Although volume depletion and a fall in GFR are commonly associated phenomena, these studies show correction of CDA by chloride by an intrarenal effect even if GFR and ECF volume are declining or, at least, persisting at a level less than normal.

The mechanism(s) by which the kidney maintains CDA is not completely understood. A reduction in GFR would serve to maintain alkalosis by a reduction in filtered bicarbonate load. Although studies by Kassirer and associates,[42, 43] Gulyassy and coworkers,[37] and Atkins and Schwartz[58] showed no evidence for a decreased GFR in humans and dogs, more recent studies that focused specifically on GFR have shown a decrease in normal men with diuretic-induced alkalosis.[20, 59] A decrease in ECF volume, which often accompanies CDA, can result in a decrease in GFR. However, with persistent decreases in ECF volume and renal blood flow, GFR does not necessarily return to normal during or immediately after complete correction of CDA by chloride administration.[20]

During euvolemia, nephron GFR in the rat with CDA also decreases as alkalosis and hypochloremia become progressively more severe.[60] However, when tubule fluid flow to the macula densa of the juxtaglomerular apparatus is blocked, this effect on single-nephron GFR is abolished, suggesting that GFR is decreased by an intrarenal mechanism, tubuloglomerular feedback.[61]

In chronic CDA, GFR appears to increase progressively and may exceed normal at least in a rat model of diuretic-induced CDA.[62, 63] Because this model was associated with progressive potassium depletion, which is a potent stimulus to kidney growth, the role of the chronicity of alkalosis versus progressive potassium depletion to effect the return of GFR to normal in prolonged experimental metabolic alkalosis is not settled.

The renin-angiotensin (ANG)-aldosterone axis has also been implicated in the maintenance of CDA[64]: chloride depletion is a potent stimulus to renin release in the rat model of CDA[65] and presumably is associated with high ANG II concentration, which has been shown to be a potent regulator of early proximal tubule bicarbonate reabsorption.[66] To examine the im-

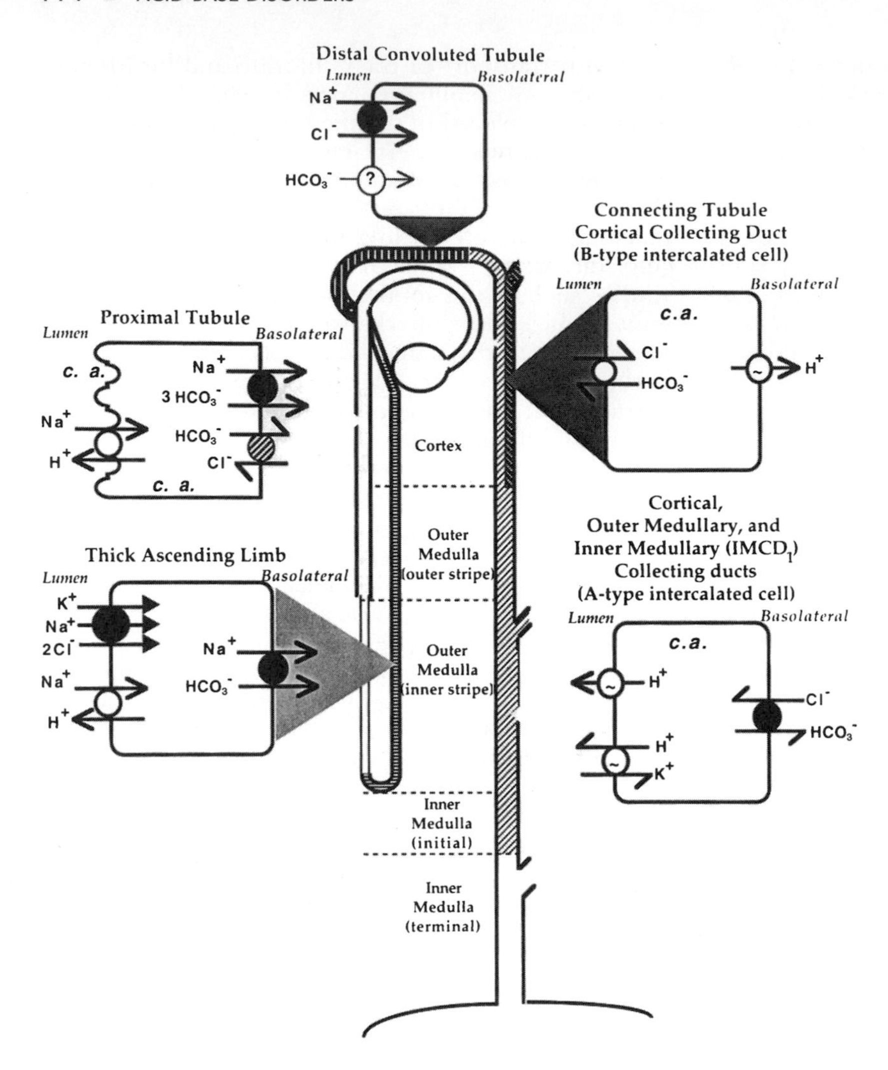


**FIGURE 7–3** ■ Transport mechanisms for chloride and bicarbonate along nephron. Several different transport mechanisms for protons, bicarbonate, and chloride are present in the various nephron segments. Other mechanisms have been proposed but are not yet widely accepted. (From Galla JH, Gifford JD, Luke RG, et al: Adaptations to chloride-depletion alkalosis. Am J Physiol 30: R771, 1991.)

portance of the effect of ANG II specifically on CDA, saralasin or enalapril in doses that modestly decreased arterial blood pressure was given to rats with maintained CDA.[67] If ANG II were important to maintenance, its blockade should promote correction; no correction was noted. In addition, ANG II in subpressor doses[67] was infused into rats in which correction was being effected by the infusion of 80 mM chloride. Again, inhibition of the corrective response would be expected, but correction was not prevented or blunted. Further, although saralasin infusion may increase bicarbonate delivery out of the proximal tubule and to the distal convolution and may also increase bicarbonaturia, alkalosis persists. Thus, ANG II does not appear to play an important role in the pathophysiology of CDA.

Kassirer and associates[68] have shown that plasma aldosterone concentrations eventually fall during CDA in humans and that exogenous administration of supraphysiologic amounts of aldosterone during the maintenance period of CDA failed to increase either net acid excretion or the degree of metabolic alkalosis. Furthermore, correction of the metabolic alkalosis occurred with NaCl replacement despite continued administration of supraphysiologic amounts of aldosterone.[68] In studies in men with chloride depletion, correction of alkalosis was achieved by KCl despite a marked increase in plasma aldosterone concentrations.[20] Thus, a change in aldosterone level appears to be unnecessary for maintenance, and chloride can correct CDA despite rising plasma aldosterone concentrations.

The absence of a clear regulatory role for GFR focuses attention on the reabsorptive mechanisms for chloride and bicarbonate along the tubule as depicted (Fig. 7–3). During maintained CDA, the proximal tubule maintains glomerulotubular balance and does not adjust chloride or bicarbonate reabsorption to effect a corrective response.[50, 69–72] When GFR and filtered bicarbonate load rise after 3 or 4 weeks, bicarbonate reabsorption is increased, which is consistent with glomerulotubular balance or, perhaps, an adaptation to load in the proximal tubule. Although the proximal tubule contributes an essential role in maintenance and correction of the alkalosis in that it must reabsorb most of the filtered load of bicarbonate and chloride, the corrective response and, thus, maintenance appears to occur at more distal nephron sites.

The thick ascending limb (TAL) of the loop of Henle absorbs bicarbonate by an apical $Na^+$-$H^+$ antiporter and basolateral $H^+$-$OH^-$-$HCO_3^-$ transport.[73] In the loop segment in acute CDA[50] and the TAL in chronic CDA,[74] bicarbonate reabsorption decreases in contrast to an increase during chronic oral $NaHCO_3$ or NaCl loading.[74] Nevertheless, fractional bicarbonate and chloride reabsorptions did not differ between normal and alkalotic rats whether alkalosis was being maintained or corrected.[50, 63, 70, 72] Thus, the reabsorption of bicarbonate in the TAL does not appear to be regulatory for CDA.

In the distal convoluted tubule (DCT), the data on bicarbonate transport are not consonant. Acute alkalosis did not influence the uptake of bicarbonate when bicarbonate delivery was controlled.[75] However, after 4 weeks of chronic alkalosis, bicarbonate delivery to and reabsorption in the DCT increased but fractional bicarbonate reabsorption did not.[63] With delivery controlled by in vivo microperfusion, alkali loading can induce bicarbonate secretion in the DCT when fluid and electrolyte deliveries are modified.[76] In this study, removal of luminal chloride inhibited bicarbonate secretion and increased bicarbonate reabsorption whereas high chloride perfusates resulted in net bicarbonate secretion in the usually reabsorbing DCT; this effect occurs in the connecting tubule and early CCD, which likely is included in these in vivo microperfused segments.[75] Thus, while this segment appears to have the capability to alter bicarbonate transport under certain conditions, the deliveries of chloride and bicarbonate to the early and late superficial distal nephron in acute CDA have been shown not to differ in rats with maintained versus correcting alkalosis.[77] In addition, in acute CDA, delivery of bicarbonate to the distal nephron determined by micropuncture of the tip of the loop of Henle of juxtamedullary nephrons was actually lower in rats with increased urinary bicarbonate excretion while correcting the alkalosis.[77] Thus, contributions from the DCT are likely to emanate from the connecting tubule or earliest portions of the CCD, which appears to play a dominant role, and both superficial and deep nephrons appear to respond to CDA in a similar qualitative manner.

The CCD, unlike any other nephron segment, can absorb or secrete bicarbonate depending on the conditions imposed and the species studied.[78–81] In the CCD, type A ICs secrete protons across the luminal membrane while reabsorbing bicarbonate in exchange for chloride across the basolateral membrane; type B ICs secrete bicarbonate in exchange for chloride into the lumen with proton absorption across the basolateral membrane.[82–85] Such a unique capability to alter the magnitude and direction of bicarbonate transport accords a potential importance to this segment for the regulation of chloride and bicarbonate excretion. Certain experimental models may not approximate clinical settings and, therefore, results from them should be interpreted cautiously. Oral bicarbonate or deoxycorticosterone loading may not produce systemic metabolic alkalosis and may be associated with alterations in either sodium delivery to or transport in the CCD. In contrast, experimental as well as clinical CDA is associated with systemic metabolic alkalosis, and, depending on conditions of the experiment, sodium avidity and volume depletion.

CCD obtained from rats with CDA and perfused in vitro show sustained bicarbonate secretion, which is dependent on luminal chloride, compared with CCDs from normal rats, which sustain bicarbonate reabsorption.[86] Furthermore, the magnitude and direction of bicarbonate transport in vitro correlates with in vivo serum bicarbonate and chloride concentration and chloride balance and not with potassium balance.[87] These data suggest that the mechanisms for regulating transport can "sense" the degree of alkalosis or chloride balance in vivo. The factors that are responsible for this regulation of bicarbonate transport in the CCD remain poorly understood at this time. The $K_m$ for chloride in the CCD luminal anion exchanger in the rabbit has been estimated to be between 20 and 55 mEq/L.[88] These concentrations are within the range that would allow changes in chloride delivery to the CCD to regulate bicarbonate secretion.

The OMCD, which possesses type A ICs, only absorbs bicarbonate[89] and luminal chloride removal increases net bicarbonate absorption in the rabbit OMCD[90]; in rats with acute CDA, $HCO_3$ uptake is decreased.[91] In the inner medullary collecting duct (IMCD), the initial segment of which also possesses type A ICs, bicarbonate absorption decreases in acute and chronic metabolic alkalosis.[91, 92] In the papillary collecting duct, chloride is intensely conserved on a low chloride diet.[93] In the medullary collecting duct, Wall and colleagues[94] have demonstrated in both control and deoxycorticosterone-loaded rats that net bicarbonate absorption occurs in the terminal portion of the IMCD (ICs are not identified in this segment). Although the role of these medullary segments in the pathophysiology of CDA is unclear, in view of their capacity to transport chloride and bicarbonate, it seems likely that they participate in a coordinated collecting duct response with the CCD.

The potential pathways for bicarbonate reabsorption and secretion in the collecting duct are complex.[95] Protons can be secreted through either $H^+$ATPase or $H^+$,$K^+$ATPase (HKA), both of which may be heterogeneous along this nephron segment. Whereas $H^+$ ATPase is functionally present all along the collecting duct, the isoform in the IMCD differs immunohistologically from that in the more proximal segments.[96] At least two isoforms of HKA, gastric (g) and colonic (c) have been identified along the collecting duct.[95] In perfused CCD from rats with acute CDA, Schering 28080, an inhibitor of $H^+$,$K^+$ATPase, completely inhibits $HCO_3^-$ reabsorption, which suggests that this transport protein is primarily responsible for bicarbonate secretion and that it resides on the basolateral membrane.[86] In the OMCD, IMCDi, and IMCDt, $HCO_3^-$ reabsorption is decreased in tubules obtained from rats with CDA.[97] In all of these studies, tubules were perfused and bathed in 100 mM $Cl^-$. Northern hybridization studies show that the cHKA isoform is expressed in the OMCD and the IMCDt in tubules from rats with CDA.[98] Morphologic studies[99] show hypertrophy and increased staining for proton ATPase of the basolateral area in the type B IC of the CCD in CDA rats. Simultaneously, proton ATPase is diminished in the luminal membrane of type A ICs but increased in subapical vesicles both in the CCD and OMCD, suggesting removal from the cell membrane.

A current overview of the proposed pathophysiology of the maintenance and correction of CDA follows. Whereas the proximal tubule and Henle's loop, which reabsorb the vast proportion of the filtered loads of chloride and bicarbonate, clearly must function normally, the primary regulatory adjustments to chloride and bicarbonate transport to maintain or correct CDA appear to occur in the more distal nephron. Before the administration of chloride, the type B IC is "poised to secrete" bicarbonate via the luminal anion exchanger with maintenance of bicarbonate secretion facilitated by increasing proton ATPase activity at the basolateral membrane. When chloride is given, chloride corrects CDA without a necessary change in volume or GFR by an effect on the CCD and probably the DCT[63, 75, 100] to lead to bicarbonate secretion, and by an effect on the OMCD to diminish reabsorption of bicarbonate that is not reabsorbed at more distal sites. Urinary chloride excretion in CDA remains low until plasma chloride concentration approaches normal[60] and, in chloride depletion, chloride uptake in the collecting duct is greatly accelerated.[92, 101] In in vivo studies, chloride delivery to the CCD increased[102]—albeit not statistically significantly—by an amount consistent in magnitude with the increase in net bicarbonate secretion seen in CCD harvested from CDA animals.[86] The magnitude of bicarbonate secretion in vitro, in turn, is comparable with the increase in urinary bicarbonate excretion.[50] Whereas the collecting duct possesses an array of anion and proton transporters that respond to acid-base disorders in general and CDA in particular, the integrated response of the several segments to maintain and then correct CDA is not yet understood. A major unresolved question is how the kidney recognizes that chloride is being repleted at concentrations at or less than that in ambient plasma.[103]

## PATHOPHYSIOLOGY OF POTASSIUM DEPLETION–MINERALOCORTICOID EXCESS ALKALOSIS

### Generation/Maintenance

**General.** Potassium depletion or, at least, hypokalemia occurs universally in metabolic alkalosis but, as discussed earlier, is not necessarily the proximate cause of the alkalosis. Because it is associated clinically and experimentally with both metabolic alkalosis and metabolic acidosis, the pathophysiologic mechanisms by which potassium depletion is generated and maintained are critical determinants of the resultant acid-base disorder.

Experimental dietary potassium depletion is associated with modest metabolic alkalosis and increases in intracellular sodium and proton concentrations in both humans[104, 105] and rats.[106–108] In contrast, in dog and rabbit[109, 110] metabolic acidosis ensues. In the dog, mild metabolic acidosis has been attributed to a low plasma aldosterone concentration secondary to potassium depletion combined with a putatively more important role for aldosterone in distal bicarbonate reabsorption.[109] In the rat, the generation of alkalosis has been attributed to the intracellular shift of protons[106] and to a shift in the set point for the maintenance of plasma bicarbonate concentration.[107] Net acid excretion does not increase during generation or change during correction by potassium.[111] In renal tubular cells, accompanying intracellular acidosis would facilitate bicarbonate reabsorption and thus maintain alkalosis. An important role of intracellular acidosis is supported by correction of the alkalosis by infusion of potassium without any suppression of renal net acid excretion[107]; correction is assumed to occur by intracellular movement of potassium, with movement of protons into the ECF where bicarbonate is titrated. Furthermore, during potassium depletion alkalosis, the rat excretes an acid load completely while maintaining an elevated plasma bicarbonate concentration.[106] Thus, evidence from the rat model suggests that the kidney does not generate alkalosis but does maintain it.

In humans with selective potassium restriction with other electrolytes maintained, an approximate 300-mM potassium deficit induced about a 2-mM stable increase in serum bicarbonate concentration and a reduction in net acid excretion within 2 days[105] (Fig. 7–4). However, when NaCl intake is also restricted, net acid excretion does increase during generation of alkalosis by potassium depletion.[104] In the NaCl-restricted group, the degree of potassium depletion was similar but the increase in serum bicarbonate concentration was considerably higher (7.5 mM). In addition, body weight and creatinine clearance were decreased; excretion of urine chloride was nonexistent; and urine aldosterone was fivefold higher compared with the high NaCl group. These features of volume and chloride restriction are not typical of clinical potassium depletion, and the extent to which they play an additional role in the pathophysiology of the alkalosis in the NaCl-restricted group is problematic.

As with CDA, either reduced GFR, augmented bicarbonate reabsorption, or both, account for maintenance of potassium-depletion alkalosis. In the rat, both renal blood flow and GFR decrease probably due to an effect of potassium depletion to increase vasoconstrictive eicosanoids and ANG II.[112, 113]

Enhanced bicarbonate reabsorption in several nephron segments also contributes to the maintenance of metabolic alkalosis. In the rat, potassium depletion accelerates renal reabsorption of bicarbonate in the proximal[114] and DCTs[115] independently of load and at physiologic or increased perfusion rates. This increase in reabsorption may be secondary to intracellular acidosis with facilitated proton secretion.

Potassium depletion is associated with enhanced renal ammonia production.[111] The principal mechanism by which this occurs is an increase in ammonia transport into the lumen due to increased ammonia production by the kidney. The reverse of this relationship also occurs in that enhanced ammonia production

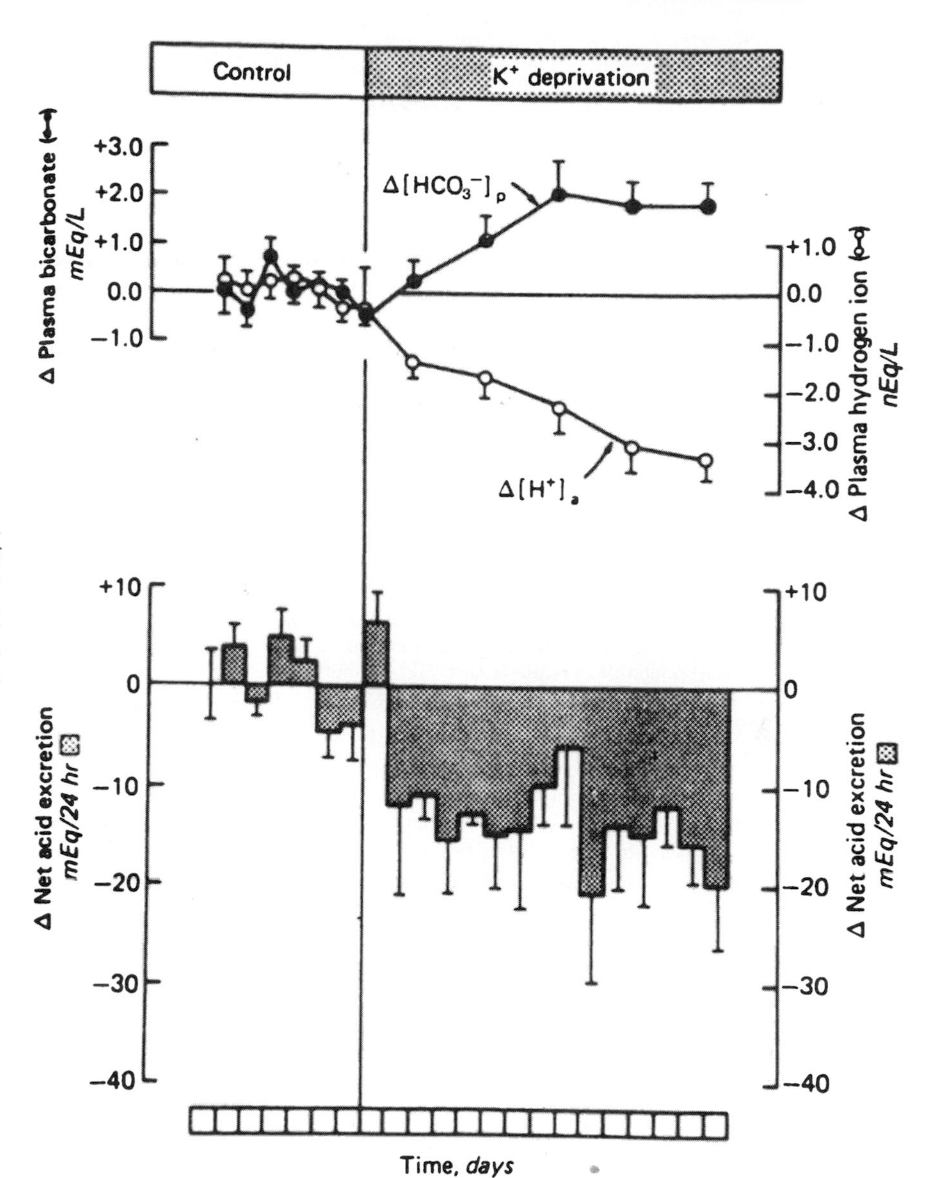


**FIGURE 7–4** ■ Effect of dietary potassium restriction in humans. After 3 days of potassium restriction, plasma bicarbonate concentration rises and net acid excretion falls. (From Jones JW, Sebastian A, Hulter HN, et al: Systemic and renal acid-base effects of chronic dietary potassium depletion in humans. Kidney Int 21:402, 1982.)

decreases urinary potassium excretion, the mechanism of which is unknown.

As with CDA, the collecting duct may play a particularly important role. Whereas the ICs are primarily responsible for proton and bicarbonate transport, the principal cells of the collecting duct are responsible primarily for sodium, potassium, and water transport. However, in the potassium-depleted rat, the ICs of the OMCD are strikingly hypertrophied.[116, 117] These cells possess a functional $H^+,K^+$ATPase, which may be greatly stimulated during potassium depletion and account for augmented bicarbonate reabsorption.[118] $NH_4^+$ secretion is also augmented in this segment.[119] An integrated view of the contribution of the various nephron segments to the generation and maintenance of potassium depletion alkalosis has not yet emerged.

**Mineralocorticoid Excess.** Excesses of aldosterone and other mineralocorticoids are commonly associated with metabolic alkalosis, and it is difficult to dissociate their specific role from that of associated potassium depletion, which per se actually suppresses aldosterone[120] while it increases plasma renin activity and, presumably, ANG II concentrations.[121] Experimentally, administration of aldosterone causes only a slight degree of metabolic alkalosis if potassium depletion is absent.[122] Moreover, the severity of the alkalosis is inversely related to the degree of hypokalemia and directly to the degree of potassium depletion (Fig. 7–5). Escape from the sodium-retaining effect of mineralocorticoids occurs at the expense of persistent vascular and ECF volume expansion and resultant hypertension, but escape does not occur from the potassium-wasting effect, which is relentless. Acting at its receptor in the main cell of the collecting duct, mineralocorticoid stimulates the apical sodium channel and basolateral $Na^+,K^+$ATPase, and increased sodium reabsorption promotes potassium secretion through the apical potassium channel. Associated sodium retention usually leads to hypertension, as in primary aldosteronism, or often to edema, as in secondary aldosteronism (e.g., in cardiac failure).

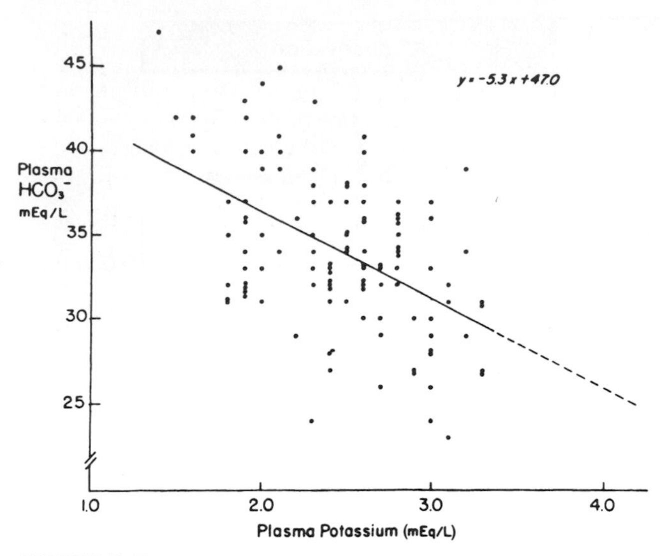


**FIGURE 7–5** ■ Correlation between plasma potassium and bicarbonate concentrations in patients with primary hyperaldosteronism. An inverse relationship is shown between the magnitudes of hypokalemia and hyperbicarbonatemia. (From Kassirer JP, London AM, Goldman DM, et al: On the pathogenesis of metabolic alkalosis in hyperaldosteronism. Am J Med 49:306, 1970.)

Although any increase in GFR due to the associated volume expansion would increase filtered bicarbonate load and thus tend to blunt an alkalosis, mineralocorticoids also have important effects on tubule reabsorption. Aldosterone stimulates sodium reabsorption and potassium and proton secretion in the CCD and, either directly or indirectly via an increased lumen-negative potential, proton secretion and, hence, bicarbonate reabsorption.[123] Aldosterone also stimulates sodium reabsorption in the ascending limb of the loop of Henle.[124] In the rabbit, the OMCD possesses a sodium-independent mineralocorticoid-sensitive proton secretory mechanism.[21] The integrated effect of mineralocorticoid action is to retain sodium, deplete potassium, and produce extracellular alkalosis with intracellular acidosis.

Potassium depletion may maintain metabolic alkalosis as follows: both proximal and distal bicarbonate reabsorptions are enhanced. In the collecting duct, the synergistic effects of potassium depletion and mineralocorticoid excess may result in intracellular acidosis due to the potassium depletion, aldosterone stimulation of sodium-dependent and sodium-independent proton secretion, and the hypertrophy of ICs in the OMCD. Hypertrophy of OMCD cells may stimulate or indicate stimulation of $H^+,K^+$ATPase activity as a mechanism to conserve potassium but thus promote bicarbonate reabsorption. Accompanying excess aldosterone would further promote potassium wasting and proton secretion through sodium-independent mechanisms by which aldosterone excess could at least theoretically generate and maintain metabolic alkalosis, even on a low sodium intake. Although a low-sodium diet appears to intensify alkalosis in potassium depletion alone, a low-sodium diet blocks the kaluretic and alkalotic effects of high-dose exogenous mineralocorticoid administration.[125, 126] Finally, it should be reemphasized that potassium depletion directly depresses aldosterone production[120] and for severe metabolic alkalosis due to potassium depletion–mineralocorticoid excess to occur, this relationship must be disturbed.

**Specific Disorders.** Mineralocorticoid excess has numerous causes. Aldosterone excess may be primary as a result of an adrenal adenoma or carcinoma[127] or hyperplasia of several varieties determined by responsiveness to other hormones.[128] Secondary mineralocorticoid excess with an increase in plasma renin activity may occur because of severe accelerated or malignant hypertension or renin from a unilateral source such as tumor of the kidney or renal artery stenosis or an increase in renin substrate, as in Cushing syndrome.[129]

Low plasma renin and high circulating aldosterone characterize these primary disorders whereas high plasma renin and aldosterone characterize the secondary causes. Almost all of the primary disorders are caused by adrenal neoplasia or hyperplasia, except the glucocorticoid-suppressible variety. This autosomal dominant disease is caused by a chimeric gene formed by the overlap of the gene for 11β-hydroxylase with that for aldosterone synthase.[130] The former is regulated by adrenocorticotropic hormone (ACTH) whereas the latter normally is not. As a consequence of this chimera, aldosterone secretion becomes responsive to ACTH and aldosterone excess results.

Apparent mineralocorticoid excess syndromes have more complex pathophysiologies and are associated with low circulating aldosterone and low plasma renin. Some of these involve genetic alterations in the enzymatic pathway for adrenosteroid biosynthesis; others are drug-induced. Licorice, found in confections, chewing tobacco, some soft drinks, and herbal preparations, and carbenoxolone, a drug used for the treatment of peptic ulcer, contain glycyrrhetinic acid or its derivative, either of which potently inhibits the renal isoform of 11β-hydroxysteroid dehydrogenase present only in the main cell of the collecting duct of the kidney.[131, 132] This enzyme normally shunts cortisol, which exceeds the concentration of aldosterone by a ratio of 100:1, to the inactive cortisone. Thus, under the influence of these inhibitors, cortisol acts at the mineralocorticoid receptor. In contrast, Liddle syndrome, an autosomal dominant disorder with variable clinical expression, is characterized by mutations in either the beta or gamma subunit of the apical sodium channel in the principal cell of the collecting duct that lead to unregulated sodium reabsorption with the cascade of events as earlier.[133]

**Mixed Disorders.** The pathophysiology of the metabolic alkalosis may be mixed. Severe potassium depletion in animals and humans is associated with renal chloride wasting,[107, 134] which would intensify metabolic alkalosis via chloride depletion. Severe potassium depletion in the rat has been shown to produce decreased chloride reabsorption in the proximal tubule, the loop segment, and the collecting duct.[135] With diuretics and other disorders,[10, 134] chloride depletion and potassium depletion, when they are sufficiently severe, may have independent roles, such as in Bartter syndrome.

In Bartter syndrome, the pathophysiology of alkalosis is likely dependent on potassium depletion with mineralocorticoid excess and chloride depletion, each of which may occur by one of several possible defects in tubule transport: a defect in NaCl transport in the ascending limb of Henle's loop,[136, 137a] isolated potassium transport defect,[138] or a defect in a chloride channel.[136, 137] A primary hereditary defect in coupled $Na^+$-$2Cl^-$-$K^+$, reabsorption in the thick ascending limb of the loop of Henle can explain the tendency to renal sodium, potassium, magnesium,[139] and chloride wasting, macula densa–, and baroreceptor-stimulated activation of the renin-aldosterone system, and high renal production of prostaglandin $E_2$.[140, 141] Both medullary interstitial prostaglandin $E_2$ excess[140] and severe potassium depletion[142] can further impair reabsorption by the $Na^+$-$2Cl^-$-$K^+$, transporter in the ascending limb. Bartter syndrome is rare, but its pathophysiology is important because it is similar to some commonly concealed causes of metabolic alkalosis.

In Gitelman syndrome, which is a similar disorder, the primary defect appears to be due to mutations of the NaCl cotransporter that reside in the DCT[143, 144]; Gitelman syndrome mimics the effect of thiazide diuretics. Thus, like thiazide diuretics, it is associated with hypocalciuria, a feature that distinguishes it from Bartter syndrome.

## HYPERCALCEMIC STATES

Hypercalcemia in humans has been associated with both metabolic acidosis and metabolic alkalosis.[145, 146] In rats, either multiple grafts of autologous parathyroid gland or 1,25-(OH)-vitamin D loading, which suppresses parathyroid hormone (PTH), produces hypercalcemia and mild metabolic alkalosis with increased net acid excretion.[147] Several lines of evidence also show that PTH inhibits bicarbonate uptake in the proximal tubule.[148] These observations suggest that hypercalcemia rather than hyperparathyroidism is necessary to generate the alkalosis.[149] In normal humans, infusion of PTH produces hypercalcemia with an initial decrease followed by a sustained increase in net acid excretion and a modest increase in serum bicarbonate concentration[150]; the role of PTH versus that of hypercalcemia was not examined in that study. Finally, in treated or untreated hypoparathyroidism, metabolic alkalosis is the rule, whereas in primary hyperparathyroidism, hyperchloremic metabolic acidosis is more common.[151] Taken together, these studies suggest that hypercalcemia and the presence of suppressed PTH levels are the circumstances in which metabolic alkalosis is most likely to occur, such as in hypercalcemia of malignancy.[152] Considering the principles of acid-base chemistry,[1] the maintained alkalosis may be due, at least in part, to the increase in strong ion difference (increased ionized $Ca^+$ per se) combined with an enhancement of bicarbonate uptake in the proximal tubule due to suppressed PTH.

The generation of metabolic alkalosis in milk-alkali syndrome is multifactorial[153]; vomiting, hypercalcemia, which directly increases bicarbonate reabsorption,[149] a high intake of alkali and a reduced GFR, which may be secondary to volume depletion, chloride depletion, hypercalcemia, and nephrocalcinosis, can all play a role.

## MISCELLANEOUS

Treatment with congeners of penicillin including ampicillin and carbenicillin have been associated with mild metabolic alkalosis.[154] The pathophysiology has not been elucidated, but a hypothesis derives from studies of sodium salts of ineffectively reabsorbed anions such as sulfate.[155] The observation that sodium sulfate does not sustain an increase in net acid excretion leaves this question open, however. These "nonreabsorbable" anionic antibiotics may simply obligate potassium and proton excretion by the kidney.[156]

Hypoproteinemic states by virtue of the decrease in the weak acid concentration, which is predominantly albumin,[157] may also result in a modest degree of metabolic alkalosis.[158] This cause of metabolic alkalosis was recognized initially as a decreased anion gap in association with gammopathies.[159]

Because the normal kidney is so efficient at excreting bicarbonate, base loading, whether exogenous or endogenous (as in bone dissolution), is rarely a sole cause of significant sustained metabolic alkalosis. Transient acute states of metabolic alkalosis commonly occur during and immediately after an oral or intravenous infusion of $NaHCO_3$ or base equivalent (e.g., citrate in transfused blood or fresh frozen plasma).[160] The ingestion of bicarbonate (baking soda) or its metabolic precursors (e.g., citrate) does not produce sustained metabolic alkalosis unless intake is massive—in the range of 1000 mEq/day—and prolonged,[161, 162] GFR is impaired, or dietary NaCl is low.[163] Typically, the alkalosis resolves spontaneously when bicarbonate administration ceases. Chloride intake may be protective against the development of metabolic alkalosis during base loading.[163] A state of transient metabolic alkalosis may also occur after the successful treatment of ketoacidosis or lactic acidosis as these organic anions are metabolized to bicarbonate. The pathophysiologic responses of the kidney to alkali loading compared with chloride depletion have underlined their fundamentally different natures. For example, in the ascending limb of the loop of Henle, bicarbonate reabsorption decreases with chloride depletion but increases with bicarbonate loading.[74]

Nonreabsorbable antacids have also been associated with alkalosis when used together with cation-exchange resins in the setting of renal insufficiency.[164] The proposed mechanism is that magnesium or aluminum hydroxides, which normally bind HCl, are bound by the resin in exchange for sodium. Because the sodium carbonates formed are soluble, bicarbonate is readily reabsorbed by the intestine[165] and alkalosis ensues because the kidney is unable to excrete the bicarbonate.

## CLINICAL AND DIAGNOSTIC ASPECTS

The clinical features of metabolic alkalosis per se are difficult to separate from those of the associated, or causative, deficits of chloride, magnesium, plasma volume, and potassium as well as changes in ionized calcium. However, apathy, confusion, and neuromuscular irritability (related in part, perhaps, to a low ionized plasma calcium) are common when alkalosis is severe. Although neuromuscular irritability may be readily evident, Chvostek and Trousseau signs are seen uncommonly.[166] Alkalosis per se has a mild positive inotropic effect on the heart and little or no effect on cardiac rhythm.[167] Cardiac arrhythmias occur primarily as a consequence of hypokalemia and encompass a variety of disturbances: atrial and ventricular premature beats, paroxysmal atrial and junctional tachycardias, atrioventricular block, and ventricular tachycardia and fibrillation.[168] Coronary insufficiency, left ventricular hypertrophy, and digitalis therapy make these more likely. Alkalosis also intensifies digitalis toxicity.[169] Electrocardiogram changes simulating acute myocardial infarction, which are rarely associated with hyperkalemia, have also been reported during hypokalemia and attributed to a reduction in the intracellular-to-extracellular ratio for potassium during replacement.[170] Compensatory hypoventilation may contribute to hypoxia or pulmonary infection in very ill or immunocompromised patients.

With severe potassium depletion, muscle weakness may dominate the clinical picture. Polyuria and polydipsia may be present because of a urinary concentrating defect.[171] Prolonged hypokalemia and alkalosis, particularly but not exclusively associated with primary aldosteronism, is associated with cortical and medullary renal cysts, which can resolve with treatment.[172] Whether the renal scarring associated with hypokalemic nephropathy can also resolve is unclear.

The cause of chronic metabolic alkalosis (see Table 7–1) is often evident on the initial assessment of the patient with a careful history and physical examination. In the absence of blood gas measurements, an increase in the anion gap favors metabolic alkalosis over respiratory acidosis in the setting of an increased serum bicarbonate concentration, which is the characteristic plasma anion pattern of both disorders. This occurs because of the following reasons: (1) an elevation of the negative charge on plasma albumin; (2) if volume contraction is present, an increased albumin concentration; and (3) in many cases, an elevation of plasma lactate,[3] which can be considerable with severe alkalosis.[173, 174] Lactate production in alkalosis may be enhanced by decreased oxygen delivery due to vasoconstriction and resultant shunting away from the capillaries,[167] decreased consumption because of impaired mitochondrial metabolism,[173] and impaired tissue extraction by increased oxygen-hemoglobin binding, which probably resolves promptly because of an increase in 2,3-DPG.[175]

Urine pH varies depending on the nature and phase of the disorder. Disequilibrium alkalosis, a phase during or immediately after generation, is characterized by an "alkaline" urine (pH > 6.2) with a urinary sodium greater than 10 mEq/L, urinary potassium greater than 30 mEq/L, and bicarbonaturia; urinary chloride concentration remains low. The use of the term "paradoxical aciduria" to describe a normally acidic urinary pH in a setting of a chronic metabolic alkalosis is inappropriate. Because renal reabsorption of bicarbonate is complete, the alkalosis is maintained: an alkaline urine suggests either correcting alkalosis during chloride repletion or disequilibrium alkalosis.

The algorithm (Fig. 7–6) presents an approach to diagnosing the numerous causes of metabolic alkalosis. The hierarchy of the proposed tests is not related to the prevalence of the disorders nor are the tests intended to be comprehensive or definitive for the causes that they suggest. The possibility of multiple causes should be kept in mind, such as surreptitious diuretic and laxative abuse combined with bulimia,[176] hyperaldosteronism secondary to severe hypertension treated with chloruretic diuretics, and hypercalcemia of malignancy with vomiting.

Urinary electrolyte determinations prior to therapy, especially chloride and potassium concentrations, can have considerable diagnostic value before treatment, particularly when the diagnosis is not obvious or the patient is concealing information (e.g., bulimia, diuretic abuse, laxative abuse). A urinary potassium concentration of less than 20 mEq/L indicates an extrarenal route of potassium loss or a substantial severity of chronic potassium deprivation. Conversely, a urine potassium excretion of greater than 30 mEq/day in the

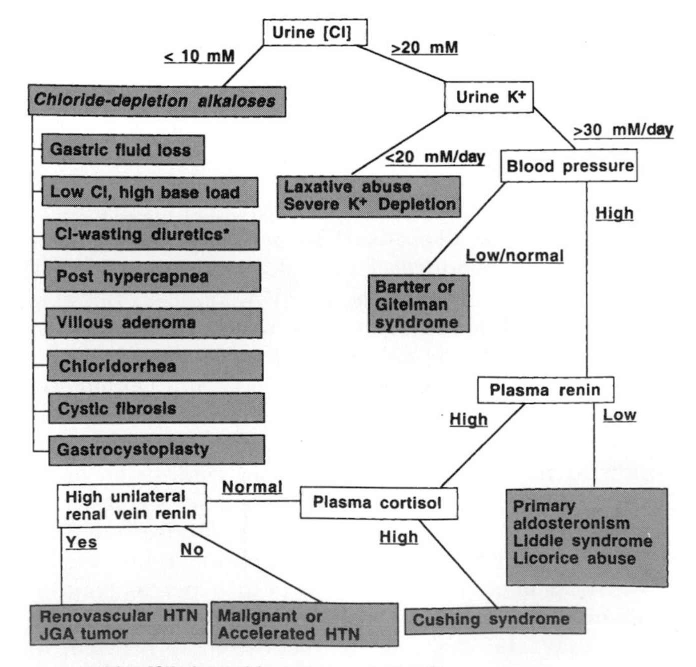


FIGURE 7–6 ■ Diagnostic algorithm for metabolic alkalosis.

presence of hypokalemia defines urinary potassium wasting and is highly suggestive of excess circulating mineralocorticoid or recent surreptitious diuretic abuse. The transtubular potassium gradient (TTKG) is also helpful particularly because a timed collection is unnecessary, thus giving an expeditious determination of the role of the kidney. This index of CCD potassium secretion is calculated as follows:

$$\text{TTKG} = (\text{urine } K^+/\text{serum } K^+) \times (\text{serum osmolality}/\text{urine osmolality})$$

In the setting of hypokalemia, a value less than 3.0 is expected.[177] Greater values suggest that the kidney is the cause or route of potassium depletion; however, clinical studies with this index are limited to date. A urine specimen should also be screened for diuretics, especially if urinary chloride is high and no cause is immediately apparent.

Alkalosis associated with gastric HCl loss, the pathophysiology of which has been discussed, is one of the most common clinical causes. In gastric achlorhydria, metabolic alkalosis can occur because of chloride loss with sodium and potassium as the major cations. In Zollinger-Ellison syndrome, alkalosis can be severe and, in the presence of pyloric obstruction, a significant ECF deficit of chloride and fluid may exist because of gastric dilatation. The diagnosis is self-evident unless the vomiting is surreptitious. In this case, bulimia[178] is often associated with a metabolic alkalosis of fluctuating severity and with episodes of disequilibrium alkalosis.

Bartter syndrome is characterized by normotension, elevated plasma renin activity, and secondary hyperaldosteronism. This syndrome has been understandably confused with several other forms of metabolic alkalosis, particularly when the patient deliberately conceals the cause. In such cases, patients with these surreptitious causes are most often women. Aggressive and persistent probing may be needed to establish the diagnosis and underlying psychiatric abnormality. The salient differences merit reiteration (Table 7–2). Bartter syndrome is familial and mainly, but not exclusively, diagnosed before adult life. Urinary chloride and potassium excretions are high because of the primary defect. Patients with surreptitious vomiting with or without bulimia may have blackened tooth enamel due to repeated exposure to gastric HCl; their renal conservation of chloride remains normal. Other uncommon clues to bulimia are scarring of the dorsum of the hand and salivary gland hypertrophy.[178] An intermittently alkaline urine can occur with acute or chronic vomiting and disequilibrium alkalosis. If it is easy for the patient to obtain diuretics, for example, by health care workers, the suspicion of abuse is heightened. Abuse of diuretics usually leads to more severe potassium depletion than vomiting; urinary potassium and chloride concentrations both will be low unless the diuretic effect is still active; in this setting, random urine sampling may reveal widely fluctuating electrolyte concentrations. With laxative abuse, the urinary potassium excretion is low unless sodium depletion is severe, in which case secondary hyperaldosteronism may occur and increase kaliuresis.[179]

**TABLE 7–2.** Differential Diagnosis of Bartter Syndrome

**Diuretic Abuse**

Urinary sodium and chloride high with recent ingestion or low after the diuretic has been excreted

**Bulimia with Vomiting**

Urinary chloride low but sodium high if vomiting is recent and bicarbonaturia is occurring with disequilibrium

**Magnesium Depletion**

May also complicate Bartter syndrome

**Laxative Abuse**

Urinary potassium $< 30$ mEq/L, mild alkalosis with severe hypokalemia, and urinary chloride $> 20$ mEq/L in the absence of volume depletion

In diarrheal states, the usual tendency is to lose rather than retain base; in secretory diarrhea such as cholera, metabolic acidosis is the rule. Thus, when metabolic alkalosis is present, the causes are few: Some villous adenomas can secrete chloride in the stool greater than 90 mEq/L, particularly those associated with alkalosis. Most are within a few centimeters of the anus but can be higher in the descending colon. Because of their soft, often sessile nature, they may be difficult to palpate and may be passed over on digital examination. Proctoscopy and colonoscopy should be performed with painstaking care.

Congenital chloridorrhea is associated with copious watery diarrhea (1 to 3 L/day) and a stool chloride concentration greater than 90 mEq/L (often as high as 145 mEq/L). If sodium and volume losses are extreme, the stool chloride concentration may be as low as 40 mEq/L. However, when these volume losses are restored, stool chloride rises promptly to typical concentrations.[34] Stool sodium and potassium concentrations are usually normal, and their sum is less than chloride concentration, unlike normal stool. Urinary chloride and potassium concentrations remain low.

Laxative abuse is not associated with severe alkalosis despite usually profound hypokalemia.[180, 181] This disparity between the degrees of hypokalemia and alkalosis is a clinical clue to the diagnosis. Urinary potassium concentration and excretion is uniformly low in laxative abuse, and plasma bicarbonate concentration is rarely above 30 to 34 mEq/L. The diagnosis may be supported by the findings of phenolphthalein in the feces and urine or melanosis coli on colonoscopy.[182]

Metabolic alkalosis associated with hypertension is most likely associated with an effect of diuretics. On the other hand, unprovoked hypokalemic alkalosis (i.e., without diuretic exposure) combined with hypertension, which is not malignant or accelerated, is associated 40% of the time with primary hyperaldosteronism.[183] Primary hyperaldosteronism can usually be conclusively diagnosed by demonstrating an elevated aldosterone excretion after oral NaCl loading and KCl supplementation; the age-adjusted normal ranges should be used for interpretation.[128, 184] The plasma renin activity is usually low, but it is not specific. Once primary aldosteronism is established, several tests are helpful to separate the multiple etiologies, such as a computed tomography scan or magnetic resonance imaging of the adrenal glands, the effect of saline infusion or posture on serum aldosterone and 18-hydroxycorticosterone, an iodocholesterol scintiscan, dexamethasone suppression, and adrenal venous sampling.

Unless there is marked renal insufficiency, metabolic alkalosis often accompanies hypokalemia and secondary hyperaldosteronism in accelerated or malignant hypertension, especially during diuretic therapy. Compared with other cases of mineralocorticoid excess, ectopic ACTH syndrome may be associated with quite severe metabolic alkalosis even though hypertension is not prominent.

# CORRECTION

## Chloride-Responsive Forms

For full correction of these forms of metabolic alkalosis, the chloride deficit must be replaced. Judicious selection of the accompanying cation—sodium, potassium, or proton—is dependent on assessment of: (1) ECF volume status by clinical examination; (2) the presence and degree of associated potassium depletion; and (3) the degree and reversibility of any depression of GFR. If the kidney is capable of excreting sodium and potassium, bicarbonate and base equivalents are excreted with either of those cations and metabolic alkalosis rapidly corrected as chloride is made available. When renal function is severely depressed by acute or chronic intrinsic renal disease, or in the presence of intractable congestive cardiac failure, or when hyperkalemia is present, it may be necessary to avoid the administration of sodium or potassium.

If, as is most commonly the case, depletion of chloride and ECF volume coexist, the administration of isotonic NaCl is the appropriate therapy and will simultaneously correct both deficits as well as any associated depression in GFR. In patients with overt signs of volume contraction such as hypotension, tachycardia, and diminished skin turgor, the administration of a minimum of 3 to 5 L of 0.15 M NaCl is usually necessary to correct both volume deficits and metabolic alkalosis. Fluid therapy should be pressed aggressively until the clinical signs of hypovolemia are reversed.

The replacement of continuing losses of fluid and electrolytes must be included in the regimen. As the chloride deficit is corrected, a brisk alkaline diuresis should occur with a fall in plasma bicarbonate concentration. If, on the other hand, the ECF volume is assessed as normal, total body chloride deficit can be estimated by the formula: body weight (kg) $\times$ 0.2 $\times$ the desired increment in the plasma chloride concentration (mEq/L). Although not essential for correction of alkalosis, correction of potassium depletion is indicated. High urinary potassium excretion may also continue as plasma volume and GFR are restored to normal. Potassium can be provided conveniently by adding KCl, usually in a concentration of 10 to 20 mEq/L of infused fluid to the regimen; serum potassium concentration should be followed carefully.

In the clinical setting of volume overload or congestive heart failure in association with chloride depletion and metabolic alkalosis, administration of NaCl is clearly inadvisable. The presence of hypokalemia then favors KCl for repletion of chloride. If concurrent hyperkalemia is present or the ability to excrete a potassium load in the presence of renal insufficiency is of concern, various therapeutic options are available: infuse chloride as HCl[185] or $NH_4Cl$; provide chloride by peritoneal dialysis, hemodialysis, or hemodiafiltration so that potassium balance, sodium balance, and plasma volume can be corrected; and add acetazolamide to the diuretic regimen.

The use of intravenous HCl is indicated if there is an immediate need for correction, the arterial pH is greater than 7.55, and both NaCl and KCl are contraindicated. The presence of hepatic encephalopathy, cardiac arrhythmia, digitalis cardiotoxicity, or altered mental status all would require emergent treatment. HCl in a 0.1 or 0.2 M solution is appropriate; higher concentrations of HCl have been associated with deterioration of some catheter materials and should be avoided. The amount of HCl needed to correct alkalosis is calculated by the formula: 0.5 $\times$ body weight (kg) $\times$ desired decrement in plasma bicarbonate concentration (mEq/L); this formula does not allow for continuing losses. The use of 50% of body weight as the volume of distribution of infused protons relates mainly to the prior buffering of alkali, including those in intracellular sites; infused protons must restore these buffers as well as titrating extracellular bicarbonate. Because the goal of such aggressive therapy is to rescue the patient from severe alkalosis, it is prudent to plan initially to restore the plasma bicarbonate concentration halfway toward normal. HCl must be given through a catheter placed in the vena cava or in a large vein draining into it. The placement of the catheter should be confirmed radiographically, because leakage of HCl can lead to sloughing of perivascular tissue; in the mediastinum, this would likely be catastrophic. The rate of infusion should not normally exceed 0.2 mEq/kg body weight/hr. The patient is best managed in an intensive care unit with frequent measurement of arterial blood gases and electrolytes.

An alternative to HCl is $NH_4Cl$, which may be given into a peripheral vein; the rate of infusion should not exceed 300 mEq/24 hr. $NH_4Cl$ should be avoided in the presence of renal or hepatic insufficiency.[186] In concurrent renal failure, azotemia would be worsened and, in hepatic failure, acute ammonia intoxication with coma could result. Lysine or arginine HCl should be avoided because these agents have been associated with dangerous hyperkalemia.[187]

If the GFR is adequate (with serum creatinine $< 4$ mg/dL), the use of acetazolamide 250 to 500 mg/day, which produces a diuresis of primarily $NaHCO_3$ by inhibition of carbonic anhydrase, can be considered.[188, 189] If hyperkalemia is absent as is usual, serum potassium concentration should be followed closely and KCl added as necessary because of the high likelihood of developing hypokalemia during the ensuing alkaline diuresis.

When the kidney is incapable of responding to chloride repletion or dialysis is necessary for the control of renal failure, exchange of bicarbonate for chloride by hemodialysis[190] or peritoneal dialysis[191] has also effectively corrected metabolic alkalosis. The usual dialysates for both peritoneal dialysis (including continuous ambulatory peritoneal dialysis) and hemodialysis contain concentrations of bicarbonate or its metabolic precursors, such as acetate, equivalent to 35 mEq/L and, thus, must be modified by substituting chloride for bicarbonate or its precursor in circumstances of metabolic alkalosis. Hemodiafiltration either intermittent or continuous with high volumes of normal saline replacement fluid with a high flux dialyzer is also effective[192] and seems the most straightforward, fastest, and likely the least expensive technique to effect correction. In an emergency, peritoneal dialysis could be performed against sterile solutions of 0.15 M NaCl with appropriate maintenance of plasma potassium, calcium, and magnesium concentration by intravenous infusion.

Additional interventions are appropriate in certain specific clinical situations associated with CDA. In the presence of pernicious vomiting or the need for the continuous removal of gastric secretions, metabolic alkalosis will continue to be generated and replacement of pre-existing deficits will be impeded by these losses. In such circumstances, the administration of an $H_2$ receptor blocker, such as cimetidine[193] or ranitidine, or an $H^+$,$K^+$ATPase inhibitor, such as omeprazole, will blunt acid production by the stomach and thus decrease gastric HCl losses.[194] Even in the presence of these agents, gastric secretions may contain significant amounts of sodium, potassium, and chloride.

Villous adenomas require surgical removal after correction of the sodium, chloride, potassium, and volume deficits; a few show malignant change. Chloridorrhea has been responsive only to continued repletion of fluid, chloride, and potassium losses by supplementation of the dietary intake, and when antidiarrheal agents are ineffective. Omeprazole has been shown to decrease stool electrolyte losses in patients with congenital chloridorrhea.[195] With diuretic-induced losses, KCl may be needed when deficits are clinically significant. The role of hypokalemia in the genesis of cardiac arrhythmias[196] and the need to supplement potassium for the amelioration of essential hypertension[197, 198] must be balanced against the risks of hyperkalemia; these issues have been the topic of vigorous debate and controversy.[134, 199] When chloruretic diuretics are being abused, the patient will probably require intensive counseling to effect a behavioral change.

## Chloride-Resistant Alkaloses

Severe potassium depletion is associated with a mild-to-moderate metabolic alkalosis in humans unless mineralocorticoid excess or exogenous base administration or additional chloride depletion is complicating, in which circumstances severe metabolic alkalosis may occur. Oral KCl 40 to 60 mEq four or five times per day usually will suffice for correction. However, if a cardiac arrhythmia or generalized weakness is present, intravenous KCl may be given at rates as high as 40 mEq/hr in concentrations not to exceed 60 mEq/L. These extraordinarily high rates should be employed only where life-threatening situations are encountered. The patient should be monitored continuously by electrocardiogram and frequent—hourly is not excessive—determinations of plasma potassium concentration. Glucose should be omitted initially from the solution used to administer potassium, because stimulated insulin secretion may cause plasma potassium concentration to decrease even further. However, once potassium repletion is begun, the presence of glucose in the infusion may facilitate cellular potassium repletion. Because hypokalemic nephropathy may impair free water excretion, plasma sodium should be monitored if hypotonic fluids are administered. When laxative abuse is responsible, the patient should be counseled to stop and should be offered psychiatric care when appropriate.

Because Bartter syndrome may comprise several disorders with different pathophysiologies, the contribution of solute deficiencies other than potassium such as sodium, chloride, magnesium, or calcium deficiencies varies. The principal goal of therapy is to prevent urinary potassium loss. Converting enzyme inhibitors, such as captopril or enalapril, which reduce ANG II production and decrease aldosterone secretion, are effective[200] and should probably be tried first. Potassium-sparing diuretics, such as amiloride 5 or 10 mg/day, triamterene 100 mg twice a day, or spironolactone 25 to 50 mg four times a day, will also blunt the urinary losses, but dietary potassium supplementation may also be needed. Because renal prostaglandin production is increased in Bartter syndrome and may contribute to sodium, chloride, and potassium wasting, prostaglandin synthetase inhibitors, such as indomethacin or ibuprofen, may ameliorate, but usually will not completely correct, the hypokalemic alkalosis.[201] Finally, magnesium depletion, which may also increase urinary potassium wasting, should be corrected. However, the degree to which magnesium repletion corrects alkalosis is uncertain, and magnesium salts often produce an unacceptable degree of gastrointestinal irritation that may compound the patient's problems.[139]

When mineralocorticoid excess is the cause, therapy is directed at either removal of the source or its blockade. Hypertension, occasionally severe, may complicate many of these disorders and should be treated aggressively. The administration of potassium-sparing diuretics will effectively reverse the adverse effects of mineralocorticoid excess on sodium, potassium, and bicarbonate excretion. Restriction of sodium and the addition of potassium to the diet will also ameliorate alkalosis and hypertension.[126]

Many primary disorders of mineralocorticoid excess are definitively treated by tumor ablation. ACTH-secreting pituitary tumors may be removed by transsphenoidal resection or by irradiation. With adrenal tumors, adrenalectomy, either unilateral or bilateral as appropriate, may be curative. In the ectopic ACTH syndrome, the ideal treatment of the secreting tumor can rarely be accomplished. In this case and with metastatic adrenal tumors, metyrapone, which inhibits the final step in cortisol synthesis, and aminoglutethimide, which inhibits the initial step in steroid biosynthesis, will blunt the myriad manifestations of hypercortisolism. In those disorders in which curative surgery cannot be carried out, mitotane, which produces selective destruction of the zona fasciculata and reticularis and leaves aldosterone production intact, has also been used to control effectively many of the manifestations of the disease. However, to the extent that severe fluid and electrolyte disturbances are due solely to aldosterone production, this drug may not suffice when hypokalemic alkalosis is present; metyrapone or aminoglutethimide would be better choices. Cisplatin has also been used in the treatment of adrenal malignancies. Detailed discussion of the use of these drugs is beyond the scope of this chapter.

Among the alkaloses produced by massive exogenous base administration, the milk-alkali syndrome is now infrequently seen. Cessation of alkali ingestion and the calcium sources (often milk and calcium carbonate) and chloride and volume repletion for the commonly associated vomiting, will usually lead to the prompt resolution of all abnormalities except for, perhaps, residual renal insufficiency.

## REFERENCES


1. Stewart PA: Modern quantitative acid-base chemistry. Can J Physiol Pharmacol 61:1444, 1983.
2. Javaheri S, Kazemi H: Metabolic alkalosis and hypoventilation in humans. Am Rev Respir Dis 136:1101, 1987.
3. Aquino HC, Luke RG: Respiratory compensation to potassium-depletion and chloride-depletion alkalosis. Am J Physiol 225:1444, 1973.
4. Hodgkin JE, Soeprono FF, Chan DM: Incidence of metabolic alkalemia in hospitalized patients. Crit Care Med 8:725, 1980.
5. Wilson RF, Gibson D, Percinel AK, et al: Severe alkalosis in critically ill surgical patients. Arch Surg 105:197, 1972.
6. Anderson LE, Henrich WL: Alkalemia-associated morbidity and mortality in medical and surgical patients. South Med J 80:729, 1987.
7. Adrogue HJ, Madias NE: Changes in plasma potassium concentration during acute acid-base disturbances. Am J Med 71:456, 1981.
8. Kassirer JP, Schwartz WB: Correction of metabolic alkalosis in man without repair of potassium deficiency. Am J Med 40:19, 1966.
9. Garella S, Chazan JA, Cohen JJ: Saline-resistant metabolic alkalosis or "chloride-wasting nephropathy." Ann Intern Med 73:31, 1970.
10. Wall BM, Williams HH, Cooke CR: Chloride-resistant metabolic alkalosis in an adult with congenital chloride diarrhea. Am J Med 85:570, 1988.
11. Luke RG, Levitin H: Impaired renal conservation of chloride and the acid-base changes associated with potassium depletion in the rat. Clin Sci 32:511, 1967.
12. Seldin DW, Rector FC Jr: The generation and maintenance of metabolic alkalosis. Kidney Int 1:306, 1972.
13. Johnson LR: Physiology of the Gastrointestinal Tract. New York, Raven Press, 1987.
14. Wallmark B, Larsson H, Humble L: The relationship between gastric acid secretion and gastric $H^+,K^+$-ATPase activity. J Biol Chem 260:13681, 1985.
15. Plawker MW, Rabinowitz SS, Etwaru DJ, et al: Hypergastrinemia, dysuria-hematuria and metabolic alkalosis: Complications associated with gastrocystoplasty. J Urol 154:546, 1995.
16. Kassirer JP, Harrington JT: Diuretics and potassium metabolism: A reassessment of the need, effectiveness and safety of potassium therapy. Kidney Int 11:505, 1977.
17. Ellison DH: The physiologic basis of diuretic synergism: Its role in treating diuretic resistance. Ann Intern Med 114:886, 1991.
18. Hropot M, Fowler N, Karlmark B, et al: Tubular action of diuretics: Distal effects on electrolyte transport and acidification. Kidney Int 28:477, 1985.
19. Puschett JB, Goldberg M: The acute effects of furosemide on acid and electrolyte excretion in man. J Lab Clin Med 71:666, 1968.
20. Rosen RA, Julian BA, Dubovsky EA, et al: On the mechanism by which chloride corrects metabolic alkalosis in man. Am J Med 84:449, 1988.
21. Stone DK, Seldin DW, Kokko JP, et al: Mineralocorticoid modulation of rabbit medullary collecting duct acidification. J Clin Invest 72:77, 1983.
22. Chan YL, Biagi B, Giebisch G: Control mechanism of bicarbonate transport across the rat proximal convoluted tubule. Am J Physiol 242:F532, 1982.
23. Carter NW, Seldin DW, Teng HC: Tissue and renal response to chronic respiratory acidosis. J Clin Invest 78:949, 1959.
24. Levitin H, Branscome W, Epstein FH: The pathogenesis of hypochloremia in respiratory acidosis. J Clin Invest 37:1667, 1958.
25. Cogan MG: Effects of acute alterations in $P_{CO_2}$ on proximal $HCO_3^-$, $Cl^-$, and $H_2O$ reabsorption. Am J Physiol 246:F21, 1984.
26. Wingo CS: Effect of acidosis on chloride transport in the cortical thick ascending limb of Henle perfused in vitro. J Clin Invest 78:1324, 1986.
27. Madsen KM, Tisher CC: Cellular response to acute respiratory acidosis in rat medullary collecting duct. Am J Physiol 245:F670, 1983.
28. Verlander JW, Madsen KM, Tisher CC: Effect of acute respiratory acidosis on two populations of intercalated cells in the rat cortical collecting duct. Am J Physiol 253:F1142, 1987.
29. Laski ME, Kurtzman NA: Collecting tubule adaptation to respiratory acidosis induced in vivo. Am J Physiol 258:F15, 1990.
30. Teixeira da Silva JC, Perrone RD, Johns CA, et al: Rat kidney band 3 mRNA modulation in chronic respiratory acidosis. Am J Physiol 260:F204, 1991.
31. Babior BM: Villous adenoma of the colon. Am J Med 41:615, 1966.
32. Shnitka TK, Freidman MHW, Kidd EG, et al: Villous tumors of the rectum and colon characterized by severe fluid and electrolyte loss. Surg Gynecol Obstet 112:609, 1961.
33. Bieberdorf FA, Gorden P, Fordtran JS: Pathogenesis of congenital alkalosis with diarrhea: Implications for the physiology of normal ileal electrolyte absorption and secretion. J Clin Invest 51:1958, 1972.
34. Holmberg C, Perheentupa J, Launiala K, et al: Congenital chloride diarrhea: Clinical analysis of 21 Finnish patients. Arch Dis Child 52:255, 1977.
35. Hogland P, Haila S, Socha J, et al: Mutations of the down-regulated in adenoma (DRA) gene cause congenital chloride diarrhoea. Nat Genet 14:316, 1996.
36. Pedroli G, Liechti-Gallati S, Birrer P, et al: Chronic metabolic alkalosis: Not uncommon in young children with severe cystic fibrosis. Am J Nephrol 15:245, 1995.
37. Gulyassy PF, van Ypersele de Strihou C, Schwartz WB: On the mechanism of nitrate-induced alkalosis: The possible role of selective chloride depletion in acid-base regulation. J Clin Invest 41:1850, 1962.
38. Needle MA, Kaloyanides GJ, Schwartz WB: The effects of selective depletion of hydrochloric acid on acid-base and electrolyte equilibrium. J Clin Invest 43:1836, 1964.

39. Polak A, Haynie GD, Hays RM, et al: Effects of chronic hypercapnia on electrolyte and acid-base equilibrium. I: Adaptation. J Clin Invest 40:1223, 1961.
40. Schwartz WB, Hays RM, Polak A, et al: Effects of chronic hypercapnia on electrolyte and acid-base equilibrium. II: Recovery, with special reference to the influence of chloride intake. J Clin Invest 40:1238, 1961.
41. van Ypersele de Strihou C, Gulyassy PF, Schwartz WB: Effects of chronic hypercapnia on electrolyte and acid-base equilibrium. III: Characteristics of the adaptive and recovery process as evaluated by provision of alkali. J Clin Invest 41:2246, 1962.
42. Kassirer JP, Berkman PM, Lawrenz DR, et al: The critical role of chloride in the correction of hypokalemic alkalosis in man. Am J Med 38:172, 1965.
43. Kassirer JP, Schwartz WB: The response of normal man to selective depletion of hydrochloric acid: Factors in the genesis of persistent gastric alkalosis. Am J Med 40:10, 1966.
44. Schwartz WB, van Ypersele de Strihou C, Kassirer JP: Role of anions in metabolic alkalosis and potassium deficiency. N Engl J Med 279:630, 1968.
45. Cohen JJ: Correction of metabolic alkalosis by the kidney after isometric expansion of extracellular fluid. J Clin Invest 47: 1181, 1968.
46. Cohen JJ: Selective Cl retention in repair of metabolic alkalosis without increasing filtered load. Am J Physiol 218:165, 1970.
47. Emmett M, Seldin DW: Clinical syndromes of metabolic acidosis and metabolic alkalosis. In Seldin DW, Giebisch G (eds): The Kidney, Physiology and Pathophysiology. New York, Raven Press, 1985, p 1611.
48. Galla JH, Bonduris DN, Luke RG: Correction of acute chloride-depletion alkalosis in the rat without volume expansion. Am J Physiol 244:F217, 1983.
49. Craig DM, Galla JH, Bonduris DN, et al: Importance of the kidney in the correction of chloride-depletion alkalosis in the rat. Am J Physiol 250:F54, 1986.
50. Galla JH, Bonduris DN, Luke RG: Effects of chloride and extracellular fluid volume on bicarbonate reabsorption along the nephron in metabolic alkalosis in the rat. J Clin Invest 80: 41, 1987.
51. Norris SH, Kurtzman NA: Does chloride play an independent role in the pathogenesis of metabolic alkalosis? Semin Nephrol 8:101, 1988.
52. Schwartz WB, Cohen JJ: The nature of the renal response to chronic disorders of acid-base equilibrium. Am J Med 64: 417, 1978.
53. Borkan S, Northrup TE, Cohen JJ, et al: Renal responses to metabolic alkalosis induced by isovolemic hemofiltration in the dog. Kidney Int 32:322, 1987.
54. Chamberlin ME, Strange K: Anisotonic cell volume regulation: A comparative view. Am J Physiol 257:C159, 1989.
55. Eveloff J, Warnock D: Activation of ion transport systems during cell volume regulation. Am J Physiol 252:F1, 1987.
56. Hoffman EK, Simonsen LO: Membrane mechanisms in volume and pH regulation. Physiol Rev 69:315, 1989.
57. Macknight ADC: Volume maintenance in isoosmotic conditions. In Kleinzeller A (ed): Current Topics in Membranes and Transport, vol 30. New York, Academic Press, 1987, p 3.
58. Atkins EA, Schwartz WB: Factors governing correction of the alkalosis associated with potassium deficiency: The critical role of chloride in the recovery process. J Clin Invest 41:218, 1961.
59. Berger BE, Cogan MG, Sebastian A: Reduced glomerular filtration and enhanced bicarbonate reabsorption maintain metabolic alkalosis in humans. Kidney Int 26:205, 1984.
60. Galla JH, Bonduris DN, Sanders PW, et al: Volume-independent reductions in glomerular filtration rate in acute chloride-depletion alkalosis in the rat. J Clin Invest 74:2002, 1984.
61. Wright FS, Briggs JP: Feedback regulation of glomerular filtration rate. Am J Physiol 233:F1, 1977.
62. Maddox DA, Gennari FJ: Load dependence of proximal tubular bicarbonate reabsorption in chronic metabolic alkalosis in the rat. J Clin Invest 77:709, 1986.
63. Wesson DE: Augmented bicarbonate reabsorption by both the proximal and distal nephron maintains chloride-deplete metabolic alkalosis in rats. J Clin Invest 84:1460, 1989.
64. Luke RG, Galla JH: Chloride-depletion alkalosis with a normal extracellular fluid volume. Am J Physiol 245:F419, 1983.
65. Abboud HE, Luke RG, Galla JH, Kotchen TA: Stimulation of renin by acute selective chloride depletion in the rat. Circ Res 44:815, 1979.
66. Liu F-Y, Cogan MG: Role of angiotensin II in glomerulotubular balance. Am J Physiol 259:F72, 1990.
67. Walters EA, Rome L, Luke RG, et al: Absence of a regulatory role of angiotensin II in acute chloride-depletion alkalosis in the rat. Am J Physiol 261:F741, 1991.
68. Kassirer JP, Appleton FM, Chazan JA, et al: Aldosterone in metabolic alkalosis. J Clin Invest 46:1558, 1967.
69. Cogan MG, Liu F-Y: Metabolic alkalosis in the rat: Evidence that reduced glomerular filtration rate rather than enhanced tubular bicarbonate reabsorption is responsible for maintaining the alkalotic state. J Clin Invest 71:1141, 1983.
70. Galla JH, Bonduris DN, Dumbauld SL, et al: Segmental chloride and fluid handling during correction of chloride-depletion alkalosis without volume expansion in the rat. J Clin Invest 73: 96, 1984.
71. Maddox DA, Gennari FJ: Proximal tubular bicarbonate reabsorption and $P_{CO_2}$ in chronic metabolic alkalosis in the rat. J Clin Invest 72:1385, 1983.
72. Mello Aires M, Malnic G: Micropuncture study of acidification during hypochloremic alkalosis in the rat. Pfleugers Arch 331: 13, 1972.
73. Krapf R: H/OH/$HCO_3$ transport in the rat cortical thick ascending limb: Evidence for an electrogenic Na/$HCO_3$ cotransporter in parallel with a Na/H antiporter. J Clin Invest 82: 234, 1988.
74. Good DW: Bicarbonate absorption by the thick ascending limb of Henle's loop. Semin Nephrol 10:132, 1990.
75. Lucci MS, Pucacco LR, Carter NW, et al: Evaluation of bicarbonate transport in rat distal tubule: Effects of acid-base status. Am J Physiol 243:F335, 1982.
76. Levine DZ, Vandorpe D, Iacovitti M: Luminal chloride modulates rat distal tubule bidirectional bicarbonate flux in vivo. J Clin Invest 85:1793, 1990.
77. Galla JH, Bonduris DN, Luke RG: Superficial distal and deep nephrons in the correction of metabolic alkalosis. Am J Physiol 257:F107, 1989.
78. Atkins JL, Burg MB: Bicarbonate transport by isolated perfused rat collecting ducts. Am J Physiol 249:F485, 1985.
79. Garcia-Austt J, Good DW, Burg MB, et al: Deoxycorticosterone-stimulated bicarbonate secretion in rabbit cortical collecting ducts: Effects of luminal chloride removal and in vivo acid loading. Am J Physiol 249:F205, 1985.
80. McKinney TD, Burg MB: Bicarbonate transport by rabbit cortical collecting tubules. J Clin Invest 77:766, 1977.
81. Tomita K, Piasona JJ, Burg MB, et al: Effects of vasopressin and bradykinin on anion transport by the rat cortical collecting duct: Evidence for an electroneutral sodium chloride transport pathway. J Clin Invest 77:136, 1986.
82. Laski ME, Warnock DG, Rector FC Jr: Effects of chloride gradients on total $CO_2$ flux in the rabbit cortical collecting tubule. Am J Physiol 244:F112, 1983.
83. Schuster VL: Cyclic adenosine monophosphate-stimulated bicarbonate secretion in rabbit cortical collecting tubules. J Clin Invest 75:2056, 1985.
84. Schuster VL: Bicarbonate reabsorption and secretion in the cortical and outer medullary collecting tubule. Semin Nephrol 10:139, 1990.
85. Star RA, Burg MB, Knepper MA: Bicarbonate secretion and chloride absorption by rabbit cortical collecting ducts: Role of chloride/bicarbonate exchange. J Clin Invest 76:1123, 1985.
86. Gifford JD, Sharkins K, Work J, et al: Total $CO_2$ transport in rat cortical collecting duct in chloride-depletion alkalosis. Am J Physiol 258:F848, 1990.
87. Gifford JD, Ware MW, Luke RG, et al: $HCO_3$ transport in rat CCD: rapid adaptation by in vivo but not in vitro alkalosis. Am J Physiol 264:F435, 1993.
88. Furuya H, Breyer M, Jacobson H: Functional characterization of $\alpha$ and $\beta$ intercalated cell types in the rabbit cortical collecting duct. Am J Physiol 261:F377, 1991.

89. Madsen KM, Tisher CC: Structural-functional relationships along the distal nephron. Am J Physiol 250:F1, 1986.
90. Stone DK, Seldin DW, Kokko JP, et al: Anion dependence of rabbit medullary collecting duct acidification. J Clin Invest 71: 1505, 1983.
91. Galla JH, Rome L, Luke RG: Bicarbonate transport in collecting duct segments during chloride-depletion alkalosis. Kidney Int 48:52, 1985.
92. Ullrich KJ, Papavassiliou F: Bicarbonate reabsorption in the papillary collecting duct of rats. Pfleugers Arch 389:271, 1981.
93. Diezi J, Michoud P, Aceves J, et al: Micropuncture study of electrolyte transport across papillary collecting duct of the rat. Am J Physiol 224:623, 1973.
94. Wall SM, Sands JM, Flessner M, et al: Net acid transport by isolated perfused inner medullary collecting ducts. Am J Physiol 258:F75, 1990.
95. Silver RB, Soleimani M: $H^+K^+$ATPase: Regulation and role in pathophysiological states. Am J Physiol 276:F799, 1999.
96. Brown D, Hirsch S, Gluck S: Localization of a proton-pumping ATPase in rat kidney. J Clin Invest 82:2114, 1988.
97. Gifford JD, Rome L, Galla JH: $H^+$-$K^+$-ATPase activity in rat collecting duct segments. Am J Physiol 262:F692, 1992.
98. Nakamura S, Wang Z, Soleimani M, et al: Colonic H-K-ATPase (cHKA) mediates ouabain-sensitive $HCO_3^-$ reabsorption in outer medullary collecting duct (OMCD) in rats with chloride-depletion alkalosis (CDA). J Am Soc Nephrol 9:10a, 1998.
99. Verlander JW, Madsen KM, Galla JH, et al: Response of intercalated cells to chloride depletion metabolic alkalosis. Am J Physiol 262:F309, 1992.
100. Wesson DE: Depressed distal tubule acidification corrects chloride-deplete metabolic alkalosis in rats. Am J Physiol 259: F636, 1990.
101. Kirchner KA, Galla JH, Luke RG: Factors influencing chloride reabsorption in the collecting duct segment of the rat. Am J Physiol 239:F552, 1980.
102. Galla JH, Bonduris DN, Luke RG: Effects of chloride and extracellular fluid volume on bicarbonate reabsorption along the nephron in metabolic alkalosis in the rat. J Clin Invest 80: 41, 1987.
103. Galla JH, Gifford JD, Luke RG, et al: Adaptations to chloride-depletion alkalosis. Am J Physiol 30:R771, 1991.
104. Hernandez RE, Schambelan M, Cogan MG, et al: Dietary NaCl determines severity of potassium depletion-induced metabolic alkalosis. Kidney Int 31:1356, 1987.
105. Jones JW, Sebastian A, Hulter HN, et al: Systemic and renal acid-base effects of chronic dietary potassium depletion in humans. Kidney Int 21:402, 1982.
106. Kaufman AM, Kahn T: Potassium-depletion alkalosis in the rat. Am J Physiol 255:F763, 1988.
107. Luke RG, Levitin H: Impaired renal conservation of chloride and the acid-base changes associated with potassium depletion in the rat. Clin Sci 32:511, 1967.
108. Struyvenberg A, DeGraeff J, Lameijer LDF: The role of chloride in hypokalemic alkalosis in the rat. J Clin Invest 44:326, 1965.
109. Hulter HN, Sebastian A, Sigala JF, et al: Pathogenesis of renal hyperchloremic acidosis resulting from dietary potassium restriction in the dog: Role of aldosterone. Am J Physiol 28: F79, 1980.
110. McKinney TD, Davidson KK: Effect of potassium depletion and protein intake in vivo on renal bicarbonate transport in vitro. Am J Physiol 252:F509, 1987.
111. Tannen RL: Effect of potassium on renal acidification and acid-base homeostasis. Semin Nephrol 7:263, 1987.
112. Linas SL, Dickman D: Mechanism of the decreased renal blood flow in the potassium-depleted rat. Kidney Int 21:757, 1982.
113. Tannen RL: Effect of $K^+$ depletion on renal and systemic hemodynamics. Contrib Nephrol 41:167, 1984.
114. Chan YL, Biagi B, Giebisch G: Control mechanism of bicarbonate transport across the rat proximal convoluted tubule. Am J Physiol 242:F532, 1982.
115. Capasso G, Jaeger P, Giebisch G, et al: Renal bicarbonate reabsorption. II: Distal tubule load dependence and effect of hypokalemia. J Clin Invest 80:409, 1987.
116. Hansen GT, Tisher CC, Robinson RR: Response of the collecting duct to disturbances of acid base and potassium balance. Kidney Int 17:326, 1980.
117. Stetson DL, Wade JB, Giebisch G: Morphologic alterations in the rat medullary collecting duct following potassium depletion. Kidney Int 17:45, 1980.
118. Wingo CS: Active proton secretion and potassium absorption in the rabbit outer medullary collecting duct: Functional evidence for proton-potassium-activated adenosine triphosphatase. J Clin Invest 84:361, 1989.
119. Nakamura S, Amlal H, Galla JH, et al: $NH_4^+$ secretion in inner medullary collecting duct in potassium deprivation: Role of colonic $H^+$-$K^+$-ATPase. Kidney Int 56:2160, 1999.
120. Cannon PJ, Ames RP, Laragh JH: Relation between potassium balance and aldosterone secretion in normal subjects and in patients with hypertensive and renal tubular disease. J Clin Invest 45:865, 1966.
121. Brunner HR, Baer RL, Sealy JE, et al: The influence of potassium administration and potassium deprivation on plasma renin in normal and hypertensive subjects. J Clin Invest 49: 2128, 1970.
122. Kassirer JP, London AM, Goldman DM, et al: On the pathogenesis of metabolic alkalosis in hyperaldosteronism. Am J Med 49:306, 1970.
123. Koeppen BM, Giebisch G: Segmental hydrogen ion transport. In Seldin DW, Giebisch G (eds): The Regulation of Acid-Base Balance. New York, Raven Press, 1989, p 139.
124. Work J, Jamison RL: Effect of adrenalectomy on transport in the rat medullary thick ascending limb. J Clin Invest 80: 1160, 1987.
125. Relman AS, Schwartz WB: The effect of DOCA on electrolyte balance in normal man and its relation to sodium chloride intake. Yale J Biol Med 24:540, 1952.
126. Seldin DW, Welt LG, Cort JH: The role of sodium salts and adrenal steroids in the production of hypokalemic alkalosis. Yale J Biol Med 29:229, 1956.
127. Arteaga E, Biglieri EG, Kater CE, et al: Aldosterone-producing adrenocortical carcinoma. Ann Intern Med 101:316, 1984.
128. Levi M: Southwestern Internal Medicine Conference: Primary hyperaldosteronism. Am J Med Sci 300:189, 1990.
129. Krakoff LR: Measurement of plasma renin substrate by radioimmunoassay of angiotensin I: Concentration in syndromes associated with steroid excess. J Clin Endocrinol Metab 37:110, 1973.
130. Lifton RP, Dhuly RG, Powers M, et al: A chimaeric 11β-hydroxylase/aldosterone synthase gene causes glucocorticoid-remediable aldosteronism and human hypertension. Nature 355:262, 1992.
131. Edwards C, Walker B: Cortisol and hypertension: What was not so apparent about "apparent mineralocorticoid excess." J Lab Clin Med 122:632, 1993.
132. Young WF Jr, Hogan MJ: Renin-independent hypermineralocorticoidism. Trends Endocrinol Metab 5:97, 1994.
133. Oh YS, Warnock DG: Disorders of the epithelial $Na^+$ channel in Liddle's syndrome and autosomal recessive pseudohypoaldosteronism type 1. Exp Nephrol 8:320, 2000.
134. Kassirer JP, Harrington JT: Fending off the potassium pushers. N Engl J Med 312:785, 1985.
135. Luke RG, Wright FS, Fowler N, et al: Effects of potassium depletion on tubular chloride transport in the rat. Kidney Int 14:414, 1978.
136. Kurtz I: Molecular pathogenesis of Bartter's and Gitelman's syndromes. Kidney Int 34:1396, 1998.
137. Bettinelli A, Ciarmatori S, Cesareo L, et al: Phenotypic variability in Bartter syndrome type I. Pediatr Nephrol 14:940, 2000.
138. Feldmann D, Alessandri JL, Deschenes G: Large deletion on the 5′ end of the ROMK1 gene causes antenatal Bartter syndrome. J Am Soc Nephrol 9:2357, 1998.
139. Baehler RW, Work J, Kotchen TA, et al: Studies on the pathogenesis of Bartter's syndrome. Am J Med 69:933, 1980.
140. Gill JR, Frolich JC, Bowden RE, et al: Bartter's syndrome: A disorder characterized by high urinary prostaglandins and a dependence of hyperreninemia on prostaglandin synthesis. Am J Med 61:43, 1976.

141. Gill JR Jr, Bartter FC: Evidence for a prostaglandin-independent defect in chloride reabsorption in the loop of Henle as a proximal cause of Bartter's syndrome. Am J Med 65:766, 1978.
142. Luke RG, Booker BB, Galla JH: Effect of potassium depletion on chloride transport in the loop of Henle in the rat. Am J Physiol 248:F682, 1985.
143. Simon DB, Lifton RP: Ion transporter mutations in Gitelman's and Bartter's syndromes. Curr Opin Nephrol Hypertens 7: 43, 1998.
144. Monkawa T, Kurihara I, Kobayashi K, et al: Novel mutations in thiazide-sensitive Na-Cl cotransporter gene of patients with Gitelman's syndrome. J Am Soc Nephrol 11:65, 2000.
145. Barzel US: Acid-base balance in disorders of calcium metabolism. N Y State J Med 76:234, 1976.
146. Heinemann HO: Metabolic alkalosis in patients with hypercalcemia. Metabolism 14:1137, 1965.
147. Mitnick P, Greenberg A, Coffman T, et al: Effects of two models of hypercalcemia on renal acid base metabolism. Kidney Int 21:613, 1982.
148. Sasaki S, Marumo F: Mechanisms of inhibition of proximal acidification by PTH. Am J Physiol 260:F833, 1991.
149. Crumb CK, Martinez-Maldonado M, Eknoyan G, et al: Effects of volume expansion, purified parathyroid extract and calcium on renal bicarbonate reabsorption in the dog. J Clin Invest 54: 1287, 1974.
150. Hulter HN, Peterson JC: Acid-base homeostasis during chronic PTH excess in humans. Kidney Int 28:187, 1985.
151. Mallette LE, Bilezikian JP, Heath DA, et al: Primary hyperparathyroidism: Clinical and biochemical features. Medicine 53: 127, 1974.
152. Mundy GR, Yates AJP: Recent advances in pathophysiology and treatment of hypercalcemia of malignancy. Am J Kidney Dis 14:2, 1989.
153. Schuman CA, Jones HW III: The "milk-alkali" syndrome: Two case reports with discussion of pathogenesis. Q J Med 55: 119, 1985.
154. Stapleton FB, Nelson B, Vats TS, et al: Hypokalemia associated with antibiotic treatment. Am J Dis Child 130:1104, 1976.
155. Lipner HI, Ruzany F, Dasgupta M, et al: The behavior of carbenicillin as a nonreabsorbable anion. J Lab Clin Med 86: 183, 1975.
156. Brunner FP, Frick PG: Hypokalemia, metabolic alkalosis, and hypernatremia due to "massive" sodium penicillin therapy. BMJ 4:550, 1968.
157. Figge J, Rossing TH, Fencl V: The role of serum proteins in acid-base equilibria. J Lab Clin Med 117:453, 1991.
158. McAuliffe JJ, Lind LJ, Leith DE, et al: Hypoproteinemic alkalosis. Am J Med 81:86, 1986.
159. Frohlich J, Adam W, Golbey MJ, et al: Decreased anion gap associated with monoclonal and pseudomonoclonal gammopathy. J Can Med Assoc 114:231, 1976.
160. Pearl RG, Rosenthal MH: Metabolic alkalosis due to plasmapheresis. Am J Med 79:391, 1985.
161. Lowder SC, Brown RD: Hypertension corrected by discontinuing chronic sodium bicarbonate ingestion: Subsequent transient hypoaldosteronism. Am J Med 58:272, 1975.
162. van Goidsenhoven GMT, Gray OV, Price AV, et al: The effect of prolonged administration of large doses of sodium bicarbonate in man. Clin Sci 13:383, 1954.
163. Cogan MG, Carneiro J, Tatsumo J: Normal diet NaCl variation can affect the renal set point for plasma pH ($HCO_3$) maintenance. J Am Soc Nephrol 1:193, 1990.
164. Madias NE, Levey AS: Metabolic alkalosis due to absorption of "nonabsorbable" antacids. Am J Med 74:155, 1983.
165. Schroeder ET: Alkalosis resulting from combined administration of a "nonsystemic" antacid and a cation-exchange resin. Gastroenterology 56:869, 1969.
166. Harrington JT, Kassirer JP: Metabolic alkalosis. In Cohen JJ, Kassirer JP (eds): Acid/Base. Boston, Little Brown, 1982, p 242.
167. Mitchell JH, Wildenthal K, Johnson RL Jr: The effects of acid-base disturbances on cardiovascular and pulmonary function. Kidney Int 1:375, 1972.
168. Helfant RW: Hypokalemia and arrhythmias. Am J Med 80 (suppl 4A):13, 1986.
169. Warren MC, Gianelly RE, Cutler RL, et al: Digitalis toxicity. II: The effect of metabolic alkalosis. Am Heart J 75:358, 1968.
170. Madias JE, Madias NE: Hyperkalemia-like ECG changes simulating acute myocardial infarction in a patient with hypokalemia undergoing potassium replacement. J Electrocardiol 22:93, 1989.
171. Schwartz WB, Relman AS: Effects of electrolyte disorders on renal structure and function. N Engl J Med 276:383, 1967.
172. Torres VE, Young WF, Offord KP, et al: Association of hypokalemia, aldosteronism and renal cysts. N Engl J Med 322:345, 1990.
173. Bersin RM, Arieff AI: Primary lactic alkalosis. Am J Med 85: 867, 1988.
174. Madias NE, Ayus JC, Adrogue HJ: Increased anion gap in metabolic alkalosis. N Engl J Med 300:1421, 1979.
175. Bellingham AJ, Detter JC, Lenfant C: Regulatory mechanisms of hemoglobin oxygen affinity in acidosis and alkalosis. J Clin Invest 50:700, 1971.
176. Oster JR: The binge-purge syndrome: A common albeit unappreciated cause of acid-base and fluid-electrolyte disturbances. South Med J 80:58, 1987.
177. Ethier JH, Kamel KS, Magner PO, et al: The transtubular potassium gradient in patients with hypokalemia and hyperkalemia. Am J Kidney Dis 15:309, 1990.
178. Mitchell JE, Seim HC, Colon E, et al: Medical complications and medical management of bulimia. Ann Intern Med 107: 71, 1987.
179. Fleischer N, Brown H, Graham DY, et al: Chronic laxative-induced hyperaldosteronism and hypokalemia simulating Bartter's syndrome. Ann Intern Med 70:791, 1969.
180. Cummings JH, Sladen GE, James OFW, et al: Laxative-induced diarrhoea: A continuing clinical problem. BMJ 1:537, 1974.
181. Schwartz WB, Relman AS: Metabolic and renal studies in chronic potassium depletion resulting from overuse of laxatives. J Clin Invest 32:258, 1953.
182. LaRusso NF, McGill DS: Surreptitious laxative ingestion. Delayed recognition of a serious condition: A case report. Mayo Clin Proc 50:706, 1975.
183. Kotchen TA, Mulrow PJ, Morrow LB, et al: Renin and aldosterone in essential hypertension. Clin Sci 41:321, 1971.
184. Young WF Jr, Hogan MJ, Klee GG, et al: Primary aldosteronism: Diagnosis and treatment. Mayo Clin Proc 65:96, 1990.
185. Wagner CW, Nesbit RR, Mansberger AR Jr: Treatment of metabolic alkalosis with intravenous hydrochloric acid. South Med J 72:1241, 1979.
186. Warren SE, Swerdlin ARH, Steinberg SM: Treatment of alkalosis with ammonium chloride. Clin Pharmacol Ther 25:624, 1979.
187. Bushinsky DA, Gennari FJ: Life-threatening hyperkalemia induced by arginine. Ann Intern Med 89:632, 1978.
188. Fraley DS, Adler S, Bruns F: Life-threatening metabolic alkalosis in a comatose patient. South Med J 72:1024, 1979.
189. Mazur JE, Devlin JW, Peters MJ, et al: Single versus multiple doses of acetazolamide for metabolic alkalosis in critically ill medical patients: A randomized double-blind trial. Crit Care Med 27:1257, 1999.
190. Swartz RD, Rubin JE, Brown RS, et al: Correction of postoperative metabolic alkalosis and renal failure by hemodialysis. Ann Intern Med 86:52, 1977.
191. Vilbar RM, Ing TS, Shin KD, et al: Treatment of metabolic alkalosis with peritoneal dialysis in a patient with renal failure. Artif Organs 2:421, 1978.
192. Kheirbek AO, Ing TS, Viol GW, et al: Treatment of metabolic alkalosis with hemofiltration in patients with renal insufficiency. Nephron 24:91, 1979.
193. Rowlands BJ, Tindall SF, Elliot DJ: The use of dilute hydrochloric acid and cimetidine to reverse severe metabolic alkalosis. Postgrad Med J 54:118, 1978.
194. Barton CH, Vaziri ND, Ness RL, et al: Cimetidine in the management of metabolic alkalosis induced by nasogastric suction. Arch Surg 114:70, 1979.
195. Aichbichler BW, Zerr CH, Santa Ana CA, et al: Proton-pump inhibition of gastric chloride secretion in congenital chloridorrhea. N Engl J Med 336:106, 1997.

196. Kassirer JP, Harrington JT: Diuretics and potassium metabolism: A reassessment of the need, effectiveness and safety of potassium therapy. Kidney Int 11:505, 1977.
197. Cappuccio FP, MacGregor GA: Does potassium supplementation lower blood pressure? A meta-analysis of published trials. J Hypertens 9:465, 1991.
198. Kaplan NM, Carnegie A, Raskin P, et al: Potassium supplementation in hypertensive patients with diuretic-induced hypokalemia. N Engl J Med 312:746, 1985.
199. Suki WN: Dietary potassium and blood pressure. Kidney Int 34 (Suppl 25):S175, 1988.
200. Hene RJ, Boer P, Koomans HA, et al: Correction of hypokalemia in Bartter's syndrome by enalapril. Am J Kidney Dis 9: 200, 1987.
201. Verberkmoes R, van Damme B, Clement J, et al: Bartter's syndrome with hyperplasia of renomedullary cells: Successful treatment with indomethacin. Kidney Int 9:302, 1976.
202. Severance HW, Holt T, Patrone NA, et al: Profound muscle weakness and hypokalemia due to clay ingestion. South Med J 81:272, 1988.
203. Schwartz WB, Hays RM, Polak A, Haynie GD: Effects of chronic hypercapnia on electrolyte and acid-base equilibrium. II: Recovery, with special reference to the influence of chloride intake. J Clin Invest 40:1238, 1961.

CHAPTER 8

# Respiratory Acidosis

Galen B. Toews, MD

Respiratory and renal regulatory mechanisms normally maintain blood pH within a narrow range (7.35 to 7.43). Respiratory and renal processes in conjunction with chemical buffers dispose of approximately 15,000 mmol (>300 L) of $CO_2$ per day under basal conditions. Although blood pH is rigorously defended in normal circumstances, acid-base disorders occur commonly in both medical and surgical patients. They may be particularly complex in critically ill, hospitalized patients. Acid-base disorders may present as single disorders or as a mixed acid-base disturbance. Pathophysiologic disruptions of systems regulating the level of $Pa_{CO_2}$ can lead to increases in $Pa_{CO_2}$ (hypercapnia), which acidifies body fluids and initiates the acid-base disturbance of respiratory acidosis.

## PHYSIOLOGIC DETERMINANTS OF $CO_2$ BALANCE

$CO_2$ balance is achieved by pulmonary excretion of $CO_2$ produced by cellular metabolism. No other excretory route for $CO_2$ exists. $CO_2$ gas exchange by the lungs is responsible for the bulk of acid excretion; more than 99.5% of the normal daily acid load produced by metabolism is eliminated by this route. $CO_2$ balance is determined by an interaction of physiologic processes of $CO_2$ production, transport, and excretion.

### $CO_2$ Production

$CO_2$ production is remarkably constant from day to day under basal conditions in normal individuals (~15,000 mmol); $CO_2$ production may increase by as much as 20-fold during maximal exercise.[1, 2]

### $CO_2$ Transport

The $CO_2$ produced in tissues must be transported by the blood to the pulmonary capillaries, where it is excreted into the atmosphere.[2] Diffusion is the driving force responsible for the steady flow of $CO_2$ from the tissues to the blood and from the blood to the alveolar spaces of the lung. The transport of $CO_2$ from the tissues to the lungs is accomplished with a remarkably small gradient for $Pa_{CO_2}$ because of the efficiency with which gaseous $CO_2$ is converted to other molecular forms. The $Pa_{CO_2}$ gradient between the tissues and the alveoli averages only 6 mm Hg; the mean $P_{CO_2}$ of the tissues is approximately 46 mm Hg, and the alveolar $P_{CO_2}$ is approximately 40 mm Hg.

The $CO_2$ produced by metabolism is transported in both the plasma and the red blood cells (Fig. 8–1). Only a small fraction of $CO_2$ is transported as dissolved $CO_2$. Most of the $CO_2$ produced by metabolism is transported to the lungs for excretion in the form of bicarbonate ions. $CO_2$, which diffuses from the tissues to venous blood, passes freely into red blood cells where carbonic anhydrase catalyzes the rapid formation of carbonic acid.[2–5]

$$CO_2 + H_2O \underset{\text{anhydrase}}{\overset{\text{carbonic}}{\rightleftharpoons}} H_2CO_3 \rightleftharpoons H^+ + HCO_3^- \quad \text{(Equation 1)}$$

The hydrogen ions formed by the dissociation of carbonic acid are buffered by intracellular proteins, predominately hemoglobin. The bicarbonate ions generated during the process of dissociation of carbonic acid diffuse readily into the plasma in exchange for chloride ions, a process known as "the chloride shift."[6–10] In the absence of the chloride shift, the hydration reaction of $CO_2$ to carbonic acid within the red blood cell would soon be inhibited by an increasing intracellular bicarbonate ion concentration limiting the capacity of red blood cells to transport $CO_2$. Bicarbonate is transported from the intracellular space to the extracellular space by a $HCO_3^-$-$Cl^-$ exchanger.[11] Accordingly, most of the $CO_2$ converted to bicarbonate ions within the red blood cells is conveyed to the lungs by the plasma. A lesser portion of the $CO_2$, which enters the red blood cell, combines directly with amino groups on the hemoglobin molecule to form carb-

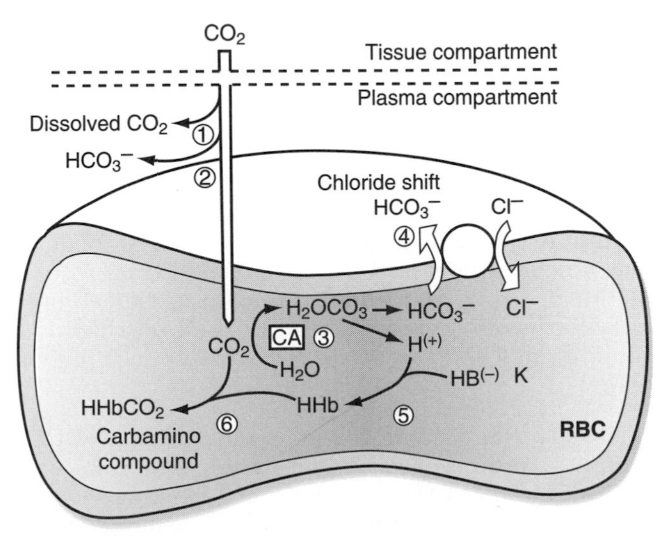


FIGURE 8–1 ■ $CO_2$ transport. See the text for details.

amino compounds. At normal body temperatures, 8% of $CO_2$ is transported as dissolved $CO_2$; 63% as bicarbonate; and 29% as carbamino-bound $CO_2$.[2, 12]

## $CO_2$ Excretion

The four determinants of $CO_2$ excretion from blood into the atmosphere are: (1) blood flow through aerated portions of the lung; (2) diffusion of $CO_2$ across the capillary endothelium and alveolar epithelium into the alveolar space; (3) alveolar ventilation; and (4) physiologic dead space.

**Blood Flow Through Aerated Lung.** Total $CO_2$ excretion may be increased by an increase in the venous to arterial $CO_2$ difference or by an increase in the cardiac output. Cardiac output that traverses the lung includes the portion that perfuses aerated portions of the lungs and allows gas exchange and the portion that traverses unventilated portions of the lung and does not participate in gas exchange. The ratio of blood traversing unventilated portions of the lung to the blood traversing both ventilated and unventilated portions of the lung is the shunt fraction.[13–18] An increased shunt fraction affects arterial oxygenation dramatically, but as ventilation-perfusion mismatch increases, it can also inhibit the release of $CO_2$ to the air. The shunt fraction is not fixed, but changes during certain physiologic states. During intense exercise, the need to excrete $CO_2$ increases because the production of $CO_2$ by exercising muscles increases. Although the increase in $CO_2$ excretion is mainly attributed to an increase in heart rate, ventilation-perfusion mismatching also decreases with the onset of exercise.[19–21] The decrease in ventilation-perfusion mismatching occurs because greater portions of the lung are aerated and accordingly more of the total cardiac output traverses areas of well-ventilated lung. Patients with underlying pulmonary disease have very abnormal ventilation-perfusion ratios with increased shunting through diseased, unaerated portions of lung. During exercise, these individuals do not experience the normal decline in ventilation-perfusion inequality; an increase in ventilation-perfusion inequality with exercise may further compromise their ability to excrete $CO_2$.[21, 22]

**Diffusion of $CO_2$.** Diffusion of $CO_2$ from whole blood to expired air does not significantly impede the transfer of $CO_2$ to the environment under normal conditions.[23–25] This process follows a reverse path to that which resulted in the uptake of $CO_2$ from tissues. In the presence of carbonic anhydrase, $CO_2$ rapidly diffuses across the capillary endothelium reaching equilibrium with gases in the alveolar space within less than 0.01 seconds.[26–28]

**Alveolar Ventilation.** The main determinant of $CO_2$ excretion under normal circumstances is alveolar ventilation. Alveolar $CO_2$ concentration is essentially equal to arterial $CO_2$ concentration. The alveolar gas equation relates $P_{ACO_2}$ to ventilation.[1]

$$P_{ACO_2} = \frac{\dot{V}_{CO_2} \times 0.863}{\dot{V}_A} \qquad \text{(Equation 2)}$$

$P_{ACO_2}$ equals alveolar $CO_2$ tension; $\dot{V}_{CO_2}$ equals $CO_2$ production expressed in liters per minute, and $\dot{V}_A$ equals alveolar ventilation in liters per minute. Accordingly, plasma $CO_2$ tension is determined by the interaction of the rate of $CO_2$ production and the rate of alveolar ventilation. $P_{ACO_2}$ varies inversely with alveolar ventilation if $CO_2$ production is stable, which is usually the case.

**Physiologic Dead Space.** Decreases in alveolar ventilation result from decreased minute ventilation, increased dead space ventilation, or a combination of the two.

$$\dot{V}_A = \dot{V}_E - \dot{V}_D \qquad \text{(Equation 3)}$$

Physiologic dead space provides a small but measurable barrier to $CO_2$ excretion under normal circumstances.[13, 14] Physiologic dead space represents the portion of expired volume from the lung that is not involved in blood to alveolar gas exchange. Physiologic dead space includes major airways, unperfused alveoli, and perfused alveoli with an abnormal block to $CO_2$ diffusion. The normal $V_D/V_T$ ratio is 0.3; this ratio must generally exceed 0.6 before increased dead space ventilation can serve as the sole cause of hypercapnia. The volume of physiologic dead space changes as a function of depth and frequency of respiration (dead space increases with shallow and rapid respiration). Under normal physiologic conditions, the dead space impedes $CO_2$ excretion minimally, but dead space can profoundly impair $CO_2$ excretion in certain pathologic states. Increases in dead space occur when large areas of the lung are left without circulation (e.g., pulmonary embolus); during marked pulmonary hypoperfusion (e.g., shock); or in severe, generalized ventilation-perfusion abnormalities (e.g., advanced chronic pulmonary disease). Dead space ventilation also increases with rapid, shallow ventilation. This breathing pattern is commonly observed in neuromuscular disease, disorders of the chest wall (e.g., kyphoscoliosis), and also in chronic obstructive pulmonary disease (COPD), pulmonary edema, or pulmonary fibrosis.

# CENTRAL NERVOUS SYSTEM CONTROL OF VENTILATION

Control of ventilation involves central rhythm generation with the depth and rate of breathing being adjusted by chemical and mechanical stimuli and higher central nervous system (CNS) neural inputs. A feedback loop exists in which ventilation influences the level of $CO_2$ and oxygen in the blood, and these levels modulate neural inputs to the respiratory centers. Receptors that sense changes in levels of $CO_2$, oxygen, and pH are located in the aortic and carotid bodies and the brain side of the blood-brain barrier.

The carotid bodies are located close to the carotid

bifurcation, and the aortic bodies lie near the aortic arch. Arterial oxygen partial pressure is the main chemical stimulus to these receptors. Receptor output is minimal above a $PaO_2$ of 200 mm Hg and increases gradually until levels of $PaO_2$ of 60 mm Hg or less are sensed. Increases are much more rapid below $PaO_2$ of 60 mm Hg. Peripheral chemoreceptors are also sensitive to arterial pH. $PaCO_2$ stimulates peripheral receptors in addition to its pH effects. Chemoreceptors have been demonstrated near the ventrolateral surface of the medulla. This receptor appears to be primarily sensitive to the pH content of brain extracellular fluid. The ventilatory response to an acute rise in $PaCO_2$ results largely from the central chemoreceptors. The ventilatory response to the same arterial pH change due to respiratory acidosis is greater than that seen with metabolic acidosis. $CO_2$ readily crosses the blood-brain barrier so that brain extracellular $PaCO_2$ is similar to blood $CO_2$. Conversely, ions including $[H^+]$ and $HCO_3^-$ cross the blood-brain barrier more slowly. Respiratory acidosis, therefore, stimulates both central chemoreceptors as the $CO_2$ crosses the blood-brain barrier and peripheral receptors. The ventilatory response reflects the sum of the signals. In metabolic acidosis, peripheral chemoreceptor stimulation is similar to that with $CO_2$, but the hydrogen ion is not able to readily reach the central chemosensor and central stimulation does not occur. Ventilation rises by 1 to 4 L/min for every 1 mm Hg rise in $PaCO_2$.[29, 30]

## FUNCTIONAL CONSEQUENCES OF HYPERCAPNIA AND RESPIRATORY ACIDOSIS

Respiratory acidosis affects many physiologic functions. The consequences of respiratory acidosis result from an interplay between local effects of $CO_2$ and effects mediated by activation of adrenergic nerves. The bulk of studies investigating consequences of hypercapnia and respiratory acidosis have utilized anesthetized animals. Few studies have been performed in conscious humans. Available studies should be interpreted cautiously because adrenergic function exhibits interspecies variation and is influenced by anesthesia.

### Effects of Hypercapnia on the Cardiovascular System

**Cardiac Mechanics.** Acute respiratory acidosis causes an impairment in myocardial contractility that is entirely reversible.[31] Respiratory acidosis alters left ventricular pressure-volume relationships to produce a decrease in left ventricular contractility and a parallel increase in end-diastolic and end-systolic volumes. Despite this, cardiac output rises due to an increase in heart rate. β-Blockade induces a larger impairment in left ventricular contractility. Thus, while hypercapnia depresses myocardial contractility, this effect is offset by the stimulating action of $CO_2$ on central and autonomic systems in an intact animal.[32]

The mechanism responsible for the fall in cardiac contractility is the rapid diffusion of $CO_2$ into cells with consequent intracellular acidosis which interferes with myofilament responses to calcium. Intracellular acidosis may have a greater effect on myofibrillar force production in low inotropic states.[33]

**Coronary Circulation.** $CO_2$ is a potent coronary vasodilator.[34] The effects of hypercapnia cause a substantial increase in coronary artery flow; a rise in coronary sinus $PaCO_2$ is noted. The beneficial effects of hypercapnia on myocardial oxygen supply may be different in the presence of heart failure or diminished coronary reserve. The response of ischemic areas of myocardium to increased $PaCO_2$ is uncertain. Vasodilatation induced by hypercapnia might improve blood flow through normal myocardium and reduce perfusion through ischemic areas.

**Arrhythmias.** The presence of both acidosis and increased adrenergic output would be expected to generate ventricular arrhythmias. In fact, rats, dogs, and Rhesus monkeys all tolerate extreme normoxic hypercapnia with only a few benign cardiac arrhythmias.

**Integrated Hemodynamic Response.** The hemodynamic response to inhalation of $CO_2$ is characterized by an increase in heart rate, stroke volume, and cardiac output and a decrease in systemic vascular resistance. Increased $PaCO_2$ increases ventricular filling. Hypercapnia improves left ventricular ejection by reducing arteriolar tone and thus decreases afterload. Hypercapnia adversely affects right ventricular performance in patients with impaired right ventricular systolic function. Respiratory acidosis induces pulmonary arteriolar vasoconstriction, thus leading to pulmonary hypertension.

**Oxygen Delivery.** An increase in $PaCO_2$ produces a rightward shift of the oxygen dissociation curve. Increases in $[H^+]$ and carbamino compounds increase P50, which promotes the release of oxygen to tissues. The decreased affinity of hemoglobin for oxygen also compromises $O_2$ loading in alveolar capillaries. This shift has minimal significance if $PaCO_2$ is normal, but severe hypercapnia can produce a decrease in $SaO_2$ in the presence of hypoxemia. This reduction in arterial oxygen content is usually compensated by an increase in cardiac output. Human data suggest that the usual endpoint is augmented $O_2$ delivery with an increased mixed-venous $PaO_2$ and improved tissue oxygenation.[36]

### Effects of Hypercapnia on the Central Nervous System

**Cerebral Blood Flow.** Acute changes in $PaCO_2$ greatly increase cerebral blood flow.[37] The effects of hypercapnia on cerebral blood flow are mediated by arterial hypertension, which increases cerebral perfusion pressure, and by cerebral vasodilatation, which reduces cerebral vascular resistance. Hypercapnia dilates arterioles throughout the brain and also increases the diameter of cerebral capillaries and venules.[38] Prolonged changes in $PaCO_2$ lead to chronic adaptation; after 1 to 2 days, cerebral blood flow returns to normal.[39] Nitrous oxide may be involved in the cerebral vasodilatation caused by hypercapnia.

**Intracranial Pressure.** Hypercapnia reversibly increases intracranial pressure.[40] This effect may be substantial. Alveolar hypoventilation secondary to inhalation of oxygen in patients with COPD has been observed to cause two- to threefold increases in intracranial pressures; values as high as 50 cm $H_2O$ have been observed.[41] Intracranial pressure is increased because of enlargement of cerebral blood volume secondary to vasodilatation and increased vascular pressure. Hypercapnia does not affect the production of cerebrospinal fluid. Although the permeability of the blood-brain barrier is minimally altered, only minimal cerebral edema results.[42] The increases in intracranial pressure are well tolerated in the absence of pre-existing intracranial abnormalities. Headache, nausea, drowsiness, and papilledema may be observed.[40] In the presence of cerebral edema, head trauma, or intracranial space-occupying lesions, increases in intracranial pressure may cause distortion of brain structures.

### Effect of Hypercapnia on Skeletal Muscle

Acute hypercapnia reduces the contractility of skeletal muscle, in particular that of the diaphragm.[43] Acute hypercapnia also reduces endurance. Little is known of the effects of chronic hypercapnia, although patients with COPD demonstrate more muscular weakness than do those who are normocapnic.[44] The abnormalities in skeletal muscle contractility are believed to be quickly reversible.

### Effects of Hypercapnia in the Gastrointestinal System

Acute and chronic hypercapnia increase the production of gastric acid.[45] Whether hypercapnia increases the risk of acute gastrointestinal bleeding in the intensive care unit (ICU) setting remains to be established. The effects of hypercapnia on the perfusion of the gut and liver could be a special concern in critically ill patients; only data from anesthetized dogs are available. Local addition of $CO_2$ to portal venous blood reduces total hepatic blood flow. Systemic acute hypercapnia increases mesenteric portal and total hepatic blood flow.[46, 47] The effect of respiratory acidosis on splanchnic perfusion is unknown.

### Effects of Hypercapnia on Renal Circulation

Mild, acute normoxic elevations of $PaCO_2$ have relatively little effect on renal blood flow and glomerular filtration rate. More severe respiratory acidosis ($PaCO_2$ $\geq$ 100 mm Hg) results in renal vasoconstriction, with concomitant fall in renal blood flow, glomerular filtration rate and urine output.[48]

### Effect of Hypercapnia on the Endocrine System

Acute normoxemic hypercapnia leads to massive release of epinephrine and norepinephrine and may increase secretion of ACTH, cortisol, aldosterone, and antidiuretic hormone.[49, 50] Chronic hypercapnia may stimulate secretion of renin-angiotensin-aldosterone and antidiuretic hormone.[51]

## SECONDARY PHYSIOLOGIC RESPONSE

Physiologic responses to acute hypercapnia have been described earlier. If hypercapnia persists, renal adaptive responses lead to further increases in plasma bicarbonate concentration. Renal responses involve an augmentation of hydrogen ion secretion by the renal tubule.[52, 53] A more complete discussion of this process can be found in Chapter 4. Net acid secretion, mainly in the form of ammonium, leads to negative hydrogen ion balance and the generation of new bicarbonate ions.[54–59] These new bicarbonate ions are conserved by an augmented rate of bicarbonate reabsorption within the kidney. Both proximal and distal acidification mechanisms contribute to the adaptive response, which requires 3 to 5 days for completion. Plasma bicarbonate concentration ceases to rise and a new steady-state of acid-base equilibrium is established.[60, 61] As bicarbonate stores are being increased, chloride stores are correspondingly depleted.

Mild hypernatremia (2 to 4 mEq/L) is typically seen in both acute and chronic hypercapnia.[62–64] Hypochloremia is a consistent finding in chronic hypercapnia; it reflects both a shift of chloride into erythrocytes and a loss of chloride in the urine during the adaptive process.[64] Plasma potassium does not change appreciably during chronic hypercapnia.[64] Hyperphosphatemia is a characteristic feature of acute hypercapnia; no notable rise in plasma phosphate occurs during chronic hypercapnia.[62] No consistent changes in plasma calcium or magnesium have been noted in response to hypercapnia.

## APPROACH TO THE DIAGNOSIS OF ACID-BASE DISORDERS

Appropriate diagnosis of acid-base disorders involves collection, analysis, and synthesis of relevant clinical information from the patient's history, physical examination, and laboratory data. An acid-base disturbance should be expected from the history and physical examination. Venous electrolytes and arterial blood

**TABLE 8–1.** Etiology of Acute Respiratory Acidosis

| |
|---|
| Failure of $CO_2$ transport from tissues to the lung |
| Cardiac arrest |
| Cardiogenic shock |
| Sepsis |
| Massive pulmonary embolus |
| Fat embolus |
| Air embolus |
| Failure to excrete $CO_2$ from the lung |
| Airway obstruction |
| Severe bronchospasm—acute severe asthma |
| Aspiration of vomitus |
| Sleep apnea |
| Laryngospasm |
| Aspiration of foreign body |
| Restrictive defects |
| Pneumothorax |
| Hemothorax |
| Flail chest |
| Impaired diaphragmatic function (e.g., ascites, obesity) |
| Acute respiratory distress syndrome |
| Severe pneumonia |

gases should be obtained. Formulas or acid-base maps are useful to determine the limits of compensation.

Careful review of the patient's history may reveal commonly encountered clinical conditions that are associated with respiratory acidosis (Table 8–1). The physical examination may reveal cyanosis. Clinical hypercapnia is almost invariably associated with some degree of hypoxemia. Accordingly, it is difficult to determine whether specific clinical manifestations are the consequence of elevations in $Paco_2$ or reductions in $Pao_2$. Despite this caveat, several clinical manifestations are characteristic of clinical hypercapnia.

CNS disturbances are among the most important clinical manifestations of hypercapnia. Marked anxiety, confusion, disorientation, combativeness, and severe dyspnea are usually present. Psychotic behavior can occur with delirium, hallucinations, maniacal behavior, and episodes of euphoria. Stupor or coma can result from severe hypercapnia. Hypercapnic coma is most common when acute respiratory failure is superimposed on chronic respiratory failure in patients with COPD. These patients can manifest minimal CNS dysfunction with $CO_2$ levels as high as 110 mm Hg, but it is not uncommon for these patients to manifest decreased alertness, confusion, drowsiness, inattentiveness, forgetfulness, and somnolence. Motor disturbances include asterixis, tremors, and myoclonic jerks. Sustained myoclonus or seizures can develop. Signs and symptoms of increased intracranial pressure may be present. Headache is a frequent complaint. Funduscopic examination often reveals blurring of the optic discs and papilledema. Deep tendon reflexes are often increased in mild-to-moderate hypercapnia but are usually decreased in severe hypercapnia. The plantar reflexes are often extensor in nature.

Mild-to-moderate acute hypercapnia is usually characterized by a prominent pulse, a normal or increased blood pressure, diaphoresis, and warm skin. Cardiovascular manifestations of acute hypercapnia may be altered significantly if the concomitant hypoxemia is severe or if congestive heart failure is present. The use of vasoactive medications such as β-adrenergic receptor blockers will also significantly alter cardiovascular manifestations. Cardiac arrhythmias are often present in patients with acute or chronic hypercapnia; they are especially common in individuals with cor pulmonale. Supraventricular tachyarrhythmias with ventricular rates of 120 to 160 beats/min are common; these arrhythmias are not associated with major hemodynamic compromise. The relative contribution of hypercapnia, hypoxemia, electrolyte abnormalities, and underlying cardiac disease is uncertain.

Salt and water retention is usually present in patients with chronic hypercapnia. Salt and water retention may be the result of cor pulmonale or may be the end result of stimulation of the renin-angiotensin-aldosterone axis and elevated levels of antidiuretic hormone.

Careful analysis of the routine laboratory data provides useful quantitative information enabling the identification of the possible predominant acid-base disturbance and clues to the potential presence of other disorders. The Davenport diagram is a commonly used visual display of acid-base relationships. It is a graphic representation of the Henderson-Hasselbalch equation. Rapid development of hypoventilation in which $CO_2$ partial pressure rises from 40 to 70 mm Hg would follow the sloping line that passes through the center, which indicates the expected values for pH and $HCO_3^-$ as the $Paco_2$ rises (1, Fig. 8–2). If this level of hypoventilation is maintained for several days, metabolic compensation would increase $HCO_3^-$ and the pH would accordingly improve (2, see Fig. 8–2). In many respiratory disorders, the course of chronic

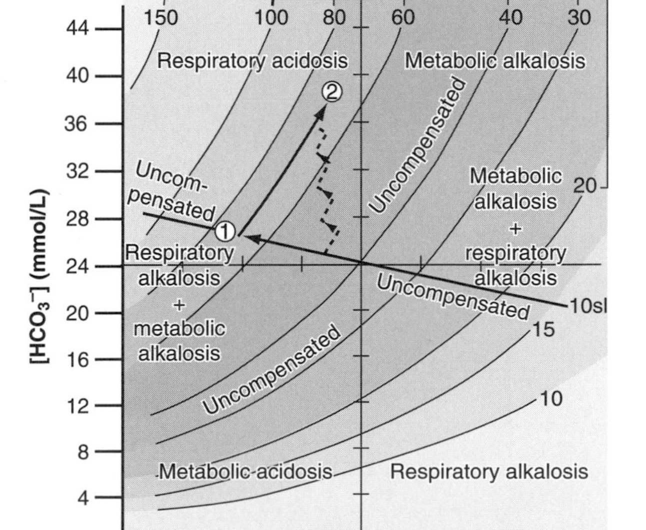


**FIGURE 8–2** ■ Compensation for respiratory acidosis. (From Culver BH: Physiology. In Albert R, Spiro S [eds]: Comprehensive Respiratory Medicine. St. Louis, Mosby International Press, 1999.)

respiratory acidosis might well follow the stuttering dotted line to the same point (see Fig. 8–2). Figure 8–3 shows the range of values seen in common acid-base disorders and outlines limits of compensation. Many mixed acid-base disorders can be diagnosed using arterial blood values in conjunction with maps or formulas (see Fig. 8–3), but the final diagnosis must include clinical data as well. The use of a map alone will not identify triple mixed acid-base disorders. The presence of a normal $Pa{CO_2}$, normal pH, and a normal plasma $HCO_3^-$ does not rule out a mixed disorder.[65, 66]

## CLINICAL SYNDROMES OF RESPIRATORY ACIDOSIS

Respiratory acidosis is the consequence of hypercapnia caused by divergent etiologies. The magnitude of hypercapnia, the rapidity with which hypercapnia develops, the severity of the acidemia, and the degree of hypoxemia differ depending on the etiology of the respiratory acidosis. An understanding of the etiology of the hypercapnic syndrome is the foundation of an appropriate therapeutic approach to respiratory acidosis. Therapeutic regimens must always address the pathologic state generating the acidosis.

The etiologies of respiratory acidosis can be divided into syndromes that cause primarily acute respiratory acidosis and those that cause predominantly chronic respiratory acidosis. The syndromes can also be divided according to the pathophysiologic alterations that cause hypercapnia (Table 8–2; see also Table 8–1).

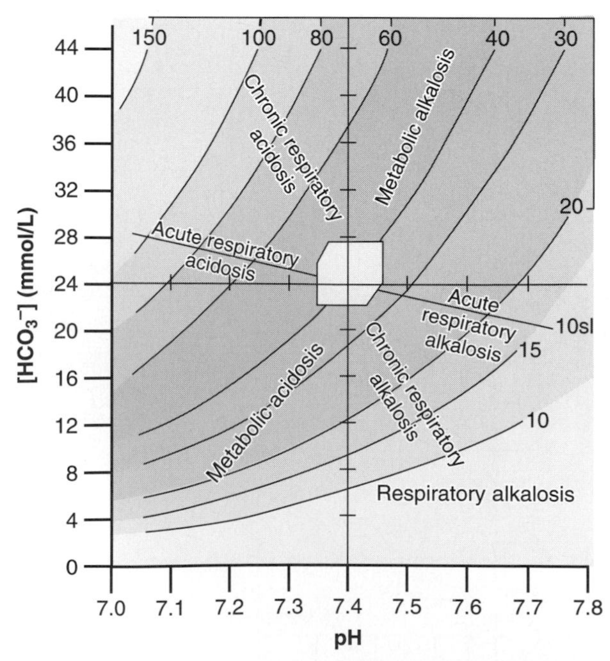


FIGURE 8–3 ■ Typical limits of compensation for acid-base abnormalities. (From Culver BH: Physiology. In Albert R, Spiro S [eds]: Comprehensive Respiratory Medicine. St. Louis, Mosby International Press, 1999; data from Goldberg M, Greene SB, Man ML, et al: Computer-based inoculation and diagnosis of acid-base disorders. JAMA 223:269, 1973.)

**TABLE 8–2.** Etiology of Chronic Respiratory Acidosis

| |
|---|
| Failure to excrete $CO_2$ from the lungs |
| Airway obstruction |
| Chronic bronchitis |
| Emphysema |
| Sleep apnea |
| Tracheal stenosis |
| Restrictive defects |
| Kyphoscoliosis |
| Fibrotic lung diseases |
| Obesity |
| Fibrothorax |
| Impaired diaphragmatic function (e.g., obesity, ascites) |
| Neuromuscular disease |
| Poliomyelitis |
| Multiple sclerosis |
| Muscular dystrophies |
| Amyotrophic lateral sclerosis |
| Diaphragmatic paralysis |
| Myxedema |
| Polymyositis |
| Failure of the CNS—respiratory drive |
| Primary alveolar hypoventilation (Ondine's curse) |
| CNS neoplasm |
| CNS infection/inflammation |
| Methadone use |
| Heroin addiction |

CNS, central nervous system.

## CLINICAL SYNDROMES OF ACUTE RESPIRATORY ACIDOSIS

### Failure of $CO_2$ Transport from the Tissues to the Lung

**Cardiac Arrest/Cardiogenic Shock.** Abrupt cessation of ventilation (cardiorespiratory arrest, cardiac arrest) in patients breathing room air leads to death from hypoxemia in 5 to 7 minutes. Hypoxemia, rather than hypercapnia, poses the main threat to life. This physiologic relationship is described by the alveolar air equation.

$$P_{A}O_2 = F_{I}O_2\,(P_B - P_{H_2O}) - \frac{Pa{CO_2}}{RQ}$$

(Equation 4)

where $P_AO_2$ equals partial pressure of oxygen in the alveolus; $F_IO_2$ equals the fraction of inspired $O_2$; $P_B$ equals barometric pressure; $P_{H_2O}$ equals the partial pressure of water; $Pa{CO_2}$ equals partial pressure of $CO_2$ in arterial blood; and RQ equals the respiratory quotient.

This equation can be simplified under conditions of breathing room air.

$$P_AO_2 = 150 - 1.2\ Pa{CO_2}$$

(Equation 5)

From this latter equation, it is apparent that in the absence of supplemental oxygen, patients develop severe hypoxemia when $Pa{CO_2}$ reaches values of 80 mm Hg. Studies in humans following ventilatory paralysis have shown that $PaCO_2$ rises 3 to 5 mm Hg per minute[67]; thus, 10 to 15 minutes are required to develop levels of $PaCO_2$ greater than 90 mm Hg.

Obviously, the ideal treatment for cardiorespiratory arrest is prevention. This can often be achieved through aggressive stabilization of critically ill patients and anticipation of deterioration in those patients at particular risk. The goal of resuscitation is to halt the hypoxic and ischemic damage to the CNS and cardiovascular system. Establishing and securing a patent airway with provision of 100% $FIO_2$, early chest compressions, rapid defibrillation, and the administration of epinephrine are the cornerstones for treatment of cardiopulmonary arrest.[68–70]

Cardiac resuscitation differs from the normal internal medicine paradigm of history gathering, physical examination, and generation of a differential diagnosis. Restoration of a patent airway can be achieved by hyperextending the head and displacing the mandible forward in all except trauma patients. Any visualized foreign body obstruction should be removed by suctioning or by use of a forceps. If complete foreign body obstruction exists, a series of alternating back blows or an attempt to increase intrathoracic pressure and expel the object (Heimlich maneuver) should be attempted. Establishment of a surgical airway requires training before this procedure is attempted. Ventilation must be immediately restored by mouth-to-mouth breathing, the use of an Ambu bag, or endotracheal intubation and mechanical ventilation. Endotracheal intubation is the standard for securing and stabilizing an airway. Ventilation should be performed with 100% oxygen if possible. Arterial blood gases should be utilized to reduce the inspired oxygen to the lowest level that provides adequate saturation of hemoglobin.

Circulatory status should be assessed following the establishment of an airway. A feeble, carotid pulse indicates a systemic blood pressure of at least 50 mm Hg. Complete circulatory arrest should prompt closed chest compression. Intravenous (IV) access should be secured with two large-bore lines, and chest leads should be placed for continuous cardiac monitoring. An initial fluid bolus of 250 to 1000 mL of normal saline or Ringer lactate should be infused rapidly. Cardiac monitoring and physical examination should provide the specific cardiac diagnosis in many cases. Cardiovascular abnormalities leading to cardiopulmonary arrest can be generically divided into rhythm disturbances, volume depletion, and pump abnormalities. The treatment of each of these abnormalities is beyond the scope of this chapter. Life-threatening arrhythmias can be approached through algorithms established by the American Heart Association.[69] Pulseless ventricular tachycardia and ventricular fibrillation require rapid defibrillation.

Complex issues surround the withholding of cardiopulmonary resuscitation (CPR). It is reasonable to attempt resuscitation in patients who have a chance of meaningful survival. Patients with poor baseline cardiovascular status, terminal malignancy, or inexorable progression of multiorgan failure often cannot be resuscitated. Physicians caring for patients in the ICU should present a fair appraisal of the likely outcome of resuscitative efforts to the patient or family at the time of admission to the ICU and then request their input on whether CPR should be initiated if a cardiopulmonary arrest occurs.

**Massive Pulmonary Embolus.** Massive pulmonary embolus is a dramatic and life-threatening complication of underlying deep venous thrombosis.[71, 72] Pulmonary embolus continues to cause substantial morbidity and mortality. Pulmonary embolism occurs when thrombi detach and are carried through the great veins to the pulmonary circulation. Physical obstruction of the pulmonary artery creates dead space in the segments served by the affected arteries. If minute ventilation does not change, which often occurs in mechanically ventilated patients in the ICU, $PaCO_2$ will rise in the context of massive pulmonary embolus. Most nonventilated patients augment minute ventilation more than necessary to maintain $CO_2$ excretion so that the $PaCO_2$ typically falls in most patients with pulmonary embolus. A widened alveolar to arterial gradient for oxygen is present in most patients with pulmonary embolus, but $PaO_2$ is not decreased in all patients. Sixty-three percent of patients with proven pulmonary embolus demonstrate a $PaO_2$ less than 70.[73]

Heparin is the mainstay for therapy for pulmonary embolus.[74–76] Thrombolytic therapy should be reserved for patients with shock duc to pulmonary embolus.[77] Right ventricular function assessed echocardiographically improves more rapidly in patients treated with thrombolytic therapy than in those treated with heparin.[78] The optimal regimen for thrombolytic therapy has not been established.

## FAILURE TO EXCRETE $CO_2$ FROM THE LUNG

### Airway Obstruction

**Acute Severe Asthma.** Status asthmaticus is defined as asthma that is severe at its outset or asthma that progresses rapidly despite standard therapy. It may result in ventilatory failure and death. Although most patients with asthma are managed uneventfully in the ambulatory care setting, all asthma patients are at risk of developing an asthma attack that is severe at its outset or progresses rapidly despite pharmacologic therapy. Patients with status asthmaticus typically decompensate over several days. The importance of this presentation is that it will allow sufficient time for intervention with appropriate pharmacologic therapy. The best treatment of status asthmaticus is to "treat it 3 days before it occurs" with corticosteroids.[79] Airway obstruction in status asthmaticus is the consequence of airway wall inflammation, airway mucus plugging of both large and small airways, and the development of sudden and unexpected increases in airflow obstruction resulting primarily from smooth muscle–mediated bronchospasm.[80–82]

Severe acute airway obstruction raises airway resistance so that inspiratory transpulmonary pressure increases between 5 and 7 cm $H_2O$ during quiet tidal breathing to 50 cm $H_2O$ or more. Expiratory muscle contraction is ineffective in increasing expiratory airflow rates because of effort independence of forced expiration. A consequence of severe expiratory airflow obstruction is incomplete emptying of alveolar gas. Airway obstruction results in maldistribution of alveolar ventilation relative to perfusion (V/Q mismatch). The intrapulmonary shunt in status asthmaticus is trivial; accordingly, correction of hypoxemia requires only modest enrichment with inspired oxygen. Dead space increases substantially in asthma due to hypoperfusion of regions of hyperinflated lung.[83, 84] Despite this increase in dead space, the early stages of status asthmaticus are characterized by mild respiratory alkalosis. As the severity of airflow obstruction increases, $Pa_{CO_2}$ increases due to inadequate alveolar ventilation. The inadequate alveolar ventilation reflects an increase in the dead space–tidal volume ratio and a decrease in minute ventilation as the patient nears respiratory arrest. $CO_2$ production may also be elevated in severe airway obstruction due to intense muscular activity. Hypercapnia does not occur unless the forced expiratory volume in 1 second ($FEV_1$) is less than 25% of predicted; however, the absence of hypercapnia does not exclude severe airflow obstruction and impending respiratory arrest.[85–87]

Characteristics of prior episodes of asthma predict fatal or near-fatal episodes. These characteristics include prior intubation, hypercapnia, or hospitalization despite chronic oral corticosteroid use. Prior intubation is the greatest single predictor of subsequent asthma death.[88–90] Survivors of near-fatal asthma have been shown to have diminished ventilatory drive in the face of hypoxemic or mechanical stimuli, suggesting these patients are less aware of progression to severe airflow obstruction.[91] The distinction between left ventricular dysfunction and airway obstruction can be difficult, particularly in elderly patients.[92] The presence of a foreign body must be considered in all children with dyspnea and wheezing and in adults with an abnormal swallowing mechanism, altered mentation, or recent dental work.

Wheezing correlates poorly with the degree of airflow obstruction.[93] Severely obstructed patients have decreased breath sounds if there is insufficient flow for wheezing to occur. Patients with status asthmaticus usually sit upright and have tachycardia, tachypnea, and pulsus paradoxus. The presence of accessory muscle use and pulsus paradoxus indicates severe airflow obstruction; the absence of these findings does not rule out severe airflow obstruction.[86, 94] Objective physiologic measurements of the degree of airflow obstruction must be made because physician estimates are often wrong, with errors equally distributed between over- and underestimates of actual airflow obstruction.[95] Physiologic assessments can utilize either peak expiratory flow rates or the measurement of $FEV_1$. Severe exacerbations are characterized by a peak expiratory flow rate (PEFR) or $FEV_1$ less than 30% to 50% of the predicted or the patient's personal best (PEFR <120 L/min, $FEV_1$ <1 L).[96]

Inhaled β-agonists should be initiated immediately.[96, 97] Large and frequent drug doses are needed in status asthmaticus. β-Agonists should be administered by inhalation. Inhaled β-agonists may be delivered equally well by a metered-dose inhaler with a spacer or by a hand-held nebulizer. Four puffs of albuterol delivered by metered dose inhaler with a spacer is as effective as albuterol delivered by nebulization.[98] Corticosteroids should be administered immediately. Failure to treat episodes of acute severe asthma with corticosteroids contributes to asthma deaths.[99] Both oral and IV routes are effective. Oral drug administrations should be avoided in patients with gastrointestinal upset or in patients at risk for intubation. The administration of 60 to 125 mg methylprednisolone (Solu-Medrol) IV every 6 hours during the initial 24 hours of treatment is reasonable.[100, 101]

Although hypercapnia indicates severe disease and the possible need for mechanical ventilation, hypercapnia alone is not an indication for intubation. Hypercapnic patients often respond to aggressive drug therapy and may have clinical courses similar to eucapnic patients. Nevertheless, $CO_2$ retention in patients with asthma should always be managed clinically as an acute emergency because it portends imminent respiratory failure. Noninvasive positive-pressure ventilation (NPPV) by facemask is a potentially useful option for patients with hypercapnic acute respiratory failure. Advantages of NPPV over intubation and mechanical ventilation include decreased need for sedation and paralysis, decreased incidence of nosocomial pneumonia, decreased incidence of otitis and sinusitis, and improved patient comfort. Disadvantages include a small increased risk of aspiration of gastric contents, skin necrosis from a tight-fitting mask, and diminished control over the patient's ventilatory status. Although controlled studies have documented the efficacy of NPPV in patients with acute exacerbations of COPD, the efficacy of NPPV in avoiding intubation in patients who have acute respiratory failure from causes other than COPD has been assessed in too few patients to draw firm conclusions. Uncontrolled studies suggest that success rates in patients with severe asthma may approach those obtained in patients who have COPD.[102–104] The use of NPPV in acute severe asthma improves dyspnea, decreases respiratory rate and heart rate, and improves arterial $Pa_{CO_2}$ and pH. Randomized trials of this modality in acute asthma are needed.

Intubation is indicated for patients who present in cardiorespiratory arrest, for obtunded patients, and for patients with impending ventilatory failure. Changes in posture, accessory muscle use, respiratory rate, mental status, and speech pattern all indicate progressive ventilatory failure. The decision to intubate relies on the judgment of a seasoned clinician as well as on arterial blood gas and pulmonary function analysis.

Severe dynamic hyperinflation usually occurs if patients with status asthmaticus are ventilated to eucapnia.[105, 106] Expired volumes above a functional residual capacity (FRC) as large as 3 to 4 L are commonly encountered. Sufficient exhalation time must exist to avoid significant lung hyperinflation. The use of high inspiratory flow rates, controlled hypoventilation, reduced inspiratory times with fast inspiratory flow rates, and square inspiratory flow waveform ventilation are necessary in many patients. Initial minute ventilations between 8 and 10 L/min, achieved by a tidal volume between 8 and 10 mL/kg and a respiratory rate between 11 and 14 breaths/min, combined with an inspiratory flow rate of 80 to 100 L/min, are unlikely to result in a dangerous degree of lung hyperinflation.[107–111] Indirect evidence suggests that mechanical ventilation in asthma should involve hypoventilation strategies that minimize lung hyperinflation. Death rates are higher in series that do not employ permissive hypercapnia.[97]

Bicarbonate therapy may have a role in patients with severe bronchospasm by restoring the responsiveness of the bronchial musculature to β-adrenergic agents. Bicarbonate administration in patients with blood pH less than 7.0 to raise pH to greater than 7.20 has been reported to be beneficial in these severely ill patients.[112, 113]

**Sleep Apnea.** Sleep-disordered breathing, a more general term used to encompass both sleep apneas and hypopnea, is common. Sleep-disordered breathing that lcads to symptomatic discasc is prcscnt in 4% of men and 2% of women. Sleep study abnormalities with no clinical symptoms have been found in 9% of men and 4% of women.[114] Apneas during sleep may be classified as central, which result from inadequate neural output to the respiratory muscle or as obstructive resulting from closure of the upper airway. A mixed pattern with both central and obstructive episodes is present in many patients; obstruction is the dominant underlying mechanism. Several conditions are predisposed to sleep apnea; sleep apnea increases with obesity, male gender, age, increased neck circumference, hypothyroidism, and use of alcohol or sedatives/hypnotic medications.[115] The pathophysiology of obstructive sleep apnea is complex and incompletely understood. Anatomic features of the upper airway interact with neuromuscular factors such as resting muscle tone of the pharyngeal dilator muscle group and the effects of sleep to determine upper airway patency.[116, 117] Hypoventilation related to hypopneic or apneic episodes results in respiratory acidosis and hypoxemia. Hypoxemia is often exacerbated by ventilation-perfusion mismatch in obese patients or in patients with underlying COPD. These metabolic disturbances may result in myocardial failure, ischemia, or arrhythmias.[118] Intermittent hypoxemia and respiratory acidosis cause pulmonary arterial vasoconstriction, potentially leading to pulmonary artery hypertension. Pulmonary hypertension and right heart failure probably occur mostly in patients with underlying COPD and patients with daytime hypoxemia and hypercapnia.[119–121]

Patients with sleep-disordered breathing frequently present the complaints of daytime sleepiness and snoring. Morning headaches, personality changes, and spousal complaints of snoring are also common presenting complaints. Unexplained obtundation or delirium may also be a presenting feature of sleep-disordered breathing. Obesity is almost invariably present in patients with sleep apnea. The diagnosis of sleep apnea requires measurements of the abnormal sleeping patterns and associated abnormalities that define the syndrome in an overnight sleep study.

Treatment of sleep apnea involves treatment of associated conditions, which may hasten the resolution of sleep-disordered breathing. Withdrawal of respiratory depressants and sedatives, treatment of underlying hypothyroidism, and vigorous regimens of weight loss should be initiated. Nasal continuous positive airway pressure (CPAP) is an effective long-term therapeutic modality.[122] Positive inspiratory pressures need to be individually titrated for each patient during sleep studies; the amount of pressure required is generally 10 to 12 cm $H_2O$.[123] Compliance studies show that only those who suffer the most severe daytime somnolence use the equipment regularly. The average nighttime use is 4 to 5 hours and about 20% to 40% of patients stop using CPAP within 3 months. Many patients claim good symptomatic improvement with 5 hours' use per night.[124] Bilevel positive airway pressure (BiPAP) is an alternative to CPAP. The use of this device is based on the principle that a higher level of positive airway pressure is required to open the obstructed pharyngeal airway segment than is required to maintain its patency. The inspiratory pressure is thus higher than the expiratory pressure. Some patents find BiPAP more comfortable to use.

## Restrictive Defects

Structural abnormalities of the lung that inhibit the movement of gases in and out of the lungs result in ventilation-perfusion abnormalities. Structural causes of acute $CO_2$ retention include acute pneumothorax, hemothorax, and flail chest with severe chest wall injury. The decrease in alveolar ventilation is overcome by an increase in tidal minute ventilation. An acute pneumothorax will result in respiratory acidosis if the shunt induced by the pneumothorax is of sufficient magnitude to offset the centrally driven hyperventilation.

Flail chest occurs with severe chest wall injuries. This condition usually results from blunt chest trauma in which several adjacent ribs are fractured on both sides of the sternum or at two locations on each of the ribs involved. The degree of pulmonary and hemodynamic disability that arises is related to the extent of the flail, the degree of underlying lung contusion, and the restrictive defect from chest wall pain.

In patients with severe alveolar hypoventilation and severe hypoxemia or hemodynamic instability, immediate endotracheal intubation, and positive-pressure ventilation are indicated. Many patients are able to maintain adequate oxygenation and ventilation with supplemental oxygen, particularly if adequate pain control can be achieved. This may require frequent or continuous IV analgesia.[125, 126] Discontinuation of the ventilator is not dependent on the disappearance of paradoxical movement of the chest wall; rather, discontinuation is usually dependent on the resolution of gas exchange abnormalities associated with the underlying lung contusion.

Tension pneumothoraces occur in the context of mechanical ventilation. Hyperventilation is not possible in this circumstance because the pneumothorax limits the ability to increase tidal volume and the respiratory frequency is constant. Prompt chest tube insertion on the involved side to relieve the pneumothorax is required.

**Acute Cardiogenic Pulmonary Edema.** The severity and duration of cardiogenic pulmonary edema determine whether hypocapnia or hypercapnia is observed. With mild or moderate pulmonary edema, hyperventilation driven by systemic hypoxia results in a respiratory alkalosis. In more severe cases, the edema increasingly interferes with the ability of the lungs to transport $CO_2$ from blood to the alveolar space. In contrast to acute respiratory distress syndrome (ARDS), as many as a third of patients with cardiogenic pulmonary edema will exhibit modest elevations of $Paco_2$ despite obvious increased drive to breathe.[127, 128] The reasons for this are obscure but may relate to intrapulmonary shunting of mixed venous blood with a high $CO_2$ content or, alternatively, to increased work of breathing caused by airway obstruction. The respiratory acidosis seen in severe pulmonary edema forewarns eminent respiratory failure and should alert the clinician to the potential need for intubation and mechanical ventilation.

## Acute Respiratory Distress Syndrome

ARDS is a common, devastating clinical syndrome of noncardiogenic pulmonary edema that results from acute damage to the alveoli.[129, 130] A consensus definition of ARDS includes: (1) acute onset; (2) bilateral infiltrates on chest radiography; and (3) pulmonary artery occlusion pressure less than 18 mm Hg or the absence of clinical evidence of left atrial hypertension. Acute lung injury is considered to be present if $Pao_2/Fio_2$ is 300 or less; ARDS is considered to be present if $Pao_2/Fio_2$ is less than 200.[131] The syndrome is usually progressive and characterized by distinct stages with different clinical, histopathologic, and radiographic manifestations.[132–135] The acute phase is manifest by the rapid onset of respiratory failure in a patient with a risk factor for the condition. Arterial hypoxemia that is refractory to treatment with supplemental oxygen is a characteristic feature. $Paco_2$ is usually normal or reduced. Radiographically, the findings are indistinguishable from those of cardiogenic pulmonary edema. Computed tomography scanning has demonstrated that atelectasis, alveolar filling, and consolidation occur predominantly in dependent lung zones.[136, 137] After the onset of acute symptoms, there is usually rapid worsening of gas exchange with decreasing lung compliance and functional residual capacity. Subsequently, lung compliance decreases further and increases occur in $V_D/V_T$. It is not uncommon for $V_D/V_T$ to exceed 0.7 in ARDS.[138] Increased dead space ventilation accounts for the majority of the minute ventilation requirements in the terminal phases of acute hypoxemic respiratory failure. $CO_2$ retention is often seen during the late phase of ARDS. The pathology responsible for increasing dead space in ARDS is complex. In ARDS, regional compliance and ventilation time constants vary greatly so that some alveolar units receive disproportionate ventilation when a constant pressure is applied to the airway. Overexpansion of compliant units by pressures delivered by mechanical ventilation redirects blood flow to more compromised regions, thus increasing $V_D/V_T$.

**Low Tidal Volume Ventilation.** Most patients with ARDS require mechanical ventilation and supplemental oxygen. Historically, physicians ventilated patients to achieve normal values for the partial pressure of arterial $CO_2$ and pH.[139] In these patients with severe lung disease, tidal volumes of 10 to 12 mL/kg of body weight have often been required to achieve these goals. Because atelectasis and edema reduced aerated lung volumes in patients with acute lung injury, it was believed that a population of alveoli could be recruited only at high transpulmonary pressures, thus high tidal volumes were believed to have beneficial effects on excretion of $CO_2$, the maintenance of pH, and oxygen delivery. Several crucial pieces of evidence led to a reconsideration of appropriate methods of mechanical ventilation. First, computed tomography has shown that the lung injury in ARDS is remarkably inhomogeneous.[140, 141] Some alveoli are normally compliant and fragile, whereas others are flooded or atelectatic. The ventilator-delivered breath expands normal aerated regions. The loss of functional alveoli necessitates that the tidal volume is distributed to fewer aerated alveoli, thus placing them at risk for alveolar overdistention. These data led to two fundamental changes in how patients with ARDS are ventilated: (1) end-inspiratory lung volume was limited to avoid alveolar overdistention; (2) sufficient positive-end expiratory pressure (PEEP) was applied to prevent end-expiratory derecruitment.[142–144]

Experimental studies also support the validity of this concept. Ventilation with use of large tidal volumes causes the disruption of the alveolar unit, the release of inflammatory mediators, lung inflammation, atelectasis, and hypoxemia.[145–149] It was reasoned that the release of inflammatory mediators could increase lung inflammation and cause injury to other organs (multiple organ failure). Thus, in patients with severe lung disease, ventilatory strategies to achieve a normal $Paco_2$ likely result in the amplification of lung injury. During the past decade, a shift in the priority of the care of these patients occurred. With the traditional approach, the attainment of normal $Paco_2$ and pH is given a higher priority than protection of the lung from excessive stretch. More recently, an approach that involves lower tidal volumes and permissive hypercapnia give higher priority to protection of the lung from excessive stretch. One prospective, multicenter, randomized trial demonstrated that decreasing tidal volume in order to lower end-inspiratory pressure substantially reduced mortality in ARDS.[150] In the group receiving lower tidal volumes, plateau pressure could not exceed 30 cm of water. The in-hospital mortality rate was 40% in the group treated with traditional tidal volumes and 31% in the group treated with lower tidal volumes, which is a reduction of mortality by 22%.

Positive results in this trial differed from those of two previous studies of low tidal volumes.[151, 152] The differences may be related to differential strategies in treating respiratory acidosis associated with alveolar hypoventilation. The most recent study corrected acidosis by infusions of bicarbonate and by increasing ventilator rates. The mean arterial pH in the beneficial study was 7.38 on day 1 after enrollment compared with a mean arterial pH of 7.28 and 7.29 in negative trials. A deleterious effect of acidosis in the previous studies may have counteracted a protective effect of the lower tidal volumes. A high priority should be given to preventing excessive lung stretch during adjustments to mechanical ventilation, and this lower tidal volume protocol should be used in patients with acute lung injury and ARDS.[150] Contraindications to permissive hypercapnic ventilation include patients with increased intracranial pressure, such as cerebral trauma or hemorrhage, space-occupying intracranial lesions, and severe hypertensive diseases.

## Neuromuscular Diseases

A wide variety of neuromuscular diseases cause weakness or paralysis of respiratory muscles and lead to hypercapnic respiratory failure. Quadriplegia resulting from acute cervical spinal cord trauma, spinal artery infarction, or spinal cord compression by tumor above cord segments C3 to C5 involves the phrenic nerves and causes partial or complete bilateral diaphragmatic paralysis. As a result of their profound respiratory muscle dysfunction, high cervical quadriplegic patients are unable to generate an adequate vital capacity during inspiration and develop a high $Pa_{CO_2}$ and a low $Pa_{O_2}$. Hypoxemia results both from hypoventilation and from microatelectesis.[153] Patients with cervical spinal cord lesions at any level cannot exhale forcefully to residual volume. Accordingly, these patients have ineffective cough and clear secretions poorly. These patients require chronic mechanical ventilation via a tracheotomy.[154]

**Guillain-Barré Syndrome.** Guillain-Barré syndrome is the most frequently encountered polyneuropathy.[155] Characteristic features include progressive symmetric weakness that often includes facial and bulbar paresis. Distal paresthesia and autonomic dysfunction including tachycardia, arrhythmias, and postural hypotension are often noted. Clinical manifestations are generally complete within 2 to 4 weeks.

Not all patients with Guillain-Barré syndrome develop respiratory failure, but all should be followed closely with daily bedside evaluation of vital capacity and respiratory muscle strength. Patients with Guillain-Barré syndrome should be electively intubated and ventilated when signs of respiratory distress are present and before $Pa_{CO_2}$ becomes elevated. Intubation should be considered when vital capacity approaches 10 mL/kg. Plasmapheresis may reduce hospital stay and time spent on the ventilator. Recovery usually begins within 2 to 4 weeks after progression ceases. Most patients recover completely, but 15% remain significantly handicapped by weakness.

**Myasthenia Gravis Crisis.** Myasthenia gravis is the prototypical myoneural junction disorder.[156] It results from circulating antibodies directed against acetylcholine receptors in the myoneural junction. Sensitized lymphocytes are also involved in the pathogenesis of this disease. The most common presenting symptom is weakness of the eye muscles manifested by diplopia or ptosis. Dysarthria and dysphasia are common. Respiratory impairment is usually secondary to weakness in the diaphragm and chest wall muscles.[157]

Myasthenia can be diagnosed on clinical grounds and by giving short-acting acetylcholinesterase-inhibiting agents such as edrophonium (Tensilon). Transient increased strength should be achieved within seconds following administration of edrophonium. Antibodies to the acetylcholine receptor can be detected in 90% of patients. Myasthenia is treated with long-acting anticholinesterase agents such as pyridostigmine (Mestinon). Plasmapheresis may improve motor function.[158] Thymectomy leads to complete remission or substantial improvement in 85% of myasthenia patients. Corticosteroids and immunosuppressive agents are utilized in patients with generalized disease. Exacerbations are usually precipitated by infection, administration of aminoglycosides, neuromuscular blocking agents, cholinergic agents, or surgery. Exacerbations require mechanical ventilation in 10% of patients.[159]

**Drugs.** Antibiotics can induce alveolar hypoventilation and precipitate acute hypercarbic respiratory failure.[160] Aminoglycosides are the class of antibiotics that most commonly cause neuromuscular blockade. Gentamicin, tobramycin, kanamycin, and streptomycin have all been implicated. Fluoroquinolones, ampicillin, tetracycline, and polymyxins have also been reported to cause this toxicity rarely. Toxicity is potentiated by conditions such as renal insufficiency that decrease aminoglycoside clearance. Cholinesterase inhibitors such as pyridostigmine can be utilized as treatment. Intubation and mechanical ventilation are sometimes required.

**Sedative Drug Overdose.** Barbiturates, benzodiazepines, and opioids can all cause hypoventilation. These patients usually present with an altered level of consciousness but can present with severe hypoventilation or apnea. Initial physician responsibilities are to identify and treat life-threatening problems. An airway should be established, and adequate ventilation should be achieved. Hypoxia should be corrected quickly to avoid anoxic brain injury, myocardial ischemia, and cardiac arrhythmia. Circulatory status of the patient should then be addressed.

**Barbiturates.** Clinical manifestations of mild-to-moderate barbiturate overdose include a reduced level of consciousness, slurred speech, and ataxia. At higher doses, hypothermia, hypotension, hypoventilation, bradycardia, coma, and apnea may be noted. Patients with severe overdose may appear to be dead.[161] Respiratory depression with hypercarbia and hypoxemia are common. In deep coma, the usual acid-base disturbances are mixed respiratory and metabolic acidosis.[162] The diagnosis of sedative overdose is usually made on clinical grounds. Confirmation of barbiturate ingestion is readily available by routine toxicology screening.

Gastric lavage is useful in acute massive overdose. Ipecac-induced vomiting is useful immediately after ingestion. Activated charcoal with a cathartic decreases further drug absorption and increases drug elimination.[163, 164] Alkalinization of the urine increases elimination of phenobarbital but not other barbiturates.[165]

**Benzodiazepines.** Clinical manifestations of benzodiazepine overdose range from slurred speech to lethargy to respiratory arrest and coma. Most patients have small mid-position pupils that do not respond to naloxone administration. The diagnosis of benzodiazepine overdose depends on a history of ingestion or a high suspicion for drug overdose. Confirmation of ingestion is rapidly available by urine toxicology screening.

Treatment of benzodiazepine overdose consists of supportive measures, gastric emptying, and flumazenil therapy. Flumazenil is a specific benzodiazepine antagonist that is useful in reversing sedation and respiratory depression.[166, 167] Flumazenil does not antagonize the CNS effects of alcohol, barbiturates, tricyclic antidepressants, or narcotics and thus may provide useful diagnostic information. Flumazenil may unmask seizures; it should be used cautiously if a mixed tricyclic antidepressant–benzodiazepine overdose is suspected. The initial dose of flumazenil is 0.2 mg IV over 30 seconds. An additional 0.3 mg can be given over 30 seconds if the desired clinical effect is not seen within 30 seconds. Additional 0.5-mg doses can be administered over 30 seconds at 1-minute intervals as needed to a total dose of 3 mg.

**Opioids.** Clinical manifestations of opioid overdose range from lethargy to respiratory arrest and coma. Other features of opioid intoxication include hypotension, decreased heart rate, muscle flaccidity, and occasionally seizures. Seizures are most common with propoxyphene and meperidine. Pupils are commonly pinpoint and respond to naloxone administration. The diagnosis of opioid overdose depends on a history of ingestion or clinical features, such as needle marks suggestive of heroin addiction.

Naloxone, a specific opioid antagonist, reverses opioid-induced sedation, hypotension, and respiratory depression.[168] It is administered intravenously at an initial dose of 0.2 to 0.4 mg. If naloxone does not produce a clinical response in 2 to 3 minutes, an additional 1 to 2 mg IV may be administered to a total dose of 10 mg. In general, opioid antagonism occurs within minutes of naloxone administration and lasts for 1 to 4 hours. Repeated boluses may be needed every 20 to 60 minutes to maintain an adequate clinical response. Noncardiogenic pulmonary edema may occur. Supplemental oxygen and mechanical ventilatory support may be required.

## CLINICAL MANIFESTATIONS OF CHRONIC RESPIRATORY ACIDOSIS

### Failure to Excrete $CO_2$ from the Lungs

**Chronic Obstructive Pulmonary Disease.** Two specific diseases that often coexist comprise the COPD syndrome. Chronic bronchitis is defined clinically by chronic cough and sputum production for at least 3 months for 2 successive years without other known causes. Emphysema is an anatomic, pathologic condition with abnormal permanent enlargement of air spaces distal to terminal bronchioles, which is accompanied by destruction of walls but without fibrosis. COPD is a major cause of death and disability. Approximately 12 million patients have chronic bronchitis, and 2 million patients have emphysema. The impact of COPD on morbidity is even greater than on mortality. COPD accounts for 5% of all doctors' office visits and more than 13% of all hospitalizations.[169, 170]

A subset of patients with COPD develop abnormal gas exchange with hypoxemia or hypercapnia. Two characteristic clinical patterns of diseases may be defined by blood gas findings.[171] Patients with severe dyspnea, mild hypoxemia, and normal or low arterial $Pa_{CO_2}$ have been called "pink puffers" (type A COPD). Patients with severe hypoxemia, $CO_2$ retention, right-sided heart failure, and little dyspnea have been called "blue bloaters" (type B COPD). These differences likely reflect variations in ventilation-perfusion mismatching and central respiratory drive. Most patients with COPD fall between these two extremes. In mild cases of COPD, hypoxemia and hypercapnia may not be apparent at rest. With exercise, however, patients with mild COPD may not be able to increase minute ventilation to meet the increased metabolic demands, and clinically apparent hypoxemia and hypercapnia may develop.[172] Patients with COPD often generate a greater percentage of increase in physiologic dead space with an increased respiratory rate that accompanies exercise.[173]

Chronic respiratory acidoses are by definition those forms of respiratory acidosis that have been present for sufficient periods of time to permit renal compensatory changes that tend to restore a more normal pH. Thus, stable, well-compensated patients with COPD may have elevated $Pa_{CO_2}$ levels, but their systemic pH may be only minimally acidic because of normal compensatory mechanisms that elevate the patients' bicarbonate levels. Thus, chronic respiratory acidosis is recognizable clinically by the existence of an elevated

$Pa_{CO_2}$ with an elevated bicarbonate concentration with a slightly acid pH.

The primary goals of management should be directed toward preventive health strategies to slow progression and reduce complications. Controlling smoking behavior is the most important preventive strategy at all phases of the disease. Smoking cessation should have a high priority for all patients with COPD.[169, 170] For patients with recognized COPD, medical treatment is directed toward the reversible component of airway obstruction. Bronchodilators used to increase airway caliber and improve symptoms include sympathomimetic β-agonists and anticholinergics.[169, 170, 174] The preferred method of administration is by inhalation with a metered-dose inhaler.[175] Anticholinergics have gained prominence in the treatment of COPD because of their selectivity and relatively low side effect profile. Corticosteroids can be beneficial for some patients with COPD. A meta-analysis of 16 clinical trials of oral steroid therapy for stable patients found that a 20% improvement in $FEV_1$ occurred in about 10% more patients on steroids than on placebo.[176] For patients with chronic cough and sputum, techniques to control secretions are important. For acute exacerbations when sputum changes color and changes in volume, treatment with antibiotics is indicated.[177, 178] Oral antibiotics such as trimethoprim-sulfamethoxazole, ampicillin, amoxicillin-clavulanate, tetracycline, and erythromycin are commonly used to eradicate pathogens colonizing the respiratory tract. These pathogens include *Haemophilus influenzae, Streptococcus pneumoniae,* and *Moraxella catarrhalis.* In patients who have chronic, stable hypoxemia, oxygen therapy prolongs life; the more continuous the therapy, the larger is the effect.[179]

## Acute or Chronic Respiratory Failure

Patients with COPD often suffer acute deterioration, which is superimposed on their stable but precariously balanced ventilatory state. These patients usually present with dyspnea that has been worsening over days, often with increased cough and sputum production. Physical findings include respiratory distress, prolonged expiratory time, use of accessory muscles, and wheezing. The chest radiograph usually only reflects COPD but may reveal a cause for the patient's acute deterioration, such as pneumonia or pneumothorax. Typical initial arterial blood gas values on room air reveal a $Pa_{O_2}$ of 35 to 45 mm Hg and a $Pa_{CO_2}$ of 60 to 70 mm Hg. The 1-year survival for patients with acute on chronic respiratory failure is approximately 50%, but only 26% of patients rate their quality of life as good or better when surveyed at 6 months.[180–182]

The alveolar hypoventilation noted in these patients is due to loss of adequate drive, muscular weakness, and excessive respiratory load. Relatively few patients develop respiratory failure from loss of drive. This occurs most commonly in the setting of physician-directed sedation. Skeletal inspiratory muscle fatigue possibly plays an important role in the alveolar hypoventilation.[183] In health, muscle function far exceeds that necessary to sustain ventilation against a normal small respiratory load. In COPD, however, the respiratory system load, as judged by the oxygen cost of breathing, is elevated to between 17% and 46% of the total body oxygen consumption, owing to abnormal airway resistance and increased elasticity. Electrolyte disturbances might contribute to the muscular weakness. Hypokalemia, hypomagnesemia, and hypophosphatemia are often present.[184, 185] Malnutrition can cause respiratory muscle weakness, and even short-term fasting depresses diaphragmatic strength and endurance.[186–188] Additionally, a flattened diaphragm generates less transmural pressure for a given tension than a normally curved diaphragm.[189] Excessive respiratory load is due to increasing airway resistance and increased elasticity. The increase in airway resistance is caused by bronchospasm, airway inflammation, and obstruction by mucus. Sleep apnea, which normally coexists with COPD, must be excluded. The most significant contributor to elastic load is dynamic hyperinflation. Airway obstruction compounded by decreased elastic recoil leads to prolongation of expiration; accordingly, expiration cannot be completed before the ensuing inspiration begins. Expiration terminates at a higher FRC. Thus, alveolar pressure remains positive with respect to end-expiratory pressure at the airway opening, and a greater effort must be generated by the end-expiratory muscle on a subsequent breath. The presence of heart failure, pneumonia, or atelectasis all contribute to increased elastic load. Increased chest wall elastic load may also be present. Obesity, pneumothorax, pleural effusion, ascites, and cough-induced rib fractures all increase chest wall elastic load.

The goals of management in a patient with acute on chronic respiratory failure are to forestall mechanical ventilation if possible and to recognize progressive respiratory failure when it is not. Bronchodilators are an essential part of the early management of these patients. Inhaled β-selective agents (albuterol) should be given by metered-dose inhaler. The addition of ipratropium to a regimen containing an inhaled β-agonist yields incremental benefit in patients with COPD. Patients with acute or chronic respiratory failure given methylprednisolone, 0.5 mg/kg every 6 hours in addition to standard bronchodilators show greater improvements in spirometric values than do patients who do not receive this drug. Beneficial effects are noted as early as 12 hours.[190, 191]

NPPV has a major role in this illness; its use can avert mechanical ventilation in 75% of patients with acute on chronic respiratory failure.[192] NPPV consists of a positive-pressure ventilator connected by way of tubing to a mask that applies positive air pressure to the nose or mouth or both. Nasal masks are the most commonly used interfaces; they are convenient and permit normal speech and swallowing. The ventilators utilized for noninvasive ventilation can include critical care ventilators, but the most commonly used ventilators are bilevel devices (BiPAP). These devices deliver a positive inspiratory airway pressure that can be combined with a positive end-expired pressure. The difference between these two pressures is the level of inspiratory assistance or pressure support.

The physiologic effects of noninvasive ventilation include avoidance of intubation, improvement in oxygenation and alveolar ventilation, reduction in work of breathing, and relief of dyspnea. Two randomized controlled studies both found nearly identical reductions in the percentage of patients needing intubations.[192, 193] In control patients, between 73% and 74% of patients require intubation, whereas only 26% of patients receiving NPPV require intubation. In patients with chronic $CO_2$ retention admitted for acute exacerbations, improvements in oxygenation are often noted without any worsening of $CO_2$ retention. $PaO_2$ improves promptly, whereas $PaCO_2$ and pH improve more gradually. A 2-hour blood gas response appears to predict ultimate success or failure of this technique.[194] Successful noninvasive ventilation is usually accompanied by improvement in both the pH and the partial pressure of arterial oxygen and a fall in the respiratory rate from approximately 34 to 24 breaths/min at 1 hour. The sensation of dyspnea is reduced in patients who are successfully managed with NPPV. Short periods of noninvasive ventilation appear to be sufficient to break the cycle of respiratory muscle insufficiency. Perhaps most important, patients randomized to receive NPPV had lower rates of complications (16% compared with 48%) and mortality (9% compared with 29%) and shorter hospital stays (23 days compared with 35 days) than conventionally treated patients.[192] Thus, NPPV therapy in acute or chronic respiratory failure improves morbidity and mortality and has the potential of reducing cost. The exact time at which noninvasive ventilation should be introduced is not clear. It should possibly be used sooner rather than later. NPPV should be instituted if the respiratory rate is higher than 30 breaths/min and the pH is less than 7.35.

If an improvement and a fall in respiratory rate do not occur within the first hour of treatment, intubation or increased ventilatory support should be considered. If patients are intubated, life-threatening alkalosis can be a common complication. Severe alkalosis is related to overzealous ventilation. Physicians commonly choose ventilator settings with a higher tidal volume and a correspondingly lower ratio of dead space to tidal volume than that found in most patients with acute or chronic respiratory failure. In addition, a minute ventilation higher than 10 L/min is often employed. As work of breathing is assumed by the ventilator, $CO_2$ production may fall by as much as 20%. All of these factors interact to dramatically lower the patients $PaCO_2$. Because pre-existing compensatory metabolic alkalosis is the rule, alkalemia with pH greater than 7.7 can easily be achieved. Attempts to normalize pH serve only to waste bicarbonate that has been vigorously conserved during the evolution of respiratory failure.

Ventilation should use the assist-control mode with tidal volumes of 5 to 7 mL/kg (350 to 500 mL) with a respiratory rate of 20 to 24 breaths/min. The triggering sensitivity setting on the ventilator should be lowered to decrease the effort required to trigger the ventilator.

# RESTRICTIVE DEFECTS

## Kyphoscoliosis

Kyphoscoliosis is a prototypical cause of severe thoracic deformity. Clinical symptoms and pathophysiologic consequences of kyphoscoliosis correlate with the degree of spinal curvature. In patients with kyphoscoliosis, a scoliotic curve less than 70 degrees rarely results in cardiopulmonary sequelae, whereas angles greater than 70 degrees place the patient at risk of developing respiratory failure. Angles greater than 100 degrees are associated with dyspnea, and angles of 120 degrees or more result in alveolar hypoventilation and cor pulmonale.[196, 197]

Significant arterial hypoxemia is usually absent in patients with kyphoscoliosis until the late development of hypercapnia. Alveolar hypoventilation results in these patients from an increase in the $V_D/V_T$. This ratio is increased because $V_T$ is reduced, whereas anatomic and alveolar dead space are usually normal. Minute ventilation is generally normal but is maintained by higher respiratory rates.[195]

Acute respiratory failure is usually precipitated by pneumonia, upper respiratory tract infection, or congestive heart failure.[198] Patients admitted with acute respiratory failure for the first time evidenced severe arterial hypoxemia ($PaO_2$ of 35), acute or chronic hypercapnia ($PaCO_2$ of 63), and mild arterial acidemia (pH of 7.34). Seven of these patients required intubation and mechanical ventilation, whereas the other 13 patients were managed without mechanical ventilation. On discharge, the mean $PaO_2$ was 63 mm Hg and the mean $PaCO_2$ was 55 mm Hg. The median survival for patients after the first episode of acute respiratory failure is approximately 9 years.[198]

## Neuromuscular Disease

**Amyotrophic Lateral Sclerosis.** Amyotrophic lateral sclerosis (ALS) is the most common lower motor neuron disorder. The etiology is unknown. The clinical course of ALS varies, but most patients present with progressive muscle weakness and wasting involving distal muscles initially.[199]

The prognosis of patients with ALS is poor. Fifty percent of patients die of complications such as aspiration and pneumonia within 3 years of the diagnosis. Progressive decreases in vital capacity are noted reflecting widespread weakness of inspiratory and expiratory muscles. Severe hypercapnia and hypoxemia are present and can be corrected only by mechanical ventilatory support. Prognosis must be individualized, because some patients with ALS stabilize after years of illness.[200]

## REFERENCES


1. Otis AB: Quantitative relationships in steady-state gas exchange. In Fenn WO, Rahn H (eds): American Physiological Society: Handbook of Physiology. Section 3: Respiration, vol 1. Baltimore, Williams & Wilkins, 1964, p 681.
2. Roughton FIW: Transport of oxygen and carbon dioxide. In Fenn WO, Rahn H (eds): American Physiological Society: Handbook of Physiology. Section 3: Respiration, vol 1. Baltimore, Williams & Wilkins, 1964, p 767.
3. Farhi LE: Gas stores of the body. In Fenn WO, Rahn H (eds): American Physiological Society: Handbook of Physiology. Section 3: Respiration, vol 1. Baltimore, Williams & Wilkins, 1964, p 873.
4. Crandall ED: Kinetics of $CO_2$ in blood. In Piiper J, Scheid P (eds): Progress in Respiration Research, vol 16, Gas Exchange Function of Normal and Diseased Lungs. Basel, Karger, 1981, p 181.
5. Forster RE, Crandall ED: Time course of exchanges between red cells and extracellular fluid during $CO_2$ uptake. J Appl Physiol 38:710, 1975.
6. Hamburger HJ: Ueber den Einfluss von Saure aund alkali auf defibrinirtes Blut. Arch Anat Physiol Lpz :513, 1893.
7. Van Slyke DD: The carbon dioxide carriers of the blood. Physiol Rev 1:141, 1921.
8. Dirken MNJ, Mook HW: The rate of gas exchange between blood cells and serum. J Physiol (Lond) 73:349, 1931.
9. Chow EI, Crandall ED, Forster RE: Kinetics of bicarbonate-chloride exchange across the human red blood cell membrane. J Gen Physiol 68:633, 1976.
10. Klocke RA: Rate of bicarbonate-chloride exchange in human red cells at 37°C. J Appl Physiol 40:707, 1976
11. Klocke RA: Velocity $CO_2$ exchange in blood. Ann Rev Physiol 50:625, 1988.
12. Dill DB, Edwards HT, Consalazio WV: Blood as a physiochemical system: Man at rest. J Biol Chem 118:635, 1937.
13. West J: Respiratory Physiology: The Essentials. Baltimore, Williams & Wilkins, 1974.
14. Murray JF: The normal lung. In The Basis for Diagnosis and Treatment of Pulmonary Diseases. Philadelphia, WB Saunders, 1976.
15. Riley RL, Cournand A: Analysis of factors affecting partial pressures of oxygen and carbon dioxide in gas and blood of lungs: Theory. J Appl Physiol 4:77, 1951.
16. West JB: Ventilation/Blood Flow and Gas Exchange. Oxford, Blackwell Press, 1970.
17. Lenfant C: Measurement of ventilation-perfusion distribution with alveolar-arterial differences. J Appl Physiol 18:1090, 1963.
18. West JB: Causes of carbon dioxide retention in lung disease. N Engl J Med 284:1232, 1971.
19. Stone HL, Liang IYS: Cardiovascular response and control during exercise. Am Rev Respir Dis 129:S13, 1984.
20. Casaburi R, Whipp BJ, Wasserman K, et al: Ventilatory and gas exchange dynamics in response to sinusoidal work. J Appl Physiol 42:300, 1977.
21. Diamond LB, Casaburi R, Wasserman K, et al: Kinetics of gas exchange and ventilation in transitions from rest or prior exercise. J Appl Physiol 43:704, 1977.
22. Jones NL, Berman LB: Gas exchange in chronic airflow obstruction. Am Rev Respir Dis 129:581, 1984.
23. Hill EP, Enns T: $CO_2$ diffusing capacity in isolated lungs. In Piiper J, Scheil P (eds): Progress in Respiration Research, vol 16, Gas Exchange Function of Normal and Diseased Lungs. Basel, Karger, 1981, p 172.
24. Forster RE: Interpretation of measurements of pulmonary diffusing capacity. In Fenn WO, Rahn H (eds): American Physiological Society: Handbook of Physiology. Section 3: Respiration, vol 2. Baltimore, Williams & Wilkins, 1965, p 1453.
25. Rahn H, Farhi LE: Ventilation, perfusion and gas exchange—the $V_A/Q$ concept. In Fenn WO, Rahn H (eds): American Physiological Society: Handbook of Physiology. Section 3: Respiration, vol 1. Baltimore, Williams & Wilkins, 1964, p 735.
26. Crandall ED, O'Brasky JE: Direct evidence for participation of rat lung carbonic anhydrase in $CO_2$ reactions. J Clin Invest 62: 618, 1978.
27. Effros RM, Chang RS, Silverman P: Acceleration of plasma bicarbonate conversion to carbon dioxide by pulmonary carbonic anhydrase. Science 199:427, 1978.
28. Klocke RA: Catalysis of $CO_2$ reactions by lung carbonic anhydrase. J Appl Physiol 44:882, 1978.
29. Berger AJ, Mitchell RA, Severinghaus JW: Regulation of respiration. N Engl J Med 297:92, 138, 194, 1977.
30. Kazemi H, Johnson DC: Regulation of cerebrospinal fluid acid-base balance. Physiol Rev 66:954, 1986.
31. Tang WC, Weil MH, Gazmuri RJ, et al: Reversible impairment of myocardial contractility due to hypercarbic acidosis in the isolated perfused rat heart. Crit Care Med 19:218, 1991.
32. Foex P, Prys-Roberts C: Interactions of beta-receptor blockade and levels in the anaesthetized dog. Br J Anaesth 46:397, 1974.
33. Orchard C, Kentish J: Effects of changes of pH on the contractile function of cardiac muscle. Am J Physiol 258:C967, 1990.
34. Case RB, Greenberg H, Moskowitz R: Alterations in coronary sinus $P_{O_2}$ and $O_2$ saturation resulting from $P_{CO_2}$ changes. Cardiovasc Res 9:167, 1975.
35. Nunn JF: Applied respiratory physiology. In The Effects of Changes in Carbon Dioxide Tension, 3rd ed. London, Butterworths, 1987, p 460.
36. Boekstegers P, Weiss M: Tissue oxygen partial pressure distribution within the human skeletal muscle during hypercapnia. Adv Exp Med Biol 277:525, 1990.
37. Kety S, Schmidt CF: The effects of altered arterial tensions of carbon dioxide and oxygen on cerebral blood flow and cerebral oxygen consumption of normal young men. J Clin Invest 27:484, 1948.
38. Atkinson JLD, Anderson RE, Sundt TM: The effect of carbon dioxide on the diameter of brain capillaries. Brain Res 517: 333, 1990.
39. Miller JD: Cerebral blood flow variations with perfusion pressure and metabolism. In Wood JH (ed): Cerebral Blood Flow: Physiologic and Clinical Aspects. New York, McGraw-Hill, 1987, p 119.
40. Miller JD, Sullivan HG: Severe intracranial hypertension. In Trubuhovich RV (ed): Management of Acute Intracranial Disasters. Boston, Little Brown, 1979, p 119.
41. Davies CE, Mackinnon J: Neurological effects of oxygen in chronic cor pulmonale. Lancet 2:883, 1949.
42. Paljarvi L, Soderfeldt B, Kalimo H, et al: The brain in extreme respiratory acidosis: A light and electron-microscopic study in the rat. Acta Neuropathol (Berl) 58:87, 1982.
43. Juan G, Calverley P, Talamo C, et al: Effect of carbon dioxide on diaphragmatic function in human beings. N Engl J Med 310:874, 1984.
44. Rochester DF, Braun NMT, Arora NS: Respiratory muscle strength in chronic obstructive pulmonary disease. Am Rev Respir Dis 119:S151, 1979.
45. Pihl BG, Pohl AL, Dickens RA, et al: Effect of chronic hypercapnia on gastric acid secretion in the dog. Ann Surg 165:254, 1967.
46. Gelman S, Ernst EA: Role of pH, $P_{CO_2}$ and $O_2$ content of portal blood in hepatic circulatory autoregulation. Am J Physiol 233: E255, 1977.
47. Mathie RT, Blumgart LH: Effect of denervation on the hepatic haemodynamic response to hypercapnia and hypoxia in the dog. Pflugers Arch 397:152, 1983.
48. Bersentes TJ, Simmons DH: Effects of acute acidosis on renal hemodynamics. Am J Physiol 212:633, 1967.
49. Chen HG, Wood CE: The adrenocorticotropic hormone and arginine vasopressin responses to hypercapnia in fetal and maternal sheep. Am J Physiol 264:R324, 1993.
50. Raff H, Raorty TP: Renin, ACTH and aldosterone during acute hypercapnia and hypoxemia in conscious rates. Am J Physiol 238:F119, 1998.
51. Colice GL: Fluid balance in acute and chronic lung disease. Am Rev Respir Dis 138:1052, 1988.
52. Rector FC Jr: Acidification of the urine. In Orloff J, Berliner RW (eds): American Physiological Society: Handbook of Physiology. Section 8: Renal Physiology. Baltimore, Waverly Press, 1973, p 431.
53. Berry CA, Wamock DG: Acidification in the in vitro perfused tubule. Kidney Int 22:507, 1982.

54. Breyer MD, Jacobson HR: Mechanisms and regulation of renal $H^+$ and $HCO_3^-$ transport. Am J Nephrol 7:150, 1987.
55. Hamm LL, Simon EE: Roles and mechanisms of urinary buffer excretion. Am J Physiol 253:F595, 1987.
56. Pitts RF: Production and excretion of ammonia in relation to acid-base regulation. In Orloff J, Berliner RW (eds): American Physiological Society: Handbook of Physiology. Section 8, Physiology. Baltimore, Williams & Wilkins, 1973, p 455.
57. Tannen RL: Ammonia metabolism. Am J Physiol 235:F265, 1978.
58. Tannen RL: Ammonia and acid-base balance. Med Clin North Am 67:781, 1983.
59. Tannen RL, Sastrasinh S: Response of ammonia metabolism to acute acidosis. Kidney Int 25:1, 1984.
60. Polak A, Haynie GD, Hays RM, et al: Effects of chronic hypercapnia on electrolyte and acid-base equilibrium. I: Adaptation. J Clin Invest 40:1223, 1961.
61. Schwartz WB, Brackett NC Jr, Cohen JJ: The response of extracellular hydrogen ion concentration to graded degrees of chronic hypercapnia: The physiologic limits of defense of pH. J Clin Invest 44:291, 1965.
62. Brackett NC Jr, Cohen JJ, Wingo CF, et al: Carbon dioxide titration curve of normal man: Effect of increasing degrees of acute hypercapnia on acid-base equilibrium. N Engl J Med 272: 6, 1965.
63. Elkington JR, Singer RB, Barker ES, et al: Effects in man of acute experimental respiratory alkalosis and acidosis on ionic transfers in the total body fluid. J Clin Invest 34:1671, 1955.
64. Sapir DG, Levine DZ, Schwartz WB: The effects of chronic hypoxemia on electrolyte and acid-base equilibrium: An examination of normocapneic hypoxemia and of the influence of hypoxemia on the adaptation to chronic hypercapnia. J Clin Invest 46:369, 1967.
65. Culver BH: Physiology. In Albert R, Spiro S (eds): Comprehensive Respiratory Medicine. St. Louis, CV Mosby, 1999, pp 4.1–4.42.
66. Goldberg M, Greene SB, Man ML, et al: Computer based inoculation and diagnosis of acid-base disorders. JAMA 223: 269, 1973.
67. Frumin MJ, Epstein RM, Cohen G: Apneic oxygenation in man. Anesthesiology 20:789, 1959.
68. Niemann JT: Cardiopulmonary resuscitation. N Engl J Med 327:1075, 1992.
69. Cummins RO (ed): Textbook of Advanced Cardiac Life Support. Chicago, American Heart Association, 1994.
70. Alexander RH (ed): Advanced Trauma Life Support Course for Physicians. New York, American College of Surgeons, 1997.
71. Goldhaber SZ: Pulmonary embolism. N Engl J Med 339:93, 1998.
72. Tapson VF, Witty LA: Massive pulmonary embolism: Diagnostic and therapeutic strategies. Clin Chest Med 16:329, 1995.
73. D'Alonzo GE, Dantzker DR: Gas exchange alterations following pulmonary thromboembolism. Clin Chest Med 5:411, 1984.
74. Ginsberg JS: Management of venous thromboembolism. N Engl J Med 335:1816, 1996.
75. Hull RD, Raskob GB, Rosenbloom D, et al: Heparin for 5 days as compared with 10 days in the initial treatment of proximal venous thrombosis. N Engl J Med 322:1260, 1990.
76. Weitz JL: Low-molecular-weight heparins. N Engl J Med 337: 688, 1997.
77. Urokinase Pulmonary Embolism Trial: A national cooperative study. Circulation 47(Suppl II):1, 1973.
78. Goldhaber SZ, Haire WD, Feldstein ML, et al: Alteplase versus heparin in acute pulmonary embolism: Randomized trial assessing right-ventricular function and pulmonary perfusion. Lancet 341:507, 1993.
79. Petty TL: Treat status asthmaticus three days before it occurs. J Intensive Care Med 4:135, 1989.
80. Hogg JC: The pathology of asthma. Clin Chest Med Chest 5: 567, 1984.
81. Sur S, Crotty TB, Kephart GM, et al: Sudden-onset fatal asthma: A distinct clinical entity with few eosinophils and relatively more neutrophils in the airway submucosa. Am Rev Respir Dis 148:713, 1993.
82. Ried LM: The presence or absence of bronchial mucus in fatal asthma. J Allerg Clin Immunol 80:415, 1987.
83. Rodriguez-Roisin R, Ballester E, Roca I, et al: Mechanisms of hypoxemia in patients with status asthmaticus requiring mechanical ventilation. Am Rev Respir Dis 139:732, 1989.
84. Roca J, Ramis L, Rodriguez-Roisin R, et al: Serial relationships between ventilation perfusion inequality and spirometry in acute severe asthma requiring hospitalization. Am Rev Respir Dis 137:1055, 1988.
85. Nowak RM, Tomlanovich MC, Sarker DD, et al: Arterial blood gases and pulmonary function testing in acute bronchial asthma: Predicting patient outcomes. JAMA 249:2043, 1983.
86. McFadden ER Jr, Lyons HA: Arterial-blood gas tension in asthma. N Engl J Med 278:1027, 1968.
87. Ferrer A, Roca J, Wagner PO, et al: Airway obstruction and ventilation-perfusion relationships in acute severe asthma. Am Rev Respir Dis 147:579, 1993.
88. Rea HH, Scragg R, Jackson R, et al: A case-controlled study of deaths from asthma. Thorax 41:833, 1986.
89. Suissa S, Ernst P, Boivin JF, et al: A cohort analysis of excess mortality in asthma and the use of inhaled beta-agonists. Am Respir Crit Care Med 149:604, 1994.
90. Levenson T, Greenberger PA, Donoghue ER, et al: Asthma death confounded by substance abuse: An assessment of fatal asthma. Chest 110:604, 1996.
91. Kikuchi Y, Okabe S, Tamura G, et al: Chemosensitivity and perception of dyspnea in patients with a history of near-fatal asthma. N Engl J Med 330:1329, 1994.
92. Fishman AP: Cardiac asthma—a fresh look at an old wheeze. N Engl J Med 320:1346, 1989.
93. Shim CS, Williams MH: Relationship of wheezing to the severity of obstruction in asthma. Arch Intern Med 143:890, 1983.
94. Rebuck AS, Read J: Assessment and management of severe asthma. Am J Med 51:788, 1971.
95. Shim CS, Williams MH Jr: Evaluation of the severity of asthma patients versus physicians. Am J Med 68:11, 1980.
96. National Asthma Education Program: Expert Panel Report Guidelines for the diagnosis and management of asthma (Publication No. 91-3042, August 1991). Bethesda, Md, Department of Health and Human Services.
97. Corbridge T, Hall IB: State of the art: The assessment and management of adults with status asthmaticus. Am J Respir Crit Care Med 151:1296, 1995.
98. Idris AH, McDermott MF, Raucci JC, et al: Emergency department treatment of severe asthma: Metered-dose inhaler plus holding chamber is equivalent in effectiveness to nebulizer. Chest 103:665, 1993.
99. Rowe BH, Keller JL, Oxman AD: Effectiveness of steroid therapy in acute exacerbations of asthma: A meta-analysis. Am J Emerg Med 10:301, 1992.
100. Benatar SR: Fatal asthma. N Engl J Med 314:423, 1986.
101. McFadden ER Jr: Clinical commentary: Dosages of corticosteroids in asthma. Am Rev Respir Dis 147:1306, 1993.
102. Shivaram U, Miro AM, Cash ME, et al: Cardiopulmonary responses to continuous positive airway pressure in acute asthma. J Crit Care 8:87, 1993.
103. Meduri GU, Cook TR, Turner RE, et al: Noninvasive positive pressure ventilation in status asthmaticus. Chest 110:767, 1996.
104. Meduri GU, Aboushala N, Fox RC, et al: Noninvasive face mask mechanical ventilation in patients with acute hypercapnic respiratory failure. Chest 100:445, 1991.
105. Tuxen DV, Williams TJ, Scheinkestel CD, et al: Use of a measurement of pulmonary hyperinflation to control the level of mechanical ventilation in patients with acute severe asthma. Am Rev Respir Dis 146:1136, 1992.
106. Tuxen DV, Lane S: The effects of ventilatory pattern on hyperinflation, airway pressures, and circulation in mechanical ventilation of patients with severe airflow obstruction. Am Rev Respir Dis 136:872, 1987.
107. Williams TJ, Tuxen DV, Scheinkestel CD, et al: Risk factors for morbidity in mechanically ventilated patients with acute severe asthma. Am Rev Respir Dis 146:607, 1992.
108. Tuxen DV: Detrimental effects of positive end-expiratory pressure during controlled mechanical ventilation of patients with severe airflow obstruction. Am Rev Respir Dis 140:5, 1989.
109. Darioli R, Perret C: Mechanical controlled hypoventilation in status asthmaticus. Am Rev Respir Dis 129:385, 1984.

110. Feihl F, Perret C: State of the art: Permissive hypercapnia: How permissive should we be? Am J Respir Crit Care Med 150: 1722, 1994.
111. Tuxen DY: Permissive hypercapnic ventilation. Am J Respir Crit Care Med 150:870, 1994.
112. Mithoefer JC, Porter WF, Karetzky MS: Indications for the use of sodium bicarbonate in the treatment of intractable asthma. Respiration 25:201, 1968.
113. Mithoefer JC, Runser RH, Karetzky MS: The use of sodium bicarbonate in the treatment of acute bronchial asthma. N Engl J Med 272:1200, 1965.
114. Young T, Palta M, Dempsey J, et al: The occurrence of sleep disordered breathing among middle-aged adults. N Engl J Med 328:1230, 1993.
115. Orr WC, Males JL, Imes NK: Myxedema and obstructive sleep apnea. Am J Med 70:1061, 1981.
116. Onal E, Lopata M: Periodic breathing and the pathogenesis of occlusive sleep apnea. Am Rev Respir Dis 126:676, 1982.
117. Hudgel DW, Chapman KR, Faulks C, et al: Changes in inspiratory muscle electrical activity and upper airway resistance during periodic breathing induced by hypoxia during sleep. Am Rev Respir Dis 135:899, 1987.
118. Hoffstein V, Mateika S: Cardiac arrhythmias, snoring and sleep apnea. Chest 106:466, 1994.
119. Chaouat A, Weitzenblum E, Krieger J, et al: Pulmonary hemodynamics in the obstructive sleep apnea syndrome: Results in 220 consecutive patients. Chest 109:380, 1996.
120. Fletcher EC, Schaff JW, Miller J, et al: Long-term cardiopulmonary sequelae in patients with sleep apnea and chronic lung disease. Am Rev Respir Dis 135:525, 1987.
121. Weitzenblum E, Krieger J, Apprill M, et al: Daytime pulmonary hypertension in patients with obstructive sleep apnea syndrome. Am Rev Respir Dis 138:345, 1988.
122. Remmers IE, Sterling IA, Thorarinsson B, et al: Nasal aim positive airway pressure in patients with occlusive sleep apnea. Am Rev Respir Dis 130:1152, 1984.
123. Series F, Marc I, Cormier Y, et al: Required levels of nasal continuous positive airway pressure during treatment of obstructive sleep apnea. Eur Respir 17:1776, 1994.
124. Reeves-Hoche MK, Hudgel DW, Meck R, et al: Continuous versus bilevel positive airway pressure for obstructive sleep apnea. Am J Respir Crit Care Med 151:443, 1995.
125. Shackford SR, Virgilio RW, Peters RW: Selective use of ventilatory therapy in flail chest injuries. J Thor Cardiovasc Surg 81: 194, 1981.
126. Trinkle JF, Richarson RD, Franz JL, et al: Management of flail chest without mechanical ventilation. Ann Thorac Surg 19: 355, 1975.
127. Avery WG, Samet P, Sackner MA: The acidosis of pulmonary edema. Am J Med 48:320, 1970.
128. Aberman A, Fulop M: The metabolic and respiratory acidosis of acute pulmonary edema. Ann Intern Med 76:173, 1972.
129. Ware LB, Matthay MA: The acute respiratory distress syndrome 342:1334, 2000.
130. Kollef MH, Schuster DP: The acute respiratory distress syndrome. N Engl J Med 332:27, 1995.
131. Bernard GR, Artigas A, Brigham KT, et al: The American-European Consensus Conference on ARDS: Definitions, mechanisms, relevant outcomes, and clinical trial coordination. Am J Respir Crit Care Med 149:818, 1994.
132. Pratt PC, Vollmer RT, Shelburne JD, et al: Pulmonary morphology in a multihospital collaborative extracorporeal membrane oxygenation project. I: Light microscopy. Am J Pathol 95:191, 1979.
133. Bachofen M, Weibel ER: Structural alterations of lung parenchyma in the adult respiratory distress syndrome. Clin Chest Med 3:35, 1982.
134. Anderson WR, Thielen K: Correlative study of adult respiratory distress syndrome by light, scanning, and transmission electron microscopy. Ultrastruct Pathol 16:615, 1992.
135. Bachofen A, Weibel ER: Alterations of the gas exchange apparatus in adult respiratory insufficiency associated with septicemia. Am Rev Respir Dis 116:589, 1977.
136. Goodman LR: Congestive heart failure and adult respiratory distress syndrome: New insights using computed tomography. Radiol Clin North Am 34:33, 1996.
137. Gattinoni L, Bombino M, Pelosi P; et al: Lung structure and function in different stages of severe adult respiratory distress syndrome. JAMA 271:1772, 1994.
138. Marini JJ, Truuwit J: Monitoring the respiratory system. In Hall JB, Schmidt GA, Wood LDH (eds): Principles of Critical Care. New York, McGraw-Hill, 1988, p 131.
139. Marini JJ: Evolving concepts in the ventilatory management of acute respiratory distress syndrome. Clin Chest Med 17: 555, 1996.
140. Gattinoni L, Presenti A, Torresin A, et al: Adult respiratory distress syndrome profiles by computed tomography. J Thorac Imaging 1:25, 1986.
141. Maunder RJ, Shuman WP, McHugh JW, et al: Preservation of normal lung regions in the adult respiratory distress syndrome: Analysis by computed tomography. JAMA 255:2463, 1986.
142. Muscedere JG, Mullen JBM, Gan K, et al: Tidal ventilation at low airway pressures can augment lung injury. Am J Respir Crit Care Med 149:1327, 1994.
143. Slutsky AS: Consensus conference on mechanical ventilation, part 1. Intensive Care Med 20:64, 1994.
144. Amato MRP, Barbas CSV, Medeiros DM, et al: Beneficial effects of the "open lung approach" with low distending pressures in acute respiratory distress syndrome. Am J Respir Crit Care Med 152:1835, 1995.
145. Dreyfuss D, Soler P, Basset G, et al: High inflation pressure pulmonary edema: Respective effects of high airway pressure, high tidal volume, and positive end-expiratory pressure. Am Rev Respir Dis 137:1159, 1988.
146. Parker JC, Townsley MJ, Rippe B, et al: Increased microvascular permeability in dog lungs due to high peak airway pressures. J Appl Physiol 57:1809, 1984.
147. Corbridge TC, Wood LDH, Crawford GP, et al: Adverse effects of large tidal volumes and low PEEP in canine acid aspiration. Am Rev Respir Dis 142:311, 1990.
148. Slutsky AS, Tremblay LN: Multiple system organ failure: Is mechanical ventilation a contributing factor? Am J Respir Crit Care Med 157:1721, 1998.
149. Ranieri VM, Suter PM, Tortorella C, et al: Effect of mechanical ventilation on inflammatory mediators in patients with acute respiratory distress syndrome: A randomized controlled trial. JAMA 282:54, 1999.
150. Acute Respiratory Distress Syndrome Network: Ventilation with lower tidal volumes as compared with traditional tidal volumes for acute lung injury and the acute respiratory distress syndrome. N Engl J Med 342:1301, 2000.
151. Stewart TE, Meade MO, Cook DL, et al: Evaluation of a ventilation strategy to prevent barotrauma in patients at high risk of acute respiratory distress syndrome. N Engl J Med 338: 355, 1998.
152. Brochard L, Roudot-Thoraval F, Roupie E, et al: Tidal volume reduction for prevention of ventilator-induced lung injury in acute respiratory distress syndrome. Am J Respir Crit Care Med 158:1831, 1998.
153. Schmidt-Nowara WW, Altman AR: Atelectasis and neuromuscular respiratory failure. Chest 85:792, 1984.
154. Luce JM: Medical management of spinal cord injury. Crit Care Med 13:126, 1985.
155. Gracey DR, McMichan JC, Divertie MB, et al: Respiratory failure in Guillain-Barré syndrome. Mayo Clin Proc 57:742, 1982.
156. Drachman DB: Myasthenia gravis. N Engl J Med 330:1797, 1994.
157. Mier-Jedrzejowicz AK, Brophy C, Green M: Respiratory muscle function in myasthenia gravis. Am Rev Respir Dis 138:867, 1988.
158. Dau PC, Lindstrom JM, Cassel CK, et al: Plasmapheresis and immunosuppressive drug therapy in myasthenia gravis. N Engl J Med 297:1134, 1977.
159. Gracey DR, Divertie MB, Howard FM: Mechanical ventilation for respiratory failure in myasthenia gravis. Mayo Clin Proc 58: 597, 1983.
160. Argiu Z, Martag FL: Disorders of neuromuscular transmission caused by drugs. N Engl J Med 301:409, 1979.
161. Lindberg MC, Cunningham A, Lindberg NH: Acute phenobarbital intoxication. South Med J 85:803, 1992.
162. Sutherland GR, Park J, Proudfoot AT: Ventilation and acid-

base changes in deep coma due to barbiturate or tricyclic antidepressant poisoning. Clin Toxicol 11:403, 1977.
163. Berg MJ, Berlinger WG, Goldberg MJ, et al: Acceleration of the body clearance of phenobarbital by oral activated charcoal. N Engl J Med 307:642, 1982.
164. Pond SM, Olson KR, Osterloh JD, et al: Randomized study of the treatment of phenobarbital overdose with repeated doses of activated charcoal. JAMA 251:3104, 1984.
165. Linton AL, Luke RG, Briggs JD: Methods of forced diuresis and its application in barbiturate poisoning. Lancet 2(512): 377, 1967.
166. The Flumazenil in Benzodiazepine Intoxication Multicenter Study Group: Treatment of benzodiazepine overdose with flumazenil. Clin Ther 14:978, 1992.
167. Weinbroum A, Halpern P, Geller E: The use of flumazenil in the management of acute drug poisoning—a review. Intensive Care Med 17(Suppl 1):S32, 1991.
168. Handal KA, Schauben JL, Salamone FR: Naloxone. Ann Emerg Med 12:438, 1983.
169. American Thoracic Society Standards for the Diagnosis and Care of Patients with Chronic Obstructive Pulmonary Disease. Am J Respir Crit Care Med 152:577, 1995.
170. British Thoracic Society: British guidelines for the management of chronic obstructive pulmonary disease. Thorax 52:51, 1997.
171. Dornhorst AC: Respiratory insufficiency. Lancet 1:1185, 1955.
172. Oliven A, Kelsen SG, Deal EC, et al: Mechanisms underlying $CO_2$ retention during low-resistive loading in patients with chronic obstructive pulmonary disease. J Clin Invest 871:1442, 1983.
173. Brown SE, King RR, Temerlin SM, et al: Exercise performance with added dead space in chronic airflow obstruction. J Appl Physiol: Respir Environ Exercise Physiol 56:1020, 1984.
174. Ferguson GT, Chormack RM: Management of chronic obstructive pulmonary disease. N Engl J Med 328:1017, 1993.
175. Gross NJ, Petty TL, Friedman M, et al: Dose response to ipratropium as a nebulized solution in patients with chronic obstructive pulmonary disease. Am Rev Respir Dis 139:1188, 1989.
176. Lucasse Y, Wong E, Guyatt GH, et al: Meta-analysis of respiratory rehabilitation in chronic obstructive lung disease. Lancet 348:1115, 1996.
177. Anthonisen NR, Manfreda J, Warren CP, et al: Antibiotic therapy in exacerbation of chronic obstructive lung disease. Ann Intern Med 106:196, 1987.
178. Saint SS, Bent S, Vittinghof E, et al: Antibiotics in chronic obstructive pulmonary disease exacerbations: A meta-analysis. JAMA 272:957, 1995.
179. Nocturnal Oxygen Therapy Trial Groups: Continuous or nocturnal oxygen therapy in hypoxemic chronic obstructive pulmonary disease. Ann Intern Med 93:391, 1980.
180. Sukumalchantra Y, Dinakara P, Williams M: Prognosis of patients with chronic obstructive pulmonary disease after hospitalization for acute ventilatory failure: A three-year follow-up study. Am Rev Respir Dis 93:215, 1966.
181. Hudson LD: Survival data in patients with acute and chronic lung disease requiring mechanical ventilation. Am Rev Respir Dis 140(Suppl):S19, 1989.
182. Connors AF, Dawson NV, Thomas C, et al: Outcomes following acute exacerbation of severe chronic obstructive lung disease. Am J Respir Crit Care Med 154:959, 1966.
183. Zakynthinos SG, Vassilakopoulos T, Roussos C: The load of inspiratory muscles in patients needing mechanical ventilation. Am J Respir Crit Care Med 152:1248, 1995.
184. Aubier M, Murciano D, Lecocguic Y, et al: Effect of hypophosphatemia on diaphragmatic contractility in patients with acute respiratory failure. N Engl J Med 313:420, 1985.
185. Dhingra S, Solven F, Wilson A, et al: Hypomagnesemia and respiratory muscle power. Am Rev Respir Dis 129:497, 1984.
186. Openbrier D, Irwin M, Rogers RM, et al: Nutritional status and lung function in patients with emphysema and chronic bronchitis. Chest 83:17, 1983.
187. Arora NS, Rochester DF: Respiratory muscle strength and maximal voluntary ventilation in undernourished patients. Am Rev Respir Dis 126:5, 1982.
188. Shindoh C, Dimarco A, Supinski G: Effect of acute fasting on diaphragm strength and endurance. Am Rev Respir Dis 144: 488, 1991.
189. Polkey MI, Kyroussis D, Hamnegard CH, et al: Diaphragm strength in chronic obstructive pulmonary disease. Am J Respir Crit Care Med 154:1310, 1996.
190. Albert RK, Martin TR, Lewis SW: Controlled clinical trial of methylprednisolone in patients with chronic bronchitis and acute respiratory insufficiency. Ann Intern Med 92:753, 1980.
191. Rubini F, Rampulla C, Nava S: Acute effect of corticosteroids on respiratory mechanics in mechanically ventilated patients with chronic airflow obstruction and acute respiratory failure. Am J Respir Crit Care Med 149:306, 1994.
192. Brouchard L, Mancebo J, Wysocki M, et al: Non-invasive ventilation for acute exacerbations of chronic obstructive pulmonary disease. 333:817, 1995.
193. Kramer N, Meyer TJ, Mehang J: Randomized prospective trial of non-invasive positive pressure ventilation in acute respiratory failure. Am J Respir Crit Care Med 151:1799, 1995.
194. Soo Hoo GW, Santiago S, William J: Nasal mechanical ventilation for hypercapnic respiratory failure in chronic obstructive pulmonary disease: Determinants of success and failure. Crit Care Med 27:417, 1994.
195. Bergofsky EH: Respiratory failure in disorders of the thoracic cage. Am Rev Respir Dis 119:643, 1979.
196. Caro CG, DuBois AB: Pulmonary function in kyphoscoliosis. Thorax 16:282, 1961.
197. Collins DK, Ponseti IV: Long term follow-up of patients with idiopathic kyphoscoliosis not treated surgically. J Bone Joint Surg 51A:425, 1969.
198. Libby DM, Briscoe WA, Boyce B, et al: Acute respiratory failure in scoliosis and kyphosis: Prolonged survival and treatment. Am J Med 73:532, 1982.
199. Tandan R, Bradley WG: Amyotrophic lateral sclerosis. Part 1: Clinical features, pathology, and ethical issues in management. Ann Neurol 18:271, 1985.
200. Kreitzer SM, Saunders NA, Tyler HR, et al: Respiratory muscle function in amyotrophic lateral sclerosis. Am Rev Respir Dis 117:437, 1978.

CHAPTER 9

# Respiratory Alkalosis

Nicolaos E. Madias, MD ▪ Horacio J. Adrogué, MD

Respiratory alkalosis is the acid-base disturbance initiated by a reduction in carbon dioxide tension of body fluids, and it entails alkalinization of body fluids. The term primary hypocapnia is synonymous. Hypocapnia elicits secondary decrements in plasma bicarbonate concentration, known as secondary physiologic responses, that should be viewed as an integral part of the respiratory alkalosis. Whole body carbon dioxide stores are decreased, and the level of $Paco_2$ is less than 35 mm Hg in patients with simple respiratory alkalosis, who are at rest and at sea level. An element of respiratory alkalosis may still occur with higher levels of $Paco_2$ in patients with metabolic alkalosis in whom a normal $Paco_2$ is inappropriately low for this primary metabolic disorder.

## PATHOPHYSIOLOGY

Primary hypocapnia usually results from transient or persistent alveolar hyperventilation that leads to negative carbon dioxide balance, thus decreasing carbon dioxide stores. The excretion rate of carbon dioxide exceeds its production rate during the period of hyperventilation, accounting for the negative balance. Primary hypocapnia might also originate from the extrapulmonary elimination of carbon dioxide by a dialysis device or extracorporeal circulation (e.g., heart-lung machine).

Primary decreases in carbon dioxide production, such as in hypothermia or hypothyroidism, are generally accompanied by parallel decreases in alveolar ventilation, thus preventing expression of respiratory alkalosis. However, in the presence of constant alveolar ventilation (i.e., mechanical ventilation), a reduction in physical activity (e.g., sedation, skeletal muscle paralysis) or a reduction in the basal metabolic rate (e.g., hypothermia) represents potential mechanisms of primary hypocapnia due to decreased carbon dioxide production.

In most cases, primary hypocapnia reflects alveolar hyperventilation due to increased ventilatory drive. The latter might be secondary to signals arising from the lung, the peripheral chemoreceptors (carotid and aortic), the brainstem chemoreceptors, or influences originating in other centers of the brain.[1] The response of the brainstem chemoreceptors to carbon dioxide can be augmented by systemic diseases (e.g., liver disease, sepsis), pharmacologic agents, volition, and other influences. Hypoxemia is a major stimulus of alveolar ventilation, but $Pao_2$ values lower than 60 mm Hg are required to elicit this effect consistently. Not uncommonly, alveolar hyperventilation is the result of maladjusted mechanical ventilators.

**Pseudorespiratory Alkalosis.** Arterial hypocapnia does not necessarily imply respiratory alkalosis or the secondary response to metabolic acidosis but can be observed in an idiotypic form of respiratory acidosis.[2] This entity, which we have called pseudorespiratory alkalosis, occurs in patients with profound depression of cardiac function and pulmonary perfusion but with relative preservation of alveolar ventilation, including patients with advanced circulatory failure and those undergoing cardiopulmonary resuscitation.[3–6] The severely reduced pulmonary blood flow limits the carbon dioxide delivered to the lungs for excretion, thus increasing the mixed venous carbon dioxide tension. By contrast, the increased ventilation-perfusion ratio causes the removal of a larger-than-normal amount of carbon dioxide per unit of blood traversing the pulmonary circulation, thus creating arterial eucapnia or frank hypocapnia (Fig. 9–1). Nonetheless, the absolute excretion of carbon dioxide is decreased and the carbon dioxide balance of the body is positive—the hallmark of respiratory acidosis. Such patients may have severe venous acidemia (often caused by mixed respiratory and metabolic acidosis) accompanied by an arterial pH that ranges from the mildly acidic to the frankly alkaline. Furthermore, the extreme oxygen deprivation prevailing in the tissues may be completely disguised by the reasonably preserved values of arterial oxygen tension (Fig. 9–2). To rule out pseudorespiratory alkalosis in a patient with circulatory failure, blood gas monitoring must include sampling of mixed (or central) venous blood.[4–6] The management of pseudorespiratory alkalosis must be directed toward optimizing systemic hemodynamics.

## SECONDARY PHYSIOLOGIC ADJUSTMENTS

The hydrogen ion concentration of blood (expressed in nEq/L) at any moment is a function of the prevailing ratio of the carbon dioxide tension ($Pco_2$, expressed in mm Hg) and the plasma bicarbonate concentration ($[HCO_3^-]$, expressed in mEq/L), as indicated by the Henderson equation,

$$[H^+] = 24 \times Pco_2/[HCO_3^-]$$

which describes the equilibrium relationship of the carbonic acid-bicarbonate system.[7] Therefore, one can estimate with ease the immediate effect on blood pH of extreme hypocapnia in the theoretical absence of a secondary physiologic response. If, for example, $Paco_2$

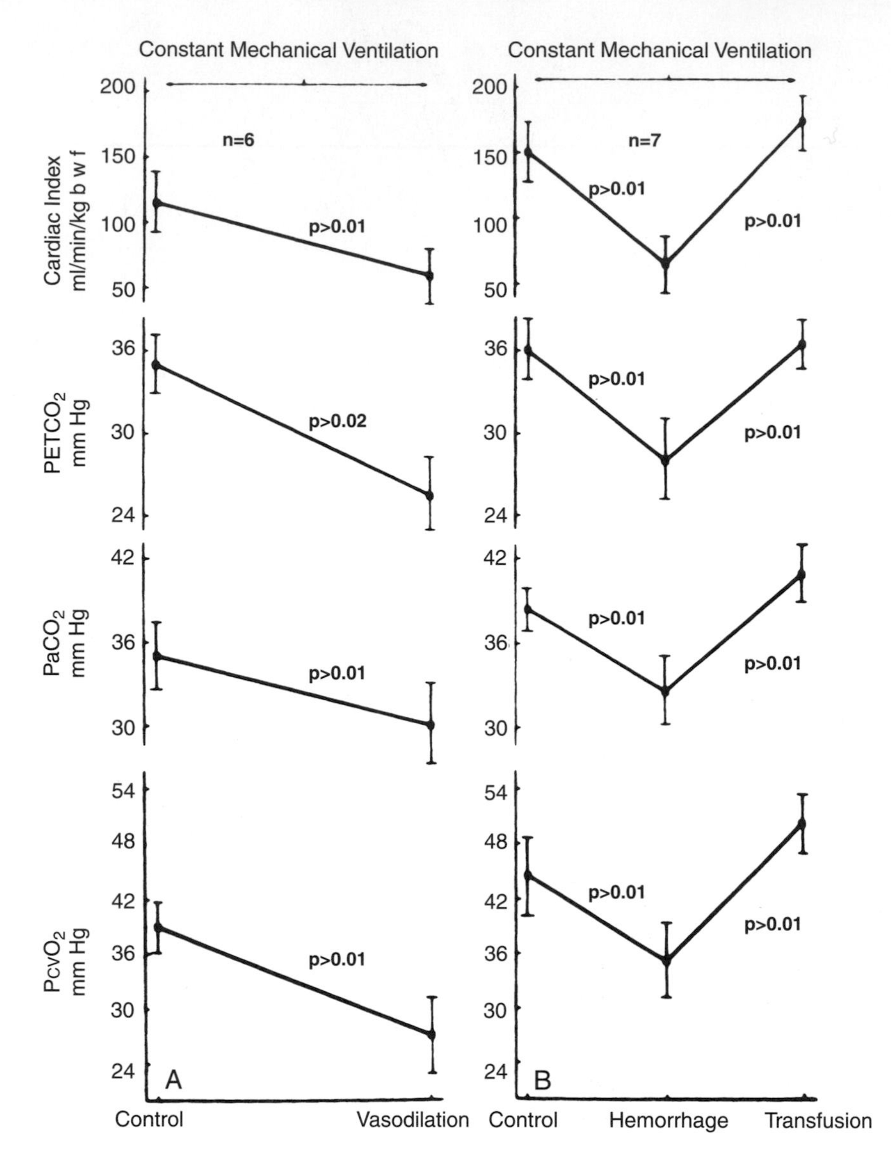


**FIGURE 9–1** ■ Reduction in end-tidal $P_{CO_2}$ ($P_{ETCO_2}$), arterial $P_{CO_2}$ ($Pa_{CO_2}$), and central venous $P_{O_2}$ ($P_{CVO_2}$) as a result of diminished cardiac index because of pharmacological vasodilatation (A) or hemorrhage (B, changes reversed by transfusion) in the presence of constant pulmonary ventilation in anesthetized dogs. In both cases, arterial hypocapnia occurred in the presence of fixed mechanical ventilation, thus discounting pulmonary hyperventilation as an obligatory mechanism for its pathogenesis. Moreover, the reduction in $Pa_{CO_2}$ was associated with a reduction in pulmonary $CO_2$ excretion, as indicated by the large and significant decrement in $P_{ETCO_2}$. (From Adrogué HJ, Rashad MN, Gorin AB, et al: Arteriovenous acid-base disparity in circulatory failure: Studies on mechanism. Am J Physiol 257: F1087, 1989.)

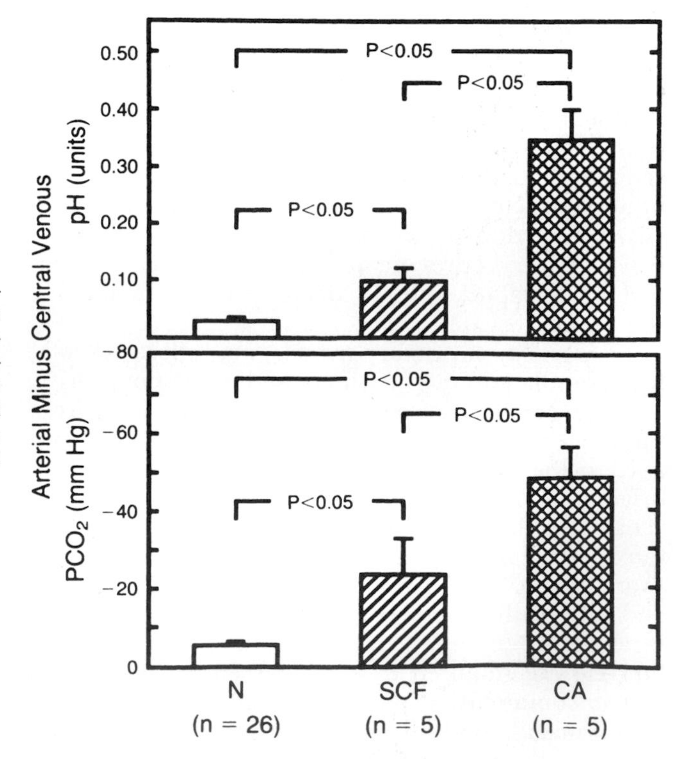


**FIGURE 9–2** ■ Arteriovenous differences in pH and $P_{CO_2}$ in patients with different hemodynamic conditions. CA, cardiac arrest in the presence of constant mechanical ventilation; N, normal hemodynamic status; SCF, severe circulatory failure. Patients with severe circulatory failure or cardiac arrest had a significant widening of the arteriovenous difference in pH and $P_{CO_2}$. (From Adrogué HJ, Rashad MN, Gorin AB, et al: Assessing acid-base status in circulatory failure: Differences between arterial and central venous blood. N Engl J Med 320:1312, 1989.)

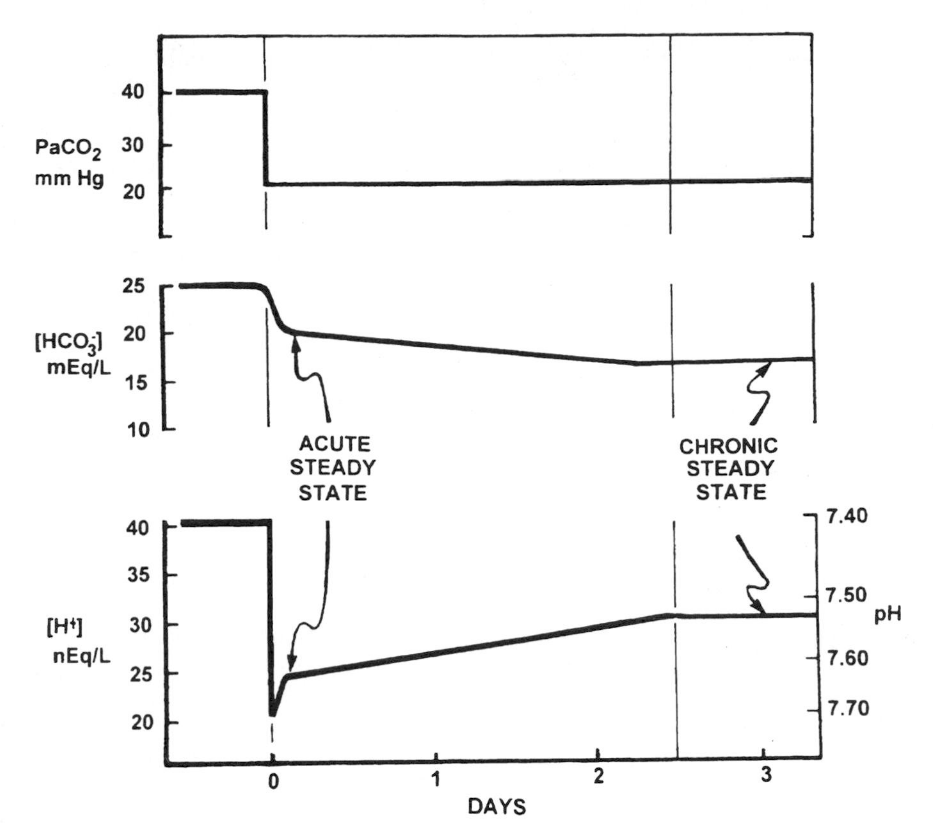


**FIGURE 9–3** ■ Schematic time course of the changes in plasma acid-base equilibrium during the generation of respiratory alkalosis. In this scheme, it is assumed that a $\Delta Pa_{CO_2}$ of 20 mm Hg is produced abruptly and maintained unchanged thereafter.

were to decrease to 10 mm Hg while plasma $[HCO_3^-]$ remained unchanged, blood pH would be:

$$[H^+] = 24 \times 10/24$$

$$[H^+] = 10 \text{ nEq/L or pH} = 8.0$$

The level of alkalemia projected to occur under this theoretical condition is incompatible with life.

Fortunately, hypocapnia elicits adaptive decrements in the plasma bicarbonate concentration that serve to ameliorate the resultant alkalemia. The time course of the changes in acid-base equilibrium associated with respiratory alkalosis is shown in Figure 9–3. An immediate decrement in plasma bicarbonate occurs in response to hypocapnia. This acute adaptation is complete within 5 to 10 minutes from the onset of hypocapnia. No further detectable changes in acid-base equilibrium occur for a period of several hours, thus establishing an operational "acute steady state."[8–11] The acute adaptation is accounted for mainly by alkaline titration of the body's nonbicarbonate buffers acting in concert with changes in the activity of cell membrane acid-base transporters and, to a lesser extent, by increased production of organic acids, notably lactic acid. When hypocapnia is sustained, renal adjustments cause an additional decrease in plasma bicarbonate further ameliorating the resulting alkalemia.[1, 12]

**Acute Respiratory Alkalosis.** The adjustment in acid-base equilibrium following the induction of acute hypocapnia and the resultant alkalemia originates totally from nonrenal mechanisms that acidify body fluids by decreasing the bicarbonate concentration in the extracellular and intracellular compartments. As noted earlier, the buffering response, changes in cell membrane transporters, and increased production of organic acids participate in the defense of body acidity.

Evidence indicates that approximately one third of the secondary acidifying response to acute respiratory alkalosis, as reflected by the decrease in extracellular bicarbonate concentration, can be ascribed to red blood cell and extracellular protein buffering; the remainder is attributed to tissue buffering and other cellular processes.[7, 13, 14] The hypocapnia-induced alkalemia results in the immediate release of protons from hemoglobin and plasma proteins that decrease plasma bicarbonate levels, as follows:

$$HBuf \rightarrow H^+ + Buf^-$$

$$HCO_3^- + H^+ \rightarrow H_2CO_3 \rightarrow H_2O + CO_2$$

As a result, a gradient that favors the transfer of bicarbonate from the interstitial compartment to the blood develops, which diminishes the net acidifying effect of blood buffers. The contribution of tissue buffering and other cellular processes to the secondary decrement in extracellular bicarbonate concentration, although large, remains incompletely defined.

When examining the effects of changes in $CO_2$ tension in body fluids, it is assumed that $CO_2$ and $HCO_3^-$ are essentially always at equilibrium in both the extracellular and intracellular compartments. This assumption is reasonable, because carbonic anhydrase is present in most cells and greatly speeds up the hydration of $CO_2$; although slower, even the uncatalyzed reaction achieves equilibrium in only a few seconds.[15] Observations in intracellular pH transients of a barnacle muscle fiber during $CO_2$ loading and unloading have shown wide fluctuations in cell acidity (decreases and increases in cell pH, respectively) that challenge the intracellular buffers.[16] Upon removal of $CO_2/HCO_3^-$ from the bathing solution, $CO_2$ passively diffuses out of the fiber, whereas most of the intracellular $HCO_3^-$ combines with $H^+$ (released during the alkaline titration of the intracellular nonbicarbonate buffers) and also leaves the cell as $CO_2$. The prompt increase in intracellular pH in response to hypocapnia (and its decrease in hypercapnia) reflects the high permeability of cell plasma membranes to carbon dioxide and the low permeability to bicarbonate. However, such permeabilities are not universally present, as demonstrated in the apical membranes of parietal and chief cells of gastric glands that are almost impermeable to both carbon dioxide and bicarbonate.[17]

Changes in the activity of cell membrane acid-base transporters, including the cation-$H^+$ exchangers and the $HCO_3^-$-dependent transporters, occur in response to an acid-base stress and are aimed at restoring the intracellular pH.[18] Several of these transporters must participate in the cellular response to acute hypocapnia, including the defense of intracellular pH and the transferring of a sizable net load of protons to the extracellular compartment. Two types of cation-$H^+$ exchangers have been described: (1) the alkalinizing $Na^+$-$H^+$ exchanger, and (2) the acidifying $K^+$-$H^+$ exchanger. In vivo, the $Na^+$-$H^+$ exchanger (NHE-1, which has a ubiquitous localization) promotes cellular $H^+$ exit in association with $Na^+$ entry. Most $Na^+$-$H^+$ exchangers normally operate at near saturation with respect to external sodium, such that changes in $Na^+$ concentration hardly change their activity.[19] On the other hand, the pH of the cell is the most important regulator of the activity of the $Na^+$-$H^+$ exchanger, because protons, independently of their role as substrate, also bind the exchanger allosterically.[20] Hypocapnia-induced intracellular alkalinization inhibits the $Na^+$-$H^+$ exchange, thus promoting the retention of protons within the cell and limiting the increase of intracellular pH by lowering the intracellular bicarbonate concentration. It is, therefore, unlikely that this transporter contributes substantially to the net transfer of protons to the extracellular compartment.

The $K^+$-$H^+$ exchanger in vivo promotes cellular entry of $H^+$ in association with $K^+$ exit. Limited information is available about the distribution of this transporter and its role in the whole-body response to an acid-base stress. In corneal epithelial cells, the $K^+$-$H^+$ exchanger mediates the cell pH recovery from an alkaline load.[21] The role of this transporter in the cellular response to acute hypocapnia remains undefined.

Several $HCO_3^-$-dependent transporters are involved in cell pH regulation. The $Na^+$-independent $Cl^-$-$HCO_3^-$ exchanger, present in various cells (known as band 3 protein in erythrocytes), promotes the cellular entry of $Cl^-$ in association with $HCO_3^-$ exit, thus resulting in acidification of the cytoplasm.[22] Because this exchanger is activated by an alkaline intracellular pH, it might participate in the defense of cell pH during acute hypocapnia.[23] Conversely, the $Na^+$-dependent $Cl^-$-$HCO_3^-$ exchanger promotes cellular alkalinization (e.g., skeletal muscle), because it mediates the net influx of $HCO_3^-$ with $Na^+$ and efflux of chloride.[24–27] It is conceivable that this transporter contributes to the transfer of extracellular bicarbonate to the intracellular compartment during acute respiratory alkalosis (a process equivalent to proton entry into the extracellular compartment).

Finally, $Na^+$-$HCO_3^-$ and $K^+$-$HCO_3^-$ cotransporters exist in many cells and serve different acid-base functions depending on the particular cell in which they reside.[28–30] Although no information is available, these cotransporters might variably participate in the recovery of cell pH and the cellular entry of extracellular bicarbonate during acute hypocapnia.

"Whole-body" intracellular hydrogen ion concentration, as assessed by the 5,5-dimethyl-2,4-oxazolidinedione (DMO) method, has been found to fall in parallel with extracellular hydrogen ion concentration when healthy human subjects hyperventilate voluntarily to achieve a $Pa_{CO_2}$ of 15 to 20 mm Hg.[31] Similar results have been obtained from studies in dog and rat muscle[13, 32, 33] and rat brain.[34] On the other hand, $^{31}$P-nuclear magnetic resonance (NMR) spectroscopy has revealed much smaller changes in canine heart intracellular pH in response to acute hypocapnia compared with the extracellular compartment.[35]

Several investigators have attributed a major component (on the order of 50% to 75%) of the reduction in plasma bicarbonate during acute hypocapnia to the accumulation of organic acids, notably lactic acid; this conclusion was based on studies in anesthetized animals subjected to sufficient mechanical ventilation to achieve severe hypocapnia ($Pa_{CO_2}$ <15 mm Hg).[14, 36–40] By contrast, studies in unanesthetized animals and in humans subjected to milder degrees of hypocapnia ($Pa_{CO_2}$ of 20 to 30 mm Hg) have failed to support this contention; these studies report only a mild (in the range of 0.5 to 1.5 mEq/L) and short-lived elevation in plasma lactate concentration.[8–10, 41–43] In all probability, the large increase in lactate observed by some reflects a degree of circulatory insufficiency consequent to the cardiovascular effects of anesthesia and vigorous mechanical ventilation. Plasma lactate concentration increased by 2 mEq/L when a hypoxia-induced acute decrement in $Pa_{CO_2}$ of 10 mm Hg was superimposed on chronic, diuretic-induced metabolic alkalosis in the dog; hyperlactatemia persisted during the chronic phase of this mixed disorder.[44] That some elevation in lactate might be induced by hypocapnia per se is a reasonable expectation in view of the enhanced net production of lactic acid known to occur when intracellular pH increases sufficiently to stimulate 6-phosphofructokinase activity. This is an expression of a homeostatic system that was presumably designed to limit deviations in systemic acidity by pH-mediated changes in organic-acid production.[45]

Figure 9–4 depicts the 95% confidence limits for

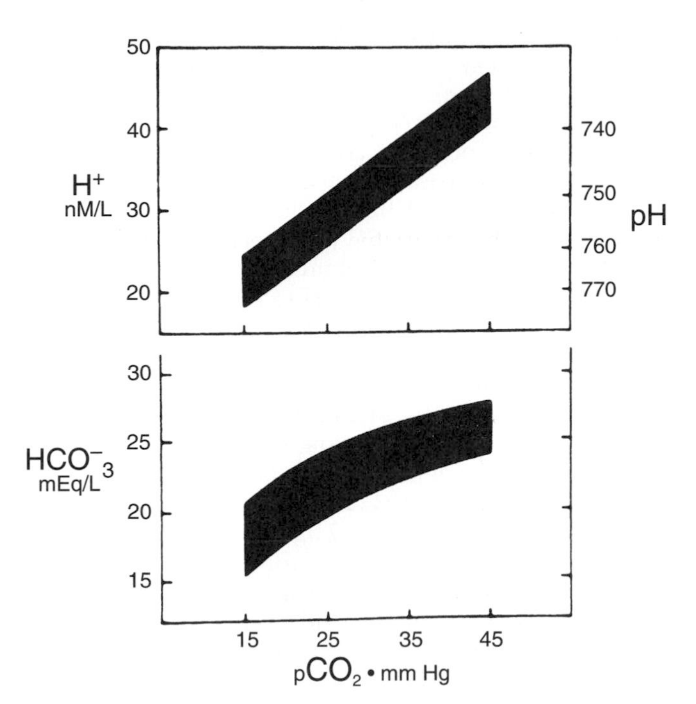


**FIGURE 9–4** ■ Ninety-five percent confidence limits for plasma bicarbonate concentration *(lower panel)* and plasma hydrogen ion concentration *(upper panel)* in acute respiratory alkalosis. The limits were calculated from data obtained in anesthetized patients who were passively hyperventilated during minor surgical procedures. (From Arbus GS, Hebert LA, Levesque PR, et al: Characterization and clinical application of the "significance band" for acute respiratory alkalosis. N Engl J Med 280:117, 1969.)

plasma bicarbonate concentration and hydrogen ion concentration in uncomplicated acute respiratory alkalosis of graded severity. These limits represent the range of responses within which acid-base equilibrium would be expected to fall if an acute reduction in $Pa_{CO_2}$ were the only factor disturbing plasma acidity. The data from which these limits were calculated were obtained during the course of acute, "whole-body" titration experiments using passive hyperventilation of anesthetized human subjects undergoing minor surgical procedures.[8] The acute, secondary change in plasma bicarbonate concentration is substantially greater in magnitude than that observed during acute hypercapnia of comparable degree, falling by approximately 0.2 mEq/L for each 1 mm Hg acute decrement in $Pa_{CO_2}$; thus, a reduction in plasma bicarbonate of approximately 3 to 4 mEq/L occurs within minutes after $Pa_{CO_2}$ is lowered to 20 to 25 mm Hg. The resultant change in blood hydrogen ion concentration, however, is strikingly similar to that observed during acute hypercapnia. On average, blood hydrogen ion concentration decreases by approximately 0.75 nEq/L for each 1 mm Hg acute reduction in $Pa_{CO_2}$. Thus, acute adaptation to a $Pa_{CO_2}$ of 20 mm Hg in a subject with a normal acid-base equilibrium at baseline will yield, on average, a plasma bicarbonate level of 20 mEq/L and a hydrogen ion concentration of 24 nEq/L (pH 7.62) (see Fig. 9–4).

**Chronic Respiratory Alkalosis.** If hypocapnia persists, plasma bicarbonate concentration falls further as a consequence of renal adaptive responses, which entail a dampening of hydrogen ion secretion by the renal tubule. As a result, a transient suppression of net acid excretion occurs, manifested mainly by a fall in ammonium excretion and, early on, by an increase in bicarbonate excretion. Transient bicarbonaturia and a rise in urinary pH occur when hypocapnia develops abruptly but not in response to gradually evolving hypocapnia. These changes in net acid excretion, in turn, lead to positive hydrogen ion balance and a reduction in the body's bicarbonate stores. Maintenance of the resultant hypobicarbonatemia is ensured by the gradual suppression in the rate of renal bicarbonate reabsorption, which is itself a reflection of the hypocapnia-induced decrease in tubular hydrogen ion secretory rate.[1, 10, 12, 46–48] A new, chronic steady state emerges when the reduced filtered load of bicarbonate is precisely balanced by the dampened rate of bicarbonate reabsorption and net acid excretion has returned to the level required to offset daily endogenous acid production.[1, 10, 12, 46–48]

Micropuncture and microperfusion studies have documented suppressed proximal and distal acidification during acute hypocapnia, including decreased proximal bicarbonate reabsorption and depressed formation and delivery of ammonium and titratable acid.[49–52] Reduced proximal bicarbonate reabsorption was also demonstrated by micropuncture in chronic hypocapnia,[53] but distal acidification has not been examined with these techniques in the chronic form of the disorder. A reduction in systemic $P_{CO_2}$ also leads to a disproportionate reduction in renal cortical $P_{CO_2}$ and augmentation of proximal chloride reabsorption.

Regarding the cellular mechanisms mediating the downregulation of renal acidification during chronic hypocapnia, parallel decreases in the rates of the luminal $Na^+$-$H^+$ exchanger (presumably the NHE-3) (Fig. 9–5) and the basolateral $Na^+$-$3HCO_3^-$ cotransporter in the proximal tubule have been found reflecting a decrease in $V_{max}$ of each transporter but no change in the Km for sodium.[54, 55] Moreover, hypocapnia induces endocytotic retrieval of $H^+$-ATPase pumps from the luminal membrane of the proximal tubule cells as well as type A intercalated cells of cortical and medullary collecting tubules.[56] In tubule microdissection studies in the rat, the activity of the $H^+$-ATPase along the entire nephron and that of the $H^+$-$K^+$-ATPase in the cortical and medullary collecting tubules were decreased by 6 hours of hypocapnia and thereafter.[57] The inhibitory effect of hypocapnia on the renal proton ATPases appears to be independent of potassium and aldosterone.[57]

The adaptive acid retention during sustained hypocapnia is normally accompanied by a loss of sodium into the urine.[10, 46, 47, 58] The resultant loss of extracellular fluid has been proposed as being responsible for the hyperchloremia that typically attends chronic respiratory alkalosis. When a new steady state emerges, renal net acid excretion returns to control levels and the altered anionic picture of the extracellular fluid, namely, hypobicarbonatemia and hyperchloremia, is maintained by a reduced bicarbonate reabsorption and

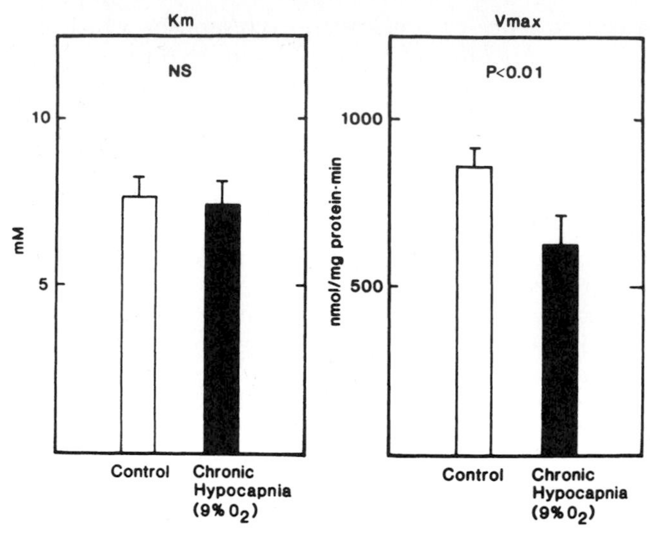


**FIGURE 9–5** ■ Kinetic characteristics of rabbit renal cortical brush-border membrane vesicle $Na^+$-$H^+$ exchanger in animals adapted to chronic hypocapnia (9% $O_2$) *(shaded bars)* or in paired, contemporaneous controls *(open bars)*. Data on Km for sodium are depicted on the left, and those on Vmax are shown on the right. Data represent means ± SE for seven paired sets of rabbits. Chronic hypocapnia resulted in a significant decrease in the Vmax of the exchanger, whereas the Km for sodium remained unaltered. (From Hilden SA, Johns CA, Madias NE: Adaptation of rabbit renal cortical $Na^+$-$H^+$ exchange activity in chronic hypocapnia. Am J Physiol 257: F615, 1989.)

an enhanced chloride reabsorption. In the presence of dietary sodium restriction, acid retention is achieved in the company of increased potassium, rather than increased sodium, excretion. If both sodium and potassium are restricted, phosphate retention rather than cation loss accompanies the renal acid retention during adaptation to hypocapnia.[46, 47] There is no appreciable change in plasma lactate during chronic hypocapnia even in the presence of moderate hypoxemia.[10, 46, 58–62]

Evidence suggests that the renal adaptation to persistent hypocapnia is likely to be mediated not by changes in blood or "whole-body" intracellular pH but by some direct effect of reduced $Pa_{CO_2}$ itself.[63–65] Thus, animals in which plasma bicarbonate had been substantially reduced before adaptation to sustained hypocapnia (by means of the chronic administration of a large HCl load) evidenced the same renal response to a primary reduction in $Pa_{CO_2}$ as normal animals, even though the net effect of such adaptation was an overt fall in blood pH (Fig. 9–6).[64]

Approximately 2 to 3 days are required for the completion of the renal response to hypocapnia (see Fig. 9–3). These adaptive mechanisms serve to produce and maintain the reduction in plasma bicarbonate characteristic of the new, chronic steady state and result in a highly predictable relationship between the degree of chronic hypocapnia and the level at which plasma bicarbonate stabilizes; it has been shown in the dog that each 1 mm Hg chronic reduction in $Pa_{CO_2}$ is associated with a fall in plasma bicarbonate concentration averaging 0.4 to 0.5 mEq/L.[46, 64, 65] Similarly, limited data in humans (patients subjected to chronic hypocapnia, high-altitude dwellers, volunteers studied at high altitude or at simulated altitude) have indicated that plasma bicarbonate decreases, on average, by approximately 0.4 mEq/L for each 1 mm Hg chronic decrease in $Pa_{CO_2}$.[58, 60, 62, 66–68] Despite the similarity in the magnitude of the secondary response of plasma bicarbonate to chronic hypocapnia between dogs and humans, the resultant impact on blood hydrogen ion concentration is substantially disparate: Whereas in the dog blood hydrogen ion concentration falls by only 0.17 nEq/L for each 1 mm Hg chronic reduction in $Pa_{CO_2}$,[46] the corresponding decrease in humans is on the order of 0.4 nEq/L.[58] The main reason for this discrepancy is the higher baseline level of plasma bicarbonate in humans (24 to 25 mEq/L versus 21 mEq/L in the dog). Thus, chronic adaptation to a $Pa_{CO_2}$ of 20 mm Hg in humans will yield, on average, a plasma bicarbonate of 16 mEq/L and a hydrogen ion concentration of 30 nEq/L (pH 7.52) (see Fig. 9–3). Currently no sufficient data exist for constructing confidence limits for chronic respiratory alkalosis in humans over a reasonably wide range of $Pa_{CO_2}$. The response of intracellular acidity to chronic hypocapnia has not been studied.

## PLASMA AND EXTRACELLULAR FLUID VOLUME

Plasma volume remains unchanged or decreases in animals with acute respiratory alkalosis; the decrease might be due to a rise in either capillary hydrostatic pressure or capillary permeability.[69, 70] Humans with hypocapnia caused by voluntary hyperventilation experience a reduction in plasma volume that results from fluid shifts into extravascular compartments.[71] When hypocapnia is sustained, plasma and interstitial fluid volumes decrease by 10% to 25%, presumably the consequence of the urinary sodium losses that occur during adaptation to the disorder.[10, 46, 58] A chronic decrease in $Pa_{CO_2}$ of 8 mm Hg in humans who ascended to high altitude resulted in a sodium deficit of about 150 mmol over a 6-day period.[58] Hypovolemia occurs irrespective of whether hypoxemia accompanies chronic hypocapnia. During prolonged exposure to high altitude, the hypoxemia-induced increase in red blood cell mass returns blood volume to normal or even a slightly expanded state despite the persistent reduction in plasma volume.

## PLASMA ELECTROLYTE COMPOSITION DURING RESPIRATORY ALKALOSIS

Mild hyponatremia ($\Delta[Na^+]$, 2 to 4 mEq/L) has been noted in acute hypocapnia,[8, 14] but plasma sodium concentration remains normal during chronic hypocapnia.[46, 58] Hyperchloremia, which is a consistent finding in respiratory alkalosis, reflects largely the chloride shift from erythrocytes during the acute state[8, 14] and the volume contraction accompanying the renal response during the chronic stage.[46]

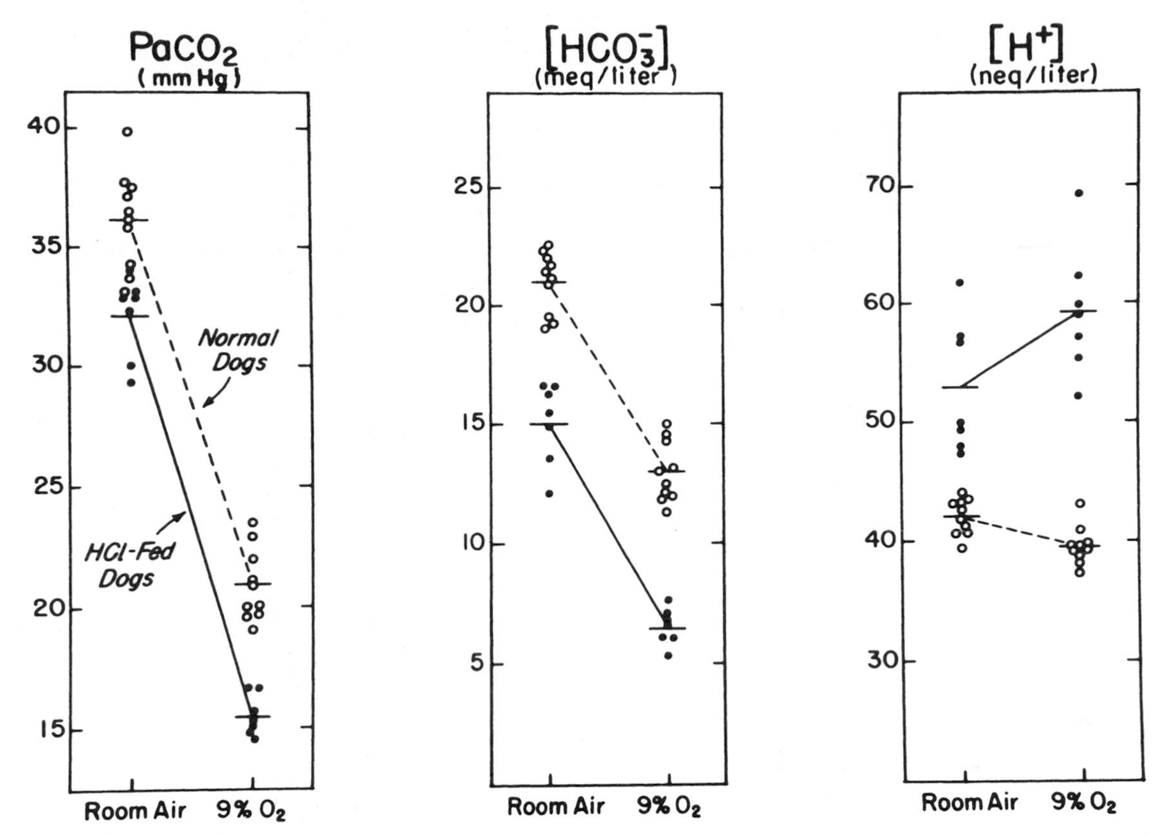


**FIGURE 9–6** ■ Changes in plasma bicarbonate concentration and hydrogen ion concentration during prolonged exposure to hypocapnia in normal dogs *(dashed lines)* and in dogs with chronic HCl-acidosis *(solid lines)*. Similar decrements in $Pa{CO_2}$ in the two groups produced nearly equivalent reductions in plasma bicarbonate concentration, despite divergent effects on hydrogen ion concentration. (From Cohen JJ, Madias NE, Wolf CJ, et al: Regulation of acid-base equilibrium in chronic hypocapnia: Evidence that the response of the kidney is not geared to the defense of extracellular [$H^+$]. J Clin Invest 57:1483, 1976.)

Acute respiratory alkalosis induced by mechanical hyperventilation under general anesthesia leads to a decrement in plasma potassium concentration in both animals and humans. Under these conditions, plasma potassium concentration decreases by approximately 0.1 to 0.4 mEq/L for each 0.1 unit rise in pH.[72, 73] The mechanism of the observed hypokalemia most likely involves both a shift of potassium into the cells and transient kaliuresis accompanying bicarbonaturia.[10, 72–74] The augmented bicarbonate excretion lasts only hours and becomes more evident when hypocapnia develops abruptly.[10, 74] When acute respiratory alkalosis is induced by voluntary hyperventilation in normal humans a mild (~0.3 mEq/L) but significant increase in plasma potassium is observed.[75] This hyperkalemic response appears paradoxic, because it occurs in association with alkalemia; it is likely to be the result of increased α-adrenergic activity. A concomitant increase in β-adrenergic activity is observed under these conditions, and the response appears to ameliorate the resultant hyperkalemia.[75]

No appreciable changes in serum potassium occur during chronic hypocapnia in the dog or in humans at sea level.[1, 46] On the other hand, a persistent reduction in plasma potassium concentration (on the order of 0.5 mEq/L) was detected in human subjects during chronic hypocapnia induced by exposure to high altitude (Δ $Pa{CO_2}$, 8 mm Hg).[58] In the new steady state, renal potassium excretion was at the baseline level, despite the reduction in plasma potassium, and no change occurred in urinary aldosterone and cortisol excretion rates. The mechanism of this apparent renal potassium wasting remains unexplained.

Mild hypophosphatemia is a characteristic feature of acute hypocapnia and reflects translocation of phosphate into cells; however, no consistent changes in serum phosphate have been noted in chronic hypocapnia.[8, 46, 76–79] Despite the hypophosphatemia, acute respiratory alkalosis decreases the fractional excretion of phosphate, and this response is blunted by β-adrenoreceptor blockers.[80] Mild reduction in ionized calcium occurs in acute hypocapnia because of an alkalemia-induced increase in protein binding of serum calcium; although this decrease could not account by itself for the tetany and seizures that occasionally attend acute hypocapnia,[81] it might play a contributory role. Serum total calcium and magnesium concentrations remain normal during persistent hypocapnia.[77, 82, 83] However, one study has identified several changes in divalent ion homeostasis during chronic hypocapnia in humans induced by exposure to high altitude.[77] Hyperphosphatemia and decreased serum ionized calcium concentration were observed in the company of decreased phosphate clearance and increased fractional excretion of calcium. Serum intact parathyroid hormone (PTH) and 1,25 $(OH)_2$ $D_3$ levels remained unchanged, but the excretion of nephrogenous cyclic adenosine 3′,5′-monophosphate (cAMP) decreased. It was concluded that chronic hypocapnia induced impaired renal tubular responsiveness to PTH and defective PTH secretion (as defined by the failure of the hormone levels to rise in response to the prevailing decrease in serum ionized calcium). Serum magnesium levels were unchanged but sustained hypomagnesuria and decreased fractional excretion of magnesium occurred during chronic hypocapnia.[77]

As noted earlier, only a mild and transient elevation in plasma lactate concentration occurs during acute hypocapnia,[8–10, 41–43] and there is no appreciable change in plasma lactate during chronic hypocapnia.[10, 46, 59–62] Plasma unmeasured anions do not change notably in acute hypocapnia, but small increases (on the order of 3 mEq/L for a 20 mm Hg chronic reduction in $Pa_{CO_2}$) have been observed in chronic respiratory alkalosis.[46, 58, 60, 62] The source of this increase remains unidentified.

## CEREBROSPINAL FLUID COMPOSITION DURING RESPIRATORY ALKALOSIS

The acidity of the cerebrospinal fluid (CSF) is in equilibrium with the brain interstitial fluid and plays a critical role in the regulation of respiration; therefore, the changes in pH in the CSF have been the subject of intensive investigation.[84] CSF hydrogen ion and bicarbonate concentrations fall in parallel with those of arterial blood during induction of acute hypocapnia.[59, 84–89] The magnitude of the reduction in hydrogen ion concentration in the CSF of the dog is similar to that observed in the arterial blood.[86–88]

The fall in CSF bicarbonate concentration is accompanied by an increase in CSF chloride concentration, which accounts for 75% of the change in the level of bicarbonate, and a mild rise in CSF lactate concentration that accounts for the remaining 25%.[90] Several investigators have noted a widening of the CSF-arterial $P_{CO_2}$ difference during acute hypocapnia, resulting from a lesser fall of $P_{CO_2}$ in CSF than in blood.[84, 89, 91–94] This effect is thought to be secondary to the decrease in cerebral blood flow associated with hypocapnia.[91, 95]

Studies of the response of CSF acidity during chronic hypocapnia have yielded variable results. Earlier studies demonstrated that CSF pH during chronic respiratory alkalosis deviated minimally from control despite systemic alkalemia.[96–98] More recent studies, however, have shown reductions in CSF hydrogen ion and bicarbonate concentrations that are similar to those of arterial blood.[59, 61, 99, 100]

## PATHOPHYSIOLOGIC CONSEQUENCES AND CLINICAL MANIFESTATIONS OF RESPIRATORY ALKALOSIS

**Respiratory System.** A primary decrease in $Pa_{CO_2}$ and the attendant increase in pH characteristic of acute respiratory alkalosis cause a shift to the left in the oxyhemoglobin dissociation curve (Bohr effect), resulting in an impediment of oxygen unloading to the tissues but an enhancement of oxygen loading in the lungs.[101–103] During chronic alkalosis, however, these effects are offset by a shift of the curve to the right produced by an increased intracorpuscular concentration of 2,3-diphosphoglycerate (2,3-DPG).[101, 104–106] Despite the impediment of oxygen unloading to the tissues in acute hypocapnia, oxygen consumption ($\dot{V}O_2$) was found to increase by approximately 12% in anesthetized and paralyzed patients during hyperventilation-induced alkalosis.[107] The mechanism of this response remains undetermined. Acute respiratory alkalosis induces a substantial bronchial constrictive effect that is eliminated by nicardipine, a calcium channel blocker.[108] In addition, the control of pulmonary vascular resistance is altered during hypocapnia. Whereas acute respiratory alkalosis attenuates the pulmonary vasoconstriction induced by hypoxemia, prolonged hypocapnia (~100 minutes) has the opposite effect.[109] It has been proposed that the enhanced vascular reactivity after prolonged respiratory alkalosis reflects increased cytosolic free calcium concentration secondary to augmented extracellular calcium influx and/or calcium released from intracellular stores.[109]

**Cardiovascular and Renal Systems.** Myocardial contractility assessed in isolated perfused hearts increases initially but rapidly returns to control levels in acute respiratory alkalosis.[110–112] The switch from the state of augmented contractility is not dependent on the activity of the myocardial $Na^+$-$H^+$ exchanger or the $Cl^-$-$HCO_3^-$ exchanger, because blockers of these transporters (amiloride, SITS) did not prevent the biphasic mechanical response.[113] Changes in both cytosolic pH and calcium concentration appear to play a major role in this response.[114] In the isolated rat heart, hypocapnia enhances postischemic calcium gain, an effect that is considered nonsalutary.[115]

The induction of acute hypocapnia in anesthetized subjects results in a decrease in cardiac output, an increase in peripheral resistance, and a fall in the systemic blood pressure.[116–118] By contrast, active hyperventilation in humans does not change, or might even increase, cardiac output and leaves systemic blood pressure virtually unchanged.[119–122] The discrepant response of cardiac output during passive compared with active hyperventilation probably reflects the decrement in venous return due to the effects of mechanical ventilation in the former and the reflex tachycardia consistently observed in the latter. Sustained hypocapnia induced by exposure to high altitude for several weeks results in a cardiac output equal to or higher than control values.[123–125] Although acute hypocapnia does not lead to cardiac arrhythmias in normal volunteers, it appears that it contributes to the generation of both atrial and ventricular tachyarrhythmias in patients with ischemic heart disease[126]; such arrhythmias are frequently resistant to standard forms of therapy. Chest pain and ischemic ST-T wave changes have been observed in acutely hyperventilating subjects with no evidence of fixed lesions on coronary angiography.[127–132]

The pathogenesis of these manifestations remains unknown, although myocardial ischemia secondary to hypocapnia-induced vasoconstriction and an alkalemia-induced shift to the left of the oxyhemoglobin dissociation curve have been proposed. Indeed, acute hypocapnia has been shown to induce coronary artery spasm and Prinzmetal angina in susceptible patients.[133, 134]

Hypocapnia produces variable effects on regional blood flows. Acute respiratory alkalosis decreases myocardial, cerebral, dermal, and renal blood flows, but it increases muscle blood flow.[92, 119–122, 135–137] Insufficient data exist with regard to the effects of persistent hypocapnia on the distribution of blood flow, but it appears that dermal and renal blood flow remain depressed, whereas muscle and liver perfusion are increased.[138–141] For reasons that remain unknown, chronic hypocapnia leads to increased responsiveness of the kidney to antidiuretic hormone administration; water retention exceeds that of normocapnic animals, resulting in the rapid development of severe hyponatremia.[142]

**Neurologic System and the Cerebral Circulation.** Acute changes in $Pa_{CO_2}$ between 20 and 80 mm Hg result in parallel changes in cerebral blood flow of 1 to 2 $mL \cdot 100\ g^{-1} \cdot min^{-1} \cdot mm\ Hg\ P_{CO_2}^{-1}$ in humans.[143–155] Such an effect indicates a substantial responsiveness of the cerebral circulation to changes in $CO_2$ tension. Because decreased $CO_2$ tension constricts cerebral arteries in vitro, the resultant increased vascular tone must be mediated by mechanisms located in the blood vessel wall itself.[156–158] The $CO_2$-induced vascular response appears to be triggered by changes in the pH of vascular smooth muscle and not by the altered $CO_2$ tension.[156, 157, 159, 160] Removal of the endothelium in vitro or endothelial damage in vivo does not alter the vascular response to acute changes in $CO_2$ tension in adult animals.[161, 162] In neonates, however, the endothelium contributes to the effects of $CO_2$ on the cerebral circulation.[163, 164] Hypotension to less than the lower limit of autoregulation can abolish the response of the cerebral blood flow to acute hypocapnia.[165, 166]

Vascular smooth muscle tone is ultimately controlled by the intracellular calcium concentration.[167] During acute respiratory alkalosis, cerebrovascular smooth muscle calcium levels increase by mechanisms that might include changes in potassium channels, nitric oxide, cyclic nucleotides, and prostanoids; the end result is augmentation in cerebrovascular tone.[167]

The open-state probability of adenosine triphosphate (ATP)-sensitive potassium ($K_{ATP}$) channels in cerebral arteries is pH dependent, and alkalemia deactivates these channels.[168–170] The closure of $K_{ATP}$ channels reduces the diffusion of potassium out of the cell, making the vascular smooth muscle cytosol less electronegative (depolarized). Upon depolarization, voltage-gated calcium channels increase the influx of extracellular calcium, thus increasing intracellular calcium concentration and augmenting vascular smooth muscle tone.

Nitric oxide of neuronal origin also participates in the effects of $CO_2$ on cerebral vessels.[167] Acute respiratory alkalosis can reduce production of nitric oxide, a potent vasodilator that controls the concentration of a vasodilatory cyclic nucleotide (cGMP) and the activity of $K_{ATP}$ channels. In addition, nitric oxide increases the concentration of cAMP, another vasodilatory compound; thus, the decrease in nitric oxide in acute respiratory alkalosis can depress cAMP levels, which in turn promote vasoconstriction.[171, 172]

In awake humans, active hyperventilation to a $Pa_{CO_2}$ of 16 mm Hg reduced cerebral blood flow by 40% initially, but blood flow recovered to within 10% of baseline after 4 hours of sustained hypocapnia.[173] Furthermore, acute termination of sustained hyperventilation can result in cerebral hyperemia and increased intracranial pressure. To avoid these complications, $Pa_{CO_2}$ should be normalized over a period of hours after sustained hypocapnia. Under normal conditions, $P_{CO_2}$ in brain interstitial fluid is slightly higher, and pH and bicarbonate levels are slightly lower than arterial values.[173, 174] When acute hyperventilation is induced, brain alkalosis results in cerebral vasoconstriction, with consequent reduction in cerebral blood flow, cerebral blood volume, and intracranial pressure. After 6 to 12 hours of sustained hypocapnia, brain extracellular pH recovers almost to baseline levels due to a reduction in bicarbonate concentration.[167] At that time, cerebral vascular tone has recovered to baseline, thus restoring cerebral blood flow, cerebral blood volume, and intracranial pressure to normal levels. If hyperventilation is acutely terminated, marked brain extracellular acidosis occurs due to both an acute rise in $P_{CO_2}$ and a persistent reduction in bicarbonate concentration; the resultant cerebral vasodilatation leads to increases in cerebral blood flow, cerebral blood volume, and possibly intracranial pressure.

The reduction in cerebral blood volume induced by hyperventilation in humans is 0.049 $ml^{-1} \cdot 100\ g^{-1} \cdot mm\ Hg\ P_{CO_2}^{-1}$. This process is responsible for the decreased intracranial pressure observed with hypocapnia.[175] Hyperventilation (i.e., $Pa_{CO_2}$ 20 to 25 mm Hg) can reduce cerebral blood flow to a level associated with mild cerebral ischemia, impairing mental function and slowing electroencephalogram (EEG).[176–179] In addition, mild alkalosis shifts the oxyhemoglobin dissociation curve to the left, further limiting oxygen delivery to the brain. In fact, many investigators consider the hypocapnia-induced changes in mental activity and EEG to result from cerebral ischemia. However, hypocapnia (i.e., $Pa_{CO_2}$ 10 to 20 mm Hg) does not change the cerebral metabolic rate or brain levels of high-energy compounds, such as ATP and phosphocreatine.[180–182] Consequently, in the normal brain, hypocapnia does not lead to gross disturbances in brain oxidative metabolism, although the long-term effect of hyperventilation (e.g., permanent functional disturbances, loss of neurons) remains unknown.

Manipulation of $Pa_{CO_2}$ is commonly used in both the operating room and the intensive care unit to treat increased intracranial pressure or correct cerebral ischemia. Intraoperative hyperventilation might help to control increased intracranial pressure, offset the effect of inhaled anesthetics (i.e., agents that tend to increase intracranial pressure), and enhance operative exposure. However, intraoperative hyperventilation has not been evaluated rigorously, and the effect on patient outcome is unknown. After head injury, acute hyperventilation can reduce increased intracranial pressure and, as a result, cerebral perfusion can increase. However, this effect is countered by the direct property of acute alkalosis to reduce cerebral blood flow. There is no objective evidence that hyperventilation improves outcome in patients with head injury.[183] Current recommendations are to avoid prophylactic hyperventilation in brain-injured patients and to reserve hyperventilation to treat increased intracranial pressure that cannot be controlled by other methods.

Various clinical manifestations frequently occur in acute hypocapnia, but these are seldom evident in the chronic phase of the disorder. A rapid decrement in $PaCO_2$ to half-normal values or lower is typically accompanied by numbness and paresthesias of the extremities, chest oppression, circumoral numbness, lightheadedness, and mental confusion; muscle cramps, increased deep-tendon reflexes, carpopedal spasm, and generalized seizures occur infrequently.[1, 79, 83, 120, 184–186] The neurologic manifestations of acute respiratory alkalosis have been attributed largely to the attendant cerebral hypoperfusion, although additional factors have been implicated, including alkalemia, the pH-induced shift to the left of the oxyhemoglobin dissociation curve, and the decrements in the levels of ionized calcium and potassium. A characteristic electroencephalographic picture consisting of generalized slowing and high-voltage wave forms has been described.[120, 187, 188] Brain and CSF lactate concentrations have been found to increase by amounts greater than those in the systemic circulation and to remain slightly increased during persistent hypocapnia.[39, 59, 61, 88, 98, 189, 190] Increased synthesis of lactate is consequent to cerebral hypoxia resulting from the intense vasoconstricting effects of hypocapnia and, probably, to alkalemia-induced acceleration of anaerobic glycolysis.

**TABLE 9–1.** Causes of Respiratory Alkalosis

|  |  |
| --- | --- |
| **Hypoxemia or Tissue Hypoxia** | Decreased inspired $O_2$ tension |
| | High altitude |
| | Bacterial or viral pneumonia |
| | Aspiration of food, foreign body, or vomitus |
| | Laryngospasm |
| | Drowning |
| | Cyanotic heart disease |
| | Severe anemia |
| | Left shift deviation of the $HbO_2$ curve |
| | Hypotension |
| | Severe circulatory failure |
| | Pulmonary edema |
| | Pseudorespiratory alkalosis |
| **Central Nervous System Stimulation** | Voluntary |
| | Pain |
| | Anxiety-hyperventilation syndrome |
| | Psychosis |
| | Fever |
| | Subarachnoid hemorrhage |
| | Cerebrovascular accident |
| | Meningoencephalitis |
| | Tumor |
| | Trauma |
| **Pulmonary Diseases with Stimulation of Chest Receptors** | Pneumonia |
| | Asthma |
| | Pneumothorax |
| | Hemothorax |
| | Flail chest |
| | Acute respiratory distress syndrome |
| | Cardiogenic and noncardiogenic pulmonary edema |
| | Pulmonary embolism |
| | Pulmonary fibrosis |
| **Drugs and Hormones** | Nikethamide, ethamivan |
| | Doxapram |
| | Xanthines |
| | Salicylates |
| | Catecholamines |
| | Angiotensin II |
| | Vasopressor agents |
| | Progesterone |
| | Medroxyprogesterone |
| | Dinitrophenol |
| | Nicotine |
| **Miscellaneous** | Pregnancy |
| | Gram-positive septicemia |
| | Gram-negative septicemia |
| | Hepatic failure |
| | Mechanical hyperventilation |
| | Heat exposure |
| | Recovery from metabolic acidosis |
| | Hemodialysis with acetate dialysate |

## CAUSES OF RESPIRATORY ALKALOSIS

Respiratory alkalosis is the most frequent acid-base disorder encountered, because it occurs in normal pregnancy and with high-altitude residence. It is also the most common acid-base abnormality in critically ill patients, occurring either as the simple disorder or as a component of mixed disturbances[4, 191–194]; indeed, in such patients, its presence constitutes a grave prognostic sign, especially if $PaCO_2$ levels are below 20 to 25 mm Hg. Table 9–1 lists the major causes of respiratory alkalosis. Most are associated with the abrupt appearance of hypocapnia, but in many cases the process might be sufficiently prolonged to permit full, chronic adaptation to occur. Consequently, no attempt has been made to separate these conditions into acute and chronic categories.

In sharp contrast with respiratory acidosis, which always reflects a serious condition, some causes of respiratory alkalosis are benign. Because blood pH levels do not exceed 7.55 in most cases of primary hypocapnia, severe manifestations of decreased systemic acidity are usually absent. Severe alkalemia, however, may be produced, particularly with maladjusted ventilators, some psychiatric conditions, and lesions involving the central nervous system.

The mechanisms by which the processes listed in Table 9–1 lead to hyperventilation differ greatly.[1, 184, 195, 196] Hypoxia stimulates ventilation through activation of peripheral chemoreceptors and might result in hypocapnia if $CO_2$ excretion is unimpeded. Such situations of hypoxia include decreased inspired oxygen tension (e.g., high-altitude residence) and conditions producing increased venous admixture and marked ventilation-perfusion inequality (e.g., bronchopulmonary disease, pulmonary edema). A reduction in $PaO_2$ below 60 mm Hg is required for hyperventilation to develop.[197]

The respiratory alkalosis observed after ascent to higher altitude has received great attention by physiologists.[198] Pulmonary ventilation increases over several days and then it reaches a new steady state. Yet, long-term residents have higher $Pa_{CO_2}$ (and lower ventilation) for a given oxygen level than those residing for a short period.[199, 200] The human tolerance to hypoxia (and the resultant extreme hyperventilation) has been evaluated in an expedition to the Himalayas.[198] Ascending to the summit of Mt. Everest (altitude 8848 m, 29,028 ft) without supplemental oxygen caused the climber to experience extreme respiratory alkalosis with $Pa_{CO_2}$ of 7.5 mm Hg (assuming that $Pa_{CO_2}$ is equal to the alveolar value), pH ranging between 7.70 and 7.80 (calculated by the Henderson-Hasselbalch equation), $Pa_{O_2}$ of 28 mm Hg, and $Sa_{O_2}$ of 70%. The corresponding levels of inspired $P_{O_2}$ and alveolar $P_{O_2}$ were 43 and 35 mm Hg, respectively. Notably, at altitudes exceeding 7000 m, the alveolar $P_{O_2}$ remained at a value of about 35 mm Hg despite the progressive reduction in inspired $P_{O_2}$; this is because of the associated progressive decrease in alveolar $P_{CO_2}$ as a result of advancing hyperventilation.[198] Furthermore, the alkalemia that the climber exhibited at extreme altitude greatly increases the oxygen affinity of the hemoglobin, thus securing a greater oxygen loading in the pulmonary capillaries. The maximal oxygen consumption at the summit of Mt. Everest is approximately 1 L/min, which is a very low value that allows slow-paced walking at that level.[198] Yet, it is sufficient to allow a climber to reach the summit.

Hypotension, especially when associated with sepsis, often causes respiratory alkalosis even in the absence of a reduced $PaO_2$.[192, 201] This phenomenon occurs because the stimulus to peripheral chemoreceptor activation is decreased oxygen delivery rather than decreased $Pa_{O_2}$. Severe anemia (hemoglobin level lower than 30% of normal) can lead to respiratory alkalosis by the same mechanism.[193] As noted earlier, severe circulatory failure in the presence of substantial pulmonary ventilation can give rise to "pseudorespiratory alkalosis," a distinct pattern of arteriovenous acid-base disparity characterized by arterial hypocapnia and alkalemia in association with venous (and tissue) hypercapnia and acidemia.[4–6]

Central nervous system–mediated hypocapnia can result from a wide variety of causes. Respiratory alkalosis can be produced through voluntary hyperventilation. The anxiety-hyperventilation syndrome can result in severe hypocapnia and alkalemia leading to the development of chest oppression, circumoral numbness, and paresthesias in the extremities. Early recognition is important, because appropriate measures might produce prompt relief.[131, 186, 202, 203] Various neurologic diseases of vascular, infectious, traumatic, or neoplastic origin can also produce hypocapnia, presumably by enhancing stimulatory inputs to ventilation or by interrupting normal inhibitory pathways.[192, 204, 205] Central hyperventilation is a distinct, extremely regular ventilatory pattern accompanying neurologic injury in the midbrain and upper pontine area that is characterized by an increase in both the depth of breathing and the respiratory rate.[204] Because these neurologic lesions are usually lethal, central hyperventilation is of grave prognostic significance.[204–207] Other ventilatory patterns accompany some equally grave lesions located in different areas. Those at the lower pontine level usually feature apneustic breathing, and lesions in the medulla are attended by irregular respiration. Yet another ventilatory pattern, known as Cheyne-Stokes respiration, is exhibited by patients with bifrontal or massive cerebral lesions,[204, 208, 209] as well as patients with cardiac failure or obesity associated with diffuse brain disease.[208, 210] A characteristic waxing-waning respiration is found in which periods of hyperventilation alternate with periods of apnea.[208] This pattern is thought to reflect isolation of the respiratory center in the brainstem from the control exerted by higher cerebral areas; the result is increased sensitivity to $CO_2$ and a respiratory rhythm in which a burst of hyperventilation causes hypocapnia, which in turn leads to a period of apnea and hypercapnia, the latter initiating a new ventilatory cycle.[208, 209, 211]

A number of pharmacologic agents can induce hyperventilation and respiratory alkalosis. Aspirin and other salicylates in doses exceeding a few grams per day can produce primary hypocapnia by direct stimulation of medullary chemoreceptors.[212–218] In cases of salicylate intoxication, respiratory alkalosis often coexists with metabolic acidosis, which arises from an accumulation of organic acids. Nikethamide, a respiratory stimulant acting directly on the respiratory center of the brainstem and, in addition, increasing the center's sensitivity to $CO_2$ and activating peripheral chemoreceptors, has been used in the treatment of $CO_2$-retaining disorders; however, the results obtained with this drug as well as other ventilatory stimulants (e.g., ethamivan, doxapram, almitrine, progesterone, and medroxyprogesterone) have been modest at best.[2, 219–224] Other drugs known to stimulate alveolar ventilation include nicotine, dinitrophenol, xanthines, and pressor hormones (e.g., epinephrine, norepinephrine, and angiotensin II[1, 225–231]). Progesterone and medroxyprogesterone are also respiratory stimulants that are presumed to act centrally.[232–234] This property of progesterone is most likely responsible for the $Pa_{CO_2}$ of normal women being lower by 2 to 3 mm Hg than that of normal men[235] and for the chronic hypocapnia characteristic of normal pregnancy (see later discussion). Progesterone is considered to be the basis of the hyperventilation that occurs during the luteal phase of the normal menstrual cycle ($\Delta Pa_{CO_2}$ of ~3 to 6 mm Hg) that is attended by a rise in blood pH and a fall in renal acid excretion.[236–239] In fact, in both pregnant and nonpregnant women, the $Pa_{CO_2}$ value is inversely related to the blood progesterone level.[238] However, estrogens may enhance the effects of progesterone on ventilation. As noted, therapeutic use of the stimulatory effect of these agents on ventilation has been made in various $CO_2$-retaining states.[220, 222, 223, 240–242]

Patients with various pulmonary diseases, including interstitial lung disease, pneumonia, pulmonary embolism, and pulmonary edema, can develop respiratory alkalosis as a result of stimulation of pulmonary receptors that signal the brainstem through ascending pathways in the vagus nerve; these receptors might be triggered by irritants (nociceptive receptors), pulmonary expansion or collapse (stretch receptors), or pulmonary capillary congestion (juxtacapillary or J receptors).[243–248] Accompanying hypoxemia, acting on peripheral arterial chemoreceptors, might also play a contributory role. Prolonged hiccuping in a patient with a tracheostomy has been reported to result in severe respiratory alkalosis.[249]

As noted previously, the chronic hypocapnia that is characteristically associated with normal pregnancy has been attributed to the physiologic effects of the high circulating levels of progesterone.[250] Measurable increases in alveolar ventilation appear early in pregnancy and, subsequently, are augmented further. On average, $Paco_2$ falls to approximately 34 mm Hg in the first trimester, to about 32 mm Hg in the second trimester, and to approximately 28 mm Hg in the third trimester, when circulating progesterone attains its highest levels.[235, 238, 251–255] The associated changes in plasma bicarbonate and, therefore, pH are consistent with adaptation to chronic respiratory alkalosis. An element of acute hypocapnia is often superimposed during parturition; $Paco_2$ occasionally falls by an additional 10 to 12 mm Hg during uterine contractions. Ventilation and acid-base values return to control levels several days postpartum.

Septicemia due to either gram-positive or gram-negative organisms commonly results in respiratory alkalosis, possibly secondary to fever, hypotension, or hypoxemia.[192, 201, 256–258] Whereas the concomitant hypoxemia and circulatory failure might account for the genesis of hypocapnia in gram-positive sepsis, direct stimulation of central chemoreceptors by bacterial toxins (lipopolysaccharides) has been shown to account, at least in part, for the respiratory alkalosis of gram-negative sepsis.[192, 201, 258] Furthermore, this effect is sufficiently consistent to call for evaluation for the presence of gram-negative sepsis when a hospitalized patient develops unexplained respiratory alkalosis.

Respiratory alkalosis in hepatic failure is an almost constant finding.[192, 193, 259–262] The specific mechanisms responsible for the hyperventilation remain uncertain, possibly including brain hypoxia and increased progesterone levels, but the extent of hypocapnia correlates best with the level of blood ammonia.[259, 262] When the respiratory alkalosis is severe, it is indicative of a poor prognosis.[192, 193]

Mechanical hyperventilation might induce respiratory alkalosis if the mechanical apparatus is improperly adjusted.[2, 194] This complication can be avoided only by assessing acid-base equilibrium frequently in patients undergoing assisted or controlled ventilation. Abrupt cessation of mechanical hyperventilation, especially in anesthetized patients or those who had received sedatives, might result in critical hypoxemia due to apnea or severe respiratory depression; the prevailing low level of $Paco_2$ fails to provide a stimulus for ventilatory drive and apnea or depressed respiration will persist until $Paco_2$ rises sufficiently to stimulate ventilation.[263–265] This mechanism accounts for a substantial number of cardiorespiratory arrests during recovery from general anesthesia. Despite claims to the contrary, cessation of voluntary hyperventilation might also result in severe hypoxemia due to depressed ventilation or apnea.[265]

Heat exhaustion, heat stroke, fever, and delirium tremens might also produce respiratory alkalosis by mechanisms that remain undefined.[1, 196, 266, 267] Thyrotoxicosis increases both oxygen and $CO_2$ production, and these processes might explain the respiratory alkalosis observed in this condition. Finally, a postmetabolic-acidosis hypocapnia can develop following rapid correction of a large bicarbonate deficit by alkali administration[268]; this persistent hyperventilation, which can last for 24 to 48 hours, is attributed to a delay in correcting the acidity at the central chemoreceptor site.

## DIAGNOSIS

Evaluation of the patient's history, physical examination, and ancillary laboratory data is required to establish the diagnosis of respiratory alkalosis. Careful observation can detect abnormal patterns of breathing in some patients, yet marked hypocapnia can occur without a clinically evident increase in respiratory effort.[2, 269] Arterial blood gas determinations are required to confirm the presence of hyperventilation.

The diagnosis of respiratory alkalosis, especially the chronic form, is often missed; physicians often misinterpret the electrolyte pattern of hyperchloremic hypobicarbonatemia as indicative of normal anion gap metabolic acidosis. A differentiating clue is the fact that plasma potassium concentration is typically within the normal range in chronic hypocapnia, whereas hypokalemia or hyperkalemia often accompanies the various types of hyperchloremic metabolic acidosis. If the patient's acid-base profile reveals hypocapnia in association with alkalemia, at least an element of respiratory alkalosis must be present. Yet hypocapnia might be associated with a normal or an acidic pH due to the concomitant presence of additional acid-base disorders. One should also note that mild degrees of chronic hypocapnia leave blood pH within the high-normal range. Careful examination of the patient's history, physical examination, and ancillary laboratory data are required to assess whether part or all of a given decrement in $Paco_2$ reflects an adaptive response to metabolic acidosis rather than being primary in nature. Once the diagnosis of respiratory alkalosis is made, a search for its cause should be carried out. The diagnosis of respiratory alkalosis can have important clinical implications. It often provides a clue to the presence of an unrecognized, serious disorder or signals the gravity of a known underlying disease.

## TREATMENT

Because chronic respiratory alkalosis poses little risk to health and produces few or no symptoms, measures at treating the acid-base disorder itself are not required. On the other hand, severe alkalemia caused by acute primary hypocapnia requires corrective measures that depend on whether serious clinical manifestations are present. Such measures can be directed at reducing plasma bicarbonate concentration, increasing $Pa_{CO_2}$, or both. Even if baseline plasma bicarbonate is moderately decreased, reducing it further can be particularly rewarding in this setting, because this maneuver combines effectiveness with relatively little risk.[196] For patients with the anxiety-hyperventilation syndrome in addition to reassurance or sedation, rebreathing into a closed system (e.g., a paper bag) might prove helpful by interrupting the vicious cycle that can result from the reinforcing effects of the symptoms of hypocapnia.[186]

Respiratory alkalosis resulting from severe hypoxemia requires oxygen therapy. The oral administration of 250 to 500 mg of acetazolamide (Diamox) can be beneficial in the management of signs and symptoms of high-altitude sickness, a syndrome characterized by hypoxemia and respiratory alkalosis.[270] Of course, patients undergoing mechanical ventilation lend themselves to an effective correction of hypocapnia (whether due to maladjusted ventilator or other causes) by resetting the device.

## MIXED ACID-BASE DISORDERS ASSOCIATED WITH RESPIRATORY ALKALOSIS

Respiratory alkalosis is frequently associated with other acid-base disorders. We describe here some of the more common clinical examples of mixed acid-base disturbances in which respiratory alkalosis is a component.[191]

**Respiratory Alkalosis and Metabolic Acidosis.** This mixed acid-base disorder is commonly encountered during the rapid correction of severe metabolic acidosis. During treatment, plasma bicarbonate concentration often returns toward normal more swiftly than the secondary hypocapnia (originally induced by the acidosis) can abate. As a consequence, the degree of hypocapnia often remains inappropriately great with respect to the then-current decrement in plasma bicarbonate concentration for a period of several hours or more; hydrogen ion concentration during such intervals is often normal or even frankly low.

Patients with salicylate intoxication commonly manifest elements of both metabolic acidosis and respiratory alkalosis, reflecting the independent effects of the salicylate molecule on both cellular metabolism (uncoupling of oxidative phosphorylation) and ventilation (stimulation of central chemoreceptors). Patients with gram-negative sepsis can also develop this mixed disturbance, reflecting the frequent occurrence of primary hyperventilation, on the one hand, and of lactic acidosis and/or renal failure, on the other. This combination also occurs occasionally in the setting of combined hepatic and renal failure. Additionally, patients undergoing "high mass transfer" hemodialysis with acetate dialysate can develop mixed respiratory alkalosis and metabolic acidosis; the former reflects rapid loss of $CO_2$ into the dialysate, and the latter reflects the removal of bicarbonate by the dialyzer at a rate faster than the body's alkali stores can be replenished by tissue metabolism of the circulating acetate.[271]

Patients with sustained respiratory alkalosis of recent onset, in whom renal adaptation to hypocapnia is as yet incomplete (i.e., if hypocapnia has been present for only a day or so), might have acid-base values indistinguishable from those characteristic of patients with this mixed disturbance. Other laboratory data and relevant historical information should serve to differentiate between these alternatives.

**Respiratory Alkalosis and Metabolic Alkalosis.** Although these two disturbances do not coexist often, when they do exist, hydrogen ion concentration might, of course, be driven to extremely low levels.[1, 272, 273] Patients with hepatic insufficiency, who often have persistent hyperventilation, might develop this combination of acid-base disturbances if they are treated with potent diuretics or if they lose gastric fluid. Pregnant patients who develop metabolic alkalosis from any cause will exhibit this mixed acid-base disorder because they typically feature chronic hypocapnia. Similarly, patients with an underlying metabolic alkalosis might develop such a picture if ventilation is stimulated (e.g., pulmonary embolus, pulmonary edema, sepsis).

Because adaptation to chronic hypocapnia requires renal function, severe alkalemia can develop in patients who have end-stage renal disease and who are receiving dialysis therapy. In consideration of the fact that peritoneal dialysis therapy maintains plasma bicarbonate levels at about 26 mEq/L regardless of the prevailing $Pa_{CO_2}$, patients receiving this treatment are at particular risk of alkalemia.[274]

This mixed disturbance can be diagnosed readily if the level of $Pa_{CO_2}$ is less than normal and if plasma bicarbonate concentration is frankly elevated. The disorder should be treated as a medical emergency, because extreme alkalemia carries a serious prognosis.[4] With the exception of patients undergoing mechanical ventilation (and the consequent ability to increase $Pa_{CO_2}$ promptly), measures should be taken to reduce rapidly the elevated plasma bicarbonate concentration.

ACKNOWLEDGMENT

We would like to thank Linda Sue Seals for her assistance in the preparation of the manuscript.

## REFERENCES

1. Gennari FJ, Kassirer JP: Respiratory alkalosis. In Cohen JJ, Kassirer JP (eds): Acid-Base. Boston, Little Brown, 1982, p 349.
2. Adrogué HJ, Tobin MJ: Blackwell's Basics of Medicine: Respiratory Failure. Boston, Blackwell Science, 1997.
3. Adrogué HJ, Madias NE: Management of life-threatening acid-base disorders (first of two parts). N Engl J Med 338:26, 1998.

4. Adrogué HJ, Madias NE: Management of life-threatening acid-base disorders (second of two parts). N Engl J Med 338:107, 1998.
5. Adrogué HJ, Rashad MN, Gorin AB, et al: Assessing acid-base status in circulatory failure: Differences between arterial and central venous blood. N Engl J Med 320:1312, 1989.
6. Adrogué HJ, Rashad MN, Gorin AB, et al: Arteriovenous acid-base disparity in circulatory failure: Studies on mechanism. Am J Physiol 257:F1087, 1989.
7. Adrogué HJ, Wesson DE: Blackwell's Basics of Medicine: Acid-Base. Boston, Blackwell Science, 1994.
8. Arbus GS, Hebert LA, Levesque PR, et al: Characterization and clinical application of the "significance band" for acute respiratory alkalosis. N Engl J Med 280:117, 1969.
9. Eldridge F, Salzer J: Effect of respiratory alkalosis on blood lactate and pyruvate in humans. J Appl Physiol 22:461, 1967.
10. Gledhill N, Beirne GJ, Dempsey JA: Renal response to short-term hypocapnia in man. Kidney Int 8:376, 1975.
11. Markello R, Cutter JA, King BD: Hyperventilation studies during nitrous oxide-narcotic-relaxant anesthesia. Anesthesiology 24:225, 1963.
12. Madias NE, Cohen JJ: Adaptation to respiratory acidosis and alkalosis. In Fishman AP (ed): Pulmonary Diseases and Disorders, 2nd ed. New York, McGraw-Hill, 1988, p 289.
13. Adler S, Roy A, Relman A: Intracellular acid-base regulation. I: Response of muscle cells to changes in $CO_2$ tension or extracellular bicarbonate concentration. J Clin Invest 44:8, 1965.
14. Giebisch G, Berger L, Pitts RF: The extrarenal response to acute acid-base disturbances of respiratory origin. J Clin Invest 34:231, 1955.
15. Sly WS, Hu PY: Human carbonic anhydrases and carbonic anhydrase deficiencies. Annu Rev Biochem 64:375, 1995.
16. Boron WF: Intracellular pH transients in giant barnacle muscle fibers. Am J Physiol 233:C61, 1977.
17. Waisbren SJ, Geibel JP, Modlin IM, et al: Unusual permeability properties of gastric gland cells. Nature 368:332, 1994.
18. Putnam RW, Roos A: Intracellular pH. In Hoffman JF, Jamieson JD (eds): Handbook of Physiology, Section 14: Cell Physiology. Oxford University Press, 1997, p 389.
19. Aronson PS: Kinetic properties of the plasma membrane $Na^+$-$H^+$ exchanger. Annu Rev Physiol 47:545, 1985.
20. Aronson PS, Nee J, Suhm M: Modifier role of internal $H^+$ in activating the $Na^+$-$H^+$ exchanger in renal microvillus membrane vesicles. Nature 299:161, 1982.
21. Bonanno JA: $K^+$-$H^+$ exchange, a fundamental cell acidifier in corneal epithelium. Am J Physiol 260 (Cell Physiol 29): C618, 1991.
22. Restrepo D, Kozody DJ, Spinelli LJ, et al: pH homeostasis in promyelocytic leukemic HL60 cells. J Gen Physiol 92:489, 1988.
23. Mugharbil A, Knickelbein RG, Aronson PS, et al: Rabbit ileal brush-border membrane Cl-$HCO_3$ exchanger is activated by an internal pH-sensitive modifier site. Am J Physiol 259 (Gastrointest Liver Physiol 22):G666, 1970.
24. Boron WF, Russell JM: Stoichiometry and ion dependencies of the intracellular-pH-regulating mechanism in squid giant axons. J Gen Physiol 81:373, 1983.
25. Roos A, Boron WF: Intracellular pH. Physiol Rev 61:296, 1981.
26. Boron WF, McCormick WC, Roos A: pH regulation in barnacle muscle fibers; dependence on intracellular and extracellular pH. Am J Physiol 237 (Cell Physiol 6):C185, 1979.
27. Boron WF, McCormick WC, Roos A: pH regulation in barnacle muscle fibers; dependence on extracellular sodium and bicarbonate. Am J Physiol 240 (Cell Physiol 9):C80, 1981.
28. Gleeson D, Smith ND, Boyer JL: Bicarbonate-dependent and -independent intracellular pH regulatory mechanisms in rat hepatocytes. Evidence for $Na^+$-$HCO_3^-$ cotransport. J Clin Invest 84:312, 1989.
29. Boron WF, Boulpaep EL: Intracellular pH regulation in the renal proximal tubule of the salamander: Basolateral $HCO_3^-$ transport. J Gen Physiol 81:53, 1983.
30. Lee HC, Forte JG, Epel D: The use of fluorescent amines for the measurement of pHi: Applications in liposomes, gastric microsomes, and sea urchin gametes. In Nuccitelli R, Deamer D (eds): Intracellular pH: Its Measurement, Regulation, and Utilization in Cellular Functions. New York, Alan R Liss, 1982, p 135.
31. Manfredi F: Effects of hypocapnia and hypercapnia on intracellular acid-base equilibrium in man. J Lab Clin Med 69:304, 1967.
32. Brown EB Jr, Goott B: Intracellular hydrogen ion changes and potassium movement. Am J Physiol 204:765, 1963.
33. Heisler N, Piiper J: Determination of intracellular buffering properties in rat diaphragm muscle. Am J Physiol 222:747, 1972.
34. Kjällquist A, Nardini M, Siesjö BK: The regulation of extra- and intracellular acid-base parameters in the rat brain during hyper- and hypocapnia. Acta Physiol Scand 76:485, 1969.
35. Katz LA, Swain JA, Portman MA, et al: Intracellular pH and inorganic phosphate content of heart in vivo: A $^{31}P$-NMR study. Am J Physiol 255:H189, 1988.
36. Eichenholz A: Respiratory alkalosis. Arch Intern Med 116:699, 1965.
37. Eichenholz A, Mulhausen RO, Anderson WE, et al: Primary hypocapnia: A cause of metabolic acidosis. J Appl Physiol 17: 283, 1962.
38. Engel K, Kildeberg P, Winters RW: Quantitative displacement of blood acid-base status in acute hypocapnia. Scand J Clin Lab Invest 23:5, 1969.
39. Plum F, Posner JB: Blood and cerebrospinal fluid lactate during hyperventilation. Am J Physiol 212:864, 1967.
40. Zborowska-Sluis DT, Dossetor JB: Hyperlactatemia of hyperventilation. J Appl Physiol 22:746, 1967.
41. Cain SM, Dunn JE II: Transient arterial lactic acid changes in unanesthetized dogs at 21,000 feet. Am J Physiol 206:1437, 1964.
42. Sykes MK, Cooke PM: The effect of hyperventilation on "excess lactate" production during anaesthesia. Br J Anaesth 37:372, 1965.
43. Takano N: Blood lactate accumulation and its causative factors during passive hyperventilation in dogs. Jpn J Physiol 16:481, 1966.
44. Madias NE, Cohen JJ, Adrogué HJ: Influence of acute and chronic respiratory alkalosis on preexisting chronic metabolic alkalosis. Am J Physiol 258:F479, 1990.
45. Hood VL, Tannen RL: Protection of acid-base balance by pH regulation of acid production. N Engl J Med 339:819, 1998.
46. Gennari FJ, Goldstein MB, Schwartz WB: The nature of the renal adaptation to chronic hypocapnia. J Clin Invest 51:1722, 1972.
47. Gougoux A, Kaehny WD, Cohen JJ: Renal adaptation to chronic hypocapnia: Dietary constraints in achieving $H^+$ retention. Am J Physiol 229:1330, 1975.
48. Stanbury SW, Thomson AE: The renal response to respiratory alkalosis. Clin Sci 11:357, 1952.
49. Bengele H, McNamara ER, Schwartz JH, et al: Acidification adaptation along the inner medullary collecting duct. Am J Physiol 255:F1155, 1988.
50. Cogan M: Effects of acute alterations in $P_{CO_2}$ on proximal $HCO_3$, $Cl^-$, and $H_2O$ reabsorption. Am J Physiol 246:F21, 1984.
51. Jacobson HR: Effects of $CO_2$ and acetazolamide on bicarbonate and fluid transport in rabbit proximal tubules. Am J Physiol 240:F54, 1981.
52. Jacobson HR: Medullary collecting duct acidification: Effects of potassium, $HCO_3$ concentration, and $P_{CO_2}$. J Clin Invest 74: 2107, 1984.
53. Santella RN, Maddox DA, Gennari FJ: Delivery dependence of early proximal bicarbonate reabsorption in the rat in respiratory acidosis and alkalosis. J Clin Invest 87:631, 1991.
54. Hilden SA, Johns CA, Madias NE: Adaptation of rabbit renal cortical $Na^+$-$H^+$ exchange activity in chronic hypocapnia. Am J Physiol 257:F615, 1989.
55. Ruiz O, Arruda JAL, Talor Z: Na-$HCO_3$ cotransport and Na-H antiporter in chronic respiratory acidosis and alkalosis. Am J Physiol 256:F414, 1989.
56. Al-Awqati Q: The cellular renal response to respiratory acid-base disorders. Kidney Int 28:845, 1985.
57. Eiam-Ong S, Laski ME, Kurtzman NA, et al: Effect of respiratory acidosis and respiratory alkalosis on renal transport enzymes. Am J Physiol 267:F390, 1994.
58. Krapf R, Beeler I, Hertner D, et al: Chronic respiratory alkalosis: the effect of sustained hyperventilation on renal regulation of acid-base equilibrium. N Engl J Med 324:1394, 1991.

59. Dempsey JA, Forster HV, DoPico GA: Ventilatory acclimatization to moderate hypoxemia in man. J Clin Invest 53:1091, 1974.
60. Dill DB, Talbott JH, Consolazio WV: Blood as a physicochemical system. XII: Man at high altitude. J Biol Chem 118:649, 1937.
61. Forster HV, Dempsey JA, Chosy LW: Incomplete compensation of CSF [$H^+$] in man during acclimatization to high altitude (4300 m). J Appl Physiol 38:1067, 1975.
62. Gennari FJ, Kaehny WD, Levesque PR, et al: Acid-base response to chronic hypocapnia in man. Clin Res 28:533A, 1980.
63. Clark DD, Chang BS, Garella SG, et al: Secondary hypocapnia fails to protect "whole body" intracellular pH during chronic HCl-acidosis in the dog. Kidney Int 23:336, 1983.
64. Cohen JJ, Madias NE, Wolf CJ, et al: Regulation of acid-base equilibrium in chronic hypocapnia: Evidence that the response of the kidney is not geared to the defense of extracellular [$H^+$]. J Clin Invest 57:1483, 1976.
65. Madias NE, Schwartz WB, Cohen, JJ: The maladaptive renal response to secondary hypocapnia during chronic HCl acidosis in the dog. J Clin Invest 60:1393, 1977.
66. Chiodi H: Respiratory adaptations to chronic high altitude hypoxia. J Appl Physiol 10:81, 1957.
67. Houston CS, Riley RL: Respiratory and circulatory changes during acclimatization to high altitude. Am J Physiol 149:565, 1947.
68. Lahiri S, Milledge JS: Acid-base in Sherpa altitude residents and lowlanders at 4880 m. Respir Physiol 2:323, 1967.
69. Stäubli M, Rohner F, Kammer P, et al: Plasma volume and proteins in voluntary hyperventilation. J Appl Physiol 60:1549, 1986.
70. Steurer J, Schiesser D, Stey C, et al: Hyperventilation enhances transcapillary diffusion of sodium fluorescein. Int J Microcirc Clin Exp 16:266, 1996.
71. Straub PW, Buhlmann AA: Reduction of blood volume by voluntary hyperventilation. J Appl Physiol 29:816, 1970.
72. Adrogué HJ, Madias NE: Changes in plasma potassium concentration during acute acid-base disturbances. Am J Med 71: 456, 1981.
73. Suzuki H, Hishida A, Ohishi K, et al: Role of hormonal factors in plasma K alterations in acute respiratory and metabolic alkalosis in dogs. Am J Physiol 258:F305, 1990.
74. Barker ES, Singer RB, Clark JK, et al: The renal response in man to acute experimental respiratory alkalosis and acidosis. J Clin Invest 36:515, 1957.
75. Krapf R, Caduff P, Wagdi P, et al: Plasma potassium response to acute respiratory alkalosis. Kidney Int 47:217, 1995.
76. Brautbar N, Leibovici H, Massry, SG: On the mechanism of hypophosphatemia during acute hyperventilation: Evidence for increased muscle glycolysis. Miner Electrolyte Metab 9:45, 1983.
77. Krapf R, Jaeger P, Hulter HN: Chronic respiratory alkalosis induces renal PTH-resistance, hyperphosphatemia and hypocalcemia in humans. Kidney Int 42:727, 1992.
78. Mostellar ME, Tuttle EP Jr: The effects of alkalosis on plasma concentration and urinary excretion of inorganic phosphate in man. J Clin Invest 43:138, 1964.
79. Okel BB, Hurst JW: Prolonged hyperventilation in man: Associated electrolyte changes and subjective symptoms. Arch Intern Med 108:157, 1961.
80. Tucker RR, Berndt TJ, Thotharthri V, et al: Propranolol blocks the hypophosphaturia of acute respiratory alkalosis in human subjects. J Lab Clin Med 128:423, 1996.
81. Edmondson JW, Brashear RE, Li T: Tetany: Quantitative interrelationships between calcium and alkalosis. Am J Physiol 228: 1082, 1975.
82. Kjeldsen K, Damgaard F: Influence of prolonged carbon monoxide exposure and high altitude on the composition of blood and urine in man. Scand J Clin Lab Invest 22 (Suppl 103): 20, 1968.
83. Saltzman HA, Heyman A, Sieker HO: Correlation of clinical and physiological manifestations of sustained hyperventilation. N Engl J Med 268:1431, 1963.
84. Merwarth CR, Sieker HO, Manfredi F: Acid-base relations between blood and cerebrospinal fluid in normal subjects and patients with respiratory insufficiency. N Engl J Med 265:310, 1961.
85. Dempsey JA, Forster HV, Gledhill N, et al: Effects of moderate hypoxemia and hypocapnia on CSF [$H^+$] and ventilation in man. J Appl Physiol 38:665, 1975.
86. Hornbein TF, Pavlin EG: Distribution of $H^+$ and $HCO_3^-$ between CSF and blood during respiratory alkalosis in dogs. Am J Physiol 228:1149, 1975.
87. Kazemi H, Shannon DC, Carvallo-Gil E: Brain $CO_2$ buffering capacity in respiratory acidosis and alkalosis. J Appl Physiol 22: 241, 1967.
88. Kazemi H, Valenca LM, Shannon DC: Brain and cerebrospinal fluid lactate concentration in respiratory acidosis and alkalosis. Respir Physiol 6:178, 1969.
89. Lambertsen CJ: Carbon dioxide and respiration in acid-base homeostasis. Anesthesiology 21:642, 1960.
90. Javaheri S, Corbett W, Wagner K, et al: Quantitative cerebrospinal fluid acid-base balance in acute respiratory alkalosis. Am J Respir Crit Care Med 150:78, 1994.
91. Fisher VJ, Christianson LC: Cerebrospinal fluid acid-base balance during a changing ventilatory state in man. J Appl Physiol 18:712, 1963.
92. Kety SS, Schmidt CF: The effects of altered arterial tensions of carbon dioxide and oxygen on cerebral blood flow and cerebral oxygen consumption of normal young men. J Clin Invest 27:484, 1948.
93. Pontén U, Siesjö BK: Gradients of $CO_2$ tension in the brain. Acta Physiol Scand 67:129, 1966.
94. Posner JB, Swanson AG, Plum F: Acid-base balance in cerebrospinal fluid. Arch Neurol 12:479, 1965.
95. Reivich M: Arterial $P_{CO_2}$ and cerebral hemodynamics. Am J Physiol 206:25, 1964.
96. Mitchell RA, Carman CT, Severinghaus JW, et al: Stability of cerebrospinal fluid pH in chronic acid-base disturbances in blood. J Appl Physiol 20:443, 1965.
97. Pauli HG, Vorburger C, Reubi F: Chronic derangements of cerebrospinal fluid acid-base components in man. J Appl Physiol 17:993, 1962.
98. Severinghaus JW, Mitchell RA, Richardson BW, et al: Respiratory control at high altitude suggesting active transport regulation of CSF pH. J Appl Physiol 18:1155, 1963.
99. Dempsey JA, Forster HV, Birnbaum ML, et al: Control of exercise hyperpnea under varying durations of exposure to moderate hypoxia. Respir Physiol 16:213, 1972.
100. Orr JA, Bisgard GE, Forster HV, et al: Cerebrospinal fluid alkalosis during high altitude sojourn in unanesthetized ponies. Respir Physiol 25:23, 1975.
101. Hsia CCW: Respiratory function of hemoglobin. N Engl J Med 338:239, 1998.
102. Lawson WH Jr: Interrelation of pH, temperature and oxygen on deoxygenation rate of red cells. J Appl Physiol 21:905, 1966.
103. Severinghaus JW: Oxyhemoglobin dissociation curve correction for temperature and pH variation in human blood. J Appl Physiol 12:485, 1958.
104. Bellingham AJ, Detter JC, Lenfant C: Regulatory mechanisms of hemoglobin oxygen affinity in acidosis and alkalosis. J Clin Invest 50:700, 1971.
105. Klocke RA, Bauer C, Forster RE: The kinetics of the oxygen-hemoglobin reactions: Influence of 2,3-diphosphoglycerate (2,3-DPG) and pH. Physiologist 13:242, 1970.
106. Lenfant C, Torrance J, English E, et al: Effect of altitude on oxygen binding by hemoglobin and on organic phosphate levels. J Clin Invest 47:2652, 1968.
107. Slater RM, Symreng T, Sum Ping, et al:. The effect of respiratory alkalosis on oxygen consumption in anesthetized patients. J Clin Anesth 4:462, 1992.
108. Combes P, Fauvage B: Combined effects of hypocapnia and nicardipine on airway resistance: A pilot study. Eur J Clin Pharmacol 51:385, 1997.
109. Gordon JB, Martinez FR, Keller PA, et al: Differing effects of acute and prolonged alkalosis on hypoxic pulmonary vasoconstriction. Am Rev Respir Dis 148:1651, 1993.
110. McElroy WT Jr, Gerdes AJ, Brown EB Jr: Effects of $CO_2$, bicarbonate and pH on the performance of isolated perfused guinea pig hearts. Am J Physiol 195:412, 1958.
111. Vaughan William EM: The individual effects of $CO_2$, bicarbonate and pH on the electrical and mechanical activity of isolated rabbit auricles. J Physiol 129:90, 1955.

112. Wead WB, Little RC: Effect of hypocapnia and respiratory alkalosis on cardiac contractility. Proc Soc Exp Biol Med 126: 606, 1967.
113. Mosca SM, Gelpi RJ, Borelli R, et al: The effects of hypocapnic alkalosis on the myocardial contractility of isovolumic perfused rabbit hearts. Arch Int Physiol Biochem Biophys 101:179, 1993.
114. Kusuoka H, Back PH, Camilion de Hurtado M, et al: Relative roles of intracellular $Ca^+$ and pH in shaping myocardial contractile response to acute respiratory alkalosis. Am J Physiol 265:H1696, 1993.
115. Panagiotopoulos S, Daly M, Nayler WG: Effect of acidosis and alkalosis on postischemic Ca gain in isolated rat heart. Am J Physiol 258:H821, 1990.
116. Combes P, Fauvage B: Systemic vasomotor interaction between nicardipine and hypocapnic alkalosis in man. Intensive Care Med 18:89, 1992.
117. Kety S, Schmidt CF: The effects of active and passive hyperventilation on cerebral blood flow, cerebral oxygen consumption, cardiac output and blood pressure of normal young men. J Clin Invest 25:107, 1946.
118. Prys-Roberts C, Kelman G, Greenbaum, et al: Circulatory influences of artificial ventilation during nitrous oxide anaesthesia in man. II: Results: The relative influence of mean intrathoracic pressure and arterial carbon dioxide tension. Br J Anaesth 39:533, 1967.
119. Burnum JF, Hickam JB, McIntosh HD: The effect of hypocapnia on arterial blood pressure. Circulation 9:89, 1954.
120. Gotoh F, Meyer JS, Takagi Y: Cerebral effects of hyperventilation in man. Arch Neurol 12:410, 1965.
121. Richardson DW, Wasserman AJ, Patterson JL: General and regional circulatory response to changes in blood pH and carbon dioxide tension. J Clin Invest 40:31, 1961.
122. Rowe GG, Castillo CA, Crumpton CW: Effects of hyperventilation on systemic and coronary hemodynamics. Am Heart J 63: 67, 1962.
123. Asmussen E, Consolazio FC: The circulation in rest and work on Mount Evans. Am J Physiol 132:555, 1941.
124. Klausen K: Cardiac output in man in rest and work during and after acclimatization to 3800 m. J Appl Physiol 21:609, 1966.
125. Vogel JA, Harris CW: Cardiopulmonary responses of resting man during early exposure to high altitude. J Appl Physiol 22: 1124, 1967.
126. Ayres SM, Grace WJ: Inappropriate ventilation and hypoxemia as causes of cardiac arrhythmias. Am J Med 46:495, 1969.
127. Bass C, Wade C, Gardner WN, et al: Unexplained breathlessness and psychiatric morbidity in patients with normal and abnormal coronary arteries. Lancet 1:605, 1983.
128. Evans DW, Lum LC: Hyperventilation: An important cause of pseudoangina. Lancet 1:155, 1977.
129. Jacobs WF, Battle WE, Ronan JA: False-positive ST-T-wave changes secondary to hyperventilation and exercise. Ann Intern Med 81:479, 1974.
130. Lary D, Goldschlager N: Electrocardiographic changes during hyperventilation resembling myocardial ischemia in patients with normal coronary arteriograms. Am Heart J 87:383, 1974.
131. Magarian GJ: Hyperventilation syndromes: Infrequently recognized common expressions of anxiety and stress. Medicine (Baltimore) 61:219, 1982.
132. McHenry PL, Cogan OJ, Elliott WC, et al: False positive ECG response to exercise secondary to hyperventilation: Cineangiographic correlation. Am Heart J 79:683, 1970.
133. Ardissino D, De Servi S, Falcone C, et al: Role of hypocapnic alkalosis in hyperventilation-induced coronary artery spasm in variant angina. Am J Cardiol 59:707, 1987.
134. Yasue H, Nagao M, Omote S, et al: Coronary arterial spasm and Prinzmetal's variant form of angina induced by hyperventilation and tris-buffer infusion. Circulation 58:56, 1978.
135. Clarke RSJ: The effect of voluntary overbreathing on the blood flow through the human forearm. J Physiol 118:537, 1952.
136. Simmons DH, Oliver RP: Effects of acute acid-base changes on renal hemodynamics in anesthetized dogs. Am J Physiol 209: 1180, 1965.
137. Wasserman AJ, Patterson JL Jr: The cerebral vascular response to reduction in arterial carbon dioxide tension. J Clin Invest 40:1297, 1961.
138. Lenfant C, Sullivan K: Adaptation to high altitude. N Engl J Med 284:1298, 1971.
139. Pauli HG, Truniger B, Larsen JK, et al: Renal function during prolonged exposure to hypoxia and carbon monoxide. Scand J Clin Lab Invest 22 (Suppl 103):55, 1968.
140. Ramsøe K, Jarnum S, Preisig R, et al: Liver function and blood flow at high altitude. J Appl Physiol 28:725, 1970.
141. Rennie D, Lozano R, Monge C, et al: Renal oxygenation in male Peruvian natives living permanently at high altitude. J Appl Physiol 30:450, 1971.
142. Kaehny WD, Gougoux A, Cohen JJ: Influence of steady-state $Pa_{CO_2}$ on escape from ADH-induced water retention in the dog. Am J Physiol 234:F291, 1978.
143. Pickard JD, Rose JE, Cooke MBD, et al: The effect of salicylate on cerebral blood flow in man. Acta Neurol Scand 64(suppl): 422, 1977.
144. Alexander SC, Wollman H, Cohen PJ, et al: Cerebrovascular response to $Pa_{CO_2}$ during halothane anesthesia in man. J Appl Physiol 19:561, 1964.
145. Fox J, Gelb AW, Enns J, et al: The responsiveness of cerebral blood flow to changes in arterial carbon dioxide is maintained during propofol-nitrous oxide anesthesia in humans. Anesthesiology 77:453, 1992.
146. Wollman H, Alexander SC, Cohen PJ, et al: Cerebral circulation during general anesthesia and hyperventilation in man. Anesthesiology 26:329, 1965.
147. Tominga S, Strandgaard S, Uemura K, et al: Cerebrovascular $CO_2$ reactivity in normotensive and hypertensive man. Stroke 7:507, 1976.
148. Grubb RL Jr, Raichle ME, Eichling JO, et al: The effects of changes in $Pa_{CO_2}$ on cerebral blood volume, blood flow, and vascular mean transit time. Stroke 5:630, 1974.
149. Wollman H, Smith TC, Stephen GW, et al: Effects of extremes of respiratory and metabolic alkalosis on cerebral blood flow in man. J Appl Physiol 24:60, 1968.
150. Artru AA: Cerebral vascular responses to hypocapnia during nitroglycerin-induced hypotension. Neurosurgery 16:468, 1985.
151. Wilkinson IMS, Browne, DRG: The influence of anaesthesia and of arterial hypocapnia on regional blood flow in the normal human cerebral hemisphere. Br J Anaesth 42:472, 1970.
152. Waltz AG: Effect of $Pa_{CO_2}$ on blood flow and microvasculature of ischemic and nonischemic cerebral cortex. Stroke 1:27, 1970.
153. Young WL, Prohovnik I, Correll JW, et al: A comparison of the cerebral hemodynamic effects of sufentanil and isoflurane in humans undergoing carotid endarterectomy. Anesthesiology 71:863, 1989.
154. McHenry LC, Slocum HC, Bivens HE, et al: Hyperventilation in awake and anesthetized man. Arch Neurol 12:270, 1965.
155. Young WL, Prohovnik I, Correll JW, et al: A comparison of cerebral blood flow reactivity to $CO_2$ during halothane versus isoflurane anesthesia for carotid endarterectomy. Anesth Analg 73:416, 1991.
156. Kontos HA, Wei EP, Raper AJ, et al: Local mechanism of $CO_2$ action on cat pial arterioles. Stroke 8:226, 1977.
157. Wahl M, Deetjen P, Thurau K, et al: Micropuncture evaluation of the importance of perivascular pH for the arteriolar diameter on the brain surface. Pflugers Arch 316:152, 1970.
158. Betz E, Enzenrob HG, Vlahov V: Interaction of $H^+$ and $Ca^+$ in the regulation of local pial vascular resistance. Pflugers Arch 343:79, 1973.
159. Severinghaus JW, Chiodi H, Eger EI II, et al: Cerebral blood flow in man at high altitude: Role of cerebrospinal fluid pH in normalization of flow in chronic hypocapnia. Circ Res 19: 274, 1966.
160. Kontos HA, Raper J, Patterson JL Jr: Analysis of vasoactivity of local pH, $P_{CO_2}$ and bicarbonate on pial vessels. Stroke 8: 358, 1977.
161. You JP, Wang Q, Zhang W, et al: Hypercapnic vasodilation in isolated rat basilar arteries is exerted via low pH and does not involve nitric oxide synthase stimulation or cyclic GMP production. Acta Physiol Scand 152:391, 1994.
162. Wang Q, Pelligrino D, Koenig HM, et al: The role of endothelium and nitric oxide in rat pial arteriolar dilatory responses to $CO_2$ in vivo. J Cereb Blood Flow Metab 14:944, 1994.

163. Leffler CW, Fedinec Al, Shibata M: Prostacyclin receptor activation and pial arteriolar dilation after endothelial injury in piglets. Stroke 26:2103, 1995.
164. Leffler CW, Mirro R, Shanklin DR, et al: Light/dye microvascular injury selectively eliminates hypercapnia-induced pial arteriolar dilation in newborn pigs. Am J Physiol 266:H623, 1994.
165. Harper AM, Glass HI: Effect of alterations in the arterial carbon dioxide tension on the blood flow through the cerebral cortex at normal and low arterial blood pressures. J Neurol Neurosur Psychiatry 28:449, 1965.
166. Whitelaw A, Karisson BR, Haaland K, et al: Hypocapnia and cerebral ischaemia in hypotensive newborn piglets. Arch Dis Child 66:I110, 1991.
167. Brian JE Jr: Carbon dioxide and the cerebral circulation. Anesthesiology 88:1365, 1998.
168. Kitazono T, Faraci FM, Taguchi H, et al: Role of potassium channels in cerebral blood vessels. Stroke 26:1713, 1995.
169. Davies NW: Modulation of ATP-sensitive $K^+$ channels in skeletal muscle by intracellular protons. Nature 343:375, 1990.
170. Kinoshita H, Karusic ZS: Role of potassium channels in relaxations of isolated canine basilar arteries to acidosis. Stroke 28: 433, 1997.
171. Parfenova H, Shibata M, Zuckerman S, et al: $CO_2$ and cerebral circulation in newborn pigs; cyclic nucleotides and prostanoids in vascular regulation. Am J Physiol 266:HI494, 1994.
172. Faraci FM, Brian JE Jr: Nitric oxide in the cerebral circulation. Stroke 25:692, 1994.
173. Raichle ME, Posner JB, Plum F: Cerebral blood flow during and after hyperventilation. Arch Neurol 23:394, 1970.
174. Albrecht RF, Miletich DJ, Ruttle M: Cerebral effects of extended hyperventilation in unanesthetized goats. Stroke 18: 649, 1987.
175. Greenberg JH, Alavi A, Reivich M, et al: Local cerebral blood volume response to carbon dioxide in man. Circ Res 43:324, 1978.
176. Gotoh F, Meyer JS, Takagi Y: Cerebral effects of hyperventilation in man. Arch Neurol 12:410, 1965.
177. Reivich M, Cohen PJ, Greenbaum L: Alterations in the electroencephalogram of awake man produced by hyperventilation: Effects of 100% oxygen at 3 atmospheres (absolute) pressure. Neurology 16:303, 1966.
178. Balke B, Ellis JP Jr, Wells JG: Adaptive responses to hyperventilation. J Appl Physiol 12:269, 1958.
179. Gibbs EL, Gibbs FA, Lennox WG, et al: Regulation of cerebral carbon dioxide. Arch Neurol Psychiatry 47:879, 1942.
180. Granholm L, Siesjö BK: The effect of combined respiratory and nonrespiratory alkalosis on energy metabolites and acid-base parameters in the rat brain. Acta Physiol Scand 81:307, 1971.
181. Carlisson C, Nilsson L, Siesjö B: Cerebral metabolic changes in arterial hypocapnia of short duration. Acta Anaesthesiol Scand 18:104, 1974.
182. van Rijen PC, Luyten PR, van der Sprenkel JWB, et al: $^1H$ and $^{31}P$ NMR measurement of cerebral lactate, high-energy phosphate levels, and pH in humans during voluntary hyperventilation: Associated EEG, capnographic, and doppler findings. Magn Reson Med 10:182, 1989.
183. Yundt KD, Dirringer MN: The use of hyperventilation and its impact on cerebral ischemia in the treatment of traumatic brain injury. Crit Care Clin 13:163, 1997.
184. Elliott GG, Morris AH: Clinical syndromes of respiratory acidosis and alkalosis. In Seldin DW, Giebisch G (eds): The Regulation of Acid-Base Balance. New York, Raven Press, 1989, p 483.
185. Kilburn KH: Shock, seizures and coma with alkalosis during mechanical ventilation. Ann Intern Med 65:977, 1966.
186. Rice RL: Symptom patterns of the hyperventilation syndrome. Am J Med 8:691, 1950.
187. Brown EB Jr: Physiological effects of hyperventilation. Physiol Rev 33:445, 1953.
188. Swanson AG, Stavney LS, Plum F: Effects of blood pH and carbon dioxide on cerebral electrical activity. Neurology 8: 787, 1958.
189. Plum F, Posner JB, Smith, WW: Effect of hyperbaric-hyperoxic hyperventilation on blood, brain and CSF lactate. Am J Physiol 215:1240, 1968.
190. Van Vaerenbergh PJJ, Demeester G, Leusen I: Lactate in cerebrospinal fluid during hyperventilation. Arch Intern Physiol Biochem 73:738, 1965.
191. Adrogué HJ, Madias NE: Mixed acid-base disorders. In Jacobson HR, Striker GE, Klahr S (eds): The Principles and Practice of Nephrology, 2nd ed. St. Louis, Mosby-Year Book, 1995, p 953.
192. Mazzara JT, Ayres SM, Grace WJ: Extreme hypocapnia in the critically ill patient. Am J Med 56:450, 1974.
193. Møller B: The hydrogen ion concentration in arterial blood. Acta Med Scand 165(Suppl 348):11, 1959.
194. Wilson RF, Gibson D, Percinel AK, et al: Severe alkalosis in critically ill surgical patients. Arch Surg 105:197, 1972.
195. Fishman AP: Alveolar ventilation and its disorders. In Fishman AP (ed): Pulmonary Diseases and Disorders, 2nd edition. New York, McGraw-Hill, 1988, p 299.
196. Madias NE, Adrogué HJ: Acid-base disturbances in pulmonary medicine. In Arieff AI, DeFronzo RA (eds): Fluid, Electrolyte, and Acid Base Disorders. New York, Churchill Livingstone, 1995, p 223.
197. Wade JG, Larson CP, Hickey RF, et al: Effect of carotid endarterectomy on carotid chemoreceptor and baroreceptor function in man. N Engl J Med 282:823, 1970.
198. West JB: Human limits for hypoxia: The physiological challenge of climbing Mt. Everest. Ann N Y Acad Sci 899:15, 2000.
199. Milledge JS, Lahiri S: Respiratory control in lowlanders and Sherpa highlanders at altitude. Respir Physiol 2:310, 1967.
200. Severinghaus JW, Bainton CR, Carcelen A: Respiratory insensitivity to hypoxia in chronically hypoxic man. Respir Physiol 1: 308, 1966.
201. Winslow EJ, Loeb HS, Rahimtoola SH, et al: Hemodynamic studies and results of therapy in 50 patients with bacteremic shock. Am J Med 54:421, 1973.
202. Soley MH, Shock NW: The etiology of effort syndrome. Am J Med Sci 196:840, 1938.
203. Tobin MJ: Dyspnea: Pathophysiologic basis, clinical presentation, and management. Arch Intern Med 150:1604, 1960.
204. Plum F, Swanson AG: Central neurogenic hyperventilation in man. Arch Neurol Psychiatry 81:535, 1959.
205. Rout MW, Lane DJ, Wollner L: Prognosis in acute cerebrovascular accidents in relation to respiratory pattern and blood gas tensions. BMJ 3:7, 1971.
206. Lange LS, Laszlo G: Cerebral tumor presenting with hyperventilation. J Neurol Neurosurg Psychiatry 28:317, 1965.
207. Plum F: Hyperpnea, hyperventilation, and brain dysfunction. Ann Intern Med 76:328, 1972.
208. Brown HW, Plum F: The neurologic basis of Cheyne-Stokes respiration. Am J Med 30:849, 1961.
209. Heyman A, Birchfield RI, Sieker HO: Effects of bilateral cerebral infarction on respiratory center sensitivity. Neurology 8: 694, 1958.
210. Karp HR, Sieker HO, Heyman A: Cerebral circulation and function in Cheyne-Stokes respiration. Am J Med 30:861, 1961.
211. Hoff HE, Breckenridge CG: Intrinsic mechanism in periodic breathing. Arch Neurol Psychiatry 72:11, 1954.
212. Anderson RJ, Potts DE, Gabow PA, et al: Unrecognized adult salicylate intoxication. Ann Intern Med 85:745, 1976.
213. Cameron IR, Semple SJG: The central respiratory stimulant action of salicylates. Clin Sci 35:391, 1968.
214. Farber HR, Yiengst MJ, Shock NW: The effect of therapeutic doses of aspirin on the acid-base balance of the blood in normal adults. Am J Med Sci 217:256, 1949.
215. Gabow PA, Anderson R, Potts DE, et al: Acid-base disturbances in the salicylate-intoxicated adult. Arch Intern Med 138:1481, 1978.
216. Riley DJ, Legawiec BA, Santiago TV, et al: Ventilatory responses to hypercapnia and hypoxia during continuous aspirin ingestion. J Appl Physiol 43:971, 1977.
217. Tenney SM, Miller RM: The respiratory and circulatory actions of salicylate. Am J Med 19:498, 1955.
218. Winters RW, White JS, Hughes MC, et al: Disturbances of acid-base equilibrium in salicylate intoxication. Pediatrics 23: 260, 1959.
219. Dull WL, Polu JM, Sadoul P: The pulmonary hemodynamic effects of almitrine infusion in men with chronic hypercapnia. Clin Sci 64:25, 1983.

220. Lyons HA, Huang CT: Therapeutic use of progesterone in alveolar hypoventilation associated with obesity. Am J Med 44: 881, 1968.
221. Madias NE, Cohen JJ: Respiratory acidosis. In Cohen JJ, Kassirer JP (eds): Acid-Base. Boston, Little Brown, 1982, p 307.
222. Moser KM, Luchsinger PC, Adamson JS, et al: Respiratory stimulation with intravenous doxapram in respiratory failure: A double-blind co-operative study. N Engl J Med 288:427, 1973.
223. Skatrud JB, Dempsey JA, Bhansali P, et al: Determinants of chronic carbon dioxide retention and its correction in humans. J Clin Invest 65:813, 1980.
224. Skatrud JB, Dempsey JA, Iber C, Berssenbrugge A: Correction of $CO_2$ retention during sleep in patients with chronic obstructive pulmonary diseases. Am Rev Respir Dis 124:260, 1981.
225. Barcroft H, Basnayake V, Celander O, et al: The effect of carbon dioxide on the respiratory response to noradrenaline in man. Am J Physiol 137:365, 1957.
226. Miller LC, Schilling AF, Logan DL, et al: Potential hazards of rapid smoking as a technic for the modification of smoking behavior. N Engl J Med 297:590, 1977.
227. Mitchell RA, Loeschcke HH, Severinghaus JW, et al: Regions of respiratory chemosensitivity on the surface of the medulla. Ann N Y Acad Sci 109:661, 1963.
228. Potter EK, McCloskey DI: Respiratory stimulation by angiotensin II. Respir Physiol 36:367, 1979.
229. Sanders JS, Berman TM, Bartlett MM, et al: Increased hypoxic ventilatory drive due to administration of aminophylline in normal men. Chest 78:279, 1980.
230. Wechsler RL, Kleiss LM, Kety SS: The effects of intravenously administered aminophylline on cerebral circulation and metabolism in man. J Clin Invest 29:28, 1950.
231. Whelan RF, Young IM: The effect of adrenaline and noradrenaline infusions on respiration in man. Br J Pharmacol 8:98, 1953.
232. Lyons HA, Antonio R: The sensitivity of the respiratory center in pregnancy and after the administration of progesterone. Trans Assoc Am Physicians 72:173, 1959.
233. Skatrud JB, Dempsey JA, Kaiser DG: Ventilatory response to medroxyprogesterone acetate in normal subjects: Time course and mechanism. J Appl Physiol 44:939, 1978.
234. Zwillich CW, Natalino M., Sutton FD, et al: Effects of progesterone on chemosensitivity in normal men. J Lab Clin Med 92: 262, 1978.
235. Gennari FJ, Cohen JJ, Kassirer JP: Normal acid-base values. In Cohen JJ, Kassirer JP (eds): Acid-Base. Boston, Little Brown, 1982, p 107.
236. Goodland RL, Pommerenke WT: Cyclic fluctuations of the alveolar carbon dioxide tension during the normal menstrual cycle. Fertil Steril 3:394, 1952.
237. Griffith FR Jr, Pucher GW, Brownell KA, et al: Studies in human physiology. III: Alveolar air and blood gas capacity. Am J Physiol 89:449, 1929.
238. Machida H: Influence of progesterone on arterial blood and CSF acid-base balance in women. J Appl Physiol 51:1433, 1981.
239. Takano N, Kaneda T: Renal contribution to acid-base regulation during the menstrual cycle. Am J Physiol 244:F320, 1983.
240. Cullen JH, Brum VC, Reidt WU: The respiratory effects of progesterone in severe pulmonary emphysema. Am J Med 27: 551, 1959.
241. Sutton FD Jr, Zwillich CW, Creagh CE, et al: Progesterone for outpatient treatment of Pickwickian syndrome. Ann Intern Med 83:476, 1975.
242. Tyler JJ: The effect of progesterone on the respiration of patients with emphysema and hypercapnia. J Clin Invest 39: 34, 1960.
243. Kornbluth RS, Turino GM: Respiratory control in diffuse interstitial lung disease and diseases of the pulmonary vasculature. Clin Chest Med 1:91, 1980.
244. Lourenço RV, Turino GM, Davidson LAG, et al: The regulation of ventilation in diffuse pulmonary fibrosis. Am J Med 38: 199, 1965.
245. Madias NE, Cohen JJ: Determinants of arterial carbon dioxide tension and carbon dioxide balance. In Cohen JJ, Kassirer JP (eds): Acid-Base. Boston, Little Brown, 1982, p 41.
246. Stein M, Levy SE: Reflex and humoral responses to pulmonary embolism. Progr Cardiovasc Dis 17:167, 1974.
247. Szucs MM Jr, Brooks HL, Grossman W, et al: Diagnostic sensitivity of laboratory findings in acute pulmonary embolism. Ann Intern Med 74:161, 1971.
248. Trenchard D, Gardner D, Guz A: Role of pulmonary vagal afferent nerve fibers in the development of rapid shallow breathing in lung inflammation. Clin Sci 42:251, 1972.
249. Campbell LA, Schwartz SH: An unusual cause of respiratory alkalosis. Chest 100:1159, 1991.
250. Hasselbalch KA, Gammeltoft SA: Die Neutralitats—regulation des graviden Organismus. Biochem Z 68:206, 1915.
251. Blechner JN, Cotter JR, Stenger VG, et al: Oxygen, carbon dioxide and hydrogen ion concentrations in arterial blood during pregnancy. Am J Obstet Gynecol 100:1, 1968.
252. Goodland RL, Reynolds JG, Pommerenke WT: Alveolar carbon dioxide tension levels during pregnancy and early puerperium. J Clin Endocrinol 14:522, 1954.
253. Lucius H, Gahlenbeck H, Kleine H-O, et al: Respiratory functions, buffer system and electrolyte concentrations of blood during human pregnancy. Respir Physiol 9:311, 1970.
254. Marx GF, Orkin LR: Physiological changes during pregnancy: A review. Anesthesiology 19:258, 1958.
255. Pernoll ML, Metcalfe J, Kovach PA, et al: Ventilation during rest and exercise in pregnancy and postpartum. Respir Physiol 25:295, 1975.
256. Blair E: Acid-base balance in bacteremic shock. Arch Intern Med 127:731, 1971.
257. MacLean LD, Mulligan GW, McLean APH, et al: Alkalosis in septic shock. Surgery 62:655, 1967.
258. Simmons DH, Nicoloff J, Guze LB: Hyperventilation and respiratory alkalosis as signs of gram-negative bacteremia. JAMA 174:2196, 1960.
259. Karetzky MS, Mithoefer JC: The cause of hyperventilation and arterial hypoxia in patients with cirrhosis of the liver. Am J Med Sci 254:797, 1967.
260. Mulhausen R, Eichenholz A, Blumentals A: Acid-base disturbances in patients with cirrhosis of the liver. Medicine (Baltimore) 46:185, 1967.
261. Prytz H, Thomsen AC: Acid-base status in liver cirrhosis: Disturbances in stable, terminal and porta-caval shunted patients. Scand J Gastroenterol 11:249, 1976.
262. Vanamee P, Poppell JW, Glicksman AS, et al: Respiratory alkalosis in hepatic coma. Arch Intern Med 97:762, 1956.
263. Fink BR, Hanks EC, Holaday DA, et al: Monitoring of ventilation by integrated diaphragmatic electromyogram: Determination of carbon dioxide ($CO_2$) threshold in anesthetized man. JAMA 172:1367, 1960.
264. Plum F, Brown HW, Snoep E: Neurologic significance of post-hyperventilation apnea. JAMA 181:1050, 1962.
265. Raimondi AC, Raimondi GA, Adrogué HJ, et al: Hypoxemia after voluntary hyperventilation [Abstract]. Medicina (Buenos Aires) 33:621, 1973.
266. Boyd AE, Beller GA: Heat exhaustion and respiratory alkalosis. Ann Intern Med 83:835, 1975.
267. Sprung CL, Portocarrero CJ, Fernaine AV, et al: The metabolic and respiratory alterations of heat stroke. Arch Intern Med 140:665, 1980.
268. Pontén U: Consecutive acid-base changes in blood, brain tissue and cerebrospinal fluid during respiratory acidosis and baseosis. Acta Neurol Scand 42:455, 1966.
269. Mithoefer JC, Bossman OG, Thibeault DW, et al: The clinical estimation of alveolar ventilation. Am Rev Respir Dis 98:868, 1968.
270. Larson EB, Roach RC, Schoene RB, et al: Acute mountain sickness and acetazolamide: Clinical efficacy and effect on ventilation. JAMA 248:328, 1982.
271. Tolchin N, Roberts JL, Havashi J, et al: Metabolic consequences of high mass-transfer hemodialysis. Kidney Int 11:366, 1977.
272. Anderson LE, Henrich WL: Alkalemia-associated morbidity and mortality in medical and surgical patients. South Med J 80: 729, 1987.
273. Voyce SJ, Goldfine HL, Gore JM: Severe metabolic and respiratory alkalosis associated with the treatment of congestive heart failure. Arch Intern Med 147:2211, 1987.
274. Wüthrich RP: Occurrence of respiratory alkalosis in continuous ambulatory peritoneal dialysis patients with pulmonary disease. Am J Kidney Dis 25:79, 1995.

CHAPTER 10

# Acid-Base Disorders in the Critical Care Setting

Gina M. Whitney, MD ▪ Harold M. Szerlip, MD

Because of the nature of the intensive care unit, it is understandable that both simple and mixed acid-base disturbances are commonly encountered. Hypotension, drug overdose, diabetes, respiratory failure, sepsis, renal failure, and hepatic dysfunction all disturb acid-base homeostasis. In addition, the therapeutic interventions used in the critical care setting further complicate acid-base equilibrium. Disturbances of pH affect a wide variety of physiologic functions with clinically significant consequences. Timely and accurate characterization of these disturbances is therefore an essential component of critical care medicine and is often a means of appraising the severity of the underlying disease process. Identification of an acid-base disturbance should prompt a search for the cause of the disturbance itself. A thoughtful evaluation of all acid-base disturbances is of primary importance, and efforts to normalize pH should be cause-specific and based on proven therapeutic efficacy.

The normal blood pH is between 7.38 and 7.42, corresponding to a hydrogen ion concentration of 38 to 42 nanomoles/liter. A decrease in serum pH is termed *acidemia,* and any abnormal rise in pH is termed *alkalemia.* The individual processes that result in the net pH may be multiple and are termed *acidoses* or *alkaloses.* Therefore, a patient whose blood pH is 7.3 is acidemic, although he or she may simultaneously have both a metabolic acidosis and a respiratory alkalosis. The classic approach to acid-base chemistry relates the concentration of protons ($H^+$) to the concentration of bicarbonate ($HCO_3$) and the $P_{CO_2}$ via the Henderson-Hasselbalch equation ($pH = pK + \log([HCO_3^-]/[0.03 \times P_{CO_2}])$). Using this approach, all disturbances can be characterized as either metabolic, reflected by a primary change in $HCO_3$, or respiratory, resulting from an abnormality in the patient's handling of carbon dioxide ($CO_2$).

Although the Henderson-Hasselbalch approach to acid-base physiology is correct in its ability to calculate pH, acid-base homeostasis can be approached using the "strong ion difference," as expounded by Stewart.[1] Because $HCO_3$ does not vary independently of $P_{CO_2}$, it is not an independent determinant of pH. According to Stewart, $H^+$ in an aqueous fluid is determined by three independent variables: $P_{CO_2}$, net strong ion difference (ions with high dissociation constants such as Na, Cl, and K), and total weak acids (in particular, proteins). Each of these three variables, and not the gain or loss of $H^+$ or $HCO_3^-$, independently determines the dissociation of water and thus pH. For all practical purposes, clinicians can still use the Henderson-Hasselbalch equation to dissect most acid-base disturbances. In the critical care setting, however, there are circumstances such as dilutional acidosis caused by NaCl infusion or metabolic alkalosis caused by hypoproteinemia in which the Stewart approach is more explanatory. A review of the strong ion difference is beyond the scope of this chapter, and the reader is referred to several excellent reviews.[2–5]

## ACID-BASE DETERMINATION AND MONITORING

Evaluation of the acid-base status of a patient always requires a routine electrolyte panel and a blood gas analysis. From the electrolyte panel the anion gap can be calculated, thus uncovering the presence of an acidosis even if it is hidden by a normal total $CO_2$. This, combined with the $P_{CO_2}$ and pH obtained from the blood gas analysis, allows proper interpretation of the underlying disorder.

In adult patients or in those with arterial access, a sample of arterial blood is routinely used for blood gas analysis. In children, however, analysis of capillary or venous blood is common, although there are certain limitations to its routine use. Collection of a blood gas sample must be done with a low-friction syringe designed to use arterial pressure as the driving force. Excess gas in the syringe equilibrates with the gas in the blood; therefore, any air bubbles in the syringe must be removed. Laboratory analysis should be done immediately. Because red blood cells rely on anaerobic metabolism, any delay can cause an increase in sample acidity. Furthermore, excess heparin in the syringe may result in low values secondary to hemodilution.[6]

The use of capillary blood gases is also an acceptable means of evaluating both pH and $P_{CO_2}$, provided the samples are collected properly. Capillary blood gases have been shown to provide an accurate assessment of both pH and $P_{CO_2}$, with the important caveat that samples be collected after 5 minutes of "arterialization" by warming the collection site.[7] Adequacy of capillary blood gas values in emergent situations has not been evaluated.

The use of mixed venous blood gas values is emerging as an important means of assessing global tissue perfusion and cardiac output.[8–11] An increased dissociation between arterial and venous $P_{CO_2}$ has been observed in pigs with decreased cardiac output secondary to severe hemorrhagic shock and in patients during cardiac arrest.[12] Venous pH and $P_{CO_2}$ have also been shown to change earlier and to a greater extent than arterial values during periods of circulatory insufficiency.[13]

Although capnography and end-tidal $CO_2$ monitoring is commonplace in the operating room, their use in the intensive care unit is just beginning to become standard. Cardiac arrest results in an abrupt fall in end-tidal $CO_2$ to near zero, and return of a spontaneous heartbeat correlates with an increase in end-tidal $CO_2$ values.[14, 15] End-tidal $CO_2$ has been shown to correlate with cardiac output, coronary perfusion pressures, and the likelihood of successful resuscitation.[16, 17] A recent study by Levine and colleagues found that an end-tidal $CO_2$ of less than 10 mm Hg 20 minutes after the initiation of resuscitation was associated with death in 100% of patients.[18]

# ACIDOSIS

## Effects of Acidemia

The effects of acidemia are multiple (Table 10–1); however, the severity and reversibility of dysfunction are largely dependent on the underlying cause and magnitude of the derangement. Unfortunately, although a multitude of studies have looked at the effects of the acidemia on isolated cells or organs, little is known about the effects of changes in pH on whole body physiology. This is especially true in critically ill patients, in whom the underlying disorder makes it difficult to distinguish the effects of acidosis from the effects of the illness itself. Although it intuitively makes sense that severe acidosis should have adverse effects on cell function, evidence clearly supporting this supposition is difficult to find.

The effects of changes in pH on cellular function are most likely mediated by intracellular pH. Yet the effect of decreases in arterial pH on intracellular pH has not been well elucidated, especially in whole body models. Clouding the picture even further is the effect of arterial pH on mitochondrial pH, possibly a more important determinant of cellular function. In both isolated livers and hepatocytes, decreasing extracellular pH had little influence on the pH gradient across the mitochondrial membrane.[19, 20] In hepatocytes, myocytes, and renal proximal tubule cells, extracellular acidosis may actually be protective against anoxic injury.[20–22]

**TABLE 10–1.** Effects of Acidemia

| |
|---|
| **Neurologic** |
| Obtundation and coma |
| Increased cerebral blood flow |
| Increased sympathetic discharge |
| Decreased responsiveness to circulating catecholamines (severe acidemia) |
| Decreased cerebral metabolism |
| **Cardiovascular** |
| Decreased systolic contractile function |
| Centralization of blood volume (venoconstriction and arteriolar dilatation) |
| Decreased renal and hepatic blood flow |
| Decreased fibrillation threshold |
| Decreased cardiac sensitivity to catecholamines (severe acidemia) |
| No change in likelihood of conversion to sinus rhythm once fibrillation is established |
| Tachycardia |
| **Respiratory** |
| Increased minute ventilation |
| Dyspnea |
| Decreased diaphragmatic contractility and endurance |
| Respiratory muscle fatigue |
| **Metabolic** |
| Inhibition of anaerobic metabolism |
| Hyperkalemia (inorganic acidemias) |
| Hyperphosphatemia |
| Increased metabolic rate |
| Increased protein catabolism |

The role of intracellular pH in the central nervous system, in the cardiovascular system, and in oxygen delivery and utilization is only beginning to be elucidated. Because $CO_2$ quickly diffuses across cell membranes, respiratory disturbances more rapidly affect intracellular pH and have a more immediate consequence than do metabolic disturbances. The effects of acidemia mediated by $CO_2$ are highly dependent on the duration of the disturbance as well; the human body has an astounding ability to adapt to chronic abnormalities in $P_{CO_2}$.

### NEUROLOGIC EFFECTS OF ACIDEMIA

The neurologic consequences of hypercarbia have been known for some time and are dependent on the chronicity of the disturbance. Acute elevations in $P_{CO_2}$ often result in confusion, lethargy, and headache when $P_{CO_2}$ reaches approximately 60 mm Hg. Chronic increases of $P_{CO_2}$ are surprisingly well tolerated, and levels as high as 150 mm Hg may be present without apparent consequence.[23]

The importance of $P_{CO_2}$ in the regulation of cerebral blood flow (CBF) is of utmost clinical importance, and there is evidence that these changes in cerebral vascular tone are regulated by pH rather than by $CO_2$ itself.[24, 25] CBF is linearly regulated between a $P_{CO_2}$ of 20 and 80 mm Hg. Ventilation to a $P_{CO_2}$ of 30 mm Hg results in a 40% to 50% reduction in CBF.[26] The dependence of CBF on pH has important clinical implications in the management of closed head injuries and in many patients who require mechanical ventilation.

### CARDIOVASCULAR EFFECTS OF ACIDEMIA

The effects of acidemia on cardiac function have been strongly debated. Data on the effects of pH on cardiac output often conflict and vary, depending on the chronicity of the acidosis, the use of general anesthesia, and the method of data collection.[27] Cardiac output is determined by multiple components, and it is the sum of the effects on these individual components that determines the overall effect of acidemia on cardiac function. Because of differing effects of acidosis on contractile force, vascular tone, and sympathetic discharge, it is difficult to predict what happens to cardiac output from studies using isolated myocytes or perfused hearts.

A fall in pH results in an increase in sympathetic discharge but simultaneously causes a decrease in the responsiveness of the cardiac myocytes and vascular smooth muscle to the effects of catecholamines. In mildly acidemic conditions (pH >7.2), the effects of increased sympathetic stimulation predominate and result in a small increase in heart rate and cardiac output.[28] During continuous infusion of lactic acid, cardiac output and the rate of development of left ventricular contractile force increase and then stabilize at new high-performance baselines. If the acidosis develops more rapidly, left ventricular performance may actually decrease.[27] More severe acidemia (pH <7.2) results in a decreased responsiveness to circulating catecholamines, which is thought to result from a decrease in the influx and use of extracellular calcium. Increasing the concentration of extracellular calcium may therefore moderate the negative inotropic effect of severe acidemia on a temporary basis.[28] Despite the apparent pH dependence of catecholamine sensitivity, infusion of sodium bicarbonate does not appear to improve sensitivity to adrenergic agonists.[29] Both metabolic and respiratory acidosis result in the same degree of cardiac depression, although the effects of respiratory acidosis occur more rapidly in experimental models, supporting the notion that the cardiovascular effects of pH are mediated by $CO_2$.[30, 31] In studies of permissive hypercapnia, however, in which pH is deliberately allowed to decrease below 7.2, cardiac output is either unaffected or actually improves.[32, 33] Furthermore, even pH below 7.0 appears to be well tolerated in diabetic acidosis.[34, 35]

The increased sympathetic tone observed in mild metabolic acidemia increases the incidence of ventricular dysrhythmias. The likelihood of recovering a sinus rhythm once resuscitation is begun, however, is not pH dependent.[36] As a result, guidelines for the management of cardiac arrest do not advocate the routine use of sodium bicarbonate.[37] Although QT dispersion (an electrocardiographic phenomenon associated with ventricular arrhythmias) is increased in normal subjects breathing gas enriched with $CO_2$, respiratory acidosis does not appear to result in the same predisposition for ventricular irritability as does metabolic acidosis.[38] Patients with hypercapnic respiratory failure have not been shown to have a greater tendency toward dysrhythmia than that attributable to their hypoxia alone.[39, 40]

Mild acidemia causes vasodilatation in isolated vessel preparations. More severe acidemia (pH <7.15), however, has been associated with a mild increase in vessel tone.[41] The significance of this finding in the clinical setting is unclear. At the bedside, myocardial performance and changes in vascular tone determine overall cardiovascular performance, and the relative contributions of each in the context of acid-base abnormalities remain to be clarified.

### EFFECTS OF ACIDEMIA ON OXYGEN DELIVERY

A fundamental principle of critical care medicine is the necessity of maximizing the delivery of oxygen to peripheral tissues in the presence of physiologic obstacles. The dissociation of oxygen from oxyhemoglobin is dependent in part on serum pH (the Bohr effect), as illustrated by the rightward shift of the oxyhemoglobin dissociation curve in the presence of acidemia (Fig. 10–1). Acidosis thus helps to unload oxygen to tissues. This seemingly beneficial effect of acute acidosis is offset in chronic acidosis by a decrease in red cell 2,3-diphosphoglycerate (2,3-DPG), which counteracts the Bohr effect.[42] Theoretically, acutely raising the pH would increase the affinity of oxygen for hemoglobin at a time when 2,3-DPG levels remain low, thus worsening tissue hypoxia.

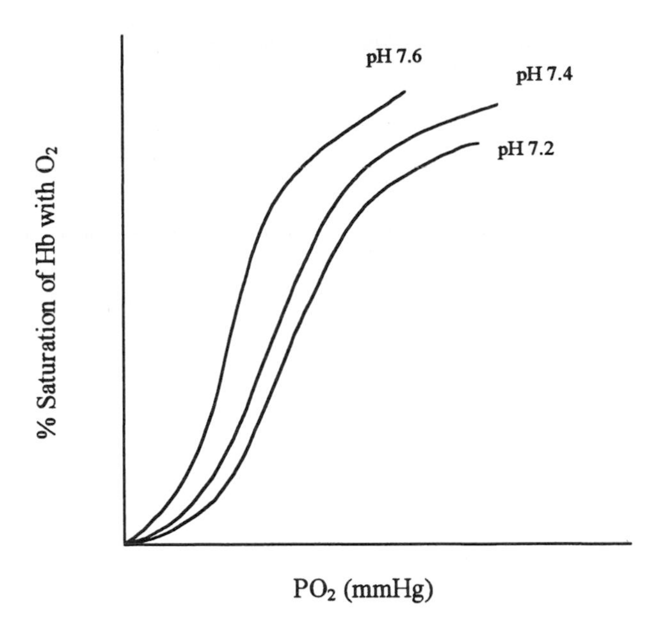


**FIGURE 10–1** ■ Effects of pH on oxyhemoglobin dissociation: the Bohr effect. The decreased affinity of hemoglobin for oxygen at low pH favors the unloading of oxygen in peripheral tissues.

## Metabolic Acidosis

Metabolic acidosis is a common acid-base disturbance in the intensive care unit (Table 10–2). A metabolic acidosis is a process whose net effect would be the lowering of body pH were it unopposed. Conceptually, a metabolic acidosis is the result of the accumulation of nonvolatile acid or the loss of serum bicarbonate, usually through the gastrointestinal or genitourinary system. In classic acid-base physiology, an acidosis is classified according to whether there is an increase in the serum anion gap (an indicator of unmeasured anions in a system) or a normal anion gap with hyperchloremia (Fig. 10–2). The usual anion gap is 10 ± 4, and elevations above 20 are generally indicative of a significant metabolic acidosis, regardless of the serum pH.[43–45] In most cases, anion gap acidoses tend to develop rapidly, as the accumulation of hydrogen ions quickly exceeds the kidney's acid excretory capacity. An acidosis with a normal serum anion gap, so-called hyperchloremic metabolic acidosis, results

**TABLE 10–2.** Causes of Metabolic Acidosis

| |
|---|
| **Anion Gap** |
| Lactic acidosis |
| Ketoacidosis |
|   Diabetic |
|   Alcoholic |
| Uremia |
| Toxins |
|   Ethylene glycol |
|   Propylene glycol |
|   Methanol |
|   Salicylates |
| **Hyperchloremic** |
| Renal tubular acidosis |
| Hyperalimentation |
| Renal failure |
| Dilutional |
| Posthypocapnic |
| Diarrhea |
| Toluene |

from a net loss of serum bicarbonate or the addition of HCl; this process generally develops more slowly.

Metabolic acidosis results in a compensatory increase in minute ventilation; near-complete respiratory compensation can be expected within hours. A decrease in pH sensitizes peripheral chemoreceptors, which triggers an increase in minute ventilation. This compensatory hyperventilation is relatively slow and is not complete for 12 to 24 hours.[46] The expected $P_{CO_2}$ for any given degree of metabolic acidosis can be predicted using the formula: $P_{CO_2} = (1.5 \times [HCO_3]) + 8 \pm 2$.[47] In mechanically ventilated patients, inadequate minute ventilation prevents this compensation.

## ANION GAP ACIDOSIS

The anion gap is the difference between the measured serum cations and anions and denotes unmeasured anions in the blood. These unmeasured anions include proteins, sulfate, phosphate, and organic anions. The anion gap is equal to (Na) − (Cl + $HCO_3$), and the normal value is 10 ± 4 (see Fig. 10–2).

### *Lactic Acidosis*

Lactic acidosis is the most common and the most serious of all anion gap acidoses. Approximately 1% of all nonsurgical inpatients develop a lactic acidosis at some point during their hospital admission.[48] There is substantial debate whether lactic acidosis represents a separate entity or is merely a consequence of a variety of other conditions common to the intensive care unit. A serum lactate level greater than 5 mmol/L is thought to represent a clinically significant lactic acidosis. Many patients in the intensive care unit maintain serum lactate levels between 2 and 5 mmol/L (denoted as hyperlactinemia), and it is unclear which patients progress to develop a frank lactic acidosis.

Lactic acid is the product of the anaerobic metabolism of pyruvate. Pyruvate is derived from glucose by means of the Embden-Meyerhof pathway (Fig. 10–3). Under normal aerobic conditions, pyruvate is oxidized and results in the production of acetyl coenzyme A. In the absence of oxygen, however, pyruvate is reduced to lactate. Lactate is converted back to pyruvate by both the liver and the kidney via the Cori cycle. Hepatic dysfunction, therefore, predisposes to the development of lactic acidemia in the presence of tissue hypoperfusion.

Early inquiries into the nature of metabolic acidosis resulted in the classification of lactic acidoses into types A (hypoxic) and B (nonhypoxic).[49] Type A lactic acidosis results from an imbalance in oxygen supply and demand, and it is commonly the result of impaired oxygen delivery, such as when there is cardiopulmonary compromise or severe hypoxemia. Type A lactic acidosis may also arise from an impaired oxygen balance in regional tissue beds, as is observed in patients with splanchnic ischemia.[50] Major sources of serum lactic acid during periods of hypoperfusion include the skin, red blood cells, brain, lung, skeletal muscle, and intestinal mucosa.[51, 52] Type B lactic acidosis is the

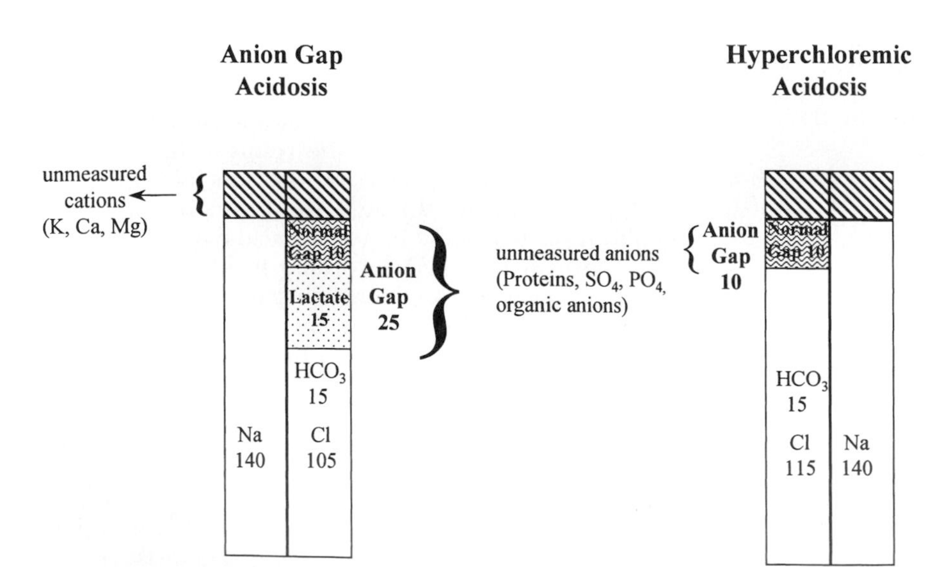


**FIGURE 10–2** ■ The anion gap is equal to $Na^+ - (Cl^- + HCO_3)$, which is equal to the unmeasured anions minus the unmeasured cations. In an anion gap acidosis, there is a decrease in $HCO_3$ and an increase in organic anions (e.g., lactate), which results in an elevated anion gap. In a hyperchloremic acidosis, there is a decrease in $HCO_3$ and an increase in $Cl^-$, with no change in anion gap.

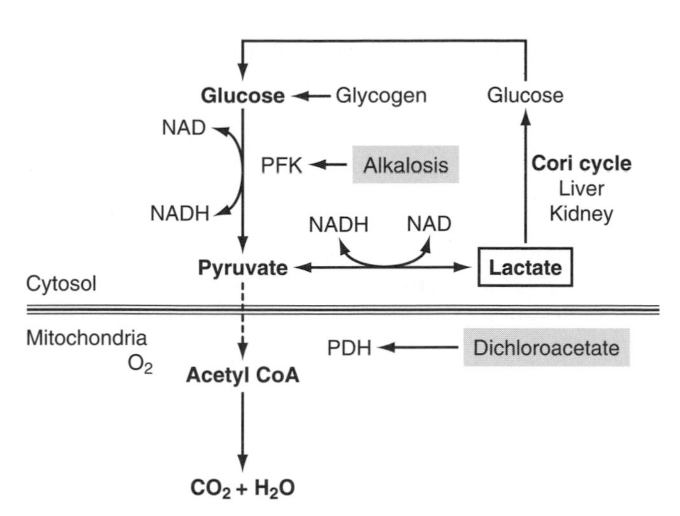


**FIGURE 10–3** ■ Metabolism of lactate. Under anaerobic conditions, pyruvate is converted to lactate. Lactate can be metabolized back to glucose in the Cori cycle. Alkalosis increases the activity of phosphofructokinase (PFK), the rate-limiting enzyme in the Embden-Meyerhof pathway. Dichloroacetate increases the activity of pyruvate dehydrogenase complex (PDH). NAD, nicotinamide adenine dinucleotide; NADH, reduced form of NAD.

result of nonhypoxic conditions such as inborn errors of metabolism or ingestion of drugs or toxins. It has become increasingly clear, however, that lactic acidosis is often the result of the simultaneous existence of both hypoxic and nonhypoxic factors, and in many cases it is difficult to separate one from the other. In a patient in shock, for example, decreased oxygen delivery to peripheral tissues results in hypoxic lactic acid accumulation. The severe acidemia decreases portal blood flow and therefore decreases hepatic clearance of lactic acid.[53] Similarly, in sepsis there is both a decrease in tissue perfusion and a decrease in the ability to use oxygen. Therefore, the classification of lactic acidosis based on cause is largely of historical and conceptual interest.

The numerous causes of lactic acidosis are outlined in Table 10–3.. As can be seen, a growing number of drugs have been implicated in the precipitation of lactic acidosis. Of particular note is the newer biguanide (metformin) and the antiretrovirals. The reader is referred to Chapter 6 for a more detailed review of the causes of lactic acidosis.

Findings of lactic acidosis on physical examination are often subtle and may consist of only hyperpnea or tachypnea. Critically ill patients with a significantly elevated anion gap or low serum bicarbonate should be suspected of having a lactic acidosis, particularly in the presence of hepatic insufficiency. A high index of suspicion must be maintained, however, because the anion gap is a relatively insensitive reflection of lactic acidosis. Iberti and coworkers found a poor correlation among arterial pH, calculated anion gap, and serum lactate levels, even in those patients with serum lactic acid levels greater than 5 mmol/L.[54] Fifty percent of patients with serum lactate levels between 5 and 9.9 mmol/L had anion gaps less than 12.

Several investigators have sought to characterize the

**TABLE 10–3.** Causes of Lactic Acidosis

**Inadequate Oxygen Delivery**

Generalized seizures
Extreme exercise
Shock
Cardiac arrest
Low cardiac output
Severe anemia
Severe hypoxemia
Carbon monoxide poisoning

**Impaired Oxygen Utilization or Defective Lactate Metabolism**

Sepsis
Thiamine deficiency
Carbon monoxide poisoning
Uncontrolled diabetes mellitus
Malignancy
Hypoglycemia
Drugs/toxins
- Ethanol
- Methanol
- Ethylene glycol
- Metformin
- Salicylate
- Aspirin
- Niacin
- Isoniazid
- Zalcitabine
- Zidovudine
- Didanosine
- Stavudine
- Lamivudine
- Nitroprusside
- Cyanide
- Catecholamines
- Cocaine
- Acetaminophen
- Streptozotocin

Pheochromocytoma
Sorbitol/fructose
Malaria
Hepatic failure
Respiratory or metabolic alkalosis
Inborn errors of metabolism
D-Lactic acidosis

prognostic value of serum lactic acid levels. Studies have found that as lactate levels rise above 2.0 to 2.5 mmol/L, the probability of survival falls precipitously.[55–57] It remains unclear, however, whether serum lactate level is an independent contributor to mortality or whether it represents an epiphenomenon confounded by the severity of the patient's illness. Just as important to prognosis as the absolute lactate concentration is the body's ability to handle a lactic acid load after a resuscitative effort. Falk and colleagues found that patients able to clear 50% of serum lactate 18 hours after a resuscitative effort had a significantly greater chance of survival.[58] Other studies reinforced these findings, revealing both significantly lower lactate levels and increased ability to clear lactate in survivors over nonsurvivors.[59] In all likelihood, the ability to clear lactate is a surrogate marker for organ dysfunction. Supporting the conclusion that the degree of hyperlactinemia is an epiphenomenon is the finding that the prognostic utility of serum lactate is dependent on whether the patient is in a clinically apparent shock state, as opposed to there being other, nonhypotensive reasons for the accumulation of lactate.[60, 61] Furthermore, dichloroacetate, which stimulates pyruvate dehydrogenase and therefore decreases lactic acidosis, has not been shown to affect survival.[62]

**Treatment of Lactic Acidosis.** The ongoing discussion of whether lactic acidosis itself contributes to mortality or is merely an indicator of the severity of the patient's underlying illness has resulted in continued debate about the proper use of buffers in the management of lactic acidosis. Participants on both sides of the clinical debate agree that the primary means of management of lactic acidosis is the reversal of those processes that led to its development. Optimizing cardiac output and tissue oxygenation by the use of supportive therapies should be of primary consideration in the management of these patients. Mechanical ventilation is instituted to reduce the metabolic work of breathing and optimize ventilation; fluids and inotropes are helpful in restoring adequate cardiac output. Vasoactive drugs should be used, based on an understanding of the underlying hemodynamics and a knowledge of the drugs' mechanisms of action. Careful consideration should be given to the heart's ability to maintain adequate cardiac output in the face of increasing afterload.

***Sodium Bicarbonate.*** Traditionally, sodium bicarbonate ($NaHCO_3$) has been the buffer of choice in the treatment of metabolic acidosis. The use of $NaHCO_3$ in the management of lactic acidosis is an attempt to normalize pH and buffer the effects of acidemia. Proponents of $NaHCO_3$ argue that the acidosis itself is detrimental to normal physiologic function. Although severe acidosis *may* have a deleterious effect on cardiopulmonary performance, some studies have actually shown an improvement in cardiac performance in the presence of a mild to moderate acidosis.[32] Because of this, the pH at which most clinicians feel obligated to use $NaHCO_3$ has fallen. Many physicians use $NaHCO_3$ in the treatment of severe acidosis when the pH is less than 7.1. At this pH, as predicted by the Henderson-Hasselbalch equation, minor changes in bicarbonate or $PCO_2$ will result in a large decrease in pH.[63] Unfortunately, there are no data that point to a specific pH at which therapy must be instituted. To avoid hypertonicity, $NaHCO_3$ should be given as an isotonic infusion rather than a bolus, and re-evaluation of acid-base status should be delayed for 30 minutes to allow for equilibration.[64] Several anecdotal case reports purport to show a benefit to treating lactic acidosis with bicarbonate-based peritoneal dialysis.[65–67] Until such therapy is studied in a prospective, randomized manner, no conclusions about the possible benefit of peritoneal dialysis can be made.

The results of several animal and human studies under a variety of experimental conditions argue against the routine use of bicarbonate. In animal studies, the use of $NaHCO_3$ resulted in an increase in lactate production in the splanchnic vascular beds, an increase in circulating lactate levels, decreased intracellular pH, a decrease in arterial pH, and a smaller increase in cardiac output relative to a normal saline infusion.[68–70] Studies in humans showed results consistent with those of the animal studies. A prospective study evaluating the use of $NaHCO_3$ in patients with lactic acidosis showed an increase in serum pH but no improvement in hemodynamics when compared with normal saline.[71] The use of $NaHCO_3$ also failed to increase hemodynamic responsiveness to circulating catecholamines, perhaps due to the observed decrease in serum ionized calcium.[72] $NaHCO_3$ may also result in impaired use of circulating oxygen and actually increase anaerobic metabolism. $NaHCO_3$ generates $CO_2$ ($HCO_3^- + H^+ \rightarrow H_2O + CO_2$). With depressed cardiac output, $CO_2$ can build up in the venous circulation, causing intracellular acidosis and depressing cardiac output even more. Administration of $NaHCO_3$ to patients with New York Heart Association class III and IV congestive heart failure resulted in a 10 mm Hg decrease in oxygen, decreased systemic oxygen consumption by 21%, decreased myocardial oxygen consumption by 17%, and caused an overall increase in serum lactate.[73]

***Dichloroacetate.*** Dichloroacetate was developed as a "rational therapy" for lactic acidosis based on its mechanism of action. It stimulates the activity of pyruvate dehydrogenase, thereby increasing the rate of oxidation of pyruvate and limiting the generation of lactate. Initial results of animal studies showed improved aerobic glucose utilization and an increase in intracellular adenosine triphosphate. A positive inotropic effect has also been shown and is thought to be due to improved glucose utilization. A large multicenter trial in humans showed a significant reduction in serum lactate, an increase in arterial pH, and an increase in the percentage of patients who were able to resolve their hyperlactinemia from 43% to 58%.[62] This study did not find any significant improvement in blood pressure in either hypotensive or normotensive patients. Furthermore, although dichloroacetate was effective in improving lactic acidosis, there was no change in mortality. Chronic use of dichloroacetate has been associated with neurologic toxicity, including limb paralysis and neuropathies.[74]

***Carbicarb.*** Carbicarb is an equimolar mixture of sodium bicarbonate and sodium carbonate designed to decrease the $CO_2$ burden that results from the administration of sodium bicarbonate (Fig. 10–4).[75] It is theoretically superior to sodium bicarbonate, in that it has an equal buffering capacity but does not result in the generation of $CO_2$.[76] Animal studies examining the effects of Carbicarb administration showed a stabilization of serum lactate levels, as well as an improved acid-base profile relative to sodium bicarbonate, which increased lactate, lowered intracellular pH, and increased $PCO_2$.[77] Carbicarb administration also resulted in a significant increase in the cardiac index when compared with normal saline and sodium bicarbonate. The improved hemodynamic parameters observed with the use of Carbicarb have been attributed to

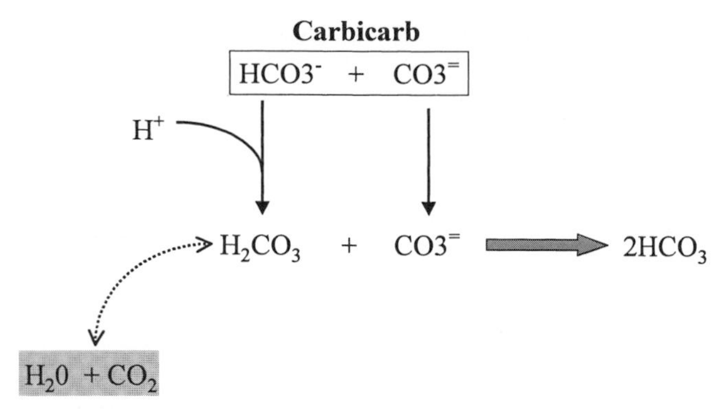


**FIGURE 10–4** ■ Carbicarb is an equimolar mixture of sodium bicarbonate and sodium carbonate. It buffers without the production of carbon dioxide.

improved myocyte intracellular pH.[78] Controlled studies examining the effectiveness of Carbicarb in the clinical setting have not yet been done, and this buffer is not presently available for use.

***Tromethamine.*** Tromethamine (Tham) is a biologically inert amino alcohol that buffers both $CO_2$ and nonvolatile acids. It is available in the United States as Tham acetate 0.3 mol/L; it has a pK of 7.8 and is therefore a good buffer at a pH of 7.4. In vivo, Tham acts as a proton acceptor. It is therefore able to buffer both respiratory and metabolic acidoses and, unlike bicarbonate, does not require an open system to exert its effects. The protonated form of Tham is excreted in the urine, so Tham administration should be avoided in patients with renal insufficiency. Potential side effects of Tham administration include hyperkalemia, hypoglycemia, ventilatory depression, and hepatic necrosis in neonates.[79] Improvement in patient outcome after the administration of Tham has not been shown. Given the risk of serious side effects, Tham should be used only after careful consideration.

The correct dose of Tham acetate (in milliliters of 0.3 mol/L solution) is equal to lean body weight multiplied by base deficit in mmol/L. The maximum daily dose of Tham in a 70-kg patient is 3.5 L, or 15 mmol/kg. Due to reduced glomerular filtration in neonates, the maximum daily dose of Tham in neonates is 7 mmol/kg.

***Tribonat.*** Tribonat is mixture of Tham, sodium bicarbonate, acetate, and phosphate designed to minimize the previously reported negative consequences of using other buffers. Initial data on the use of Tribonat demonstrated only a transient, minor intracellular acidification, as opposed to a much more significant drop in intracellular pH induced by the administration of sodium bicarbonate.[80–82] In contrast to sodium bicarbonate, Tribonat has minimal effects on either plasma sodium or osmolality. Although its use is common in Scandinavian countries, to date there have been no human studies demonstrating an improved outcome with the use of Tribonat.

### *D-Lactic Acidosis*

When there is overgrowth of gut bacteria, an overproduction of D-lactate may occur.[83] Although this disorder is more common in unguents, cases are occasionally seen in humans. Therefore, clinicians must be able to recognize this syndrome. Patients present with an anion gap acidosis and normal lactate levels. They typically have neurologic findings such as confusion, ataxia, and loss of memory. Symptoms are worsened after high-carbohydrate meals. The D-isomer of lactate cannot be metabolized by lactate dehydrogenase, which is specific for the L form, but must be cleared by D-α-hydroxy acid dehydrogenase. This enzyme can metabolize up to 2500 mEq of D-lactate a day. In patients with short bowel syndrome or who have undergone jejunal-ileal bypass, there is an overgrowth of bacteria; in addition, carbohydrates that normally do not reach the colon now readily do. Enough D-lactate can be produced to overwhelm enzymatic clearance.

Because the laboratory assay for lactate uses lactate dehydrogenase specific for L-lactate, elevated lactate levels are not measured in this disorder. D-Lactic acidosis should be considered in patients with a history of intestinal disease who present with confusion and an anion gap metabolic acidosis. D-Lactate can be measured using gas chromatography or by substituting D-lactate dehydrogenase when running the assay. Treatment is aimed at decreasing the overgrowth of bacteria with antibiotics and the avoidance of high-carbohydrate meals.

### *Diabetic Ketoacidosis*

Diabetic ketoacidosis (DKA) is responsible for 16% of diabetes-related mortality and is the most common cause of death in diabetic children. Of those patients who are found to have DKA, 10% are new-onset diabetics, and 90% have previously been diagnosed with diabetes.[84] Presentation may be one of mental status changes, shock, or severe gastroenteritis-like symptoms. Patients often have a history of polyuria, polydipsia, noncompliance with their insulin regimen, or concomitant illness. In one study, 27% of patients presenting with DKA were type 2 diabetics, and infection was identified as the most common precipitating factor in this group of patients.[85] Patients with type 2 diabetes may occasionally have a more indolent presentation, experiencing mild symptoms for weeks to months before developing DKA.[86] Physical examination is usually significant for signs of intravascular volume depletion, Kussmaul respiration, or the fruity odor of acetone on the breath. By definition, the laboratory diagnosis of DKA requires glucose greater than 250 mg/dL, pH less than 7.35, decreased serum bicarbonate, anion gap acidosis, and positive serum ketones.

It is important to recognize and treat any superimposed infections that may have contributed to the development of DKA. Although leukocytosis is common in DKA, a white blood cell count greater than 25,000 should intensify the search for an infectious source. Careful analysis of arterial blood gas values may reveal a primary respiratory alkalosis in addition to the metabolic acidosis, which may indicate sepsis or an underlying pulmonic process.

Although the acidosis is most commonly an anion gap acidosis, a mixed anion gap–hyperchloremic acidosis or, rarely, a pure hyperchloremic acidosis may be present.[87] The type of acidosis depends on the volume status of the patient. If fluid intake has been adequate, the kidneys will excrete ketones, reducing the unmeasured anions without affecting the acidosis.

DKA is a consequence of relative insulin deficiency and a simultaneous increase in counter-regulatory hormones (epinephrine, glucagon, norepinephrine, cortisol, and growth hormone). This results in an elevated extracellular glucose concentration that cells are unable to use, secondary to the deficiency of insulin. With a deficiency of intracellular glucose, cells shift to a state of catabolic and ketogenic metabolism. Rates of lipolysis, gluconeogenesis, and glycogenolysis are all increased, and glycolysis decreases. (See Chapter 5.)

As a result of insulin deficiency, extracellular hyperkalemia is often present, although because of the osmotic diuresis, total body potassium is invariably low.[88] Similar to potassium, the serum phosphate is frequently elevated, despite total body phosphate depletion. Serum glucose is commonly elevated between 200 and 500 mg/dL. Euglycemic DKA, however, has been reported in the presence of decreased oral intake and pregnancy.[89] Measured serum sodium is low and must be corrected for hyperglycemia: corrected serum Na = measured Na + 0.016 (glucose − 100).

If there is concomitant tissue hypoperfusion—a condition that commonly occurs in DKA—β-hydroxybutyrate will be the primary ketone formed. Because β-hydroxybutyrate is not detected by the nitroprusside reaction used in standard serum and urine tests, laboratory analysis for ketones may on occasion be negative. Theoretically, adding a small amount of hydrogen peroxide to the urine sample will oxidize β-hydroxybutyrate to acetoacetate, enabling detection by the nitroprusside test. With time, however, β-hydroxybutyrate will be converted naturally to acetoacetate. As a result, treatment of DKA may actually result in an initial increase in detected ketones in the urine or serum. It is thus more important to follow the closure of the anion gap than the serum ketones when monitoring the appropriateness of therapy.

**Management of Diabetic Ketoacidosis.** The efficient management of DKA relies on the prompt initiation of fluid resuscitation with an isotonic solution, followed by intravenous (IV) insulin infusion, often in accordance with institutional protocols.[90] In the absence of hemodynamically significant intravascular volume depletion, a moderate regimen of fluid replacement has been shown to result in less acid-base derangement.[91] In the presence of clinically apparent volume depletion, however, 0.9% saline should be infused more rapidly, with 1 to 2 L given within the first hour. After initial volume resuscitation, 0.45% saline should be administered with an appropriate amount of potassium replacement. When serum potassium falls below 4.5 mEq/L, potassium chloride should be added to the IV fluids at a concentration of 10 to 20 mEq/L. Controlled studies have failed to show any benefit in replacing phosphate during the treatment of DKA.[92] Many practitioners, however, often replace some of the potassium in the form of $KPO_4$ in order to replete both ions simultaneously. Because the total body potassium deficit in DKA far exceeds the phosphate depletion, the sole use of $KPO_4$ to replace depleted potassium stores may result in iatrogenic hyperphosphatemia.

After initial volume replacement, insulin therapy should be initiated. Premature administration of insulin before intravascular volume expansion may result in hypotension and cardiovascular collapse as water moves into cells from the extracellular space. Therapy with regular insulin is begun at the rate of 0.1 U/kg/hr continuous IV infusion. A bolus of regular insulin (0.1 U/kg IV) should be given before initiation of the infusion. For regular insulin, the IV route is preferred; its half-life of 5 minutes allows for close titration of the fall in serum glucose. For every hour that the glucose does not fall by 50 to 100 mg/dL, the rate of insulin infusion should be increased by 50% to 100%. When glucose reaches 250 mg/dL, IV fluids should be changed to include 5% dextrose. At this point, both IV dextrose and insulin infusions should be maintained *until the ketosis has resolved.* As the insulin decreases the production of ketoacids and as the kidney excretes those already present in the serum, the anion gap will normalize, and a hyperchloremic metabolic acidosis may emerge. Bicarbonate stores are regenerated over the next 12 to 24 hours. After closure of the anion gap and suppression of ketogenesis, the IV insulin can be discontinued. At least 1 hour before stopping the insulin infusion, subcutaneous regular insulin should be given. Serum electrolytes should continue to be monitored after the transition to a subcutaneous insulin regimen.

The use of sodium bicarbonate in the management of DKA has not been shown to improve patient outcome, even in the presence of an initial serum pH less than 7.0.[34, 35] The routine use of $NaHCO_3$ therefore cannot be recommended.

In the management of DKA in children, it is critical that the physician monitor the patient for any change in neurologic status. Cerebral edema, which occurs more frequently in children, typically presents 4 to 16 hours after the initiation of treatment and is thought to be secondary to rapid correction of the hyperglycemia.[93–95] The acute development of headache, a change in the patient's level of consciousness, or signs of increased intracranial pressure should be treated promptly with mannitol (10 to 20 gm/$m^2$ IV), and management of the ketoacidosis should be slowed. When the patient's condition allows, a computed tomography scan of the head is required to rule out an intracranial event such as thrombosis of a cerebral artery or the sagittal sinus, which can occur in these patients.

It is essential to closely monitor patients being treated for DKA. Cardiopulmonary or renal insufficiency may result in clinically significant volume overload. The use of a flowsheet combined with frequent

**Diabetic Ketoacidosis Flowsheet**

Patient Name Number Weight Height
Date of Admission

|  |  |  |  |  |  |  |  |  |  |  |  |  |  |
|---|---|---|---|---|---|---|---|---|---|---|---|---|---|
| Date |  |  |  |  |  |  |  |  |  |  |  |  |  |
| Time |  |  |  |  |  |  |  |  |  |  |  |  |  |
|  |  |  |  |  |  |  |  |  |  |  |  |  |  |
| **Clinical Data** |  |  |  |  |  |  |  |  |  |  |  |  |  |
| HR |  |  |  |  |  |  |  |  |  |  |  |  |  |
| RR |  |  |  |  |  |  |  |  |  |  |  |  |  |
| BP |  |  |  |  |  |  |  |  |  |  |  |  |  |
| Temp |  |  |  |  |  |  |  |  |  |  |  |  |  |
|  |  |  |  |  |  |  |  |  |  |  |  |  |  |
| **Laboratory Data** |  |  |  |  |  |  |  |  |  |  |  |  |  |
| Glucose |  |  |  |  |  |  |  |  |  |  |  |  |  |
| Na |  |  |  |  |  |  |  |  |  |  |  |  |  |
| K |  |  |  |  |  |  |  |  |  |  |  |  |  |
| Cl |  |  |  |  |  |  |  |  |  |  |  |  |  |
| $CO_2$ |  |  |  |  |  |  |  |  |  |  |  |  |  |
| BUN |  |  |  |  |  |  |  |  |  |  |  |  |  |
| Cr |  |  |  |  |  |  |  |  |  |  |  |  |  |
| Calcium |  |  |  |  |  |  |  |  |  |  |  |  |  |
| Phosphorus |  |  |  |  |  |  |  |  |  |  |  |  |  |
|  |  |  |  |  |  |  |  |  |  |  |  |  |  |
| Anion Gap |  |  |  |  |  |  |  |  |  |  |  |  |  |
| Corrected Na |  |  |  |  |  |  |  |  |  |  |  |  |  |
|  |  |  |  |  |  |  |  |  |  |  |  |  |  |
| **Blood Gas Data** |  |  |  |  |  |  |  |  |  |  |  |  |  |
| pH |  |  |  |  |  |  |  |  |  |  |  |  |  |
| $pCO_2$ |  |  |  |  |  |  |  |  |  |  |  |  |  |
| $HCO_3$ |  |  |  |  |  |  |  |  |  |  |  |  |  |
| Base Excess |  |  |  |  |  |  |  |  |  |  |  |  |  |
|  |  |  |  |  |  |  |  |  |  |  |  |  |  |
| Urine ketones |  |  |  |  |  |  |  |  |  |  |  |  |  |
|  |  |  |  |  |  |  |  |  |  |  |  |  |  |
| **Interventions** |  |  |  |  |  |  |  |  |  |  |  |  |  |
| IVF rate |  |  |  |  |  |  |  |  |  |  |  |  |  |
| Dextrose % |  |  |  |  |  |  |  |  |  |  |  |  |  |
| Na mmol /l |  |  |  |  |  |  |  |  |  |  |  |  |  |
| KCl mmol/l |  |  |  |  |  |  |  |  |  |  |  |  |  |
| $KPO_4$ mmol/l |  |  |  |  |  |  |  |  |  |  |  |  |  |
| Insulin gtt (units / hour) |  |  |  |  |  |  |  |  |  |  |  |  |  |
|  |  |  |  |  |  |  |  |  |  |  |  |  |  |
|  |  |  |  |  |  |  |  |  |  |  |  |  |  |

**FIGURE 10–5** ■ Use of a flowsheet allows for optimal management of patients with diabetic ketoacidosis.

monitoring is an efficient and logical way to manage these patients (Fig. 10–5). Such a record enables all participants in the patient's care to monitor trends in clinical and laboratory parameters and detect clinical decompensation early in the course of treatment.

### *Alcoholic Ketoacidosis*

Alcoholic ketoacidosis (AKA), first described in 1940, is an increasingly recognized cause of ketoacidosis. AKA is diagnosed in nondiabetic alcohol abusers who present with an anion gap acidosis and ketonemia without significant hyperglycemia. Typically, the patient has been on an alcohol binge and, because of the development of abdominal pain or nausea and vomiting, has stopped taking in nutrition. Patients with AKA usually present 24 to 48 hours into their fast with the chief complaints of nausea, vomiting, abdominal pain, and shortness of breath. Alcohol levels are unmeasurable, or alcohol is present only in nonintoxicating levels.[96] When evaluating someone with suspected AKA, it is important to consider other causes of anion gap acidosis, such as ingestion of methanol, ethylene glycol, or salicylates. In addition, because of the frequency of lactic acidosis in alcoholics, lactate levels should be measured.

Although an anion gap acidosis is always present, it is not unusual for patients with AKA to have mixed acid-base disturbances. Metabolic alkalosis from vomiting and respiratory alkalosis from liver disease or underlying infection are commonly present. In fact, frank alkalemia may exist. Wrenn and coworkers found that only 58% of patients were acidemic, and 78% of patients had a mixed acid-base disturbance.[97] β-Hydroxybutyrate is the primary ketoacid seen in AKA and therefore may be undetectable by nitroprusside testing.

Hypoglycemia is seen in those patients who have not recently eaten or in whom alcohol consumption has continued until the time of admission. Electrolyte abnormalities are frequent and include hypokalemia, hypophosphatemia, and hypomagnesemia. Approximately 10% of patients with AKA have a serum glucose value greater than 250 mg/dL, and distinguishing between DKA and AKA may prove difficult. Fasting blood glucose should be checked in these patients after the acute episode and any superimposed illnesses have resolved.

**Treatment of Alcoholic Ketoacidosis.** The treatment of AKA consists of volume repletion with 0.9% saline, glucose infusion in those patients who are not hyperglycemic, and correction of all electrolyte abnormalities. Before the administration of glucose, however, thiamine must be given to avoid precipitating Wernicke encephalopathy. The optimal rate of fluid replacement in the management of AKA has not been established. Restoration of adequate intravascular volume promotes renal excretion of ketones, and glucose administration decreases both ketone body formation and the level of circulating counter-regulatory hormones. With ketogenesis turned off, the regeneration of bicarbonate can begin. In those patients who are hyperglycemic, insulin should be administered. Similar to DKA, a hyperchloremic metabolic acidosis may develop during the recovery phase of AKA, although it generally resolves within 24 hours.

***Toxins***

Ingestions account for 5% to 10% of all intensive care unit admissions, and 64% of all pediatric ingestions result in admission to a pediatric intensive care unit.[98] Toxin ingestion is an important cause of anion gap acidosis and should always be considered when evaluating a patient with anion gap acidosis. Although measurement of the serum osmolal gap may support the diagnosis of ingestion of low-molecular-weight toxins such as methanol or ethylene glycol, serum toxicology screens specifically looking for these substances should serve as the gold standard. Even before the correct diagnosis is made, treatment to support the patient's vital signs should be initiated. Intoxication with methanol or ethylene glycol should be strongly suspected in the presence of an anion gap acidosis, particularly in conjunction with mental status changes or in the absence of ketosis.

The serum osmolal gap is the difference between the calculated and the measured serum osmolality. A normal serum osmolality is 285 to 295 mOsm, and a normal serum osmolal gap is 5 to 10 mOsm/kg. An increased osmolal gap may help identify osmotically active low-molecular-weight molecules more rapidly than toxicology screening can. Because of several pitfalls, however, it is important for the clinician not to misinterpret the absence of an osmolal gap as indicating that the acidosis is *not* secondary to toxic ingestion. If the serum osmolality is measured using vapor pressure methodology, as opposed to freezing point depression, volatile substances such as methanol and ethylene glycol that remain in the vapor phase may not be detected.[99] Furthermore, it is the metabolism of these toxins into osmotically inactive acids that produces the acidosis. Thus, shortly after ingestion, the osmolal gap will be elevated without an acidosis; later, when the acidosis is most pronounced, there may not be an osmolal gap.[100]

**Ethylene Glycol.** Ethylene glycol is a viscous, sweet liquid and is therefore a common accidental ingestion in children and a frequent substitute for ethanol in alcohol abusers. Ethylene glycol ingestion should be suspected in the presence of an acidosis with a low blood alcohol level and acute intoxication. Ethylene glycol is not detected on routine toxicology screens, and gas chromatography is required for identification. Laboratory requests should specify ethylene glycol as the suspected toxin.

Ethylene glycol is a low-molecular-weight toxin whose metabolites are far more toxic than the parent compound.[101] It is rapidly absorbed and hepatically metabolized by alcohol dehydrogenase to glycolic acid and subsequently to oxalic acid. A small amount is converted to glycine and then hippurate. These metabolic processes generate the reduced form of nicotinamide adenine dinucleotide, consequently favoring lactate production from pyruvate. The anion gap acidosis results from the accumulation of the various acid metabolites of ethylene glycol and lactate.[102] Laboratory analysis reveals a severe anion gap acidosis. With clinically significant ingestions (serum levels of approximately 50 mg/dL), in the early stages the osmolar gap is elevated; however, as ethylene glycol is metabolized, the osmolar gap narrows.[103] Pleocytosis and elevated protein are often noted on examination of the cerebrospinal fluid. Urinalysis frequently reveals calcium oxalate crystals and, more rarely, hippurate crystals. These classic findings may initially be missed and may never be noted if anuric renal failure supervenes.

Antifreeze preparations of ethylene glycol commonly contain sodium fluorescein as a colorant. The urine of a patient with suspected antifreeze ingestion may fluoresce under Wood lamp examination for several hours after ingestion. Traditional methods of identifying ethylene glycol ingestion should still be pursued, regardless of the result of Wood lamp fluorescence.[104]

Fatalities occur with ingestion of approximately 100 mL of ethylene glycol.[105] Patients typically pass through three stages of toxicity.[106,107] The initial stage is characterized by central nervous system depression, stupor, and eventually coma. This stage lasts about 12 hours. It is during this early period that the acidosis becomes evident. The second stage is heralded by cardiopulmonary failure. Oliguric acute renal failure develops in the last stage. Recovery of renal function occurs if the patient survives. The acute renal failure is probably secondary to calcium oxalate deposition.[108] Not only can these crystals be seen in the urine, but they can also be found in the brain and liver on postmortem examination.

***Management of Ethylene Glycol Intoxication.*** Although there are no supportive data, gastric lavage with activated charcoal is recommended within 1 to 2 hours of ingestion. Promoting a diuresis with saline and a loop diuretic enhances renal clearance.[109] Therapy should be directed toward preventing the metabolism of ethylene glycol to its toxic intermediates and removal of ethylene glycol from the body. Because alcohol dehydrogenase, the enzyme responsible for the metabolism of ethylene glycol, has a much higher affinity for ethanol, IV ethanol infusion has been the mainstay of therapy. Ethanol is supplied as a 10% solution in D-5-W. A loading dose of 0.8 to 1.0 g/kg of ethanol should be given, followed by a continuous infusion of approximately 100 mg/kg/hr to maintain a blood alcohol level of 100 to 150 mg/dL. In ethanol-tolerant patients, the infusion may need to be increased to as high as 200 mg/kg/hr. In patients undergoing hemodialysis, the rate of ethanol infusion should be doubled.[110]

Recent clinical practice has evolved to include the use of 4-methylpyrazole (fomepizole) in the management of ethylene glycol intoxication rather than ethanol infusion. 4-Methylpyrazole is a competitive inhibitor of alcohol dehydrogenase that does not cause the central nervous system depression seen with ethanol infusion. Side effects include rash, eosinophilia, nausea, dizziness, and headache.[111] An initial loading dose of 15 mg/kg is followed in 12 hours by a dose of 10 mg/kg every 12 hours for four doses, which is then increased to 15 mg/kg every 12 hours for four doses. It is necessary to increase the dose administered because 4-methylpyrazole induces the enzymes that result in its metabolism.[112] The dose of 4-methylpyrazole must also be increased if hemodialysis is initiated. Growing evidence suggests that in patients without renal failure or significant acidosis, 4-methylpyrazole may be used as monotherapy without the need for hemodialysis.[113, 114] Patients with ethylene glycol toxicity should also be given pyridoxine and thiamine. Both these cofactors may help shunt the metabolism of glycolic acid away from oxalate and theoretically prevent organ toxicity.[106]

Once the metabolism of ethylene glycol is blocked, it can be removed from the body by hemodialysis. Although presently in a state of flux, the accepted indications for hemodialysis in the management of ethylene glycol intoxication include a serum level of greater than 50 mg/dL, end-organ damage, and refractory metabolic acidosis (pH <7.15). Hemodialysis should be continued until serum levels decrease to less than 20 mg/dL. Hemodialysis effectively removes the acid intermediates and resolves the metabolic acidosis resulting from ethylene glycol ingestion. The patient's acid-base status should be monitored hourly during therapy.

**Methanol.** Methanol or wood alcohol is the simplest of all alcohols. It is a commonly used solvent and has a growing role as an alternative fuel for gasoline. Because it is inexpensive, it has been used as an illegal adulterant to ethanol—a practice responsible for periodic outbreaks of methanol poisoning. Legally, it is used as a "denaturant" added to ethanol, rendering it theoretically undrinkable and therefore tax free. Interestingly, methanol was frequently added to alcoholic beverages in the early part of the 20th century. Although the usual route of toxicity is by ingestion, toxicity has also been reported through inhalation.[115]

Methanol is metabolized by alcohol dehydrogenase to formaldehyde and then to formic acid at a slower rate than ethanol. Methanol produces less intoxication than both ethanol and ethylene glycol. Methanol, itself, is nontoxic. Its metabolites, however, can be fatal. There is usually a latent period of 12 to 16 hours before signs and symptoms of toxicity appear. The ingestion of as little as 30 mL can cause death. The hallmark of methanol ingestion is a profound anion gap acidosis caused by formic acid accumulation, as well as the buildup of other organic acids, including ketoacids and lactic acid.[116] Because of respiratory depression, hyperventilation is usually absent, thus exacerbating the acidosis. The most characteristic clinical sign of methanol toxicity is acute visual disturbance. Ocular symptoms usually do not appear until the methanol levels are greater than 100 mg/dL. Patients complain of blurry vision, as if viewing objects through a snowstorm. Examination of the retina usually reveals optic disc edema. Blindness frequently occurs and is usually permanent.[117] Other symptoms include gastrointestinal manifestations such as nausea, vomiting, and abdominal pain. Up to two thirds of patients may develop pancreatitis as well.[118]

The successful treatment of methanol toxicity depends on rapid diagnosis. Methanol intoxication should be considered in any patient with an anion gap acidosis and central nervous system disturbance. Because of methanol's low molecular weight, initially the measured serum osmolality is elevated, and the osmolal gap is usually greater than 20 mOsm.[119, 120] Each 10 mg/dL of methanol adds 3.4 mOsm/L to the serum osmolality. Treatment of suspected methanol ingestion should never await confirmation by toxicology results. Treatment should be begun promptly when the clinical suspicion is high and laboratory analysis reveals a metabolic acidosis and the presence of an osmolal gap.

***Management of Methanol Ingestion.*** If the patient is asymptomatic, gastric lavage should be performed with activated charcoal to minimize any further absorption. Similar to ethylene glycol, the treatment of methanol toxicity is aimed at preventing the metabolism of methanol to its toxic intermediates and removal of methanol from the body. Because alcohol dehydrogenase has a 100-fold greater affinity for ethanol than for methanol, infusion of ethanol serves as a high-affinity competitive substrate that blocks the metabolism of methanol.[121] Ethanol levels should be maintained at 100 mg/dL (approximately 10 g/hr). Ethanol infusion should be continued until serum methanol levels fall below 20 mg/dL. Ethanol infusion, however, prolongs the half-life of methanol.[122] Fomepizole can be substituted for ethanol.[123]

Hemodialysis using a bicarbonate bath helps remove the methanol and improve the acidosis. Care should be taken, however, to minimize the risk of hemorrhage by performing hemodialysis without heparinization. In a retrospective study examining the outcome of methanol ingestion, 13.5% of patients who had a head computed tomography scan had evidence of putamenal hemorrhage—perhaps a complication of heparinization during hemodialysis.[124] Indications for hemodialysis are a serum methanol concentration greater than 50 mg/dL, metabolic acidosis that does not correct easily, formate levels greater than 20 mg/dL, renal insufficiency, and visual impairment.[125]

Folate, which is necessary for the oxidation of formic acid to $CO_2$ and water, may be a beneficial adjuvant to therapy.[126] Therapy should be monitored with frequent acid-base analysis, electrolyte monitoring, and calculation of anion and osmolal gaps.[127]

**Propylene Glycol.** Propylene glycol is a common vehicle for many drugs used in the critical care setting, including topical silver sulfadiazine and IV preparations of nitroglycerin, diazepam, lorazepam, phenytoin, etomidate, and trimethoprim-sulfamethoxazole, among others. Although it is considered relatively safe, many case reports have appeared demonstrating toxicity.[128, 129] Approximately 40% to 50% of administered propylene glycol is oxidized by alcohol dehydrogenase to lactic acid.[130] Toxic patients commonly develop an unexplained anion gap acidosis with increased serum osmolality. Considering that patients receiving many of the medications solubilized with propylene glycol frequently have other possible causes for their acidosis, intensivists must be aware of this iatrogenic cause of the acidosis. Correction of the metabolic abnormalities usually occurs quickly following discontinuation of the medication. Competitive inhibition of alcohol dehydrogenase by ethanol or fomepizole would theoretically be beneficial, but their use has not been reported.

## Non–Anion Gap Acidosis

### RENAL TUBULAR ACIDOSIS

Renal tubular acidosis (RTA) comprises a group of disorders that result in a non–anion gap acidosis in the presence of adequate glomerular function. The current understanding of RTA is an evolving one, with implications for classification of the various subtypes. RTA is associated with myriad other diseases and therapies and is therefore commonly encountered in the intensive care unit (Table 10–4). The presence of a normal anion gap acidosis in the absence of obvious causes should prompt an initial investigation.[131]

**TABLE 10–4.** Causes of Renal Tubular Acidosis

**Proximal Renal Tubular Acidosis**

- Idiopathic
- Genetic
  - Cystinosis
  - Tyrosinemia
  - Galactosemia
  - Wilson disease
- Sporadic (may be transient in children)
- Acquired disorders
  - Multiple myeloma
  - Vitamin D deficiency
  - Amyloidosis
  - Renal transplant rejection
  - Renal transplantation
- Toxins and drugs
  - Heavy metals—lead, copper, cadmium, mercury
  - Acetazolamide
  - Ifosfamide

**Distal Renal Tubular Acidosis with Hypokalemia**

- Idiopathic
- Genetic
  - Familial
  - Ehler-Danlos syndrome
  - Wilson disease
- Marfan syndrome
- Nephrocalcinosis
- Hypergammaglobulinemic states
- Drugs and toxins
  - Amphotericin B
  - Aminoglycosides
  - Ifosfamide
  - Analgesics
  - Vanadate
  - Lithium carbonate
  - Toluene
- Autoimmune disease
  - Sjögren syndrome
  - Rheumatoid arthritis
  - Thyroiditis
  - Chronic active hepatitis
  - Primary biliary cirrhosis
- Cirrhosis
- Medullary sponge kidney
- Renal transplantation

**Distal Renal Tubular Acidosis with Hyperkalemia**

- Sickle cell anemia
- Urinary tract obstruction
- Systemic lupus erythematosus
- Renal transplantation

**Type IV Renal Tubular Acidosis**

- Aldosterone deficiency
  - Adrenal insufficiency
  - Hyporenin-hypoaldosteronism
  - Drugs and toxins
    - Angiotensin-converting enzyme inhibitors
    - Angiotensin receptor blockers
    - Nonsteroidal anti-inflammatory drugs
    - Heparin
- Aldosterone resistance
  - Drugs and toxins
    - Spironolactone
    - Pentamidine
    - Trimethoprim
    - Amiloride
  - Gordon syndrome (chloride shunt)

### RENAL INSUFFICIENCY

The excretion of nonvolatile acids is one of the primary functions of the nephron; with a decline in renal function, the kidney's ability to maintain acid-base homeostasis is compromised. With deteriorating renal function, the nephron loses its ability to generate ammonia.[132] Although surrounding nephrons offer some compensation by increasing ammoniagenesis, a decline in acid excretion ensues. With mild to moderate renal failure, a hyperchloremic metabolic acidosis develops. As the glomerular filtration rate falls below 25 mL/min, the excretion of phosphates, sulfates, and organic anions declines. It is these unmeasured anions that contribute to the anion gap. It has recently been noted that as many as 50% to 80% of patients with chronic renal failure may never develop an anion gap acidosis despite very low glomerular filtration rates (<10 mL/min).[133] The reasons for this have not been established. It is possible that better control of phosphate and decreased protein intake may help limit phosphate and sulfate accumulation.

The acidosis associated with renal failure is generally mild. Bicarbonate usually does not fall below 12 mEq/L. Because patients with chronic renal failure are theoretically in daily net positive acid balance, it is interesting that a more serious acidosis does not occur. This may result from buffering of hydrogen ions by bone. The buffering of retained acids by bone results in the leaching of calcium and a negative calcium balance.[134] Another possible explanation for the mild acidosis is that with a falling glomerular filtration rate, the kidney retains not only organic acids but also organic anions, which serve as base equivalents. If this latter theory is true, the extent of positive hydrogen balance and its deleterious effect on bone may not be as great as previously believed.[135]

The maintenance of normal pH in patients with renal failure may theoretically improve the condition of the skeletal system. Even though the use of sodium bicarbonate in patients with chronic renal failure is common, there are no clinical data to support its use.

## TOTAL PARENTERAL NUTRITION AND AMINO ACID–ASSOCIATED ACIDOSIS

Hyperchloremic metabolic acidosis has been reported to occur in patients receiving total parenteral nutrition containing synthetic L-amino acid preparations. This effect is thought to be secondary to an excess of cationic amino acids as compared with anionic amino acids in these formulas. The severity of the acidosis associated with the use of protein solutions is less than that encountered with the use of the older protein hydrolysate formulations.[136] To minimize the possibility of inducing acidosis, parenteral nutrition solutions should be buffered with acetate or another organic anion.

## DILUTIONAL ACIDOSIS

Dilutional acidosis was first described by Peters and Van Slyke in 1931.[137] An acute increase in extracellular fluid volume can result in the development of a hyperchloremic metabolic acidosis. This phenomenon is thought to occur as a result of a change in the volume distribution of bicarbonate, which leads to a decrease in its serum concentration. Recent studies, however, have shown a much more modest decrease than would be predicted by a change in bicarbonate volume distribution alone.[138] Garella and colleagues showed that serum bicarbonate is only modestly diluted by large increases in extracellular volume.[139] Thus, a clinically significant metabolic acidosis would occur only with massive fluid administration. Dilutional acidosis, however, is not uncommon in the critical care setting. This is best explained by returning to the concept of the strong ion difference (SID). Because critically ill patients are frequently hypoproteinemic (or, in physical chemistry terms, have a decrease in total weak acid), in order to maintain pH, their SID is usually decreased. Infusion of 0.9% NaCl increases the chloride concentration and therefore further reduces the SID, producing an increase in $[H^+]$. Furthermore, it is not unusual for patients in intensive care units to receive rather large volumes of IV fluid. The intensivist needs to recognize this phenomenon and consider using solutions with lower chloride concentrations if massive amounts of IV fluids are to be given.

## POSTHYPOCAPNIC METABOLIC ACIDOSIS

Alveolar hyperventilation in excess of $CO_2$ production results in hypocapnia and increases serum pH. Renal compensation for hypocapnia includes a decrease in net acid excretion, as well as a decrease in bicarbonate reabsorption.[140] This serves to normalize pH within 24 to 72 hours of the development of a respiratory alkalosis. Acute hypocapnia produces a decrease in serum bicarbonate of 2 mEq/L for every 10 mm Hg decrease in $P_{CO_2}$, whereas chronic hypocapnia results in a decrease of 5 mEq/L for every 10 mm Hg decrease in $P_{CO_2}$.[141]

If normocapnia is restored abruptly, as may occur in a mechanically ventilated patient, a hyperchloremic metabolic acidosis ensues. Within days of resolution of hypocapnia, ammonium and titratable acid excretion increase, and bicarbonate generation by the tubules normalizes, returning pH to normal.

## DIARRHEA

Diarrhea is a common clinical scenario in the intensive care unit, although the frequency of various causes of diarrhea remains unknown in this subset of patients. Diarrhea is often associated with enteral tube feedings, particularly in the presence of villous atrophy, which is frequently present in critically ill patients.[142] In addition, an increased incidence of *Clostridium difficile* toxin–related colitis has been observed in critically ill patients.[143]

Fecal losses from diarrhea may approach 2 to 10 L/day, and as many as 70% of patients with diarrhea develop acid-base disturbances.[144] Hyperchloremic metabolic acidosis results from the loss of large amounts of bicarbonate or organic anions (which are potential precursors of alkali) in the stool. If, however, the loss of chloride is greater than that of bicarbonate, as may occur with congenital chloride diarrhea, a metabolic alkalosis will develop.

Loss of other bicarbonate-rich fluids from ileostomies or pancreatic fistulas may cause a hyperchloremic metabolic acidosis as well. The key to therapy is the recognition of the cause of the acidosis. If the gastrointestinal losses cannot be diminished, therapy with sodium bicarbonate or other equivalent base should be instituted.

### TOLUENE

Inhalation of paint and glue, which contain toluene, is known to result in a metabolic acidosis. The precise pathophysiologic explanation for the metabolic acidosis has not been clearly elucidated. Toluene may induce a distal RTA through an unknown mechanism.[145] Alternatively, the acidosis may be caused by metabolism of toluene to hippurate, generating a proton.[146] The rapid renal clearance of the organic anion produces the hyperchloremic acidosis. If renal failure supervenes, the accumulation of hippurate will transform the hyperchloremic metabolic acidosis into an anion gap acidosis.[147] Urinalysis often reveals hematuria, pyuria, and proteinuria, suggesting possible glomerular or tubulointerstitial damage.[148] Hypophosphatemia and hyperkalemia are commonly observed as well. Management of toluene-induced metabolic acidosis includes restoration of intravascular volume and correction of abnormal serum electrolytes. Many clinicians supplement bicarbonate to restore plasma bicarbonate to a level of 10 to 12 mEq/L.

## Respiratory Acidosis

Respiratory acidosis is caused by accumulation of $CO_2$ secondary to inadequate alveolar ventilation. Decreased ventilation can be secondary to numerous disease processes, from altered states of consciousness to primary pulmonary disorders to neuromuscular diseases (Table 10–5). Because of the frequency of pulmonary and neuromuscular disease in the critical care setting, respiratory acidosis is one of the most common acid-base disorders seen in the intensive care unit. In addition, as a result of emerging ventilation strategies, hypercapnia is becoming even more widespread. Recent studies confirming the survival benefit of permissive hypercapnic ventilation ensure that respiratory acidosis will continue to be a common clinical scenario in the intensive care unit.[149]

**TABLE 10–5.** Causes of Respiratory Acidosis

|  |
|---|
| **Central Respiratory Depression** |
| Primary hypoventilation |
| Drug overdose |
| Cerebrovascular accident |
| Brain tumor |
| Head trauma |
| Encephalitis, meningitis |
| **Musculoskeletal** |
| Scoliosis |
| Chest wall deformities |
| Muscle paralysis |
| Myasthenia gravis |
| Poliomyelitis |
| Guillain-Barré syndrome |
| Hypokalemia |
| Hypophosphatemia |
| Paralytic drugs |
| **Pulmonary** |
| Chronic obstructive lung disease |
| Acute asthma |
| Acute respiratory distress syndrome |
| Obstructive sleep apnea |
| Ventilator malfunction |

When severe, acute respiratory acidosis may result in confusion, anxiety, lethargy, and seizures. Hypercarbia results in myocardial depression, increased pulmonary vascular resistance, and increased CBF. As predicted by the alveolar gas equation, the increase in alveolar $CO_2$ must be accompanied by a decrease in alveolar oxygen and hypoxia. Acute increases in $CO_2$ result in a small increase in serum $HCO_3$ (a 1 mEq/L increase in $HCO_3$ for every 10 mm Hg increase in $CO_2$). Severe elevations in $CO_2$ or significant hypoxemia is indicative of respiratory failure and must be managed with either invasive or noninvasive ventilation.

In contrast, chronic hypercapnia is well tolerated by most patients, although some may develop symptoms of daytime somnolence or confusion. Chronic elevations in $CO_2$ lead to a blunting of the hypercapnia-mediated respiratory drive, secondary to decreased sensitivity of the carotid sinus to elevations in $CO_2$ tension.[150] To preserve a near normal pH, chronic elevation in the $PCO_2$ results in renal conservation of bicarbonate. This compensation takes approximately 5 days to be complete, and serum bicarbonate may exceed 40 mEq/L. An increase of 4 mEq/L in serum bicarbonate can be expected for every 10 mm Hg elevation in $PCO_2$. In patients who chronically retain $CO_2$, acute exacerbations of their underlying pulmonary disease often result in worsening respiratory acidosis and the need for noninvasive or invasive ventilation, with the goal of achieving near normal serum pH. Attempting to reach normocapnia unnecessarily prolongs the need for ventilation.

Assessment of a critically ill patient who develops a respiratory acidosis should include a thorough physical examination, looking for factors that might be contributing to alveolar hypoventilation. Careful neurologic examination may reveal a new central neurologic event. Most important, the ventilator needs to be checked for a malfunction. The endotracheal tube, if present, should be suctioned and proper placement verified. An air leak around the tube needs to be ruled out. A chest x-ray should be ordered to look for a pneumothorax or new pulmonary infiltrate. An increasing A-a gradient indicates either excessive $CO_2$ production (i.e., a recent increase in carbohydrate intake) or, more probably, a pulmonary disorder. An A-a gradient that is unchanged from previous values points to alveolar hypoventilation.

**Management of Respiratory Acidosis.** Restoring normocapnia has historically been a primary goal in the management of critically ill patients; however, practice standards are quickly changing in this respect. Elevations in $CO_2$, if they are to be corrected, should be corrected slowly. Rapid decreases in $CO_2$ tension result in changes similar to those seen in acute respiratory alkalosis and may include arrhythmias, decreased CBF, and seizures.

Increasing alveolar ventilation is the primary means of restoring normocapnia, and this can be accomplished in several ways. Optimizing airway patency via mild hyperextension of the neck is often effective. If necessary, noninvasive or invasive mechanical ventilation should be initiated. In a patient with upper airway edema resulting in inefficient ventilation, IV or inhaled steroids in addition to nebulized racemic epinephrine may be helpful.[151, 152] Inhaled $\beta_2$ agonists and anticholinergics such as ipratropium bromide are often beneficial in a patient with bronchoconstriction.

***Permissive Hypercapnia.*** Permissive hypercapnia is emerging as a promising new strategy for providing ventilatory support while minimizing lung injury caused by exposure to alveolar overdistention. Until recently, patients have been ventilated with the goal of achieving normocapnia. This often required significant tidal volumes, which resulted in both volu- and barotrauma. Permissive hypercapnic ventilation reduces ventilator-associated lung injury by establishing less rigid parameters for arterial $CO_2$. It has been used primarily in ventilating patients with reactive airway disease and acute lung injury.[153–155]

Increased morbidity and mortality have been associated with ventilator-related lung injury.[156, 157] A recent multicenter study by the Acute Respiratory Distress Syndrome Network showed a 22% decrease in overall mortality when patients with acute lung injury were ventilated with reduced tidal volumes.[155] Mean plateau pressures required to ventilate patients in the low-tidal-volume group were only 25 cm of water, compared with 33 cm of water in the group ventilated with higher tidal volumes. Although patients ventilated permissively did require a higher level of positive end-expiratory pressure, their overall tidal volumes were reduced. The use of positive end-expiratory pressure with reduced tidal volumes is believed to reduce lung injury by minimizing shear stress caused by repeated recruitment of alveoli.

Ventilation is targeted to achieve $P_{CO_2}$ in the range of 60 to 100 and maintain a pH greater than 7.05. The precise degree of acidosis that is tolerated is highly dependent on the clinician, and many use sodium bicarbonate to maintain serum pH greater than 7.0. As previously discussed, the respiratory acidosis that accompanies permissive hypercapnia has not been associated with any adverse cardiovascular effects.[32, 33] In fact, in animal studies, buffering the acidosis may worsen lung injury.[158] $SaO_2$ should be maintained at greater than 85% to 90%. Tidal volumes are initially set at 5 to 7 mL/kg and are adjusted to maintain plateau pressures less than 30 cm $H_2O$. Breath frequency should be maintained at less than 30 per minute to allow for adequate exhalation times and to avoid "breath stacking." The primary goal is to provide adequate tissue oxygenation with lower tidal volumes. If possible, an $F_{IO_2}$ less than 70% should be used. In the event that tissue oxygenation is inadequate, inspiratory time may be increased to allow for "reverse ratio ventilation." If there is no evidence of tissue hypoxia (i.e., lactic acidosis), a lower saturation may be acceptable. Finally, positive end-expiratory pressure may have to be increased to provide adequate oxygenation. Permissive hypercapnia does require increased sedation relative to traditional modes of ventilation in order to overcome the hypercapnia-induced respiratory drive. Some patients may even require neuromuscular blockade.

# ALKALOSIS

## Effects of Alkalemia

Increases in serum pH have the potential for adverse effects (Table 10–6). Although both metabolic and respiratory alkaloses are common disturbances, the changes in pH are rarely as great as those seen in acidoses.

### CARDIOVASCULAR EFFECTS

Mild alkalemia appears to increase myocardial contractility and produces vasoconstriction. Severe alkalemia (pH >7.6) results in decreased blood flow to the cerebral and coronary circulations. Hyperventilation has been used in the past as a provocative test for anginal chest pain, based on its ability to induce coronary artery vasospasm.[159, 160] Although alkalemia is thought to increase the likelihood of both supraventricular and ventricular arrhythmias, particularly in those with pre-existing ischemic heart disease, the data supporting this belief are difficult to verify. In animals, respiratory alkalosis depresses conduction in the Purkinje tissue and ventricles while decreasing the ventricular excitability threshold.[161] The presumed proarrhythmic effect of alkalosis more likely reflects the hypokalemia that is often present concurrently.

### EFFECTS ON IONIZED CALCIUM

Alkalemia increases the binding of calcium to albumin, thereby reducing serum ionized calcium. The resultant hypocalcemia may result in headache, seizures, perioral numbness, and tetany. When an alka-

**TABLE 10–6.** Adverse Effects of Severe Alkalemia

| |
|---|
| **Cardiovascular** |
| Arteriolar vasoconstriction |
| Decreased coronary blood flow |
| Decreased threshold for angina |
| Arrhythmias |
| **Respiratory** |
| Hypoventilation resulting in hypercapnia and hypoxemia |
| **Cerebral** |
| Decrease in cerebral blood flow |
| Tetany, seizures |
| Lethargy, delirium, and stupor |

lemia is metabolic in origin, it is often accompanied by hypokalemia. Care must be taken to maintain normal serum potassium to avoid compounding the proarrhythmic effects of alkalemia with those of extracellular hypokalemia.

### EFFECTS ON OXYGEN DELIVERY

The affinity of hemoglobin for oxygen is increased in the presence of an alkalotic pH (see Fig. 10–1). Alkalemia thus favors oxygen loading in the lung and reduces unloading in the peripheral tissues. This effects lasts only 1 to 2 days, however, secondary to the body's increased production of 2,3-DPG, which results in improved tissue oxygenation.[162]

## Metabolic Alkalosis

Metabolic alkalosis is the presence of an elevated serum bicarbonate level in the absence of a primary respiratory process. It is the most common acid-base disturbance seen in hospitalized patients. Seventy percent of these disturbances are solely metabolic, and the remaining 30% occur in conjunction with a concomitant respiratory disorder.[163] Metabolic alkalosis results in compensatory hypoventilation in an attempt to restore normal serum pH. Serum $P_{CO_2}$ should increase by 6 mm Hg for every increase of 10 mEq/L in serum bicarbonate.

Because of the enormous capacity of the kidney to excrete bicarbonate, metabolic alkalosis is conceptualized as a two-step process requiring the generation of excess bicarbonate and the maintenance of the hyperbicarbonatemia.[164] Bicarbonate can be increased by the loss of hydrogen, as occurs with vomiting, or by the gain of bicarbonate, as occurs with the administration of exogenous bicarbonate. Underlying volume depletion, chloride depletion, hyperaldosteronism, and hypokalemia help maintain elevated bicarbonate levels by both increasing bicarbonate reabsorption and decreasing bicarbonate secretion. Many of the disorders occurring in the intensive care unit, as well as the therapies used, are commonly associated with a metabolic alkalosis (Table 10–7).

**TABLE 10–7.** Causes of Metabolic Alkalosis

| |
|---|
| Vomiting |
| Loss of intestinal secretions |
| Congenital chloride diarrhea |
| Primary or secondary hyperaldosteronism |
| Loop or thiazide diuretics |
| Syndromes of apparent mineralocorticoid excess |
| 11 β-hydroxysteroid dehydrogenase deficiency |
| Liddle syndrome |
| Excess bicarbonate intake (usually requires renal insufficiency) |
| Posthypercapnic metabolic alkalosis |
| Refeeding after starvation |
| Bartter syndrome |
| Hypokalemia |
| Hypoproteinemia |
| Contraction alkalosis |

### EVALUATION OF METABOLIC ALKALOSIS

Metabolic alkaloses are classified according to their relative responsiveness to the administration of volume (or chloride).

#### *Volume (Chloride)–Responsive Metabolic Alkalosis*

The majority of metabolic alkaloses are volume responsive and result from the loss of sodium or chloride.[165] Although chloride depletion independent of volume depletion can help maintain a metabolic alkalosis, except in experimental models, it is difficult to separate volume depletion from chloride depletion; for all practical purposes, they are one and the same. Both conditions increase bicarbonate reabsorption in the nephron. These patients generally have urine chloride concentrations lower than 10 to 15 mEq/L before treatment.[166] Volume expansion with 0.9% saline promptly induces bicarbonaturia and rapid correction of the alkalosis.

**Loss of Gastric Fluid.** Loss of gastric fluid by nasogastric suction or vomiting results in the loss of both protons and chloride from the body. Pharmacologic agents that result in decreased proton excretion may minimize such losses. Both $H_2$-receptor antagonists and gastric proton pump inhibitors help prevent metabolic alkalosis in this setting.[167]

**Diuretic-Induced Metabolic Alkalosis.** Diuretic-induced metabolic alkalosis is common in the intensive care unit and is usually attributable to the use of loop or thiazide diuretics. These diuretics produce urine that is bicarbonate poor and chloride rich, contracting the extracellular fluid around a fixed content of bicarbonate.[168] In nonedematous patients, the acute administration of diuretics causes only a mild increase in serum bicarbonate; however, in patients with edema, in whom massive diuresis is not uncommon, significant metabolic alkalosis may occur.[169] Treatment is aimed at minimizing the use of diuretics, replacing chloride losses with NaCl and KCl, and maintaining normal serum potassium levels. The judicious use of the carbonic anhydrase inhibitor acetazolamide may help moderate the alkalosis by promoting bicarbonaturia. Care must be taken, however, to avoid hypokalemia. Acetazolamide is particularly useful in those patients who cannot tolerate volume expansion.[170, 171]

**Posthypercapnic Metabolic Alkalosis.** Because patients with chronic respiratory acidosis have a compensatory increase in their serum bicarbonate, rapid correction of the hypercapnia produces a metabolic alkalosis. In turn, the alkalosis decreases ventilation, raising the $CO_2$. As long as the patient is not hypokalemic or intravascularly volume contracted, renal excretion of bicarbonate will increase, correcting the metabolic alkalosis over approximately 24 to 48 hours. This phenomenon can be avoided if the respiratory acidosis is corrected gradually, with careful monitoring of arterial blood gas values. Because potassium is the primary cation that accompanies bicarbonate excretion in the urine, it is important to maintain normal serum values, or the correction of alkalosis will be impaired.[172] In those patients with chronic hypercapnia and serum bicarbonate levels greater than 35 mEq/L, the judicious use of acetazolamide usually increases urinary losses of bicarbonate and improves the alkalosis.[173]

#### *Volume (Chloride)–Resistant Metabolic Alkalosis*

Volume-resistant metabolic alkaloses are considerably less common in the intensive care unit and occur in a variety of relatively rare conditions. These patients continue to secrete increased chloride, even in the presence of volume expansion. Hyperaldosteronism (either primary or secondary), usually in combination with hypokalemia, may result in a clinically significant metabolic alkalosis. In addition, corticosteroids with significant mineralocorticoid activity may result in hyperbicarbonatemia. The aldosterone antagonist spironolactone or other potassium-sparing diuretics are useful in the management of aldosterone-mediated metabolic alkalosis.

### HYPOKALEMIA

Hypokalemia can both help maintain an established metabolic alkalosis and, if severe enough, generate an alkalosis. A decrease in serum potassium results in the movement of potassium out of cells. This outward movement of a positively charged species is associated with an inward movement of hydrogen ions, with subsequent intracellular acidification.[174] Intracellular acidification stimulates hydrogen ion secretion and bicarbonate reabsorption.[175] In addition, potassium depletion stimulates potassium reabsorption by H, K ATPase, with the resultant loss of hydrogen ions into the urine.[176] Because of these effects of potassium depletion, it is difficult to correct a metabolic alkalosis without repletion of potassium stores.

### HYPOPROTEINEMIC METABOLIC ALKALOSIS

Patients who are critically ill are frequently hypoalbuminemic. Because albumin is a weak acid, it contributes to serum pH. Theoretically, hypoalbuminemia can produce a metabolic alkalosis. In a group of critically ill surgical patients with metabolic alkalosis, hypoproteinemia in the range of 4 to 5.5 g/dL was the only nonrespiratory metabolic disturbance present.[177] In vitro data demonstrating that lowering the plasma protein concentration increases pH support this finding.[178] Therapy of this metabolic disorder should be directed toward providing nutritional support to increase serum protein levels.

### ACTIVE MANAGEMENT OF METABOLIC ALKALOSIS

Correction of a metabolic alkalosis is often accomplished by eliminating the specific cause that helped generate and maintain the condition. Occasionally, if conservative management has failed to correct a severe metabolic alkalosis, a more active approach must be taken. The use of dilute hydrochloric acid (0.1 to 0.2 N) is an effective means of resolving a metabolic alkalosis. It must be administered via a central venous catheter at an infusion rate less than 0.2 mmol/kg/hr. Dosing of HCl should be calculated based on a volume distribution of 50% of body weight. To reduce serum bicarbonate from 50 to 40 mEq/L in a 70-kg patient, the amount of HCl given should be $10 \times 70 \times 0.5$, or 350 mmol.[179] Amino acid solutions containing arginine monohydrochloride have been used as well, but they carry a risk of life-threatening hyperkalemia and are therefore not recommended. Finally, dialysis may be used to correct a resistant metabolic alkalosis.

**TABLE 10–8.** Causes of Respiratory Alkalosis

| |
|---|
| Hypoxemia |
| Stimulation of pulmonary or pleural receptors |
| Pneumonia |
| Pulmonary embolism |
| Pulmonary edema |
| Asthma |
| Psychogenic hyperventilation |
| Medications |
| Theophylline |
| Catecholamines |
| Salicylates |
| Progesterone |
| Central nervous system disorders |
| Subarachnoid hemorrhage |
| Cheyne-Stokes respirations |
| Increased intracranial pressure |
| Fever |
| Early sepsis |
| Increased minute ventilation secondary to ventilator management |

## Respiratory Alkalosis

Respiratory alkalosis is characterized by a low $P_{CO_2}$ in the absence of a primary metabolic acidosis. It is caused by an increase in alveolar ventilation or, more rarely, a decrease in tissue production of $CO_2$ (Table 10–8). Acute compensation for a respiratory alkalosis results in a decrease in serum bicarbonate concentration, and a new bicarbonate steady-state level is reached in approximately 10 minutes. This effect is not accounted for by changes in urinary bicarbonate excretion.[180] Acute respiratory alkalosis results in a 2 to 4 mEq/L decrease in serum bicarbonate for every 10 mm Hg change in $P_{CO_2}$. Chronic respiratory alkalosis results in a decrease in serum bicarbonate of 6 mEq/L for every 10 mm Hg decrease in $P_{CO_2}$ and is the only simple acid-base disturbance that can be completely compensated.

Alveolar hyperventilation often results from an increase in the central drive to breathe and is commonly the result of hypoxemia, stimulation of mechanoreceptors and chemoreceptors in the lungs by pulmonary disease, or direct stimulation of the respiratory center. Hypoxemia increases ventilatory drive via stimulation of chemoreceptors in the carotid body or the aortic arch. Hypoxemic respiratory drive increases for any decline in $Po_2$ but becomes increasingly significant as $Po_2$ falls below 60 mm Hg. Respiratory alkalosis, particularly in the absence of respiratory distress, is often an early indicator of sepsis. Other conditions that should be considered are primary central nervous system disorders and aspirin ingestion.

### CEREBRAL BLOOD FLOW AND CARBON DIOXIDE

Hypercarbia vasodilates cerebral arteries both in vitro and in vivo. This effect on cerebral vascular tone appears to be regulated by pH itself, rather than by $Pco_2$. Severinghaus and coworkers demonstrated normal CBF in patients with a compensated respiratory alkalosis.[24] In vitro studies have also demonstrated a pH dependence of cerebral vascular tone, regardless of the $Pco_2$.[25, 181] These effects are mediated by a variety of signaling mechanisms, including prostaglandins, potassium, intracellular calcium stores, cyclic mononucleotides, and nitric oxide. The relative contributions and degree of redundancy in regulation are unknown.[182]

The pH dependence of CBF is of primary importance in the acute management of increased intracranial pressure and is a consideration in permissive hypercapnic ventilation as well. CBF is well regulated within a range of $Pco_2$ between 20 and 80 mm Hg; a $Pco_2$ of 25 results in a 40% to 50% reduction in CBF.[26, 183] An increase in $Pco_2$ to 80 mm Hg results in a CBF that is sixfold higher than baseline in awake animals. Approximately 50% of this effect is mediated by catecholamines.[184]

The effect of hyperventilation on CBF is short-lived. In awake humans hyperventilated to a $Pco_2$ of 16, CBF was decreased by 40%, but within 4 hours, blood flow had returned to within 10% of baseline.[185] Additionally, the effects of hyperventilation are attenuated by hypotension and augmented by inhalational anesthetics such as isoflurane or halothane.[186–188] The ephemeral effect of hyperventilation on CBF is believed to be secondary to a compensatory decrease in the concentration of bicarbonate within the cerebrospinal fluid.[189] Discontinuation of therapeutic hyperventilation should therefore be done slowly, over a period of hours. Otherwise, hyperemia and a resultant increase in intracranial pressure may be observed.

The use of hyperventilation in the management of closed head injuries is based on the responsiveness of CBF, and therefore intracranial volume, to pH. Although hyperventilation results in a substantial decrease in intracranial pressure in these patients, it is unclear whether hyperventilation results in any improvement in neurologic outcome. One study identified a slightly higher 1-year survival in patients treated with hyperventilation and an even further decrease in mortality in patients treated with hyperventilation and Tham. These data have been criticized, however, for a lack of precision in outcome measurement.[190] Because decreasing CBF by hyperventilation worsens ischemia in patients with traumatic brain injury, it has recently been recommended that hyperventilation not be initiated in these patients.[191]

## MIXED ACID-BASE DISTURBANCES

Because of their subtle nature, mixed acid-base disturbances are often overlooked unless there is a high index of suspicion. Important clues to their existence can be obtained from the history and physical examination (Table 10–9). In addition, a careful review of information obtained from the standard electrolyte panel and arterial blood gas analysis can uncover previously unrecognized acid-base disorders. Mixed acid-base disturbances are always present when there is a normal pH with an abnormal $Pco_2$, abnormal bicarbonate, or elevated anion gap. Another clue to a mixed disturbance is the presence of a delta anion gap.

### Delta Anion Gap

Theoretically, the increase in the anion gap above normal, the so-called delta anion gap, should be equivalent to the decrease in the serum bicarbonate. Thus the ratio of the delta anion gap to the decrease in bicarbonate (delta bicarbonate) should be 1. Any variance implies an additional metabolic process. A ratio greater than 1 indicates that a concomitant metabolic alkalosis is present, whereas a ratio less than 1 indicates the presence of a hyperchloremic metabolic acidosis.

For this 1:1 relationship to be true, buffering of protons would have to be done exclusively by bicarbonate, the volume distribution of the unmeasured anion and bicarbonate would have to be equal, and the excretion and metabolism of the unmeasured anion would have to be equal to the regeneration of bicarbonate. Considering these prerequisites, it is remarkable that the ratio is as close to 1 as it typically is. Because of these uncertainties, the normal ratio of the delta anion gap to the delta bicarbonate more closely approximates 0.6 to 1.8. Thus, additional disturbances should not be sought unless the ratio falls outside these bounds.

### Salicylate Toxicity

The ingestion of salicylates is an important cause of mixed acid-base disturbances, producing both a respi-

**TABLE 10–9.** Clues in the History and Physical Examination to Underlying Acid-Base Disorders

| Findings | Acid-Base Disorder |
|---|---|
| Vomiting | Metabolic alkalosis |
| Diarrhea | Metabolic acidosis |
| Diabetes | Metabolic acidosis |
| Obstructive lung disease | Respiratory acidosis |
| Renal failure | Metabolic acidosis |
| Liver disease | Respiratory alkalosis |
| Orthostasis | Metabolic alkalosis |
| Hypotension | Metabolic acidosis |

ratory alkalosis and a metabolic acidosis. Despite recent decreases in the incidence of aspirin poisoning secondary to the institution of childproof-cap laws, the ready availability of salicylate or its congeners in numerous products still makes salicylate toxicity a major cause of toxin-induced metabolic disturbance. Salicylate toxicity is usually easily diagnosed in children because a history of ingestion is often obtained. The diagnosis may be less apparent in adults, especially the elderly, who may be on chronic aspirin therapy for a variety of diseases.[192] The common presenting sign is tachypnea. The patient may also complain of tinnitus. Tinnitus may progress to hearing loss when serum concentrations of salicylic acid are 20 to 45 mg/dL or higher.[193] Other central nervous system manifestations are agitation, seizures, and even coma. Noncardiogenic pulmonary edema may develop, as may upper gastrointestinal bleeding. Hypoglycemia may occur in children but is rare in adults. Other symptoms include nausea, vomiting, and hyperpyrexia.

Evidence of salicylate ingestion can be rapidly obtained by adding 10% ferric chloride to urine in a 1:4 dilution. A purple color indicates the presence of salicylate. Unfortunately, because of the sensitivity of this test, it is positive even after ingesting a single tablet. In the setting of salicylate overdose, peak serum concentrations are achieved 4 to 6 hours after ingestion. The severity of the ingestion can be predicted using the Done nomogram, which uses salicylate levels at varying time points following ingestion.[194] It cannot be used with chronic ingestions or with the ingestion of enteric-coated aspirin.

As already mentioned, a mixed acid-base disturbance is commonly present. Salicylate directly increases ventilation through an unclear central nervous system mechanism, causing a respiratory alkalosis. A high anion gap acidosis may also exist. Part of this gap is secondary to the unmeasured salicylate anion. In addition, lactate production is increased by the respiratory alkalosis. In animal models, lactate production does not increase if the respiratory alkalosis is prevented.[195] High serum levels of salicylates can uncouple oxidative phosphorylation and may contribute to the lactic acidosis. Ketoacids have also been implicated in salicylate toxicity. It is unclear, however, whether this is a direct effect of salicylate or secondary to underlying disease. Although it has been suggested that metabolic acidosis is a much more common finding in children than in adults, this observation has not been validated. In a study by Gabow and colleagues, 80% of adults demonstrated a metabolic acidosis.[196] In this study, 33% of the adults had ingested drugs in addition to salicylate and were less likely to have a respiratory alkalosis. Of note, the adults with combined drug ingestion also had lower anion gaps than those who had taken salicylate alone. It is possible that the respiratory depression caused by these other substances prevented the alkalosis-induced increase in lactic acid. Although many clinicians use the Done nomogram to direct therapy, the toxic effects of salicylate overdose have poor correlation with serum concentrations.[197] Serial determinations of arterial pH in addition to careful clinical examination should be primary in guiding therapy. Acidemia increases the penetration of acetylsalicylic acid (ASA) into the cerebrospinal fluid, and there appears to be a close correlation between cerebrospinal fluid levels of salicylate and mortality.[198]

In all suspected cases of salicylate toxicity, gastric lavage and activated charcoal should be instituted. The use of bicarbonate lavage has been recommended in cases of overdoses with enteric-coated aspirin to help dissolve the tablets.[199] In patients with serum salicylate levels greater than 35 mg/dL, alkalinization of the blood and urine with sodium bicarbonate not only decreases salicylate entry into the cerebrospinal fluid but also increases renal excretion of ASA.[200] Care must be taken to correct hypokalemia in order to facilitate urinary alkalinization. Increasing urine pH from 5 to 8 results in a 10- to 20-fold increase in urine salicylate clearance.[201] Hemodialysis may be used as well in the presence of severe salicylate poisoning, a very high serum concentration of ASA (>100 mg/dL), or an inability to clear the drug renally.

## REFERENCES


1. Stewart PA: How to understand acid-base. In Stewart PA (ed): Quantitative Acid-Base Primer for Biology and Medicine. New York, Elsevier, 1981, pp. 1–286.
2. Kellum JA: Metabolic acidosis in the critically ill: Lessons from physical chemistry. Kidney Int 53:S81–S86, 1998.
3. Morfei JM: Stewart's strong ion difference approach to acid-base analysis. Respir Care 44:45–52, 1999.
4. Gilfix BM, Bique M, Magder S: A physical chemical approach to the analysis of acid-base balance in the clinical setting. J Crit Care 8:187–197, 1993.
5. Wilkes P: Hypoproteinemia, strong-ion difference and acid-base status in critically ill patients. J Appl Physiol 84:1740–1748, 1998.
6. Wuillemin WA, Gerber AU: [Sources of error in the preanalytic phase of blood gas analysis]. Schweiz Rundsch Med Prax 84: 200–203, 1995.
7. Harrison AM, Lynch JM, Dean JM, Witte MK: Comparison of simultaneously obtained capillary and arterial blood gases in pediatric intensive care unit patients. Crit Care Med 25:1904–1908, 1997.
8. Bakker J, Vincent JL, Gris P, et al: Veno-arterial carbon dioxide gradient in human septic shock. Chest 101:509–515, 1992.
9. Benjamin E, Paluch TA, Berger SR, et al: Venous hypercarbia in canine hemorrhagic shock. Crit Care Med 15:516–518, 1987.
10. Weil MH, Rackow EC, Trevino R, et al: Difference in acid-base state between venous and arterial blood during cardiopulmonary resuscitation. N Engl J Med 315:153–156, 1986.
11. Zhang H, Vincent J-L: Arteriovenous differences in $pCO_2$ and pH are good indicators of critical hypoperfusion. Am Rev Respir Dis 148:867–871, 1993.
12. Grundler W, Weil MH, Rackow EC: Arteriovenous carbon dioxide and pH gradients during cardiac arrest. Circulation 74: 1071–1074, 1986.
13. Oropello JM, Manasia A, Hannon E, et al: Continuous fiberoptic arterial and venous blood gas monitoring in hemorrhagic shock. Chest 109:1049–1055, 1996.
14. Falk JL, Rackow EC, Weil MH: End-tidal carbon dioxide concentration during cardiopulmonary resuscitation. N Engl J Med 318:607–611, 1988.
15. Sanders AB, Kern KB, Otto CW, et al: End tidal carbon dioxide monitoring during cardiopulmonary resuscitation. JAMA 262: 1347–1351, 1989.
16. Sanders AB, Atlas M, Ewy GA, et al: Expired $pCO_2$ as an index of coronary perfusion pressure. Am J Emerg Med 3: 147–149, 1985.

17. Gudipati CV, Weil MH, Bisera J, et al: Expired carbon dioxide: A non-invasive measure of cardiopulmonary resuscitation. Circulation 77:234–239, 1988.
18. Levine RL, Wayne MA, Miller CC: End-tidal carbon dioxide and outcome of out-of-hospital cardiac arrest. N Engl J Med 337:301–306, 1997.
19. Durand T, Delmas-Beauvieux MC, Canioni P, Gallis JL: Role of intracellular buffering power on the mitochondria-cytosol pH gradient in the rat liver perfused at 4 degrees C. Cryobiology 38:68–80, 1999.
20. Bonventre JV, Cheung JY: Effects of metabolic acidosis on viability of cells exposed to anoxia. Am J Physiol 249:C149–C159, 1985.
21. Gores GJ, Nieminen AL, Wray BE, et al: Intracellular pH during "chemical hypoxia" in cultured rat hepatocytes. J Clin Invest 83:386–396, 1989.
22. Pentilla A, Trump BF: Extracellular acidosis protects Ehrlich tumor cells and rat renal cortex against anoxic injury. Science 185:277–278, 1974.
23. Neff TA, Petty TL: Tolerance and survival in severe chronic hypercapnia. Arch Intern Med 129:59–66, 1972.
24. Severinghaus JW, Chiodi H, Eger EI II, et al: Cerebral blood flow in man at high altitude: Role of cerebrospinal fluid pH in normalization of flow in chronic hypocapnia. Circ Res 19: 274–282, 1966.
25. Kontos HA, Raper J, Patterson JL Jr: Analysis of vasoactivity of local pH, $pCO_2$ and bicarbonate on pial vessels. Stroke 8: 358–360, 1977.
26. Reivich M: Arterial $pCO_2$ and cerebral hemodynamics. Am J Physiol 206:25–35, 1964.
27. Wildenthal K, Mierzwiak DS, Myers RW, Mitchell JH: Effects of acute lactic acidosis on left ventricular performance. Am J Physiol 214:1352–1359, 1968.
28. Mehta PM, Kloner RA: Effects of acid base disturbance, septic shock, and calcium and phosphorus abnormalities on cardiovascular function. Crit Care Clin 3:747–758, 1987.
29. Orchard CH, Cingolani HE: Effects of changes in pH on the contractile function of heart muscle. Am J Physiol 258:C967–C981, 1990.
30. Smith HW: The actions of acids on turtle heart muscle with reference to the penetration of anions. Am J Physiol 76:411–447, 1926.
31. Ellis D, Thomas RC: Direct measurement of the intracellular pH of mammalian cardiac muscle. J Physiol (Lond) 262:755–771, 1976.
32. Thorens J-B, Jolliet B, Ritz M, et al: Effects of rapid permissive hypercapnia on hemodynamics, gas exchange, and oxygen transport and consumption during mechanical ventilation for acute respiratory distress syndrome. Intensive Care Med 22: 182–191, 1996.
33. Carvalho CR, Barbas CS, Medeiros DM, et al: Temporal hemodynamic effects of permissive hypercapnia associated with ideal PEEP in ARDS. Am J Respir Crit Care Med 156:1458–1466, 1997.
34. Lever E, Jaspan JB: Sodium bicarbonate therapy in severe diabetic ketoacidosis. Am J Med 75:263–268, 1983.
35. Morris LR, Murphy MB, Kitabchi AE: Bicarbonate therapy in severe diabetic ketoacidosis. Ann Intern Med 105:836–840, 1986.
36. Kerber RE, Pandian NG, Hoyt R, et al: Effect of ischemia, hypertrophy, hypoxia, acidosis, and alkalosis on canine defibrillation. Am J Physiol 244:II825, 1983.
37. American Heart Association: Guidelines for cardiopulmonary resuscitation and emergency cardiac care. JAMA 268:2171–2295, 1992.
38. Kiely DG, Cargill RI, Lipworth BJ: Effects of hypercapnia on hemodynamic, inotropic, lusitropic, and electrophysiologic indices in humans. Chest 109:1215–1221, 1996.
39. Sideras DA, Katsadorus DP, Valianos G, Assioura A: Type of cardiac dysrhythmias in respiratory failure. Am Heart J 89: 32, 1975.
40. Orchard CH, Cingolani HE: Acidosis and arrhythmias in cardiac muscle. Cardiovasc Res 28:1312–1319, 1994.
41. Carrier O, Cowsert M, Hancock J, Guyton AC: Effect of hydrogen ion on vascular resistance in isolated artery segments. Am J Physiol 207:169, 1964.
42. Mines AH: Oxygen carriage by blood. In Johnson LR (ed): Essential Medical Physiology. New York, Raven Press, 1992, pp 267–272.
43. Winter SD, Pearson JR, Gabow PA: The fall of the serum anion gap. Arch Intern Med 150:311–313, 1990.
44. Gabow PA, Kaehny WD, Fennessey PV, et al: Diagnostic importance of an increased serum anion gap. N Engl J Med 303: 854–858, 1980.
45. Gabow PA: Disorders associated with an altered anion gap. Kidney Int 27:472–483, 1985.
46. Asch MJ, Dell RB, Williams GS, et al: Time course for development of respiratory compensation in metabolic acidosis. J Lab Clin Med 73:610–615, 1969.
47. Albert MS, Dell RB, Winters RW: Quantitative displacement of acid-base equilibrium in metabolic acidosis. Ann Intern Med 66:312–322, 1967.
48. Luft D, Deischel G, Schmulling RM, et al: Definition of a clinically relevant lactic acidosis in patients with internal diseases. Am J Clin Pathol 80:484–489, 1983.
49. Huckabee WE: Abnormal resting blood lactate. Am J Med 30: 833–848, 1961.
50. Borden EB: Early diagnosis of acute mesenteric ischemia. J Crit Illness 1:17–24, 1986.
51. Cohen RD, Woods HF: Clinical and Biochemical Aspects of Lactic Acidosis. London, Biochemical Scientific Publishing, 1976, p 276.
52. Brown S, Gutierrez G, Clark C, et al: The lung as a source of lactate in sepsis and ARDS. J Crit Care 11:2–8, 1996.
53. Cohen RD: The Production and Removal of Lactate in Acute Conditions: International Symposium. Basel, Karger, 1979, pp 10–19.
54. Iberti TJ, Leibowitz AB, Papadakos PJ, et al: Low sensitivity of the anion gap as a screen to detect hyperlactinemia in critically ill patients. Crit Care Med 18:275–277, 1990.
55. Peretz DI, Scott HM, Duff J, et al: The significance of lactic acidemia in the shock syndrome. Ann N Y Acad Sci 119: 1133–1141, 1965.
56. Cady LD Jr, Weil MH, Afifi AA, et al: Quantitation of severity of critical illness with special reference to blood lactate. Crit Care Med 1:75–80, 1973.
57. Kruse JA, Mehta KC, Carlson RW: Definition of clinically significant lactic acidosis [abstract]. Chest 92:S100, 1987.
58. Falk JL, Rackow EC, Leavy J: Delayed lactate clearance in patients surviving circulatory shock. Acute Care 11:212–215, 1985.
59. Parker MM, Schelhammer J, Natanson C: Serial cardiovascular variables in survivors and non-survivors of human septic shock: Heart rate as an early predictor of prognosis. Crit Care Med 15:923–929, 1987.
60. Anderson CT, Westgard JO, Schlimgen K, et al: Contribution of arterial blood lactate measurement to the care of critically ill patients. Am J Clin Pathol 68:63–67, 1977.
61. Mizock BA, Falk JL: Lactic acidosis in critical illness. Crit Care Med 20:80–93, 1992.
62. Stacpoole PW, Wright EC, Baumgartner TG, et al: A controlled clinical trial of dichloroacetate for treatment of lactic acidosis in adults. The Dichloroacetate–Lactic Acidosis Study Group. N Engl J Med 327:1564–1569, 1992.
63. Narins RG, Cohen JJ: Bicarbonate therapy in severe acidosis [letter]. Ann Intern Med 108:311, 1988.
64. Adrogue HJ, Brensilver JJ, Cohen JJ, Madias NE: Influence of steady state alterations in acid base equilibrium on the fate of administered bicarbonate in the dog. J Clin Invest 71:867–883, 1983.
65. Vaziri ND, Ness R, Wellikson L, et al: Bicarbonate-buffered peritoneal dialysis: An effective adjunct in the treatment of lactic acidosis. Am J Med 67:392–396, 1979.
66. Foulks CJ, Wright LF: Successful repletion of bicarbonate stores in ongoing lactic acidosis: A role for bicarbonate-buffered peritoneal dialysis. South Med J 74:1162–1163, 1981.
67. Schmidt R, Horn E, Richards J, Stamatakis M: Survival after metformin-associated lactic acidosis in peritoneal dialysis–dependent renal failure. Am J Med 102:486–488, 1997.
68. Arieff AI, Park R, Leach W: Pathophysiology of experimental lactic acidosis in dogs. Am J Physiol 239:7135–7142, 1980.

69. Arieff AI, Gertz EW, Park R, et al: Lactic acidosis and the cardiovascular system in the dog. Clin Sci 64:573–580, 1983.
70. Bersin RM: Effects of sodium bicarbonate on myocardial metabolism and circulatory function during hypoxia. In Arieff A (ed): Hypoxia, Metabolic Acidosis, and the Circulation. Oxford, Oxford University Press, 1992, pp 139–174.
71. Mathieu D, Neviere R, Billard V, et al: Effects of bicarbonate therapy on hemodynamics and tissue oxygenation in patients with lactic acidosis: A prospective controlled clinical trial. Crit Care Med 19:1352–1356, 1991.
72. Cooper DJ, Walley KR, Wiggs BR, Russell JA: Bicarbonate does not improve hemodynamics in critically ill patients who have a lactic acidosis. Ann Intern Med 112:492–498, 1990.
73. Bersin RM, Chatterjee K, Arieff AI: Metabolic and hemodynamic consequences of sodium bicarbonate administration in patients with heart disease. Am J Med 87:7–13, 1989.
74. Stacpoole PW, Moore GW, Kornhauser DM: Toxicity of chronic dichloroacetate. N Engl J Med 300:372, 1979.
75. Filley GF, Kindig NB: Carbicarb, an alkalinizing ion generating agent of possible clinical usefulness. Trans Am Clin Climatol Assoc 96:141–153, 1984.
76. Sun JH, Filley GF, Hord K, et al: Carbicarb: An effective substitute for sodium bicarbonate for the treatment of metabolic acidosis. Surgery 102:835–838, 1987.
77. Bersin RM, Arieff AI: Improved hemodynamic function during hypoxia with Carbicarb, a new agent for the management of acidosis. Circulation 77:227–233, 1988.
78. Rhee KH, Toro LO, McDonald GG, et al: Carbicarb, sodium bicarbonate, and sodium chloride in hypoxic lactic acidosis. Chest 104:913–918, 1993.
79. Nahas GG, Sutin KM, Fermon C, et al: Guidelines for the treatment of acidemia with Tham. Drugs 55:191–224, 1998.
80. Bjeneroth G, Sammeli O, Li Y-C, et al: Effects of alkaline buffers on the cytoplasmic pH in lymphocytes. Crit Care Med 22:1550–1556, 1994.
81. Li Y-C, Wiklund L, Tarkkila P, et al: Influence of alkaline buffers on cytoplasmic pH in myocardial cells exposed to metabolic acidosis. Resuscitation 32:33–44, 1996.
82. Li Y-C, Wiklund L, Bjeneroth G: Influence of alkaline buffers on the cytoplasmic pH in myocardial cells exposed to hypoxia. Resuscitation 34:71–77, 1997.
83. Halperin ML, Kamel KS: D-Lactic acidosis: Turning sugar into acids in the gastrointestinal tract. Kidney Int 49:1–8, 1996.
84. Krentz AJ, Nattrass M: Diabetic ketoacidosis, non-ketotic hyperosmolar coma and lactic acidosis. In Pickup JC, Williams G (eds): Textbook of Diabetes, vol 1. London, Blackwell Scientific, 1991, pp 480–481.
85. Westphal S: The occurrence of diabetic ketoacidosis in non-insulin dependent diabetes and newly diagnosed diabetic adults. Am J Med 101:19–24, 1996.
86. Schreiber M, Steele A, Gogven J, et al: Can a severe degree of ketoacidosis develop overnight? J Am Soc Nephrol 7:192, 1996.
87. Adrogue HJ, Wilson H, Boyd AE III, et al: Plasma acid base patterns in diabetic ketoacidosis. N Engl J Med 307:1603–1610, 1982.
88. Adrogue HJ, Lederer ED, Suki WN, et al: Determinants of plasma potassium levels in diabetic ketoacidosis. Medicine (Baltimore) 65:163–172, 1986.
89. Munro JF, Campbell IW, McCuish AC, Duncan LJP: Euglycaemic diabetic ketoacidosis. BMJ 2:578–580, 1973.
90. Fleckman AM: Diabetic ketoacidosis. Endocrinol Metab Clin North Am 22:181–206, 1993.
91. Adrogue HJ, Barrero J, Eknoyan G: Salutary effects of modest fluid replacement in the treatment of adults with diabetic ketoacidosis. JAMA 262:2108–2113, 1989.
92. Fisher JN, Kitabchi AE: A randomized study of phosphate therapy in the treatment of diabetic ketoacidosis. J Clin Endocrinol Metab 57:177–180, 1983.
93. Harris GD, Fiordalisi I, Harris WI, et al: Minimizing the risk of brain herniation during the treatment of diabetic ketoacidemia: A retrospective and prospective study. J Pediatr 117:22–31, 1990.
94. Duck SC, Wyatt DT: Factors associated with brain herniation in the treatment of diabetic ketoacidosis. J Pediatr 113:10–14, 1988.
95. Rosenbloom AL: Intracerebral crises during diabetic ketoacidosis. Diabetes Care 13:22–33, 1990.
96. Miller PD, Heinig RE, Waterhouse C: Treatment of alcoholic acidosis. Arch Intern Med 138:67–72, 1978.
97. Wrenn KD, Slovis CM, Minion GE, et al: The syndrome of alcoholic ketoacidosis. Am J Med 91:119–129, 1991.
98. Pearson-Sharer AL, Steinhart CM: Evaluation of the poisoned child. In Holbrook PR (ed): Textbook of Pediatric Critical Care. Philadelphia, WB Saunders, 1993, pp 982–997.
99. Walker JA, Krause EA, Eisinger RP: The missing gap: A pitfall in the diagnosis of alcohol intoxication by osmometry. Arch Intern Med 146:1843–1844, 1986.
100. Glaser DS: Utility of the serum osmol gap in the diagnosis of methanol or ethylene glycol ingestions. Ann Emerg Med 27: 343–346, 1996.
101. Clay KL, Murphy RC: On the metabolic acidosis of ethylene glycol intoxication. Toxicol Appl Pharmacol 39:39–49, 1977.
102. Gabow PA, Clay K, Sullivan JB, et al: Organic acids and ethylene glycol intoxication. Ann Intern Med 105:16–20, 1986.
103. Hewlett TP, McMartin KE: Ethylene glycol poisoning: The value of glycolic acid determinations for diagnosis and treatment. Clin Toxicol 24:389–402, 1986.
104. Winter ML, Ellis MD, Snodgrass WR: Urine fluorescence using a Wood's lamp to detect antifreeze additive sodium fluorescein: A qualitative adjunctive test in suspected ethylene glycol ingestion. Ann Emerg Med 19:663–667, 1990.
105. Gordon HL, Hunter JM: Ethylene glycol poisoning: A case report. Anaesthesia 37:332–338, 1982.
106. Ford MD, McMartin K: Ethylene glycol and methanol. In Ford M, Delaney K, Ling L, Erickson T (eds): Clinical Toxicology. Philadelphia, WB Saunders, 2001, pp 757–767.
107. Friedman EA: Consequences of ethylene glycol poisoning. Am J Med 32:891–902, 1962.
108. Collins JM, Hennes DM, Holzgang CR, et al: Recovery after prolonged oliguria due to ethylene glycol intoxication: The prognostic value of serial, percutaneous renal biopsy. Arch Intern Med 125:1059–1062, 1970.
109. Cheng JT, Beysolow TD, Kaul B, et al: Clearance of ethylene glycol by kidneys and hemodialysis. J Toxicol Clin Toxicol 25: 95–108, 1987.
110. McCoy HG, Cipolle RJ, Ehlers SM: Severe methanol poisoning: Application of a pharmacokinetic model for ethanol therapy and hemodialysis. Am J Med 67:804–807, 1979.
111. Brent J, McMartin K, Phillips SP, et al: 4-Methylpyrazole therapy of methanol poisoning: Preliminary results of the meta trial. J Toxicol Clin Toxicol 351:567, 1997.
112. Wu DF, Clejan L, Potter B, et al: Rapid decrease of cytochrome P-45011E1 in primary hepatocyte culture and its maintenance by added 4-methylpyrazole. Hepatology 12:1379–1389, 1990.
113. Borron SW, Megarbane B, Baud FJ: Fomepizole in treatment of uncomplicated ethylene glycol poisoning [letter]. Lancet 354:831, 1999.
114. Sivilotti MLA, Burns MJ, McMartin KE, et al: Toxicokinetics of ethylene glycol during fomepizole therapy: Implications for management. Ann Emerg Med 36:114–125, 2000.
115. Frenia ML, Schauben JL: Methanol inhalation toxicity. Ann Emerg Med 22:1919–1923, 1993.
116. McMartin KE, Ambre JJ, Tephly TR: Methanol poisoning in human subjects: Role for formic acid accumulation in the metabolic acidosis. Am J Med 68:414–418, 1980.
117. Ingemansson S-O: Clinical observations in ten cases of methanol poisoning with particular reference to ocular manifestations. Acta Ophthalmol 62:15–24, 1984.
118. Swartz RD, Millman RP, Billi JE, et al: Epidemic methanol poisoning: Clinical and biochemical analysis of a recent episode. Medicine 60:373–382, 1982.
119. Glaser DS: Utility of the serum anion gap in the diagnosis of methanol or ethylene glycol ingestion. Ann Emerg Med 27: 343–346, 1996.
120. Kruse JA, Cadnapaphornchai P: The serum osmole gap. J Crit Care 8:185–197, 1994.
121. Pappas SC, Silverman M: Treatment of methanol poisoning with ethanol and hemodialysis. Can Med Assoc J 126:1391–1394, 1982.
122. Palatnick W, Redman LW, Sitar DS, et al: Methanol half-life

during ethanol administration: Implications for management of methanol poisoning. Ann Emerg Med 26:202–207, 1995.
123. Burns MJ, Graudins A, Aaron CK, et al: Treatment of methanol poisoning with intravenous 4-methylpyrazole. Ann Emerg Med 30:829–832, 1997.
124. Phang PT, Passerini L, Mielke B, et al: Brain hemorrhage associated with methanol poisoning. Crit Care Med 16:137–140, 1988.
125. Gonda A, Gault H, Churchill D, et al: Hemodialysis for methanol intoxication. Am J Med 64:749–758, 1978.
126. Johlin FC, Fortman CS, Nghiem DD, et al: Studies on the role of folic acid and folate-dependent enzymes in human methanol poisoning. Mol Pharmacol 31:557–561, 1987.
127. King ML: Acute methanol poisoning: A case study. Heart Lung 21:260–264, 1992.
128. Reynolds HN, Teiken P, Regan ME, et al: Hyperlactatemia, increased osmolar gap, and renal dysfunction during continuous lorazepam infusion. Crit Care Med 28:1631–1634, 2000.
129. Fligner CL, Jack R, Twiggs GA, Raisys VA: Hyperosmolality induced by propylene glycol. JAMA 253:1606–1609, 1985.
130. Ruddick JA: Toxicology, metabolism, and biochemistry of 1,2-propanediol. Toxicol Appl Pharmacol 21:102–111, 1972.
131. Smulders YM, Frissen PHJ, Slaats H, Silberbusch J: Renal tubular acidosis: Pathophysiology and diagnosis. Arch Intern Med 156:1629–1636, 1996.
132. Goodman AD, Lemann J Jr, Lennon RJ, et al: Production, excretion and net balance of fixed acid in patients with renal acidosis. J Clin Invest 44:495–506, 1965.
133. Wallia R, Greenburg A, Piraino B, et al: Serum electrolyte patterns in end stage renal disease. Am J Kidney Dis 8:98–104, 1986.
134. Litzow JR, Lemann J Jr, Lennon EJ: The effect of treatment of acidosis on calcium balance in patients with chronic azotemic renal disease. J Clin Invest 46:280–286, 1967.
135. Cohen RM, Feldman GM, Fernandez PC: The balance of acid, base, and charge in health and disease. Kidney Int 52:287–293, 1997.
136. Heird WC, Dell RB, Driscoll JM: Metabolic acidosis resulting from IV alimentation mixtures containing synthetic amino acids. N Engl J Med 287:943–948, 1972.
137. Peters JP, Van Slyke DD: Quantitative Clinical Chemistry: Interpretations, vol 1. Baltimore, Williams & Wilkins, 1931, pp 971–972.
138. Rosenbaum BJ, Makoff DL, Maxwell MH: Acid base and electrolyte changes induced by acute isotonic saline infusion in nephrectomized dogs. J Lab Clin Med 74:427–435, 1969.
139. Garella S, Chang BS, Kahn SI: Dilution acidosis and contraction alkalosis: Review of a concept. Kidney Int 8:279–283, 1975.
140. Gennari FJ, Goldstein MB, Schwartz WB: The nature of renal adaptation to chronic hypercapnia. J Clin Invest 51:1722, 1972.
141. Bidani A, DuBose TD Jr: Acid base regulation: Cellular and whole body. In Arieff AI, DeFronzo RA (eds): Fluid, Electrolyte and Acid-Base Disorders, 2nd ed. New York, Churchill Livingstone, 1995, pp 69–103.
142. Guenter PA, Settle RG, Perlmutter S, et al: Tube feeding-related diarrhea in acutely ill patients. J Parenter Enteral Nutr 15:277–280, 1991.
143. Brown E, Talbot GH, Axelrod P, et al: Risk factors for *Clostridium difficile* toxin-associated diarrhea. Infect Control Hosp Epidemiol 11:283–290, 1990.
144. Caprilli R, Frieri G, Vernia P, Colaneri O: Acid base disturbances in diarrhea. In Barany FR, Shields R, Caprilli R (eds): Gastrointestinal Emergencies 2. Oxford, Pergamon Press, 1980, pp 9–16.
145. Taher S, Anderson R, McCartney R, et al: Renal tubular acidosis associated with toluene "sniffing." N Engl J Med 290:765–768, 1974.
146. Carlisle EJF, Donnelly SM, Vasuvattakul S, et al: Glue-sniffing and distal renal tubular acidosis: Sticking to the facts. J Am Soc Nephrol 1:1019–1027, 1991.
147. Fischman DM, Oster JR: Toxic effects of toluene: A new cause of high anion gap acidosis. JAMA 241:1713–1715, 1979.
148. Voigts A, Kaufman CE Jr: Acidosis and other metabolic abnormalities associated with paint sniffing. South Med J 76:433–437, 1983.
149. Acute Respiratory Distress Syndrome Network: Ventilation with lower tidal volumes as compared with traditional tidal volumes for acute lung injury and the acute respiratory distress syndrome. N Engl J Med 342:18, 1301–1308, 2000.
150. Whipp BJ, Wasserman K: Carotid bodies and ventilatory control dynamics in man. Fed Proc 39:2668–2673, 1980.
151. Fitzgerald D, Mellis C, Johnson M, et al: Nebulized budesonide is as effective as nebulized adrenaline in moderately severe croup. Pediatrics 97:722–725, 1996.
152. MacDonnell SP, Timmins AC, Watson JD: Adrenaline administered via a nebulizer in adult patients with upper airway obstruction. Anaesthesia 50:35–36, 1995.
153. Georgopoulos D, Kondili E, Prinianakis G: How to set the ventilator in asthma. Monaldi Arch Chest Dis 55:74–83, 2000.
154. Tuxen DV: Permissive hypercapneic ventilation. Am J Respir Crit Care Med 150:870–874, 1994.
155. Acute Respiratory Distress Syndrome Network: Ventilation with lower tidal volumes as compared with traditional tidal volumes for acute lung injury and the acute respiratory distress syndrome. N Engl J Med 342:18, 1301–1308, 2000.
156. Pingleton SK: Barotrauma in acute lung injury: Is it important? Crit Care Med 23:223, 1995.
157. Schnapp LM, Chin DP, Szaflarski N, et al: Frequency and importance of barotrauma in 100 patients with acute lung injury. Crit Care Med 23:272, 1995.
158. Laffey JG, Engelberts D, Kavanagh BP: Buffering hypercapnic acidosis worsens acute lung injury. Am J Respir Crit Care Med 161:141–146, 2000.
159. Sueda S, Saeki H, Otani T, et al: Investigation of the most effective provocation test for patients with coronary spastic angina: Usefulness of accelerated exercise following hyperventilation. Jpn Circ J 63:85–90, 1999.
160. Savonitto S, Ardissino D: Different significance of hyperventilation-induced electrocardiographic changes in healthy subjects and patients with coronary artery disease Eur Heart J 17: 1302–1304, 1996.
161. Cline RE, Wallace AG, Young WG, Sealy WC: Electrophysiologic effects of respiratory and metabolic alkalosis on the heart. J Thorac Cardiovasc Surg 52:769–776, 1966.
162. Bellingham AJ, Detter JC, Lenfant C: Regulatory mechanisms of hemoglobin oxygen affinity in acidosis and alkalosis. J Clin Invest 50:700–706, 1971.
163. Hodgkin JE, Soeprono FF, Chan DM: Incidence of metabolic alkalemia in hospitalized patients. Crit Care Med 8:725–728, 1980.
164. Seldin DW, Rector FC Jr: The generation and maintenance of metabolic alkalosis. J Clin Invest 51:1722, 1972.
165. Rimmer JM, Gennari FJ: Metabolic alkalosis. J Intensive Care Med 2:137–150, 1987.
166. Koch SM, Taylor RF: Chloride ion in intensive care medicine. Crit Care Med 20:227–239, 1992.
167. Barton CH, Vaziri ND, Ness RL, et al: Cimetidine in the management of metabolic alkalosis induced by nasogastric drainage. Arch Surg 114:70–74, 1979.
168. Puschett JB, Goldberg M: The acute effects of furosemide on acid and electrolyte excretion in man. J Lab Clin Med 71: 666–677, 1968.
169. Kassirer JP, Harrington JT: Diuretics and potassium metabolism: A reassessment of the need, effectiveness, and safety of potassium therapy. Kidney Int 11:505–515, 1977.
170. Miller PD, Berns AS: Acute metabolic alkalosis perpetuating hypercarbia: A role for acetazolamide in chronic obstructive pulmonary disease. JAMA 238:2400–2401, 1977.
171. Leaf A, Schwartz WB, Relman AS: Oral administration of a potent carbonic anhydrase inhibitor. I. Changes in electrolyte and acid base. N Engl J Med 250:18, 759–764, 1954.
172. Turino GM, Goldring RM, Heinemann HO: Renal response to mechanical ventilation in patients with chronic hypercapnia. Am J Med 56:151–156, 1974.
173. Schwartz WB, Hays RM, Polak A, Haynie GD: Effects of chronic hypercapnia on electrolyte and acid-base equilibrium. II. Recovery, with special reference to the influence of chloride intake. J Clin Invest 40:1238–1249, 1961.
174. Adam WR, Koretsky AP, Weiner MW: 31P-NMR in vivo measurement of renal intracellular pH: Effects of acidosis and $K^+$ depletion in rats. Am J Physiol 251:F904–910, 1986.

175. Capasso G: Renal bicarbonate absorption in the rat. J Clin Invest 80:409–414, 1987.
176. Cheval L, Barlet-Bas C, Khadouri C, et al: K(+)-ATPase-mediated Rb+ transport in rat collecting tubule: Modulation during K+ deprivation. J Physiol 260:F800–F805, 1991.
177. Fencl V, Rossing TH: Acid-base disorders in critical care medicine. Annu Rev Med 40:17–29, 1989.
178. Rossing TH, Maffeo N, Fencl V: Acid-base effects of altering plasma protein concentration in human blood in vitro. J Appl Physiol 61:2260–2265, 1986.
179. Adrogue HJ, Madias NE: Management of life-threatening acid base disorders. N Engl J Med 338:2, 107–111, 1998.
180. Arbus GS, Herbert LA, Levesque PR, et al: Characterization and clinical application of the "significance band" for acute respiratory alkalosis. N Engl J Med 280:117–123, 1969.
181. Ian R, Vogel P, Lassen NA, et al: Role of extracellular and intracellular acidosis from hypercapnia-induced inhibition of tension of isolated rat cerebral arteries. Circ Res 76:269–275, 1995.
182. Brian JE: Carbon dioxide and the cerebral circulation. Anesthesiology 88:1365–1386, 1998.
183. Alexander SC, Smith TC, Strobel G, et al: Cerebral carbohydrate metabolism of man during respiratory and metabolic alkalosis. J Appl Physiol 24:66–72, 1968.
184. Berntman L, Dahlgren N, Siesjo BK: Cerebral blood flow during and oxygen consumption in the rat brain during extreme hypercarbia. Anesthesiology 50:299–305, 1979.
185. Raichle ME, Posner JB, Plum F: Cerebral blood flow during and after hyperventilation. Arch Neurol 23:394–403, 1970.
186. Phelps ME, Grubb RL Jr, Ter-Pogossian MM: Correlation between $pCO_2$ and regional cerebral blood volume by X-ray fluorescence. J Appl Physiol 35:274–280, 1973.
187. Strebel S, Kaufmann M, Baggi M, Zenklusen U: Cerebrovascular carbon dioxide reactivity during exposure to equipotent isoflurane and isoflurane in nitrous oxide anaesthesia. Br J Anaesth 71:272–276, 1993.
188. Drummond JC, Todd MM: The response of the feline cerebral circulation to $PaCO_2$ during anesthesia with isoflurane and halothane and during sedation with nitrous oxide. Anesthesiology 62:268–273, 1985.
189. Hansen NB, Nowicki PT, Miller RR, et al: Alterations in cerebral blood flow and oxygen consumption during prolonged hypocarbia. Pediatr Res 20:147–150, 1986.
190. Schierhout G, Roberts I: Hyperventilation therapy for acute traumatic brain injury. Cochrane Database of Systematic Reviews 2, 2000.
191. Brain Trauma Foundation, American Association of Neurological Surgeons, Joint Section on Neurotrauma and Critical Care: Hyperventilation. J Neurotrauma 17:513, 2000.
192. Anderson RJ, Potts DE, Gabow PA, et al: Unrecognized adult salicylate intoxication. Ann Intern Med 85:745–748, 1976.
193. Brien J: Ototoxicity associated with salicylates. Drug Saf 9: 143–148, 1993.
194. Done AK: Aspirin overdosage: incidence, diagnosis, and management. Pediatrics 62:890–897, 1978.
195. Eichenholz A, Mulhausen RO, Redleaf PS: Nature of acid-base disturbance in salicylate intoxication. Metabolism 12:164–175, 1963.
196. Gabow PA, Anderson RJ, Potts DE, et al: Acid-base disturbances in the salicylate-intoxicated adult. Arch Intern Med 138:1481–1484, 1978.
197. Dugandzic RM, Tierney MG, Dickinson GE, et al: Evaluation of the validity of the Done nomogram in the management of acute salicylate intoxication. Ann Emerg Med 18:1186–1190, 1989.
198. Hill JB: Salicylate intoxication. N Engl J Med 288:1110–1113, 1973.
199. Kwong TC, Laczin J, Baum J: Self-poisoning with enteric-coated aspirin. Am J Clin Pathol 80:888–890, 1983.
200. Prescott LF, Balali-Mood M, Critchley JA, et al: Diuresis or urinary alkalinization for salicylate poisoning. BMJ 285:1383–1386, 1982.
201. Morgan AG, Polack A: The excretion of salicylate in salicylate poisoning. Clin Sci 41:475–484, 1971.

CHAPTER 11

# Renal Tubular Acidosis

Thomas D. DuBose Jr., MD ▪ Glenn A. McDonald, MD

Renal tubular acidosis (RTA) is a clinical syndrome characterized, in part, by hyperchloremic metabolic acidosis that occurs as a result of a defect in urinary acidification. The decrease in net $H^+$ ion secretion can be localized to the nephron segment in which the defect occurs. Examples of specific defects involved in the pathogenesis of classical distal RTA include acquired or inherited abnormalities of the $H^+$-ATPase, the $HCO_3^-$-$Cl^-$ exchanger, and the enzyme carbonic anhydrase. Classical distal RTA (type 1 RTA) and proximal RTA (type 2 RTA) are associated with hypokalemia. In contrast, a more generalized abnormality in the distal nephron, type 4 RTA, is associated with hyperkalemia.

## DIFFERENTIAL DIAGNOSIS OF HYPERCHLOREMIC ACIDOSIS

A low plasma $HCO_3^-$ and an elevated plasma $Cl^-$ concentration, in the presence of acidemia, represent the salient features of hyperchloremic acidosis. The presence of acidemia must be confirmed by measuring arterial pH to distinguish hyperchloremic acidosis from chronic respiratory alkalosis. The clinical disorders that cause hyperchloremic metabolic acidosis are displayed in Table 11–1. The two most important disorders to distinguish include bicarbonate loss from the gastrointestinal (GI) tract and a renal acidification defect.

### Loss of $HCO_3^-$ From the Gastrointestinal Tract Versus Renal Tubular Acidosis

Diarrhea is a common cause of hyperchloremic metabolic acidosis. Diarrheal stools contain a large amount of $HCO_3^-$ decomposed by reaction with organic acids. The $HCO_3^-$ loss and the ensuing volume depletion cause hyperchloremic metabolic acidosis. Hypokalemia develops due to direct $K^+$ loss in the stool and increased renal $K^+$ secretion (in the cortical collecting tubule [CCT]) due to a secondary increase in elaboration of renin and aldosterone in response to volume depletion. Both hypokalemia and nonrenal metabolic acidosis increase renal ammonium ($NH_4^+$) synthesis, which increases urinary buffering capacity and urinary pH. The presence of $NH_4^+$ in the urine can be used clinically to distinguish hyperchloremic metabolic acidosis due to diarrhea from RTA. In the latter, $NH_4^+$ excretion is invariably low.[1] Urine pH, although a time-honored method to distinguish these disorders, is less reliable because urinary ammonium excretion is augmented in chronic metabolic acidosis due to diarrhea, causing urine pH to increase over time.

Therefore, in the evaluation of hyperchloremic metabolic acidosis, it is important to determine whether the kidney is responding normally to the acidosis by increasing urinary $NH_4^+$ excretion. The kidney responds to chronic metabolic acidosis primarily by increasing $NH_4^+$ production and excretion adaptively. In contrast, ammonium production and excretion are impaired with chronic renal insufficiency, hyperkalemia, and all forms of RTA.

Because the measurement of urinary $NH_4^+$ concentrations may be problematic for the routine hospital clinical pathology laboratory, it is helpful to estimate the urinary ammonium concentration by consideration of the electrolytes present in urine. Because $NH_4^+$ is a cation, its presence in urine, especially when in large amounts as expected in nonrenal forms of hyperchloremic metabolic acidosis, should be denoted by an increase in urinary anions ($Cl^-$) in excess of the usual cations ($Na^+ + K^+$). The urine anion gap (UAG) is calculated on a "spot" urine sample as follows[2]:

$$UAG = (Na^+ + K^+)_u - (Cl^-)_u \quad \text{(Equation 1)}$$

**TABLE 11–1.** Differential Diagnosis of Hyperchloremic Metabolic Acidosis

| |
|---|
| **Gastrointestinal Bicarbonate Loss** |
| Diarrhea |
| External pancreatic or small bowel drainage |
| Ureterosigmoidostomy, jejunal loop |
| Drugs |
|   Calcium chloride |
|   Magnesium sulfate |
|   Cholestyramine |
| **Renal Acidosis** |
| Proximal RTA (type 2) |
| Distal ("classical") RTA (type 1) |
| Generalized distal nephron dysfunction (type IV) |
|   Mineralocorticoid deficiency |
|   Mineralocorticoid resistance |
|   Nonmineralocorticoid voltage defects |
| Renal insufficiency |
| **Others** |
| Acid loads (ammonium chloride, arginine hydrochloride, hyperalimentation, sulfur) |
| Loss of potential bicarbonate |
|   Ketosis with ketone excretion |
|   Dilutional acidosis |
|   Posthypocapnic state |

RTA, renal tubular acidosis.

Urinary $NH_4^+$ is present if the sum of the major cations ($Na^+$ + $K^+$) is less than the concentration of the major anion ($Cl^-$). Therefore, a negative anion gap denotes the presence of ammonium in the urine and signals a "normal" renal response to acidosis of nonrenal origin (i.e., diarrhea). Hyperchloremic metabolic acidosis of renal origin (i.e., RTA) is supported by the presence of a positive UAG. A positive UAG confirms a deficiency of $NH_4^+$ and occurs when the sum of the major cations ($Na^+$ + $K^+$) in the urine exceeds the major urinary anion ($Cl^-$). A positive UAG, therefore, denotes an "abnormal" renal response to acidosis and is consistent with a defect in net acid secretion. The presence of urinary anions other than chloride can invalidate the UAG. Examples of urinary anions that invalidate this shorthand method of estimating urinary ammonium concentrations include drug anions, ketones, and toxins such as toluene. If these constituents are suspected, urinary ammonium $NH^+$ may be estimated reliably by measuring urine osmolality ($U_{Osm}$) and the concentrations of $Na^+$ plus $K^+$, urine urea, and glucose. Urinary ammonium ($U_{NH4^+}$) is calculated as follows:

$$U_{NH4^+} = 0.5\ (U_{Osm} - (2[Na^+ + K^+] + \text{urea} + \text{glucose})\ \text{(all expressed in mmol/L)}$$

(Equation 2)

The fractional excretion of sodium may also be helpful to differentiate hyperchloremic metabolic acidosis due to diarrhea from RTA. The fractional excretion of sodium is typically low (<1% to 2%) in patients with diarrhea compared with RTA (2% to 3%).

## Other Causes of Hyperchloremic Acidosis

In addition to diarrhea and RTA, there are other less common causes of hyperchloremic metabolic acidosis (see Table 11–1). External pancreatic and biliary diversion may lead to the loss of $HCO_3^-$-rich fluid and result in hyperchloremic metabolic acidosis. The excretion of sodium salts of ketones, during the recovery phase of ketoacidosis, represents the loss of potential $HCO_3^-$ and may result in hyperchloremic metabolic acidosis. Ureteral diversion is commonly associated with hyperchloremic metabolic acidosis, because the ileum and colon are both endowed with an apical $HCO_3^-$-$Cl^-$ exchanger. When chloride from urine comes into contact with the gut, chloride is absorbed in exchange for bicarbonate, which leads to excretion of bicarbonate, absorption of chloride, and hyperchloremic metabolic acidosis.[3] The degree of acidosis is magnified by stasis and prolonged contact of urine with the $HCO_3^-$-$Cl^-$ exchanger in the pouch. Because of bicarbonate secretion, potassium secretion is also stimulated and leads to hypokalemia. Finally, the administration of acid or acid equivalent (arginine HCl, lysine HCl, or $NH_4Cl$) or medications such as cholestyramine, calcium chloride, and magnesium sulfate are associated with hyperchloremic metabolic acidosis.[4] Dilutional acidosis occurs in conjunction with rapid infusion of isotonic saline. In these latter examples, the serum potassium is usually normal.

Progressive renal failure is associated with metabolic acidosis. Hyperchloremic metabolic acidosis is commonly seen when the glomerular filtration rate (GFR) is between 20 and 50 mL/min.[5] As renal failure progresses to a GFR of less than 10 to 15 mL/min, the acidosis converts to the typical high anion gap acidosis of "uremic" acidosis. The main defect in advanced renal failure is impaired ammoniagenesis and ammonium excretion.[5] The latter is a result of impaired medullary ammonium transport and trapping of $NH_3$/$NH_4^+$ in the outer and inner medulla.

In summary, the defect in renal acidification in RTA may be manifest by either an acid urine and low UAG with acidosis or frank bicarbonaturia during $NaHCO_3$ therapy (proximal RTA); an inappropriately alkaline urine pH and positive UAG (classical distal RTA); or hyperkalemia and a positive UAG with aldosterone deficiency, aldosterone resistance, or a "voltage" defect in the collecting tubule (generalized defect in distal nephron).

# PROXIMAL RENAL TUBULAR ACIDOSIS

## $Na^+$-$H^+$ Exchanger

The kidney employs two fundamental mechanisms to maintain acid-base homeostasis: $HCO_3^-$ absorption and $H^+$ secretion. Of the 4000 mEq of $HCO_3^-$ filtered by the kidney each day, 80% to 90% is reabsorbed in the proximal tubule. Effective $HCO_3^-$ absorption in the proximal tubule is mediated by $H^+$ secretion.[6] Even though the distal tubule is responsible for the secretion of 50 to 80 mEq of $H^+$ and final acidification of the urine, the vast majority of $H^+$ secretion obviously occurs in conjunction with $HCO_3^-$ reclamation in the proximal tubule.

Bicarbonate absorption is dependent on $H^+$ secretion across the apical membrane of the proximal tubule in exchange for $Na^+$ entry into the cell via the $Na^+$-$H^+$ exchanger.[7–12] The specific $Na^+$-$H^+$ exchanger located on the apical membrane of the proximal tubule is the NHE-3. A low intracellular $Na^+$ concentration is maintained by the active extrusion of $Na^+$ across the basolateral membrane via the $Na^+,K^+$-ATPase. The enzyme carbonic anhydrase present in the cytoplasm (type II) and on the apical and basolateral membrane (type IV) is critical to accelerate the following reaction:

$$H^+ + HCO_3^- \longleftrightarrow H_2CO_3 \overset{CA}{\longleftrightarrow} CO_2 + H_2O$$

(Equation 3)

The active secretion of $H^+$ into $HCO_3^-$-rich glomerular filtrate by the NHE-3 results in the formation of $H_2CO_3$. Luminal carbonic anhydrase (type IV) facilitates the conversion of $H_2CO_3$ to $CO_2$ and $H_2O$. $CO_2$ freely diffuses through the luminal membrane. Under the influence of cytoplasmic carbonic anhydrase (type II), $CO_2$ forms $H_2CO_3$, which dissociates rapidly to $H^+$ and $HCO_3^-$, which are transported, respectively, across the apical and basolateral membranes. $HCO_3^-$ exits the cell via the electrogenic $Na^+/HCO_3^-/CO_3^{2-}$ symporter. The negative cell potential is the primary driving force for this transport process. In addition to $H^+$ secretion via the $Na^+$-$H^+$ exchanger, an apical $H^+$-ATPase is also responsible for a small but significant fraction of bicarbonate reclamation in the proximal tubule.

## Other Proximal Tubular Functions

In addition to its role in $H^+$ secretion and $HCO_3^-$ absorption, the proximal tubule is the primary site for glucose, amino acid, phosphate, and organic anion reclamation. Each of these solutes is transported across the apical membrane via a $Na^+$-cotransport process. $Na^+$ enters the apical membrane down its electrochemical gradient. Low intracellular $Na^+$ concentrations and the negative intracellular potential are maintained via the basolateral $Na^+,K^+$-ATPase. Once inside the cell, these solutes are either metabolized or diffuse passively across the basolateral membrane. Citrate is reabsorbed in the proximal tubule in parallel with $Na^+$ via the $Na^+$ dicarboxylate cotransporter-1 (NaDC-1).[13] The metabolism of citrate within the cell leads to the generation of $HCO_3^-$. The presence of citrate in tubular fluid and urine has been proved to be protective in the prevention of calcium oxalate stones and nephrocalcinosis. In the presence of all forms of metabolic acidosis, except proximal RTA, citrate is preferentially reabsorbed, resulting in hypocitruria and predisposing patients to nephrolithiasis. In proximal RTA, because this $Na^+$-coupled transport system is impaired, urinary citrate remains high—even with metabolic acidosis—and nephrolithiasis rarely, if ever, occurs.

## Lessons from Animal and Naturally Occurring Models of Generalized and Isolated Proximal Tubular Transport Defects

RTA involving the proximal tubule can be divided into two major categories: (1) generalized disorders of proximal tubule reabsorption, and (2) precise abnormalities in renal acidification (Table 11–2). Generalized dysfunction of the proximal tubule could occur through three possible mechanisms: (1) an increase in paracellular permeability resulting in backleak of all reabsorbed solutes into the lumen; (2) a generalized defect in proximal tubule absorption, such as adenosine triphosphate (ATP) depletion; and (3) a defect in basolateral $Na^+,K^+$-ATPase activity. Specific cellular abnormalities, which may lead to selective defects in proximal tubule acidification, include abnormalities in: (1) the $Na^+$-$H^+$ exchanger (NHE-3); (2) the $H^+$-ATPase; (3) the $Na^+/HCO_3^-/CO_3^{2-}$ symporter; (4) the enzymes carbonic anhydrase type II or IV; and (5) abnormalities in cell depolarization.

**TABLE 11–2.** Disorders Associated with Proximal Renal Tubular Acidosis

**Isolated Bicarbonate Transport Defect**

- Primary (sporadic or familial)
- Carbonic anhydrase
  - Inhibition
    - Acetazolamide
    - Mafenide (Sulfamylon)
  - Deficiency
    - Osteopetrosis with carbonic anhydrase II deficiency (Sly syndrome)
- Pryuvate carboxylase deficiency
- York-Yendt syndrome
- Cyanotic congenital heart disease

**Generalized Proximal Tubular Transport Defect**

- Proximal (sporadic or familial)
- Genetically transmitted systemic diseases
  - Cystinosis
  - Lowe syndrome
  - Hereditary fructose intolerance (during fructose ingestion)
  - Tyrosinemia
  - Galactosemia
  - Wilson disease
  - Miotochondrial phosphoenolpyruvate carboxykinase deficiency
  - Metachromatic leukodystrophy
  - Glycogen storage disease
  - Cytochrome-*c* oxidase deficiency
  - Acyl-CoA dehydrogenase deficiency
  - Silver-Russell syndrome
- Dysproteinemic states
  - Multiple myeloma
  - Light chain disease
- Amyloidosis
- Vitamin D deficiency, dependence, or resistance
- Other renal diseases
  - Sjögren syndrome
  - Medullary cystic disease
  - Early rejection of kidney transplant
  - Balkan nephropathy
  - Chronic renal vein thrombosis
  - Nephrotic syndrome
  - Paroxysmal nocturnal hemoglobinuria
- Toxins/drugs (historic)
  - Lead
  - Gentamicin
  - Cadmium
  - Maleic acid
  - Coumarin
  - Streptozocin
  - Ifosfamide
  - Tacrolimus
  - Outdated tetracycline

Generalized dysfunction of the proximal tubule, which is the more common of the two examples appreciated by the co-occurrence of RTA, glycosuria, aminoaciduria, phosphaturia, and hypercitraturia, is referred to collectively as Fanconi syndrome. The recognition of this syndrome in both animal models and human subjects has allowed a better understanding of $Na^+$-coupled transport in the proximal tubule. A classic animal model of generalized proximal tubular dysfunction is maleic acid nephropathy.[14] Most studies suggest that the generalized defect and the defect in transcellular $HCO_3^-$ absorption are due to depletion of intracellular ATP, with inhibition of the $Na^+,K^+$-

ATPase. Disruption of active $HCO_3^-$, amino acid, and solute absorption in the proximal tubule due to ATP depletion and inhibition of $Na^+,K^+$-ATPase has also been observed in an experimental model of cystinosis.[15] Hereditary fructose intolerance is associated with Fanconi syndrome upon exposure to dietary fructose. Patients with this disorder lack the enzyme fructose-1-aldolase, which results in sequestration of intracellular phosphate and is associated with ATP depletion.[16] Severe vitamin D deficiency, also associated with Fanconi syndrome, is characterized by low levels of vitamin D, a low serum calcium concentration, and increased levels of parathyroid hormone.[17, 18] Whereas each of these substances has been shown to affect the proximal tubule, the mechanism responsible for proximal tubular dysfunction is unclear but, nevertheless, resolves with the administration of vitamin D.

Isolated abnormalities of proximal tubular renal acidification in the absence of Fanconi syndrome are less common but may be associated with depolarization abnormalities or genetic mutations. One model—the infusion of L-lysine in dogs—results in marked bicarbonaturia due to inhibition of $HCO_3^-$ absorption.[19] The presence of luminal L-lysine has been shown to depolarize proximal tubular cells, which could alkalinize the cell by decreasing $HCO_3^-$ extrusion across the basolateral membrane. Mice—in which the gene encoding the renal $Na^+$-$H^+$ exchanger (NHE-3) has been knocked out—have metabolic acidosis with a proximal RTA.[20]

Sly and associates have described a group of patients with inherited carbonic anhydrase II deficiency. These patients develop osteopetrosis, cerebral calcification, and combined proximal and distal RTA.[21, 22] This observation is not unexpected considering the role that carbonic anhydrase plays in $HCO_3^-$ reclamation.

## Clinical Features of Proximal Renal Tubular Acidosis

Patients with proximal RTA commonly present with hyperchloremic metabolic acidosis, an acid urine pH (pH $<5$), and minimal $HCO_3^-$ excretion. As $HCO_3^-$ is administered to correct the metabolic acidosis, bicarbonaturia occurs and the fractional excretion of $HCO_3^-$ often exceeds 10% to 15%. This response to alkali therapy, the ensuing increase in potassium excretion in response to the bicarbonate leak into the distal tubule, and the difficulty with which the plasma bicarbonate is corrected are unique features of proximal RTA. Sebastian and associates demonstrated that the level of $K^+$ excretion correlates directly with $HCO_3^-$ excretion.[23] Decreased NaCl absorption associated with proximal tubular dysfunction enhances $K^+$ excretion by increasing delivery of $Na^+$ to the distal nephron and the increase in aldosterone elaboration in response to volume depletion.

Most cases of proximal RTA are associated with generalized proximal tubule dysfunction (Fanconi syndrome) so that glycosuria, aminoaciduria, proteinuria, hyperphosphaturia, hypophosphatemia, hyperuricosuria, hypouricemia, and hypercitraturia are observed commonly. Hypercalciuria, a common feature of metabolic acidosis, is absent in proximal RTA, presumably as a result of enhanced calcium absorption in the distal nephron in response to increased bicarbonate delivery. Rickets, a frequent manifestation of Fanconi syndrome, is a result of phosphate wasting and not of proximal RTA or acidosis. Of particular concern in children with proximal RTA is growth retardation, which is a direct consequence of acidosis. Because growth retardation will correct with alkali therapy, this complication becomes one of the major indications for correction of the serum bicarbonate concentration.

## Management

The primary therapeutic objective in the management of patients with proximal RTA is to maintain a near-normal serum $HCO_3^-$ concentration and arterial pH. The bicarbonaturia associated with this disorder, which amplifies potassium excretion, requires administration of a mixture of sodium and potassium salts (e.g., K-Shohl solution) (Table 11–3). A feature of proximal RTA is the large amount of $HCO_3^-$ required to correct the acidosis. As an adjunct, the administration of thiazide diuretics has been used to decrease GFR from chronic volume depletion. Sequelae of proximal RTA vary according to cause (generalized versus isolated). Nevertheless, in children with isolated proximal RTA, stunted growth is normalized by correction of the acidosis. Additionally, the manifestations of isolated proximal RTA in children tend to improve with age.

**TABLE 11–3.** Forms of Alkali Replacement

| | |
|---|---|
| **Shohl Solution** | |
| $Na^+$ citrate 500 mg | Each 1 mL contains 1 mEq sodium and is equivalent to 1 mEq of bicarbonate |
| Citric acid 334 mg/5 mL | |
| **$NaHCO_3$ Tablets** | 3.9 mEq/tablet (325 mg)<br>7.8 mEq/tablet (650 mg) |
| **Baking Soda** | 60 mEq/tsp |
| **K-Lyte** | 25 or 50 mEq/tablet |
| **Polycitra (K-Shohl solution)** | |
| $Na^+$ citrate 500 mg | Each mL contains 1 mEq potassium and 1 mEq sodium and is equivalent to 2 mEq bicarbonate |
| $K^+$ citrate 550 mg | |
| Citric acid 334 mg/5 mL | |
| **Polycitra Crystals** | |
| $K^+$ citrate 3300 mg | Each packet contains 30 mEq potassium and is equivalent to 30 mEq bicarbonate |
| Citric acid 1002 mg per packet | |
| **Urocit-K Tablets** | |
| Potassium citrate | 5 or 10 mEq per tablet |

# DISTAL RENAL TUBULAR ACIDOSIS

## Mechanism and Regulation of Distal Acidification

The role of the distal nephron in maintaining acid-base homeostasis occurs through $HCO_3^-$ absorption and net acid secretion. As discussed previously, the proximal tubule absorbs approximately 90% of the filtered $HCO_3^-$ load, with the distal nephron accounting for the remaining 10%. In addition, the distal nephron is responsible for secreting daily approximately 50 to 80 mEq of $H^+$, which matches daily net acid production from metabolism. Thus, excretion of net acid replaces the $HCO_3^-$ lost in extracellular buffering of those acids gained from metabolism of dietary protein. Proton secretion in the distal nephron generates large pH gradients between the blood and the lumen. The kidney utilizes an elaborate buffering system to avoid unsustainably large transepithelial $H^+$ concentration gradients and the ensuing tubular toxicity associated with the expected local acidity that would be necessary to secrete 50 to 80 mEq $H^+$/day without buffering. This buffering system is divided into two categories: (1) $NH_4^+$, and (2) titratable acid. Titratable acids in urine include phosphate, creatinine, and other miscellaneous buffers. Total net acid excretion (NAE) is represented by the sum of titratable acid and $NH_4^+$ excretion (minus minimal $HCO_3^-$ excretion, if any). Therefore, to maintain acid-base balance, NAE must approximate net acid production.

## $H^+$ Secretion/ $HCO_3^-$ Absorption and the Pathophysiologic Basis of Classical Distal Renal Tubular Acidosis

### ANATOMIC AND PHYSIOLOGIC SEGREGATION OF THE COLLECTING DUCT

The collecting duct can be divided into three functional segments: (1) the CCT, (2) the outer medullary collecting tubule (OMCT), and (3) the inner medullary collecting duct (IMCD). The CCT is a low-capacity $H^+$ secretory segment where the rate of $H^+$ secretion is modulated by aldosterone, $Na^+$, and $K^+$ absorption and systemic acid-base balance. The CCT has the capacity for both $H^+$ and $HCO_3^-$ secretion.[24–27] The former function is accomplished by type A intercalated cells; the latter function is achieved by type B intercalated cells. The OMCT, in contrast, has a high capacity for $H^+$ secretion, which is regulated by systemic acid-base homeostasis, the serum $K^+$ concentration, and aldosterone.[28–30] Finally, the IMCD is a low-capacity proton secretory system. In this segment, ammonium transport is regulated by acid-base homeostasis and also by the serum $K^+$ concentration.[31]

In each segment of the distal nephron, $HCO_3^-$ absorption is mediated by apical membrane $H^+$ secretion.[32, 33] Because of the negative cell potential, $H^+$ secretion must occur by an active transport process.[34–36] Two ATP-dependent proton pumps, the $H^+$-ATPase and the $H^+,K^+$-ATPase, have been identified in the distal nephron and together are responsible for $H^+$ secretion.[37, 38] Immunohistochemical studies have localized the $H^+$-ATPase to the apical membrane of acid secreting cells (type A intercalated cells) in the CCT and OMCT. The $H^+,K^+$-ATPase is present in intercalated cells of the cortical collecting duct and outer medullary collecting duct.[37, 38] There are at least two isoforms of $H^+,K^+$-ATPase expressed in the kidney, $HK\alpha_1$ ("gastric") and $HK\alpha_2$ ("colonic"). $HK\alpha_1$ is identical to the $H^+,K^+$-ATPase in gastric parietal cells, whereas $HK\alpha_2$ is homologous to the $H^+,K^+$-ATPase in the distal colon. Several studies have demonstrated that $HK\alpha_2$ mRNA and protein (but not $HK\alpha_1$) are dramatically upregulated by chronic hypokalemia and chronic acidosis.[39] Furthermore, increased $H^+,K^+$-ATPase activity in the outer and IMCD results in enhanced $HCO_3^-$ absorption.[40] Apical proton secretion generates $HCO_3^-$ intracellularly, which then exits the cell via the $HCO_3^-$-$Cl^-$ exchanger (AE-1) present on the basolateral membrane.[41–43] Thus, these three transporters, the apical $H^+$-ATPase and $H^+,K^+$-ATPase and the basolateral $HCO_3^-$-$Cl^-$ exchanger, could be involved, if defective, in the development of an acidification defect in the distal nephron. Additionally, defective net $H^+$ secretion could occur by the insertion of a "leak" pathway for $H^+$ into the collecting duct. This abnormality, also referred to as a "gradient lesion," occurs most commonly with amphotericin B nephrotoxicity but is also seen in other forms of inherited or acquired distal RTA.

## $HCO_3^-$ Secretion

Whereas $HCO_3^-$ secretion is mediated by a basolateral $H^+$-ATPase in series with an apical membrane $HCO_3^-$-$Cl^-$ exchanger in type B intercalated cells in the CCT, its role in distal RTA has not been established. This transporter and $HCO_3^-$ secretion are upregulated by metabolic alkalosis and downregulated by metabolic acidosis. It has been suggested that trafficking of a genetically defective *AE-1* gene product—the basolateral $HCO_3^-$-$Cl^-$ exchanger—to the apical membrane of type A intercalated cells could contribute to the development of an acidification defect in families with autosomal dominant classical distal RTA.[44]

## Ammonium Production and Excretion

Whereas ammonium is secreted in several segments of the nephron, most ammonium secretion occurs in the proximal tubule and is regulated by acid-base homeostasis. Ammonium transport involves both $NH_3$ diffusion and $NH_4^+$ transport. $NH_4^+$ secretion into the proximal tubule lumen occurs via the apical membrane $Na^+$-$H^+$ exchanger (NHE-3) through substitution of $NH_4^+$ for $H^+$. Ammonium secretion is augmented dramatically by systemic metabolic acidosis.

At physiologic pH, α-ketoglutarate, a major metabolic product of ammoniogenesis, is converted to $HCO_3^-$ ions, which are transported across the basolateral membrane to the ECF. This end-product of ammoniagenesis represents, therefore, "new bicarbonate" when returned to the systemic circulation via the renal vein. As mentioned earlier, "new bicarbonate" restores the $HCO_3^-$ lost in the ECF from buffering the acid products of metabolism.

After ammonium enters the proximal tubule lumen, an elaborate system exists to generate high medullary interstitial concentrations of ammonium.[45] First, the $HCO_3^-$ concentration and pH of tubular fluid increase progressively along the thin descending limb of Henle's loop as a result of water abstraction.[46, 47] This alkaline environment favors $NH_3$ diffusion out of the tubule lumen. In addition, direct transport of $NH_4^+$ is accomplished via the $Na^+$-$2Cl^-$-$K^+$ transporter (through competition for the $K^+$ site) in the medullary thick ascending limb of the loop of Henle.[45] Ammonium absorption at this site is stimulated by acidosis and hypokalemia and is impaired by hyperkalemia.[48–52] $NH_3$ is capable of reentering the proximal straight tubule from the interstitium.[45] Active absorption of $NH_4^+$ in the thick ascending limb of the loop of Henle allows for trapping of $NH_4^+$ in the medullary countercurrent multiplication system.[53] The end result of this system is a medullary-to-cortical concentration gradient for ammonium with medullary concentrations exceeding cortical concentrations several-fold.[54] This corticomedullary ammonium gradient is augmented by metabolic acidosis.[48] Ammonium is trapped in the medullary collecting duct by a combination of $NH_3$ diffusion from the interstitium and active $H^+$ secretion by the medullary collecting duct ($H^+$-ATPase and the $H^+$,$K^+$-ATPase).[48, 55] This process generates high concentrations of ammonium in the final urine. Because $NH_4^+$ transport is accomplished by the $Na^+$,$K^+$-ATPase and $Na^+$-2Cl,$K^+$ cotransporter, competition between $K^+$ and $NH_4^+$ helps to explain the association between hyperkalemia and metabolic acidosis.[56]

## Regulation of Distal Acidification

Apical proton secretion and basolateral $HCO_3^-$ transport regulate, in concert, net $HCO_3^-$ absorption in the distal nephron. The responsible transporters include the electrogenic $H^+$-ATPase, and the electroneutral $H^+$,$K^+$-ATPase on the apical membrane and the $HCO_3^-$-$Cl^-$ exchanger on the basolateral membrane. Alteration in the negative transepithelial potential difference, which is dependent on the rate of $Na^+$ absorption, has a significant secondary impact on proton secretion by the electrogenic $H^+$-ATPase.[57] Thus, a decline in $Na^+$ delivery or $Na^+$ avidity, through either impairment of epithelial $Na^+$ channel (ENaC) function or through absence of mineralocorticoid, will secondarily impair $H^+$ secretion. A defect in $H^+$ secretion in the CCT in response to a decline in $Na^+$ transport–dependent transepithelial voltage has been called a "voltage defect." Mineralocorticoids have been demonstrated to be a potent determinant of proton secretion. In the CCT, mineralocorticoids stimulate $Na^+$ absorption (ENaC). Mineralocorticoids increase the lumen negative transepithelial potential, which stimulates electrogenic proton secretion secondarily.[58, 59] This early effect of aldosterone on ENaC is reinforced after 24 hours to upregulate the basolateral $Na^+$,$K^+$-ATPase as well. Taken together, mineralocorticoids increase the negative transepithelial potential, thus enhancing $Na^+$ absorption. Mineralocorticoids have also been shown to stimulate $H^+$-ATPase in the cortical outer and inner medullary collecting tubule in the absence of $Na^+$.[34, 60, 61] Thus, in summary, both mineralocorticoids and $Na^+$ absorption in the CCT have important regulatory effects on net $H^+$ secretion in the collecting duct.

Potassium homeostasis also plays a significant role in the regulation of renal acidification. Clearance studies have suggested that potassium deficiency stimulates distal proton secretion.[62] It has now been established that this regulatory response occurs, at least in part, through upregulation of the $H^+$,$K^+$-ATPase. Potassium status can also affect renal acidification indirectly. Potassium is an important determinant of aldosterone and, as discussed earlier, aldosterone is an important determinant of $H^+$ secretion. Potassium also affects ammonium synthesis and excretion.[52] Chronic hypokalemia stimulates ammonium production, whereas hyperkalemia suppresses ammoniagenesis.[51] Alterations in ammonium production may also affect the medullary interstitial gradient and buffer availability. Hyperkalemia impairs ammonium absorption in the thick ascending limb and also decreases medullary concentrations of total ammonium and secretion of $NH_3$ into the medullary collecting duct.[49, 51, 63]

# PATHOGENESIS OF DISTAL RENAL TUBULAR ACIDOSIS

## Classical Hypokalemic Distal Renal Tubular Acidosis

The mechanisms involved in the pathogenesis of hypokalemic distal RTA are not yet completely resolved. The occurrence of hypokalemia demonstrates that generalized CCT dysfunction or aldosterone deficiency is not causative. The inability to acidify the urine maximally (to $<$pH 5.5) has resulted in the designation of classical hypokalemic distal RTA as a "gradient lesion" or "rate defect" and has suggested the possibility of an abnormal leak pathway or defect in proton secretion, respectively.[64, 65] The last characteristic that helps to elucidate the pathogenesis of the acidification defect in these patients is the response of the urine $P_{CO_2}$ to $NaHCO_3$ infusion. Infusions of $NaHCO_3$ to produce a high $HCO_3^-$ excretion rate result normally in distal nephron hydrogen secretion and the generation of a high $CO_2$ tension in the urine. The magnitude of the urinary $P_{CO_2}$ (referred to as the urine-minus-blood $P_{CO_2}$, or U-B $P_{CO_2}$) is quantitatively related to distal nephron hydrogen ion secretion.[32, 66] A decrease in the rate of hydrogen ion secretion as a result of a defect of one of the $H^+$ transporters on the apical membrane ($H^+$- or $H^+,K^+$-ATPase) or the basolateral $HCO_3^-$-$Cl^-$ exchanger will lead to a low U-B $P_{CO_2}$. In contrast, a backleak of $H^+$, which occurs with a "gradient" defect, is associated with a normal U-B $P_{CO_2}$. In patients with classical hypokalemic distal RTA, the U-B $P_{CO_2}$ is usually subnormal, except in amphotericin B–induced distal RTA.[66–68] This finding supports the view that most patients with distal RTA have a "rate" or "pump" defect.

### GRADIENT DEFECT

A gradient defect or "leak" pathway in the collecting tubule would provide a pathway for acid efflux from the lumen, which would greatly decrease net proton secretion. In the absence of a transepithelial pH gradient, the effect of such a leak would be minimal or absent but would interfere with normal acidification when the filtered $HCO_3^-$ is low and the need to excrete an acidic urine is high. During infusion of $NaHCO_3$ for measurement of urinary $P_{CO_2}$ at a time of high bicarbonate delivery to the distal nephron, the leak pathway would be overcome because $H^+$ would be trapped. The characteristic clinical features of a gradient defect would include an inability to acidify the urine below a pH of 5.5.

### $H^+$ SECRETORY DEFECTS

Alternatively, the rate of proton secretion could be affected by abnormalities in a specific transporter or mechanism involved in proton secretion. These abnormalities include the apical $H^+$-ATPase or $H^+,K^+$-ATPase and the basolateral $HCO_3^-$-$Cl^-$ exchanger. Impairment of the $H^+$-ATPase in classical distal RTA has been documented in both acquired and inherited disorders. Acquired defects of $H^+$-ATPase have been demonstrated in renal biopsy specimens of patients with Sjögren syndrome with evidence of classical hypokalemic distal RTA. These biopsy specimens revealed an absence of $H^+$-ATPase protein in the apical membrane of α-intercalated cells. To further emphasize the importance of $H^+$-ATPase in classical RTA, Karet and associates described two different mutations in the *ATP6B1* gene encoding the B-subunit of the $H^+$-ATPase. One defect is associated with normal hearing; the other defect is associated with sensorineural deafness.[69, 70]

Abnormalities in the $H^+,K^+$-ATPase could result in both hypokalemia and metabolic acidosis. A role for $H^+,K^+$-ATPase involvement in classical distal RTA was suggested by the observation that chronic administration of vanadate in rats decreased $H^+,K^+$-ATPase activity and was associated with metabolic acidosis, hypokalemia, and an inappropriately alkaline urine.[71] Additionally, an unusually high incidence of hypokalemic distal RTA (endemic RTA) in Thailand has been associated with drinking water contaminated with vanadate.[71] Environmental vanadate toxicity seems to be an unlikely explanation for these manifestations, however. Alternatively, the striking association between chronic hypokalemia and the acidification defect in patients in this region suggests that chronic hypokalemia could be responsible for chronic tubulointerstitial disease, which could, in time, cause the acidification defect. This hypothesis for this form of "endemic" classical distal RTA is also attractive because chronic hypokalemia has been shown to be a potent stimulus for upregulation of the $H^+,K^+$-ATPase in the collecting tubule. It would be logical to assume a role for chronic hypokalemia and tubulointerstitial involvement in the development of some forms of classical distal RTA through compromise of the $H^+,K^+$-ATPase. Nevertheless, to date, there has been no documented genetic linkage between $H^+,K^+$-ATPase genes and inherited forms of classical distal RTA.

### DEFECTS IN THE $HCO_3^-$-$Cl^-$ EXCHANGER

Three groups have demonstrated independently an association between mutations in the *AE-1* gene, which encodes the basolateral $HCO_3^-$-$Cl^-$ exchanger in the collecting duct, and the occurrence of autosomal dominant classical distal RTA.[44, 72, 73] The typical clinical manifestations of classical distal RTA were associated with heterozygosity for the *AE1* point mutation, G1766A.[44, 72, 73] This mutation encodes an amino acid substitution, R598H, which is located at the cytoplasmic end of the *AE1* protein in transmembrane span 6. Surprisingly, however, when these point mutations were expressed in vitro, abnormalities in the $HCO_3^-$-$Cl^-$ exchanger were not observed. It was hypothesized that misdirection of the $HCO_3^-$-$Cl^-$ exchanger to the *apical* membrane rather than to the *basolateral* membrane might cause this disorder, resulting in impaired net $H^+$ secretion. If correct, enhanced $HCO_3^-$-$Cl^-$ exchange on the apical membrane would increase rather than decrease urinary $P_{CO_2}$ during bicarbonate infusion. The fact that an increase in the U-B $P_{CO_2}$ was demonstrated in patients with inherited classical distal RTA supports this view.

Therefore, in summary, evidence exists for impaired function of the $H^+$-ATPase and $H^+,K^+$-ATPase, mistrafficking of the $HCO_3^-$-$Cl^-$ exchanger to the apical membrane, and a leak pathway for $H^+$ as underlying defects in several examples of inherited and acquired classical distal RTA. As already discussed, another rare mechanism for inherited distal RTA includes carbonic anhydrase II deficiency (Sly syndrome). The diverse pathophysiology of the various inherited and acquired forms of classical distal RTA are outlined in Table 11–4.

## Impaired $NH_4^+$ Production and Excretion

Patients with abnormalities in $H^+$ secretion by the collecting duct in classical distal RTA also exhibit uniformly low excretory rates of ammonium.[2, 68] In the

**TABLE 11–4.** Molecular Basis of Distal Renal Tubular Acidosis

| | |
|---|---|
| **Classical Distal RTA** | |
| *Inherited* | |
| Autosomal dominant | Defect in *AE-1* gene encodes for single missense mutation (R589H) in the $HCO_3^-$-$Cl^-$ exchanger (band 3 protein)<br>Transporter may be mistargeted to the apical membrane<br>Other missense mutations reported in some families (R589C and S613F) |
| Autosomal recessive | |
| With deafness | Mutations in *ATP6B1,* encoding B-subunit of the collecting duct apical $H^+$-ATPase, maps to chromosome 7q33-34; progressive sensorineural hearing loss |
| With normal hearing | Linkage to the segment of 7q33-34 distinct from *ATP6B1* (rd RTA2) |
| Carbonic anhydrase II deficiency | Defect in enzyme carbonic anhydrase II in RBCs, bone, kidney |
| *Endemic (Northeastern Thailand)* | Possible abnormality in $H^+$,$K^+$-ATPase? |
| *Acquired* | Reduced expression of $H^+$-ATPase |
| **Generalized Distal Nephron Dysfunction** | |
| *Pseudohypoaldosteronism Type I* | |
| Autosomal recessive | Missense mutation with the loss of function of ENaC maps to chromosome 16p12.2-13.11 in six families and to 12p13.1-pter in five additional families |
| Autosomal dominant | Heterozygous mutations of MLR<br>Two frameshift mutations, two premature termination codons, and one splice donor mutation of the mineralocorticoid receptor gene |
| *Pseudohypoaldosteronism Type II* | Linkage to 1q31-42 and 17p11-q21; transporter not yet identified |

ENaC, epithelial sodium channel; RBC, red blood cell; RTA, renal tubular acidosis.

face of hyperchloremic metabolic acidosis, low ammonium excretion demonstrates that the kidney is causing or perpetuating the metabolic acidosis. Defective ammonium excretion may occur because of an inability to trap ammonium in the medullary collecting duct as a result of a higher than normal tubular fluid pH, which is obtained when $H^+$ secretion is impaired (e.g., a defect in $H^+$-ATPase, $H^+$,$K^+$-ATPase, or the basolateral $HCO_3^-$-$Cl^-$ exchanger). Moreover, urinary concentrating defects from the medullary interstitial disease are common in patients with classical distal RTA and may interfere with the medullary countercurrent multiplier and reduce the corticomedullary concentration gradient for ammonium, thus reducing ammonium excretion.[1, 48] Because classical distal RTA is associated with hypokalemia, it would be anticipated that ammonium production and excretion would be enhanced. Nevertheless, ammonium excretion remains low for the prevailing systemic acidosis and urine pH, most likely as a result of failure of the corticomedullary countercurrent system.

## Clinical Presentation of Classical Distal Renal Tubular Acidosis

Classical hypokalemic distal RTA is associated, therefore, with positive acid balance, a hyperchloremic metabolic acidosis, and volume depletion. Hyperchloremia is augmented by volume depletion. The positive acid balance and progressive acidosis cause calcium, magnesium, and phosphate wasting and may culminate in metabolic bone disease. Stunted growth is common in prepubertal children. Both hypercalciuria, which is associated with distal RTA, and hypocitraturia, which accompanies chronic metabolic acidosis, provide a favorable environment for urinary stone formation and nephrocalcinosis.[74, 75] Nephrocalcinosis associated with hyperchloremic metabolic acidosis strongly implicates classical distal RTA, because this does not occur with either proximal RTA or generalized distal nephron dysfunction with hyperkalemia.[76] Pyelonephritis commonly complicates distal RTA and is not only seen in association with nephrocalcinosis but is also more difficult to eradicate in the presence of nephrocalcinosis.

## Clinical Examples of Classical Distal Renal Tubular Acidosis

Classical distal RTA may occur as an autosomal dominant or autosomal recessive inherited defect (primary distal RTA) or in association with a systemic illness (secondary distal RTA). Overwhelmingly, most patients with classical distal RTA have secondary distal RTA. The different etiologies of classical distal RTA are displayed in Table 11–5.

### INHERITED CLASSICAL DISTAL RENAL TUBULAR ACIDOSIS

More than 300 individuals from 30 families have been identified with primary distal RTA.[72–74, 77–80] Males and females are equally affected. Although autosomal dominant and X-linked modes of inheritance have been reported, most patients appear to have an autosomal dominant mode of inheritance.[22, 74, 78, 79, 81] A candidate gene for this disorder is *AE-1.* This gene encodes for the $HCO_3^-$-$Cl^-$ exchanger (band 3 protein) in red blood cells and in type A intercalated cells in the collecting duct.[72] Investigators have reported that af-

**TABLE 11–5.** Disorders Associated with Classical Hypokalemic Distal Renal Tubular Acidosis

| | |
|---|---|
| **Primary** | |
| Familial | |
| 1. Autosomal dominant | |
| a. *AE1* gene | |
| 2. Autosomal recessive | |
| a. With deafness *(ATP6B1)* | |
| b. Without deafness (rd RTA2) | |
| Sporadic | |
| **Endemic** | |
| Northeastern Thailand | |
| **Secondary to Systemic Disorders** | |
| *Autoimmune Diseases* | |
| Hyperglobulinemic purpura | Fibrosing alveolitis |
| Cryoglobulinemia | Chronic active hepatitis |
| Sjögren syndrome | Primary biliary cirrhosis |
| Thyroiditis | Polyarteritis nodosa |
| HIV nephropathy | |
| *Hypercalciuria and Nephrocalcinosis* | |
| Primary hyperparathyroidism | Idiopathic hypercalciuria |
| Hyperthyroidism | Wilson disease |
| Medullary sponge kidney | Hereditary fructose intolerance |
| Fabry disease | |
| X-linked hypophosphatemia | Hereditary sensorineural deafness |
| Vitamin D intoxication | |
| *Drug and Toxin-Induced Disease* | |
| Amphotericin B | Toluene |
| Cyclamate | Mercury |
| Vanadate | Lithium |
| Hepatic cirrhosis | Classic analgesic nephropathy |
| Ifosfamide | Foscarnet |
| *Tubulointerstitial Diseases* | |
| Balkan nephropathy | Renal transplantation |
| Chronic pyelonephritis | Leprosy |
| Obstructive uropathy | Jejunoileal bypass with hyperoxaluria |
| Vesicoureteral reflux | |
| *Associated with Genetically Transmitted Diseases* | |
| Ehlers-Danlos syndrome | Hereditary elliptocytosis |
| Sickle cell anemia | Marfan syndrome |
| Medullary cystic disease | Jejunal bypass with hyperoxaluria |
| Hereditary sensorineural deafness | |
| Osteopetrosis with carbonic anhydrase II deficiency | Carnitine palmitoyltransferase I |

HIV, human immunodeficiency virus.

fected patients from several families are heterozygous for a single missense mutation in the *AE-1* gene.[72, 73] In vitro functional assays have failed to convincingly delineate the transport defect responsible for the development of acidosis.[72, 73] Loss of polarized targeting of a functional $HCO_3^-$-$Cl^-$ exchanger into the apical, rather than the basolateral, membrane has been suggested. If this theory is correct, it would be anticipated that enhanced $HCO_3^-$ secretion by a misdirected $HCO_3^-$-$Cl^-$ exchanger would *increase* the U-B $P_{CO_2}$ with $HCO_3^-$ diuresis. Preliminary studies have suggested that this may indeed be the case. Most patients with inherited distal RTA have associated hypercalciuria and hypocitraturia that predispose to nephrocalcinosis and bone disease.[80]

The features of autosomal recessive distal RTA include severe metabolic acidosis, an inappropriately alkaline urine, growth failure, rickets, and renal calcification. This constellation of findings may occur with or without sensorineural deafness. Progressive bilateral sensorineural hearing loss (SNHL) occurs with mutations in *ATP6B1*, encoding the B-subunit of the collecting duct apical electrogenic proton pump ($H^+$-ATPase) and the $H^+$-ATPase in the cochlea.[70] In patients with normal hearing and autosomal recessive distal RTA (rd RTA2), studies have demonstrated linkage to another region of 7q33-34 in a 14-cM region flanked by D7S500 and D7S688.[69] Thus, two separate genes cause autosomal recessive distal RTA with normal and impaired hearing.

Carbonic anhydrase II deficiency results in an autosomal recessive syndrome characterized by osteopetrosis, RTA, and cerebral calcifications.[21, 22] Whereas the type of RTA has not been clearly delineated, patients exhibit frank bicarbonate wasting that is consistent with proximal tubular dysfunction and an inability to acidify the urine during a sustained systemic acidosis. Therefore, inherited defects of the $HCO_3^-$-$Cl^-$ exchanger, the $H^+$-ATPase, and carbonic anhydrase II are clearly associated with various forms of inherited distal RTA. Association, in some cases with the $H^+$,$K^+$-ATPase, while possible, have not been proved by linkage analysis.

## ENDEMIC DISTAL RENAL TUBULAR ACIDOSIS

A high incidence of distal RTA has been reported in northeast Thailand.[82, 83] This disorder has a female-to-male ratio of 3:1 and ranges in age from 18 to 76 years of age. Associated features include severe hypokalemia resulting in profound muscle weakness, nephrocalcinosis, renal stones, hypocitraturia, osteomalacia, and nocturia. The hypokalemia and the accompanying features are more severe in the summer and are most prevalent in impoverished groups whose diet consists almost entirely of rice. Therefore, dietary hypokalemia may be causative. Although the precise mechanism involved remains unclear, chronic tubulointerstitial renal disease as a result of chronic hypokalemia appears to be a better explanation than vanadate toxicity, which was initially suggested.[71, 84]

## SECONDARY DISTAL RENAL TUBULAR ACIDOSIS

The disorders associated with acquired classical distal RTA are outlined in Table 11–5. Hyperglobulinemia is commonly associated with acquired classical distal RTA. Up to 50% of patients with Sjögren syndrome and hyperglobulinemic purpura eventually exhibit an acidification defect.[85, 86] These patients may sometimes have profound hypokalemia. Other autoimmune and hyperglobulinemic states that are associated with distal RTA include cryoglobulinemia, thyroiditis, Graves' disease, primary biliary cirrhosis, chronic active hepatitis, systemic lupus erythematosus, and human immunodeficiency virus (HIV) nephropathy.[87–90]

Abnormalities in calcium homeostasis, particularly when nephrocalcinosis is present, are commonly seen in patients with acquired distal RTA. Examples of the co-occurrence of distal RTA and nephrocalcinosis include: primary hyperparathyroidism, vitamin D intoxication, hyperthyroidism, idiopathic hypercalciuria, medullary sponge kidney, X-linked hypophosphatemia, and type 1 glycogen storage disease.[91–98]

Distal RTA can also be caused by various drugs or toxins. Examples include amphotericin B,[99–102] lithium carbonate,[103] toluene,[104, 105] analgesics,[106, 107] ifosfamide, foscarnet,[108] and vanadate.[71] Distal RTA occurs in the chronic rejection of renal transplantation.[109–112] Distal RTA with renal transplantation is attributed to defective ammonium excretion and generalized distal tubular malfunction.[111] Renal tubulointerstitial disease can be associated with distal RTA. Prominent examples include hyperoxaluria,[113] obstructive uropathy,[114] vesicoureteral reflux,[115] lupus nephritis, leprosy, and pyelonephritis with nephrolithiasis.[116] Distal RTA is also associated with a variety of inherited disorders not discussed earlier, including Ehlers-Danlos syndrome, hereditary elliptocytosis, hereditary spherocytosis, sickle cell disease, medullary cystic disease, type I glycogen storage disease, and carnitine palmitoyltransferase I deficiency.[22, 93, 117–120]

## Treatment of Classical Distal Renal Tubular Acidosis

The primary therapeutic objective in patients with classical distal RTA is to correct chronic metabolic acidosis. This can be achieved by administration of alkali in an amount sufficient to neutralize the daily acid load or approximately 1 to 3 mEq/kg/day. The various forms of alkali replacement are displayed in Table 11–3. Shohl solution is more readily tolerated than $NaHCO_3$ tablets (325 or 650 mg or 3.9 and 7.8 mEq/tablet, respectively). Compliance is often limited by taste fatigue with Shohl solution and GI discomfort with $NaHCO_3$ tablets. Correction of the acidosis reduces urinary potassium and sodium excretion, thus decreasing the need for potassium supplementation.[121–123] If required, potassium can be administered as potassium bicarbonate (K-Lyte 25 or 50 mEq), potassium citrate (Urocit-K), or Polycitra (K-Shohl).

Rarely, patients present with flaccid paralysis due to severe hypokalemia, metabolic acidosis, and hypocalcemia requiring immediate therapy. Because hypokalemia may result in respiratory depression, increasing systemic pH with alkali therapy may worsen the hypokalemia. Therefore, immediate intravenous potassium replacement should be achieved before alkali administration.

### PROGNOSIS

The goal of alkali therapy in distal RTA is to prevent the relentless progression of renal disease. The GFR should be expected to stabilize with normalization of the serum bicarbonate (into the range of 22 to 24 mEq/L). This requires modest amounts (1 to 3 mEq/kg/day) of alkali therapy. Hypercalciuria usually subsides when the acidosis is corrected and urinary citrate excretion increases, thus reducing the incidence of urolithiasis. Similarly, nephrocalcinosis may subside over many years. Potassium homeostasis improves or normalizes in most adult patients, and the renal phosphate clearance also improves. In children, growth is usually restored. Therefore, most, if not all, of the accompanying abnormalities are corrected with sustained correction of the serum bicarbonate.

# RENAL TUBULAR ACIDOSIS ASSOCIATED WITH HYPERKALEMIA: GENERALIZED DISTAL NEPHRON DYSFUNCTION

## Pathophysiology of Voltage Defect

When a decrease in the negative transepithelial potential difference in the collecting tubule impairs proton secretion in this segment, it is referred to as "voltage defect." Any process that inhibits sodium transport in the CCT would be expected to cause such a defect because translocation of the cation $Na^+$ from the lumen to the interstitium is the main determinant of transepithelial voltage in the CCT. A decrease in negative voltage decreases the electrical gradient $K^+$ and $H^+$ secretion by the CCT. The traditional model of such a transport defect is that observed after amiloride administration. Amiloride occupies the ENaC on the apical membrane of the CCT inhibiting sodium transport, decreasing negative transepithelial voltage, and secondarily inhibiting both $K^+$ and $H^+$ secretion (in the principal and type A intercalated cells, respectively). Therefore, with a "voltage" lesion, both hyperkalemia and metabolic acidosis may develop. It is now appreciated that the mechanism for the generation of acidosis and hyperkalemia in patients receiving trimethoprim and pentamidine is identical to that observed with amiloride.[56] Point mutations in the ENaC have been shown to cause autosomal recessive pseudohypoaldosteronism type 1 (PHA I).[124] This defect in ENaC impairs $Na^+$ absorption, reduces transepithelial voltage, and subsequently impairs $K^+$ and $H^+$ transport. Therefore, autosomal recessive PHA I represents an example of an inherited "voltage" defect.

## Role of Aldosterone Deficiency in Generation of Hyperkalemic Acidosis

Aldosterone enhances the lumen negative transepithelial potential difference in the CCT through upregulation of $Na^+$ absorption. Initially, aldosterone upregulates ENaC (and subsequently the basolateral $Na^+,K^+$-ATPase) to stimulate $Na^+$ absorption, $K^+$ secretion, and $H^+$ secretion. Therefore, it is not surprising that a deficiency in aldosterone would result in the development of hyperkalemia and metabolic acidosis.[125] In contrast to the CCT, aldosterone stimulates potassium and hydrogen ion secretion in the medullary collecting tubule independently of sodium transport.[43, 61, 125] Therefore, a relative decrease in the amount of aldosterone, or decrease in responsiveness of the collecting tubule to aldosterone, could result in a reduction in distal sodium absorption. Such a reduction would be expected to impair both potassium and hydrogen ion secretion. Aldosterone also plays a significant role in ammonium absorption and excretion by the IMCD.[60] In the rat, selective aldosterone deficiency has been reported to be associated with impaired ammonium excretion and reduced papillary $P_{CO_2}$ during bicarbonate loading, thus verifying a defect in proton secretion. Both of these processes lead to a decrease in proton secretion, which favors the development of metabolic acidosis. The importance of mineralocorticoids in the regulation of NAE has been documented in mineralocorticoid-deficient animals and humans.[126, 127] In patients who have undergone an adrenalectomy, NAE and plasma total $CO_2$ decline if a mineralocorticoid is selectively discontinued but increase with the reinitiation of the mineralocorticoid.[126, 128] The change in plasma total $CO_2$ correlated directly, in these studies, with changes in ammonium excretion and inversely with corresponding changes in potassium balance.

## Role of Hyperkalemia in the Generation of Hyperchloremic Metabolic Acidosis

Hyperkalemia has an independent effect on NAE through inhibition of renal ammoniagenesis. Hyperkalemia is associated, in addition, with a decrease in ammonium transport and, thus, excretion. This contributes significantly to the development of metabolic acidosis.[63, 129] DuBose and associates have shown that hyperkalemia decreases ammonium excretion and production in the proximal tubule.[52, 60] Hyperkalemia greatly impaired ammonium absorption in the thick ascending limb, reducing inner medullary concentrations of total $NH_3$ and decreasing secretion of $NH_3$ into the IMCD.[49, 51, 52, 63] The mechanism for impaired absorption of $NH_4^+$ in the medullary thick ascending limb of the loop of Henle is competition between $K^+$ and $NH_4^+$ for the $K^+$ secretory site on the $Na^+$-$2Cl^-$-$K^+$ transporter. The importance of hyperkalemia as a cause of metabolic acidosis is underscored by the observation that correction of hyperkalemia is associated with a significant increase in NAE and a parallel correction of the acidosis.

## Clinical Examples of Voltage Defects and Mineralocorticoid Deficiency and Resistance

Hyperkalemic hyperchloremic metabolic acidosis can occur as a result of one of three abnormalities: (1) deficiency of mineralocorticoid, (2) resistance to mineralocorticoid, or (3) renal tubular dysfunction. The causes of voltage defects (tubular dysfunction) and deficiency or resistance to mineralocorticoid are outlined in Table 11–6. Mineralocorticoid deficiency may occur in concert with general adrenal failure (Addison disease) when a decrease in elaboration of both glucocorticoid and mineralocorticoid occurs. Addison disease can be caused by destruction of the adrenal cortex with hemorrhage, infection, invasion by tumors, or autoimmune disease. Patients have hypoglycemia, anorexia, weakness, hyperpigmentation, relative or frank hypotension, and a failure to respond to stress.

**TABLE 11–6.** Generalized Abnormality of Distal Nephron with Hyperkalemia

**Mineralocorticoid Deficiency**

***Primary Mineralocorticoid Deficiency***

- Combined deficiency of aldosterone, deoxycorticosterone, and cortisol
  - Addison disease
  - Bilateral adrenalectomy
  - Bilateral adrenal destruction
    - Hemorrhage or carcinoma
- Congenital enzymatic defects
  - 21-Hydroxylase deficiency
  - 3β-Hydroxydehydrogenase deficiency
  - Desmolase deficiency
- Isolated (selective) aldosterone deficiency
  - Chronic idiopathic hypoaldosteronism
  - Heparin in the critically ill patient
  - Familial hypoaldosteronism
    - Corticosterone methyloxidase deficiency, types 1 and 2
  - Primary zona glomerulosa defect
  - Transient hypoaldosteronism of infancy
  - Persistent hypotension and/or hypoxemia in critically ill patient
- Angiotensin II–converting enzyme inhibition
  - Endogenous
  - Angiotensin-converting enzyme inhibitors and $AT_1$ receptor antagonists

***Secondary Mineralocorticoid Deficiency***

- Hyporeninemic hypoaldosteronism
  - Diabetic nephropathy
  - Tubulointerstitial nephropathies
  - Nephrosclerosis
  - Nonsteroidal anti-inflammatory agents
  - Acquired immunodeficiency syndrome
  - IgM monoclonal gammopathy

**Mineralocorticoid Resistance**

- Pseudohypoaldosteronism type I (PHA I)—autosomal dominant

**Renal Tubular Dysfunction (Voltage Defect)**

- Pseudohypoaldosteronism type I (PHA I)—autosomal recessive
- Pseudohypoaldosteronism type II (PHA II)—autosomal recessive
- Drugs that interfere with $Na^+$ channel function in CCT
  - Amiloride
  - Triamterene
  - Trimethoprim
  - Pentamidine
- Drugs that interfere with $Na^+$,$K^+$-ATPase in CCT
  - Cyclosporin A
- Drugs that inhibit aldosterone effect on CCT
  - Spironolactone
- Disorders associated with tubulointerstitial nephritis and renal insufficiency
  - Lupus nephritis
  - Methicillin nephrotoxicity
  - Obstructive nephropathy
  - Kidney transplant rejection
  - Sickle cell disease
  - Williams syndrome with uric acid nephrolithiasis

CCT, cortical collecting tubule.

Renal salt wasting, hyponatremia, hyperkalemia, and metabolic acidosis coexist.[130, 131] Typically, serum aldosterone levels are low and the plasma renin level is high. Metabolic acidosis occurs because of a decrease in $H^+$ secretion in the collecting tubule from decreased $H^+$-ATPase number and function. Hyperkalemia further aggravates the acidosis by depression of ammonium production and excretion.

Selective or isolated hypoaldosteronism can occur in critically ill patients, particularly in the setting of sepsis or cardiogenic shock.[132] Heparin, often administered in this setting, impairs aldosterone synthesis as a result of direct toxicity to the zona glomerulosa with direct inhibition of the enzyme aldosterone synthase.[133] Moreover, hypoxia and cytokines may contribute to aldosterone synthesis failure in the critically ill patient.[132, 134]

One of the best examples of resistance to mineralocorticoid is autosomal dominant PHA I. This disorder, which is clinically less severe than autosomal recessive PHA I (discussed later), is associated with hyperkalemia, renal salt wasting, metabolic acidosis, elevated renin and aldosterone levels, and hypotension. The autosomal dominant disorder has been shown to be the result of a mutation in the intracellular mineralocorticoid receptor in the collecting tubule.[124] Unlike the autosomal recessive disorder, this defect is not expressed in organs other than the kidney and becomes less severe with advancing age. Carbenoxolone raises the intracellular concentration of cortisol, thus overcoming the functional defect in the mutant receptor and improving mineralocorticoid resistance. Because the decrease in mineralocorticoid reduces apical $Na^+$ absorption and activity of ENaC, transepithelial potential difference declines and $K^+$ secretion is impaired.[135]

The prototype for a "voltage" defect is autosomal recessive PHA I. This disorder is the result of a loss of function point mutation of the gene, which encodes the ENaC on the apical membrane of the CCT.[136–138] Children with this disorder have severe hyperkalemia and renal salt wasting because of a functional block of ENaC. In addition, the hyperchloremic metabolic acidosis may be severe and is associated with hypotension and marked elevations of plasma renin and aldosterone. These children also manifest vomiting, hyponatremia, failure to thrive, and respiratory distress. The latter is due to involvement of ENaC in the alveoli, preventing $Na^+$ and water absorption in the lungs. Patients with this disease respond to a high salt intake and correction of the hyperkalemia. Unlike the autosomal dominant form, autosomal recessive PHA I persists throughout life.

Another "voltage defect," but with unknown pathogenesis, is pseudohypoaldosteronism type II (PHA II) or Gordon syndrome. This disorder, which occurs in adults, results in hyperkalemia, hyperchloremic metabolic acidosis, hypertension, mild volume expansion, and suppressed renin and aldosterone levels.[135, 139, 140] These patients typically respond to thiazide diuretics, suggesting a disorder of the distal tubule $Na^+$-$Cl^-$ cotransporter.[141, 142] Nevertheless, linkage analysis has not supported this relationship, and the etiology is unknown at present. Genetic analysis of these patients has revealed linkage to chromosomes 1q31-42 and 17p11-q21 (see Table 11–4). The response of these patients to $Na_2SO_4$ infusion validates the presence of a voltage defect, perhaps as a result of preferential absorption ("shunting") of chloride in the distal tubule.

In addition to inherited voltage defects, there are examples of acquired voltage defects due to drugs or tubulointerstitial disease.[143, 144] Examples of the former include amiloride and the structurally related compounds trimethoprim and pentamidine. As discussed earlier, this explains the occurrence of hyperkalemic-hyperchloremic acidosis in patients who receive higher doses of these agents. Trimethoprim and pentamidine occupy the $Na^+$ channel as does amiloride and cause hyperkalemia, which contributes to the acidosis.[145–147] Spironolactone and triamterene are more likely to cause hyperkalemia in patients with renal insufficiency or hyporeninemic hypoaldosteronism.[148–150] Those tubulointerstitial diseases, which may be associated with impairment or destruction of collecting duct function, includes obstructive uropathy, lupus nephritis, sickle cell nephropathy, analgesic nephropathy, and multiple myeloma.[112, 143, 151, 152]

## Hyporeninemic-Hypoaldosteronism

The pathogenesis of the metabolic acidosis in hyporeninemic-hypoaldosteronism is complex and multifactorial. Proximal $HCO_3^-$ absorption has been shown to be mildly decreased in the presence of normal plasma $HCO_3^-$ concentrations. The ability to acidify the urine during metabolic acidosis is intact, but typically a reduced rate of NAE and ammonium excretion occurs. In contrast to selective hypoaldosteronism, levels of aldosterone are reduced but can respond to ACTH and angiotensin II.[153] The GFR is typically low, unlike PHA I or PHA II.

In hyporeninemic-hypoaldosteronism both the metabolic acidosis and the hyperkalemia are out of proportion to the level of reduction in GFR. Many patients have congestive heart failure, diabetic nephropathy, or tubulointerstitial renal disease, cardiac arrhythmias, and hypertension. Ammonium excretion is impaired because of hyperkalemia and improves with correction to a normal potassium. Many of these patients have progressive renal disease and with end-stage renal disease develop the typical high anion gap acidosis of renal failure.

## Identification and Treatment of Generalized Defect

The first priority in the treatment of hyperkalemic hyperchloremic metabolic acidosis is to identify the underlying disorder. To this end, a careful dietary and drug history is critical and can identify unsuspected sources of exogenous $K^+$ intake. It is also important

**TABLE 11–7.** Treatment of Generalized Dysfunction of the Nephron with Hyperkalemia

Alkali therapy
Loop diuretic (furosemide, bumetanide)
Sodium polystyrene sulfonate (Kayexalate)
Fludrocortisone (0.1–0.3 mg/day)
  Avoid in hypertension, volume expansion, heart failure
  Combine with loop diuretic
Avoid drugs associated with hyperkalemia
In pseudohypoaldosteronism type I—add NaCl supplement

to identify contributing or precipitating factors that include: low urine flow, decreased distal $Na^+$ delivery, acute renal failure, hyperglycemia, and hyperosmolality. Treatment is summarized in Table 11–7. The workup should consist of an evaluation of $K^+$ excretion by the transtubular $K^+$ gradient or the fractional excretion of $K^+$, an estimate of renal ammonium excretion (UAG), urine pH, the U-B $P_{CO_2}$, and an evaluation of plasma renin activity and aldosterone secretion (Table 11–8). Aldosterone secretion, if evaluated, should be obtained under stimulated conditions with dietary salt restriction and furosemide-induced volume depletion. Drugs associated with hyperkalemia, such as triamterene, spironolactone, amiloride, pentamidine, trimethoprim, nonsteroidal anti-inflammatory drugs, angiotensin-converting enzyme-I, or $K^+$ supplements, should be discontinued. Salt substitutes and herbal preparations should be avoided, and a diet low in $K^+$ should be emphasized.

The severity of the hyperkalemia is the primary determinant in the decision to treat patients with this disorder. Patients with combined glucocorticoid and mineralocorticoid deficiency should receive both steroids in replacement dosages. Mineralocorticoids should be avoided in the face of hypertension or congestive heart failure. If supraphysiologic doses of mineralocorticoids are needed, patients should be monitored closely for volume overexpansion, hypertension, and hypokalemia. If the serum potassium level is reduced effectively with either cation-exchange resin or loop diuretics, the result will often be an improvement in the metabolic acidosis by increasing ammonium excretion. Volume depletion should be avoided unless the patient is volume overexpanded or hypertensive. Children with PHA I should receive a NaCl supplement; adults with PHA II should be treated with thiazide diuretics. In summary, because hyperkalemia interferes with the kidney's response to metabolic acidosis, treatment consists of correction of hyperkalemia, restoration of euvolemia, alkali therapy, loop diuretics, and dietary potassium restriction. In severe hypoaldosteronism, the effect of loop diuretics can be enhanced by the addition of replacement mineralocorticoids.

## A STEPWISE APPROACH TO THE DIAGNOSIS OF RENAL TUBULAR ACIDOSIS

### Overview

A defect in urinary acidification should be suspected in any patient with chronic hyperchloremic metabolic acidosis that cannot be attributed to GI bicarbonate loss. The diagnostic studies that distinguish the various causes of RTA are summarized in Table 11–8. A positive urine net charge or anion gap in the presence of metabolic acidosis represents inappropriately low urinary ammonium excretion and strongly suggests a renal tubular origin or RTA. The serum potassium may provide a clue to the type of defect. Patients with either classical distal RTA or proximal RTA usually have hypokalemia, whereas patients with generalized dysfunction of the distal nephron due to aldosterone deficiency or resistance usually have hyperkalemia. A urine pH of less than 5.5 in the presence of spontaneous metabolic acidosis, or after an ammonium chloride challenge, suggests a proximal tubular defect or a generalized defect in the distal nephron with associated hyperkalemia and reduced ammoniagenesis. A urine pH above 5.5 usually denotes a defect in distal nephron $H^+$ ion secretion, which can be further examined by evaluating the U-B $P_{CO_2}$ during bicarbonate infusion. Generalized distal nephron

**TABLE 11–8.** Diagnostic Studies in Renal Tubular Acidosis

| | Type of RTA | | |
|---|---|---|---|
| **Finding** | ***Proximal (II)*** | ***Classical Distal I*** | ***Generalized Distal Dysfunction (IV)*** |
| Plasma $[K^+]$ | Low | Low | High |
| Urine pH with acidosis | <5.5 | >5.5 | <5.5 or >5.5 |
| Urine net charge | | | Positive |
| Fanconi lesion | Positive | Positive | Absent |
| Fractional bicarbonate excretion | Present | Absent | <5–10% |
| | >10–15% | <5% | |
| U-B $P_{CO_2}$ | Normal | Low* | Low |
| Response to therapy | Least readily | Readily | Less readily |
| Associated features | Fanconi syndrome | Nephrocalcinosis/hyperglobulinemia | Renal insufficiency |

*Except with amphotericin B.
RTA, renal tubular acidosis.

dysfunction is associated with the low U-B $P_{CO_2}$, whereas in proximal RTA the U-B $P_{CO_2}$ is normal. Hyperkalemia in association with a low U-B $P_{CO_2}$ and an inappropriately low transtubular $K^+$ gradient or $FE_K\%$ suggests simultaneous defects in hydrogen ion and potassium secretion. This combination is seen with a generalized defect in CCT function or with mineralocorticoid deficiency or resistance. Response to alkali therapy may help elucidate the diagnosis of RTA. Proximal RTA is particularly difficult to correct, whereas classical hypokalemic distal RTA responds readily to bicarbonate administration. Finally, accompanying features of the disorder help categorize the general type of lesion. Fanconi syndrome is associated with proximal RTA, nephrocalcinosis, and nephrolithiasis with classical hypokalemic distal RTA. Diabetic nephropathy, obstructive uropathy, and tubulointerstitial disease are associated with a generalized dysfunction of the distal nephron that is associated with hyperkalemia.

## Detailed Description of Tests of Urinary Acidification

The paradigms for each of those studies described earlier are summarized later in more detail and are displayed in Table 11–8.

### URINARY ANION GAP AND AMMONIUM EXCRETION

All forms of RTA are associated with an inappropriately low excretion of ammonium. Urinary ammonium excretion can be estimated on a spot urine specimen by measuring the urinary net charge or UAG.[1, 2, 154] This approach is described at the beginning of this chapter.

### MINIMAL URINE pH AND MAXIMAL ACID EXCRETION

The measurement of urine pH is the most common first step in accessing the ability to acidify the urine. The urine pH should be below 5.5 and is usually below 5.0 in the presence of metabolic acidosis. A urine pH consistently above 5.5 in the presence of systemic acidosis implies that an acidification defect involving the more distal portions of the nephron exists. However, caution is urged because the urine pH is not always a reliable means of distinguishing renal from nonrenal hyperchloremic acidosis. A urine pH below 5.5 is also seen in patients with proximal RTA when systemic acidosis is present and the filtered load of bicarbonate is low (i.e., <15 mEq/L).[121] The explanation for this finding is that when the distal nephron is not impaired, reduced filtered loads of $HCO_3^-$ can be absorbed in the more distal segments, thus limiting $HCO_3^-$ delivery into the final urine. A urine pH below 5.5 is also characteristic of patients with selective aldosterone deficiency. In this disorder, low urinary buffer excretion allows the urine pH to become acidic. Taken together, these findings emphasize that although urine pH is the most commonly used test of renal acidification, it does not measure hydrogen ion excretion. Patients with chronic metabolic acidosis and normal renal function (as seen with chronic diarrhea) may have a higher urine pH as a result of excretion of large quantities of ammonium and other urinary buffers. A low urine pH, therefore, does not ensure that the proton secretory mechanism is either intact or appropriate for the level of acidosis, and a high urine pH does not prove an abnormality in acidification.

If the urine pH is measured promptly on freshly voided "first morning" urine, it is not necessary to collect urine under mineral oil.[155] In the presence of systemic acidosis, there is no need to perform an ammonium chloride loading test. If systemic acidosis is not present at the time of the study, ammonium chloride powder (not enteric coated) may be given as a single oral dose of 0.1 g/kg in gelatin capsules along with food, followed by hourly determinations of urine pH for 2 to 8 hours. The total $CO_2$ concentration in plasma should decrease by at least 3 to 5 mEq/L, and the urine pH should fall below 5.5.

### U-B $P_{CO_2}$

The increment in urinary $P_{CO_2}$ during sodium bicarbonate ($NaHCO_3$) infusion or oral $NaHCO_3$ administration in amounts that result in excretion of a highly alkaline urine is a reliable and sensitive index of proton secretion by the distal nephron.[32, 66, 68, 156] After $NaHCO_3$ loading, the urine $P_{CO_2}$ is expected to reach a value approximately 25 mm Hg higher than systemic arterial blood levels. The test is performed by infusing a solution that contains 500 mEq $NaHCO_3$ at a rate of 3 mL/min into a peripheral vein. Timed urine collections of approximately 15 to 30 minutes' duration are obtained by having the patient void spontaneously while in the upright position. The test may be terminated after completion of at least three clearance periods when the urine pH is consistently 7.5 or greater. A steady state is usually achieved within 180 to 260 minutes after initiation of the $NaHCO_3$ infusion. Urine should always be collected under mineral oil for measurement of urine $P_{CO_2}$ and pH. This test may also be performed by administration of acetazolamide, thus avoiding problems inherent with $NaHCO_3$ loading.[157] However, $HCO_3^-$ should be given orally (two 650-mg tablets tid) for 2 days before the administration of acetazolamide 250 mg po to ensure the presence of sufficient bicarbonate in the urine. Patients with decreased rates of distal hydrogen secretion are expected to display subnormal values with high $HCO_3^-$ excretion, because the U-B $P_{CO_2}$ gradient is less than 10 to 15 mm Hg.[68, 156] In contrast, patients with a gradient or "backleak" defect retain the ability to generate high urinary $CO_2$ tensions during $NaHCO_3$ loading.[66, 158–161]

## REFERENCES

1. Halperin ML, et al: Distal renal tubular acidosis syndromes: A pathophysiological approach. Am J Nephrol 5(1):1–8, 1985.

2. Goldstein MB, et al: The urine anion gap: A clinically useful index of ammonium excretion. Am J Med Sci 292(4):198–202, 1986.
3. Kleinman PK: Cholestyramine and metabolic acidosis [Letter]. N Engl J Med 290(15):861, 1974.
4. Heird WC, et al: Metabolic acidosis resulting from intravenous alimentation mixtures containing synthetic amino acids. N Engl J Med 287(19):943–948, 1972.
5. Widmer B, et al: Serum electrolyte and acid base composition. The influence of graded degrees of chronic renal failure. Arch Intern Med 139(10):1099–1102, 1979.
6. Vieira FL, Malnic G: Hydrogen ion secretion by rat renal cortical tubules as studied by an antimony microelectrode. Am J Physiol 214(4):710–718, 1968.
7. Alpern RJ, Chambers M: Cell pH in the rat proximal convoluted tubule: Regulation by luminal and peritubular pH and sodium concentration. J Clin Invest 78(2):502–510, 1986.
8. Kinsella JL, Aronson PS: Properties of the $Na^+$-$H^+$ exchanger in renal microvillus membrane vesicles. Am J Physiol 238(6): F461–F469, 1980.
9. Murer H, Hopfer U, Kinne R: Sodium/proton antiport in brush-border-membrane vesicles isolated from rat small intestine and kidney. Biochem J 154(3):597–604, 1976.
10. Sasaki S, Shigai T, Takeuchi J: Intracellular pH in the isolated perfused rabbit proximal straight tubule. Am J Physiol 249(3 Pt 2):F417–F423, 1985.
11. Schwartz GJ: $Na^+$-dependent $H^+$ efflux from proximal tubule: Evidence for reversible $Na^+$-$H^+$ exchange. Am J Physiol 241(4): F380–F385, 1981.
12. Warnock DG, Reenstra WW, Yee VJ: $Na^+/H^+$ antiporter of brush border vesicles: Studies with acridine orange uptake. Am J Physiol 242(6):F733–F739, 1982.
13. Pajor AM: Sequence and functional characterization of a renal sodium/dicarboxylate cotransporter. J Biol Chem 270(11):5779–5785, 1995.
14. Al-Bander HA, et al: Dysfunction of the proximal tubule underlies maleic acid-induced type II renal tubular acidosis. Am J Physiol 243(6):F604–F611, 1982.
15. Coor C, et al: Role of adenosine triphosphate (ATP) and $Na^+K^+$-ATPase in the inhibition of proximal tubule transport with intracellular cystine loading. J Clin Invest 87(3):955–961, 1991.
16. Burch HB, et al: Metabolic effects of large fructose loads in different parts of the rat nephron. J Biol Chem 255(17):8239–8244, 1980.
17. Bank N, Aynediian HS: A micropuncture study of the effect of parathyroid hormone on renal bicarbonate reabsorption. J Clin Invest 58(2):336–344, 1976.
18. Iino Y, Burg MB: Effect of parathyroid hormone on bicarbonate absorption by proximal tubules in vitro. Am J Physiol 236(4):F387–F391, 1979.
19. Chan YL, Kurtzman NA: Effects of lysine on bicarbonate and fluid absorption in the rat proximal tubule. Am J Physiol 242(6):F604–F609, 1982.
20. Schultheis PJ, et al: Targeted disruption of the murine $Na^+$-$H^+$ exchanger isoform 2 gene causes reduced viability of gastric parietal cells and loss of net acid secretion. J Clin Invest 101(6): 1243–1253, 1998.
21. Sly WS, et al: Carbonic anhydrase II deficiency identified as the primary defect in the autosomal recessive syndrome of osteopetrosis with renal tubular acidosis and cerebral calcification. Proc Natl Acad Sci U S A 80(9):2752–2756, 1983.
22. Sly WS, et al: Carbonic anhydrase II deficiency in 12 families with the autosomal recessive syndrome of osteopetrosis with renal tubular acidosis and cerebral calcification. N Engl J Med 313(3):139–145, 1985.
23. Sebastian A, McSherry E, Morris RC Jr: On the mechanism of renal potassium wasting in renal tubular acidosis associated with the Fanconi syndrome (type 2 RTA). J Clin Invest 50(1): 231–243, 1971.
24. Iacovitti M, et al: Distal tubule bicarbonate accumulation in vivo: Effect of flow and transtubular bicarbonate gradients. J Clin Invest 78(6):1658–1665, 1986.
25. Levine DZ: An in vivo microperfusion study of distal tubule bicarbonate reabsorption in normal and ammonium chloride rats. J Clin Invest 75(2):588–595, 1985.
26. Lucci MS, et al: Evaluation of bicarbonate transport in rat distal tubule: Effects of acid-base status. Am J Physiol 243(4): F335–F341, 1982.
27. Schwartz GJ, Barasch J, Al-Awqati Q: Plasticity of functional epithelial polarity. Nature 318(6044):368–371, 1985.
28. Lombard WE, Kokko JP, Jacobson HR: Bicarbonate transport in cortical and outer medullary collecting tubules. Am J Physiol 244(3):F289–F296, 1983.
29. Peraino RA, Suki WN: Urine $HCO_3^-$ augments renal $Ca^{2+}$ absorption independent of systemic acid-base changes. Am J Physiol 238(5):F394–F398, 1980.
30. Stokes JB: Na and K transport across the cortical and outer medullary collecting tubule of the rabbit: Evidence for diffusion across the outer medullary portion. Am J Physiol 242(5): F514–F520, 1982.
31. Graber ML, et al: pH and $PCO_2$ profiles of the rat inner medullary collecting duct. Am J Physiol 241(6):F659–F668, 1981.
32. DuBose TD Jr: Hydrogen ion secretion by the collecting duct as a determinant of the urine to blood $PCO_2$ gradient in alkaline urine. J Clin Invest 69(1):145–156, 1982.
33. DuBose TD Jr, Pucacco LR, Carter NW: Determination of disequilibrium pH in the rat kidney in vivo: Evidence of hydrogen secretion. Am J Physiol 240(2):F138–F146, 1981.
34. Koeppen BM, Helman SI: Acidification of luminal fluid by the rabbit cortical collecting tubule perfused in vitro. Am J Physiol 242(5):F521–F531, 1982.
35. McKinney TD, Burg MB: Bicarbonate absorption by rabbit cortical collecting tubules in vitro. Am J Physiol 234(2):F141–F145, 1978.
36. Stone DK, Xie XS: Proton translocating ATPases: Issues in structure and function. Kidney Int 33(4):767–774, 1988.
37. Kaunitz JD, Gunther RD, Sachs G: Characterization of an electrogenic ATP and chloride-dependent proton translocating pump from rat renal medulla. J Biol Chem 260(21):11567–11573, 1985.
38. Wingo CS, et al: $H^+,K^+$-ATPase immunoreactivity in cortical and outer medullary collecting duct. Kidney Int 38(5):985–990, 1990.
39. DuBose TD Jr, et al: Regulation of $H^+,K^+$-ATPase expression in kidney. Am J Physiol 269(4 Pt 2):F500–F507, 1995.
40. Wall SM: $NH_4^+$ augments net acid secretion by a ouabain-sensitive mechanism in isolated perfused inner medullary collecting ducts. Am J Physiol 270(3 Pt 2):F432–F439, 1996.
41. Fischer JL, Husted RF, Steinmetz PR: Chloride dependence of the $HCO_3^-$ exit step in urinary acidification by the turtle bladder. Am J Physiol 245(5 Pt 1):F564–F568, 1983.
42. Schuster VL, Bonsib SM, Jennings ML: Two types of collecting duct mitochondria-rich (intercalated) cells: Lectin and band 3 cytochemistry. Am J Physiol 251(3 Pt 1):C347–C355, 1986.
43. Stone DK, et al: Anion dependence of rabbit medullary collecting duct acidification. J Clin Invest 71(5):1505-1508, 1983.
44. Karet FE, et al: Mutations in the chloride-bicarbonate exchanger gene AE1 cause autosomal dominant but not autosomal recessive distal renal tubular acidosis. Proc Natl Acad Sci U S A 95(11):6337–6342, 1998.
45. Good DW, Knepper MA, Burg MB: Ammonia and bicarbonate transport by thick ascending limb of rat kidney. Am J Physiol 247(1 Pt 2):F35–F44, 1984.
46. Buerkert J, Martin D, Trigg D: Segmental analysis of the renal tubule in buffer production and net acid formation. Am J Physiol 244(4):F442–F454, 1983.
47. DuBose TD Jr, et al: Comparison of acidification parameters in superficial and deep nephrons of the rat. Am J Physiol 244(5): F497–F503, 1983.
48. Good DW, Caflisch CR, DuBose TD Jr: Transepithelial ammonia concentration gradients in inner medulla of the rat. Am J Physiol 252(3 Pt 2):F491–F500, 1987.
49. DuBose TD Jr, Good DW: Chronic hyperkalemia impairs ammonium transport and accumulation in the inner medulla of the rat. J Clin Invest 90(4):1443–1449, 1992.
50. Nagami GT, Sonu CM, Kurokawa K: Ammonia production by isolated mouse proximal tubules perfused in vitro: Effect of metabolic acidosis. J Clin Invest 78(1):124–129, 1986.
51. DuBose TD Jr, Good DW: Effects of chronic hyperkalemia on renal production and proximal tubule transport of ammonium in rats. Am J Physiol 260(5 Pt 2):F680–F687, 1991.

52. Tannen RL, McGill J: Influence of potassium on renal ammonia production. Am J Physiol 231(4):1178–1184, 1976.
53. Kurtz I, et al: Spontaneous luminal disequilibrium pH in S3 proximal tubules: Role in ammonia and bicarbonate transport. J Clin Invest 78(4):989–996, 1986.
54. Steinmetz PR, Lawson LR: Effect of luminal pH on ion permeability and flows of $Na^+$ and $H^+$ in turtle bladder. Am J Physiol 220(6):1573–1580, 1971.
55. Knepper MA, Good DW, Burg MB: Mechanism of ammonia secretion by cortical collecting ducts of rabbits. Am J Physiol 247(5 Pt 2):F729–F738, 1984.
56. DuBose TD Jr: Hyperkalemic hyperchloremic metabolic acidosis: Pathophysiologic insights. Kidney Int 51(2):591–602, 1997.
57. Laski ME, Kurtzman NA: Characterization of acidification in the cortical and medullary collecting tubule of the rabbit. J Clin Invest 72(6):2050–2059, 1983.
58. O'Neil RG, Helman SI: Transport characteristics of renal collecting tubules: Influences of DOCA and diet. Am J Physiol 233(6):F544–F558, 1977.
59. Schwartz GJ, Burg MB: Mineralocorticoid effects on cation transport by cortical collecting tubules in vitro. Am J Physiol 235(6):F576–F585, 1978.
60. DuBose TD Jr, Caflisch CR: Effect of selective aldosterone deficiency on acidification in nephron segments of the rat inner medulla. J Clin Invest 82(5):1624–1632, 1988.
61. Stone DK, et al: Mineralocorticoid modulation of rabbit medullary collecting duct acidification: A sodium-independent effect. J Clin Invest 72(1):77–83, 1983.
62. McKinney TD, Davidson KK: Effect of potassium depletion and protein intake in vivo on renal tubular bicarbonate transport in vitro. Am J Physiol 252(3 Pt 2):F509–F516, 1987.
63. Good DW: Active absorption of $NH_4^+$ by rat medullary thick ascending limb: Inhibition by potassium. Am J Physiol 255(1 Pt 2):F78–F87, 1988.
64. Arruda JA, Kurtzman NA: Mechanisms and classification of deranged distal urinary acidification. Am J Physiol 239(6): F515–F523, 1980.
65. Batlle DC, et al: Clinical and pathophysiologic spectrum of acquired distal renal tubular acidosis. Kidney Int 20(3):389–396, 1981.
66. DuBose TD Jr, Caflisch CR: Validation of the difference in urine and blood carbon dioxide tension during bicarbonate loading as an index of distal nephron acidification in experimental models of distal renal tubular acidosis. J Clin Invest 75(4):1116–1123, 1985.
67. Batlle DC: Segmental characterization of defects in collecting tubule acidification. Kidney Int 30(4):546–554, 1986.
68. Halperin ML, et al: Studies on the pathogenesis of type I (distal) renal tubular acidosis as revealed by the urinary $P_{CO_2}$ tensions. J Clin Invest 53(3):669–677, 1974.
69. Karet FE, et al: Localization of a gene for autosomal recessive distal renal tubular acidosis with normal hearing (rdRTA2) to 7q33–34. Am J Hum Genet 65(6):1656–1665, 1999.
70. Karet FE, et al: Mutations in the gene encoding B1 subunit of $H^+$-ATPase cause renal tubular acidosis with sensorineural deafness. Nat Genet 21(1):84–90, 1999.
71. Dafnis E, et al: Vanadate causes hypokalemic distal renal tubular acidosis. [Published erratum appears in Am J Physiol 1992 262:F449–F453, 1992.]
72. Bruce LJ, et al: Familial distal renal tubular acidosis is associated with mutations in the red cell anion exchanger (Band 3, AE1) gene. J Clin Invest 100(7):1693–1707, 1997.
73. Jarolim P, et al: Autosomal dominant distal renal tubular acidosis is associated in three families with heterozygosity for the R589H mutation in the AE1 (band 3) $Cl^-/HCO_3^-$ exchanger. J Biol Chem 273(11):6380–6388, 1998.
74. Buckalew VM Jr: Familial renal tubular acidosis. Ann Intern Med 69(6):1329–1330, 1968.
75. Coe FL, Parks JH: Stone disease in hereditary distal renal tubular acidosis. Ann Intern Med 93(1):60–61, 1980.
76. Brenner RJ, et al: Incidence of radiographically evident bone disease, nephrocalcinosis, and nephrolithiasis in various types of renal tubular acidosis. N Engl J Med 307(4):217–221, 1982.
77. Buckalew VM Jr, et al: Incomplete renal tubular acidosis. Physiologic studies in three patients with a defect in lowering urine pH. Am J Med 45(1):32–42, 1968.
78. Gyory AZ, Edwards KD: Renal tubular acidosis: A family with an autosomal dominant genetic defect in renal hydrogen ion transport, with proximal tubular and collecting duct dysfunction and increased metabolism of citrate and ammonia. Am J Med 45(1):43–62, 1968.
79. Hamed IA, et al: Familial absorptive hypercalciuria and renal tubular acidosis. Am J Med 67(3):385–391, 1979.
80. Randall RE Jr: Familial renal tubular acidosis revisited. Ann Intern Med 66(5):1024–1025, 1967.
81. Shapira E, et al: Enzymatically inactive red cell carbonic anhydrase B in a family with renal tubular acidosis. J Clin Invest 53(1):59–63, 1974.
82. Nimmannit S, et al: Pathogenesis of sudden unexplained nocturnal death (lai tai) and endemic distal renal tubular acidosis. Lancet 338(8772):930–932, 1991.
83. Nimmannit S, et al: Prevalence of endemic distal renal tubular acidosis and renal stone in the northeast of Thailand. Nephron 72(4):604–610, 1996.
84. Sitprija V, et al: Renal tubular acidosis, vanadium and buffaloes. Nephron 54(1):97–98, 1990.
85. Shioji R, et al: Sjögren's syndrome and renal tubular acidosis. Am J Med 48(4):456–463, 1970.
86. Talal N: Sjögren's syndrome, lymphoproliferation, and renal tubular acidosis. Ann Intern Med 74(4):633–634, 1971.
87. Bridi GS, et al: Glomerulonephritis and renal tubular acidosis in a case of chronic active hepatitis with hyperimmunoglobulinemia. Am J Med 52(2):267–278, 1972.
88. Golding PL: Renal tubular acidosis in chronic liver disease. Postgrad Med J 51(598):550–556, 1975.
89. Mason AM, Golding PL: Renal tubular acidosis and autoimmune thyroid disease. Lancet 2(7683):1104–1107, 1970.
90. Seux-Levieil ML, et al: Evaluation of renal acidification in HIV-infected patients with hypergammaglobulinemia. Nephron 75(2):196–200, 1997.
91. Deck MD: Medullary sponge kidney with renal tubular acidosis: A report of 3 cases. J Urol 94(4):330–335, 1965.
92. Osther PJ, et al: Urinary acidification and urinary excretion of calcium and citrate in women with bilateral medullary sponge kidney. Urol Int 52(3):126–130, 1994.
93. Restaino I, et al: Nephrolithiasis, hypocitraturia, and a distal renal tubular acidification defect in type 1 glycogen storage disease. J Pediatr 122(3):392–396, 1993.
94. Rochman J, et al: Renal tubular acidosis due to the milk-alkali syndrome. Isr J Med Sci 13(6):609–613, 1977.
95. Savani RC, Mimouni F, Tsang RC: Maternal and neonatal hyperparathyroidism as a consequence of maternal renal tubular acidosis. Pediatrics 91(3):661–663, 1993.
96. Seikaly M, Browne R, Baum M: Nephrocalcinosis is associated with renal tubular acidosis in children with X-linked hypophosphatemia. Pediatrics 97(1):91–93, 1996.
97. Szeto CC, et al: Thyrotoxicosis and renal tubular acidosis presenting as hypokalaemic paralysis. Br J Rheumatol 35(3):289–291, 1996.
98. Zisman E, et al: Hyperthyroidism and renal tubular acidosis. Arch Intern Med 121(2):118–122, 1968.
99. Douglas JB, Healy JK: Nephrotoxic effects of amphotericin B, including renal tubular acidosis. Am J Med 46(1):154–162, 1969.
100. McCurdy DK, Frederic M, Elkinton JR: Renal tubular acidosis due to amphotericin B. N Engl J Med 278(3):124–130, 1968.
101. Patterson RM, Ackerman GL: Renal tubular acidosis due to amphotericin B nephrotoxicity. Arch Intern Med 127(2):241–244, 1971.
102. Sawaya BP, Briggs JP, Schnermann J: Amphotericin B nephrotoxicity: The adverse consequences of altered membrane properties [editorial]. J Am Soc Nephrol 6(2):154–164, 1995.
103. Batlle D, et al: Distal nephron function in patients receiving chronic lithium therapy. Kidney Int 21(3):477–485, 1982.
104. Erramouspe J, Galvez R, Fischel DR: Newborn renal tubular acidosis associated with prenatal maternal toluene sniffing. J Psychoactive Drugs 28(2):201–204, 1996.
105. Taher SM, et al: Renal tubular acidosis associated with toluene "sniffing." N Engl J Med 290(14):765–768, 1974.
106. Steele TW, Edwards KD: Analgesic nephropathy. Changes in various parameters of renal function following cessation of analgesic abuse. Med J Aust 1(4):181–187, 1971.

107. Steele TW, Gyory AZ, Edwards KD: Renal function in analgesic nephropathy. BMJ 2(651):213–216, 1969.
108. Navarro JF, et al: Nephrogenic diabetes insipidus and renal tubular acidosis secondary to foscarnet therapy. Am J Kidney Dis 27(3):431–434, 1996.
109. Better OS, et al: Syndrome of incomplete renal tubular acidosis after cadaver kidney transplantation. Ann Intern Med 71(1): 39–46, 1969.
110. Gyory AZ, et al: Renal tubular acidosis, acidosis due to hyperkalaemia, hypercalcaemia, disordered citrate metabolism and other tubular dysfunctions following human renal transplantation. Q J Med 38(150):231–254, 1969.
111. Jordan M, et al: An immunocytochemical study of $H^+$ ATPase in kidney transplant rejection. J Lab Clin Med 127(3):310–314, 1996.
112. Wilson DR, Siddiqui AA: Renal tubular acidosis after kidney transplantation: Natural history and significance. Ann Intern Med 79(3):352–361, 1973.
113. Vainder M, Kelly J: Renal tubular dysfunction secondary to jejunoileal bypass. JAMA 235(12):1257–1258, 1976.
114. Better OS, et al: Studies on renal function after relief of complete unilateral ureteral obstruction of three months' duration in man. Am J Med 54(2):234–240, 1973.
115. Guizar JM, et al: Renal tubular acidosis in children with vesicoureteral reflux. J Urol 156(1):193–195, 1996.
116. Cochran M, et al: Renal tubular acidosis of pyelonephritis with renal stone disease. BMJ 2(607):721–729, 1968.
117. Bergman AJ, et al: Rate-dependent distal renal tubular acidosis and carnitine palmitoyltransferase I deficiency. Pediatr Res 36(5):582–588, 1994.
118. Fathallah DM, et al: Carbonic anhydrase II (CA II) deficiency in Maghrebian patients: Evidence for founder effect and genomic recombination at the CA II locus. Hum Genet 99(5): 634–637, 1997.
119. Fathallah DM, et al: A unique mutation underlying carbonic anhydrase II deficiency syndrome in patients of Arab descent. Hum Genet 94(5):581–582, 1994.
120. Sato S, Zhu XL, Sly WS: Carbonic anhydrase isozymes IV and II in urinary membranes from carbonic anhydrase II-deficient patients. Proc Natl Acad Sci U S A 87(16):6073–6076, 1990.
121. Morris RC Jr: Renal tubular acidosis: Mechanisms, classification and implications. N Engl J Med 281(25):1405–1413, 1969.
122. Sebastian A, McSherry E, Morris RC Jr: Renal potassium wasting in renal tubular acidosis (RTA): Its occurrence in types 1 and 2 RTA despite sustained correction of systemic acidosis. J Clin Invest 50(3):667–678, 1971.
123. Sebastian A, McSherry E, Morris RC Jr: Impaired renal conservation of sodium and chloride during sustained correction of systemic acidosis in patients with type 1, classic renal tubular acidosis. J Clin Invest 58(2):454–469, 1976.
124. Geller DS, et al: Mutations in the mineralocorticoid receptor gene cause autosomal dominant pseudohypoaldosteronism type I. Nat Genet 19(3):279–281, 1998.
125. Hulter HN, et al: Impaired renal $H^+$ secretion and $NH_3$ production in mineralocorticoid-deficient glucocorticoid-replete dogs. Am J Physiol 232(2):F136–F146, 1977.
126. Sebastian A, et al: Effect of mineralocorticoid replacement therapy on renal acid-base homeostasis in adrenalectomized patients. Kidney Int 18(6):762–773, 1980.
127. Wilcox CS, Cemerikic DA, Giebisch G: Differential effects of acute mineralo- and glucocorticosteroid administration on renal acid elimination. Kidney Int 21(4):546–556, 1982.
128. Sebastian A, et al: Amelioration of metabolic acidosis with fludrocortisone therapy in hyporeninemic hypoaldosteronism. N Engl J Med 297(11):576–583, 1977.
129. Tannen RL: Relationship of renal ammonia production and potassium homeostasis. Kidney Int 11(6):453–465, 1977.
130. DeFronzo RA: Hyperkalemia and hyporeninemic hypoaldosteronism [clinical conference]. Kidney Int 17(1):118–34, 1980.
131. Schambelan M, Sebastian A, Biglieri EG: Prevalence, pathogenesis, and functional significance of aldosterone deficiency in hyperkalemic patients with chronic renal insufficiency. Kidney Int 17(1):89–101, 1980.
132. Davenport MW, Zipser RD: Association of hypotension with hyperreninemic hypoaldosteronism in the critically ill patient. Arch Intern Med 143(4):735–737, 1983.
133. O'Kelly R, Magee F, McKenna TJ: Routine heparin therapy inhibits adrenal aldosterone production. J Clin Endocrinol Metab 56(1):108–112, 1983.
134. Shimizu T, et al: Site and mechanism of action of trichlormethiazide in rabbit distal nephron segments perfused in vitro. J Clin Invest 82(2):721–730, 1988.
135. Schambelan M, Sebastian A, Rector FC Jr: Mineralocorticoid-resistant renal hyperkalemia without salt wasting (type II pseudohypoaldosteronism): Role of increased renal chloride reabsorption. Kidney Int 19(5):716–727, 1981.
136. Chang SS, et al: Mutations in subunits of the epithelial sodium channel cause salt wasting with hyperkalaemic acidosis, pseudohypoaldosteronism type 1. Nat Genet 12(3):248–253, 1996.
137. Grunder S, et al: A mutation causing pseudohypoaldosteronism type 1 identifies a conserved glycine that is involved in the gating of the epithelial sodium channel. EMBO J 16(5):899–907, 1997.
138. Schild L: The ENaC channel as the primary determinant of two human diseases: Liddle syndrome and pseudohypoaldosteronism. Nephrologie 17(7):395–400, 1996.
139. Arnold JE, Healy JK: Hyperkalemia, hypertension and systemic acidosis without renal failure associated with a tubular defect in potassium excretion. Am J Med 47(3):461–472, 1969.
140. Spitzer A, et al: Short stature, hyperkalemia and acidosis: A defect in renal transport of potassium. Kidney Int 3(4):251–257, 1973.
141. Gordon RD, et al: Hypertension and severe hyperkalaemia associated with suppression of renin and aldosterone and completely reversed by dietary sodium restriction. Australas Ann Med 19(4):287–294, 1970.
142. Lee MR, et al: Hypertension and hyperkalaemia responding to bendrofluazide. Q J Med 48(190):245–258, 1979.
143. Mehta BR, et al: Hyporeninemic hypoaldosteronism in a patient with multiple myeloma. Am J Kidney Dis 4(2):175–178, 1984.
144. Rodriguez-Soriano J, et al: Normokalaemic pseudohypoaldosteronism is present in children with acute pyelonephritis. Acta Paediatr 81(5):402–406, 1992.
145. Kleyman TR, Roberts C, Ling BN: A mechanism for pentamidine-induced hyperkalemia: Inhibition of distal nephron sodium transport. Ann Intern Med 122(2):103–106, 1995.
146. Schlanger LE, Kleyman TR, Ling BN: $K^+$-sparing diuretic actions of trimethoprim: Inhibition of $Na^+$ channels in A6 distal nephron cells. Kidney Int 45(4):1070–1076, 1994.
147. Velazquez H, et al: Renal mechanism of trimethoprim-induced hyperkalemia [see comments]. Ann Intern Med 119(4):296–301, 1993.
148. Domingo P, et al: Trimethoprim-sulfamethoxazole-induced renal tubular acidosis in a patient with AIDS [letter]. Clin Infect Dis 20(5):1435–1437, 1995.
149. Gabow PA, Moore S, Schrier RW: Spironolactone-induced hyperchloremic acidosis in cirrhosis. Ann Intern Med 90(3):338–340, 1979.
150. Hulter HN, et al: Renal and systemic acid-base effects of chronic spironolactone administration. Am J Physiol 240(5): F381–F387, 1981.
151. D'Angio CT, Dillon MJ, Leonard JV: Renal tubular dysfunction in methylmalonic acidaemia. Eur J Pediatr 150(4):259–263, 1991.
152. De Ferrari ME, et al: Type IV renal tubular acidosis and uric acid nephrolithiasis in William's syndrome—an unusual mode of renal involvement. Nephrol Dial Transplant 12(7):1484–1486, 1997.
153. Schambelan M, Stockigt JR, Biglieri EG: Isolated hypoaldosteronism in adults: A renin-deficiency syndrome. N Engl J Med 287(12):573–578, 1972.
154. Carlisle EJ, Donnelly SM, Halperin ML: Renal tubular acidosis (RTA): Recognize the ammonium defect and pHorget the urine pH. Pediatr Nephrol 5(2):242–248, 1991.
155. Chafe L, Gault MH: First morning urine pH in the diagnosis of renal tubular acidosis with nephrolithiasis. Clin Nephrol 41(3):159–162, 1994.
156. Stinebaugh BJ, et al: Control of the urine-blood $P_{CO_2}$ gradient in alkaline urine. Kidney Int 17(1):31–39, 1980.
157. Tesar V, et al: Distal renal tubular acidosis in patients with Wilson's disease. Sb Lek 93(9–10):315–323, 1991.

158. Bonilla-Felix M: Primary distal renal tubular acidosis as a result of a gradient defect. Am J Kidney Dis 27(3):428–430, 1996.
159. Garg LC: Lack of effect of amphotericin B on urine-blood $P_{CO_2}$ gradient in spite of urinary acidification defect. Pflugers Arch 381(2):137–142, 1979.
160. Lewis DW: What was wrong with Tiny Tim? Am J Dis Child 146(12):1403–1407, 1992.
161. Zawadzki J: Permeability defect with bicarbonate leak as a mechanism of immune-related distal renal tubular acidosis. Am J Kidney Dis 31(3):527–532, 1998.

CHAPTER 12

# Acidosis of Chronic Renal Failure

Philippe Gauthier, MD ▪ Eric E. Simon, MD ▪ Jacob Lemann, Jr., MD

Systemic metabolic acidosis has long been known to occur among patients with advanced kidney diseases.[1] A decrease in the titratable base [bicarbonate] of the serum was observed more than a century ago.[2] Subsequent studies have confirmed and extended these observations.[3–12] Data illustrating the decline in serum bicarbonate concentrations as glomerular filtration rates (GFRs) decrease among patients with chronic kidney diseases, in comparison with comparable data among healthy subjects, are shown in Figure 12–1. Blood pH declines in a similar fashion.

Significant quantities of hydrogen ions are produced daily by various metabolic processes. The $H^+$ is immediately buffered, mainly by bicarbonate, and eventually excreted by the kidneys. Although the lungs play an important role in the acute regulation of acid-base balance, the kidneys are responsible for the ultimate excretion of the protons formed by metabolism each day. Together with the intra- and extracellular buffer systems, these organs normally tightly regulate blood pH. When this system fails, the result can be chronic metabolic acidosis, which is known to have several adverse clinical consequences. This chapter reviews the normal physiology of acid generation and excretion by the kidney followed by a review of the perturbations of this system that occur with chronic renal insufficiency. We then discuss the clinical consequences of the resultant acidosis and, hopefully, convince the reader that these consequences are significant enough to warrant early and effective treatment, which does not necessarily have to be delayed until dialysis is begun. Finally, we discuss treatment of acidosis for both predialysis and end-stage renal disease patients.

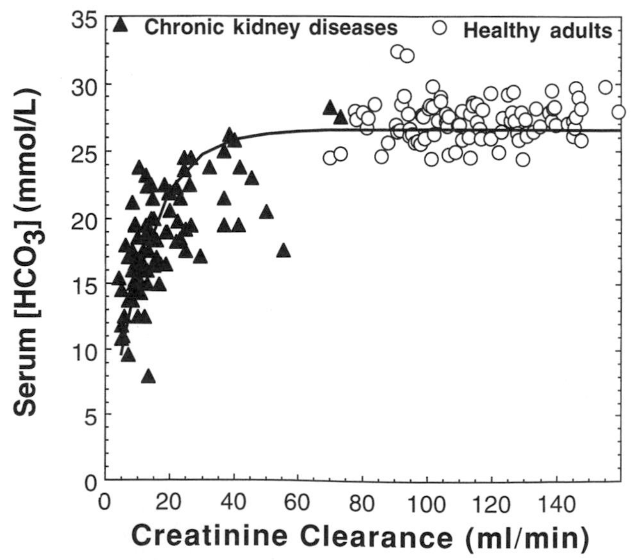


**FIGURE 12–1** ▪ The relationships between the serum $[HCO_3]$ and creatinine clearance among patients with chronic kidney diseases and healthy adults. The regression curve was $[HCO_3] = 26.6 (1 - e^{0.8787 * Ccr})$; $r^2 = 0.72$.

## NORMAL ACID-BASE METABOLISM

Daily metabolic acid production is derived primarily from dietary sources. Fat and carbohydrates are metabolized into fairly strong acids. However, these acids are usually oxidized into $CO_2$ and $H_2O$, resulting in little net acid production because the lungs exhale the $CO_2$. In pathologic states, such as lactic acidosis or diabetic ketoacidosis, strong acids may accumulate as a result of the incomplete oxidation of these substances. Another source of metabolic acids is the metabolism of nucleoproteins and nucleic acids, which results in the production of uric acid. Most amino acids contain carboxyl groups with equal numbers of amino groups. Metabolism then produces equal amounts of bicarbonate and ammonium. If the process stopped here, blood returning from the liver would be alkaline, because ammonium is not an effective acid at blood pH. However, in the urea cycle, the bicarbonate and ammonium are combined to yield $H_2O$, $CO_2$, and urea, resulting in no net acid production. The sulfur-containing amino acids methionine, cysteine, and cystine are metabolized to $CO_2$, urea, sulfate, and two $H^+$, thus resulting in net acid production. Subjects fed large amounts of methionine excrete acid and sulfate in almost equal proportions.[6] Another source of acid production is the hydrolysis of phosphoesters and phosphorylated amino acids (i.e., phosphoserine, phosphothreonine), a reaction that yields phosphate and $H^+$.[14] Thus, there are three major endogenous sources of fixed acid production[5]: (1) the incomplete oxidation of neutral foodstuffs, (2) the oxidation of organic sulfur to sulfate, and (3) the hydrolysis of phosphoesters. Additionally, the diet and the intestine play a role in fixed acid production. Most diets provide potential bicarbonate, mainly as potassium salts of metabolizable organic acids, exemplified by potassium citrate. Additionally, there is fecal excretion of potassium salts of organic acids, principally the short-chain fatty acids acetate, butyrate, and propionate, which may be considered as representing either $H^+$ gain to the body or, equivalently, $HCO_3$ loss. The contributions of the diet and the stool to overall net fixed acid production have been assessed.[15] Usual American diets result in a net production of $H^+$ of 0.5 to 1 mEq/kg/day, which is immediately buffered and ultimately secreted by the kidney.[21] However, this quantity varies with diet. A mainly vegetarian diet increases $HCO_3$ production, and net fixed acid is reduced. A diet that contains large amounts of eggs and animal proteins, which are rich in sulfur, increases the net fixed acid production.

The kidney is the organ that is chiefly responsible for excreting the daily acid or alkali load. With most Western diets, the kidney will predominately excrete acid because these diets tend to be relatively high in protein. There are three major mechanisms by which the kidney can excrete the daily acid load: (1) the reclamation of filtered bicarbonate, (2) the excretion of ammonium ions, and (3) the excretion of titratable acid.

Quantitatively, the major role of the kidney is to reclaim the 4000 mmol of bicarbonate that is filtered daily. If this large quantity of base were not absorbed, acidosis would rapidly ensue. This is accomplished along the proximal tubule through the actions of the $Na^+/H^+$ antiporter and carbonic anhydrase, as described in Chapter 2. The net process is that of reclaiming filtered bicarbonate. Early experiments demonstrated a maximum reabsorptive rate (Tm) for bicarbonate of about 2.8 mEq per minute per 100 mL GFR. However, a later study[22] showed that when care is taken to maintain euvolemia in humans receiving a bicarbonate load, this Tm disappears. This is because hypervolemia causes the proximal tubule to reabsorb less sodium. Because $H^+$ is secreted in exchange for $Na^+$, this limits hydrogen ion secretion and, in turn, bicarbonate reabsorption. Early experiments with bicarbonate loads resulted in such hypervolemia due to the accompanying sodium, thus giving the false impression that when larger amounts of bicarbonate are presented, the tubule is incapable of reabsorbing it all. When the proximal tubule continues to avidly reabsorb sodium, there seems to be no discernible limit to bicarbonate reabsorption. However, when sodium reabsorption in the proximal tubule is decreased, less bicarbonate is reabsorbed.

The second and third methods of acid clearance (i.e., excretion of ammonium and titratable acid) rely on distal hydrogen ion excretion. There are two major distal hydrogen transporters. First, an $H^+$-ATPase, is located in the intercalated cells of the collecting duct. This pump can actively secrete $H^+$ against a chemical gradient. A favorable electrical gradient is maintained via the epithelial sodium channel (ENaC). This channel allows for rapid sodium efflux from the peritubular space, creating a negative voltage in the lumen, thus favoring the secretion of positively charged ions such as $H^+$ and $K^+$. Second, an $H^+,K^+$-ATPase, is also found in intercalated cells. These two $H^+$ transporters are capable of lowering intraluminal pH to about 4.5, representing an 800-fold increase in $H^+$ concentration over that of serum at a pH of 7.4. Although this gradient is large, the concentration of $H^+$ at this pH is only $3.1 \times 10^{-5}$ mol/L or 0.03 mEq/L. Thus, if the daily load of 80 mEq is to be excreted, mechanisms must exist to greatly enhance $H^+$ ion excretion. The first of these involves the synthesis of ammonia by the proximal tubule via the deamidation and deamination of glutamine. Traditionally, it was thought that ammonia ($NH_3$), a volatile substance that easily diffuses into the tubule, was produced. The molecule is a weak base with a pKa of about 9.3. Thus, when it enters the distal tubule it is rapidly protonated to ammonium ($NH_4^+$), which is not diffusible, thus "trapping" both the ammonia molecule and a hydrogen ion. However, more recent understanding suggests that the proximal tubule produces ammonium, which remains largely protonated throughout the tubule. Despite the recognition that ammonium may be transported as $NH_4^+$, nonionic diffusion of $NH_3$ with subsequent trapping of $NH_4^+$ is still a significant mode of ammonia transport. The medullary interstitium concentrates ammonia, and the high interstitial $NH_3$ and $NH_4^+$ favor movement from the interstitium into the collecting duct. Defects in collecting duct acidification impair diffusion-trapping of ammonia, which is expected. However, defects in countercurrent multiplication (e.g., concentrating defect) impair medullary accumulation of $NH_3$ and $NH_4^+$ and thus also impair entry of ammonia into the collecting duct. As described in Chapter 1, each molecule of ammonium excreted represents the excretion of one $H^+$. As long as the urine pH is less than 7, the large majority of ammonia is protonated to $NH_4^+$, thus allowing for a pH-independent mechanism of acid excretion. An increase in cortical ammonia production is the chief mechanism by which acid excretion is augmented in acute acidosis.[23]

Another mechanism by which $H^+$ secretion is augmented is by providing a urinary proton buffer system. The major buffer is phosphate, although creatinine also contributes. At blood pH, phosphate exists as 80% $HPO_4^{2-}$ and 20% $H_2PO_4^-$, a ratio of about 4:1. However, at a urine pH of 5.8 about 90% of phosphate exists as $H_2PO_4^-$, and at a pH of 4.8 it becomes 99% $H_2PO_4^-$. The hydrogen buffered by this system is referred to as "titratable acid" because it can be measured by titrating a urine sample from its pH to blood pH. Titratable acid excretion then requires both intact distal acidification and the presence of sufficient buffer. If either is lacking, net acid excretion is reduced. In summary, the three mechanisms for net acid secretion by the kidney are (1) the reabsorption of filtered bicarbonate, (2) the secretion of ammonium, and (3) the excretion of titratable acid. Defects in any of these mechanisms can result in the inability to excrete the entire daily acid load.

## GENERATION OF ACIDOSIS IN CHRONIC RENAL FAILURE

It has long been recognized that renal insufficiency leads to acidosis (see Fig. 12–1). Even moderate degrees of renal insufficiency with serum creatinine levels from 2 to 4 mg/dL may result in a small but statistically significant decrease in serum [$HCO_3$] compared with normal levels.[12] However, the values usually remain within normal limits. In early renal failure, serum chloride increases in proportion to the fall in [$HCO_3$] so

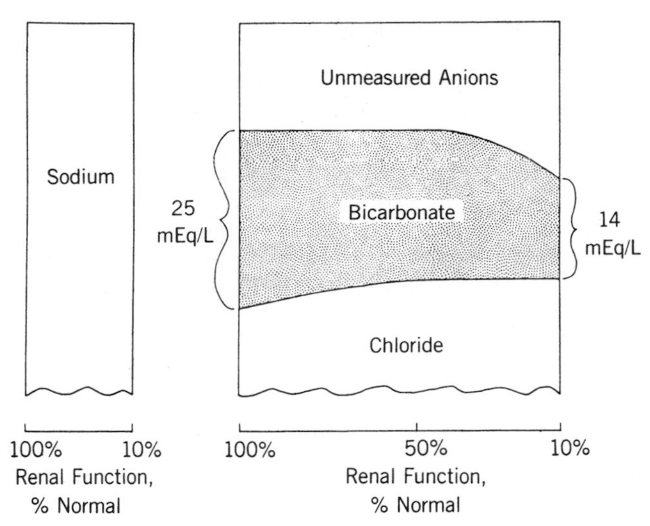


**FIGURE 12–2** ■ Changing pattern of serum electrolyte composition that occurs during the progression of chronic, uncomplicated renal failure. The vertical axis reflects the serum concentration in milliequivalents per liter. Note that the concentration of serum $Na^+$ does not change appreciably as renal function declines. By contrast, the serum anion composition changes considerably. Early in the development of progressive renal failure, a sizable reduction in serum bicarbonate occurs that is entirely offset by an increase in serum chloride; the unmeasured anion concentration remains normal. Only when renal function falls to levels less than 30% to 50% of normal does this pattern of hyperchloremic metabolic acidosis give way to a more familiar "anion gap" acidosis of azotemia. Even under these circumstances, serum chloride remains elevated at levels achieved during more moderate renal insufficiency. (From Widmer B, Gerhardt R, Harrington JJ, Cohen SJ: Serum electrolyte and acid-base composition: Influence of graded degrees of chronic renal failure. Arch Intern Med 139:1099–1102, 1979.)

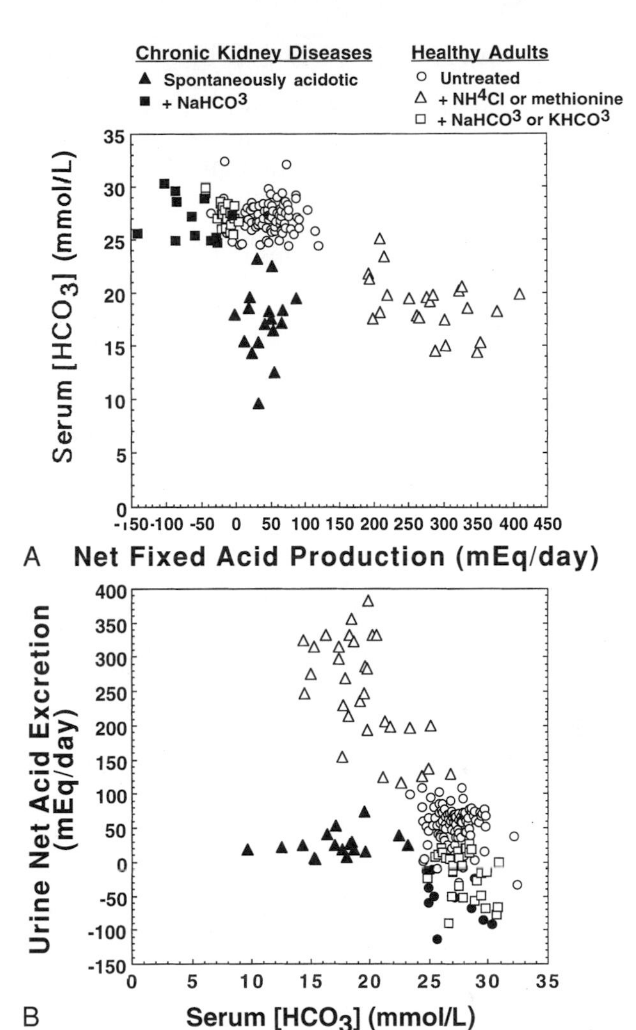


**FIGURE 12–3** ■ *A,* Serum $[HCO_3]$ in relation to rates of daily fixed acid production among (1) spontaneously acidotic patients with chronic kidney diseases, (2) patients in whom acidosis was corrected by the ongoing administration of $NaHCO_3$, and (3) healthy adults as well as healthy adults made acidotic by the ongoing administration of $NH_4Cl$, $KHCO_3$, or $NaHCO_3$. *B,* Daily rates of urinary net acid excretion in relation to serum $[HCO_3]$ among the same patient groups.

that the anion gap remains normal. As renal insufficiency becomes more severe, serum $[HCO_3]$ continues to fall with obviously low values becoming evident when GFR is in the range of 20 to 40 mL/min (see Fig. 12–1). As renal function worsens, organic and inorganic anions are retained, and the anion gap increases as serum $[HCO_3]$ falls (Fig. 12–2).

As summarized in Figure 12–3, metabolic acidosis develops with advanced kidney diseases because of a reduced capacity of the damaged kidneys to excrete net acid, not because of increased rates of fixed acid production. As illustrated in Figure 12–3*A*, serum bicarbonate concentrations are low among patients with advanced kidney diseases despite daily rates of fixed acid production that are normal, varying across a range similar to those observed among healthy adults eating comparable diets. Furthermore, increased rates of fixed acid production must be produced in healthy subjects (e.g., ammonium chloride loading) in order to cause serum bicarbonate concentrations to decrease into the range observed among patients with kidney diseases. As shown in Figure 12–3*B*, when fixed acid production is experimentally increased, net renal acid excretion increases progressively among healthy subjects as serum bicarbonate concentrations fall. By contrast, among patients with kidney diseases, net acid excretion is low and does not rise as serum bicarbonate concentrations decrease. In one of the seminal papers of this field, Wrong and Davies in 1958 performed a series of experiments with both normal subjects and those with varying types of renal insufficiency.[4] Subjects were acid loaded with ammonium chloride. Normal subjects demonstrated a decrease in urine pH to between 4.6 and 5.0, together with a proportional increase in ammonium excretion. These changes were seen even before a decrease in serum $[HCO_3^-]$ could be measured. Titratable acid excretion also increased and continued to increase after urine pH stabilized. This finding can only be explained by an increase in buffer excretion. In fact, this was the case, especially for phosphate, which accounted for a mean of 60% of titratable acid excretion. Nevertheless, ammonium excretion accounted for the majority of the augmentation in net acid excretion. Acid loading was also performed on a group of patients with renal insufficiency but no evidence of specific tubular defects. All except one patient had serum bicarbonate concentrations that were at the lower end of the normal range. After acid loading, all except one subject demonstrated reduced urine pH to 5.3 or lower, which was not significantly different from the normal group. However, ammonium excretion, although increasing with decreasing urine pH, was overall greatly reduced from that of normal subjects. Titratable acid excretion was less severely impaired. Again, this impairment in titratable acid secretion was caused by a decrease in urinary buffers, particularly phosphate.

Subsequent studies confirmed these findings and further refined our understanding of the diseased and healthy kidney's responses to chronic and acute acidosis. Figure 12–4[6–9, 13–20] summarizes studies of daily urinary pH and urinary excretion rates of bicarbonate, titratable acid, and ammonium, the components of net acid excretion, in relation to serum bicarbonate among patients with advanced kidney diseases in comparison with healthy subjects. Data are shown for patients with chronic kidney diseases with spontaneous acidosis as well as during periods when serum bicarbonate concentrations were maintained within the normal range by the ongoing administration of $NaHCO_3$. For comparison, similar observations among untreated healthy adults, adults given $NH_4Cl$, or those given either $NaHCO_3$ or $KHCO_3$ are also shown. When spontaneously acidotic, most patients with chronic kidney diseases do not excrete bicarbonate into their urine and can maximally reduce the pH of their urine (see Fig. 12–4*A*, *B*). However, a few patients continue to excrete small amounts of bicarbonate (see Fig. 12–4*A*) and are unable to maximally acidify their urine, despite the systemic metabolic acidosis (see Fig. 12–4*B*). Because most of the patients can maximally acidify their urine, they can excrete normal amounts of titratable acid in relation to the available quantity of phosphate (filtered buffer) that is present in their urine (see Fig. 12–4*C*). The main factor contributing to the low rates of net acid excretion among acidotic patients with chronic kidney diseases is the marked reduction in the capacity of their kidneys to excrete ammonium into their urine (see Fig. 12–4*D*). When serum bicarbonate concentrations are increased into the normal range in patients with kidney diseases by ongoing treat-

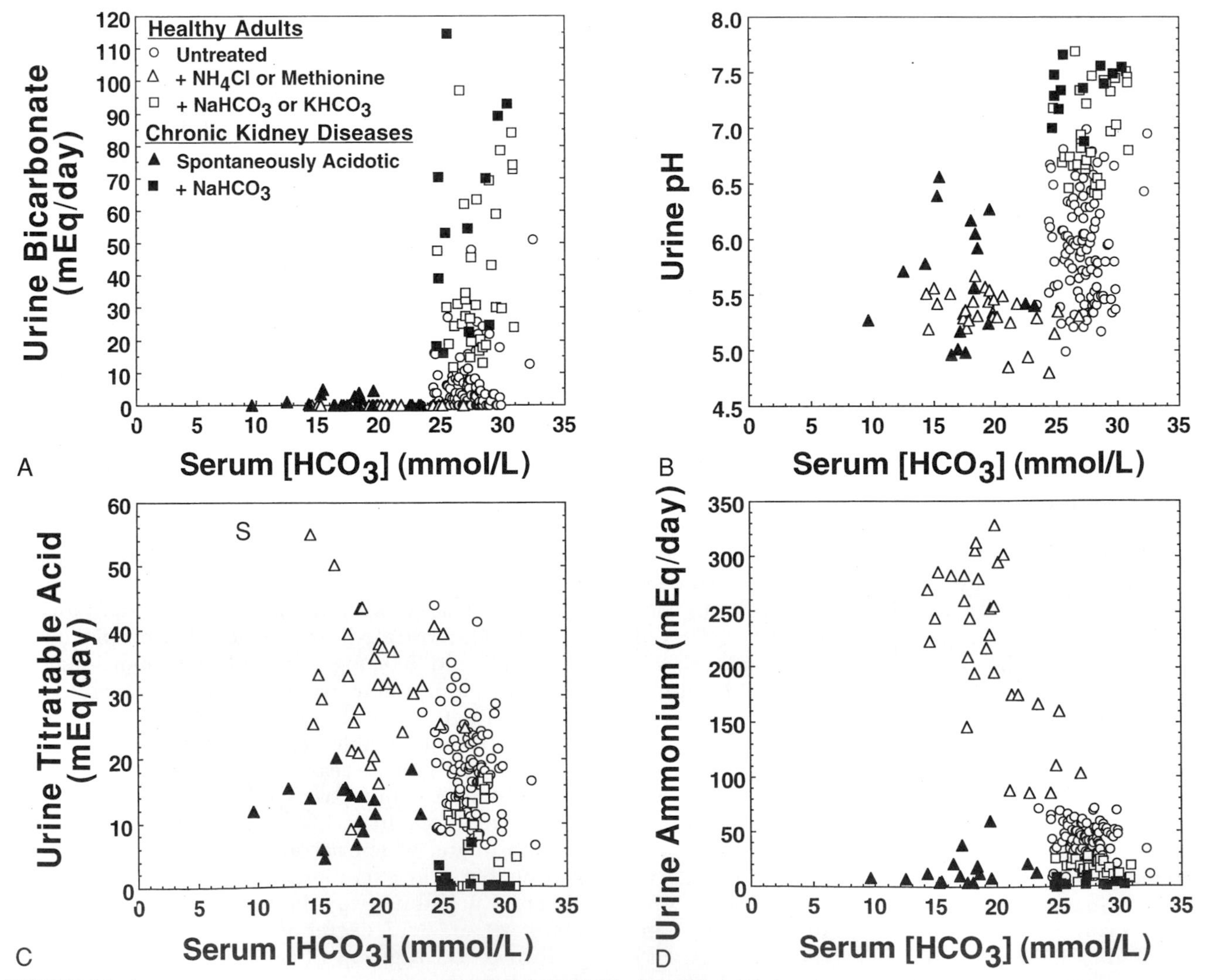


**FIGURE 12–4** ■ Daily urine $HCO_3$ excretion rates (*A*), urine pH (*B*), titratable acid excretion rates (*C*), and $NH_4^+$ excretion rates (*D*) in relation to serum [$HCO_3$] among patients with chronic kidney diseases and among healthy subjects.

ment with $NaHCO_3$, urine bicarbonate excretion increases; urine pH rises; titratable acid excretion becomes negligible; and the already low rate of ammonium excretion falls further. The patterns of these responses are comparable with those that are seen among healthy subjects given $KHCO_3$ or $NaHCO_3$. Thus, in the acidosis of chronic renal failure (CRF), as judged by the final urine, distal hydrogen ion secretion is relatively unimpaired; buffer secretion is moderately impaired; and ammonium excretion is severely impaired. This defect in ammonium excretion is emphasized in Figure 12–5. Normally, an acid load results in a several-fold increase in ammonium excretion with a more modest increase in titratable acid excretion. By contrast, in CRF, despite the prevailing systemic acidosis, there is a failure to increase ammonia excretion to the levels found in normal subjects with acidosis. Even when factored for GFR, ammonium excretion fails to increase appropriately (see Fig. 12–5*B*).

Several investigators have examined the specific nature of this defect in ammonia excretion in CRF. The first question that must be addressed is whether this phenomenon is the result of a specific tubular defect or simply the reduction in nephron mass. Oliver first formulated the "nephron dropout" theory in 1939 when he demonstrated that many nephrons were still intact in the diseased kidney.[24] This theory further states that nephrons are either "on" or "off" and that a decrease in GFR is caused by a loss of nephrons rather than a decrease in filtration within individual nephrons. One could postulate that in a case of a steadily declining nephron population, the remaining nephrons may increase ammoniagenesis to compensate. After a loss of a significant number of nephrons, acid clearance would be expected to be insufficient to account for the daily acid production, leading to a decline in serum bicarbonate. This would then stimulate the remaining nephrons to increase ammoniagenesis until a balance is again achieved and the serum bicarbonate is stabilized at a lower level. Eventually, the capacity of the remaining nephrons to excrete acid can be exceeded and systemic acidosis worsens. In 1962, Elkinton[5] addressed this issue. If acidosis results from a specific tubular defect, then the degree of acid retention shou0ld be proportional to or greater than the loss of nephron population. Conversely, if it is only caused by a loss of renal mass, then acidosis should occur at a slower rate than the loss of nephrons owing to the reserve capacity of the remainder. One cannot directly measure the number of remaining nephrons, but the estimated GFR should be a close approximation given the nephron dropout theory. Elkinton found that in most renal diseases, including glomerular diseases, the decline in bicarbonate concentration was less than predicted by the blood urea nitrogen (BUN) and suggested compensation, whereas in some cases the decline in serum bicarbonate was greater than that predicted by the BUN and suggested the presence of specific tubular defects (e.g., renal tubular acidosis [RTA]). Further experiments in dogs[25] have shown that residual nephrons do in fact increase ammonium excretion (when expressed on a per nephron basis). In these experiments unilateral renal insufficiency was produced using the pyelonephritis model, and the bladder was divided to allow for separate measurements from each kidney. Acidosis was induced us-

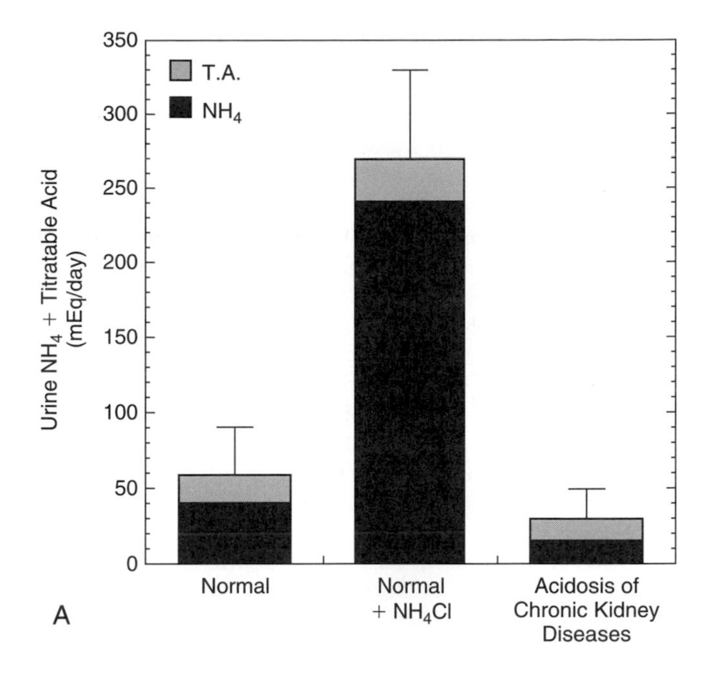


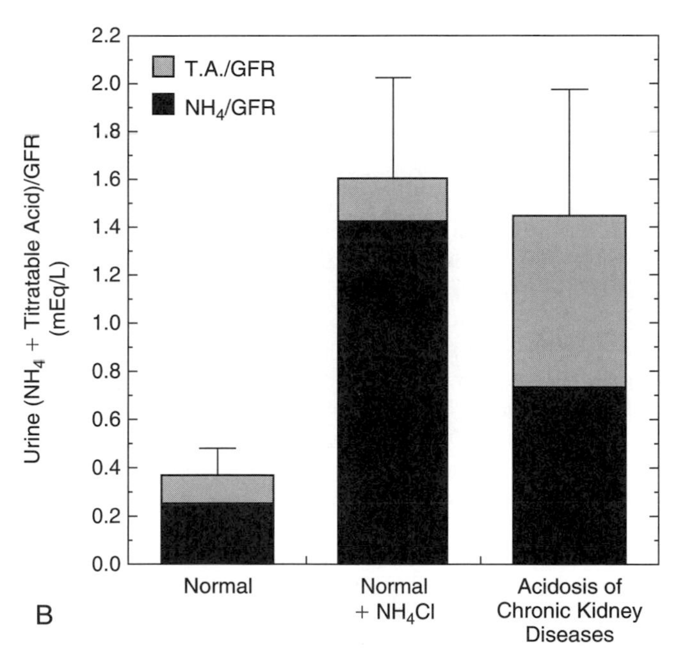


**FIGURE 12–5** ■ *A*, Sum of daily urinary excretion rates of ammonium plus titratable acid, mEq/day, among 47 normal adults (serum $[HCO_3]$ 27 ± 1 mEq/L, $C_{creatinine}$ 165 ± 28 L/day), 14 healthy adults with stable $NH_4Cl$ acidosis (individually constant doses averaging for the group 3.3 ± 0.9 mEq/kg/day; serum $[HCO_3]$ 20 ± 2 mEq/L, $C_{creatinine}$ 172 ± 34 L/day), and 17 patients with chronic kidney disease and acidosis (serum $[HCO_3]$ 17 ± 3 mEq/L, $C_{creatinine}$ 20 ± 14 L/day). *B*, Sum of daily urinary excretion rates of ammonium plus titratable acid, mEq/day, factored by $C_{creatinine}$, L/day, for the same subjects shown in *A*. GFR, glomerular filtraton rate; T.A., urine titratable acidity.

ing an ammonium chloride infusion. Initially, the GFR declined in the diseased kidney and rose slightly in the healthy one. Ammonium excretion per unit of GFR was the same in each kidney. After the unimpaired kidney was removed, ammonium excretion per unit of GFR from the remnant, diseased kidney increased by an average of 90%. This is consistent with the hypothesis that the remnant nephrons were stimulated by the acidosis to increase ammonium production. As in humans, the urine pH actually increased slightly; thus, the increment in ammonium excretion was likely caused predominantly by an increase in ammonia synthesis. However, despite this increase in ammonium excretion per nephron, the overall renal ammonium excretion was not sufficient to clear the acid load. Thus, it would appear that the decline in renal ammonium excretion in chronic renal insufficiency is proportional to the reduction in renal mass and occurs despite an increase in single (remnant) nephron ammonium excretion. In humans with mild renal insufficiency, a small decline in serum bicarbonate seems sufficient to stimulate the remnant nephrons to excrete the daily acid load. Such patients might become acidotic when given an additional acid challenge (because reserve capacity is already being utilized). However, once GFR declines into the range of 20 to 40 mL/min, the remaining nephrons lack sufficient capacity to excrete the metabolic load and clinically relevant acidosis ensues.

As noted earlier, one explanation for the decline in ammonia excretion in the face of a decline in nephron mass is simply that ammoniagenesis declines in proportion to the decrease in renal mass. In normal subjects given an acid load, net acid excretion can be augmented many times above normal (see Fig. 12–5*A*) primarily by augmentation of urinary ammonium excretion. However, as shown in Figures 12–1 and 12–2, acidosis already begins to ensue when the nephron mass is reduced to about a third of normal. Further, as shown in Figure 12–5*B*, ammonia excretion is low even when factored for GFR. Thus, although a simple decrease in nephron mass with a resultant decrease in ammoniagenesis may account for much of the failure to increase acid excretion in renal insufficiency, these considerations suggest that it is not the only factor.

Studies in humans with renal failure in which the renal artery and veins were catheterized allowed direct examination of the role of ammoniagenesis in CRF.[26] These studies showed that ammoniagenesis was indeed impaired in CRF. However, surprisingly, arterial glutamine delivery was not rate limiting and glutamine extraction was in fact greatly impaired. Glutamine extraction in normal subjects with metabolic acidosis was sevenfold higher (when factored for GFR) than in patients with CRF. The authors suggested that uremia produced a defect in glutamine uptake, perhaps into the mitochondria, and that intrarenal breakdown of peptides delivered to the kidney provided the ammonia nitrogen.

Micropuncture studies in rats with remnant kidneys have shown additional mechanisms for the defect in ammonium as well as net acid excretion. In these rats, proximal tubular hydrogen ion secretion decreases with the loss in renal mass, resulting in a gradual decrease in the proximal tubule's ability to reclaim filtered bicarbonate.[27] The intact nephron hypothesis requires that remnant nephrons handle an ever-greater proportion of the total filtered load of fluid and electrolytes. It has been well demonstrated that adaptive changes in remnant nephrons occur in rats with renal insufficiency, which result in a dramatic increase in single-nephron GFR, distal fluid delivery, and increased fractional excretion of sodium.[28] As discussed earlier, it has been shown that the capacity of the proximal tubule to reclaim bicarbonate depends on its ability to reabsorb sodium. As tubular hydrogen ion excretion depends on an $Na^+$-$H^+$ antiporter, it follows that a reduction in proximal tubule sodium reabsorption will lead to a decrease in the reclamation of filtered bicarbonate. The resultant increased delivery of bicarbonate to the distal tubule can, to some extent, be compensated by distal acidification. However, with the already augmented distal bicarbonate delivery, the quantitative capacity of the distal hydrogen pumps is near maximal; thus, all of this bicarbonate cannot be neutralized. Indeed, the pH of the urine entering the collecting duct in the rats with remnant kidneys is higher than normal, obligating continued bicarbonate reabsorption in the collecting duct rather than enhancing titratable acid excretion.[27] This may be one reason why urine pH in chronic renal insufficiency may be slightly higher than in healthy subjects. A second factor limiting net acid excretion is the defect in ammonium excretion. When measured at the end of the proximal tubule, ammonia delivery increased greatly in the remnant kidneys.[27] However, unlike the normal kidney with metabolic acidosis, much of this ammonium was not transferred to the final urine but was presumably lost in the renal veins. Thus, failure of re-entrapment of ammonium in the collecting duct was a major contributor to the defect in ammonium excretion. Of particular note was that the osmolality of the interstitium was decreased, and thus it was postulated that the decrease in medullary concentration of ammonia contributed to the failure to transfer the ammonia from the interstitium to the collecting duct. The importance of the medulla in ammonia excretion is also supported by studies in rats with papillectomy and renal failure whose ammonium excretion was actually less than nephrectomized rats despite similar GFRs.[29]

Phosphate excretion has also been shown to be disordered in chronic renal insufficiency. As we have seen, for a given urine pH, titratable acid excretion can be augmented by increasing buffer, primarily phosphate, excretion. Wrong and Davies[4] observed in normal subjects given an acid load that phosphate excretion increased, causing an increment in titratable acid excretion. However, the authors attributed this to the normal diurnal variation in phosphate excretion. Later work has demonstrated that acute acidosis produced in normal subjects causes phosphate excretion to increase. In rats, renal phosphate excretion was increased by 56% after 10 days of experimental acidosis, mainly via a decrease in proximal tubular $Na^+$-P cotransporter activity.[30] This represents an additional mechanism for clearing the acid load. These rats, however, had normal renal function. Gonick and associates addressed the question of phosphate excretion after an acid load in patients with impaired kidney function.[11] After acid loading, titratable acid and phosphate excretion were reduced among patients with renal disease compared with normal subjects. The decrement in titratable acid excretion per unit of GFR was less than that of ammonium, implying that phosphate excretion is better preserved with a loss of renal mass than is ammoniagenesis. Although phosphate excretion in chronic renal insufficiency is reduced, excretion per nephron is actually increased as renal mass is lost. This increment in phosphate excretion/GFR in dogs has been shown to be primarily the result of an increase in serum parathyroid hormone (PTH) levels,[31] with a more minor role of elevated serum phosphate levels augmenting excretion by increasing the filtered load. Serum concentrations of phosphatonin (or a substance like phosphatonin), a hormonal factor that inhibits phosphate reabsorption, have also been found to be elevated in renal failure[32] and may participate in the reduction in phosphate reabsorption. Thus, a largely pH-independent decrease in titratable acid excretion takes place in chronic renal insufficiency but is less significant than the decrease in ammonium excretion because phosphate excretion is relatively well preserved. As shown in Figure 12–5*B*, this translates into a titratable acid excretion that is actually augmented when factored for GFR.

The aforementioned considerations apply to all patients with a reduction in nephron mass. Patients with CRF may have specific tubular defects that result in RTA; conversely, many patients with RTA have renal insufficiency. Thus, sometimes the lines between acidosis of renal failure and RTA become obscured. The patients with RTA have acidosis out of proportion to the decrease in GFR. A complete discussion of RTA is found in Chapter 11.

## CONSEQUENCES OF METABOLIC ACIDOSIS

There are several clinical consequences of metabolic acidosis. Many of the symptoms associated with uremia may be the result of acidosis. Nausea, vomiting, generalized weakness, and dyspnea may present in patients with nonuremic acidosis, such as RTA, or during experimental acidosis in healthy subjects. More important, the acidosis of uremia has an important effect on both bone and nutrition.

It has long been recognized that patients with chronic acidosis are in negative calcium balance. The mineral phase of bone, primarily $Ca_{10}(PO_4)_6(OH)_2$ and $Ca_{10}(PO_4)_6CO_3$, is a reservoir of alkali. Human infants can be demonstrated to be in negative acid balance (e.g., renal net acid excretion exceeds fixed acid production), because these salts are deposited in their growing bones.[33] In humans with significant renal insufficiency, the adaptive capabilities of remnant nephrons can be exceeded and many such subjects are shown to be in persistently positive acid balance, despite low but stable serum $[HCO_3^-]$.[7] Those observations suggested buffering of the retained $H^+$ outside of body fluids, presumably by alkaline bone salts. In acid-loaded normal subjects, an equivalent negative calcium balance matched the quantity of acid retained.[16] This could represent the slow dissolution of bone salts. Such dissolution has been well demonstrated in isolated rat calvariae in which calcium enters an acidified medium (via bicarbonate reduction) accompanied by a concomitant movement of protons into the bone.[34] This does not occur when the acidity of the medium is raised by elevating the $P_{CO_2}$ (i.e., respiratory acidosis).[35] Other investigators, however, have called this concept into question. Oh points out that the skeleton contains a total of 25,300 mEq of base.[36] Assuming a persistently positive acid balance of 19 mEq/day, half of the skeleton would be dissolved in less than 2 years and the entire skeleton consumed in 3.6 years. Early metabolic studies detailing a positive acid balance may have been methodologically flawed because they did not take into account all potential sources of urinary hydrogen ion excretion. However, it is difficult to conclude that bone plays no role in buffering a chronic acidosis. A lesser degree of positive acid balance than originally postulated that is then buffered by bone has not been ruled out.

Other explanations for the contribution of chronic metabolic acidosis to bone disease exist. Some, but not all, studies have suggested that acidosis increases serum PTH levels. A mechanism for this effect, if it occurs, is unclear, but the ultimate effect may be an adaptive mechanism to inhibit renal tubular phosphate reabsorption and therefore increase both urinary phosphate and titratable acid excretion. It has been shown that optimal correction of acidosis in dialysis patients ameliorates osteodystrophy.[37] Further experiments in patients with chronic renal insufficiency, but not on hemodialysis, demonstrate that when serum ionized calcium is clamped, bicarbonate infusion significantly lowers serum PTH levels.[38] In dialysis patients, after correction of acidosis, PTH becomes more responsive to serum calcium, which results in a shift of the PTH/calcium curve downward.[39] Thus, it appears that in addition to hypocalcemia, hyperphosphatemia, and low calcitriol levels, acidosis stimulates PTH secretion in chronic renal insufficiency.

Chronic acidosis may also have an effect on nutritional status. In humans with normal renal function, the generation of a chronic acidosis, using a metabolic diet, results in a decrease in albumin synthesis and a negative nitrogen balance.[40] This same study demonstrated a suppression of insulin-like growth factor (IGF-1), free thyroxine, and tri-iodothyronine. Another study demonstrated that in humans, a diet-induced metabolic acidosis caused weight loss and whole-body protein degradation.[41] When hemodialysis using bicarbonate containing dialysate was introduced, patients exhibited an improved appetite and significant gain in dry weight compared with patients continuing dialysis using acetate-based dialysate.[42] Several other studies in both chronic renal insufficiency[43] and hemodialysis[44, 45] have shown that correction of acidosis leads to a decrease in whole-body protein degradation and increases in serum albumin levels. These findings have also been extended to patients treated by chronic ambulatory peritoneal dialysis (CAPD).[46]

Some mechanisms whereby chronic acidosis causes malnutrition have been elucidated in rats. Acidosis caused increased proteolysis in isolated muscle cells that was not prevented by the inhibition of lysosomal or calcium-dependent proteases.[47] However, when ATP production was blocked, the proteolysis resolved, suggesting an ATP-dependent pathway. Involvement of the ubiquitin-proteasome pathway was suggested by an increase in mRNA encoding this system. Other investigators have shown, again in rats, that branched-chain amino acid catabolism is increased in CRF via an acidosis-induced activation of the enzyme branched-chain ketoacid dehydrogenase.[48] Furthermore, acidosis seems to cause resistance to the action of various anabolic hormones, such as growth hormone (GH), insulin, and insulin-like growth factor.[49] Thus, it would appear that chronic acidosis is at least partially responsible for the malnutrition and catabolism of uremia. However, there is a lack of clinical studies that specifically address the role of acidosis in the malnutrition of uremia in humans.[50]

Another potentially adverse effect of chronic metabolic acidosis is the contribution to progression of renal failure. The increase in ammoniagenesis in response to acidosis results in an increase in renal cortical ammonia accumulation. In rats, ammonia accumulation in the remnant kidney model has been linked to complement activation and interstitial nephritis.[51] To date, there have been no clinical studies to evaluate this proposition.

Perhaps the most serious effect of chronic acidosis is on the growth of children. It has been recognized for some time that distal RTA (RTA type I; see Chapter 11) is associated with growth retardation in children, which can be ameliorated with alkali therapy.[52] Unlike adults, who can be shown to be in negative calcium balance during acidosis, children, even growing very slowly, maintain a positive calcium balance during acidosis.[53] Recent experiments have elucidated some of these mechanisms. In humans, experimentally induced metabolic acidosis blunts secretory pulses of GH by the anterior pituitary.[54] Furthermore, hepatic GH receptor expression and IGF-1 mRNA are also decreased.[55] In rats, it can be shown that endochondral growth can be inhibited by an acid media.[56] This appears to be the result of a reduction in IGF-1 and GH receptors on the endochondral cells.[57]

## TREATMENT OF THE ACIDOSIS OF RENAL FAILURE

Although the effects of chronic acidosis are fairly well documented and significant, it is not entirely clear to what extent treatment is beneficial, especially in predialysis patients. As noted earlier, in children, treatment to maintain normal blood pH may promote normal growth and is thus definitely indicated. Further, treatment of chronic acidosis may help to prevent bone disease and catabolism, two of the most significant complications of CRF. However, studies to demonstrate the benefit of treatment in adults have provided mixed results.

Patients with end-stage renal disease may develop severe metabolic acidosis, and in such patients treatment is necessary in the face of life-threatening acidosis (e.g., blood pH $<7.2$). The question then becomes at what point and to what extent should the acidosis be corrected? There are some fears that a high bicarbonate dialysis could lead to a metabolic alkalosis. However, patients on hemodialysis using a high bicarbonate dialysate (i.e., 40 mmol/L) have better control of acidosis and an increase in triceps skinfold thickness when compared with those using a 30-mmol/L bicarbonate dialysate.[58] Furthermore, the higher bicarbonate level is well tolerated. A reasonable goal is to achieve a predialysis serum bicarbonate concentration of 20 mEq/L or greater. If this cannot be achieved via dialysis alone, consideration should be given to the addition of oral $NaHCO_3$ supplements. The additional sodium load may, however, contribute to worsening interdialytic expansion of the extracellular fluid and weight gain.

Few studies have examined the issue of treatment of acidosis in predialysis patients. However, because of the adverse effects of chronic acidosis and the relatively benign nature of treatment, it seems prudent to consider providing oral $NaHCO_3$ supplementation to maintain serum bicarbonate concentration above 18 to 20 mEq/L. $NaHCO_3$ can be given in either tablet or powder form. A 648-mg tablet provides 7.7 mEq $HCO_3$. The goal should be to neutralize fixed acid production, starting at a dose of 0.5 mEq/kg body weight/day or about 2 tablets tid for an adult of average size. Initially, this dose may need to be increased to provide for the additional titration of body fluid buffers, thus restoring serum $[HCO_3]$ into the normal range. The dose may then require adjustment to maintain this level. Powdered $NaHCO_3$ (baking soda), which is less costly, may be used instead of tablets for patients who do not dislike the saltiness of $NaHCO_3$ when dissolved in water. One level teaspoonful equals about 5 g $NaHCO_3$ or about 60 mEq. Thus, the initial dose is a level one-quarter teaspoonful of $NaHCO_3$ (measured with a kitchen one-quarter teaspoon measure) three times a day, which provides about 15 mEq/dose or 45 mEq/day. Bicarbonate may also be administered as Shohl solution (Bicitra), a mixture containing 1 mEq of $Na_3$-citrate/mL in citric acid, the latter providing a lemon flavor to mask the saltiness of $Na_3$-citrate. The initial dose is two teaspoonfuls or 10 mL three times a day. Many patients find this solution more palatable than plain sodium bicarbonate, but others dislike taking liquid medicines. Furthermore, citrate can enhance the intestinal absorption of aluminum[59] in some patients who continue to use aluminum-containing phosphate binders. In any case, the main risk of treatment is the risk of the additional sodium load, especially in patients approaching end-stage renal disease who already may be volume over-loaded and hypertensive. However, sodium retention during $NaHCO_3$ administration appears to be less of a problem than if the sodium is given as an equivalent amount of NaCl.[60]

Finally, diet may play a role. Although the evidence is somewhat equivocal, low-protein diets may slow the progression of some types of renal disease. Also, as we have seen, a large fraction of fixed acids are produced from the metabolism of sulfur-containing amino acids. Thus, a low-protein diet can be expected to decrease the daily acid load and ameliorate chronic acidosis. It is important, however, that such a diet not contribute to malnutrition. Thus, with a few caveats, the treatment of chronic acidosis is cheap, effective, and has considerable potential benefit. However, in adults, it remains unclear at what point in the course of chronic renal insufficiency such treatment should commence. Thus, the potential benefits should be balanced by the potentially adverse effects of the sodium load.

## REFERENCES


1. Peters JP, Van Slyke DD: Quantitative Clinical Chemistry, vol 1. Baltimore, Williams & Wilkins, 1932, pp 984–989.
2. Von Jaksh R: Uber die alkalescenz des blutes bei krankheiten. Z Klin Med 13:350–362, 1888.
3. Schwartz WB, Hall PW, Hayes RM, Relman AS: On the mechanism of acidosis in chronic renal disease. J Clin Invest 38: 39–52, 1958.
4. Wrong O, Davies HEF: The excretion of acid in renal disease. Q J Med 28:259–313, 1959.
5. Elkinton JR: Hydrogen ion turnover in health and renal disease. Ann Intern Med 57:666–684, 1962.
6. Lemann J Jr, Relman AS: The relation of sulfur metabolism to acid-base balance and electrolyte excretion: the effects of dl-methionine in normal man. J Clin Invest 38:2215–2223, 1959.
7. Goodman AD, Lemann J Jr, Lennon EJ, Relman AS: Production, excretion and net balance of fixed acid in patients with renal acidosis. J Clin Invest 44:495–506, 1965.
8. Lemann J Jr, Lennon EJ, Goodman AD, et al: The net balance of acid in subjects given large loads of acid or alkali. J Clin Invest 44:507–517, 1965.
9. Litzow JR, Lemann J Jr, Lennon EJ: The effects of treatment of acidosis on calcium balance in patients with chronic azotemic renal disease. J Clin Invest 46:280–286, 1967.
10. Simpson DP: Control of hydrogen ion homeostasis and renal acidosis. Medicine 50:503–541, 1971.
11. Gonick HC, Kleeman CR, Rubini ME, Maxwell MH: Functional impairment in chronic renal disease: Studies of acid secretion. Nephron 6:28–49, 1969.
12. Widmer B, Gerhardt R, Harrington JT, Cohen JJ: Serum electrolyte and acid base composition: Influence of graded degrees of chronic renal failure. Arch Intern Med 139:1099–1102, 1979.
13. Relman AS, Lennon EJ, Lemann J Jr: Endogenous production of fixed acid production and the measurement of the net balance of acid in normal subjects. J Clin Invest 40:1621–1630, 1961.
14. Lennon EJ, Lemann J Jr, Relman AS: The effects of phosphoproteins on acid balance in normal subjects. J Clin Invest 41:637–645, 1962.
15. Lennon EJ, Lemann J Jr, Litzow JR: The effects of diet and stool composition on the net external acid balance of normal subjects. J Clin Invest 45:1601–1607, 1966.
16. Lemann J Jr, Litzow JR, Lennon EJ: The effects of chronic acid loads in normal man: Further evidence for the participation of bone mineral in the defense against chronic metabolic acidosis. J Clin Invest 45:1608–1614, 1966.
17. Lennon EJ, Lemann J Jr: The effect of a potassium deficient diet on the pattern of recovery from experimental metabolic acidosis. Clin Sci 34:365–378, 1968.
18. Weber HP, Gray RW, Dominguez JH, Lemann J Jr: The lack of effect of chronic metabolic acidosis on 25-OH-vitamin D metabolism and serum parathyroid hormone in humans. J Clin Endocrinol Metab 43:1047–1055, 1976.
19. Adams ND, Gray RW, Lemann J Jr: The calciuria of increased fixed acid production in humans: Evidence against a role for parathyroid hormone and 1,25-$(OH)_2$-vitamin D. Calcif Tissue Int 27:233–239, 1979.
20. Lemann J Jr, Gray RW, Pleuss JA: Potassium bicarbonate, but not sodium bicarbonate, reduces urinary calcium excretion and improves calcium balance in healthy men. Kidney Int 35:688–695, 1989.
21. Relman AS: Renal acidosis and renal excretion of acid in health and disease. Ann Intern Med 12:295–345, 1964.
22. Slatopolsky E, Hoffsten P, Purkerson M, Bricker NS: On the influence of extracellular fluid volume expansion and of uremia on bicarbonate reabsorption in man. J Clin Invest 49:988–998, 1970.
23. Simon E, Martin D, Buerkert J: Handling of ammonium by the renal proximal tubule during acute metabolic acidosis. Am J Physiol 245:F680–F686, 1983.
24. Oliver J (ed): Architecture of the Kidney in Chronic Bright's Disease. New York, Paul B Hoeber, 1939.
25. Dorhout-Mees EJ, Machado M, Slatopolsky E, et al: The functional adaptation of the diseased kidney: Ammonium excretion. J Clin Invest 45:289–296, 1966.
26. Tizianello A, De Ferrari G, Garibotto G, et al: Renal metabolism of amino acids and ammonia in subjects with normal renal function and in patients with chronic renal insufficiency. J Clin Invest 65:1162–1173, 1980.
27. Buerkert J, Martin D, Trigg D, Simon E: Effect of reduced renal mass on ammonium handling and net acid formation by the superficial and juxtamedullary nephron of the rat. J Clin Invest 71:1661–1675, 1983.
28. Pennell JP, Bourgoignie JJ: Adaptive changes of juxtamedullary glomerular filtration in the remnant kidney. Pflugers Arch 389: 131–135, 1981.
29. Finkelstein FO, Hayslett JP: Role of medullary structures in the functional adaptation of renal insufficiency. Kidney Int 6: 419–425, 1974.
30. Ambuhl PM, Zajicek HK, Wang H, et al: Regulation of renal phosphate transport by acute and chronic metabolic acidosis in the rat. Kidney Int 53:1288–1298, 1998.
31. Slatopolsky E, Gradowska L, Kashemsant C, et al: The control of phosphate excretion in uremia. J Clin Invest 45:672–677, 1966.
32. Kumar R: Tumor-induced osteomalacia and the regulation of phosphate homeostasis [Review]. Bone 27:333–338, 2000.
33. Kildeberg P, Engel K, Winters RW, et al: Balance of net acid in growing infants. Acta Pediatr Scand 58:321–329, 1969.
34. Bushinsky DA, Lechleider RJ: Mechanism of proton-induced bone calcium release: Calcium carbonate dissolution. Am J Physiol 253:F998–F1005, 1987.
35. Bushinsky DA: Net calcium efflux from live bone during chronic metabolic, but not respiratory, acidosis. Am J Physiol 256:F836–F842, 1989.
36. Oh MS: Irrelevance of bone buffering to acid-base homeostasis in chronic metabolic acidosis. Nephron 59:7–10, 1991.
37. Lefebvre A, de Vernejoul MC, Gueris J, et al: Optimal correction of acidosis changes progression of dialysis osteodystrophy. Kidney Int 36:1112–1118, 1989.
38. Lu K, Shieh S, Li B, et al: Rapid correction of metabolic acidosis in chronic renal failure: Effect on parathyroid hormone activity. Nephron 67:419–424, 1994.
39. Graham KA, Hoenich NA, Tarbit M, et al: Correction of acidosis in hemodialysis patients increases the sensitivity of the parathyroid glands to calcium. J Am Soc Nephrol 8:627–631, 1997.
40. Ballmer PE, McNurlan MA, Hulter H, et al: Chronic metabolic acidosis decreases albumin synthesis and induces negative nitrogen balance in humans. J Clin Invest 95:39–45, 1995.
41. Reaich D, Channon SM, Scrimgeour CM, et al: Ammonium

chloride-induced acidosis increases protein breakdown and amino acid oxidation in humans. Am J Physiol 263:E735–E739, 1992.
42. Seyffart G, Ensminger A, Scholz R, et al: Increase of body mass during long-term bicarbonate hemodialysis. Kidney Int 32(S22): S174–S177, 1987.
43. Reaich D, Channon S, Scrimgeour CM, et al: Correction of acidosis in humans with CRF decreases protein degradation and amino acid oxidation. Am J Physiol 28:E230–E235, 1993.
44. Graham KA, Reaich D, Channon S, et al: Correction of acidosis in hemodialysis decreases whole-body protein degradation. J Am Soc Nephrol 8:632–637, 1996.
45. Movilli E, Zani R, Carli O, et al: Correction of metabolic acidosis increases serum albumin concentrations and decreases kinetically evaluated protein intake in hemodialysis patients: A prospective study. Nephrol Dial Transplant 13:1719–1722, 1998.
46. Walls J: Effect of correction of acidosis on nutritional status in dialysis patients. Miner Electrolyte Metab 23:234–236, 1997.
47. Bailey JL, Wang X, England BK, et al: The acidosis of chronic renal failure activates muscle proteolysis in rats by augmenting transcription of genes encoding proteins of the ATP-dependent ubiquitin-proteasome pathway. J Clin Invest 97:1447–1453, 1996.
48. Price SR, Reaich D, Marinovic AC, et al: Mechanisms contributing to muscle wasting in acute uremia: Activation of amino acid catabolism. J Am Soc Nephrol 9:439–443, 1998.
49. Garibotto G: Muscle amino acid metabolism and the control of muscle protein turnover in patients with chronic renal failure. Nutrition 15:145–155, 1999.
50. Bergstrom J, Wang T, Lindholm B: Factors contributing to catabolism in end-stage renal disease patients. Miner Electrolyte Metab 24:92–101, 1998.
51. Nath KA, Hostetter MK, Hostetter TH: Pathophysiology of chronic tubulo-interstitial disease in rats: Interactions of dietary acid load, ammonia, and complement component C3. J Clin Invest 76:667–675, 1985.
52. Caldas A, Broyer M, Dechaux M, Kleinknecht C: Primary distal tubular acidosis in childhood: Clinical study and long-term follow-up of 28 patients. J Pediatr 121:233–241, 1992.
53. Chan JC: Renal tubular acidosis. J Pediatr 102:327–340, 1983.
54. Challa A, Chan W, Krieg RJ Jr, et al: Effect of metabolic acidosis on the expression of insulin-like growth factor and growth hormone receptor. Kidney Int 44:1224–1227, 1993.
55. Krieg RJ Jr, Santos F, Chan JC: Growth hormone, insulin-like growth factor and the kidney. Kidney Int 48:321–336, 1995.
56. Kuemmerle N, Krieg RJ, Catta K, et al: Growth hormone and insulin-like growth factor in non-uremic acidosis and uremic acidosis. Kidney Int S58:S102–S105, 1997.
57. Green J, Maor G: Effect of metabolic acidosis on the growth hormone/IGF-1 endocrine axis in skeletal growth centers. Kidney Int 57:2258–2267, 2000.
58. Williams AJ, Dittmer ID, McArley A, Clarke J: High bicarbonate dialysate in haemodialysis patients: Effects on acidosis and nutritional status. Nephrol Dial Transplant 12:2633–2637, 1997.
59. Molitoris BA, Froment BH, Mackenzie TA, et al: Citrate: A major factor in the toxicity or orally administered aluminum compounds. Kidney Int 36:949, 1989.
60. Husted FC, Nolph KD: $NaHCO_3$ and NaCl tolerance in chronic renal failure. Clin Nephrol 7:21–25, 1977.

Section II

# Water

CHAPTER 13

# Cell Biology of Vasopressin and Aquaporins

David Sheikh-Hamad, MD ▪ David Marples, MD ▪ Søren Nielsen, MD, PhD

The discovery of aquaporin membrane water channels by Agre and colleagues answered a long-standing question regarding how water crosses biologic membranes and provided the impetus for the study of physiology and pathophysiology of water balance disorders. Of nine known aquaporin isoforms, at least six are expressed in the kidney at distinct nephron sites. Aquaporin type 1 (AQP1) is abundant in the proximal tubule and descending thin limb, where it provides the chief route for proximal nephron water reabsorption. AQP2 is abundant in the collecting duct principal cells and is the chief target for vasopressin-regulated water entry through the collecting ducts. Acutely, AQP2 regulation involves vasopressin-mediated trafficking between an intracellular reservoir and the apical plasma membrane. Chronically, changes in AQP2 protein abundance provide adaptive responses for long-term regulation of water balance. Importantly, multiple studies have now identified a critical role for AQP2 in several inherited and more commonly acquired types of nephrogenic diabetes insipidus (NDI) as well as renal failure, where AQP2 expression and targeting are decreased. Conversely, AQP2 expression and targeting are increased in some water-retentive states such as pregnancy and congestive heart failure (CHF). AQP3 and AQP4 are basolateral water channels located in the collecting duct, whereas AQP6 is an intracellular water channel in intercalated cells in the collecting duct. AQP7 is expressed in the brush border of the straight proximal tubule. This chapter is based on previous reviews[1–6] and focuses mainly on the role of AQP2 in the regulation of water balance in normal and some pathophysiologic states.

## VASOPRESSIN AND ITS RECEPTORS

Vasopressin and oxytocin are cyclic nonapeptides whose actions are mediated by stimulation of specific G protein-coupled receptors currently classified into vascular ($V_1$), renal tubular ($V_2$), pituitary ($V_3$), vasopressin, and oxytocin receptors.[7] In addition, a fourth vasopressin receptor subtype, which also responds to angiotensin II, has been reported. This dual angiotensin II/arginine vasopressin (AVP) receptor is a novel angiotensin II/$V_2$ receptor, combined with adenylate cyclase, and responds with equal sensitivity to angiotensin II and AVP. Based on immunocytochemical studies, the distribution of angiotensin II/AVP receptor in the kidney is confined to the outer medullary thick ascending limbs and inner medullary collecting ducts, suggesting an important role for this receptor in renal tubular sodium and fluid reabsorption.[8] Vasopressin is secreted by the paraventricular nucleus in the hypothalamus and modulates pituitary adrenocorticotropic hormone (ACTH) secretion through a V1b-receptor–mediated process. Regulation of V1b receptors contributes to the adaptation of the hypothalamic-pituitary-adrenal axis to stress, as evidenced by the correlation between vasopressin receptor number and pituitary ACTH responsiveness.[9] Vasopressin is also synthesized and secreted by the adrenal medulla in many species including human. V1a receptors are present in the adrenal gland and are involved in the secretion of steroid hormones (aldosterone and glucocorticoids) in some species. Thus, vasopressin regulates adrenal gland function through autocrine and paracrine mechanisms.[10] The peptide sequences of vasopressin and oxytocin differ only in the amino acids at positions 3 and 8. The formation of a disulfide bond between cysteine residues at positions 1 and 6 produces a cyclic peptide with a carboxy terminal tail containing three amino acids. Although both hormones share similarities in their action, oxytocin is known for its ability to elicit uterine smooth muscle contraction, whereas the primary role of vasopressin is the facilitation of water reabsorption by the kidney. In addition, it is well recognized that vasopressin and oxytocin are involved in numerous central nervous system (CNS) processes, including higher cognitive functions such as memory and learning.[11] Systemically and centrally administered AVP improves performance in avoidance tasks in experimental animals. However, the physiologic mechanism of action for this effect and whether the cognitive enhancing actions of AVP reflect learning or performance are not well characterized. Some of the effects may be secondary to increases in blood pressure. However, centrally administered AVP can facilitate memory, in part by activating AVP systems in the lateral septum. These data suggest that the cognitive-enhancing actions of AVP may involve two parallel, but ultimately homologous, systems at the functional level. Thus, circulating AVP may facilitate memory through nonspecific (performance) effects, whereas centrally derived

AVP may facilitate memory through a direct effect on the neural substrates of memory processing in the limbic system.[12]

In the kidney, vasopressin exerts its effects through stimulation of V1a (blood vessels) and $V_2$ (tubules) receptors. In addition to its action on collecting duct cells to increase water conductance, vasopressin reduces blood flow to the inner medulla (V1a receptor-mediated nitric oxide activation) while maintaining a constant blood flow to the outer medulla. The reduction of medullary blood flow is necessary for optimization of urine osmolality during water restriction.[13] Additional actions of vasopressin include stimulation of liver glycogenolysis, platelet adhesion, and adrenal angiotensin II secretion—effects that are mediated through V1a receptor activation.[14] Antidiuretic hormone (ADH) synthesis or release may be induced by various stimuli. Most important of these are high osmolarity and decreased effective arterial blood volume (EABV). Small changes in serum osmolality, above 280 mosmol/kg $H_2O$, such as those seen with clinically relevant hypernatremia, will lead to a steep rise in serum ADH levels. Similarly, decreased EABV is the driving force for ADH release in patients with CHF and cirrhosis, hence the sodium and water retention. This driving force overrides the inhibitory effects of hyponatremia on ADH release, if hyponatremia were to coexist. In addition, ADH is released with noxious stimuli, during stress, and with nausea—conditions that are commonly encountered after surgery. Administration of hypotonic solutions under these circumstances may lead to the development of acute hyponatremia. Please review Table 13–1 for conditions associated with elevated ADH release.

Over the past several years, an orally active and specific vasopressin $V_1$ receptor antagonist—OPC-21268—became available. Administration of OPC-21268 (intravenously or orally) induces vasodilation in a dose-dependent manner and thus may have clinical potentials in certain hypertensive disorders. In addition, an orally active and specific vasopressin $V_2$ receptor antagonist—OPC-31260—was also introduced. Oral administration of OPC-31260 inhibits the antidiuretic action of AVP and may be useful in the management of hyponatremia and disorders of water overload.[15] However, judicious use of this drug is advised, owing to the potential for the development of hypernatremia and CNS complications.

**TABLE 13–1.** Stimuli for Antidiuretic Hormone Release

| Decreased Effective Arterial Blood Volume |
|---|
| **Endogenous Stimuli** |
| Pain |
| Nausea |
| Stress |
| Thirst |
| Hypertonic states: hypernatremia, hyperglycemia, contrast dye, mannitol |
| **Hormones** |
| Angiotensin II |
| Isoproterenol |
| Glucocorticoid deficiency |
| Hypothyroidism |
| **Drugs** |
| Anesthesia |
| Diuretics: thiazide diuretics, ethacrynic acid, furosemide |
| Hypoglycemic agents: sulfonylurea, chlorpropamide, tolbutamide |
| Lipid-lowering agents: clofibrate |
| Psychotropic drugs: trifluoperazine, fluphenazine, haloperidol, amitriptyline |
| Antiepileptics: carbamazepine |
| Monoamine oxidase inhibitors |
| Chemotherapeutic agents: vincristine, vinblastine |
| Opiates: morphine, demerol, methadone |
| Nicotine |
| Bromocriptine |
| **Pulmonary Diseases** |
| Asthma, pneumonia, pneumothorax, cystic fibrosis, positive-pressure breathing, acute respiratory syndrome |
| **CNS Diseases** |
| Infection, brain tumor, brain abscess, CVA, subarachnoid or subdural bleed, hydrocephalus, collagen vascular disease, schizo-affective disorders, delirium tremens, electroshock therapy, malignancy hypertension, spinal cord injury, porphyria, multiple sclerosis |
| **Malignancies** |
| Carcinoma of the lung, pancreas, duodenum, kidney, ureter, bladder, prostate, cervix, endometrium, tongue, nasopharynx |
| Lymphoma, sarcoma, mesothelioma, multiple myeloma |

## RENAL AQUAPORINS AND THEIR STRUCTURE

Of the known aquaporins, at least six are expressed in the kidney (AQP1, -2, -3, -4, -6, -7, and -8) (Tables 13–2 and 13–3). Among these, three are expressed in the collecting duct (i.e., AQP2, -3, and -4). AQP2,[16] the "vasopressin-regulated water channel," is the apical water channel of collecting duct principal cells and is the chief target for short-term regulation of water permeability by vasopressin.[1, 5, 6] Long-term regulation of AQP2 also occurs and is mediated through changes in the total abundance of AQP2 in collecting duct cells.[1, 6] In addition, studies suggest a role for aquaporins in disorders of water balance. Moreover, gene knockout studies of aquaporins have confirmed their essential role in water balance regulation.

Aquaporins have six membrane spanning domains. Both the amino and carboxy termini are cytoplasmic and have similar internal tandem repeats that are presumably the result of ancient gene duplication.[2] It is believed that the tandem repeats, which contain asparagine-proline-alanine (APA), form interacting tight-turn structures in the membrane to create the pathway for water translocation across the plasma membrane. Two of the loops in AQP1 (B and E) are believed to form "hemi-channels" that connect between the membrane leaflets to form a single pathway within a symmetric structure that resembles an "hourglass."[17] AQP1 and AQP2 (and possibly also AQP3 and AQP5) exist as tetramers,[18, 19] whereas AQP4 exists as multimeric membrane aggregates resembling square arrays.[20]

Since the discovery of aquaporins, it has become apparent that osmotic water transport across the tu-

**TABLE 13–2.** Distribution of Aquaporins 1 to 9 in the Kidney and Other Organs

| Group | Species | No. of Amino Acids | Localization in Kidney | Subcellular Distribution | Regulation | Extrarenal Localization |
|---|---|---|---|---|---|---|
| ***Renal Aquaporins*** | | | | | | |
| Aquaporin 1 | Human | 269 | Proximal tubules, descending thin limbs | APM/BLM | – | Multiple organs |
| Aquaporin 2 | Rat | 271 | Collecting duct principal cells | APM VES | + + + | Testis |
| Aquaporin 3 | Rat | 292 | Collecting duct | BLM | + | Multiple organs |
| Aquaporin 4 | Rat | 301 | Medullary collecting duct | BLM | – | Brain and multiple organs |
| Aquaporin 6 | Rat | 276 | Cortex, medulla ? | ? | ? | ? |
| Aquaporin 7 | Rat | 269 | Proximal tubule | APM ? | ? | Testis, fat, epididymis |
| ***Extrarenal Aquaporins*** | | | | | | |
| Aquaporin 5 | Rat | 265 | ? | | | Submandibular gland |
| Aquaporin 8 | Rat | 263 | ? | | | Testis, pancreas, liver, colon, heart, placenta |

APM, apical plasma membrane; BLM, basolateral plasma membrane; VES, intracellular vesicles.

bule epithelium is chiefly dependent on aquaporin water channels.[1] This is supported by the work of Schnermann and colleagues, who demonstrated larger gradients of osmolality between the proximal tubule fluid and the blood in AQP1 knockout mice compared with control mice (30 versus 10 mOsm/kg $H_2O$).[21] The archetypical member of aquaporins, AQP1, is highly abundant in the proximal tubule and descending thin limb of Henle (Figs. 13–1 and 13–2), and it constitutes almost 3% of total membrane protein in the kidney.[3] It localizes to both the apical and basolateral membranes, consistent with a role for transcellular water reabsorption in the proximal nephron.[22] A critical role for AQP1 in urinary concentration was confirmed in transgenic knockout mice that lack AQP1.[23] AQP1-deficient mice manifest polyuria and severe concentrating defect. Water deprivation in these animals leads to marked dehydration and hypernatremia, whereas tubule perfusion analysis reveals 80% to 90% reduction in water permeability of the proximal tubules and descending limbs.[24] These studies strongly suggest that the major pathway for water reabsorption in the proximal tubule and descending thin limb is transcellular (via AQP1) and not paracellular. It is interesting that the predominant phenotype in transgenic mice lacking AQP1 is a medullary-concentrating defect. This suggests the presence of compensatory mechanisms or additional pathways for water absorption in the proximal tubule in the absence of AQP1. The expression of AQP7 in proximal tubules suggests that this channel may form the entry route for proximal tubule water reabsorption in AQP1-deficient mice.

AQP2[16] is abundantly expressed in the apical plasma membrane and subapical vesicles in collecting duct principal cells (Figs. 13–3, see Color Plate, and 13–4)[25] and at lower abundance in connecting tubules.[26] This channel is the target of vasopressin-regulated water reabsorption in the collecting ducts,[1] which is a conclusion that is based on several studies. AQP2 expression correlates directly with collecting duct water permeability in humans and experimental animals.[27–29] Mutations in the human AQP2 gene[28] or 95% reduction in AQP2 expression in rats[29] are associated with profound NDI. AQP3 and AQP4 are expressed in multiple organs.[30] These channels are present in collecting duct principal cells, where they localize to the basolateral

**TABLE 13–3.** Physiologic Conditions or Water Balance Disorders Associated with Altered Expression and/or Targeting of AQP2

- Conditions with reduced AQP2 expression and polyuria
  - Genetic defects
    - Brattleboro rats (central DI)
    - DI +/+ severe mice (low cAMP)
    - AQP2 mutants (human)
    - $V_2$ receptor variants (human)
  - Acquired NDI (rat models)
    - Lithium
    - Hypokalemia
    - Hypercalcemia
    - Postobstructive NDI
      - Bilateral
      - Unilateral
  - Low-protein diet (urinary concentrating defect with no polyuria)
  - Water loading (compulsive water drinking)
  - Experimental chronic renal failure (5/6 nephrectomy model)
  - Ischemia-induced acute renal failure (polyuric phase in rat model)
  - Age-induced NDI
- Conditions with reduced AQP2 expression and altered urinary concentration and dilution without polyuria
  - Nephrotic syndrome models (rat models)
    - PAN
    - Adriamycin
    - Hepatic cirrhosis (CBL, compensated)
  - Ischemia-induced acute renal failure (oliguric phase in rat model)
- Conditions with increased AQP2 expression with expansion of extracellular fluid volume
  - Vasopressin infusion (SIADH)
  - Congestive heart failure
  - Hepatic cirrhosis ($CCL_4$-induced, noncompensated)?
  - Pregnancy

AQP2, aquaporin type 2; DI, diabetes insipidus; NDI, nephrogenic diabetes insipidus; PAN, puromycin aminonucleoside; CBL, common bile duct ligation; SIADH, syndrome of inappropriate secretion of antidiuretic hormone.

Reduced $V_2$ receptor density has profound effect on the AQP2 targeting and expression. A mild increase occurs in urine production rates.

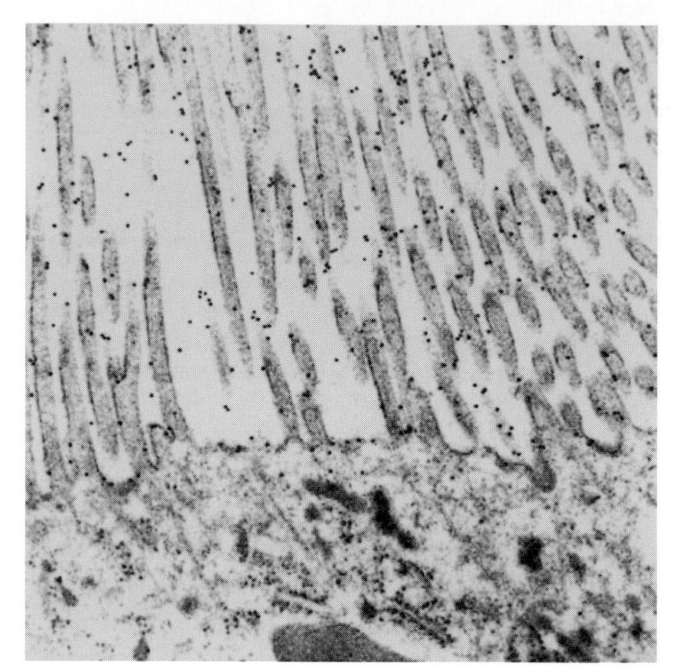

**FIGURE 13–1** ■ Immunoelectron microscopic localization of AQP1 in segment 3 proximal tubule (cryosubstituted and low-temperature Lowicryl HM20-embedded tissue). AQP1 is very abundant in the apical plasma membrane of the brush border (×390,000).

membrane, representing potential exit pathways for water from the collecting ducts. Studies on AQP4 knockout mice reveal a mild urinary concentrating defect,[23] whereas inner medulla collecting duct (IMCD) tubule perfusion analysis reveals a fourfold reduction in water permeability.[31] These findings indicate that AQP4 is responsible for basolateral membrane water movement in IMCDs. The lower abundance of AQP4 in cortical and outer medullary collecting duct basolateral membranes, together with higher abundance of AQP3 in these segments, suggest that AQP3 may play a more significant role in water exit from these sites. The severe urinary concentrating defect found in transgenic mice lacking AQP3 is consistent with that.

# REGULATION OF AQUAPORINS

## Short-Term Regulation of AQP2

On the basis of indirect biophysical evidence, it has been suspected for many years that the vasopressin-induced increase in water permeability in the collecting duct was dependent on the appearance of specific water channels in the apical plasma membrane of the vasopressin-responsive cells. Osmotic water permeability of the apical plasma membrane in collecting duct cells, the rate-limiting step in water reabsorption in this segment, may be regulated by at least two different mechanisms: (1) a post-translational modification of the channel, thus regulating the water conductance, or (2) a change in the number of functional water channels in the membrane by vasopressin-regulated AQP2 trafficking. The presence of AQP2 in small subapical vesicles favored the latter hypothesis, and several in vitro and in vivo studies have now established regulated AQP2 trafficking as the mechanism for acute changes in water conductance following vasopressin stimulation. In vitro studies in isolated perfused tubules demonstrated direct correlation between water conductance and the density of AQP2 labeling in the apical plasma membrane.[32] Furthermore, in vivo studies in vasopressin-deficient Brattleboro rats have also shown a marked increase in apical plasma membrane labeling for AQP2 in response to vasopressin or 1-deamino (8-D-arginine) vasopressin (DDAVP) treatment.[33–35] Conversely, acute treatment of rats with a vasopressin ($V_2$) receptor antagonist[36, 37] or water loading (to reduce endogenous vasopressin levels[38]) results in internalization of AQP2 from the apical plasma membrane to small intracellular vesicles (Fig. 13–5), further supporting the role of AQP2 trafficking in the regulation of collecting duct water permeability.

Cyclic adenosine monophosphate (cAMP) levels in collecting duct principal cells are increased by binding of vasopressin to $V_2$ receptors.[39, 40] The synthesis of cAMP by adenylate cyclase is stimulated by $V_2$ receptor-coupled heterotrimeric guanosine triphosphate (GTP)-binding protein, Gs. Upregulation of collecting duct water conductance by vasopressin-mediated adenylate cyclase activation suggests involvement of protein

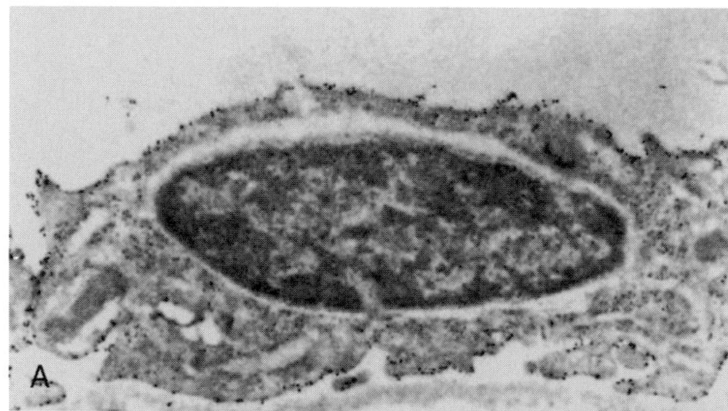


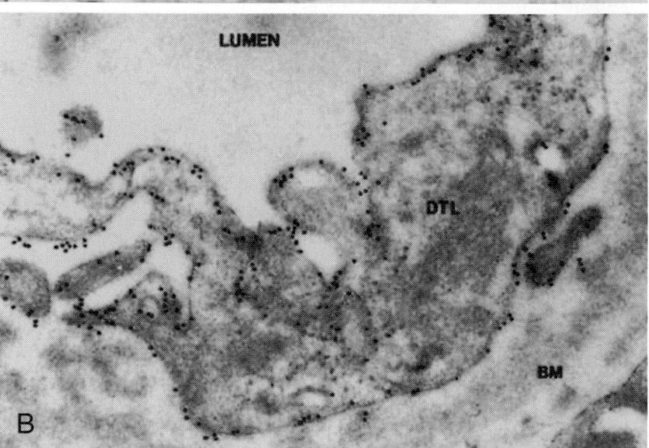


**FIGURE 13–2** ■ Immunoelectron microscopic localization of AQP1 in descending thin limbs (DTL) of the loop of Henle (cryosubstituted and low-temperature Lowicryl HM20–embedded tissue). AQP1 is very abundant in both the apical and basolateral plasma membrane. The lumen and the basement membrane (BM) are indicated.

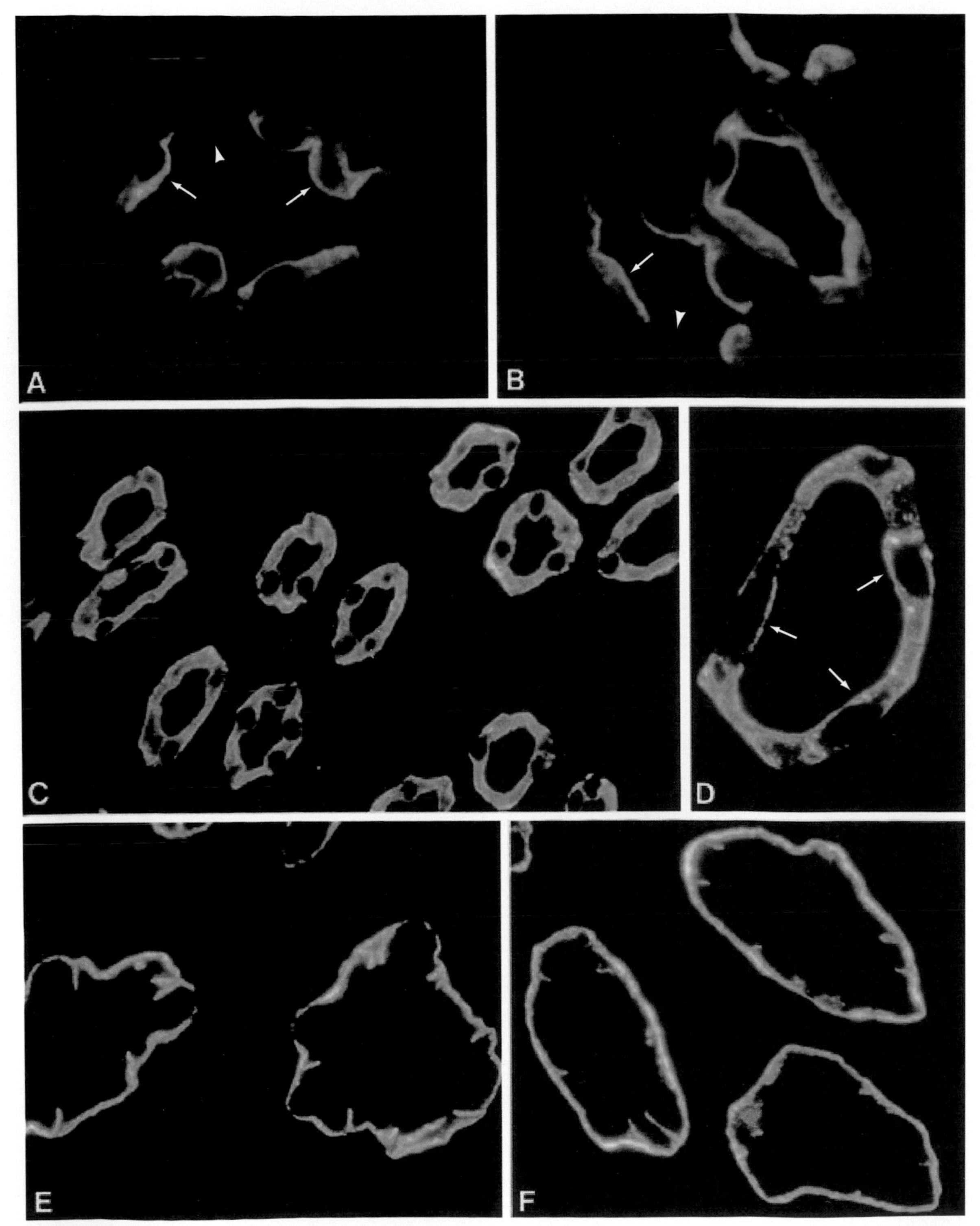


**FIGURE 13–3** ■ Immunofluorescence microscopy of AQP2 in cortical (*A*), outer medullary (*B*), and inner medullary (*C* and *D*) collecting duct, and of AQP3 (*E*) and AQP4 (*F*) in the inner medullary collecting duct. AQP2 is very abundant in the apical plasma membrane domains as well as in subapical domains (*arrows* in panels *A, B,* and *D*), whereas intercalated cells are unlabeled (*arrowheads* in panels *A* and *B*). In the inner medullary collecting duct, AQP2 is also present in the basolateral part of the cell. AQP3 is abundant in both basal and lateral plasma membranes, whereas AQP4 is expressed predominantly in the basal plasma membrane and less prominently in the lateral plasma membranes. (×31100 in *A, B,* and *D* through *F*; ×3550 in *C*.)

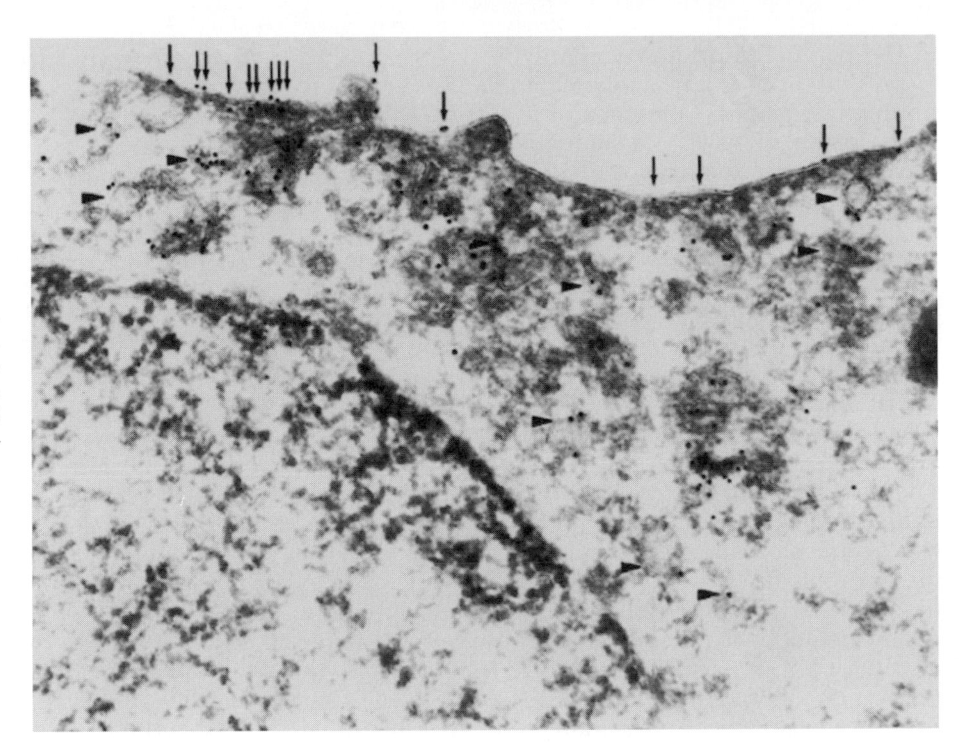

**FIGURE 13–4** ■ Immunoelectron microscopic labeling of AQP2 in an ultrathin cryosection of the inner medullary collecting duct. AQP2 is abundant both in the apical plasma membrane *(arrows)* and in small subapical vesicles *(arrowheads)*.

kinase A (PKA) in AQP2 regulation. Examination of PKA-mediated post-translational modification of AQP2 protein as a mechanism for regulation of water conductance has yielded interesting results. Although PKA-mediated AQP2 phosphorylation (serine 256) may be involved in trafficking of AQP2-containing vesicles from the subapical compartment to the plasma membrane,[41–43] it does not significantly modify water conductance of the channel.[44, 45] Thus, vasopressin-regulated trafficking of AQP2 appears to be the major regulator of collecting duct water permeability.[44, 45] Analysis of the effects of prostaglandins on water conductance has provided additional insight into the interaction between ADH and prostaglandins. Prostaglandin $E_2$ inhibits vasopressin-induced water permeability by reducing cAMP levels.[4] In addition, data from Zelenina and associates suggest that prostaglandins are involved in the retrieval of AQP2 from the plasma membrane, an effect that is independent of AQP2 phosphorylation by PKA.[46]

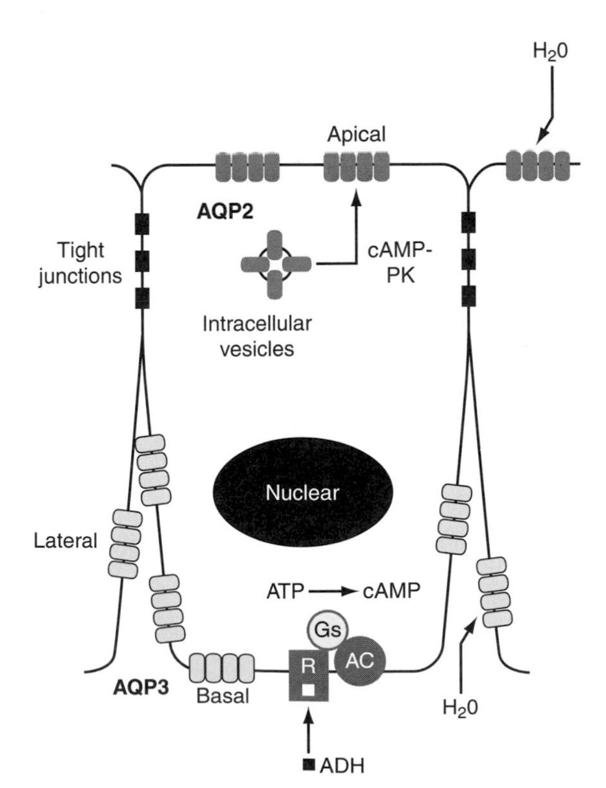


**FIGURE 13–5** ■ Diagram representing vasopressin-regulated transcellular water permeation of the apical membrane of the collecting duct principal cell via AQP2 and constitutive water permeation of the basolateral membrane via AQP3. (From Agre P: Aquaporin water channels in the kidney. J Am Soc Nephrol 11[4]:764–777, 2000.)

## Cellular Processes Underlying AQP2 Trafficking

Because the fundamentals of the shuttle hypothesis have been confirmed, interest has turned to the cellular mechanisms mediating AQP2 transfer to the apical membrane following vasopressin stimulation. The shuttle hypothesis has several features whose molecular mechanisms are poorly understood. First, AQP2-containing vesicles move from a distribution throughout the cell to the apical region of the cell in response to vasopressin; this movement is *specific, rapid,* and highly *coordinated.* Second, AQP2-bearing vesicles fuse with the apical plasma membrane in response to vasopressin, but not to a significant degree in the absence of vasopressin stimulation, despite AQP2 availability in the cell. This is clearly demonstrated in vasopressin-deficient Brattleboro rats, where baseline cellular AQP2 protein level is approximately one third of that in the parent strain; however, only 5% of total AQP2 is present in the apical plasma membrane.[47] These findings suggest the presence of a "clamp" that prevents fusion of AQP2-containing subapical vesicle to the plasma membrane in the absence of vasopressin "trigger."

The coordinated delivery of AQP2 to the apical membrane is dependent on translocation of AQP2-bearing vesicles along cytoskeletal elements, in particular, the microtubular network. Chemical disruption of microtubules inhibits the increase in permeability both in toad's bladder (a model for the study of collecting ducts) and in the mammalian collecting duct.[48, 49] However, whereas microtubule-disruptive agents inhibit the development of the hydrosmotic response to vasopressin, they have no effect on the maintenance of an established response. In addition, microtubule-disruptive agents slow the development of the response to vasopressin without affecting the final permeability in toad bladders.[50] These results suggest the involvement of microtubules in the coordinated delivery of water channels, without actual involvement in channel insertion or recycling. Lastly, the delivery of AQP2-bearing vesicles to the apical membrane resembles neuronal synaptic transmission. Although this phenomenon has not yet been proved, it is supported by the expression of a number of proteins in collecting duct cells, which are normally involved in the mechanics of neuronal transmission.[51–54]

## Long-Term Regulation of AQP2

Water permeability of the collecting duct is regulated in two distinct ways: (1) short-term vasopressin-regulated trafficking of AQP2 between intracellular vesicles and the apical plasma membrane, and (2) long-term regulation of AQP2 via mechanisms that alter the total abundance of AQP2, thus modulating the acute response. Hence, the short-term and long-term mechanisms act in concert. These conclusions are based on the following observations. First, water restriction for 24 to 48 hours, or DDAVP treatment for 5 days, result in a marked increase in AQP2 protein levels in the rat's inner medulla, an effect that is paralleled by a large increase in the acute response of collecting duct to vasopressin.[25, 27] Second, Brattleboro rats (which lack vasopressin) or normal rats treated with $V_2$ receptor antagonist for a prolonged period[55, 56] express low levels of AQP2, suggesting that vasopressin is important for the chronic adaptive changes in AQP2 levels and hence water permeability. In addition, water loading decreases the overall abundance of AQP2, presumably by decreasing vasopressin levels. The chronic adaptive change in AQP2 is ascribed to transcriptional regulation of AQP2 gene, presumably through a cAMP-responsive element in its promoter.[57–59] Conversely, downregulation of AQP2 expression (e.g., in response to water loading) is likely to be the result of reduced gene transcription or enhanced AQP2 protein degradation.

## Vasopressin-Independent Regulation of AQP2

The presence of a cAMP-responsive element in AQP2 gene promoter[60] and a PKA phosphorylation site in the protein[8, 16] are consistent with vasopressin-dependent regulation of AQP2. However, some studies have suggested the presence of vasopressin-independent signaling mechanisms in AQP2 regulation, which may play an important role in AQP2 physiology and pathophysiology. First, in a rat model of lithium-induced nephrogenic diabetes insipidus (NDI), in which AQP2 level is downregulated, Marples and associates showed that water deprivation increases AQP2 expression more than sustained DDAVP treatment, suggesting that dehydration induces AQP2 beyond the level achieved by vasopressin stimulation.[29] A second line of evidence was provided by Ecelbarger and associates,[61] using a rat model for the study of inappropriate ADH syndrome (SIADH). In this study, rats were water-loaded while receiving continuous infusion of ADH through subcutaneously implanted mini-pumps for 7 days. Surprisingly, on day 3, and despite high circulating levels of ADH, AQP2 levels in the inner medulla of water-loaded rats was only 17% of that observed in ADH-treated animals that did not receive water loading. These data suggest that although vasopressin stimulation increases total AQP2 protein in normal physiologic states (e.g., dehydration), ADH effects on AQP2 appear to be overridden in the setting of water overload, thus providing a "vasopressin escape." In a subsequent study, it became apparent that this phenomenon is related to downregulation of cAMP production in response to vasopressin stimulation, and hence AQP2 production and targeting to the plasma membrane are attenuated.[62] These studies demonstrate that reduction of AQP2 level plays a major role in "vasopressin escape" and suggest the presence of a hitherto unknown signal that provides a mechanism for downregulation of AQP2, despite high circulating vasopressin levels. Third, treatment of normal rats with OPC31260, a specific vasopressin $V_2$ receptor antagonist, causes a decrease in AQP2 expression,[37, 55] albeit only to one half the level observed in normal controls.[55] Subsequent water deprivation in OPC31260-treated animals reveals normalization of AQP2 levels despite continued blockade of $V_2$ receptors.[55] Thus, water deprivation increases AQP2 levels through a vasopressin-independent mechanism.[29] This observation was clearly demonstrated in additional studies in Brattleboro rats that lack vasopressin.[63] Despite vasopressin deficiency, during dehydration, AQP2 levels reach 30% to 60% of those seen in normal Wistar rats,[63, 64] further emphasizing the potential importance of vasopressin-independent signaling pathways in AQP2 regulation.

Long-term adaptive changes in response to vasopressin treatment or water deprivation may also induce major changes in the expression and activity of other transporters (mainly, Na transporters). These transporters are responsible for the generation of the concentration gradient in the medulla, the driving force for water reabsorption via aquaporins. The interaction between these transporters and aquaporins and its implication on water homeostasis remain to be determined.

## Alternate Mechanisms for AQP2 Regulation

A number of possible signals other than vasopressin could be involved in the control of AQP2. One possible candidate is the rate of diuresis. However, in a rat model of streptozotocin-induced diabetes mellitus with severe glycosuria and osmotic diuresis, AQP2 expression was not significantly altered.[65] Furthermore, significant polyuria, induced by furosemide treatment for 1 or 5 days, had no effect on AQP2 expression,[55] whereas in another study furosemide gave a modest increase in AQP2 expression.[56] Thus, diuresis itself does not appear to cause an alteration in AQP2 expression. Because furosemide causes washout of the medullary interstitial hypertonicity, the furosemide experiments also demonstrate that tonicity is not important in AQP2 signaling. This conclusion is supported by additional observations in lithium- and hypokalemia-induced AQP2 downregulation, where AQP2 expression in the hypertonic medulla and the isotonic cortex is inhibited to an equal extent.[66] Lastly (see later), some studies have revealed regional differences in AQP2 expression, suggesting that local factors may be important in some conditions. This is clearly the case in experiments with unilateral ureteric obstruction, where there is a profound downregulation of AQP2 in the obstructed kidney, with only a modest decrease in the nonobstructed kidney. Thus, in addition to systemic and neural factors that induce change in the *nonobstructed* kidney, the data suggest a role for local factors in AQP2 regulation in the *obstructed* kidney.[67] Such local factors might include pressure effects specific to this model and tissue accumulation of unknown metabolites.

## Regulation of Other Aquaporins

Whereas water movement across the apical plasma membrane of collecting duct principal cells is AQP2-dependent, the available data suggest involvement of AQP3 and AQP4 in water exit through the basolateral membrane. The basolateral membrane has high constitutive water permeability, obviating the need for AQP3 and AQP4 regulation. However, regulated expression of both AQP3 and AQP4, and thus water exit through the basal membrane, has been reported.[56, 68–70] AQP3 expression changes following vasopressin stimulation, as well as in several pathologic states.[68–70] However, changes in AQP3 do not appear to correlate with changes in AQP2, suggesting that the signaling mechanisms that control the expression of these two channels are not always identical.[71, 72] With the exception of Adriamycin-induced nephrotic syndrome model, in which AQP4 expression declines, this channel does not appear to be actively regulated.[69] It is constitutively expressed and appears to provide the major pathway for water exit across the collecting duct basolateral membrane, as AQP4 knockout mice demonstrate an 80% decline in collecting duct water permeability.[73]

More recently, it has become clear that AQP1 plays an important role in the generation of concentrated urine. Although urine output in AQP1 knockout mice appears normal, water deprivation studies reveal urinary concentrating defect, in association with dehydration and hypernatremia.[23] These abnormalities are likely the result of diminished water permeability in the thin descending limb of the loop of Henle, where AQP1 is expressed, with resultant impairment of the countercurrent multiplication system, which is essential for the generation of medullary osmotic gradient. Furthermore, changes in AQP1 have also been reported in several conditions in which a concentrating defect exists, including ureteric obstruction,[74] nephrotic syndrome,[68, 69] and chronic renal failure[70] (see Table 13–2). The signals involved in these changes are currently unknown and may provide future therapeutic targets for modulation of urine osmolality and output.

# ROLE OF AQUAPORINS IN THE PATHOPHYSIOLOGY OF WATER BALANCE DISORDERS

## Central and Nephrogenic Diabetes Insipidus: Role of AQP2

Central diabetes insipidus is a condition characterized by very low or undetectable levels of vasopressin. The polyuria in this condition can be reversed, and urine osmolality can be substantially increased by exogenous administration of arginine vasopressin. Using the vasopressin-deficient Brattleboro rat as a model for the study of central diabetes insipidus, the following insight was gained. Brattleboro rats express low levels of AQP2 in comparison with the parent strain, Long-Evans. As expected, due to the deficiency of vasopressin, which controls AQP2 trafficking to the plasma membrane, labeling for AQP2 in the apical plasma membrane is diminished.[27] Prolonged treatment with either vasopressin or DDAVP results in marked increase in AQP2 expression and its targeting to the apical membrane in both cortical and inner medulla collecting ducts.[27, 35] Another indirect line of evidence for vasopressin-mediated AQP2 dysregulation in diabetes insipidus comes from a mouse strain expressing high cAMP-phosphodiesterase, an important enzyme in cAMP metabolism. In this mouse, cytosolic cAMP levels remain low, and vasopressin cannot provoke a normal antidiuretic response, hence these mice manifest NDI.[75] These animals express approximately one quarter of the normal level of AQP2, and the degree of polyuria correlates with AQP2 expression in the individual mouse tested.[75] These data strongly suggest that AQP2 and cAMP dysregulation play a crucial role in the development of polyuria in diabetes insipidus.

Additional support for the latter was provided by a number of studies.[5, 76, 77] AQP2 is found in the urine at concentrations that inversely correlate with the hydration state. After water loading, AQP2 level in the urine declines and increases with water deprivation.[76] Furthermore, patients with central diabetes insipidus reveal low levels of AQP2 in the urine, which increase following vasopressin injection.[76] Thus, rather than providing a direct measure of AQP2 levels in kidney tissue, urine AQP2 levels vary as a function of vasopressin action on collecting duct principal cells. Because a lack of $V_2$ receptors underlies NDI in most cases, and $V_2$ receptors mediate the antidiuretic actions of vasopressin, the results with central diabetes insipidus predict that AQP2 levels may also be reduced in NDI. Indeed, patients with hereditary NDI reveal low urinary AQP2 levels as well.[76]

Inherited forms of NDI are rare diseases characterized by renal unresponsiveness to vasopressin. The most common form is an X-linked NDI due to mutations in the $V_2$-vasopressin receptor gene.[78] Because both AQP2 targeting and expression are regulated tightly by vasopressin, the reduction in $V_2$-mediated signaling is critical to AQP2 dysregulation, which in turn results in severe polyuria in these patients. Direct evidence for the involvement of AQP2 in this form of diabetes insipidus was provided by Deen and colleagues. Examination of patients with a rare autosomal recessive form of NDI (non–X-linked NDI) reveals mutated AQP2 gene and nonfunctional protein products.[28]

## Dysregulation of AQP2 Is a Common Feature in Multiple Forms of Renal Concentrating Defects (Nephrogenic Diabetes Insipidus)

Although collecting duct water permeability is the main determinant of urinary concentration, other factors may also play a role. Chief among these is the osmotic gradient produced by the loop of Henle. This is a regulated process in which salt uptake in the thick ascending limb is modified in both the short and the long terms by the action of factors that include vasopressin. Other important factors include tubular flow rate, renal blood flow, glomerular function, and proximal tubule reabsorptive capacity. In addition to the contribution of these factors to water balance abnormalities, recent findings suggest that long-term changes in aquaporins may be important in a wide range of pathologic conditions. These conditions include a number of acquired forms of NDI, as well as states of water excess, such as CHF and cirrhosis. A discussion of these changes follows.

The commonest drug-induced form of NDI is caused by lithium treatment. Approximately 1 American in 1000 is on lithium therapy,[79] and approximately 50% of these patients will have a significant urinary concentrating defect.[80] In a rat model of this condition, therapeutic range levels of lithium in the plasma are associated with a profound polyuria. Previously, it had been assumed that this defect was the result of impaired ability of vasopressin to stimulate adenylate cyclase.[81] However, studies suggest that despite the dehydration, which provides a stimulus for upregulation of AQP2, lithium-treated animals demonstrate diminished fraction of AQP2 in the plasma membrane and leads to 95% decline in total cellular AQP2 in comparison with untreated controls.[29] Clearly, such a decrease in AQP2 would have a profound effect on the ability of the cells to mount an antidiuretic response, hence the polyuria. Of interest, such a decrease in AQP2 is not a specific feature of lithium treatment. Decreased AQP2 levels are also seen in two other clinically important settings of NDI, hypokalemia, and hypercalcemia.[66, 82, 83] However, although decreased AQP2 level is shared among hypokalemia, hypercalcemia, and lithium treatment, the regulation of AQP2 shuttling varies between these conditions. *In hypercalcemia and lithium-treated animals, there is an additional impairment in the targeting of AQP2 to the plasma membrane, a feature that is not observed in hypokalemia.*

A major cause of morbidity among older men is urinary retention, usually as a consequence of prostate hypertrophy. This obstruction is often compounded by an impaired concentrating ability and polyuria. The involvement of AQP2 in postobstructive polyuria was studied in a rat model of reversible bilateral ureteric obstruction, induced by ligation of the ureters for 24 hours, followed by examination of urine output, urine osmolality, and renal AQP2 abundance at days 1, 2, or 7 after release of the ureteric ligature.[84] Obstructed animals manifest marked osmotic diuresis (clearance of accumulated salt and urea) during the first 24 hours after relief of obstruction, followed by persistent polyuria that was not obligated by solute excretion. Although AQP2 appeared to be efficiently targeted to the apical plasma membrane, AQP2 levels were decreased to about a quarter of control levels even at the end of the obstruction period and remained low for several days thereafter.[84] These data suggest that the concentration defect seen in ureteric obstruction is related at least partially to a reduction in the total availability of AQP2 in collecting ducts.

Various other conditions not generally considered forms of NDI are also associated with vasopressin-resistant urinary concentrating defect. Among these is a renal concentrating defect associated with protein deficient diet, where changes in both urea and water reabsorption are observed.[71] Interestingly, there is an impairment of vasopressin-induced water transport in this condition only in the terminal portion of the inner medullary collecting ducts,[71] which correlates with decreased AQP2 expression in this part of the tubule, *specifically*. This is an interesting observation, because in several other conditions where AQP2 levels are reduced, the effect spans the entire length of collecting tubule.[29, 66] These findings are consistent with previous reports suggesting the involvement of "other" local renal factors in the regulation of AQP2, in addition to vasopressin.[29, 67]

Renal failure, both acute and chronic, is associated with polyuria and a concentrating defect. Although a wide range of abnormalities contribute to the overall tubular dysfunction in renal failure, decreased AQP2 levels have been shown in models of acute (ischemic[85]) and chronic (5/6 nephrectomy[70]) renal failure, suggesting a role for AQP2 dysregulation in the tubular abnormalities observed in renal insufficiency.

## Defects in AQP2 Expression May Persist after Correction of the Primary Defect

A common feature of a number of acquired NDI forms is the extended time required for normal concentrating capacity to be re-established once the underlying condition has been corrected. This is the case in animal models of NDI following lithium treatment and ureteric obstruction.[29, 84] Resumption of lithium-free diet for 7 days is associated with only a moderate increase in urine osmolality. Interestingly, this correlates with a persistent deficit in AQP2 expression. Similar results were observed after ureteric obstruction, where at day 7 following relief of obstruction, AQP2 level was only 50% of that seen in control animals.[84] Although urine output was apparently normal in these animals, water deprivation tests revealed a significant and persistent urinary concentrating defect.[84] Such defects were observed even 1 month after relief of obstruction.[74] In contrast with the lithium and ureteric obstruction models, in the hypokalemia model, both AQP2 levels and concentrating ability return to normal levels within 1 week. Thus, chronic decline in AQP2 level appcars to corrclatc with urinary concentrating defects in some animal models of NDI and may also have clinical significance in patients with similar problems.

## Aquaporins in Cirrhosis, Nephrosis, and Congestive Heart Failure

In contrast to NDI, where renal water loss is the rule, some conditions are characterized by water retention. The presence of AQP2 dysregulation in NDI suggested that AQP2 abnormalities may exist in water-retentive states. Two studies have looked at AQP2 expression in rats with CHF, induced by coronary artery ligation.[72, 86] These studies showed a significant increase in AQP2, both at the mRNA and protein levels. Of interest, these changes were seen only in rats with hyponatremia-associated heart failure (uncompensated CHF), whereas similarly treated rats with compensated heart failure (i.e., without hyponatremia) showed no change in AQP2 expression.[72] Immunocytochemistry studies showed that AQP2 was predominantly in the apical plasma membrane, where it would be active in facilitating water reabsorption.[72] These effects could be explained by the observed rise in circulating vasopressin levels, because treatment of rats with CHF for 24 hours with OPC31260, a vasopressin $V_2$ receptor antagonist, reversed the increase in AQP2 levels and increased urine output.[86] Thus, both increased expression and enhanced targeting of AQP2 to the plasma membrane seem to be important in CHF-associated water retention.

The correlation between renal AQP2 expression and cirrhosis, however, is inconclusive. In a rat model of hepatic cirrhosis with ascites, induced by $CCl_4$ treatment, AQP2 protein and mRNA levels were increased, and the increase correlated with the amount of ascites.[87, 88] As in the rat CHF model, upregulation of AQP2 appeared to be vasopression-dependent, because treatment with OPC31260 reversed the increase in AQP2 mRNA levels.[88] However, unlike rats with CHF, rats in this model had normal serum sodium and osmolality; the significance of this variation is unclear at the present time. In a second model of cirrhosis with ascites and hyponatremia, produced by $CCl_4$ inhalation, there was no change in AQP2 expression, but AQP1 expression in the cortex was increased.[89] The authors concluded that water retention is likely to be the result of increased AQP1 expression and water reabsorption in the proximal tubule, combined with failure of the normal "vasopressin escape" phenomenon (discussed earlier). In a third model of cirrhosis without ascites (induced by ligation of the common bile duct), AQP2 expression in the renal cortex was reduced, whereas inner medullary AQP2 was unchanged.[90] Serum vasopressin levels were normal in this study, and it was suggested that downregulation of AQP2 in compensated cirrhosis without ascites may be an appropriate response to water retention.[90] In summary, although the current data suggest abnormal regulation of water channels in cirrhosis, the contribution of these abnormalities to water retention in this setting is unclear.

Nephrotic syndrome is characterized by glomerular basal membrane damage, loss of protein into the urine, serum lipid abnormalities, and salt and water retention. Except in one model of nephrotic syndrome, where vasopressin levels were found to be elevated,[68] the cumulative data suggest that vasopressin does not play a significant role in the pathogenesis of water retention in nephrosis.[69, 91]

# SUMMARY

Regulation of urine output, and hence control of water balance in the body, occurs mainly in the renal collecting duct, where acutely, water permeability is regulated by shuttling of AQP2 from a store of intracellular vesicles to the apical plasma membrane in response to vasopressin, and chronically, by changes in the total abundance of the protein. The magnitude of the acute response, however, is dependent on the total level of AQP2 in the tissue. The chronic changes appear to be important in normal water physiology as well as in pathologic disorders of water balance. One of the signals for AQP2 regulation is vasopressin itself, which acts via cAMP; however, it is now apparent that other hitherto unknown signals play a key role in its regulation. The role of changes in the expression of other aquaporins, and the signals that regulate such changes, remain to be defined and will provide a rich avenue for future research.

## REFERENCES


1. Knepper MA: Molecular physiology of urinary concentrating mechanism: regulation of aquaporin water channels by vasopressin. Am J Physiol Renal Physiol 272:F3–F12, 1997.
2. Agre P, Bonhivers M, Borgnia MJ: The aquaporins: Blueprints for cellular plumbing systems. J Biol Chem 273:14659–14662, 1998.
3. Agre P, Preston GM, Smith BL, et al: Aquaporin CHIP: The archetypal molecular water channel. Am J Physiol Renal Physiol 265:F463–F476, 1993.
4. Knepper MA, Nielsen S, Chou CL, Digiovanni SR: Mechanism of vasopressin action in the renal collecting duct. Semin Nephrol 14:302–321, 1994.
5. Nielsen S, Kwon T, Christensen BM, et al: Physiology and pathophysiology of renal aquaporins. J Am Soc Nephrol 10:647–663, 1999.
6. Marples D, Frokiaer J, Nielsen S: Long-term regulation of aquaporins in the kidney. Am J Physiol Renal Physiol 276:F331–F339, 1999.
7. Thibonnier M, Berti-Mattera LN, Dulin N, et al: Signal transduction pathways of the human V1-vascular, V2-renal, V3-pituitary vasopressin and oxytocin receptors. Prog Brain Res 119:147–161, 1998.
8. Ruiz-Opazo N: Identification of a novel dual angiotensin II/ vasopressin receptor. Nephrologie 19:417–420, 1998.
9. Aguilera G, Rabadan-Diehl C: Regulation of vasopressin V1b receptors in the anterior pituitary gland of the rat. Exp Physiol 85:19S–26S, 2000.
10. Grazzinin E, Boccara G, Joubert D, et al: Vasopressin regulates adrenal functions by acting through different vasopressin receptor subtypes. Adv Exp Med Biol 449:325–334, 1998.
11. Koob GF, Lebrun C, Bluthe RM, et al: Role of neuropeptides in learning versus performance: Focus on vasopressin. Brain Res Bull 23:359–364, 1989.
12. Koob GF, Lebrun C, Bluthe RM, et al: Role of neuropeptides in learning versus performance: Focus on vasopressin. Brain Res Bull 23:359–364, 1989.
13. Cowley AW: Control of the renal medullary circulation by vasopressin V1 and V2 receptors in the rat. Exp Physiol 85:223S–231S, 2000.
14. Zingg HH: Vasopressin and oxytocin receptors. Baillieres Clin Endocrinol Metab 10:75–96, 1996.
15. Hirai A, Uchida D, Yoshida S: Vasopressin. Nippon Rinsho 50: 2893–2900, 1992.
16. Fushimi K, Ushida S, Hara Y, et al: Cloning and expression of apical membrane water channel of rat kidney collecting tubule. Nature 361:549–552, 1993.
17. Jung JS, Preston GM, Smith BL, et al: Molecular structure of the water channel through aquaporin CHIP: The hourglass model. J Biol Chem 269:14648–14654, 1994.
18. Yang B, Brown D, Verkman AS: The mercurial insensitive water channel (AQP-4) forms orthogonal arrays in stably transfected Chinese hamster ovary cells. J Biol Chem 271:4577–4580, 1996.
19. Van Hoek AN, Yang B, Kirmiz S, Brown D: Freeze-fracture analysis of plasma membranes of CHO cells stably expressing aquaporins 1–5. J Membr Biol 165:243–254, 1998.
20. Rash JE, Yasumura T, Hudson CS, et al: Direct immunogold labeling of aquaporin-4 in square arrays of astrocyte and ependymocyte plasma membrane in rat brain and spinal cord. Proc Natl Acad Sci U S A 95:11981–11986, 1998.
21. Vallon V, Verkman AS, Schnermann J: Luminal hypotonicity in proximal tubules of aquaporin-1-knockout mice. Am J Physiol Renal Physiol 278:F1030–F1033, 2000.
22. Nielsen S, Smith B, Christensen EI, et al: CHIP28 water channels are localized in constitutively water-permeable segments of the nephron. J Cell Biol 120:371–383, 1993.
23. Ma T, Yang B, Gillespie A, et al: Severely impaired urinary concentrating ability in transgenic mice lacking aquaporin-1 water channels. J Biol Chem 273:4296–4299, 1998.
24. Schnermann J, Chou CL, Ma T, et al: Defective proximal tubule fluid reabsorption in transgenic aquaporin-1 null mice. Proc Natl Acad Sci U S A 95:9660–9664, 1998.
25. Nielsen S, Digiovanni SR, Christensen EI, et al: Cellular and subcellular immunolocalization of vasopressin-regulated water channel in rat kidney. Proc Natl Acad Sci U S A 90:11663–11667, 1993.
26. Kishore BK, Mandon B, Oza NB, et al: Rat renal arcade segment expresses vasopressin-regulated water channel and vasopressin V2 receptor. J Clin Invest 97:2763–2771, 1996.
27. Digiovanni SR, Nielsen S, Christensen EI, Knepper MA: Regulation of collecting duct water channel expression by vasopressin in Brattleboro rat. Proc Natl Acad Sci U S A 91:8984–8988, 1994.
28. Deen PM, Verdijk MA, Knoers NV: Requirement of human water channel aquaporin-2 for vasopressin-dependent concentration of urine. Science 264:92–95, 1994.
29. Marples D, Christensen S, Christensen EI, et al: Lithium-induced downregulation of aquaporin-2 water channel expression in rat kidney medulla. J Clin Invest 95:1838–1845, 1995.
30. Frigeri A, Gropper MA, Turck CW, Verkman AS: Immunolocalization of the mercurial-insensitive water channel and glycerol intrinsic protein in epithelial cell plasma membranes. Proc Natl Acad Sci U S A 92:4328–4331, 1995.
31. Chou CL, Ma T, Yang B, et al: Fourfold reduction of water permeability in inner medullary collecting duct of aquapoirin-4 knockout mice. Am J Physiol Cell Physiol 274:C549–C554, 1998.
32. Nielsen S, Chou CL, Marples D, et al: Vasopressin increases water permeability of kidney collecting duct by inducing translocation of aquaporin-CD water channels to plasma membrane. Proc Natl Acad Sci U S A 92:1013–1017, 1995.
33. Marples D, Knepper MA, Christensen EI, Nielsen S: Redistribution of aquaporin-2 water channels induced by vasopressin in rat kidney inner medulla collecting duct. Am J Physiol Cell Physiol 269:C655–C664, 1995.
34. Sabolic I, Katsura T, Verbavatz JM, Brown D: The AQP2 water channel: Effect of vasopressin treatment, microtubule disruption, and distribution in neonatal rats. J Membr Biol 145:107–108, 1995.
35. Yamamoto T, Sasaki S, Fushimi K, et al: Vasopressin increases aquaporin-CD water channel in apical membrane of collecting duct principal cells in Brattleboro rats. Am J Physiol Cell Physiol 268:C1546–C1551, 1995.
36. Christensen BM, Marples D, Jensen UB, et al: Acute effects of vasopressin V2-receptor antagonist on kidney AQP2 expression and subcellular distribution. Am J Physiol Renal Physiol 275: F285–F297, 1998.
37. Hayashi M, Sasaki S, Tsuganezawa H, et al: Expression and distribution of aquaporin of collecting duct are regulated by vasopressin V2 receptor in rat kidney. J Clin Invest 94:1778–1783, 1994.
38. Saito T, Ishikawa SE, Sasaki S, et al: Alteration in water channel AQP-2 by removal of AVP stimulation in collecting duct cells of dehydrated rats. Am J Physiol Renal Physiol 272:F183–F191, 1997.
39. Kurokawa K, Massry SG: Interaction between catecholamines and vasopressin on renal medullary cyclic AMP of rat. Am J Physiol 225:825–829, 1973.
40. Edwards RM, Jackson BA, Dousa TP: ADH-sensitive cAMP cystem in papillary collecting duct: Effect of osmolality and PGE2. Am J Physiol Renal Physiol 240:F311–F318, 1981.
41. Katsura T, Gustafson CE, Ausieelo DA, Brown D: Protein kinase A phosphorylation is involved in regulated exocytosis of aquaporin-2 in transfected LLC-PK1 cells. Am J Physiol Renal Physiol 272:F817–F822, 1997.
42. Fushimi K, SASAKI S, Marumo F: Phosphorylation of serine 256 is required for cAMP-dependent regulatory exocytosis of the aquaporin-2 water channel. J Biol Chem 272:14800–14804, 1997.
43. Christensen BM, Zelenina M, Aperia A, Nielsen S: Localization

and regulation of PKA-phosphorylated AQP2 in response to V(2)-receptor agonist/antagonist treatment. Am J Physiol Renal Physiol 278:F29–F42, 1998.
44. Kuwahara M, Fushimi K, Terada Y, et al: cAMP-dependent phosphorylation stimulates water permeability of aquaporin-collecting duct water channel protein expressed in Xenopus oocytes. J Biol Chem 270:10384–10387, 1995.
45. Lande MB, Jo I, Ziedel ML, et al: Phosphorylation of aquaporin-2 does not alter the membrane water permeability of rat papillary water channel-containing vesicles. J Biol Chem 271:5552–5557, 1996.
46. Zelenina M, Christensen BM, Nielsen S, Aperia A: Prostaglandin E(2) interaction with AVP: Effects on AQP2 phosphorylation and distribution. Am J Physiol Renal Physiol 278:F388–F394, 2000.
47. Digiovani SR, Nielsen S, Christensen EI, Knepper MA: Regulation of collecting duct water channel expression by vasopressin in Brattleboro rat. Proc Natl Acad Sci U S A 91:8984–8988, 1994.
48. Phillips ME, Taylor A: Effect of colcemid on the water permeability response to vasopressin in isolated perfused rabbit collecting tubules. J Physiol (Lond) 456:591–608, 1992.
49. Phillips ME, Taylor A: Effect of nocodazol on the water permeability response to vasopressin in rabbit collecting tubules perfused in vitro. J Physiol (Lond) 411:529–544, 1989.
50. Valenti G, Hugon JS, Bourguet J: To what extent is microtubular network involved in antidiuretic response. Am J Physiol Renal Physiol 255:F1098–F1106, 1988.
51. Rothman JE: Mechanisms of intracellular protein transport. Nature 372:55–63, 1994.
52. Nielsen S, Marples D, Birn H, et al: Expression of VAMP-2-like protein in kidney collecting duct intracellular vesicles: Colocalization with aquaporin-2 water channels. J Clin Invest 96: 1834–1844, 1995.
53. Franki N, Nacaluso F, Gao Y, Hays RM: Vesicle fusion proteins in rat inner medullary collecting duct and amphibian bladder. Am J Physiol 268:792–797, 1995.
54. Jo I, Harris HW, Amedt-Raduege AM, et al: Rat kidney papilla contains abundant synaptobrevin protein that participates in the fusion of antidiuretic hormone (ADH) water channel-containing endosomes in vitro. Proc Natl Acad Sci U S A 92:1876–1880, 1995.
55. Marples D, Christensen BM, Frokiaer J, et al: Dehydration reverses vasopressin-V2-receptor antagonist induced diuresis and aquaporin-2 downregulation in rats. Am J Physiol Renal Physiol 275:F400–F409, 1998.
56. Terris J, Ecelbarger CA, Nielsen S, Knepper MA: Long-term regulation of four renal aquaporins in rats. Am J Physiol Renal Physiol 271:F414–F422, 1996.
57. Yasui M, Zelenina SM, Celsi G, Aperia A: Adenylate cyclase-coupled vasopressin receptor activates AQP2 promoter via a dual effect on CRE and AP1 elements. Am J Physiol Renal Physiol 270:F443–F450, 1997.
58. Hozawa S, Holtzman EJ, Ausiello DA: cAMP motifs regulating transcription in the aquaporin 2 gene. Am J Physiol Cell Physiol 270:C1695–C1702, 1996.
59. Matsumura Y, Uchida S, Rai T, et al: Transcriptional regulation of aquaporin-2 water channel gene by cAMP. J Am Soci Nephrol 8:861–867, 1997.
60. Uchida S, Sasaki S, Fushimi K, Marumo F: Isolation of human aquaporin-CD gene. J Biol Chem 269:23451–23455, 1994.
61. Ecelbarger CA, Nielsen S, Olson BR, et al: Role of renal aquaporins in escape from vasopressin-induced antidiuresis in rat. J Clin Invest 99:1852–1863, 1997.
62. Ecelbarger CA, Chou CL, Lee AJ, et al: Escape from vasopressin-induced antidiuresis: Role of vasopressin resistance of the collecting duct. Am J Physiol Renal Physiol 274:F1161–F1166, 1998.
63. Promeneur D, Kwon TH, Christensen BM, et al: Vasopressin-independent regulation of collecting duct AQP2 expression in rat. Am J Physiol Renal Physiol 279:F370–F382, 1998.
64. Kishore BK, Terris JM, Knepper MA: Quantitation of aquaporin-2 abundance in microdissected collecting ducts: Axial distribution and control by AVP. Am J Physiol Renal Physiol 271:F62–F70, 1996.
65. Marples D, Rasch R, Knepper MA, Nielsen S: Decreased aquaporin-2 expression of rat kidney collecting duct in acquired diabetes insipidus is not a consequence of polyuria or medullary osmotic washout. J Physiol (Lond) 497P:P91–P92, 1996.
66. Marples D, Frokiaer J, Dorup MA, et al: Hypokalemia-induced downregulation of aquaporin-2 water channel expression in rat kidney medulla and cortex. J Clin Invest 97:1960–1968, 1996.
67. Frokiaer J, Christensen BM, Marples D, et al: Downregulation of aquaporin-2 parallels changes in renal water excretion in unilatertal ureteric obstruction. Am J Physiol Renal Physiol 273: F213–F223, 1997.
68. Apostol E, Ecelbarger CA, Teerris J, et al: Reduced renal medullary water channel expression in puromycin aminoglycoside-induced nephrotic syndrome. J Am Soc Nephrol 8:15–24, 1997.
69. Fernandez-Llama P, Andrews P, Nielsen S, et al: Impaired aquaporin and urea transporter expression in rats with adriamycin-induced nephrotic syndrome. Kidney Int 53:1244–1253, 1998.
70. Kwon T, Frokiaer J, Knepper MA, Nielsen S: Downregulation of AQP1, AQP2 and AQP3 in kidneys of rats with experimental chronic renal failure. Am J Physiol Renal Physiol 275:F724–F741, 1998.
71. Sands JM, Naruse M, Jacobs JD, et al: Changes in aquaporin-2 protein contribute to the urine concentrating defect in rats fed a low protein diet. J Clin Invest 97:2807–2814, 1996.
72. Nielsen S, Terris J, Andersen D, et al: Congestive heart failure in rats is associated with increased expression and targeting of aquaporin-2 water channel in collecting duct. Proc Natl Acad Sci U S A 94:5450–5455, 1997.
73. Ma T, Yang B, Gillespie A, et al: Generation and phenotype of transgenic knockout mouse lacking the mercurial-insensitive water channel aquaporin-4. J Clin Invest 100:957–962, 1997.
74. Frokiaer J, Kwon T, Wen J, et al: Bilateral ureteral obstruction (BUO) is associated with long-term downregulation of both aquaporin-1 (AQP1) and aquaporin-2 (AQP2) which parallels the impairment in urinary concentrating capacity. J Am Soc Nephrol 9:18, 1998.
75. Frokiaer J, Marples D, Valtin H, et al: Low aquaporin-2 protein levels in polyuric DI +/+ severe mice with constitutively high cAMP-phosphodiesterase activity. Am J Physiol Renal Physiol 276:F179–F190, 1999.
76. Kanno K, Sasaki S, Hirata Y, et al: Urinary excretion of aquaporin-2 in patients with diabetes insipidus. N Engl J Med 332: 1540–1545, 1995.
77. Saito T, Ishikawa SE, Sasaki S, et al: Urinary excretion of aquaporin-2 in the diagnosis of central diabetes insipidus. J Clin Endocrinol Metab 82:1823–1827, 1997.
78. Bichet DG: Vasopressin receptors in health and disease. Kidney Int 49:1706–1711,1996.
79. Peet M, Pratt JP: Lithium: Current status in psychiatric disorders. Drugs 46:7–17, 1993.
80. Boton R, Gaviria M, Batlle DC: Prevalence, pathogenesis and treatment of renal dysfunction associated with chronic lithium therapy. Am J Kidney Dis 10:329–345, 1987.
81. Christensen S: Vasopressin and renal concentrating ability. In Johnson FN (ed): Lithium Therapy Monographs, vol 2. Basel, Karger, 1988, pp 20–34.
82. Earm JH, Marples D, Frokiaer J, et al: Decreased aquaporin-2 expression and apical membrane delivery in kidney collecting ducts of polyuric hypercalcemic rats. J Am Soc Nephrol 9:2181–2193, 1998.
83. Sands JM, Flores FX, Kato A, et al: Vasopressin-elicited water and urea permeabilities are altered in IMCD in hypercalcemic rats. Am J Physiol Renal Physiol 274:F978–F985, 1998.
84. Frokiaer J, Marples D, Knepper MA, Nielsen S: Bilateral ureteral obstruction downregulates expression of vasopressin-sensitive AQP2 water channel in rat kidney. Am J Physiol Renal Physiol 270:F657–F668,1996.
85. Fernandez-Llama P, Andrews P, Turner R, et al: Decreased abundance of collecting duct aquaporins in post-ischemic renal failure in rats. J Am Soc Nephrol 10:1658–1668, 1999.
86. Xu DL, Schrier RW, Martin PY, et al: Upregulation of aquaporin-2 water channel expression in chronic heart failure rat. J Clin Invest 99:1500–1505, 1997.
87. Asahina Y, Izumi N, Enomoto N, et al: Increased gene expression of water channel in cirrhotic rat kidneys. Hepatology 21:169–173, 1995.

88. Fujita N, Ishikawa SE, Sasaki S, et al: Role of water channel AQP-CD in water retention in SIADH and cirrhotic rats. Am J Physiol Renal Physiol 269:F926–F931, 1995.
89. Fernandez-Llama P, Jimenez W, Bosch-Marce M, et al: Dysregulation of aquaporin-1 and aquaporin-2 in the kidneys of cirrhotic rats. J Am Soc Nephrol 9:18,1998.
90. Jonassen T, Nielsen S, Christensen S, Petersen JS: Decreased vasopressin-mediated renal water reabsorption in rats with compensated liver cirrhosis. Am J Physiol Renal Physiol 275:F216–F225, 1998.
91. Fernandez-Llama P, Andrews P, Ecelbarger CA, et al: Concentrating defect in experimental nephrotic syndrome: Altered expression of aquaporins and thick ascending limb Na transporters. Kidney Int 54:170–179,1998.

CHAPTER 14

# Hyponatremia

Michel Chonchol, MD ▪ Tomas Berl, MD

## CONTROL OF SERUM SODIUM

Serum sodium concentration or [$Na^+$] is kept in the narrow range of 138 to 142 mmol/L despite great variation in water intake. This finely tuned water balance is made possible by the countercurrent mechanism, which allows for both urinary concentration and dilution, acting in concert with the hypothalamic osmoreceptors that control secretion of antidiuretic hormone (ADH, vasopressin). A decrease in serum sodium occurs when a defect in urinary dilution is combined with water intake that exceeds the subject's diluting ability.

### Serum Sodium and Osmolality

As the predominant osmotically active constituent of the extracellular fluid, the concentration of sodium is the primary determinant of plasma osmolality. Thus, serum osmolality can be usually calculated by the formula:

$$(2 \times [Na^+]) + (\text{blood urea nitrogen (mg/dL)}/2.8) + (\text{glucose (mg/dL)}/18)$$

Whereas a decrement in serum sodium most commonly reflects a hypotonic state, this is by no means always the case. As illustrated in Figure 14–1, hyponatremia can coexist with either normal or even high osmolality. The presence of solutes that do not penetrate cell membranes such as glucose (in the absence of insulin), mannitol, and glycine,[1] which is employed in hysteroscopy, laparoscopy, and transurethral prostate resection, decreases serum sodium by translocation of water from cells to the extracellular space. Hyperglycemia accounts for 15% of hyponatremia in hospitalized patients. A decrease in [$Na^+$] of 1.6 mmol/L occurs for every 100 mg/dL (5.6 mmol/L) increase in plasma glucose. However, studies suggest that the decrease should be closer to 2.4 mmol/L, particularly when glucose is greater than 400 mg/dL.[2] Hyperlipidemia and hyperproteinemia can also depress the serum sodium level without associated extracellular fluid (ECF) hypotonicity. This laboratory artifact is called pseudohyponatremia and depends entirely on the method used to measure sodium in the serum. Forty years ago, the flame emission spectrophotometer (FES) revolutionized the measurement of serum sodium in clinical laboratories. According to this technique, the serum sample is first diluted, and an ultrafine spray of this dilution is blown across a flame. The FES measures the intensity of the light emitted at the wavelength characteristic of sodium, the intensity being directly proportional to the number of sodium atoms in the sample.[3]

Serum consists of water (93% of serum volume) and nonaqueous components—mainly lipids and proteins (7% of serum volume). Sodium is restricted to serum water. In states of hyperproteinemia or hyperlipidemia, there is an increased mass of the nonaqueous components of serum and a concomitant decrease in the proportion of serum composed of water. Thus, pseudohyponatremia results because the flame photometry method measures sodium concentration in whole plasma. A sodium-selective electrode gives the true, physiologically pertinent sodium concentration because it measures sodium activity in serum water. However, only direct reading potentiometry, in which the serum sample is not diluted (as opposed to indirect

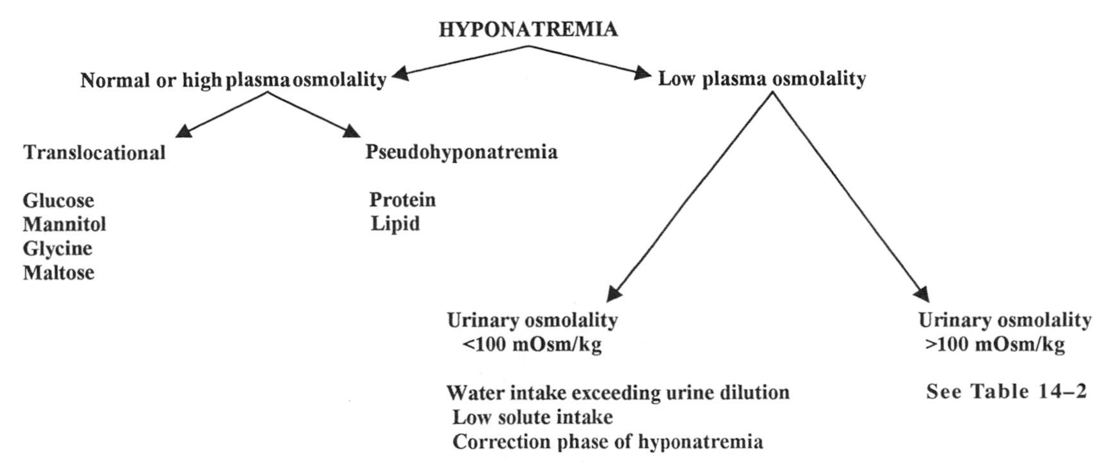


**FIGURE 14–1** ▪ Diagnostic approach for the patient with hyponatremia.

potentiometry, in which the sample is diluted) gives an accurate concentration.

It must be also noted that plasma osmolality can also be increased by a number of solutes such as urea, ethanol, methanol, and ethylene glycol (Table 14–1). These solutes are cell permeable and, therefore, do not translocate water from cells. As such, these do not themselves cause hyponatremia, but their presence can lead to a normal measured plasma osmolality in an otherwise hyponatremic patient. Such patients have a decrease in effective plasma tonicity and should be approached as having a hypotonic disorder.

**TABLE 14–1.** Substances that Increase Osmolality Without Changing Serum Sodium

| Normonatremic Hyperosmolality |
|---|
| Urea |
| Ethanol |
| Ethylene glycol |
| Isopropyl alcohol |
| Methanol |

## APPROACH TO THE HYPOTONIC HYPONATREMIC PATIENT

As noted earlier, disorders in the renal diluting mechanism frequently underlie the development of hyponatremia and hypo-osmolality. Such patients, therefore, have a less than maximally dilute urine (>100 mOsm/kg). On the other hand, the presence of hyponatremia in a patient with dilute urine reflects the intake of water in excess of normal diluting ability (see Fig. 14–1). The latter allows for very generous water intake (~20 L/day) when solute intake is normal (~600 to 900 mOsm/day). However, in the presence of very low solute intake, a positive water balance can ensue even with moderately high fluid intake (~5 L/day). This explains the hyponatremia seen in beer drinkers and in other low solute consumption states.[4] Finally, a low urinary osmolality may be seen in the correction phase of a hyponatremic state when the underlying process that caused the initial limitation in urinary dilution is either reversed or treated. In the approach to the patient with hypotonic hyponatremia whose urine is not dilute (>100 mOsm/kg), an assessment of the ECF volume provides a useful working classification of hyponatremia: (1) hyponatremia with ECF volume depletion, (2) hyponatremia with excess ECF volume, and (3) hyponatremia with normal ECF volume (Fig. 14–2).[5]

### Hyponatremia with Extracellular Fluid Volume Depletion

A patient with hypovolemic hyponatremia has both a total body $Na^+$ and a water deficit; the $Na^+$ deficit exceeds the water deficit. Serum sodium concentration is determined by:

$$(\text{Total body } Na^+) + (\text{total body } K^+/\text{total body water})$$

In the setting of hypovolemic hyponatremia, the loss of sodium and possibly potassium undoubtedly contributes to hyponatremia. However, these losses, if accompanied by parallel decrements in total body water, would cause no changes in serum sodium. Therefore, a relative retention of water is also operant.

The underlying mechanism involves a volume contraction that stimulates secretion of ADH with continued oral or parenteral hypotonic fluid intake. In addition to hypothalamic osmoreceptors, nonosmotic pathways control ADH release. Baroreceptors in the aortic arch and carotid sinus and vagal receptors located in the left atrium contribute to the release of ADH in response to volume contraction. When the osmoreceptors and volume receptors for control of ADH receive opposing stimuli, the effect of the volume receptors on ADH release generally predominates. In the presence of hypovolemia, ADH is secreted and water is retained despite hypo-osmolality. Thus, although hyponatremia in this setting clearly involves a depletion of body solutes, a concomitant failure to excrete water is critical to the process.

The decrease in ECF volume is manifested by physical findings such as flat neck veins, decreased skin turgor, dry mucous membranes, orthostatic hypotension, and tachycardia. An examination of the urinary $Na^+$ concentration is helpful in assessing whether the fluid losses are renal or extrarenal in origin. A urinary $Na^+$ concentration of less than 20 mEq/L reflects a normal renal response to volume depletion and points to an extrarenal source of fluid loss. This is seen most commonly in patients with gastrointestinal disease with vomiting or diarrhea. Hypovolemic hyponatremia in patients whose urinary $Na^+$ concentration is greater than 20 mEq/L points to the kidney as the source of the sodium losses.

**Gastrointestinal and Third-Space Losses.** In the presence of gastrointestinal losses through either vomiting or diarrhea, the kidney is extremely $Na^+$ avid, and the urinary $Na^+$ concentration tends to be very low because the kidney responds to this state of volume contraction by conserving sodium chloride (NaCl). Sequestration of fluids into third spaces such as the peritoneal cavity in peritonitis and pancreatitis or in the small bowel lumen with ileus and burns can also lead to hypovolemia. In these situations, the urinary $Na^+$ concentration is usually less than 10 mmol/L and the urine is hyperosmolar. In patients with vomiting and metabolic alkalosis, in which bicarbonaturia is present, the urinary bicarbonate anion obligates cations and, therefore, may be associated with a urinary sodium concentration greater than 20 mEq/L. The urinary chloride concentration, however, will be less than 10 mEq/L. If renal function is severely impaired, the damaged kidney may not possess the capacity for maximal conservation of sodium chloride.[6]

**Diuretics.** Use of diuretics is one of the most common situations in which hyponatremia is associated with hypovolemia. Because the kidney is the source of sodium losses, the urinary sodium concentration is

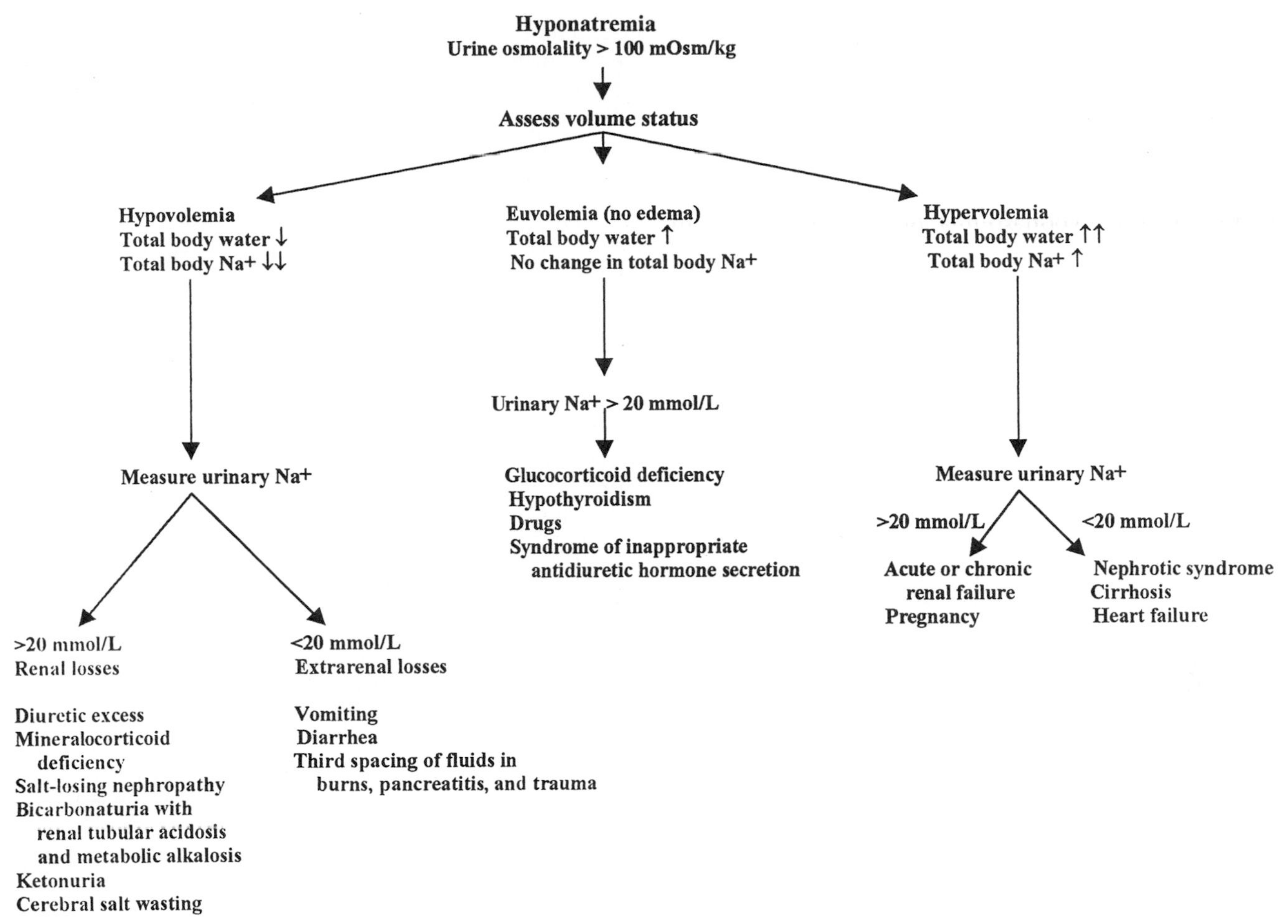


**FIGURE 14–2** ■ Diagnostic approach for the patient with hypotonic hyponatremia. (From Halterman R, Berl T: Therapy of dysnatremic disorders. In Brady H, Wilcox C [eds]: Therapy in Nephrology and Hypertension. Philadelphia, WB Saunders, 1999, pp 257–269.)

high (>20 mEq/L). Hyponatremia occurs almost exclusively with the use of thiazide diuretics. The variation in the hyponatremic risk associated with loop or thiazide diuretics relates to their site of action.[7, 8] Loop diuretics inhibit the $Na^+/Cl^-$ reabsorption in the thick ascending limb of Henle (TALH). This interferes with the generation of a hypertonic medullary interstitium. Therefore, even though volume contraction leads to increased ADH secretion, responsiveness to ADH is diminished because of the impairment in medullary hypertonicity. Thiazide diuretics, however, act in the distal tubule by interfering solely with urinary dilution rather than urinary concentration. Hyponatremia seen in the setting of thiazide use is usually evident within 14 days in most patients. Underweight women and elderly patients appear to be particularly susceptible to this complication. Several mechanisms for diuretic-induced hyponatremia have been postulated:

- Hypovolemia-stimulated ADH release and decreased fluid delivery to the diluting segment
- Impaired water excretion through interference with maximal urinary dilution in the cortical diluting segment
- $K^+$ depletion. It has been suggested that potassium depletion may alter the sensitivity of the osmoreceptor mechanism and thus cause ADH release. In addition, hypokalemia may also directly stimulate thirst.

Although the diagnosis of diuretic-induced hyponatremia is frequently obvious, surreptitious abuse of diuretics is being increasingly recognized and should be considered in patients in whom other electrolyte abnormalities and high urinary $Cl^-$ are present.

**Salt-Losing Nephropathy.** A salt-losing state sometimes occurs in patients with advanced chronic renal insufficiency (glomerular filtration rate [GFR] < 15 mL/min) and is characterized by hyponatremia and hypovolemia. In the majority of these patients, the $Na^+$ wasting tendency is not one that manifests itself at normal rates of sodium intake.

**Mineralocorticoid Deficiency.** Hyponatremia with ECF volume contraction, urine $Na^+$ higher than 20 mmol/L, and high serum $K^+$, urea, and creatinine are indicative of mineralocorticoid deficiency. The mechanism of the defect in water excretion associated with mineralocorticoid deficiency is mediated by ADH, which is activated by decrements of ECF volume, rather than by deficiency of the hormone per se.

**Osmotic Diuresis.** An osmotically active, nonreabsorbable solute obligates the renal excretion of $Na^+$ and results in volume depletion. With continuing water intake, the diabetic patient with severe glucosuria, the patient with a urea diuresis after relief of urinary tract obstruction, and the patient with mannitol diuresis all undergo urinary losses of $Na^+$ and water leading to hypovolemia and hyponatremia. The urinary $Na^+$ concentration is typically greater than 20 mmol/L. In diabetics, the $Na^+$ wasting is accentuated by ketonuria, which also causes obligatory $Na^+$ loss. The ketone bodies β-hydroxybutyrate and acetoacetate also obligate urinary electrolyte losses and aggravate the renal $Na^+$ wasting seen in diabetic ketoacidosis, starvation, and alcoholic ketoacidosis.

**Cerebral Salt Wasting.** Hyponatremia is a common electrolyte disorder seen in many patients with intracranial disease and is often attributed to the syndrome of inappropriate secretion of antidiuretic hormone (SIADH). A number of studies have shown that hyponatremia in the setting of central nervous system (CNS) disease may actually be caused by cerebral salt wasting (CSW), which is defined as the renal loss of sodium during intracranial disease, leading to hyponatremia and a decrease in ECF volume.[9] In fact, a substantial number of neurosurgical patients who develop hyponatremia and otherwise meet the clinical criteria for a diagnosis of SIADH have a volume status inconsistent with that diagnosis. Thus, the evidence of a negative salt balance and reductions in both plasma and total blood volume in these patients is more consistent with a diagnosis of CSW.[10] The exact mechanism by which CNS disease leads to renal salt wasting is not understood. The most likely process involves decreased sympathetic input resulting in decreased sodium reabsorption or central elaboration of a brain natriuretic factor. By either or both mechanism(s), increased urine volume and sodium excretion would lead to a decrease in effective arterial blood volume (EABV) and thus provide a baroreceptor stimulus for the release of ADH (Fig. 14–3*A*). In this setting, the release of ADH is an appropriate response to the volume depletion. In contrast, release of ADH in SIADH is truly inappropriate because EABV is expanded.[10] See Figure 14–3*B* for clinical differentiation of SIADH and CSW.[10] The treatment of CSW consists of vigorous sodium and volume replacement. Although not well studied, CSW tends to be transient with evidence of renal salt wasting usually resolving after 3 to 4 weeks.

## Hyponatremia with Excess Extracellular Fluid Volume

In this setting, both total body sodium and total body water are increased, but total body water is increased to a greater extent. Hyponatremia in the setting of ECF volume expansion is usually associated with edematous states, such as congestive heart failure, hepatic cirrhosis, and nephrotic syndrome. The degree of hyponatremia often correlates with the severity of the underlying condition and is an important prognostic factor. These disorders all have in common a decreased effective circulating arterial volume, leading to increased thirst and increased ADH levels. These states are characterized by avid $Na^+$ retention (urinary $Na^+$ concentration <10 mEq/L). This avid retention may be obscured by the concomitant use of diuretics, which are frequently used to treat these patients. Oliguric acute and chronic renal failure may be associated with hyponatremia if water intake exceeds the ability to excrete equivalent volumes.

**Congestive Heart Failure.** The integrity of the arterial circulation, as determined by cardiac output and peripheral vascular resistance or compliance, is the predominant determinant of renal sodium and water excretion.[11] In fact, edematous patients with heart failure have intravascularly volume contraction owing to lower systemic mean arterial pressure and the low cardiac output state. Several mechanoreceptors on the high-pressure side of the circulation can sense arterial underfilling (reduction in the "effective arterial blood volume").[12] These receptors are found in the left ventricle, carotid sinus, aortic arch, and renal afferent arterioles. Decreased activation of these receptors due to a decrease in systemic arterial pressure, stroke volume, renal perfusion, or peripheral vascular resistance leads to an increase in sympathetic outflow from the CNS, activation of the renin-angiotensin-aldosterone system, and the nonosmotic release of ADH, as well as the stimulation of thirst.[13] Stimulation of the renin-angiotensin-aldosterone system and catecholamine production will decrease the GFR, which leads to a decrease in water delivery and an increase in proximal tubular reabsorption. The neurohumoral-mediated decrease in delivery of tubular fluid to the distal nephron and an increase in ADH secretion mediate hyponatremia by limiting sodium and water excretion. The goal of these mechanisms is to return perfusion pressure to normal. There is a correlation between the degree of neurohormonal activation and the severity of left ventricular dysfunction as assessed by ejection fraction or functional class. In fact, hyponatremia has also been correlated with the severity of cardiac disease and with patient survival. When compared with eunatremic patients, survival is reduced significantly when the serum $Na^+$ decreases below 137 mmol/L. In fact, a serum $Na^+$ of 125 mmol/L reflects severe heart failure.

Levels of ADH are elevated in patients with heart failure in both the presence and the absence of diuretics. A decrease in vasopressin levels occurs once heart failure is treated clinically. It is postulated that nonosmotic pathways are operative in patients with congestive heart failure. Activation of carotid baroreceptors has been implicated in the nonosmotic release of ADH during arterial underfilling in patients with heart failure. Aquaporin type 2 (AQP2) water channels are increased in the cortex and papilla of rats with heart failure, which is an effect that is reversed by a nonpeptide $V_2$ receptor antagonist.[14]

**Hepatic Failure.** Patients with hepatic insufficiency and cirrhosis share pathophysiologic processes with heart failure patients. The hallmark of cirrhosis is peripheral and splanchnic vasodilatation, leading to renal sodium retention. However, these patients have increased cardiac output, mainly because of multiple

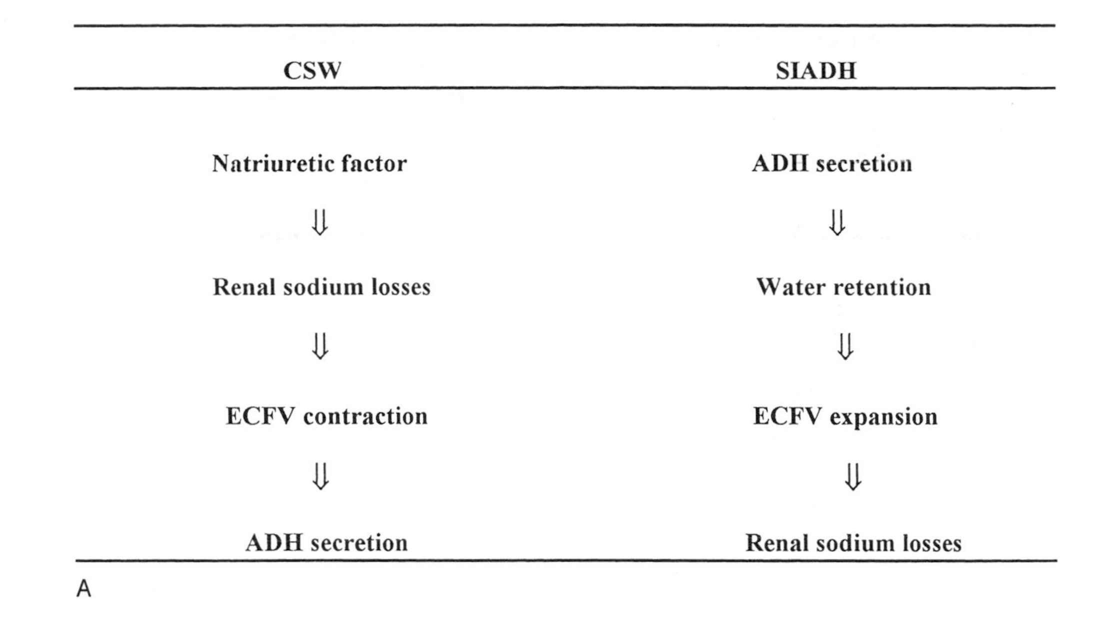


| | CSW | SIADH |
|---|---|---|
| **Extracellular fluid volume** | ⇓ | ⇑ |
| **Hematocrit** | ⇑ | **Normal** |
| **Albumin concentration** | ⇑ | **Normal** |
| **BUN/creatinine** | ⇑ | ⇓ |
| **Treatment** | **Normal saline** | **Fluid restriction** |

B

**FIGURE 14–3** ■ *A*, Differences in pathophysiologic mechanism between cerebral salt wasting (CSW) versus syndrome of inappropriate secretion of antidiuretic hormone (SIADH). *B*, Differential diagnosis of CSW versus SIADH. ADH, antidiuretic hormone; BUN, blood urea nitrogen; ECFV, extracellular fluid volume. (Modified from Palmer BF: Hyponatremia in a neurosurgical patient. Syndrome of inappropriate antidiuretic hormone secretion versus cerebral salt wasting. Nephrol Dial Transplant 15:262–268, 2000.)

arteriovenous fistulas in their alimentary tract and skin. The vasodilatation may be mediated by nitric oxide (NO). Inhibition of NO corrects the arterial hyporesponsiveness to vasoconstrictors.[15]

Splanchnic arterial vasodilatation and arteriovenous fistulas result in decreased mean arterial blood pressure and effective cardiac output. This fall in the effective arterial blood volume reduces the stimulation of the carotid and renal baroreceptors, causing increased vasopressin secretion, activation of the renin-angiotensin-aldosterone axis, and secretion of norepinephrine. The net effect is a hyperdynamic circulation and avid $Na^+$ and water retention. As the cirrhosis becomes more severe (no ascites → ascites → ascites with hepatorenal syndrome), there is a progressive increase in plasma renin, norepinephrine, and ADH activity. Mean arterial pressure, water excretion, and serum [$Na^+$] fall.

The nonosmotic secretion of vasopressin is central to the water excretory defect and has been found to relate to increased hypothalamic vasopressin mRNA content in cirrhotic rats. In fact, cirrhotic Brattleboro rats that lack vasopressin do not develop hyponatremia. Gene expression of vasopressin-regulated AQP2 has also been shown to be increased in cirrhotic rats.[16] Despite the disturbed hormonal milieu, the renal blood blow and GFR are maintained by endogenous vasodilatory prostaglandins: prostaglandin $I_2$ and prostaglandin $E_2$. This fine balance can be easily disturbed by the administration of nonsteroidal anti-inflammatory drugs (NSAIDs), and these should be avoided in patients with chronic liver disease. Other factors implicated in hyponatremia associated with cirrhosis include diuretic therapy, which can lead to intravascular volume contraction followed by nonosmotic release of antidiuretic hormone and water retention.

**Nephrotic Syndrome.** Patients with nephrotic syndrome, especially with normal renal function, usually have intravascular volume contraction through alteration in Starling's forces resulting from hypoalbuminemia and lowered plasma oncotic pressure. In contrast to the water-retaining disorders discussed above, in which increased AQP2 expression has been found, in rat models of nephrotic syndrome (i.e., treated with puromycin and Adriamycin [doxorubicin]), expression of AQP2 and AQP3 in the renal collecting duct is downregulated. Downregulation of AQP2 and AQP3, together with a decrease in the urinary concentrating ability, is a response that may be appropriate to the ECF volume expansion in these models.[17]

**Advance Chronic Renal Insufficiency.** Hyponatremia with edema can occur with either acute or chronic renal failure. It is clear that in the setting of either experimental or human renal disease, the ability to excrete free water is maintained better than the ability to reabsorb water. Nonetheless, full urinary dilution is not achieved and urinary osmolality below 200 mOsm/kg is rarely observed. Thus, a patient with a GFR of 2 mL/min (2880 mL/day) could have a fractional water excretion of 25% (720 mL/day), but of this only one third would be free water (240 mL/day). Thus, a decrement in GFR with an increase in thirst underlies the hyponatremia of patients with renal insufficiency.

**Pregnancy.** A physiologic decrease in serum sodium occurs with pregnancy, a hypervolemic state. This is mediated by a shift of the ADH-plasma osmolality relationship so that the threshold for the hormone's release is decreased by approximately 10 mOsm/kg. An increase in AQP2 expression is also observed in this setting.[18]

## Hyponatremia with Normal Extracellular Fluid Volume

Euvolemic hyponatremia is the most commonly encountered dysnatremia in hospitalized patients.[19] In these patients, no physical signs of increased total body $Na^+$ are detected. They may have slight excess of volume but are not edematous. Probable clinical causes here include the following.

**Glucocorticoid Deficiency.** Glucocorticoid deficiency is important in the impaired water excretion of primary and secondary adrenal insufficiency. Elevation of vasopressin levels accompanies the water excretory defect resulting from anterior pituitary deficiency and adrenocorticotropic hormone (ACTH) deficiency. This can be corrected by physiologic doses of glucocorticoids. In addition, vasopressin-independent factors, such as impaired renal hemodynamics and decreased distal fluid delivery to the diluting segments of the nephron, are also implicated in the defective water handling in glucocorticoid deficiency.

**Hypothyroidism.** Hyponatremia occurs in patients with hypothyroidism and myxedema. The cardiac output and GFR in severe hypothyroidism are often reduced. The decrease in cardiac output leads to nonosmotic release of vasopressin and a reduction in the GFR, which leads to diminished free water excretion through decreased delivery to the distal fluid. The exact mechanism, however, is less clear. In support of a vasopressin-independent mechanism, investigators have found normal suppression of vasopressin after water loading in patients with untreated myxedema.[20] However, elevated levels of vasopressin in the basal state and after a water load have been demonstrated in patients with advanced hypothyroidism. Although both vasopressin-dependent and vasopressin-independent factors may be operating, hyponatremia is readily reversed by treatment with levothyroxine (thyroxine).

**Psychosis.** Acutely psychotic patients, particularly those with schizophrenia, are at risk of developing hyponatremia.[21, 22] The mechanism may be multifactorial,[23] involving increased thirst perception (leading to polydipsia), a mild defect in osmoregulation that causes ADH to be secreted at lower osmolality, and enhanced renal response to ADH. Antipsychotic drugs may play a role as well.

**Postoperative Hyponatremia.** Most hospitalized hyponatremic patients are asymptomatic and euvolemic and have measurable vasopressin levels.[24] Postoperative hyponatremia occurs mainly in the setting of infusion of excessive amounts of electrolyte-free water (hypotonic saline or 5% dextrose in water) and the presence of vasopressin, which prevents the excretion of this electrolyte-free water. Hyponatremia can also occur in the postoperative setting despite near-isotonic saline infusion within 24 hours of induction of anesthesia. This occurs in the presence of vasopressin by the generation of negative electrolyte free water by the kidneys, which has the net effect of providing free water to the patient.[25] In a small subgroup of young females, hyponatremia is accompanied by cerebral edema, leading to seizures and hypoxia with catastrophic neurologic events.[26] This seems to occur primarily in premenopausal women, particularly after they undergo gynecologic surgery.

**Drugs Causing Hyponatremia.** Drug-induced hyponatremia is mediated by ADH analogues such as desmopressin or by ADH release agonists or agents potentiating the action of ADH. In other cases, the mechanism is not known. Table 14–2 lists the drugs associated with hyponatremia.[27]

**Aging-Related Hyponatremia.** Hyponatremia is a common finding in the geriatric population and may be a cause of great morbidity and mortality. If not recognized, it may lead to serious irreversible symp-

**TABLE 14–2.** Drugs Associated with Hyponatremia

| | |
|---|---|
| **Antidiuretic Hormone Analogues** | **Drugs that Potentiate Renal Action of Antidiuretic Hormone** |
| Deamino-D-arginine vasopressin | Chlorpropamide |
| Oxytocin | Cyclophosphamide |
| **Drugs that Enhance Antidiuretic Hormone Release** | Nonsteroidal anti-inflammatory drugs |
| Chlorpropamide | Acetaminophen |
| Clofibrate | **Drugs that Cause Hyponatremia by Unknown Mechanism** |
| Carbamazepine-oxycarbazepine | Haloperidol |
| Vincristine | Fluphenazine |
| Nicotine | Amitriptyline |
| Narcotics | Thioridazine |
| Antipsychotics/antidepressants | Fluoxetine |
| Ifosfamide | Sertraline |
| | Ecstasy |

Modified from Veis JH, Berl T: Hyponatremia. In Jacobson HR, Striker GE, Klahr S (eds): The Principles and Practice of Nephrology. St. Louis, CV Mosby, 1995, pp 888–893.

**TABLE 14–3.** Diagnostic Approach for the Syndrome of Inappropriate Antidiuretic Hormone Release

**Diagnostic Criteria**

Decreased extracellular fluid effective osmolality (<270 mOsm/kg $H_2O$)
Inappropriate urinary concentration (>100 mOsm/kg $H_2O$)
Clinical euvolemia
Elevated urinary sodium concentration under conditions of a normal salt and water intake
Absence of adrenal, thyroid, pituitary, or renal insufficiency or diuretic use

From Verbalis J: The syndrome of inappropriate antidiuretic hormone secretion and other hypoosmolar disorders. In Schrier RW, Gottschalk C (eds): Diseases of the Kidney, vol 3. Boston, Little Brown, 1997, pp 2392–2427.

toms and even to death. SIADH occurs commonly in the older population and may be caused by diseases and medications. Miller and associates found that a subset of older patients with hyponatremia of the SIADH type develop hyponatremia without obvious underlying cause other than the anticipated changes of aging that affect the water regulatory systems. The development of hyponatremia in persons in this age group is probably associated with age-related excess release or lack of suppression of ADH. Thus, SIADH-like hyponatremia in these patients can be considered idiopathic, with the greatest risk factor being advanced age.[28]

Thiazides are often implicated in the etiology of hyponatremia seen in the elderly population. Clark and associates observed that elderly subjects with unsuspected underlying defects in urinary dilution may present with clinically significant hyponatremia in the setting of thiazide use and water ingestion. Alterations in the distal tubular delivery of water, which are probably related to lower prostaglandin production, may contribute to susceptibility to thiazide-induced hyponatremia in the elderly.[29]

**Syndrome of Inappropriate Vasopressin Secretion.** This syndrome is the most common cause of hyponatremia in hospitalized patients. The diagnosis of the SIADH is made primarily by excluding other causes of hyponatremia. The diagnostic criteria for SIADH are summarized Table 14–3.[30] The commonest causes are malignancies, pulmonary disease, and CNS disorders. CNS bleeds, tumors, infections, and trauma cause SIADH by releasing excess ADH. In cancers (usually small cell lung, duodenum, pancreas, and olfactory neuroblastoma), there is ectopic ADH production. The cells of some of these tissues are capable of increasing vasopressin secretion in response to osmotic stimulation in vitro.

Human immunodeficiency virus (HIV) infection is now leading to a new category of patients with SIADH. Up to 35% of patients with acquired immunodeficiency syndrome (AIDS) admitted to the hospital will have SIADH; *Pneumocystis carinii* pneumonia, CNS infections, and malignancies are the likely causes. Other common causes of this syndrome are listed in Table 14–4.[31] Several patterns of abnormal vasopressin release emerge from careful studies of patients with clinical SIADH. In one third of patients with SIADH, ADH release varies appropriately with the serum sodium concentration but begins at an abnormally low threshold of serum osmolality, suggesting a "resetting of the osmostat." Any ingestion of free water above this threshold would lead to its excretion, maintaining the serum sodium concentration at the new low level, usually 125 to 130 mmol/L. The remaining patients do not demonstrate any specific pattern of ADH release and reveal no correlation with the serum sodium concentration. These patients are unable to excrete a solute-free urine and, therefore, ingested water is re-

**TABLE 14–4.** Causes of the Syndrome of Inappropriate Antidiuretic Hormone Release

| Carcinomas | Pulmonary Disorders | CNS Disorders |
|---|---|---|
| Bronchogenic carcinoma | Viral pneumonia | Encephalitis (viral or bacterial) |
| Carcinoma of the duodenum | Bacterial pneumonia | Meningitis (viral, bacterial, and fungal) |
| Carcinoma of the pancreas | Pulmonary abscess | Head trauma |
| Thyroma | Tuberculosis | Brain abscess |
| Carcinoma of the stomach | Aspergillosis | Brain tumors |
| Lymphoma | Positive-pressure breathing | Guillain-Barré syndrome |
| Ewing sarcoma | Asthma | Acute intermittent porphyria |
| Carcinoma of the bladder | Pneumothorax | Subdural hematoma |
| Prostatic carcinoma | Mesothelioma | Subarachnoid hemorrhage |
| Oropharyngeal tumor | Cystic fibrosis | Cerebellar and cerebral atrophy |
| Carcinoma of the ureter | | Cavernous sinus thrombosis |
| | | Neonatal hypoxia |
| | | Hydrocephalus |
| | | Shy-Drager syndrome |
| | | Rocky Mountain spotted fever |
| | | Delirium tremens |
| | | Cerebrovascular accident (thrombosis or hemorrhage) |
| | | Acute psychosis |
| | | Peripheral neuropathy |
| | | Multiple sclerosis |

CNS, central nervous system.
From Berl T, Schrier RW: Disorders of water metabolism. In Schrier RW (ed): Renal and Electrolyte Disorders, 5th ed. Philadelphia, Lippincott-Raven, 1997, pp 1–67.

tained, giving rise to moderate nonedematous volume expansion and dilutional hyponatremia. The degree of volume expansion and hyponatremia is limited by the phenomenon of "vasopressin escape." Animal experiments show that, despite simultaneous water and ADH infusion, urine flow rises and urine osmolality decreases. This escape from antidiuresis is caused by marked and selective decrease in the expression of the arginine-vasopressin-regulated water channel AQP2, without a concomitant fall in the expression of the basolateral AQP3 and AQP4. However, in this model, the intracellular trafficking of AQP2 to the apical membrane was intact.[32] The downregulation appears to be dependent upon the maintenance of volume expansion and independent of changes in plasma or interstitial osmolality.

# MANAGEMENT OF HYPONATREMIA

Although most hyponatremic patients are symptomatic, severe hyponatremia is a medical emergency that may lead to cerebral edema, tentorial herniation, and death.[33] The therapeutic strategy is dictated by: (1) the underlying cause of the disorder, (2) the presence or absence of symptoms, (3) the duration of the disorder, and (4) the risk of neurologic complications. Acutely hyponatremic patients (with hyponatremia developing within 48 hours) are at great risk for developing permanent neurologic sequelae from cerebral edema if hyponatremia remains uncorrected; however, patients with chronic hyponatremia are at risk for osmotic demyelination if hyponatremia is corrected by an excessive amount. The treatment approach has been described in detail.[5]

## Symptoms of Hyponatremia

Most patients with hyponatremia are asymptomatic. Although gastrointestinal complaints occur early, most manifestations of hyponatremia are of a neuropsychiatric nature and include headache, lethargy, reversible ataxia, psychosis, seizures, and coma. Elderly and young children with hyponatremia are most likely to become symptomatic. The severity of symptoms is also dependent on the rate at which serum sodium concentration is lowered. Although no predictable correlation exists between changes in sensorium and the degree of hyponatremia, most patients who have seizures and coma have plasma sodium concentrations of less than 120 mEq/L. The signs and symptoms are most likely to be related to the cellular swelling and cerebral edema that is associated with hyponatremia. These occur primarily with rapid development of hyponatremia, typically in hospitalized patients managed with hypotonic fluids in the postoperative setting and in those receiving diuretics. The mortality rate can be as high as 50% in patients with severe hyponatremia if left untreated. Neurologic symptoms in a hyponatremic patient require prompt and immediate attention and treatment.

## Cerebral Adaptation to Hypotonicity

Decreases in extracellular osmolality produce flow of water into the intracellular space, and the resultant cellular edema within the fixed volume of the cranium causes an increase in intracranial pressure (ICP), which is responsible for the symptoms in acute hyponatremia. The brain possesses adaptive mechanisms that defend against such increases in ICP, making overt neurologic manifestations infrequent compared with the overall high prevalence of hyponatremia.[34] The first line of defense (within 1 to 3 hours) appears to be an increment in the flow of fluid from the interstitial space of the brain into cerebrospinal fluid (CSF). The excess CSF then enters the systemic circulation and effectively relieves some elevation of ICP.

The second defense mechanism that becomes operative, approximately 3 hours after the onset of hypotonicity, is the loss of cell solutes, primarily potassium. This is followed over the ensuing 72 hours by the loss of organic solutes, including glutamate, taurine, myoinositol, and glutamine.[35] The failure to adapt to extracellular hypotonicity results in cerebral water gain and edema. The benefits afforded by cerebral adaptation are also the source of the problems encountered in the treatment of hyponatremia. The increase in tonicity that is associated with correction of chronic hyponatremia requires an adaptive process in order to prevent cellular dehydration. Although serum sodium and potassium concentrations return to normal in a few hours, it takes several days for the osmotically active solutes in the brain to reach normal levels. This temporary imbalance causes cerebral dehydration and can lead to a potential breakdown of the blood-brain barrier.

Extensive literature documents that correction of chronic hyponatremia with resultant cerebral dehydration, in humans, is associated with central pontine myelinolysis (CPM) or, more broadly, with demyelinating lesions in the brain as whole—the so-called "osmotic demyelination." The risk for development of CPM is related to the severity and chronicity of the hyponatremia. It rarely occurs if the serum sodium levels are initially more than 120 mmol/L and if the hyponatremia is acute in onset (<48 hours). The typical clinical presentation is for patients to show an initial improvement in mental status after the start of correction, with a subsequent deterioration and development of: (1) motor abnormalities, sometimes progressing to flaccid quadriplegia and even respiratory paralysis; (2) pseudobulbar palsy; and (3) mental status or behavioral changes, including progressive loss of consciousness. On $T_2$-weighted magnetic resonance imaging, the lesions appear hyperintense. These lesions do not enhance with gadolinium and may not appear for 2 weeks after development. Therefore, a diagnosis of myelinolysis should not be excluded during the first 2 weeks of illness if the imaging is negative. CPM frequently pursues a fatal course within 3 to 5 weeks, making this a very serious complication of therapy. Table 14–5 lists the risk factors for neurologic complications of hyponatremia and its correction.[36]

TABLE 14–5. Patients at Risk for Developing Neurologic Complications of Hyponatremia

| Acute Cerebral Edema | Osmotic Demyelination |
|---|---|
| Postoperative menstruating women | Alcoholics |
| Elderly women taking thiazides | Malnourished patients |
| Polydipsic patients | Burn patients |
| Children | Elderly women taking thiazides |
| Associated hypoxemia | |

From Lauriat S, Berl T: The hyponatremia patient: Practical focus on therapy. J Am Soc Nephrol 8:1599–1607, 1997.

## Treatment of Hyponatremia (Fig. 14–4)[5]

**Treatment of Acute Symptomatic Hyponatremia.** In patients with acute (<48 hours) symptomatic hyponatremia, treatment should be prompt because the risk of cerebral edema far exceeds the risk of treatment complications. The goal of the correction should be targeted for a rise in serum sodium concentration of approximately 2 mEq/L/hr until symptoms resolve. Although full correction is probably safe, it is not necessary to aim for it. The infusion of hypertonic saline can promptly increase serum sodium, because the concentration of sodium in the urine is likely to be lower. The administration of furosemide promotes the excretion of free water [$UNa^+ + UK^+ < PNa^+$], thus further promoting an increase in serum sodium. Correction may be obtained with administration of hypertonic saline at the rate of 1 to 2 mL/hr per kg body weight. If severe neurologic manifestations are present, such as seizures, obtundation, or coma, 3% NaCl infusion rates can be increased up to 4 to 6 mL/hr per kg body weight. In the absence of hypertonic saline, mannitol (1 g/kg) could be used.[37] In turn, the prompt excretion of mannitol also ensures the excretion of electrolyte-free water. Whenever using hypertonic saline to treat severe hyponatremia, the patient should be monitored in an intensive care unit setting and electrolytes should be measured regularly. The change in serum sodium cannot be predicted solely on the basis of the infused solution, because a variation in the volume and electrolyte content of the concomitantly produced urine can have an impact on the degree of this change.

**Treatment of Chronic Symptomatic Hyponatremia.** When patients present with symptomatic hyponatremia of an unknown duration or for longer than 48 hours, then therapy for correction of hyponatremia should be applied with great caution to avoid complications of therapy. The key question of whether it is the rate or the magnitude of correction that increases the likelihood for neurologic complication remains unanswered. At the bedside, these two variables are not readily dissociated, because a rapid correction rate is usually accompanied by a greater absolute magnitude of correction over a given period of time. Therefore, these two variables should be strongly considered when applying therapeutic regimens for patients with chronic symptomatic hyponatremia.

We have proposed the following guidelines for treating the chronic hyponatremic patient[36]:

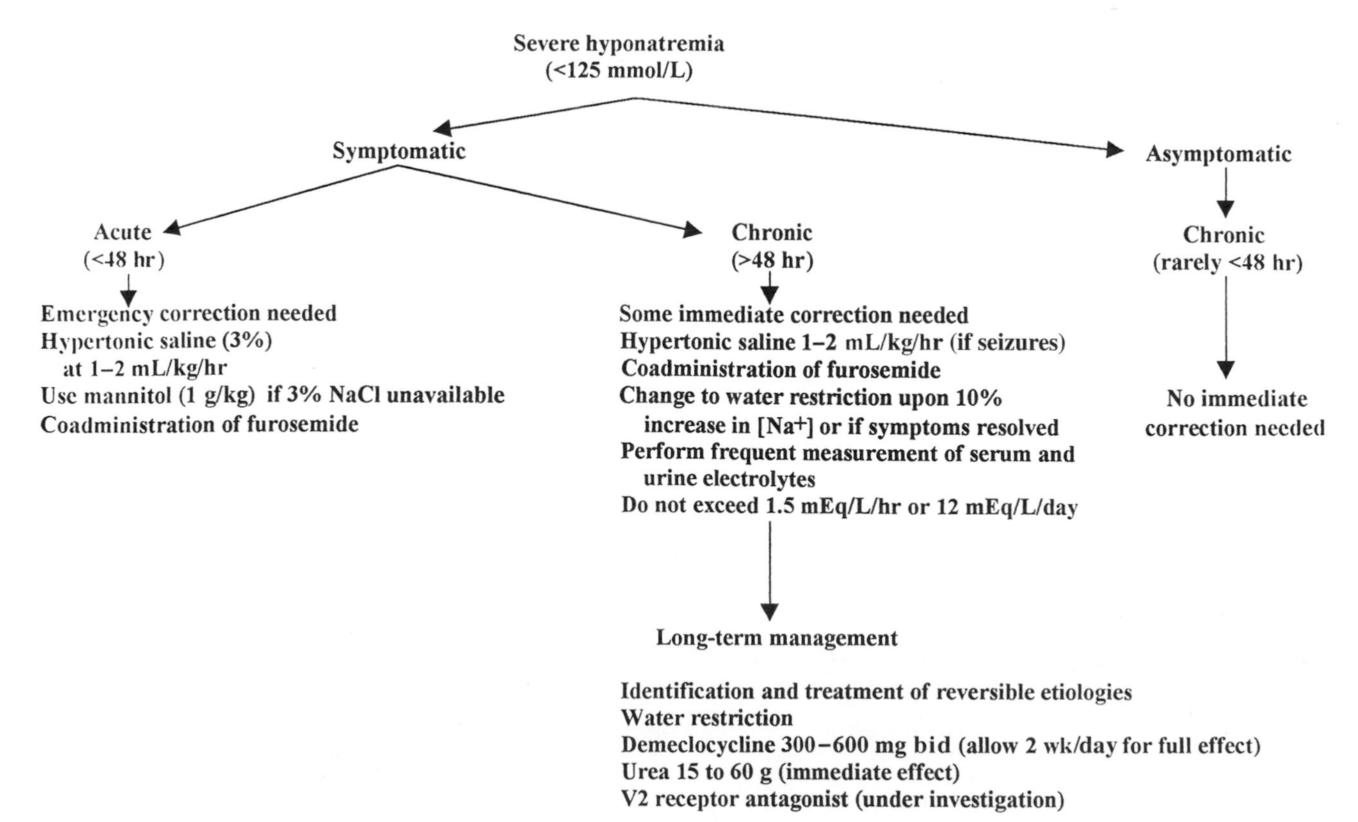


FIGURE 14–4 ■ Treatment of severe euvolemic hyponatremia. (From Halterman R, Berl T: Therapy of dysnatremic disorder. In Brady H, Wilcox C [eds]: Therapy in Nephrology and Hypertension. Philadelphia, WB Saunders, 1999, pp 257–269.)

1. Because cerebral water is increased only by approximately 10% in severe chronic hyponatremia, promptly increase the serum sodium level by 10%, or by approximately 10 mmol/L.
2. After the initial correction, do not exceed a correction rate of 1 to 1.5 mmol/L hr.
3. Do not increase the serum sodium by more than 12 mmol/L in 24 hours.

The rate and electrolyte content of infused fluids as well as the rate and electrolyte content of the urine are important variables to consider when correcting hyponatremia. There are data in experimental animals and even a human case report that suggest that if these parameters have been exceeded, the relowering of serum $Na^+$ by the administration of free water with vasopressin could prevent the development of the demyelinating syndrome.[38] After the desired increment is attained, therapy can continue in the form of water restriction.

**Treatment of Chronic Asymptomatic Hyponatremia.** The initial evaluation of patients with chronic asymptomatic hyponatremia should include looking for an underlying disorder. Hypothyroidism, adrenal insufficiency, and SIADH should all be considered as possible etiologies. A careful review of the patient's medications should always be made. The therapeutic approach for patients with SIADH of unknown etiology should be conservative, because significant changes in serum tonicity might lead to severe neurologic complications.

Fluid restriction is the first line of therapy in patients with chronic asymptomatic hyponatremia. Fluid restriction should be prescribed with an initial restriction of 1 L/day. In most patients, this is adequate to allow net free water excretion, but in some, such a volume exceeds insensible and urinary losses, with no resultant improvement. Fluid restriction of 1 L or less is difficult to attain in the outpatient setting and may necessitate pharmacologic therapy. Of these, demeclocycline is the drug of choice in the treatment of chronic hyponatremia.[39] The acute use of $V_2$ antagonists has been described in patients with SIADH. As expected, it is accompanied by decreases in urinary osmolality. Its use in a sustained manner is under investigation.[40]

**Hypovolemic Hyponatremia** (Table 14–6). Patients with hypovolemic hyponatremia have sustained a deficit in total body sodium that exceeds the deficit in water. In the presence of hypovolemia, AVP is secreted and water retained despite the hypo-osmolality perpetuating the hyponatremia. Neurologic manifestations secondary to the hyponatremia are unusual, because the losses of both sodium and water limit any osmotic shift in the brain. The main objective of therapy is the administration of isotonic saline, with treatment of the underlying disorder. Restoration of the ECF interrupts the nonosmotic release of vasopressin followed with normalization of the serum sodium. Nonetheless, there is no reason to assume that hypovolemia per se protects against the complications of excessive treatment. If replacement with isotonic NaCl is necessary for the restoration of volume, the rate of increase in serum $Na^+$ can be greatly alternated by the concomitant administration of vasopressin to ensure the excretion of a concentrated urine.

**TABLE 14–6.** Treatment of Noneuvolemic Hyponatremia

| Hypovolemic Hyponatremia | Hypervolemic Hyponatremia |
|---|---|
| Volume restoration with isotonic saline | Water restriction |
| Identify and correct etiology of water and sodium losses | Sodium restriction |
| | Loop diuretics |
| | Treatment of stimulus for sodium and water excretion |
| | $V_2$ receptor antagonist (under investigation) |

**Hypervolemic Hyponatremia** (see Table 14–6). Hypervolemic hyponatremia is observed in patients who have an increase in total body sodium content, but the rise in total body water exceeds that of sodium. This condition is very difficult to treat, because it often reflects severe dysfunction of either the liver, heart, or kidney. Nonosmotic stimulation of AVP as well as an increase in thirst secondary to decrease in effective arterial blood volume is characteristic in heart failure, cirrhosis, and nephrotic syndrome. Compliance with water restriction is essential but difficult to achieve. Diuretics are key agents to treat edematous disorders, but caution must be used in selecting the appropriate regimen. Whereas thiazide diuretics should be avoided because they impair urinary dilution and may worsen the hyponatremia, loop diuretics increase free water excretion and can improve the serum sodium. Patients with congestive heart failure should be treated with an angiotensin-converting enzyme inhibitor. The increase in cardiac output that follows decreases the neurohormonal mediated processes that limit water excretion. Oral $V_2$ receptor antagonists are being tested in hyponatremic patients with congestive heart failure and cirrhosis. In a few patients with cirrhosis, ascites, and water retention, OPC-31260 (a $V_2$ receptor antagonist) was found to be effective in causing water diuresis.[41] $V_2$ antagonists are not yet available for widespread clinical use.

## REFERENCES


1. Ayus JC, Arief AI: Glycine-induced hypo-osmolar hyponatremia. Arch Intern Med 157:223–226, 1997.
2. Hillier TA, Abbott RD, Borrett EJ: Hyponatremia: Evaluating correction factors for hyperglycemia. Am J Med 106:399–403, 1999.
3. Weisberg LS: Pseudohyponatremia: A reappraisal. Am J Med 86: 315–318, 1989.
4. Thaler SM, Teitelbaum I, Berl T: "Beer potomania" in non-beer drinkers: Effect of low dietary solute intake. Am J Kidney Dis 31:1028–1031, 1998.
5. Halterman R, Berl T: Therapy of dysnatremic disorders. In Brady H, Wilcox C (eds): Therapy in Nephrology and Hypertension. Philadelphia, WB Saunders, 1999, pp 257–269.
6. Schrier RW, Regal EM: Influence of aldosterone on sodium, water and potassium metabolism in chronic renal disease. Kidney Int 1:156, 1972.
7. Ashraf N, Locksley R, Arieff AI: Thiazide-induced hyponatremia associated with death or neurological damage in outpatients. Am J Med 70:1163, 1998.

8. Szatalowicz VL, Miller PD, Lacher JW: Comparative effect of diuretics on renal water excretion in hyponatremic edematous disorders. Clin Sci 62:235, 1982.
9. Harrigan MR: Cerebral salt wasting syndrome: A review. Neurosurgery 38:152–160, 1996.
10. Palmer BF: Hyponatremia in a neurosurgical patient: Syndrome of inappropriate antidiuretic hormone secretion versus cerebral salt wasting. Nephrol Dial Transplant 15:262–268, 2000.
11. Schrier RW: Pathogenesis of sodium and water retention in high-output and low-output cardiac failure, nephrotic syndrome, cirrhosis, and pregnancy. N Engl J Med 319:1065–1072, 1988.
12. Schrier RW, Berl T, Anderson RJ: Osmotic and nonosmotic control of vasopressin release. Am J Physiol 236:F321–F332, 1979.
13. Schrier RW, Abraham WT: Hormones and hemodynamics in heart failure. N Engl J Med 341:577–584, 1999.
14. Xu DL, Martin PY, Ohara M, et al: Upregulation of aquaporin-2 water channel expression in chronic heart failure of the rat. J Clin Invest 99:1500–1503, 1997.
15. Martin PY, Gines P, Schrier RW: Nitric oxide as mediator of hemodynamic abnormalities and sodium and water retention in cirrhosis. N Engl J Med 339:553–541, 1998.
16. Fujita N, Ishikawa SE, Sasaki S, et al: Role of water channel AQP-CD in water retention in SIADH and cirrhotic rats. Am J Physiol 269:F926–F931, 1995.
17. Berl T: Aquaporin in health and disease. Kidney Int 53:1417–1418, 1998.
18. Ohara M, Martin PY, Xu DL, et al: Upregulation of aquaporin 2 water channel expression in pregnant rats. J Clin Invest 101: 1076–1083, 1998.
19. Anderson RJ, Chung HM, Kluge R, Schrier RW: Hyponatremia: A prospective analysis of its epidemiology and the pathogenetic role of vasopressin. Ann Intern Med 102:164–168, 1985.
20. Iwasaki Y, Oiso Y, Yamauchi K, et al: Osmoregulation of plasma vasopressin in myxedema. J Clin Endocrinol Metab 70:534–539, 1990.
21. Raskind MA, Barnes RF: Water metabolism in psychiatric disorders. Semin Nephrol 4:316, 1984.
22. Russel GF, Bruce JT: Impaired water diuresis in patients with anorexia nervosa. Am J Med 40:38, 1966.
23. Goldman M; Luchins DJ, Robertson GL: Mechanism of altered water metabolism in psychotic patients with polydipsia and hyponatremia. N Engl J Med 318:397, 1988.
24. Anderson RJ: Hospital-associated hyponatremia. Kidney Int 29: 1237–1247, 1986.
25. Steele A, Gowrishankar M, Abrahamson S, et al: Postoperative hyponatremia despite near isotonic saline infusion: A phenomenon of desalination. Ann Intern Med 126:20–25, 1997.
26. Arieff AI: Hyponatremia, convulsions, respiratory arrest, and permanent brain damage after elective surgery in healthy women. N Engl J Med 314:1529–1535, 1986.
27. Veis JH, Berl T: Hyponatremia. In Jacobson HR, Striker GE, Klahr S (eds): The Principles and Practice of Nephrology. St. Louis, CV Mosby, 1995, pp 888–893.
28. Miller M, Hecker MS, Friedlander DA, Carter JM: Apparent idiopathic hyponatremia in an ambulatory geriatric population. J Am Geriatr Soc 44:404–408, 1996.
29. Clark BA, Shannon RP, Rosa RM, Epstein FH: Increased susceptibility to thiazide-induced hyponatremia in the elderly. J Am Soc Nephrol 5:1106–1111, 1994.
30. Verbalis J: The syndrome of inappropriate antidiuretic hormone secretion and other hypoosmolar disorders. In Schrier RW, Gottschalk C (eds): Diseases of the Kidney, vol 3. Boston, Little Brown, 1997, pp 2392–2427.
31. Berl T, Schrier RW: Disorders of water metabolism. In Schrier RW (ed): Renal and Electrolyte Disorders, 5th ed. Philadelphia, Lippincott-Raven, 1997, pp 1–67.
32. Ecelbarger CA, Nielsen S, Olson BR, et al: Role of renal aquaporins in escape from vasopressin-induced antidiuresis in rats. J Clin Invest 99:1852–1863, 1997.
33. Sterns RH: The management of symptomatic hyponatremia. Semin Nephrol 10:510–514, 1990.
34. Verbalis JG: Hyponatremia: Epidemiology, pathophysiology and therapy. Curr Opin Nephrol Hypertens 2:636, 1993.
35. Sterns RH, Baer J, Ebersol S, et al: Organic osmolytes in acute hyponatremia. Am J Physiol 264:F833–F836, 1993.
36. Lauriat S, Berl T: The hyponatremic patient: Practical focus on therapy. J Am Soc Nephrol 8:1599–1607, 1997.
37. Porzio P, Halberthal M, Bohn D, Halperin ML: Treatment of acute hyponatremia: Ensuring the excretion of a predictable amount of electrolyte-free water. Crit Care Med 28:1905–1910, 2000.
38. Soupart A, Ngassa M, Decaux G: Therapeutic relowering of the serum sodium in a patient after excessive correction of hyponatremia. Clinical Nephrol 51:383–386, 1999.
39. Forrest JN, Cox M, Hong C, et al: Superiority of demeclocycline over lithium in the treatment of chronic syndrome of inappropriate secretion of antidiuretic hormone. N Engl J Med 298: 173, 1978.
40. Saito T, Ishikawa SE, Abe K, et al: Acute aquaresis by the nonpeptide arginine vasopressin (AVP) antagonist OPC-31260 improves hyponatremia in patients with syndrome of inappropriate secretion of antidiuretic hormone (SIADH). J Clin Endocrinol Metab 82:1054–1057, 1997.
41. Inoue T, Ohnishi A, Matsuo A, et al: Therapeutic and diagnostic potential of a vasopressin-2 antagonist for impaired water handling in cirrhosis. Clin Pharmacol Ther 63:561–570, 1998.

CHAPTER 15

# Hypernatremia and the Polyuric Disorders

Daniel G. Bichet, MD ■ Jean-Pierre Mallié, MD

Hypertonicity ordinarily results from a high concentration of salt, which stresses animal cells because the ensuing osmotic efflux of water shrinks the cells and concentrates their contents. This shrinkage causes mechanical stresses. Concentration of intracellular salts and crowding of large intracellular molecules greatly affect the structure and activity of proteins, DNA, and other cellular macromolecules.[1]

The tonicity of body fluids is maintained within a narrow physiologic range by homeostatic mechanisms controlling water intake and excretion. The key components of this system are antidiuretic hormone (ADH), arginine vasopressin (AVP), and the renal countercurrent system. In this chapter we describe osmoreceptors located in the hypothalamus that control the secretion of vasopressin in response to changes in tonicity. In turn, vasopressin governs the excretion of water by its end-organ effect on the renal collecting system.

## HYPERNATREMIC STATES

From the clinical point of view, two primary mechanisms defend the body against water depletion and hyperosmolality of the extracellular fluid (ECF) space. These two defense mechanisms are the capacity of the kidney to excrete a concentrated urine and the stimulation of thirst to increase water intake. Each pathway is very effective, and disturbance of the urinary concentrating mechanism alone generally does not cause hyperosmolality if the thirst mechanism is intact. Hypernatremia develops when hypotonic fluid losses occur in combination with a disturbance in water intake. This combination of events is most commonly seen in the aged, with alteration in the level of consciousness; in intubated patients; in children and adults with nephrogenic diabetes insipidus and inadequate access to water; and, rarely, in a subject with a primary disturbance of thirst. As shown in Figure 15–1, hypernatremia can develop with low, normal, or high total body sodium.[2] Net water loss accounts for the majority of cases of hypernatremia.[3]

### Hypernatremia Associated with Low Total Body Sodium

When losses of both sodium and water occur, but there is a relatively greater loss of water, hypernatremia with low total body sodium develops. On physical examination, patients with low total body sodium manifest signs of hypovolemia such as orthostatic hypotension, tachycardia, flat neck veins, poor skin turgor, dry mucous membranes, and sometimes altered mental status. Hypotonic losses can occur by the renal route, as is seen with an osmotic diuresis due to mannitol, glucose, or urea excretion, or by an extrarenal route, as can occur with profuse sweating or diarrhea.

In cases of osmotic diuresis, the urine is hypotonic or isotonic, with a urinary sodium concentration greater than 20 mEq/L. When extrarenal losses of hypotonic fluid occur, the renal water- and sodium-conserving mechanisms continue to operate normally. Therefore, urinary osmolality is high (usually >800 mOsm/kg water), and urinary sodium concentration is less than 10 mEq/L.

### Hypernatremia Associated with High Total Body Sodium

Administration of exogenous hypertonic sodium–containing solutes can result in hypernatremia with a high total body sodium, the least common type of hypernatremia.[4] This type most commonly occurs secondary to the administration of hypertonic sodium bicarbonate during resuscitative efforts, intravascular infusion of hypertonic saline during therapeutic abortions, dialysis against a high-sodium-concentration dialysate, and seawater drowning. Ingesting large quantities of sodium chloride tablets in hot, humid climates can also result in hypernatremia with a high total body sodium.

Clinically insignificant elevations in serum sodium concentration occur in patients with primary hyperaldosteronism and Cushing syndrome. In these patients, urine sodium concentration reflects sodium intake.

Patients with hypernatremia associated with high total body sodium exhibit an isotonic or hypertonic urine, with a urinary sodium concentration greater than 20 mEq/L.

### Signs and Symptoms of Hypernatremia

Manifestations of hypernatremia and hyperosmolar states are usually of a neurologic nature and are related to cellular dehydration.[5–10] Neurologic symptoms associated with hypernatremia include restlessness, irritability, lethargy, muscular twitching, hyperreflexia, and spasticity. Coma, seizures, and death may ultimately occur. Morbidity and mortality of acute hypernatremia are very high. Mortality from acute hypernatremia may be as high as 45% in children and 75% in adults, especially if the serum sodium is greater than

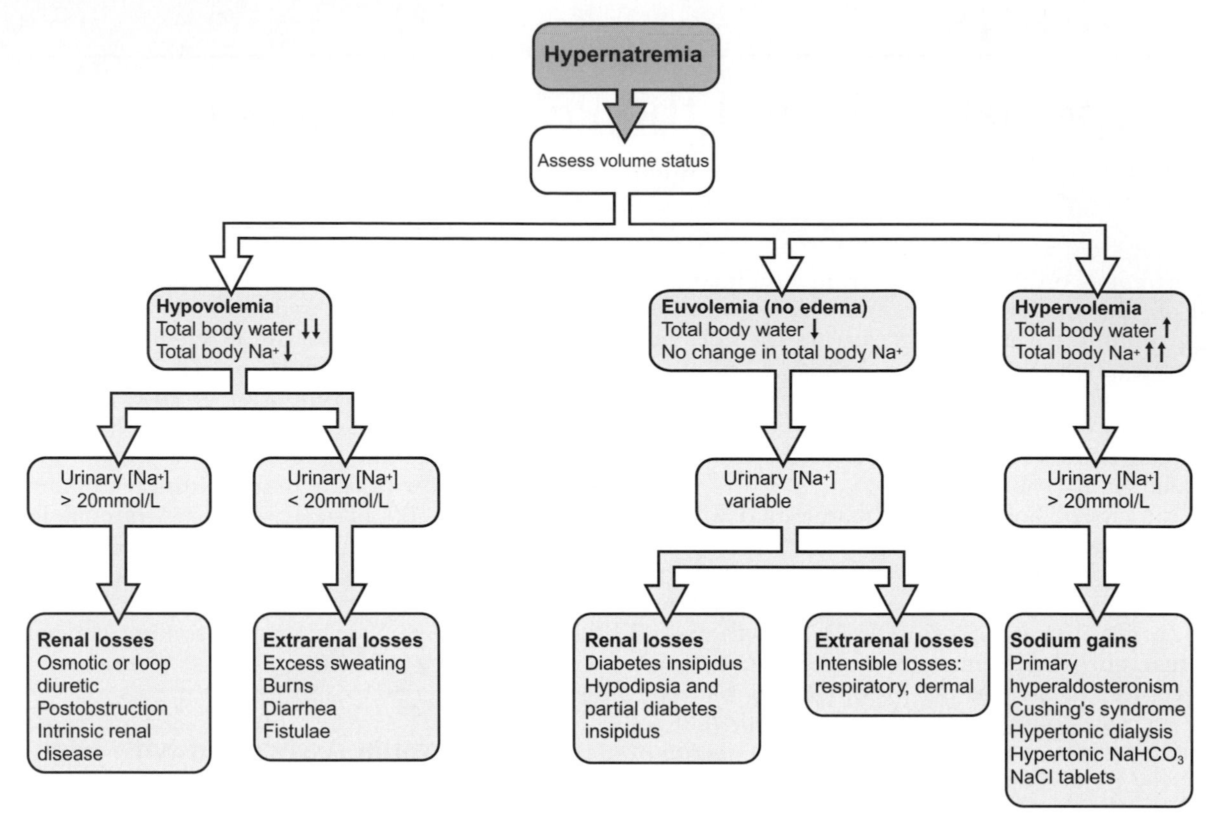


**FIGURE 15–1** ■ Diagnostic approach for the hypernatremic patient. Note that a net water loss accounts for the majority of cases of hypernatremia. In addition, a tonicity balance calculation is an accurate way to understand the basis for the change in natremia and the proper goals of therapy. This tonicity balance calculation allows the demonstration of iatrogenic sodium gains and their proper treatment.[276] (Modified from Berl T, Kumar S: Disorders of metabolism. In Johnson RJ, Feehally J [eds]: Comprehensive Clinical Nephrology. London, Mosby, 2000, p. 9.1.)

160 mEq/L.[7] In patients who were at least 60 years of age, hypernatremia was associated with a mortality of 42%, seven times that of age-matched hospitalized control patients.[11] Mortality is not predicted by the severity of hypernatremia, and mortality is slightly lower in patients with chronic hypernatremia.[7] Survivors of acute hypernatremia frequently exhibit neurologic sequelae. In adults, hypernatremia is associated with high mortality and may reflect the severity of the underlying disease.

In addition to the cellular mechanical stresses described early,[1] signs and symptoms of hypernatremia can be related to a variety of anatomic derangements. Tearing of cerebral vessels secondary to loss of volume and shrinkage of brain cells in hyperosmolar states may occur. Brain shrinkage is countered by an adaptative response that is initiated promptly and consists of solute gain by the brain, which tends to restore lost water. This response leads to the normalization of brain volume and accounts for the milder symptoms of hypernatremia that develops slowly.[12] Acute hypernatremia can result in the development of capillary and venous congestion, subcortical and subarachnoid bleeding, and venous thrombosis.[13, 14] Some of these changes may be evident on computed tomography scans of the head. Alterations in the brain water and solutes following hypernatremia have been described.[3, 15]

## Therapy for Hypernatremia

Treatment of patients with hypernatremia involves management of the hypernatremia itself and the concomitant problems that are frequently present. A close investigation of the underlying illness is always required. The primary goal in the treatment of hypernatremia is restoration of serum tonicity. The specific approach depends on the patient's ECF volume status (Fig. 15–2).

Correction of circulatory disturbances, with plasma expanders or isotonic sodium chloride, in patients with low total body sodium secondary to hypotonic fluid losses is of primary importance. Once hemodynamics are stabilized, hypernatremia can be treated by increasing free water intake with 0.45% sodium chloride, 0.2% sodium chloride (referred to as one-quarter isotonic saline), 5% dextrose, or ingestion of free water. The more hypotonic the infusate, the lower the infusion rate required; the risk of cerebral edema increases with the volume of the infusate.[3]

In patients who are hypernatremic and hypervolemic secondary to salt intoxication, removal of excess sodium is the goal. This can be accomplished by administration of a diuretic along with 5% dextrose or by dialysis in patients with impaired renal function. The amount of water necessary to dilute the sodium

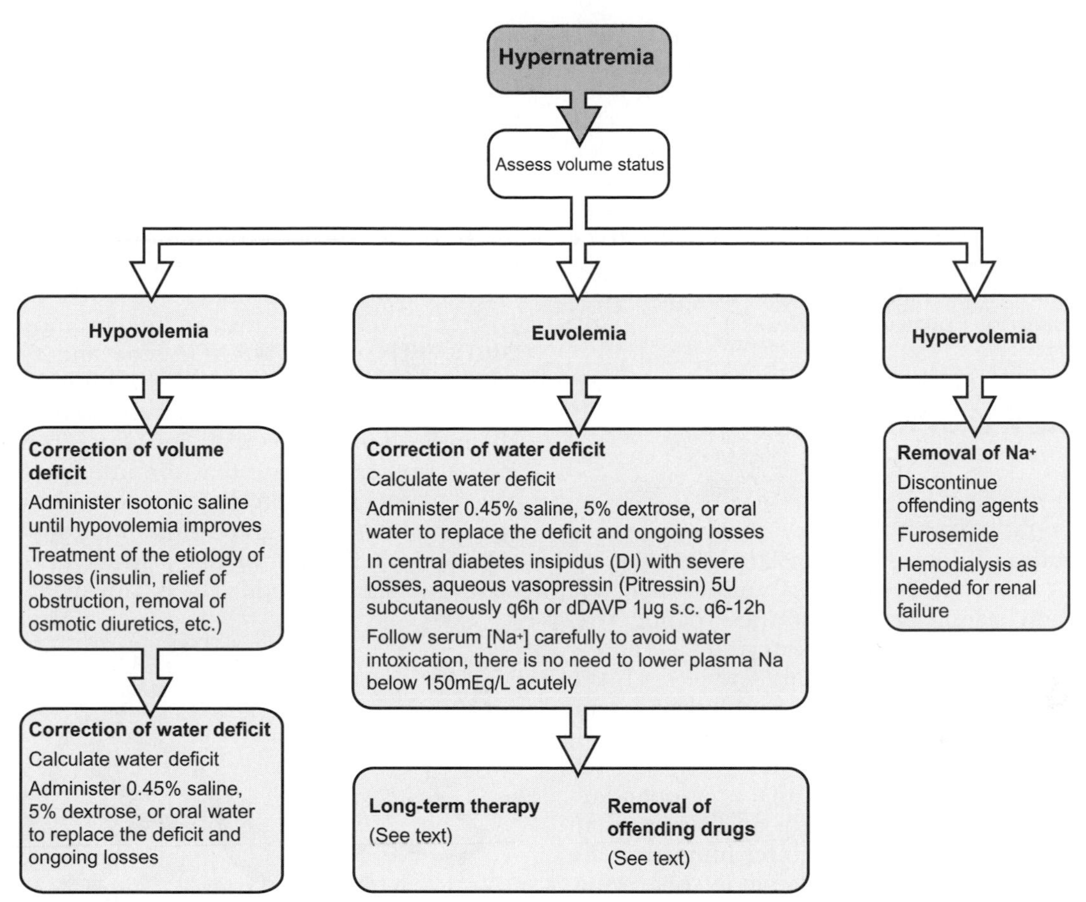


**FIGURE 15–2** ■ Management options for patients with hypernatremia. (Modified from Berl T, Kumar S: Disorders of metabolism. In Johnson RJ, Feehally J [eds]: Comprehensive Clinical Nephrology. London, Mosby, 2000, p 9.1.)

concentration back to normal can be calculated as follows:

$$\text{Water deficit (L)} = 0.6 \times \text{body weight (kg)} \times \left[1 - \frac{\text{current plasma sodium } (P_{Na})}{140}\right]$$

In this formula, the estimated total body water is calculated as a fraction of body weight. The fraction is 0.6 in children; 0.6 and 0.5 in nonelderly men and women, respectively; and 0.5 and 0.45 in elderly men and women, respectively. In a 70-kg man with a plasma sodium concentration of 158 mEq/L, using the above formula yields a water deficit of 8.4 L. This formula only estimates the water deficit, and careful patient monitoring is necessary during therapy.

A hypernatremic patient who has sustained pure water losses and who is euvolemic requires replacement of water in the form of a 5% dextrose infusion. The water deficit can be calculated using the preceeding formula. The following three assumptions may make the calculation less than totally accurate: body water is always 60% of body weight, water is lost uniformly throughout all body cells, and there is pure water loss without solute loss. Thus, the formula provides only an estimation of the water deficit, which can direct initial therapy. The total water deficit should be replaced rapidly only when symptoms are severe; there is no need to acutely "correct" a plasma sodium below 150 mEq/L. In patients with hypernatremia that has developed over a period of hours (e.g., those with accidental sodium loading), rapid correction improves the prognosis without increasing the risk of cerebral edema, because accumulated electrolytes are rapidly extruded from brain cells.[3] In such patients, reducing the serum sodium concentration by 1 mmol/L/hr is appropriate. In patients with chronic hypernatremia, a slower pace of correction is indicated, because the full dissipation of accumulated brain solutes occurs over several days.[12] Faster correction in the presence of idiogenic osmoles may result in cerebral edema by creating an osmotic gradient between brain and plasma. Slower correction of the water deficit can prevent the development of cerebral edema by allowing the solutes (idiogenic osmoles) time to dissipate.

Correction of hypernatremia over 4 to 24 hours in experimental animals was associated with the development of cerebral edema (9% increase in brain water content).[16] Brain amino acid content was still increased with this time interval for correction of hypernatremia. Experimental data investigating correction over longer periods are lacking. As a rule, extreme care must be taken to avoid excessively rapid correction of hypernatremia, which increases the risk of iatrogenic cerebral edema, with possibly catastrophic consequences. The fluid prescription should be reassessed at regular intervals in the light of laboratory values, and the patient's clinical status should be re-evaluated at frequent intervals. The treatment of hypernatremic, vomiting children with severe nephrogenic diabetes insipidus secondary to *AVPR2* or *AQP2* mutations is described later in this chapter. A "lithium patient" (with acquired nephrogenic diabetes insipidus) undergoing a routine surgical procedure with subsequent massive postoperative polyuria and hypernatremia is also described later (see "Treatment of Polyuric Disorders").

# ARGININE VASOPRESSIN

## Synthesis

Nonapeptides of the vasopressin family are the key regulators of water homeostasis in amphibians, reptiles, birds, and mammals. Because these peptides reduce urinary output, they are also referred to as antidiuretic hormones. For a detailed review of the magnocellular hypothalamoneurohypophysial system, see reference 17. Oxytocin and AVP are synthesized in separate populations of magnocellular neurons (20 to 40 μm cell body diameter) of the supraoptic and paraventricular nuclei.[18] Oxytocin and vasopressin magnocellular neurons are found intermingled in the magnocellular nuclei, although there is some topographic segregation. Oxytocin is most recognized for its key role in parturition and milk letdown in mammals.[19] The axonal projections of AVP- and oxytocin-producing neurons from supraoptic and paraventricular nuclei reflect the dual function of AVP and oxytocin as hormones and neuropeptides, in that they project their axons to several brain areas and to the neurohypophysis. Another pathway from parvocellular neurons (10 to 15 μm cell body diameter) to the hypophysial portal system transports high concentrations of AVP to the anterior pituitary gland. AVP produced by this pathway together with corticotropin-releasing hormone (CRH) are two major hypothalamic secretagogues regulating the secretion of adrenocorticotropic hormone (ACTH) by the anterior pituitary.[20]

More than half of parvocellular neurons coexpress both *CRH* and *prepro-AVP-NPII*. In addition, while passing through the median eminence and the hypophysial stalk, magnocellular axons can release AVP into the long portal system. Furthermore, a number of neuroanatomic studies have shown the existence of short portal vessels that allow communication between the posterior and anterior pituitary. Thus, in addition to parvocellular vasopressin, magnocellular vasopressin is able to influence ACTH secretion.[20, 21]

AVP and its corresponding carrier protein, neurophysin II (NPII), are synthesized as a composite precursor by the magnocellular and parvocellular neurons described previously. In contrast to conventional neurotransmitters (e.g., acetylcholine, excitatory and inhibitory amino acids, monoamines), which are synthesized in nerve terminals and can be packaged locally in recycled small vesicular membranes, the biosynthesis and secretion of neuropeptides such as oxytocin and vasopressin in the hypothalamoneurohypophysial system require continual de novo transcription and translation of peptide precursor proteins.[17] The precursor is packaged into neurosecretory granules and transported axonally in the stalk of the posterior pituitary. En route to the neurohypophysis, the precursor is processed into the active hormone. Prepro-vasopressin has 164 amino acids and is encoded by the 2.5-kb *prepro-AVP-NPII* gene located in chromosome region 20p13.[22] The *prepro-AVP-NPII* gene and the *prepro-OT-NPI* gene are located within the same chromosomal locus, at a very short distance from each other (3 to 11 kb) in head-to-head orientation. Data from transgenic mouse studies indicate that the intergenic region between the OT and AVP genes contains the critical enhancer sites for magnocellular neurons' cell-specific expression.[23] Exon 1 of the *prepro-AVP-NPII* gene encodes the signal peptide, AVP, and the $NH_2$-terminal

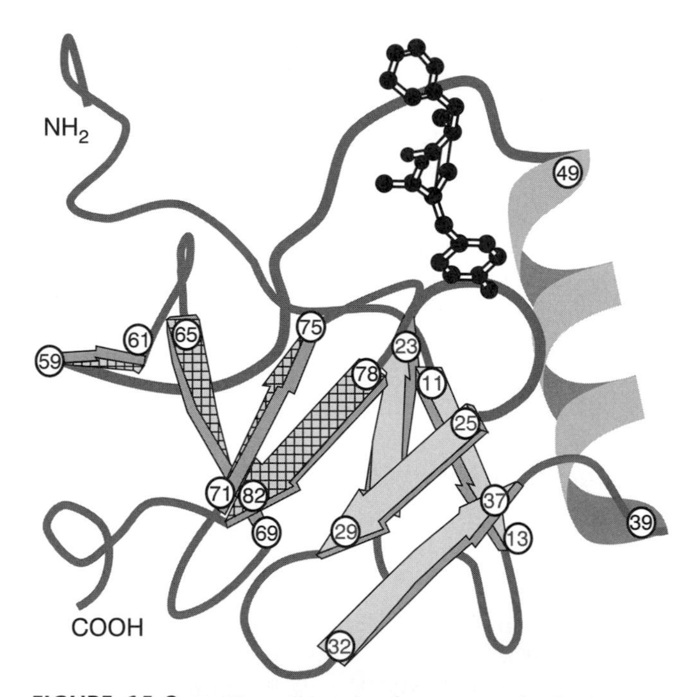


**FIGURE 15–3** ■ Three-dimensional structure of a bovine peptide-neurophysin monomer complex. The structure of each chain is 12% helix and 40% β sheet. The chain is folded into two domains, as predicted by disulfide-pairing studies. The amino-terminal domain begins in a long loop (residues 1–10), then enters a four-stranded (residues 11–13, 19–23, 25–29, and 32–37) antiparallel β sheet (sheet I; *four shaded arrows*), followed by a three-turn $3_{10}$-helix (residues 39–49) and another loop (residues 50–58). The carboxyl-terminal domain is shorter, consisting of only a four-stranded (residues 59–61, 65–69, 71–75, and 78–82) antiparallel β sheet (sheet II; *four cross-hatched arrows*).[24] The arginine vasopressin molecule (balls and sticks model) is shown in the peptide-binding pocket of the neurophysin monomer. The strongest interactions in this binding pocket are salt-bridge interactions between the $\alpha NH3^+$ group of the peptide, the $\gamma$-$COO^-$ group of $Glu^{NP47}$ (residue number 47 of the neurophysin molecule), and the side chain of $Arg^{NP8}$. The $\gamma$-$COO^-$ group of $Glu^{NP47}$ plays a bifunctional role in the peptide-binding pocket: It directly interacts with the hormone, and it interacts with other neurophysin residues to establish the correct, local structure of the peptide-neurophysin complex. $Arg^{NP8}$ and $Glu^{NP47}$ are conserved in all neurophysin sequences from mammals to invertebrates.

region of NPII. Exon 2 encodes the central region of NPII, and exon 3 encodes the COOH-terminal region of NPII and the glycopeptide. Pro-vasopressin is generated by the removal of the signal peptide from prepro-vasopressin and the addition of a carbohydrate chain to the glycopeptide. Additional post-translation processing occurs within neurosecretory vesicles during transport of the precursor protein to axon terminals in the posterior pituitary, yielding AVP, NPII, and glycopeptide. The AVP-NPII complex forms tetramers that can self-associate to form higher oligomers[24] (Fig. 15–3). Neurophysins should be seen as chaperone-like molecules serving intracellular transport in magnocellular cells.[17]

In the posterior pituitary, AVP is stored in vesicles. Exocytotic release is stimulated by minute increases in serum osmolality (hypernatremia, osmotic regulation) and by more pronounced decreases of ECF (hypovolemia, nonosmotic regulation). Oxytocin and neurophysin I are released from the posterior pituitary by the suckling response in lactating females.

## Osmotic and Nonosmotic Stimulation

The regulation of ADH release from the posterior pituitary is dependent primarily on two mechanisms involving the osmotic and nonosmotic pathways[25] (Fig. 15–4). Vasopressin release can be regulated by changes in either osmolality[26] or cerebrospinal fluid $Na^+$ concentration.[27–30] Voisin and colleagues demonstrated coincident detection of CSF $Na^+$ and osmotic pressure in magnocellular osmoregulatory neurons of the supraoptic nucleus.[31]

The concept of cerebral osmoreceptors and their role in the control of vasopressin secretion derives from the classical studies of Verney.[32] These osmoreceptors have been shown to respond to changes in blood osmolality of 1% or less, and all the available evidence leads to the conclusion that they are located in the anterior part of the brain, presumably in the anterior hypothalamus.

Three criteria must be met for cells to be identified as osmoreceptive. First, increasing the osmolality of the perfusing fluid should result in an increase in firing frequency (a specific electrophysiologic property of vasopressin-secreting magnocellular cells), but no response should be obtained if the osmolality is increased with solutes such as urea or glycerol, because these solutes can diffuse across the cell membrane. Furthermore, the osmoreceptor cells should display a sensitivity to changes in osmolality that approaches that observed in vivo. Second, the putative osmoreceptors must, if they are not the magnocellular neurons themselves, have neuroanatomic connections with the magnocellular neurons. Third, if the osmoreceptors are separated from the magnocellular neurons, alterations in vasopressin secretion secondary to changes in plasma osmolality should occur.[33] The following candidates fulfill these criteria for osmoreceptors:

- Magnocellular cells that synthesize vasopressin in the supraoptic nucleus and paraventricular nucleus

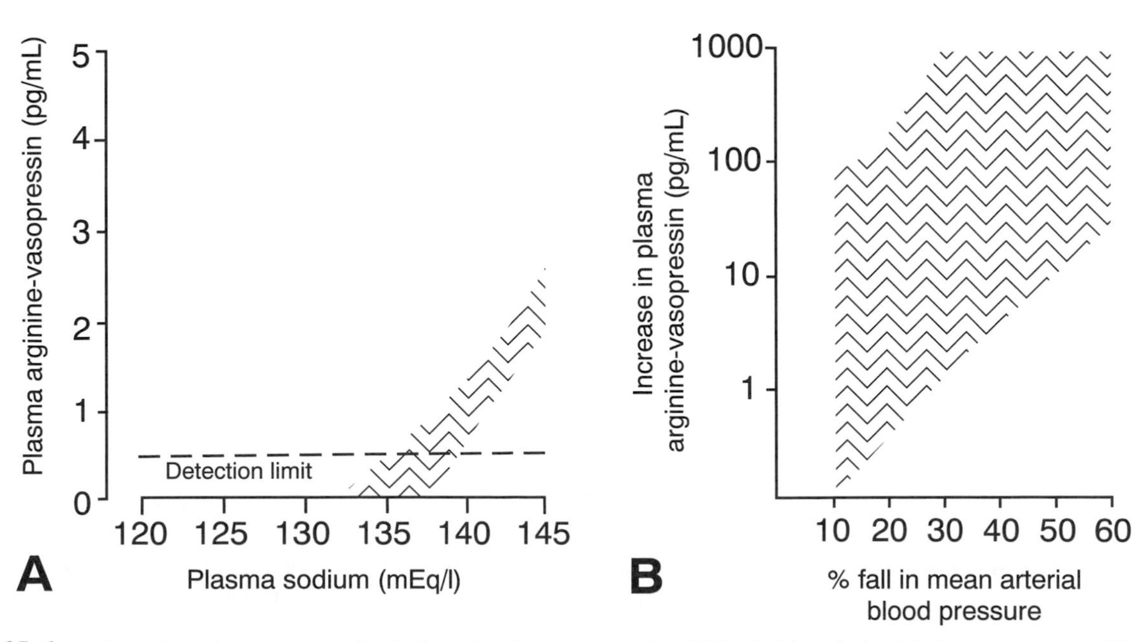


**FIGURE 15–4** ■ Osmotic and nonosmotic stimulation of arginine vasopressin (AVP). *A,* The relationship between plasma AVP ($P_{AVP}$) and plasma sodium ($P_{Na}$) in 19 normal subjects is described by the area with zagging lines, which includes the 99% confidence limits of the regression line $P_{Na}/P_{AVP}$. The osmotic threshold for AVP release is about 280 to 285 mmol/kg, or 136 mEq of sodium per liter. AVP secretion should be abolished when plasma sodium is lower than 135 mEq/L.[258] *B,* Increase in plasma AVP during hypotension (*zagging lines*). Note that a large diminution in blood pressure in normal humans induces large increments in AVP. (From Vokes T, Robertson GL: Physiology of secretion of vasopressin. In Czernichow P, Robinson AG [eds]: Diabetes Insipidus in Man. Basel, S. Karger, 1985.)

- Perinuclear zone around the supraoptic nucleus
- Cells in the subfornical organ (SFO) and organum vasculosum of the lamina terminalis (OVLT)
- Cells in the lateral preoptic area

Changes in excitatory synaptic drive, derived from osmosensitive neurons in the OVLT, combine with endogenously generated osmoreceptor potentials to modulate the firing rate of magnocellular cells and hence the release of AVP. In other words, although magnocellular neurons are themselves osmosensitive,[30, 34] they require input from the lamina terminalis to respond fully to osmotic challenges.[35, 36] Neurons in the lamina terminalis are also osmosensitive,[30] and because the SFO and OVLT lie outside the blood-brain barrier, they can integrate this information with endocrine signals borne by circulating hormones, such as angiotensin II, relaxin, and atrial natriuretic peptide.[37, 38] Whereas circulating angiotensin II and relaxin excite both oxytocin and vasopressin magnocellular neurons, atrial natriuretic peptide inhibits vasopressin neurons.[39–41] In addition to an angiotensinergic path from the SFO, the OVLT and the median preoptic nucleus provide direct glutaminergic and GABAergic projection to the hypothalamoneurohypophysial system.[42, 43] Because inputs from the lamina terminalis can be either excitatory or inhibitory, the view is that the osmoresponsive circuit increases the overall sensitivity of the hypothalamoneurohypophysial system to osmotic stimuli. Nitric oxide may also modulate neurohormone release.[44, 45]

The cellular basis for osmoreceptor potentials has been characterized using patch-clamp recordings and morphometric analysis in magnocellular cells isolated from the supraoptic nucleus of the adult rat.[30] In these cells, stretch-inactivating cationic channels transduce osmotically evoked changes in cell volume into functionally relevant changes in membrane potential (Fig. 15–5). In addition, magnocellular neurons operate as intrinsic $Na^+$ detectors.[31] A vanilloid receptor–related osmotically activated channel has been cloned and shown to be expressed in neurons of the circumventricular organs.[46] However, a full biophysical characterization of this channel has not been published.

Vasopressin release can also be caused by the nonosmotic stimulation of AVP. Large decrements in blood volume or blood pressure (>10%) stimulate ADH release (see Fig. 15–4). A fall in arterial blood pressure produces secretion of vasopressin due to an inhibition of baroreceptors in the aortic arch and activation of chemoreceptors in the carotid body.[47] Afferents from these receptors terminate in the dorsal medulla oblongata of the brainstem, including the nucleus of the tractus solitarius. The resting inhibitory effect of baroreceptor activity on vasopressin neurons is mediated indirectly via the A6 noradrenergic cell group of the locus coeruleus, the diagonal band of Broca in the forebrain, and neurons lying just outside the magnocellular nuclei.[48–50] Release from this inhibition after hemorrhage or direct electrical stimulation of the nucleus of the tractus solitarius causes the activation of vasopressin neurons via the stimulatory A1 noradrenergic cell group of the ventral medulla.[51, 52] The A1 group projects directly to vasopressin magnocellular cells to stimulate hormone release via α1-adrenoreceptors.[53] It is of note that knockout mice with loss of function of angiotensinogen (a precursor peptide of angiotensin II) or of the angiotensin receptor type 1A do not demonstrate obvious alterations in thirst or in water

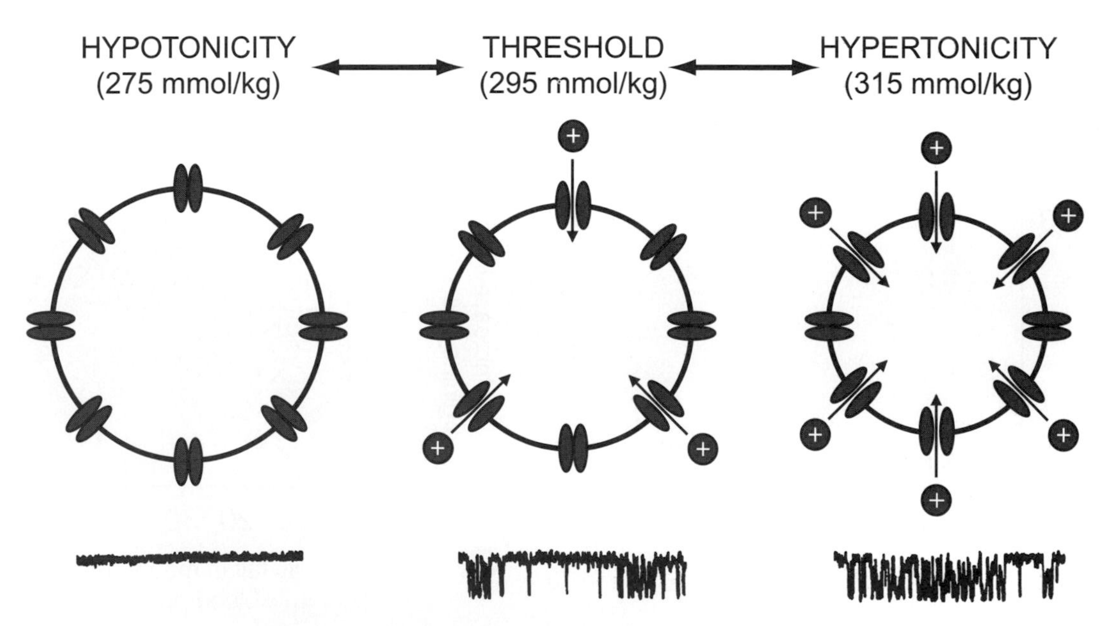


**FIGURE 15–5** ■ Stretch inactivated (SI) cationic channels transduce osmoreception. Under resting osmotic conditions (*middle panel*), a portion of the SI cationic channels is active and allows the influx of positive charge. Hypotonic stimulation (*left*) provokes cell swelling and inhibits channel activity, thereby hyperpolarizing the cell. In contrast, hypertonic stimulation (*right*) causes cell shrinking. Activation of an increased number of channels under this condition augments charge influx and results in membrane depolarization. Traces representing changes in the activity of a single SI channel are shown below. (From Bourque CW, Oliet SHR: Osmoreceptors in the central nervous system. Annu Rev Physiol 59:601, 1997.)

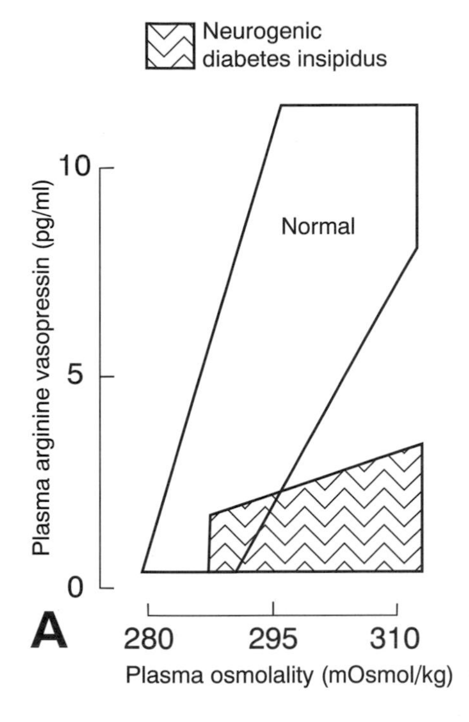


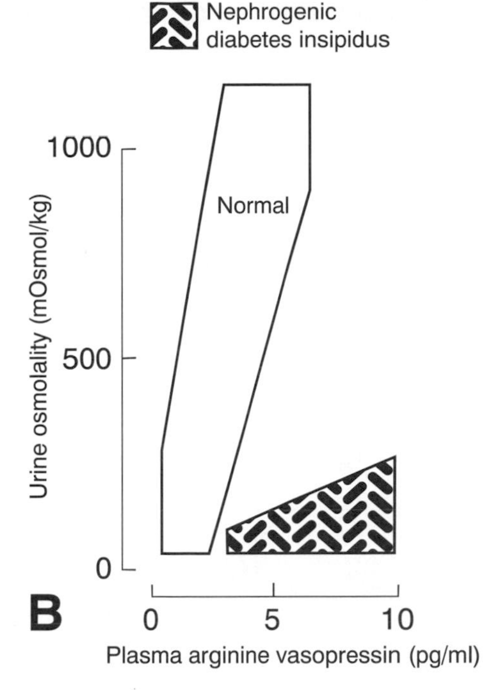


**FIGURE 15–6** ■ *A,* Relationship between plasma arginine vasopressin (AVP) and plasma osmolality during infusion of hypertonic saline solution. Patients with primary polydipsia and nephrogenic diabetes insipidus have values within the normal range (*open area*), in contrast to patients with neurogenic diabetes insipidus, who show subnormal plasma antidiuretic hormone (ADH) responses (*cross-hatched area*). *B,* Relationship between urine osmolality and plasma ADH during dehydration and water loading. Patients with neurogenic diabetes insipidus and primary polydipsia have values within the normal range (*open area*), in contrast to patients with nephrogenic diabetes insipidus, who have hypotonic urine despite high plasma ADH (*strippled area*). (From Zerbe RL, Robertson GL: Disorders of ADH. Med North Am 13:1570, 1984.)

balance.[54–56] Mice that lack the gene encoding the angiotensin receptor type 2 have a mild impairment in drinking response to water deprivation.[57]

The osmotic stimulation of AVP release by dehydration, hypertonic saline infusion, or both is regularly used to determine the vasopressin secretory capacity of the posterior pituitary. This secretory capacity can be assessed *directly* by comparing the plasma AVP concentrations measured sequentially during the dehydration procedure with the normal values[58] and then correlating the plasma AVP values with the urine osmolality measurements obtained simultaneously (Fig. 15–6).

The AVP release can also be assessed *indirectly* by measuring plasma and urine osmolalities at regular intervals during the dehydration test.[59] The maximal urine osmolality obtained during dehydration is compared with the maximal urine osmolality obtained after the administration of vasopressin (Pitressin, 5 U SC in adults, 1 U SC in children) or 1-deamino (8-D-arginine) vasopressin (desmopressin [DDAVP], 1 to 4 μg IV over 5 to 10 minutes).

The nonosmotic stimulation of AVP release can be used to assess the vasopressin secretory capacity of the posterior pituitary in a rare group of patients with the essential hyponatremia and hypodipsia syndrome.[60] Although some of these patients may have partial central diabetes insipidus, they respond normally to nonosmolar AVP release signals such as hypotension, emesis, and hypoglycemia.[60] In all other cases of suspected central diabetes insipidus, these nonosmotic stimulation tests will not give additional clinical information.[61]

## Clinically Important Hormonal Influences on Vasopressin Secretion

Angiotensin is a well-known dipsogen and has been shown to cause drinking in all the species tested.[62] Angiotensin II receptors have been described in the SFO and OVLT (reviewed in reference 63). However, knockout models for angiotensinogen[55] or for angiotensin 1A receptor[54, 56] did not alter thirst or water balance. Disruption of the angiotensin receptor induced only mild abnormalities of thirst after dehydration.[57] Earlier reports suggested that the IV administration of atrial peptides inhibits the release of vasopressin,[64] but this was not confirmed by Goetz and coworkers.[65] Furthermore, Ogawa and colleagues found no evidence that atrial natriuretic peptide, administered centrally or peripherally, was important in the physiologic regulation of plasma AVP release in conscious rats.[66] A very rapid and robust release of AVP is seen in humans after cholecystokinin injection.[67] Nitric oxide is an inhibitory modulator of the hypothalamoneurohypophysial system in response to osmotic stimuli.[68–71] Vasopressin secretion is under the influence of a glucocorticoid-negative feedback system,[72] and the vasopressin responses to a variety of stimuli (hemorrhage, hypoxia, hypertonic saline) in normal humans and animals appear to be attenuated or eliminated by pretreatment with glucocorticoids. Finally, nausea and emesis are potent stimuli of AVP release in humans and seem to involve dopaminergic neurotransmission.[73]

## Cellular Actions of Vasopressin

The neurohypophysial hormone AVP has multiple actions, including the inhibition of diuresis, contraction of smooth muscle, platelet aggregation, stimulation of liver glycogenolysis, modulation of ACTH release from the pituitary, and central regulation of somatic functions (thermoregulation, blood pres-

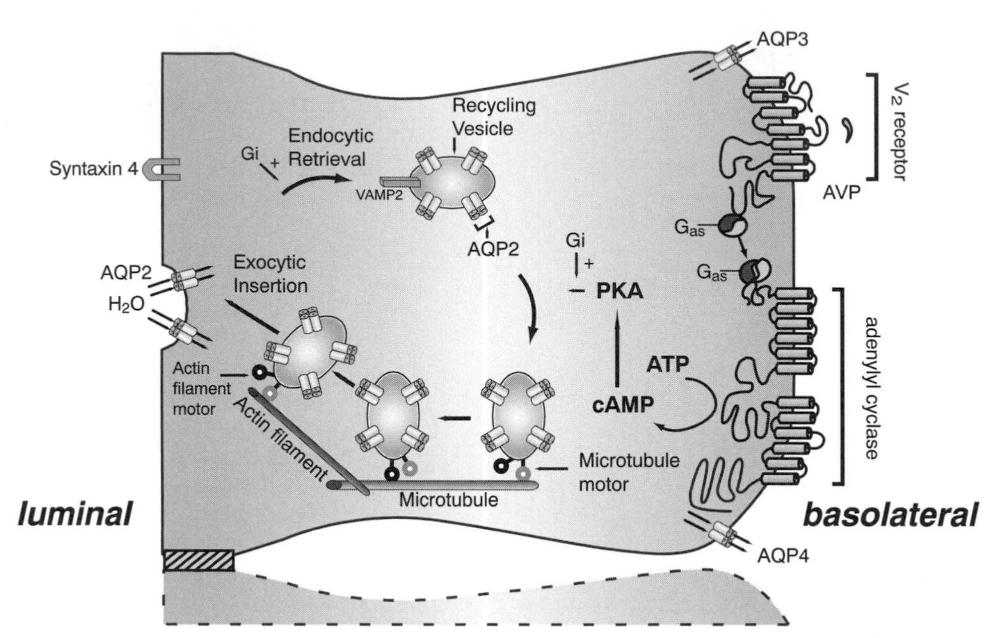


**FIGURE 15–7** ■ Schematic representation of the effect of arginine vasopressin (AVP) to increase water permeability in the principal cells of the collecting duct. AVP is bound to the $V_2$ receptor (a G protein–linked receptor) on the basolateral membrane. The basic process of G protein–coupled receptor signaling consists of three steps: a hepta-helical receptor that detects a ligand (in this case, AVP) in the extracellular milieu, a G protein that dissociates into α subunits bound to guanosine triphosphate (GTP) and βγ subunits after interaction with the ligand-bound receptor, and an effector (in this case, adenylyl cyclase) that interacts with dissociated G protein subunits to generate small-molecule second messengers. AVP activates adenylyl cyclase, increasing the intracellular concentration of cyclic adenosine monophosphate (cAMP). The topology of adenylyl cyclase is characterized by two tandem repeats of six hydrophobic transmembrane domains separated by a large cytoplasmic loop and terminates in a large intracellular tail. Generation of cAMP follows receptor-linked activation of the heteromeric G protein ($G_s$) and interaction of the free $G_{\alpha s}$-chain with the adenylyl cyclase catalyst. Protein kinase A (PKA) is the target of the generated cAMP. Cytoplasmic vesicles carrying the water channel proteins (represented as homotetrameric complexes) are fused to the luminal membrane in response to AVP, thereby increasing the water permeability of this membrane. Microtubules and actin filaments are necessary for vesicle movement toward the membrane. The mechanisms underlying docking and fusion of aquaporin type 2 (AQP2)–bearing vesicles are not known. The detection of the small GTP binding protein Rab3a, synaptobrevin 2, and syntaxin 4 in principal cells suggests that these proteins are involved in AQP2 trafficking.[91] When AVP is not available, water channels are retrieved by an endocytic process, and water permeability returns to its original low rate. AQP3 and AQP4 water channels are expressed on the basolateral membrane.

sure).[74] These multiple actions of AVP could be explained by the interaction of AVP with at least three types of G protein–coupled receptors; the $V_{1a}$ (vascular hepatic) and $V_{1b}$ (anterior pituitary) receptors act through phosphatidylinositol hydrolysis to mobilize calcium,[74] and the $V_2$ (kidney) receptor is coupled to adenylate cyclase.[75]

The first step in the action of AVP on water excretion is its binding to AVP type 2 receptors ($V_2$ receptors) on the basolateral membrane of the collecting duct cells (Fig. 15–7). The human $V_2$ receptor gene, *AVPR2,* is located in chromosome region Xq28 and has three exons and two small introns.[76, 77] The sequence of the complementary DNA (cDNA) predicts a polypeptide of 371 amino acids with a structure typical of guanine nucleotide (G) protein–coupled receptors with seven transmembrane, four extracellular, and four cytoplasmic domains[78] (Fig. 15–8). The activation of the $V_2$ receptor on renal collecting tubules stimulates adenylate cyclase via the stimulatory G protein ($G_s$) and promotes the cyclic adenosine monophosphate (cAMP)–mediated incorporation of water channels (aquaporins) into the luminal surface of these cells. This process is the molecular basis of the vasopressin-induced increase in the osmotic water permeability of the apical membrane of the collecting tubule.

Aquaporin type 1 (AQP1; also known as CHIP, a channel-forming integral membrane protein of 28 kd) was the first protein shown to function as a molecular water channel[79] and is constitutively expressed in mammalian red cells, renal proximal tubules, thin descending limbs,[80–83] and other water-permeable epithelia.[82] At the subcellular level, AQP1 is localized in both apical and basolateral plasma membranes, which may represent entrance and exit routes for transepithelial water transport.

Murata and associates described an atomic model of AQP1 at 3.8 Δ resolution from electron crystallographic data and solved a long-standing puzzle in physiology: how membranes can be freely permeable to water but impermeable to protons.[84] They confirmed the key importance of the two Asn-Pro-Ala motifs in the pore helices HB and HE (for a review on aquaporins, see reference 85). The positive charge of a proton

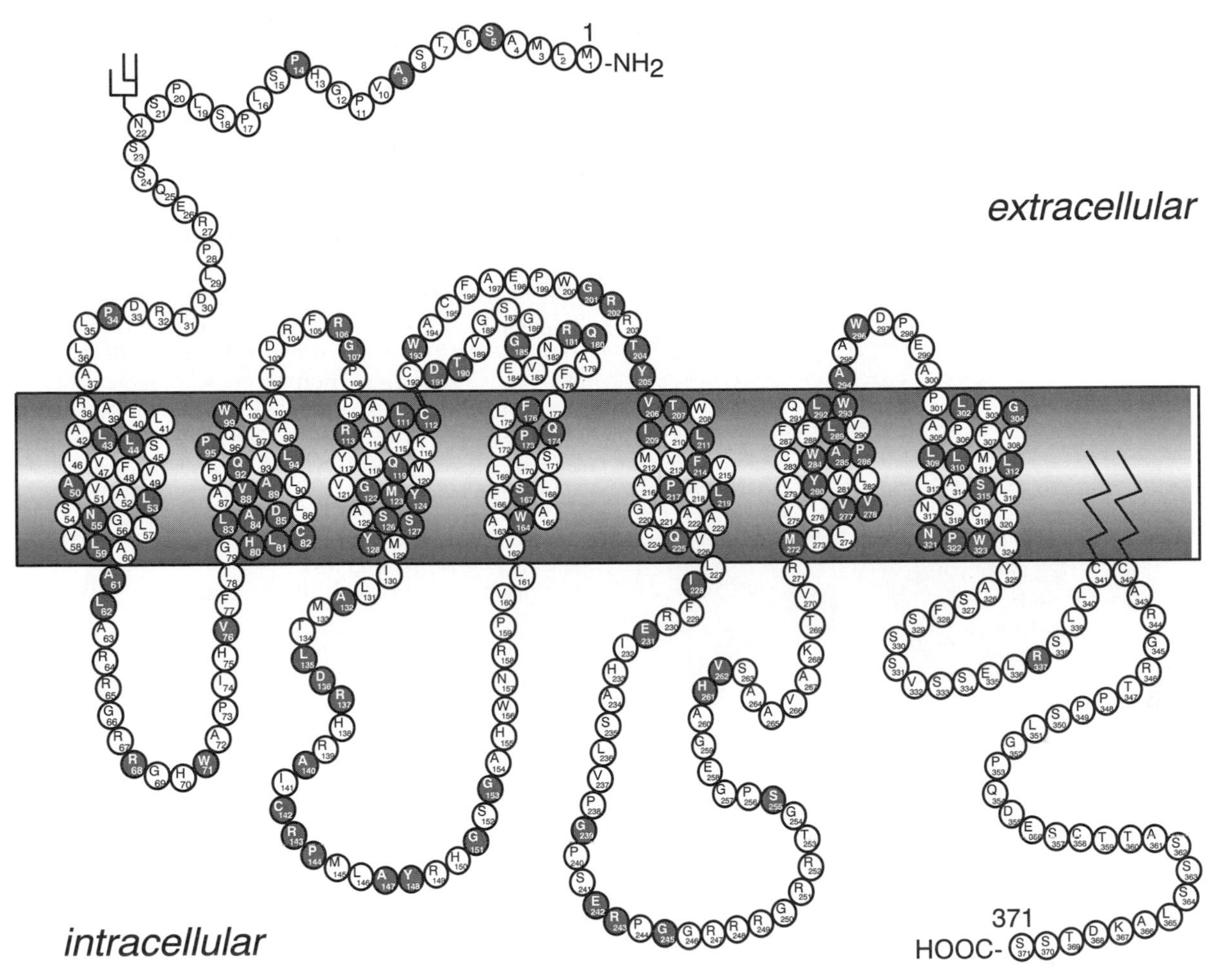


**FIGURE 15–8** ■ Schematic representation of the $V_2$ receptor and identification of 155 putative disease-causing *AVPR2* mutations. Predicted amino acids are given as the one-letter code. A solid symbol indicates the location (or the closest codon) of a mutation; a number indicates more than one mutation in the same codon. The names of the mutations were assigned according to recommended nomenclature.[273] The extracellular, transmembrane, and cytoplasmic domains are defined according to Mouillac and coworkers.[277] The common names of the mutations are listed by type. *Seventy-eight missense:* L43P, L44F, L44P, L53R, N55D, N55H, L59P, L62P, H80R, L81F, L83P, L83Q, A84D, D85N, V88L, V88M, Q92R, L94Q, P95L, W99R, R106C, G107E, C112R, R113W, G122R, M123K, S126F, S127F, Y128S, A132D, L135P, R137H, [C142W; R143G], R143P, A147V, W164S, S167L, S167T, Q174L, R181C, G185C, D191G, G201D, R202C, T204N, Y205C, V206D, T207N, I209F, F214S, P217T, L219P, L219R, M272K, V277A, Y280C, A285P, P286L, P286R, P286S, L289P, L292P, A294P, L309P, S315R(AGC>AGA), S315R(AGC>AGG), N317K, C319R, N321D, N321K, N321Y, P322H, P322S, W323R, W323S. *Seventeen nonsense:* W71X, Q119X, Y124X, W164X, S167X, Q180X, W193X(TGG>TAG), W193X(TGG>TGA), Q225X, E231X, E242X, W284X, W293X, W296X, L312X, W323X, R337X. *Forty-two frameshift:* in $E_{I}$ – 15delC, 27–54del, 46–47delCT, 54–55ins28, 102delG; in TMI – 137–138delTA; in $C_{I}$ – 185–219del, 206–207insG, [225delC; 223C>A]; in $TM_{II}$ – 247–248ins7, 268–269delCT, 295delT; in $TM_{III}$ – 331–332delCT, 335–336delGT, 340delG, 407–446del; in $C_{II}$ – 418delG, 430–442del, 442–443insG, 452delG, 457–463del, 460delG; in $E_{III}$ – 567–568insC, 572–575del, 612–613insC, 614–615delAT; in $TM_{V}$ – 631delC; $C_{III}$ – 682–683insC, 692delA, 717delG, 727–728delAG, 738delG, 738–739insG, 763delA, 784delG, 785–786insT; in $TM_{VI}$ – 838–839insT, 847–851del, 851–852ins5; in $TM_{VII}$ –, 907delG, 930delC, 969delG. *Six inframe deletions or insertions:* in $C_{I}$ – 185–193del; in $TM_{II}$ – 252–253ins9; in $TM_{III}$ – Y128del; in $TM_{IV}$ – F176del; in $E_{III}$ – R202del; in $TM_{VI}$ – V279del. *Three splice-site:* IVS2+1delG, IVS2+1G>A, IVS2-2A>G. [184, 187, 188, 190, 199, 200, 280–307] Eight large deletions and one complex mutation are not shown.[184, 190, 199, 296, 300] Please note that new and recurrent *AVPR2* mutations are identified every year (see www.medicine.mcgill.ca/nephros/).

($H_3O^+$) can move along a column of water by hydrogen bond exchange; this single-file hydrogen-bonded chain of water molecules, which conducts protons with great efficiency, has been termed "proton wire" by Pomes and Roux.[86] In the middle of the AQP1 pore, the oxygen atom of the water molecule forms hydrogen bonds with Asn 76 and/or Asn 192 by changing the hydrogen-bonding partner from the adjacent water molecule. This reorients the two hydrogen atoms of the water molecule at the pore constriction perpendicular to the channel axis (Fig. 15–9). Thus, the two hydrogen atoms of the water molecule are prevented from forming hydrogen bonds with adjacent water molecules in the single-file column.

Aquaporin type 2 (AQP2) is the vasopressin-regulated water channel in renal collecting ducts. It is exclusively present in principal cells of inner medullary collecting duct cells and is diffusely distributed in the cytoplasm in the euhydrated condition, whereas apical staining of AQP2 is intensified in the dehydrated condition or after administration of DDAVP, a synthetic structural analog of AVP. The short-term AQP2 regulation by AVP involves the movement of AQP2 from intracellular vesicles to the plasma membrane, a

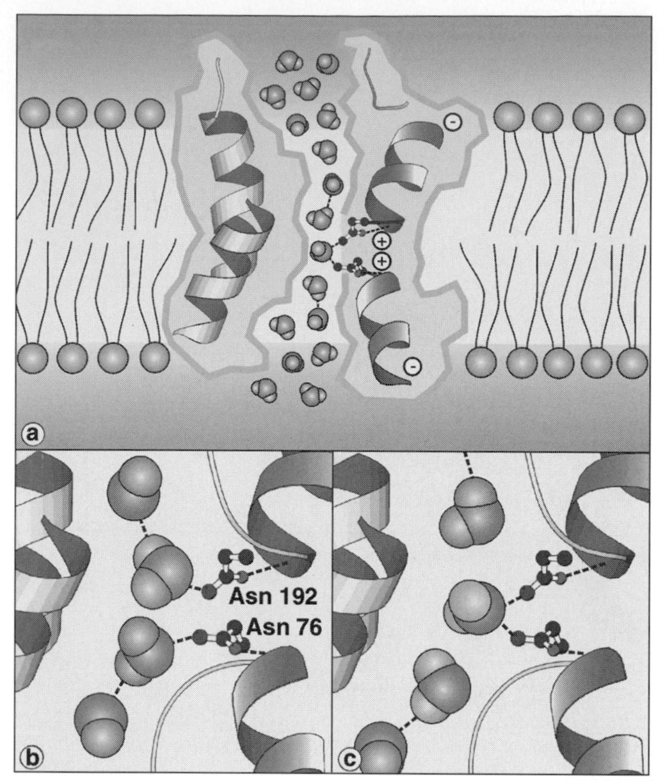


**FIGURE 15–9** ■ Schematic representations explaining the mechanism for blocking proton permeation of aquaporin type 1 (AQP1). *A,* Diagram illustrating how partial charges from the helix dipoles restrict the orientation of the water molecules passing through the constriction of the pore. *B* and *C,* Diagrams illustrating hydrogen bonding of a water molecule with Asn 76 and/or Asn 192, which extend their amido groups into the constriction of the pore. The ribbon and ball-stick models in this figure were prepared with MOLSCRIPT.[308] (From Murata K, Mitsuoka K, Hirai T, et al: Structural determinants of water permeation through aquaporin-1. Nature 407: 599, 2000.© 2000 by Macmillan Magazines Ltd.)

confirmation of the shuttle hypothesis of AVP action that was proposed 2 decades ago.[87] In the long-term regulation, which requires a sustained elevation of circulating AVP levels for 24 hours or more, AVP increases the abundance of water channels. This is thought to be a consequence of increased transcription of the *AQP2* gene.[88] The activation of PKA leads to phosphorylation of AQP2 on serine residue 256 in the cytoplasmic carboxyl terminus. This phosphorylation step is essential for the regulated movement of AQP2-containing vesicles to the plasma membrane upon elevation of intracellular cAMP concentration.[89, 90] A second G protein (the first being the cholera toxin–sensitive G protein $G_s$) has also been shown to be essential for the AVP-induced shuttling of AQP2. This G protein is sensitive to pertussis toxin and is involved in the pathway downstream of the cAMP/cAMP-dependent protein kinase signal.[91] The molecular basis for the translocation of the AQP2-containing vesicles is not completely known, but it is thought to be analogous to neuronal exocytosis.[92] This is supported by identification in the vesicles of various proteins known to be involved in regulated exocytosis, for example, Rab3a and synaptobrevin II (VAMP2) or synaptobrevin II–like protein.[93–95] In contrast to neuronal exocytosis, which is triggered by $Ca^{2+}$, cAMP and PKA appear to be crucial for the translocation process.[96, 97] Vesicle trafficking probably involves the interaction of AQP2-containing vesicles with the cytoskeleton[98] (see Fig. 15–7). Drugs that disrupt microtubules or actin filaments have long been known to inhibit the hormonally induced permeability response in target epithelia.[99] Sabolic and coworkers showed that microtubules are required for the apical polarization of AQP2 in principal cells.[100] AQP3 and AQP4 are the constitutive water channels in the basolateral membranes of renal medullary collecting ducts.

AVP also increases the water reabsorptive capacity of the kidney by regulating the urea transporter UT1, which is present in the inner medullary collecting duct, predominantly in its terminal part.[101] AVP also increases the permeability of principal collecting duct cells to sodium.[102]

In summary, as stated elegantly by Ward and colleagues, in the absence of AVP stimulation, collecting duct epithelia exhibit very low permeability to sodium urea and water.[102] These specialized permeability properties permit the excretion of large volumes of hypotonic urine formed during intervals of water diuresis. In contrast, AVP stimulation of the principal cells of the collecting ducts leads to selective increases in the permeability of the apical membrane to water ($P_f$), urea ($P_{urea}$), and sodium ($P_{Na}$).

These actions of vasopressin in the distal nephron are possibly modulated by prostaglandin $E_2$ and by the luminal calcium concentration. High levels of E-prostanoid ($EP_3$) receptors are expressed in the kidney.[103] However, mice lacking $EP_3$ receptors for prostaglandin $E_2$ were found to have quasi-normal regulation of urine volume and osmolality in response to various physiologic stimuli.[103] An apical calcium-polycation receptor protein expressed in the terminal portion of the inner medullary collecting duct of the rat has been shown to reduce AVP-elicited osmotic water permeability when luminal calcium concentration rises.[104] This possible link between calcium and water metabolism may play a role in the pathogenesis of renal stone formation.[104]

The gene that codes for the water channel of the apical membrane of the kidney collecting tubule has been designated *AQP2* and was cloned by homology to the rat aquaporin of the collecting duct.[105–107] The human *AQP2* gene is located in chromosome region 12q13 and has four exons and three introns.[106–108] It is predicted to code for a polypeptide of 271 amino acids that is organized into two repeats oriented at 180 degrees to each other and has six membrane-spanning domains, both terminal ends located intracellularly, and conserved Asn-Pro-Ala boxes (Fig. 15–10). These features are characteristic of the major intrinsic protein family.[107] AQP2 is detectable in urine, and changes in urinary excretion of this protein can be used as an index of the action of vasopressin on the kidney.[109–111]

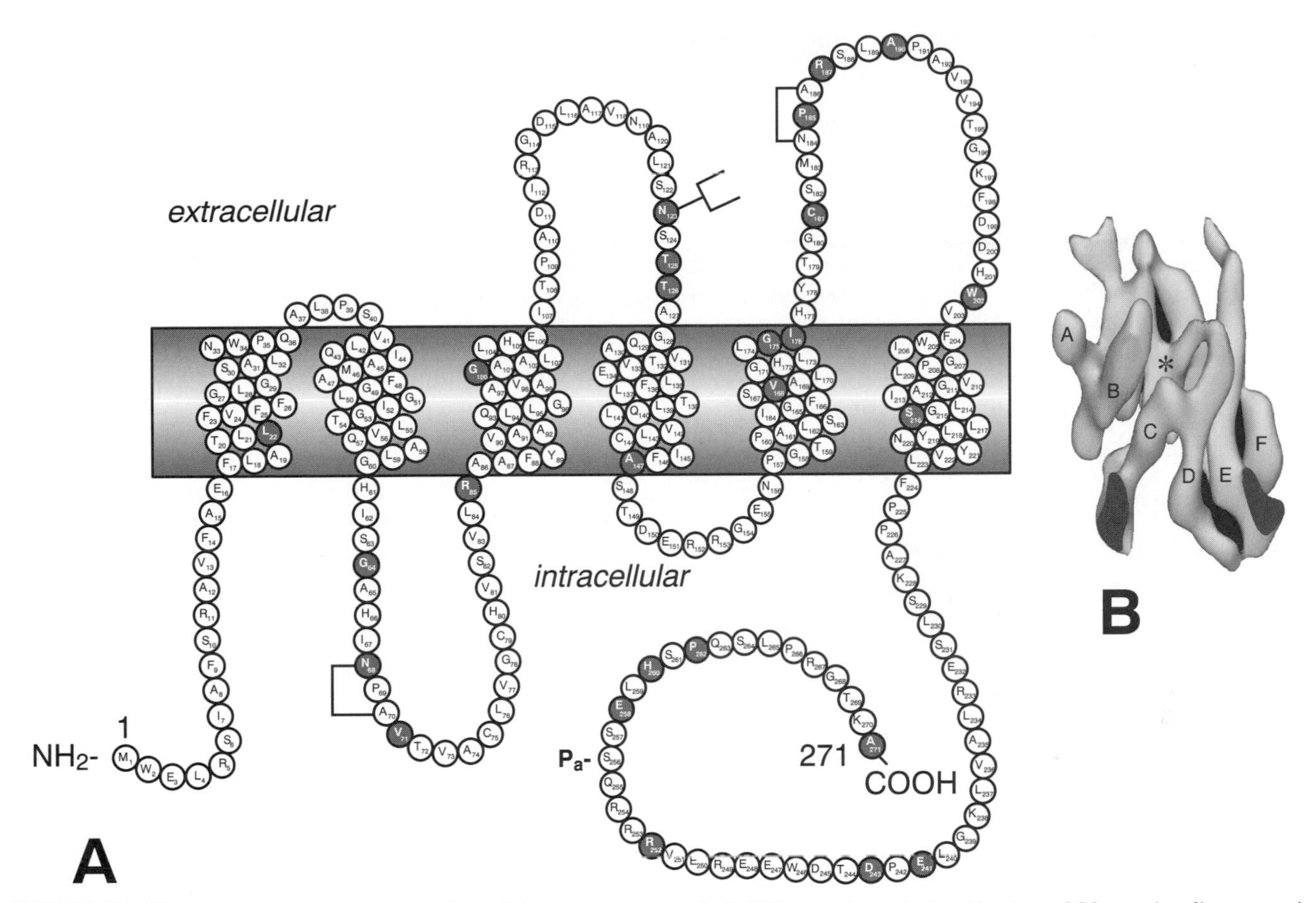


**FIGURE 15–10** ■ *A,* Schematic representation of the aquaporin type 2 (AQP2) protein and identification of 26 putative disease-causing *AQP2* mutations. A monomer is represented with six transmembrane helices. The location of the protein kinase A (PKA) phosphorylation site ($P_a$) is indicated. This site is possibly involved in the arginine vasopressin (AVP)–induced trafficking of AQP2 from intracellular vesicles to the plasma membrane and in the subsequent stimulation of endocytosis.[89, 90] The extracellular (E), transmembrane (TM), and cytoplasmic (C) domains are defined according to Deen and colleagues.[106] Solid symbols indicate the location of the mutations. The common names of the mutations are listed by domain. $TM_I$: L22V; $C_{II}$: G64R, N68S, V71M, R85X; $TM_{III}$: G100X; $E_{II}$: 369delC, T125M, T126M; $TM_{IV}$: A147T; $TM_V$: V168M, G175R, IVS2-1G>A; $E_{III}$: C181W, P185A, R187C, A190T, W202C; $TM_{VI}$: S216P; $C_{IV}$: 721delG, 727delG, 756–765del, E258K, 779–780insA, P262L, 812–816del.[106, 123, 226, 297, 302, 309–313] *B,* A surface-shaded representation of the six-helix barrel of the AQP1 protein viewed parallel to the bilayer; black lines indicate the approximate helix axes. (Modified from Cheng A, van Hoek AN, Yeager M, et al: Three-dimensional organization of a human water channel. Nature 387:627, 1997. For the identification of new *AQP2* mutations, see also Kuwahara M, Iwai K, Ooeda T, et al: Three families with autosomal dominant nephrogenic diabetes insipidus caused by aquaporin-2 mutations in the C-terminus. Am J Hum Genet 69:738–748, 2001.)

## KNOCKOUT MICE WITH URINARY CONCENTRATION DEFECTS

A useful strategy to establish the physiologic function of a protein is to determine the phenotype produced by pharmacologic inhibition of protein function or by gene disruption. Transgenic knockout mice deficient in AQP1, AQP2, AQP3, AQP4, AQP3 and AQP4, CLCNK1, NKCC2, AVPR2, or AGT have been engineered.[112–120] Angiotensinogen (AGT)–deficient mice are characterized by both concentrating and diluting defects secondary to a defective renal papillary architecture.[120]

As reviewed by Rao and Verkman, extrapolation of data in mice to humans must be done with caution.[121] For example, the maximal osmolality of mouse urine (>3000 mOsm/kg $H_2O$) is much greater than that of human urine (1000 mOsmol/kg $H_2O$), and normal serum osmolality in mice is 330 to 345 mOsmol/kg $H_2O$, substantially greater than that in humans (280 to 290 mOsm/kg $H_2O$). Protein expression patterns and thus the interpretation of phenotype studies may also be species dependent. For example, AQP4 is expressed in both the proximal tubule and the collecting duct in mice but only in the collecting duct in rats and humans.[121]

The *Aqp3, Aqp4, Clcnk-1, and Agt* knockout mice have no identified human counterparts. Of interest, AQP1 null individuals have no obvious symptoms.[122] Yang and coworkers[119] generated an AQP2-T126M knock-in mutant mouse to recapitulate the clinical features of the naturally occurring human *AQP2* mutation *T126M.*[123] The mutant mice appeared normal at 2 to 3 days after birth but failed to thrive and generally died by day 6 if not given supplemental fluid. These mice were characterized by an extremely severe concentrating defect, with urine osmolality of 225 ± 9 mOsm/kg $H_2O$, concomitant serum osmolality of 450 ± 50 mOsm/kg $H_2O$, and renal failure. Mice lacking the AVPR2 receptor also failed to thrive and died within the first week after birth due to hypernatremic dehydration.[118]

The absence of the gene coding for the Na-K-2Cl cotransport (NKCC2) in the luminal membrane of the thick ascending loop of Henle in the mouse also caused polyuria that was not compensated elsewhere in the nephron and recapitulated many features of classic Bartter syndrome in humans.[117] The absence of transcellular NaCl transport via NKCC2 probably abolished the lumen's positive transepithelial voltage that enables paracellular reabsorption of sodium and potassium accross the wall of the thick ascending tubule. The combined absence of transcellular and paracellular transport of salt accross the thick ascending limb cells prevents the establishment of the normal osmotic gradient necessary for urine concentration.

## THE BRATTLEBORO RAT WITH AUTOSOMAL RECESSIVE NEUROGENIC DIABETES INSIPIDUS

The classic animal model for studying diabetes insipidus has been the Brattleboro rat with autosomal recessive neurogenic diabetes insipidus. *di/di* Rats are homozygous for a 1-bp deletion (G) in the second exon that results in a frameshift mutation in the coding sequence of the carrier NPII.[124] The polyuric symptoms are also observed in heterozygous *di/n* rats. Homozygous Brattleboro rats may still demonstrate some $V_2$ antidiuretic effect, because the administration of a selective nonpeptide $V_2$ antagonist (SR121463A, 10 mg/kg IP) induced a further increase in urine flow rate (200 to 354 ± 42 mL/24 hr) and a decline in urinary osmolality (170 to 92 ± 8 mmol/kg).[125] Oxytocin, which is present at enhanced plasma concentrations in Brattleboro rats, may be responsible for the antidiuretic activity observed.[126, 127] Oxytocin is not stimulated by increased plasma osmolality in humans. The Brattleboro rat model is therefore not strictly comparable with the rarely observed human cases of autosomal recessive neurogenic diabetes insipidus.[128, 129]

## QUANTITATING RENAL WATER EXCRETION

Diabetes insipidus is characterized by the excretion of abnormally large volumes of hypo-osmotic urine (<250 mmol/kg). This definition excludes osmotic diuresis, which occurs when excess solute is being excreted, as with glucose in the polyuria of diabetes mellitus. Other agents that produce osmotic diuresis are mannitol, urea, glycerol, contrast media, and loop diuretics. Osmotic diuresis should be considered when solute excretion exceeds 60 mmol/hr.

## CLINICAL CHARACTERISTICS OF DIABETES INSIPIDUS DISORDERS

### Central Diabetes Insipidus

#### COMMON FORMS

Failure to synthesize or secrete vasopressin normally limits maximal urinary concentration and, depending on the severity of the disease, causes varying degrees of polyuria and polydipsia. Experimental destruction of the vasopressin-synthesizing areas of the hypothalamus (supraoptic and paraventricular nuclei) causes a permanent form of the disease. Similar results are obtained by sectioning the hypophysial hypothalamic tract above the median eminence. Sections below the median eminence, however, produce only transient diabetes insipidus. Lesions to the hypothalamic-pituitary tract are frequently associated with a three-stage response both in experimental animals and in humans.[130]

1. An initial diuretic phase lasting from a few hours to 5 to 6 days.
2. A period of antidiuresis unresponsive to fluid administration. This antidiuresis is probably due to vasopressin release from injured axons and may last from a few hours to several days. Because urinary dilution is impaired during this phase, continued water administration can cause severe hyponatremia.
3. A final period of diabetes insipidus. The extent of the injury determines the completeness of the diabetes insipidus, and, as already discussed, the site of the lesion determines whether the disease will be permanent.

A detailed assessment of water balance following transphenoidal surgery has been reported.[131] One hundred one patients who underwent transphenoidal pituitary surgery at the National Institutes of Health Clinical Center were studied. Twenty-five percent of the patients developed spontaneous isolated hyponatremia, 20% developed diabetes insipidus, and 46% remained normonatremic. Normonatremia, hyponatremia, and diabetes insipidus were associated with increasing degrees of surgical manipulation of the posterior lobe and pituitary stalk during surgery.

The causes of central diabetes insipidus in adults and in children are listed in Table 15–1.[132–134] Rare causes of central diabetes insipidus include leukemia, thrombotic thrombocytopenic purpura, pituitary apoplexy, sarcoidosis, and Wegener granulomatosis.[135] A

**TABLE 15–1.** Causes of Hypothalamic Diabetes Insipidus in Children and Adults

| | Children (%) | Children and Young Adults (%) | Adults (%) |
|---|---|---|---|
| Primary brain tumor | 49.5 | 22 | 30 |
| before surgery | 33.5 | | 13 |
| after surgery | 16.0 | | 17 |
| Idiopathic (isolated or familial) | 29.0 | 58 | 25 |
| Histiocytosis | 16.0 | 12 | — |
| Metastatic cancer† | — | | 8 |
| Trauma‡ | 2.2 | 2 | 17 |
| Post infectious disease | 2.2 | 6 | — |

* Primary malignancy: craniopharyngioma, dysgerminoma, meningioma, adenoma, glioma, astrocytoma.

† Secondary: metastatic from lung or breast, lymphoma, leukemia, dysplastic pancytopenia.

‡ Trauma could be severe or mild.

Data from references 132–135.

distinctive syndrome characterized by early diabetes insipidus with subsequent progressive spastic cerebellar ataxia has also been described.[136] Five patients who all presented with central diabetes insipidus and hypogonadism as the first manifestations of neurosarcoidosis have been reported.[137]

Circulating antibodies to vasopressin do not play a role in the development of diabetes insipidus.[138] Antibodies to vasopressin occasionally develop during treatment with ADH; when they do, this almost always results in secondary resistance to its antidiuretic effect.[138, 139] Maghnie and associates studied 79 patients with central diabetes insipidus who were seen at four pediatric endocrinology units between 1970 and 1996.[134] There were 37 male and 42 female patients whose median age at diagnosis was 7 years (range, 0.1 to 24.8). In 10 patients, central diabetes insipidus developed during an infectious illness or less than 2 months afterward (varicella in 5 patients, mumps in 2 patients, and measles, toxoplasmosis, and hepatitis B in 1 patient each). Deficits in anterior pituitary hormones were documented in 48 patients (61%) a median of 0.6 year (range, 0.1 to 18.0) after the onset of diabetes insipidus. The most frequent abnormality was growth hormone deficiency (59%), followed by hypothyroidism (28%), hypogonadism (24%), and adrenal insufficiency (22%). Seventy-five percent of the patients with Langerhans cell histiocytosis had an anterior pituitary hormone deficiency that was first detected a median of 3.5 years after the onset of diabetes insipidus. The frequency and progression of Langerhans cell histiocytosis–related anterior pituitary and other nonendocrine hypothalamic dysfunction and the response to treatment in 12 adult patients were also reviewed.[140] None of the patients with central diabetes insipidus secondary to *prepro-AVP-NPII* mutations developed anterior pituitary hormone deficiencies.

## RARE FORMS: AUTOSOMAL DOMINANT CENTRAL DIABETES INSIPIDUS AND THE DIDMOAD SYNDROME

Lacombe[141] and Weil[142] described a familial non-X-linked form of diabetes insipidus without any associated mental retardation. The descendants of the family described by Weil were later found to have autosomal dominant neurogenic diabetes insipidus.[143–145] Repaske and colleagues[146] reported in 1990 that the genetic locus for autosomal dominant central diabetes insipidus[141–145] was within or near the gene encoding for AVP. Furthermore, they suggested that a defective *AVP-NPII* gene might be the basis for this disease. Neurogenic diabetes insipidus (OMIM 125700)[147] is now a well-characterized entity, secondary to mutations in *prepro-AVP-NPII* (OMIM 192340).[147] This disorder is also referred to as central, cranial, pituitary, or neurohypophysial diabetes insipidus. Patients with autosomal dominant neurogenic diabetes insipidus retain some limited capacity to secrete AVP during severe dehydration, and the polyuro-polydipsic symptoms usually appear after the first year of life,[148] when the infant's demand for water is more likely to be understood by adults.

Thirty-four *prepro-AVP-NPII* mutations segregating with autosomal dominant or autosomal recessive neurogenic diabetes insipidus have been described.[129, 148–171] The mechanisms by which a mutant allele causes neurogenic diabetes insipidus could involve the induction of magnocellular cell death as a result of the accumulation of AVP precursors within the endoplasmic reticulum (ER).[167, 172] This hypothesis could account for the delayed onset and autosomal mode of inheritance of the disease. In addition to the cytotoxicity caused by mutant AVP precursors, the interaction between the wild-type and the mutant precursors suggests that a dominant-negative mechanism may also contribute to the pathogenesis of autosomal dominant diabetes insipidus.[173] The absence of symptoms in infancy in autosomal dominant central diabetes insipidus is in sharp contrast to nephrogenic diabetes insipidus secondary to mutations in *AVPR2* or in *AQP2,* in which the polyuro-polydipsic symptoms are present during the first week of life.

Of interest, errors in protein folding represent the underlying basis for a large number of inherited diseases[174, 175] and are also pathogenic mechanisms for *AVPR2* and *AQP2* mutants responsible for hereditary nephrogenic diabetes insipidus. Why *prepro-AVP-NPII* misfolded mutants are cytotoxic to AVP-producing neurons is an unresolved issue. The nephrogenic diabetes insipidus *AVPR2* missense mutations are likely to impair folding and lead to the rapid degradation of the affected polypeptide and not to the accumulation of toxic aggregates, because the other important functions of the principal cells of the collecting ducts (where *AVPR2* is expressed) are entirely normal.

Three families with autosomal recessive neurogenic diabetes insipidus have been identified in which the patients were homozygous or compound heterozygotes for *prepro-AVP-NPII* mutations.[128, 129] Two of these families are characterized phenotypically by severe and early onset in the first 3 months of life of polyuria, polydipsia, and dehydration. As a consequence, early hereditary diabetes insipidus can be neurogenic or nephrogenic.

The acronym DIDMOAD describes the following clinical features of a syndrome: *d*iabetes *i*nsipidus, *d*iabetes *m*ellitus, *o*ptic *a*trophy, and sensorineural *d*eafness.[176, 177] An unusual incidence of psychiatric symptoms has also been described in these subjects.[178] These symptoms included paranoid delusions; auditory or visual hallucinations; psychotic behavior; violent behavior; organic brain syndrome, typically in the late or preterminal stage of the illness; progressive dementia; and severe learning disabilities, mental retardation, or both. The syndrome is an autosomal recessive trait, the diabetes insipidus is usually partial and of gradual onset,[177] and the polyuria can be wrongly attributed to poor glycemic control. Furthermore, a severe hyperosmolar state can occur if untreated diabetes mellitus is associated with an unrecognized pituitary deficiency. The dilatation of the urinary tract observed in DIDMOAD syndrome may be secondary to chronic high urine flow rates and, perhaps, to some degenerative aspects of the innervation of the urinary tract.[176] Wolfram syndrome (OMIM 222300)[147] is secondary to mutations in the *WFS1* gene (chromosome region 4p16), which codes for a transmembrane protein expressed in various tissues, including brain and pancreas.[179–181]

### SYNDROME OF HYPERNATREMIA AND HYPODIPSIA

Some patients with hypernatremia and hypodipsia syndrome may have partial central diabetes insipidus.[182] These patients also have persistent hypernatremia, which is not due to any apparent extracellular volume loss; absence or attenuation of thirst; and a normal renal response to AVP. In almost all the patients studied to date, the hypodipsia has been associated with cerebral lesions in the vicinity of the hypothalamus. It has been proposed that in these patients there is a "resetting" of the osmoreceptor, because their urine tends to become concentrated or diluted at inappropriately high levels of plasma osmolality. However, by using the regression analysis of plasma AVP concentration versus plasma osmolality, it has been possible to show that in some of these patients the tendency to concentrate and dilute urine at inappropriately high levels of plasma osmolality is due solely to a marked reduction in sensitivity or a gain in the osmoregulatory mechanism. This finding is compatible with the diagnosis of partial central diabetes insipidus. In other patients, however, plasma AVP concentrations fluctuate randomly, bearing no apparent relationship to changes in plasma osmolality. Such patients frequently display large swings in serum sodium concentrations and exhibit hypodipsia. It appears that most patients with essential hypernatremia fit one of these two patterns. Both of these groups of patients consistently respond normally to nonosmolar AVP release signals, such as hypotension, emesis, hypoglycemia, or all three. These observations suggest that the osmoreceptor may be anatomically as well as functionally separate from the nonosmotic efferent pathways and neurosecretory neurons for vasopressin. Furthermore, a hypothalamic lesion may impair the osmotic release of AVP while the nonosmotic release of AVP remains intact, and the osmoreceptor neurons that regulate vasopressin secretion are not totally synonymous with those that regulate thirst, although they appear to be anatomically close if not overlapping.

## Nephrogenic Diabetes Insipidus

### X-LINKED NEPHROGENIC DIABETES INSIPIDUS AND MUTATIONS IN THE *AVPR2* GENE

X-linked nephrogenic diabetes insipidus (NDI) (OMIM 304800)[147] is generally a rare disease in which the affected male patients do not concentrate their urine after the administration of AVP.[183] Because it is a rare, recessive, X-linked disease, females are unlikely to be affected, but heterozygous females exhibit variable degrees of polyuria and polydipsia because of skewed X chromosome inactivation. X-linked NDI is secondary to *AVPR2* mutations that result in the loss of function or a dysregulation of the $V_2$ receptor.

#### ***Rareness and Diversity of* AVPR2 *Mutations***

We estimated the incidence of X-linked NDI in the general population from patients born in the province of Quebec during the 10-year period 1988 to 1997 to be approximately 8.8 per million (SD = 4.4 per million) male live births.[184] Thus, X-linked NDI is generally a rare disorder. By contrast, NDI was known to be a common disorder in Nova Scotia.[185] Thirty affected males who resided mainly in two small villages with a total population of 2500[186] were descendants of members of the Hopewell pedigree studied by Bode and Crawford[185] and carried the nonsense mutation *W71X*.[187, 188] This is the largest known pedigree with X-linked NDI and has been referred to as the Hopewell kindred, named after the Irish ship *Hopewell,* which arrived in Halifax in 1761.[185] Descendants of Scottish Presbyterians migrated to the Ulster province of Ireland in the 17th century; they then emigrated from Ireland in 1718 and settled in northern Massachusetts. A later group of immigrants were passengers on the *Hopewell* and settled in Colchester County, Nova Scotia. Members of the two groups were subsequently united in Colchester County.[185] Thus, it is likely that Ulster Scot immigrants, perhaps on more than one occasion, brought the *W71X* mutation to North America. To date, we have identified the *W71X* mutation in 38 affected males who reside predominantly in the maritime provinces of Nova Scotia and New Brunswick. We estimated the incidence in these two maritime provinces to be 6 per 104,063 or approximately 58 per million (SD = 24 per million) male live births for the 10-year period 1988 to 1997.

To date, 155 putative disease-causing *AVPR2* mutations have been identified in 239 NDI families (see Fig. 15–8).[189] (Additional information is available from the NDI Mutation Database at www.medicine.mcgill.ca/nephros/.) Of these, we identified 82 different mutations in 117 NDI families referred to our laboratory. Half of the mutations are missense mutations. Frameshift mutations due to nucleotide deletions or insertions (27%), nonsense mutations (11%), large deletions (5%), inframe deletions or insertions (4%), splice-site mutations (2%), and one complex mutation account for the remainder. Mutations have been identified in every domain, but on a per nucleotide basis, about twice as many mutations occur in transmembrane domains compared with the extracellular or intracellular domains. We previously identified private mutations, recurrent mutations, and mechanisms of mutagenesis.[190, 191] The 10 recurrent mutations (*D85N, V88M, R113W, Y128S, R137H, S167L, R181C, R202C, A294P,* and *S315R*) were found in 35 ancestrally independent families.[184] The occurrence of the same mutation on different haplotypes was considered evidence of recurrent mutation. In addition, the most frequent mutations—*D85N, V88N,*

*R113W, R137H, S167L, R181C,* and *R202C*—occurred at potential mutational hot spots (a C-to-T or G-to-A nucleotide substitution occurred at a CpG dinucleotide).

***Benefits of Genetic Testing***

The natural history of untreated X-linked NDI includes hypernatremia, hyperthermia, mental retardation, and repeated episodes of dehydration in early infancy.[192–196] Mental retardation, a consequence of repeated episodes of dehydration, was prevalent in the Crawford and Bode study,[195] in which only 9 of 82 patients (11%) had normal intelligence; however, data from the Nijmegen group suggest that this complication was overestimated in its NDI patients.[196, 197] Early recognition and treatment of X-linked NDI, with an abundant intake of water, allow a normal life span with normal physical and mental development.[198] Familial occurrence of NDI in males and mental retardation in untreated patients are two characteristics suggestive of X-linked NDI. Skewed X-inactivation is the most likely explanation for clinical symptoms of NDI in female carriers.[184, 199, 200]

Identification of the molecular defect underlying X-linked NDI is of immediate clinical significance, because early diagnosis and treatment of affected infants can avert the physical and mental retardation resulting from repeated episodes of dehydration. Diagnosis of X-linked NDI was accomplished by mutation testing of chorionic villous samples ($n = 4$), cultured amniotic cells ($n = 5$), or cord blood ($n = 17$). Three infants who had mutation testing done on amniotic cells ($n = 1$) or chorionic villous samples ($n = 2$) also had their diagnosis confirmed by cord blood testing. Of the 23 offspring tested, 12 were found to be affected males, 7 were unaffected males, and 4 were noncarrier girls (DG Bichet et al, unpublished data). The affected males were immediately treated with abundant water intake, a low-sodium diet, and hydrochlorothiazide. They have not experienced severe episodes of dehydration, and their physical and mental development remains normal; however, their urinary output is decreased by only 30%, and a normal growth curve is still difficult to reach during the first 2 to 3 years of life, despite treatment and intensive attention. Water should be offered every 2 hours day and night, and temperature, appetite, and growth should be monitored. Admission to the hospital may be necessary for continuous gastric feeding. The voluminous amounts of water kept in patients' stomachs exacerbate physiologic gastrointestinal reflux in infants and toddlers, and many affected boys frequently vomit and have a strong positive "Tuttle test" (esophageal pH testing). These young patients often improve with the absorption of an $H_2$ blocker and with metoclopramide (which could induce extrapyramidal symptoms) or with domperidone, which seems to be better tolerated and more efficacious.

***Most Mutant $V_2$ Receptors Retained in Intracellular Compartments***

Classification of the defects of mutant $V_2$ receptors is based on that of the low-density lipoprotein receptor, where mutations have been grouped according to the function and subcellular localization of the mutant protein whose cDNA has been transiently transfected in a heterologous expression system.[201] Following this classification, type 1 mutant receptors reach the cell surface but display impaired ligand binding and are consequently unable to induce normal cAMP production. The presence of mutant $V_2$ receptors on the surface of transfected cells can be determined pharmacologically. By carrying out saturation binding experiments using tritiated AVP, the number of cell surface mutant receptors and their apparent binding affinity can be compared with that of the wild-type receptor. In addition, the presence of cell surface receptors can be assessed directly by using immunodetection strategies to visualize epitope-tagged receptors in whole-cell immunofluorescence assays.

Type 2 mutant receptors have defective intracellular transport. This phenotype is confirmed by carrying out, in parallel, immunofluorescence experiments on cells that are intact (to demonstrate the absence of cell surface receptors) or permeabilized (to confirm the presence of intracellular receptor pools). In addition, protein expression is confirmed by Western blot analysis of membrane preparations from transfected cells. It is likely that these mutant type 2 receptors accumulate in a pre-Golgi compartment, because they are initially glycosylated but fail to undergo glycosyl trimming maturation.

Type 3 mutant receptors are ineffectively transcribed. This subgroup seems to be rare, because Northern blot analysis of transfected cells reveals that most $V_2$ receptor mutations produce the same quantity and molecular size of receptor mRNA.

Of the 12 mutants that we tested (*N55H, L59P, L83Q, V88M, 497CC->GG, ΔR202, I209F, 700delC, 908insT, A294P, P322H,* and *P322S*) only three (*ΔR202, P322S,* and *P322H*) were detected on the cell surface. Similarly, the 10 mutant receptors (*Y128S, E242X, 803insG, 834delA, ΔV278, Y280C, W284X, L292P, W293X,* and *L312Y*) tested by Schöneberg and colleagues did not reach the cell membrane and were trapped in the interior of the cell.[202, 203] Similar results for the following mutants were obtained: *L44F, L44P, W164S, S167L, and S167T*[204]; *R143P* and *ΔV278*[205]; and *Y280C, L292P,* and *R333X*.[206]

Other genetic disorders are also characterized by protein misfolding. *AQP2* mutations responsible for autosomal recessive NDI are also characterized by misrouting of the misfolded mutant proteins and trapping in the ER.[207] The *ΔF508* mutation in cystic fibrosis is also characterized by misfolding and retention in the ER of the mutated cystic fibrosis transmembrane conductance regulator, which is associated with calnexin and Hsp70 (for a review, see reference 208). The *C282Y* mutant HFE protein, which is responsible for 83% of hemochromatosis in the white population, is retained in the ER and middle Golgi compartment, fails to undergo late Golgi processing, and is subject to accelerated degradation.[209] Mutants encoding other renal membrane proteins that are responsible for

Gitelman syndrome[210] and cystinuria[211] are also retained in the ER.

Missense mutations responsible for these various diseases are often situated in regions of the protein that are not part of the active site, the binding site, or the site of interaction with other proteins. These mutations have been shown to decrease the half-life of the affected protein.[174] Missense mutations and short inframe deletions or insertions impair the propensity of the affected polypeptide to fold into its the functional conformation; thus the term *conformational diseases* has been coined.[212] The NDI missense mutations are likely to impair folding and to lead to rapid degradation of the affected polypeptide but not to accumulation of toxic aggregates, because the other important functions of the principal cells of the collecting duct (where $V_2$ receptors are expressed) are entirely normal. These cells express the epithelial sodium channel (ENac). A decreased function of this channel results in a sodium-losing state.[213] This has not been observed in patients with *AVPR2* mutations.

#### *In Vitro Adenovirus-Mediated Gene Transfer Experiments*

Schöneberg and colleagues genetically rescued truncated or missense $V_2$ receptors by coexpression of a polypeptide consisting of the last 130 amino acids of the $V_2$ receptor in COS-7 cells.[202, 203] Four of the six truncated receptors (*E242X, 804delG, 834delA,* and *W284X*) and the missense mutant *Y280C* regained considerable functional activity, as demonstrated by an increase in the number of binding sites and stimulation of adenylyl cyclase activity, but the absolute number of expressed receptors at the cell surface remained low, and the precise mechanism of the rescue phenomenon (dimerization) was unclear.[214] Most of the loss-of-function mutations secondary to *AVPR2* missense mutations are unlikely to be improved by this coexpression strategy, and delivery of the gene transfer vehicle is a major unresolved problem.

#### *Nonpeptide Vasopressin Antagonists*

Several orally active nonpeptide AVP receptor antagonists have been reported,[215, 216] and one, SR 121463, is a potent and selective $V_2$ receptor antagonist.[125] This extremely stable molecule is highly selective for $V_2$ receptors from several species, including humans, and exhibits powerful intravenous and oral aquaretic effects.[125] SR 121463 inhibits AVP-evoked cAMP formation in human kidney membranes and reverses extrarenal $V_2$ receptor antagonism of DDAVP-induced release of hemostatic factors in dogs.[217] VPA-985 is a similar aquaretic compound.[216] From a therapeutic point of view, $V_2$ receptor–specific antagonists that block the action of AVP at the level of the renal collecting duct specifically promote water excretion.

We recently assessed whether these selective $V_2$-vasopressin receptor antagonists could facilitate the folding of mutant proteins that are responsible for NDI and are retained in the ER. We monitored the biosynthesis of mutant $V_2$ receptors in the presence of SR 121463 and VPA-985. These cell-permeable antagonists were able to convert precursor forms of mutant $V_2$ receptor into fully glycosylated, mature receptor proteins that were now targeted to the cell surface, as determined by pulse-chase analysis and cell surface immunofluorescence microscopy. Once at their correct cellular location, these receptors were able to bind AVP and produce an intracellular cAMP response that was 15 times higher than that produced in cells not exposed to these antagonists.[218] This effect could not be mediated by or completed with $V_2$ receptor antagonists that are membrane-impermeable, indicating that SR 121463A was mediating its effects intracellularly.

On the basis of these data, we propose a model in which small nonpeptide $V_2$ receptor antagonists permeate the cell and bind to incompletely folded mutant receptors. This would stabilize a conformation of the receptor that allows its release from the ER quality control apparatus. The stabilized receptor would then be targeted to the cell surface, where, upon dissociation from the antagonist, it could bind vasopressin and promote signal transduction. Given that these antagonists are specific to the $V_2$ receptor and that they perform a chaperone-like function, we termed these compounds *pharmacologic chaperones.*[175, 218]

## AUTOSOMAL RECESSIVE AND DOMINANT NEPHROGENIC DIABETES INSIPIDUS DUE TO *AQP2* MUTATIONS

On the basis of desmopressin infusion studies and phenotypic characteristics of both males and females affected with NDI, a non-X-linked form of NDI with a postreceptor (post-cAMP) defect was suggested.[219–222] A patient who presented shortly after birth with typical features of NDI but who exhibited normal coagulation and normal fibrinolytic and vasodilatory responses to desmopressin was shown to be a compound heterozygote for two missense mutations (*R187C* and *S217P*) in the *AQP2* gene[106] (see Fig. 15–10). To date, 26 putative disease-causing *AQP2* mutations have been identified in 25 NDI families (see Fig. 15–10). By type of mutation, there are 65% missense, 23% frameshift due to small nucleotide deletions or insertions, 8% nonsense, and 4% splice-site mutations. (Additional information is available from the NDI Mutation Database at http://www.medicine.mcgill.ca/nephros/.)

Reminiscent of expression studies done with AVPR2 proteins, misrouting of AQP2 mutant proteins has been shown to be the major cause underlying autosomal recessive NDI.[123, 207, 223] To determine whether the severe AQP2 trafficking defect observed with the naturally occurring mutations *T126M, R187C,* and *A147T* is correctable, CHO and Madin-Darby canine kidney cells were incubated with the chemical chaperone glycerol for 48 hours. Using immunofluorescence, redistribution of AQP2 from the ER to the plasma membrane–endosome fractions was observed. This redistribution was correlated with improved water permeability measurements.[207, 224] It will be important to correct this defective AQP2 trafficking in vivo.

In contrast to the AQP2 mutations in autosomal recessive NDI, which are located throughout the gene, the dominant mutations are predicted to affect the carboxyl terminus of AQP2.[225] One dominant mutation, *E258K*, has been analyzed in detail in vitro; AQP2-E258K had reduced water permeability compared with wild-type AQP2.[226] In addition, AQP2-E258K was retained in the Golgi apparatus, which differs from mutant AQP2 in recessive NDI that is retained in the ER. The dominant action of AQP2 mutations can be explained by the formation of heterotetramers of mutant and wild-type AQP2 that are impaired in their routing after oligomerization.[226, 227]

### ACQUIRED NEPHROGENIC DIABETES INSIPIDUS

The acquired form of NDI is much more common than the congenital form of the disease, but it is rarely severe. The ability to elaborate a hypertonic urine is usually preserved, despite the impairment of the maximal concentrating ability of the nephrons. Polyuria and polydipsia are therefore moderate (3 to 4 L/day). The more common causes of acquired NDI are listed in Table 15–2.

**TABLE 15–2.** Acquired Causes of Nephrogenic Diabetes Insipidus

- Chronic renal disease
  - Polycystic disease
  - Medullary cystic disease
- Pyelonephritis
  - Ureteral obstruction
  - Far-advanced renal failure
- Electrolyte disorders
  - Hypokalemia
  - Hypercalcemia
- Drugs
  - Alcohol
  - Phenytoin
  - Lithium
  - Demeclocycline
  - Acetohexamide
  - Tolazamide
  - Glyburide
  - Propoxyphene
  - Amphotericin
  - Foscarnet
  - Methoxyflurane
  - Norepinephrine
  - Vinblastine
  - Colchicine
  - Gentamicin
  - Methicillin
  - Isophosphamide
  - Angiographic dyes
  - Osmotic diuretics
  - Furosemide and ethacrynic acid
- Sickle cell disease
- Dietary abnormalities
  - Excessive water intake
  - Decreased sodium chloride intake
  - Decreased protein intake
- Miscellaneous
  - Multiple myeloma
  - Amyloidosis
  - Sjögren disease
  - Sarcoidosis

Lithium administration has become the most common cause of NDI. Boton and coworkers reported that this abnormality was estimated to be present in at least 54% of 1105 unselected patients on chronic lithium therapy.[228] Nineteen percent of these patients had polyuria, as defined by a 24-hour urine output exceeding 3 L. Renal biopsy revealed a chronic tubulointerstitial nephropathy in all 24 patients with biopsy-proven lithium toxicity.[229]

The mechanism whereby lithium causes polyuria has been extensively studied. Lithium has been shown to inhibit adenylate cyclase in a number of cell types, including renal epithelia.[230, 231] The concentration of lithium in the urine of patients on well-controlled lithium therapy (i.e., 10 to 40 mmol/L) is sufficient to inhibit adenylate cyclase. Measurements of adenylate cyclase activity in membranes isolated from a cultured pig kidney cell line (LLC-$PK_1$) revealed that lithium in the concentration area of 10 mmol/L interfered with the hormone-stimulated guanyl nucleotide regulatory unit ($G_s$).[232]

The effect of chronic lithium therapy has been studied in rat kidney membranes prepared from the inner medulla. It caused a marked downregulation of AQP2 and AQP3,[233] which was only partially reversed by cessation of therapy, dehydration, or DDAVP treatment; this is consistent with clinical observations of slow recovery from lithium-induced urinary concentrating defects.[234] Downregulation of AQP2 has also been shown to be associated with the development of severe polyuria due to other causes of acquired NDI (hypokalemia,[235, 236] release of bilateral ureteral obstruction,[237] and hypercalciuria[238]). Thus, AQP2 expression is severely downregulated in both congenital[109] and acquired NDI.

More studies are needed to determine whether nonpeptide vasopressin agonists, permeable cAMP-like compounds, or other signaling molecules will be able to restore AQP2 expression and function. In patients receiving long-term lithium therapy, amiloride has been proposed to prevent the uptake of lithium in the collecting ducts. Amiloride may thus prevent the inhibitory effect of intracellular lithium on water transport.[239]

## Primary Polydipsia

Primary polydipsia is a state of hypotonic polyuria secondary to excessive fluid intake. Primary polydipsia was extensively studied by Barlow and de Wardener in 1959[240]; however, there has been little progress in understanding the pathophysiology of this disease over the past 30 years. Barlow and de Wardener described seven women and two men who were compulsive water drinkers; their ages ranged from 48 to 59 years, except for one patient who was 24.[240] Eight of these patients had histories of previous psychological disorders, which ranged from delusions, depression, and agitation to frank hysterical behavior. The other patient appeared normal. The consumption of water fluctuated irregularly from hour to hour or from day to day; in some patients, there were remissions and relapses lasting several months or longer. In eight of the patients, the mean plasma osmolality was significantly lower than normal. Vasopressin tannate in oil made most of these patients feel ill; in one, it caused overhydration. In four patients, the fluid intake returned to normal after electroconvulsive therapy or a period of continuous narcosis; the improvement in three was transient, but in the fourth it lasted 2 years.

Polyuric female subjects might be heterozygous for de novo or previously unrecognized *AVPR2* mutations or autosomal dominant *AQP2* mutations[226] and may be classified as compulsive water drinkers.[241] Therefore, the diagnosis of compulsive water drinking must be made with care and may represent our ignorance of yet undescribed pathophysiologic mechanisms.

Robertson used the term *dipsogenic diabetes insipidus* to describe a selective defect in the osmoregulation of thirst.[241] Three patients studied under basal conditions of ad libitum water intake had thirst, polydipsia, polyuria, and high-normal plasma osmolality. They had normal secretion of AVP, but the osmotic threshold for thirst was abnormally low. These dipsogenic diabetes insipidus cases might represent up to 10% of all patients with diabetes insipidus.[241]

## Diabetes Insipidus and Pregnancy

### PREGNANCY IN A PATIENT KNOWN TO HAVE DIABETES INSIPIDUS

An isolated deficiency of vasopressin without a concomitant loss of hormones in the anterior pituitary does not result in altered fertility, and with the exception of polyuria and polydipsia, gestation, delivery, and lactation are uncomplicated.[242] Treated patients may require increasing dosages of desmopressin. The increased thirst may be due to a resetting of the thirst osmostat.[243]

Increased polyuria also occurs during pregnancy in patients with partial NDI.[244] These patients may be obligatory carriers of the NDI gene.[245]

### DIABETES INSIPIDUS BEGINNING DURING GESTATION AND REMITTING AFTER DELIVERY

Barron and colleagues described three pregnant women in whom transient diabetes insipidus developed late in gestation and subsequently remitted postpartum.[246] In one of these patients, dilute urine was present in spite of high plasma concentrations of AVP. Hyposthenuria in all three patients was resistant to administered aqueous vasopressin. Because excessive vasopressinase activity was not excluded as a cause of this disorder, Barron and colleagues labeled the disease vasopressin-resistant rather than nephrogenic diabetes insipidus.

A well-documented case of enhanced activity of vasopressinase was described in a woman in the third trimester of a previously uncomplicated pregnancy.[247] She had massive polyuria and markedly elevated plasma vasopressinase activity. The polyuria did not respond to large IV doses of AVP but responded promptly to desmopressin, a vasopressinase-resistant analogue of AVP. The polyuria disappeared with the disappearance of the vasopressinase. The incidence of vasopressinase-mediated, desmopressin-responsive diabetes insipidus is not known. However, another case of transient desmopressin-resistant diabetes insipidus in a pregnant woman has been described.[248] It is suggested that pregnancy may be associated with several different forms of diabetes insipidus, including central, nephrogenic, and vasopressinase mediated.[244]

# DIFFERENTIAL DIAGNOSIS OF POLYURIC STATES

Plasma sodium and osmolality are maintained within normal limits (136 to 143 mmol/L for plasma sodium, 275 to 290 mmol/kg for plasma osmolality) by a thirst-ADH-renal axis. Thirst and ADH, both stimulated by increased osmolality, have been termed a "double-negative" feedback system.[249] Thus, even when the ADH limb of this double-negative regulatory feedback system is lost, the thirst mechanism still preserves the plasma sodium and osmolality within the normal range, but at the expense of pronounced polydipsia and polyuria. Thus, the plasma sodium concentration or osmolality of an untreated patient with diabetes insipidus may be slightly higher than the mean normal value, but because the values usually remain within the normal range, these small increases have no diagnostic significance.

Theoretically, it should be relatively easy to differentiate among central diabetes insipidus, NDI, and primary polydipsia. A comparison of the osmolality of urine obtained during dehydration from patients with central diabetes insipidus or NDI with that of urine obtained after the administration of AVP should reveal a rapid increase in osmolality only in the central diabetes insipidus patients. Urine osmolality should increase normally in response to moderate dehydration in primary polydipsia patients.

However, these distinctions may not be so clear, because of several factors.[250] First, chronic polyuria of any cause interferes with the maintenance of the medullary concentration gradient, and this "washout" effect diminishes the maximal concentrating ability of the kidney. The extent of the blunting varies in direct proportion to the severity of the polyuria and is independent of its cause. Hence, for any given level of basal urine output, the maximal urine osmolality achieved in the presence of saturating concentrations of AVP is depressed to the same extent in patients with primary polydipsia, central diabetes insipidus, and NDI (Fig. 15–11). Second, most patients with central diabetes insipidus maintain a small but detectable capacity to secrete AVP during severe dehydration, and urine osmolality may rise above plasma osmolality. Third, many patients with acquired NDI have an incomplete deficit in AVP action, and concentrated urine could again be obtained during dehydration testing. Finally, all polyuric states (whether central, nephrogenic, or psychogenic) can induce large dilatations of the urinary tract and bladder.[196, 251, 252] As a consequence, the uri-

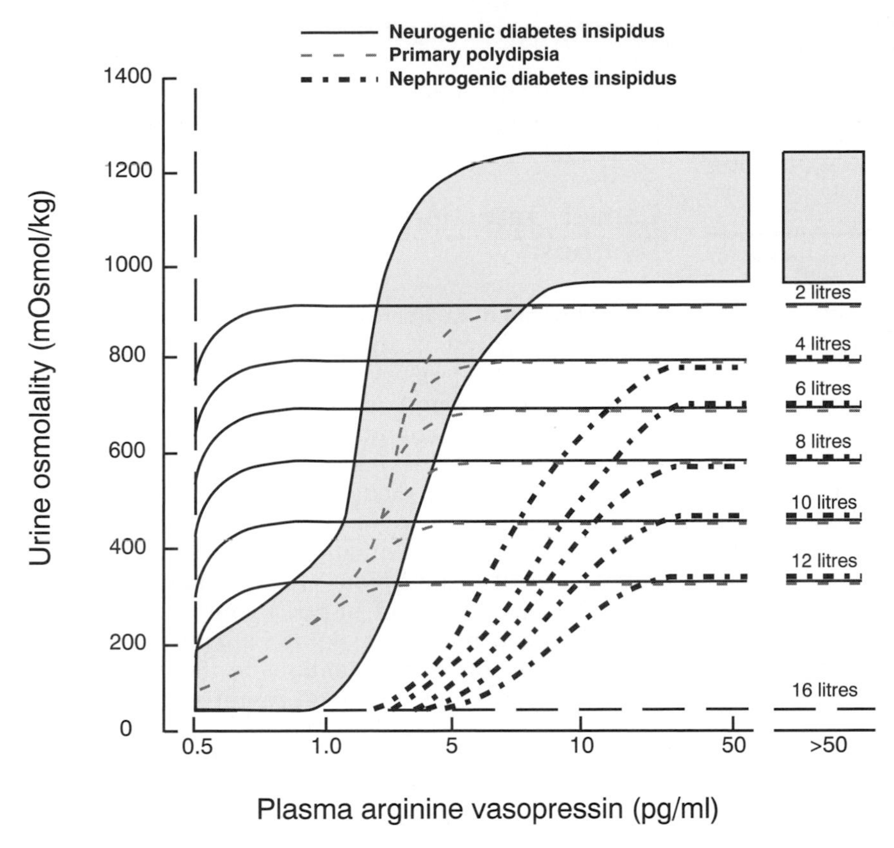


**FIGURE 15–11** ■ The relationship between urine osmolality and plasma vasopressin in patients with polyuria of diverse cause and severity. Note that for each of the three categories of polyuria (neurogenic diabetes insipidus, nephrogenic diabetes insipidus, and primary polydipsia), the relationship is described by a family of sigmoid curves that differ in height. These differences in height reflect differences in maximal concentrating capacity due to "washout" of the medullary concentration gradient. They are proportional to the severity of the underlying polyuria (indicated in liters per day at the right end of each plateau) and are largely independent of the cause. Thus, the three categories of diabetes insipidus differ principally in the submaximal or ascending portion of the dose-response curve. In patients with partial neurogenic diabetes insipidus, this part of the curve lies to the left of normal, reflecting increased sensitivity to the antidiuretic effects of very low concentrations of plasma arginine vasopressin (AVP). In contrast, in patients with partial nephrogenic diabetes insipidus, this part of the curve lies to the right of normal, reflecting decreased sensitivity to the antidiuretic effects of normal concentrations of plasma AVP. In primary polydipsia, this relationship is relatively normal. (From Robertson GL: Diagnosis of diabetes insipidus. In Czernichow P, Robinson AG [eds]: Frontiers of Hormone Research, vol 13, Diabetes Insipidus in Man. Basel, S. Karger, 1985, p 176.)

nary bladder of these patients may contain an increased residual capacity, and changes in urine osmolalities induced by diagnostic maneuvers might be difficult to demonstrate.

## Indirect Test

Measurement of urine osmolality after dehydration or vasopressin administration is usually referred to as "indirect testing," because vasopressin secretion is indirectly assessed through changes in urine osmolality. The patient is maintained on a complete fluid restriction regimen until urine osmolality reaches a plateau, as indicated by an hourly increase of less than 30 mmol/kg for at least 3 successive hours. After the plasma osmolality is measured, 5 U of aqueous vasopressin is administered subcutaneously. Urine osmolality is measured 30 and 60 minutes later. The last urine osmolality value obtained before the vasopressin injection and the highest value obtained after the injection are compared. The patients are then separated into five categories according to previously published criteria[59] (Table 15–3).

## Direct Test

The two approaches of Zerbe and Robertson are used.[58] First, during the dehydration test, plasma is collected and assayed for vasopressin. The results are plotted on a nomogram depicting the normal relationship between plasma sodium or osmolality and plasma AVP in normal subjects (see Fig. 15–6). If the relation-

**TABLE 15–3.** Urinary Responses to Fluid Deprivation and Exogenous Vasopressin in Recognition of Partial Defects in Antidiuretic Hormone Secretion

| | No. Cases | Maximal $U_{osm}$ with Dehydration (mmol/kg) | $U_{osm}$ after Vasopressin (mmol/kg) | % Change ($U_{osm}$) | $U_{osm}$ Increase after Vasopressin (%) |
|---|---|---|---|---|---|
| Normal subjects | 9 | 1068 ± 69 | 979 ± 79 | −9 ± 3 | <9 |
| Complete central diabetes insipidus | 18 | 168 ± 13 | 445 ± 52 | 183 ± 41 | >50 |
| Partial central diabetes insipidus | 11 | 438 ± 34 | 549 ± 28 | 28 ± 5 | >9 <50 |
| Nephrogenic diabetes insipidus | 2 | 123.5 | 174.5 | 42 | <50 |
| Compulsive water drinking | 7 | 738 ± 53 | 780 ± 73 | 5.0 ± 2.2 | <9 |

Data from Miller M, Dalakos, T, Moses AM, et al: Recognition of partial defects in antidiuretic hormone secretion. Ann Intern Med 73:721, 1970.

**TABLE 15–4.** Direct and Indirect Tests of Arginine Vasopressin (AVP) Function in Patients with Polyuria

Measurements of AVP cannot be used in isolation but must be interpreted in light of four other factors: (1) clinical history and concurrent measurements of (2) plasma osmolality, (3) urine osmolality, and (4) maximal urinary response to exogenous vasopressin in reference to the basal urine flow

Data from Stern P, Valtin H: Verney was right, but ... [editorial]. N Engl J Med 305:1581, 1981.

ship between plasma vasopressin and osmolality falls below the normal range, the disorder is diagnosed as central diabetes insipidus.

Second, partial NDI and primary polydipsia can be differentiated by analyzing the relationship between plasma AVP and urine osmolality at the end of the dehydration period (see Figs. 15–6 and 15–11). However, a definitive differentiation between these two disorders might be impossible, because a normal or even supranormal AVP response to increased plasma osmolality occurs in polydipsic patients. None of the patients with psychogenic or other forms of severe polydipsia studied by Robertson showed any evidence of pituitary suppression.[250]

Zerbe and Robertson found that in the differential diagnosis of polyuria, all seven cases of severe neurogenic diabetes insipidus diagnosed by the standard indirect test were confirmed when diagnosed by the plasma vasopressin assay.[58] However, two of six patients using the indirect test as having partial neurogenic diabetes insipidus had normal vasopressin secretion as measured by the direct assay; one was found to have primary polydipsia and the other NDI. Moreover, 3 of 10 patients diagnosed as having primary polydipsia by the indirect test had clear evidence of partial vasopressin deficiency by the direct assay.[58] These patients were thus wrongly diagnosed with primary polydipsia. A combined direct and indirect testing of the AVP function is described in Table 15–4.

## Therapeutic Trial

In selected patients with an uncertain diagnosis, a closely monitored therapeutic trial of desmopressin (10 μg intranasally twice a day) may be used to distinguish partial NDI from partial neurogenic diabetes insipidus and primary polydipsia. If desmopressin at this dosage causes a significant antidiuretic effect, NDI is effectively excluded. If polydipsia as well as polyuria is abolished and plasma sodium does not fall below the normal range, the patient probably has central diabetes insipidus. Conversely, if desmopressin causes a reduction in urine output without a reduction in water intake and hyponatremia appears, the patient probably has primary polydipsia. Because fatal water intoxication is a remote possibility, the desmopressin trial should be carried out with close monitoring.

## Recommendations

Table 15–5 lists recommendations for obtaining a differential diagnosis of diabetes insipidus.[253]

## Carrier Detection and Postnatal Diagnosis

As described earlier in this chapter, the identification, characterization, and mutational analysis of three different genes—*prepro-AVP-NPII, AVPR2,* and the vasopressin-sensitive water channel gene *(AQP2)*—provide the basis for understanding the different hereditary forms of diabetes insipidus: autosomal dominant or recessive neurogenic diabetes insipidus, X-linked NDI, and autosomal recessive or dominant NDI, respectively. The identification of mutations in these three genes that cause diabetes insipidus enables the early diagnosis and management of at-risk members of families with identified mutations. Some patients with Bartter syndrome secondary to mutations in the Na-K-2Cl cotransporter gene *(NKCC2)* may present with severe hypernatremia, hyperchloremia, and a low urine osmolality unresponsive to DDAVP.[254] In these cases, the antenatal period is characterized by polyhydramnios. In our experience, perinatal polyuro-polydipsic patients whose mothers' pregnancies were characterized by polyhydramnios are probably not bearing *AVPR2* or *AQP2* mutations. We encourage physicians who follow families with X-linked NDI to recommend mutation analysis before the birth of a male infant, because early

**TABLE 15–5.** Differential Diagnosis of Diabetes Insipidus

1. Measure plasma osmolality and sodium concentration under conditions of ad libitum fluid intake. If they are above 295 mmol/kg and 143 mmol/L, respectively, the diagnosis of primary polydipsia is excluded, and the work-up should proceed directly to step 5 or 6 to distinguish between neurogenic and nephrogenic diabetes insipidus. Otherwise, go to step 2.
2. Perform a dehydration test. If urinary concentration does not occur before plasma osmolality or sodium reaches 295 mmol/kg or 143 mmol/L, respectively the diagnosis of primary polydipsia is again excluded, and the work-up should proceed to step 5 or 6. Otherwise, go to step 3.
3. Determine the ratio of urine to plasma osmolality at the end of the dehydration test. If it is less than 1.5, the diagnosis of primary polydipsia is again excluded, and the work-up should proceed to step 5 or 6. Otherwise, go to step 4.
4. Perform a hypertonic saline infusion with measurements of plasma vasopressin and osmolality at intervals during the procedure. If the relationship between these two variables is subnormal, the diagnosis of diabetes insipidus is established. Otherwise, go to step 5.
5. Perform a vasopressin infusion test. If urine osmolality rises by more than 150 mOsm/kg above the value obtained at the end of the dehydration test, nephrogenic diabetes insipidus is excluded. Alternatively, go to step 6.
6. Measure urine osmolality and plasma vasopressin at the end of the dehydration test. If the relationship is normal, the diagnosis of nephrogenic diabetes insipidus is excluded.

Data from Robertson GL: Diseases of the posterior pituitary. In Felig D, Baxter JD, Broadus AE, Frohman LA (eds): Endocrinology and Metabolism. New York, McGraw-Hill, 1981, p 251.

diagnosis and treatment can avert the physical and mental retardation associated with episodes of dehydration. Diagnosis of X-linked NDI within 72 hours of birth can be accomplished by mutation testing of a sample of cord blood.[255] Early diagnosis of autosomal recessive NDI is also essential for early treatment to avoid repeated episodes of dehydration. Mutation detection in families with inherited neurogenic diabetes insipidus provides a powerful clinical tool for early diagnosis and management of subsequent cases, especially in early childhood, when diagnosis is difficult and the clinical risks are the greatest.[148]

# RADIOIMMUNOASSAY OF ARGININE VASOPRESSIN AND OTHER LABORATORY DETERMINATIONS

## Radioimmunoassay of Arginine Vasopressin

Three developments were basic to the elaboration of a clinically useful radioimmunoassay for plasma AVP[256, 257]: the extraction of AVP from plasma with petrol-ether and acetone and the subsequent elimination of nonspecific immunoreactivity, the use of highly specific and sensitive rabbit antiserum, and the use of a tracer ($^{125}$I-AVP) with high specific activity. More than 25 years later, the same extraction procedures are widely used,[258–261] and commercial tracers and antibodies are available. AVP can also be extracted from plasma by using Sep-Pak C18 cartridges.[262–264]

Blood samples collected in chilled 7-mL lavender-stoppered tubes containing EDTA are centrifuged at 4°C, 1000 *g* (3000 rpm in a usual lab centrifuge), for 20 minutes. This 20-minute centrifugation is mandatory for obtaining platelet-poor plasma samples, because a large fraction of the circulating vasopressin is associated with the platelets in humans.[259, 265] The tubes may be kept for 2 hours on slushed ice before centrifugation. Plasma is then separated, frozen at −20°C, and extracted within 6 weeks of sampling. Details for sample preparation (Table 15–6) and assay procedure (Table 15–7) can be found in the writings of Bichet and colleagues.[258, 259] An AVP radioimmunoassay should be validated by demonstrating (1) a good correlation between plasma sodium or osmolality and plasma AVP during dehydration and infusion of hypertonic saline solution (see Fig. 15–4) and (2) the inability to obtain detectable values of AVP in patients with severe central diabetes insipidus. Plasma AVP immunoreactivity may be elevated in patients with diabetes insipidus following hypothalamic surgery.[266]

**TABLE 15–6.** Arginine Vasopressin Measurements: Sample Preparation

| |
|---|
| 4°C blood in EDTA tubes |
| Centrifugation at 1000 *g* × 20 minutes |
| Plasma frozen at −20°C |
| Extraction: |
| 2 mL acetone + 1 mL plasma |
| 1000 *g* × 30 minutes at 4°C |
| Supernatant + 5 mL of petrol-ether |
| 1000 *g* × 20 minutes at 4°C |
| Freeze at −80°C. |
| Discard nonfrozen upper phase |
| Evaporate lower phase to dryness |
| Store desiccated samples at −20°C |

**TABLE 15–7.** Arginine Vasopressin (AVP) Measurements: Assay Procedure

| | |
|---|---|
| Day 1 | Assay setup<br>400 μL/tube (200 μL sample or standard + 200 μL of antiserum or buffer)<br>Incubation 80 hours, 40°C |
| Day 4 | $^{125}$I-AVP<br>100 μL/tube<br>1000 cpm/tube<br>Incubation 72 hours, 40°C |
| Day 7 | Separation dextran + charcoal |

In pregnant patients, the blood contains high concentrations of cystine aminopeptidase, which can (in vitro) inactivate enormous quantities (ng × mL$^{-1}$ × min$^{-1}$) of AVP. However, phenanthroline effectively inhibits these cystine aminopeptidases (Table 15–8).

## Aquaporin Type 2 Measurements

Urinary AQP2 excretion can be measured by radioimmunoassay[109] or quantitative Western analysis,[110] providing an additional indication of the responsiveness of the collecting duct to AVP.[110, 111]

## Plasma Sodium and Plasma and Urine Osmolality Measurements

Measurements of plasma sodium and plasma and urine osmolality should be immediately available at various intervals during dehydration procedures. Plasma sodium is easily measured by flame photometry or with a sodium-specific electrode.[267] Plasma and urine osmolalities are also reliably measured by freezing point depression instruments with a coefficient of variation at 290 mmol/kg of less than 1%.

In our clinical research unit, plasma sodium and plasma and urine osmolalities are measured at the beginning of each dehydration procedure and at regular intervals (usually hourly) thereafter, depending on the severity of the polyuric syndrome explored. In one case, an 8-year-old patient (31 kg body weight) with a

**TABLE 15–8.** Measurement of Arginine Vasopressin Levels in Pregnant Patients

| |
|---|
| 1,10-Phenanthroline monohydrate (Sigma) |
| 60 mg/mL—solubilized with several drops of glacial acetic acid |
| 0.1 mL/10 mL of blood |

Data from Davison JM, Gilmore EA, Durr J, et al.: Altered osmotic thresholds for vasopressin secretion and thirst in human pregnancy. Am J Physiol 246:F105, 1984.

clinical diagnosis of congenital NDI (later found to bear the de novo *AVPR2* mutant *274insG*[190]) continued to excrete large volumes of urine (300 mL/hr) during a short 4-hour dehydration test. During this time, the patient was suffering from severe thirst, his plasma sodium was 155 mEq/L, his plasma osmolality was 310 mmol/kg, and his urine osmolality was 85 mmol/kg. The patient received 1 μg of desmopressin IV and was allowed to drink water. Repeated urine osmolality measurements demonstrated a complete urinary resistance to desmopressin. It would have been dangerous and unnecessary to prolong the dehydration in this young patient. Thus, the usual prescription of overnight dehydration should not be used in patients—especially children—with severe polyuria and polydipsia (>4 L/day). Great care should be taken to avoid any severe hypertonic state, arbitrarily defined as a plasma sodium greater than 155 mEq/L.

At variance with published data,[58, 259] we have found that plasma and serum osmolalities are equivalent (i.e., similar values are obtained). Blood taken in heparinized tubes is easier to handle because the plasma can be more readily removed after centrifugation. The tube used (green-stoppered tube) contains a minuscule concentration of lithium and sodium, which does not interfere with plasma sodium or osmolality measurements. Frozen plasma or urine samples can be kept for further analysis of their osmolalities; the results obtained are similar to those obtained immediately after blood sampling, except in patients with severe renal failure. In the latter patients, plasma osmolality measurements are increased after freezing and thawing, but the plasma sodium values remain unchanged.

Plasma osmolality measurements can be used to demonstrate the absence of unusual osmotically active substances (e.g., glucose and urea in high concentrations, mannitol, ethanol).[268] With this information, plasma or serum sodium measurements are sufficient to assess the degree of dehydration and its relationship to plasma AVP. Nomograms describing the normal plasma sodium–plasma AVP relationship (see Fig. 15–4) are as valuable as "classic" nomograms describing the relationship between plasma osmolality and effective osmolality (i.e., plasma osmolality minus the contribution of "ineffective" solutes: glucose and urea).

## MAGNETIC RESONANCE IMAGING IN PATIENTS WITH DIABETES INSIPIDUS

Magnetic resonance imaging (MRI) permits visualization of the anterior and posterior pituitary glands and the pituitary stalk. The pituitary stalk is permeated by numerous capillary loops of the hypophysial-portal blood system. This vascular structure also provides the principal blood supply to the anterior pituitary lobe, as there is no direct arterial supply to this organ. In contrast, the posterior pituitary lobe has a direct vascular supply. Therefore, the posterior lobe can be more rapidly visualized in a dynamic mode after administration of gadolinium (gadopentetate dimeglumine) as contrast material during MRI. The posterior pituitary lobe is easily distinguished by a round, high-intensity signal (the posterior pituitary "bright spot") in the posterior part of the sella turcica on T1-weighted images. This round, high-intensity signal is usually absent in patients with central diabetes insipidus.[134] MRI is reported to be the best technique with which to evaluate the pituitary stalk and infundibulum in patients with idiopathic polyuria. Thus, the absence of posterior pituitary hyperintensity, although nonspecific, is a cardinal feature of central diabetes insipidus. In five patients who did have posterior pituitary hyperintensity at diagnosis, this feature invariably disappeared during follow-up.[134] Thickening of either the entire pituitary stalk or just the proximal portion was the second most common abnormality on MRI scans.[134]

## TREATMENT OF POLYURIC DISORDERS

In most patients with complete hypothalamic diabetes insipidus, the thirst mechanism remains intact. Thus, these patients do not develop hypernatremia and suffer only from the inconvenience associated with marked polyuria and polydipsia. If hypodipsia develops or access to water is limited, severe hypernatremia can supervene. The treatment of choice for patients with severe hypothalamic diabetes insipidus is desmopressin, a synthetic, long-acting vasopressin analogue with minimal vasopressor activity but a large antidiuretic potency. The usual intranasal daily dose is between 5 and 20 μg. To avoid the potential complication of dilutional hyponatremia, which is exceptional in these patients due to an intact thirst mechanism, desmopressin can be withdrawn at regular intervals to allow the patients to become polyuric. Aqueous vasopressin (Pitressin) or desmopressin (4 μg/1-mL ampule) can be used intravenously in acute situations, such as after hypophysectomy or for the treatment of diabetes insipidus in a brain-dead organ donor. Pitressin tannate in oil and nonhormonal antidiuretic drugs are somewhat obsolete and rarely used. Chlorpropamide (250 to 500 mg daily) appears to potentiate the antidiuretic action of circulating AVP, but the troublesome side effects of hypoglycemia and hyponatremia can occur.

The treatment of congenital NDI has been reviewed[196, 269, 270] and was described in the section "Benefits of Genetic Testing." A low-osmolar and low-sodium diet, hydrochlorothiazide (1 to 2 mg/kg/day) alone or with amiloride (20 mg/1.73m$^2$/day), and indomethacin (0.75 to 1.5 mg/kg) substantially reduce water excretion and are helpful in the treatment of children. Prostaglandin synthetase inhibitors should be used only for short periods because of possible deleterious effects with chronic administration. Initial nausea may occur in some patients who start on amiloride, but it is generally transient and rarely a reason to discontinue therapy.[196] Many adult patients receive no treatment at all.

Patients with acquired NDI secondary to long-term lithium usually benefit from a low sodium intake and, under strict surveillance, the chronic administration of hydrochlorothiazide or amiloride. A low sodium intake and a distal diuretic induce contraction of the ECF volume, cause increased proximal fluid—and lithium—reabsorption, and decrease the volume of water presented to the distal tubule. Plasma lithium should be measured frequently at the initiation of such treatment. In the postoperative care of polyuric lithium patients, indomethacin (25 mg three times a day) decreases glomerular filtration rate and decreases water excretion. The lithium dosage should be decreased and plasma lithium levels should be measured frequently if indomethacin is used and only a short treatment (4 to 7 days) is indicated.

Hypernatremic dehydration seen in breast-fed infants[271] can apparently be easily prevented by the simple habit of offering newborns water once a day.[272] In most cases the newborn refuses the offer, and the mothers are advised not to be concerned, because this means that the child is getting sufficient water in breast milk. This clinical presentation is easily differentiated from the intense thirst and continuous voiding of newborns with congenital NDI.

### ACKNOWLEDGMENTS

The authors' work cited in this chapter is supported by the Canadian Institutes of Health Research, the Canadian Kidney Foundation, the Fonds de la Recherche en Santé du Québec, and the Fondation J. Rodolphe-La Haye. Danielle Binette provided secretarial and computer graphics expertise.

## REFERENCES

1. Burg MB, Kwon ED, Kultz D: Regulation of gene expression by hypertonicity. Annu Rev Physiol 59:437, 1997.
2. Weitzman RE, Kleeman CR: The clinical physiology of water metabolism. Part III. The water depletion (hyperosmolar) and water excess (hyposmolar) syndromes. West J Med 132:16, 1980.
3. Adrogue HJ, Madias NE: Hypernatremia. N Engl J Med 342: 1493, 2000.
4. Epstein FH, Kleeman CR, Hendrikx A: The influence of bodily hydration on the renal concentrating process. J Clin Invest 36: 629, 1957.
5. Arieff AI: Effects on the central nervous system of hypernatremic and hyponatremic states. Kidney Int 10:104, 1976.
6. Arieff A, Guisado R, Lasarowitz V: Pathophysiology of hyperosmolar states. In Andreoli T, Grantham J, Rector FJ (eds): Disturbances in Body Fluid Osmolality. Bethesda, MD, American Physiological Society, 1977, p 227.
7. Covey C, Arieff A: Disorders of sodium and water metabolism and their effects on the central nervous system. In Brenner B, Stein J (eds): Sodium and Water Homeostasis, Contemporary Issues in Nephrology, vol 1. New York, Churchill Livingstone, 1978, p 213.
8. Kleeman CR: The kidney in health and disease. X. CNS manifestations of disordered salt and water balance. Hosp Pract 14: 59, 1979.
9. Pollock AS, Arieff AI: Abnormalities of cell volume regulation and their functional consequences. Am J Physiol 239:F195, 1980.
10. Shen FH, Sherrard DJ, Scollard D, et al: Thirst, relative hypernatremia, and excessive weight gain in maintenance peritoneal dialysis. Trans Am Soc Artif Intern Organs 24:142, 1978.
11. Snyder NA, Feigal DW, Arieff AI: Hypernatremia in elderly patients: A heterogeneous, morbid, and iatrogenic entity. Ann Intern Med 107:309, 1987.
12. Lien YH, Shapiro JI, Chan L: Effects of hypernatremia on organic brain osmoles. J Clin Invest 85:1427, 1990.
13. Feinberg L, Lutterell C, Redd H: Pathogenesis of lesion in the nervous system in hypernatremic states. II. Experimental studies of gross anatomic changes and alterations of chemical composition of tissues. Pediatrics 23:46, 1959.
14. Young RS, Truax BT: Hypernatremic hemorrhagic encephalopathy. Ann Neurol 5:588, 1979.
15. Gullans SR, Verbalis JG: Control of brain volume during hyperosmolar and hypoosmolar conditions. Annu Rev Med 44:289, 1993.
16. Covey CM, Arieff AI, Armstrong D, et al: Therapy of chronic hypernatremia: Changes induced in brain water, osmolality and amino acids. Clin Res 27:61, 1979.
17. Burbach JP, Luckman SM, Murphy D, et al: Gene regulation in the magnocellular hypothalamo-neurohypophysial system. Physiol Rev 81:1197, 2001.
18. Richter D: Molecular events in the expression of vasopressin and oxytocin and their cognate receptors. Am J Physiol 255: F207, 1988.
19. Williams PD, Pettibone DJ: Recent advances in the development of oxytocin receptor antagonists. Curr Pharm Design 2: 41, 1996.
20. Kalogeras KT, Nieman LN, Friedman TC, et al: Inferior petrosal sinus sampling in healthy human subjects reveals a unilateral corticotropin-releasing hormone–induced arginine vasopressin release associated with ipsilateral adrenocorticotropin secretion. J Clin Invest 97:2045, 1996.
21. Yanovski JA, Friedman TC, Nieman LK, et al: Inferior petrosal sinus AVP in patients with Cushing's syndrome. Clin Endocrinol (Oxf) 47:199, 1997.
22. Rao VV, Loffler C, Battey J, et al: The human gene for oxytocin-neurophysin I (OXT) is physically mapped to chromosome 20p13 by in situ hybridization. Cell Genet 61:271, 1992.
23. Gainer H: Molecular studies of cell-specific gene expression and secretion in the hypothalamo-neurohypohysial system. Proceedings of the World Congress on Neurohypophysial Hormones, Bordeaux, France, September 8–12, 2001, p 23.
24. Chen L, Rose JP, Breslow E, et al: Crystal structure of a bovine neurophysin II dipeptide complex at 2.8 angstrom determined from the single-wave length anomalous scattering signal of an incorporated iodine atom. Proc Natl Acad Sci U S A 88: 4240, 1991.
25. Robertson GL, Berl T: Pathophysiology of water metabolism. In Brenner BM, Rector FC (eds): The Kidney, 5th ed. Philadelphia, WB Saunders, 1996, p 873.
26. Thrasher TN, Brown CJ, Keil LC, et al: Thirst and vasopressin release in the dog: An osmoreceptor or sodium receptor mechanism? Am J Physiol 238:R333, 1980.
27. Olsson K, Kolmodin R: Dependence of basic secretion of antidiuretic hormone on cerebrospinal fluid ($Na^+$). Acta Physiol Scand 91:286, 1974.
28. Leng G, Dyball RE, Luckman SM: Mechanisms of vasopressin secretion. Horm Res 37:33, 1992.
29. Bourque CW, Oliet SHR, Richard D: Osmoreceptors, osmoreception, and osmoregulation. Front Neuroendocrinol 15:231, 1994.
30. Bourque CW, Oliet SHR: Osmoreceptors in the central nervous system. Annu Rev Physiol 59:601, 1997.
31. Voisin DL, Chakfe Y, Bourque CW: Coincident detection of CSF $Na^+$ and osmotic pressure in osmoregulatory neurons of the supraoptic nucleus. Neuron 24:453, 1999.
32. Verney E: The antidiuretic hormone and the factors which determine its release. Proc R Soc London Ser B 135:25, 1947.
33. Thrasher TN, Ramsey DJ: Anatomy of osmoreception. In Jard S, Jamison R (eds): Vasopressin, vol 208. Paris, Colloques INSERM/John Libbey Eurotext, 1991, p 267.

34. Mason WT: Supraoptic neurones of rat hypothalamus are osmosensitive. Nature 287:154, 1980.
35. Leng G, Blackburn RE, Russell JA: Role of anterior peri-third ventricular structures in the regulation of supraoptic neuronal activity and neurohypophysial hormone secretion in the rat. J Neuroendocrinol 1:35, 1989.
36. Honda K, Negoro H, Dyball RE, et al: The osmoreceptor complex in the rat: Evidence for interactions between the supraoptic and other diencephalic nuclei. J Physiol 431:225, 1990.
37. Mendelsohn FA, Quirion R, Saavedra JM, et al: Autoradiographic localization of angiotensin II receptors in rat brain. Proc Natl Acad Sci U S A 81:1575, 1984.
38. Osheroff PL, Phillips HS: Autoradiographic localization of relaxin binding sites in rat brain. Proc Natl Acad Sci U S A 88: 6413, 1991.
39. Ferguson AV, Kasting NW: Angiotensin acts at the subfornical organ to increase plasma oxytocin concentrations in the rat. Regul Pept 23:343, 1988.
40. Standaert DG, Cechetto DF, Needleman P, et al: Inhibition of the firing of vasopressin neurons by atriopeptin. Nature 329: 151, 1987.
41. Way SA, Leng G: Relaxin increases the firing rate of supraoptic neurones and increases oxytocin secretion in the rat. J Endocrinol 132:149, 1992.
42. Nissen R, Renaud LP: GABA receptor mediation of median preoptic nucleus–evoked inhibition of supraoptic neurosecretory neurones in rat. J Physiol 479:207, 1994.
43. Yang CR, Senatorov VV, Renaud LP: Organum vasculosum lamina terminalis–evoked postsynaptic responses in rat supraoptic neurones in vitro. J Physiol 477:59, 1994.
44. Luckman SM: Evidence for nitric oxide (NO) actions throughout the forebrain osmoresponsive circuit. Adv Exp Med Biol 449:187, 1998.
45. Luckman SM, Huckett L, Bicknell RJ, et al: Up-regulation of nitric oxide synthase messenger RNA in an integrated forebrain circuit involved in oxytocin secretion. Neuroscience 77:37, 1997.
46. Liedtke W, Choe Y, Marti-Renom M, et al: Vanilloid receptor–related osmotically activated channel (VR-OAC), a candidate vertebrate osmoreceptor. Cell 103:525, 2000.
47. Share L: Role of vasopressin in cardiovascular regulation. Physiol Rev 68:1248, 1988.
48. Bisset GW, Chowdrey HS: Control of release of vasopressin by neuroendocrine reflexes. Q J Exp Physiol 73:811, 1988.
49. Jhamandas JH, Raby W, Rogers J, et al: Diagonal band projection towards the hypothalamic supraoptic nucleus: Light and electron microscopic observations in the rat. J Comp Neurol 282:15, 1989.
50. Jhamandas JH, Renaud LP: A gamma-aminobutyric-acid–mediated baroreceptor input to supraoptic vasopressin neurones in the rat. J Physiol 381:595, 1986.
51. Day TA, Randle JC, Renaud LP: Opposing alpha- and beta-adrenergic mechanisms mediate dose-dependent actions of noradrenaline on supraoptic vasopressin neurones in vivo. Brain Res 358:171, 1985.
52. Raby WN, Renaud LP: Dorsomedial medulla stimulation activates rat supraoptic oxytocin and vasopressin neurones through different pathways. J Physiol 417:279, 1989.
53. Day TA, Sibbald JR: A1 cell group mediates solitary nucleus excitation of supraoptic vasopressin cells. Am J Physiol 257: R1020, 1989.
54. Ito M, Oliverio MI, Mannon PJ, et al: Regulation of blood pressure by the type 1A angiotensin II receptor gene. Proc Natl Acad Sci U S A 92:3521, 1995.
55. Nimura F, Labosky P, Kakuchi J, et al: Gene targeting in mice reveals a requirement for angiotensin in the development and maintenance of kidney morphology and growth factor regulation. J Clin Invest 96:2947, 1995.
56. Sugaya T, Nishimatsu S, Tanimoto K, et al: Angiotensin II type 1a receptor–deficient mice with hypotension and hyperreninemia. J Biol Chem 270:18719, 1995.
57. Hein L, Barsh GS, Pratt RE, et al: Behavioural and cardiovascular effects of disrupting the angiotensin II type-2 receptor gene in mice. Nature 377:744, 1995.
58. Zerbe RL, Robertson GL: A comparison of plasma vasopressin measurements with a standard indirect test in the differential diagnosis of polyuria. N Engl J Med 305:1539, 1981.
59. Miller M, Dalakos T, Moses AM, et al: Recognition of partial defects in antidiuretic hormone secretion. Ann Intern Med 73: 721, 1970.
60. Bichet DG, Kluge R, Howard RL, et al: Hyponatremic states. In Seldin DW, Giebisch G (eds): The Kidney: Physiology and Pathophysiology, 2nd ed. New York, Raven Press, 1992, p 1727.
61. Baylis PH, Gaskill MB, Robertson GL: Vasopressin secretion in primary polydipsia and cranial diabetes insipidus. QJM 50: 345, 1981.
62. Rolls B, Rolls E: Thirst (Problems in the Behavioural Sciences). Cambridge, UK, Cambridge University Press, 1982.
63. Fitzsimons JT: Angiotensin, thirst, and sodium appetite. Physiol Rev 78:583, 1998.
64. Samson WK: Atrial natriuretic factor inhibits dehydration and hemorrhage-induced vasopressin release. Neuroendocrinology 40:277, 1985.
65. Goetz KL, Wang BC, Geer PG, et al: Effects of atriopeptin infusion versus effects of left atrial stretch in awake dogs. Am J Physiol 250:R221, 1986.
66. Ogawa K, Arnolda LF, Woodcock EA, et al: Lack of effect of atrial natriuretic peptide on vasopressin release. Clin Sci 72: 525, 1987.
67. Abelson JL, Le Mellédo J-M, Bichet DG: Dose response of arginine vasopressin to the CCK-B agonist pentagastrin. Neuropsychopharmacology 24:161–169, 2001.
68. Ota M, Crofton JT, Festavan GT, et al: Evidence that nitric oxide can act centrally to stimulate vasopressin release. Neuroendocrinology 57:955, 1993.
69. Yasin S, Costa A, Trainer P, et al: Nitric oxide modulates the release of vasopressin from rat hypothalamic explants. Endocrinology 133:1466, 1993.
70. Kadowaki K, Kishimoto J, Leng G, et al: Up-regulation of nitric oxide synthase (NOS) gene expression together with NOS activity in the rat hypothalamo-hypophysial system after chronic salt loading: Evidence of a neuromodulatory role of nitric oxide in arginine vasopressin and oxytocin secretion. Endocrinology 134:1011, 1994.
71. Wang H, Morris JF: Constitutive nitric oxide synthase in hypothalami of normal and hereditary diabetes insipidus rats and mice: Role of nitric oxide in osmotic regulation and its mechanism. Endocrinology 137:1745, 1996.
72. Raff H: Glucocorticoid inhibition of neurohypophysial vasopressin secretion. Am J Physiol 252:R635, 1987.
73. Rowe JW, Shelton RL, Helderman JH, et al: Influence of the emetic reflex on vasopressin release in man. Kidney Int 16: 729, 1979.
74. Nathanson MH, Moyer MS, Burgstahler AD, et al: Mechanisms of subcellular cytosolic $Ca^{2+}$ signaling evoked by stimulation of the vasopressin $V_{1a}$ receptor. J Biol Chem 267:23282, 1992.
75. Jard S, Elands J, Schmidt A, et al: Vasopressin and oxytocin receptors: An overview. In Imura H, Shizume K (eds): Progress in Endocrinology. Amsterdam, Elsevier Science, 1988, p 1183.
76. Birnbaumer M, Seibold A, Gilbert S, et al: Molecular cloning of the receptor for human antidiuretic hormone. Nature 357: 333, 1992.
77. Seibold A, Brabet P, Rosenthal W, et al: Structure and chromosomal localization of the human antidiuretic hormone receptor gene. Am J Hum Genet 51:1078, 1992.
78. Watson S, Arkinstall S: The G Protein Linked Receptor Factsbook. London, Academic Press, 1994.
79. Preston GM, Carroll TP, Guggino WB, et al: Appearance of water channels in *Xenopus* oocytes expressing red cell CHIP28 protein. Science 256:385, 1992.
80. Denker BM, Smith BL, Kuhajda FP, et al: Identification, purification, and partial characterization of a novel Mr 28,000 integral membrane protein from erythrocytes and renal tubules. J Biol Chem 263:15634, 1988.
81. Sabolic I, Valenti G, Verbavatz JM, et al: Localization of the CHIP28 water channel in rat kidney. Am J Physiol 263:C1225, 1992.
82. Nielsen S, Smith BL, Christensen EI, et al: CHIP28 water channels are localized in constitutively water-permeable segments of the nephron. J Cell Biol 120:371, 1993.

83. Nielsen S, Agre P: The aquaporin family of water channels in kidney. Kidney Int 48:1057, 1995.
84. Murata K, Mitsuoka K, Hirai T, et al: Structural determinants of water permeation through aquaporin-1. Nature 407:599, 2000.
85. Verkman AS, Mitra AK: Structure and function of aquaporin water channels. Am J Physiol Renal Physiol 278:F13, 2000.
86. Pomes R, Roux B: Structure and dynamics of a proton wire: A theoretical study of $H^+$ translocation along the single-file water chain in the gramicidin A channel. Biophys J 71:19, 1996.
87. Wade JB, Stetson DL, Lewis SA: ADH action: Evidence for a membrane shuttle mechanism. Ann N Y Acad Sci 372:106, 1981.
88. Knepper MA: Molecular physiology of urinary concentrating mechanism: Regulation of aquaporin water channels by vasopressin. Am J Physiol 272:F3, 1997.
89. Fushimi K, Sasaki S, Marumo F: Phosphorylation of serine 256 is required for cAMP-dependent regulatory exocytosis of the aquaporin-2 water channel. J Biol Chem 272:14800, 1997.
90. Katsura T, Gustafson C, Ausiello D, et al: Protein kinase A phosphorylation is involved in regulated exocytosis of aquaporin-2 in transfected LLC-PK1 cells. Am J Physiol 272:F817, 1997.
91. Valenti G, Procino G, Liebenhoff U, et al: A heterotrimeric G protein of the Gi family is required for cAMP-triggered trafficking of aquaporin 2 in kidney epithelial cells. J Biol Chem 273: 22627, 1998.
92. Mandon B, Nielsen S, Kishore BK, et al: Expression of syntaxins in rat kidney. Am J Physiol 273:F718, 1997.
93. Jo I, Harris HW, Amendt-Raduege AM, et al: Rat kidney papilla contains abundant synaptobrevin protein that participates in the fusion of antidiuretic hormone–regulated water channel–containing endosomes in vitro. Proc Natl Acad Sci U S A 92: 1876, 1995.
94. Liebenhoff U, Rosenthal W: Identification of Rab3-, Rab5a- and synaptobrevin II–like proteins in a preparation of rat kidney vesicles containing the vasopressin-regulated water channel. FEBS Lett 365:209, 1995.
95. Nielsen S, Marples D, Birn H, et al: Expression of VAMP-2–like protein in kidney collecting duct intracellular vesicles: Colocalization with aquaporin-2 water channels. J Clin Invest 96:1834, 1995.
96. Star RA, Nonoguchi H, Balaban R, et al: Calcium and cyclic adenosine monophosphate as second messengers for vasopressin in the rat inner medullary collecting duct. J Clin Invest 81: 1879, 1988.
97. Snyder HM, Noland TD, Breyer MD: cAMP-Dependent protein kinase mediates hydrosmotic effect of vasopressin in collecting duct. Am J Physiol 263:C147, 1992.
98. Brown D, Katsura T, Gustafson CE: Cellular mechanisms of aquaporin trafficking. Am J Physiol 275:F328, 1998.
99. Taylor A, Mamelak M, Reaven E, et al: Vasopressin: Possible role of microtubules and microfilaments in its action. Science 181:347, 1973.
100. Sabolic I, Katsura T, Verbabatz JM, et al: The AQP2 water channel: Effect of vasopressin treatment, microtubule disruption, and distribution in neonatal rats. J Membr Biol 143: 165, 1995.
101. Shayakul C, Steel A, Hediger MA: Molecular cloning and characterization of the vasopressin-regulated urea transporter of rat kidney collecting ducts. J Clin Invest 98:2580, 1996.
102. Ward DT, Hammond TG, Harris HW: Modulation of vasopressin-elicited water transport by trafficking of aquaporin2-containing vesicles. Annu Rev Physiol 61:683, 1999.
103. Fleming EF, Athirakul K, Oliverio MI, et al: Urinary concentrating function in mice lacking EP3 receptors for prostaglandin $E_2$. Am J Physiol 275:F955, 1998.
104. Sands JM, Naruse M, Baum M, et al: Apical extracellular calcium/polyvalent cation–sensing receptor regulates vasopressin-elicited water permeability in rat kidney inner medullary collecting duct. J Clin Invest 99:1399, 1997.
105. Fushimi K, Uchida S, Hara Y, et al: Cloning and expression of apical membrane water channel of rat kidney collecting tubule. Nature 361:549, 1993.
106. Deen PMT, Verdijk MAJ, Knoers NVAM, et al: Requirement of human renal water channel aquaporin-2 for vasopressin-dependent concentration of urine. Science 264:92, 1994.
107. Sasaki S, Fushimi K, Saito H, et al: Cloning, characterization, and chromosomal mapping of human aquaporin of collecting duct. J Clin Invest 93:1250, 1994.
108. Deen PMT, Weghuis DO, Sinke RJ, et al: Assignment of the human gene for the water channel of renal collecting duct aquaporin 2 (AQP2) to chromosome 12 region q12->q13. Cytogenet Cell Genet 66:260, 1994.
109. Kanno K, Sasaki S, Hirata Y, et al: Urinary excretion of aquaporin-2 in patients with diabetes insipidus. N Engl J Med 332: 1540, 1995.
110. Elliot S, Goldsmith P, Knepper M, et al: Urinary excretion of aquaporin-2 in humans: A potential marker of collecting duct responsiveness to vasopressin. J Am Soc Nephrol 7:403, 1996.
111. Saito T, Ishikawa SE, Sasaki S, et al: Urinary excretion of aquaporin-2 in the diagnosis of central diabetes insipidus. J Clin Endocrinol Metab 82:1823, 1997.
112. Ma T, Yang B, Gillespie A, et al: Generation and phenotype of a transgenic knockout mouse lacking the mercurial-insensitive water channel aquaporin-4. J Clin Invest 100:957, 1997.
113. Ma T, Yang B, Gillespie A, et al: Severely impaired urinary concentrating ability in transgenic mice lacking aquaporin-1 water channels. J Biol Chem 273:4296, 1998.
114. Matsumura Y, Uchida S, Kondo Y, et al: Overt nephrogenic diabetes insipidus in mice lacking the CLC-K1 chloride channel. Nat Genet 21:95, 1999.
115. Chou C-L, Knepper MA, van Hoek AN, et al: Reduced water permeability and altered ultrastructure in thin descending limb of Henle in aquaporin-1 null mice. J Clin Invest 103:491, 1999.
116. Ma T, Song Y, Yang B, et al: Nephrogenic diabetes insipidus in mice lacking aquaporin-3 water channels. Proc Natl Acad Sci U S A 97:4386, 2000.
117. Takahashi N, Chernavvsky DR, Gomez RA, et al: Uncompensated polyuria in a mouse model of Bartter's syndrome. Proc Natl Acad Sci U S A 97:5434, 2000.
118. Yun J, Erlenbach I, Kostenis E, et al. $V_2$ vasopressin receptor function studied in mice and yeast. Proceedings of the NDI Conference, La Jolla, CA, March 10–12, 2000, p 25.
119. Yang B, Gillespie A, Carlson EJ, et al: Neonatal mortality in an aquaporin-2 knock-in mouse model of recessive nephrogenic diabetes insipidus. J Biol Chem 276:2775, 2001.
120. Okubo S, Niimura F, Matsusaka T, et al: Angiotensinogen gene null-mutant mice lack homeostatic regulation of glomerular filtration and tubular reabsorption. Kidney Int 53:617, 1998.
121. Rao S, Verkman AS: Analysis of organ physiology in transgenic mice. Am J Physiol Cell Physiol 279:C1, 2000.
122. Preston GM, Smith BL, Zeidel ML, et al: Mutations in aquaporin-1 in phenotypically normal humans without functional CHIP water channels. Science 265:1585, 1994.
123. Mulders SB, Knoers NVAM, van Lieburg AF, et al: New mutations in the AQP2 gene in nephrogenic diabetes insipidus resulting in functional but misrouted water channels. J Am Soc Nephrol 8:242, 1997.
124. Schmale H, Richter D: Single base deletion in the vasopressin gene is the cause of diabetes insipidus in Brattleboro rats. Nature 308:705, 1984.
125. Serradeil-Le Gal C, Lacour C, Valette G, et al: Characterization of SR 121463A, a highly potent and selective, orally active vasopressin $V_2$ receptor antagonist. J Clin Invest 98:2729, 1996.
126. Balment RJ, Brimble MJ, Forsling ML: Oxytocin release and renal actions in normal and Brattleboro rats. Ann N Y Acad Sci 394:241, 1982.
127. Chou CL, DiGiovanni SR, Luther A, et al: Oxytocin as an antidiuretic hormone. II. Role of $V_2$ vasopressin receptor. Am J Physiol 269:F78, 1995.
128. Bichet DG, Arthus M-F, Lonergan M, et al: Hereditary central diabetes insipidus: Autosomal dominant and autosomal recessive phenotypes due to mutations in the *prepro-AVP-NPII* gene. J Am Soc Nephrol 9:386A, 1998.
129. Willcutts MD, Felner E, White PC: Autosomal recessive familial neurohypophyseal diabetes insipidus with continued secretion of mutant weakly active vasopressin. Hum Mol Genet 8:1303, 1999.
130. Verbalis JG, Robinson AG, Moses AM: Postoperative and posttraumatic diabetes insipidus. In Czernichow P, Robinson AG (eds): Frontiers of Hormone Research, vol 13, Diabetes Insipidus in Man. Basel, S. Karger, 1985, p 247.

131. Olson BR, Gumowski J, Rubino D, et al: Pathophysiology of hyponatremia after transsphenoidal pituitary surgery. J Neurosurg 87:499, 1997.
132. Czernichow P, Pomarede R, Brauner R, et al: Neurogenic diabetes insipidus in children. In Czernichow P, Robinson AG (eds): Frontiers of Hormone Research, vol 13, Diabetes Insipidus in Man. Basel, S. Karger, 1985, p 190.
133. Greger NG, Kirkland RT, Clayton GW, et al: Central diabetes insipidus: 22 years' experience. Am J Dis Child 140:551, 1986.
134. Maghnie M, Cosi G, Genovese E, et al: Central diabetes insipidus in children and young adults. N Engl J Med 343:998, 2000.
135. Moses AM, Blumenthal SA, Streeten DHP: Acid-base and electrolyte disorders associated with endocrine disease: pituitary and thyroid. In Arieff AI, de Fronzo RA (eds): Fluid, Electrolyte and Acid-Base Disorders. New York, Churchill Livingstone, 1985, p 851.
136. Birnbaum DC, Shields D, Lippe B, et al: Idiopathic central diabetes insipidus followed by progressive spastic cerebral ataxia: Report of four cases. Arch Neurol 46:1001, 1989.
137. Bullmann C, Faust M, Hoffmann A, et al: Five cases with central diabetes insipidus and hypogonadism as first presentation of neurosarcoidosis. Eur J Endocrinol 142:365, 2000.
138. Vokes TJ, Gaskill MB, Robertson GL: Antibodies to vasopressin in patients with diabetes insipidus: Implications for diagnosis and therapy. Ann Intern Med 108:190, 1988.
139. Bichet DG, Kortas C, Manzini C, et al: A specific antibody to vasopressin in a man with concomitant resistance to treatment with Pitressin. Clin Chem 32:211, 1986.
140. Kaltsas GA, Powles TB, Evanson J, et al: Hypothalamo-pituitary abnormalities in adult patients with Langerhans cell histiocytosis: Clinical, endocrinological, and radiological features and response to treatment. J Clin Endocrinol Metab 85:1370, 2000.
141. Lacombe UL: De la polydipsie [Thesis of Medicine, no. 99]. Imprimerie et Fonderie de Rignoux, 1841.
142. Weil A: Ueber die hereditare form des diabetes insipidus. Arch Pathol Anat Physiol Klin Med (Virchows Arch) 95:70, 1884.
143. Weil A: Ueber die hereditare form des diabetes insipidus. Deutches Arch Klin Med 93:180, 1908.
144. Camerer JW: Eine ergänzung des Weilschen diabetes-insipidus-stammbaumes. Arch Rassen-und Gesellschaftshygiene Biol 28: 382, 1935.
145. Dölle W: Eine weitere ergänzung des Weilschen diabetes-insipidus-stammbaumes. Z Menschliche Vererbungs-und Konstitutionslehre 30:372, 1951.
146. Repaske DR, Phillips JAD, Kirby LT, et al: Molecular analysis of autosomal dominant neurohypophyseal diabetes insipidus. J Clin Endocrinol Metab 70:752, 1990.
147. Online Mendelian Inheritance in Man (OMIM). Center for Medical Genetics, Johns Hopkins University (Baltimore, MD), and National Center for Biotechnology Information, National Library of Medicine (Bethesda, MD), 1997. http://www.ncbi.nlm.nih.gov/omim/.
148. Rittig R, Robertson GL, Siggaard C, et al: Identification of 13 new mutations in the vasopressin-neurophysin II gene in 17 kindreds with familial autosomal dominant neurohypophyseal diabetes insipidus. Am J Hum Genet 58:107, 1996.
149. Rutishauser J, Boni-Schnetzler M, Boni J, et al: A novel point mutation in the translation initiation codon of the pre- provasopressin-neurophysin II gene: Cosegregation with morphological abnormalities and clinical symptoms in autosomal dominant neurohypophyseal diabetes insipidus. J Clin Endocrinol Metab 81:192, 1996.
150. Rittig S, Siggaard C, Ozata M, et al: Familial neurohypophyseal diabetes insipidus due to mutation that substitutes histidine for tyrosine-2 in the antidiuretic hormone. J Investig Med 44: 387A, 1996.
151. Ito M, Oiso Y, Murase T, et al: Possible involvement of inefficient cleavage of preprovasopressin by signal peptidase as a cause for familial central diabetes insipidus. J Clin Invest 91: 2565, 1993.
152. Krishnamani MRS, Phillips JAI, Copeland KC: Detection of a novel arginine vasopressin defect by dideoxy fingerprinting. J Clin Endocrinol Metab 77:596, 1993.
153. McLeod JF, Kovacs L, Gaskill MB, et al: Familial neurohypophyseal diabetes insipidus associated with a signal peptide mutation. J Clin Endocrinol Metab 77:599A, 1993.
154. Repaske DR, Summar ML, Krishnamani MR, et al: Recurrent mutations in the vasopressin-neurophysin II gene cause autosomal dominant neurohypophyseal diabetes insipidus. J Clin Endocrinol Metab 81:2328, 1996.
155. Repaske DR, Medlej R, Gultekin EK, et al: Heterogeneity in clinical manifestation of autosomal dominant neurohypophyseal diabetes insipidus caused by a mutation endocing Ala-1->Val in the signal peptide of the arginine vasopressin/neurophysin II/copeptin precursor. J Clin Endocrinol Metab 82: 51, 1997.
156. Heppner C, Kotzka J, Bullmann C, et al: Identification of mutations of the arginine vasopressin–neurophysin II gene in two kindreds with familial central diabetes insipidus. J Clin Endocrinol Metab 83:693, 1998.
157. Bahnsen U, Oosting P, Swaab DF, et al: A missense mutation in the vasopressin-neurophysin precursor gene cosegregates with human autosomal dominant neurohypophyseal diabetes insipidus. EMBO J 11:19, 1992.
158. Gagliardi PC, Bernasconi S, Repaske DR: Autosomal dominant neurohypophyseal diabetes insipidus associated with a missense mutation encoding Gly23−>Val in neurophysin II. J Clin Endocrinol Metab 82:3643, 1997.
159. Repaske DR, Browning JE: A de novo mutation in the coding sequence for neurophysin-II (Pro24−>Leu) is associated with onset and transmission of autosomal dominant neurohypophyseal diabetes insipidus. J Clin Endocrinol Metab 79:421, 1994.
160. Yuasa H, Ito M, Nagasaki H, et al: Glu-47, which forms a salt bridge between neurophysin-II and arginine vasopressin, is deleted in patients with familial central diabetes insipidus. J Clin Endocrinol Metab 77:600, 1993.
161. Ito M, Mori Y, Oiso Y, et al: A single base substitution in the coding region for neurophysin II associated with familial central diabetes insipidus. J Clin Invest 87:725, 1991.
162. Nagasaki H, Ito M, Yuasa H, et al: Two novel mutations in the coding region for neurophysin-II associated with familial central diabetes insipidus. J Clin Endocrinol Metab 80:1352, 1995.
163. Ueta Y, Taniguchi S, Yoshida A, et al: A new type of familial central diabetes insipidus caused by a single base substitution in the neurophysin II coding region of the vasopressin gene. J Clin Endocrinol Metab 81:1787, 1996.
164. Beuret N, Rutishauser J, Bider MD, et al: Mechanism of endoplasmic reticulum retention of mutant vasopressin precursor caused by a signal peptide truncation associated with diabetes insipidus. J Biol Chem 274:18965, 1999.
165. Calvo B, Bilbao JR, Urrutia I, et al: Identification of a novel nonsense mutation and a missense substitution in the vasopressin-neurophysin II gene in two Spanish kindreds with familial neurohypophyseal diabetes insipidus. J Clin Endocrinol Metab 83:995, 1998.
166. Calvo B, Bilbao JR, Rodriguez A, et al: Molecular analysis in familial neurohypophyseal diabetes insipidus: Early diagnosis of an asymptomatic carrier. J Clin Endocrinol Metab 84:3351, 1999.
167. Siggaard C, Rittig S, Corydon TJ, et al: Clinical and molecular evidence of abnormal processing and trafficking of the vasopressin preprohormone in a large kindred with familial neurohypophyseal diabetes insipidus due to a signal peptide mutation. J Clin Endocrinol Metab 84:2933, 1999.
168. Fujii H, Iida S, Moriwaki K: Familial neurohypophyseal diabetes insipidus associated with a novel mutation in the vasopressin-neurophysin II gene. Int J Mol Med 5:229, 2000.
169. Rutishauser J, Kopp P, Gaskill MB, et al: A novel mutation (R97C) in the neurophysin moiety of prepro-vasopressin-neurophysin II associated with autosomal-dominant neurohypophyseal diabetes insipidus. Mol Genet Metab 67:89, 1999.
170. Grant FD, Ahmadi A, Hosley CM, et al: Two novel mutations of the vasopressin gene associated with familial diabetes insipidus and identification of an asymptomatic carrier infant. J Clin Endocrinol Metab 83:3958, 1998.
171. Abbes AP, Bruggeman B, van Den Akker EL, et al: Identification of two distinct mutations at the same nucleotide position, concomitantly with a novel polymorphism in the vasopressin-neurophysin II gene (AVP-NP II) in two Dutch families with

familial neurohypophyseal diabetes insipidus. Clin Chem 46: 1699, 2000.
172. Ito M, Jameson JL, Ito M: Molecular basis of autosomal dominant neurohypophyseal diabetes insipidus: Cellular toxicity caused by the accumulation of mutant vasopressin precursors within the endoplasmic reticulum. J Clin Invest 99:1897, 1997.
173. Ito M, Yu RN, Jameson JL: Mutant vasopressin precursors that cause autosomal dominant neurohypophyseal diabetes insipidus retain dimerization and impair the secretion of wild-type proteins. J Biol Chem 274:9029, 1999.
174. Bross P, Corydon TJ, Andresen BS, et al: Protein misfolding and degradation in genetic diseases. Hum Mutat 14:186, 1999.
175. Welch WJ, Howard M: Commentary: Antagonists to the rescue. J Clin Invest 105:853, 2000.
176. Peden NR, Gay JD, Jung RT, et al: Wolfram (DIDMOAD) syndrome: A complex long-term problem in management. QJM 58:167, 1986.
177. Wolfram DJ: Diabetes mellitus and simple optic atrophy among siblings: Report of four cases. Mayo Clin Proc 13:715, 1938.
178. Swift RG, Sadler DB, Swift M: Psychiatric findings in Wolfram syndrome homozygotes. Lancet 336:667, 1990.
179. Inoue H, Tanizawa Y, Wasson J, et al: A gene encoding a transmembrane protein is mutated in patients with diabetes mellitus and optic atrophy (Wolfram syndrome). Nat Genet 20: 143, 1998.
180. Strom TM, Hortnagel K, Hofmann S, et al: Diabetes insipidus, diabetes mellitus, optic atrophy and deafness (DIDMOAD) caused by mutations in a novel gene (wolframin) coding for a predicted transmembrane protein. Hum Mol Genet 7:2021, 1998.
181. Hardy C, Khanim F, Torres R, et al: Clinical and molecular genetic analysis of 19 Wolfram syndrome kindreds demonstrating a wide spectrum of mutations in WFS1. Am J Hum Genet 65:1279, 1999.
182. Howard RL, Bichet DG, Schrier RW: Hypernatremic and polyuric states. In Seldin DW, Giebisch G (eds): The Kidney: Physiology and Pathophysiology, 2nd ed. New York, Raven Press, 1992, p 1753.
183. Bichet DG: Nephrogenic diabetes insipidus. In Cameron JS, Davison AM, Grünfeld JP, et al (eds): Oxford Textbook of Clinical Nephrology. New York, Oxford University Press, 1992, p 789.
184. Arthus M-F, Lonergan M, Crumley MJ, et al: Report of 33 novel *AVPR2* mutations and analysis of 117 families with X-linked nephrogenic diabetes insipidus. J Am Soc Nephrol 11:1044, 2000.
185. Bode HH, Crawford JD: Nephrogenic diabetes insipidus in North America: The Hopewell hypothesis. N Engl J Med 280: 750, 1969.
186. Bichet DG, Hendy GN, Lonergan M, et al: X-linked nephrogenic diabetes insipidus: From the ship Hopewell to restriction fragment length polymorphism studies. Am J Hum Genet 51: 1089, 1992.
187. Bichet DG, Arthus M-F, Lonergan M, et al: X-linked nephrogenic diabetes insipidus mutations in North America and the Hopewell hypothesis. J Clin Invest 92:1262, 1993.
188. Holtzman EJ, Kolakowski LF, O'Brien D, et al: A null mutation in the vasopressin $V_2$ receptor gene (AVPR2) associated with nephrogenic diabetes insipidus in the Hopewell kindred. Hum Mol Genet 2:1201, 1993.
189. Bichet DG, Fujiwara TM: Nephrogenic diabetes insipidus. In Scriver CR, Beaudet AL, Sly WS, et al (eds): The Metabolic and Molecular Bases of Inherited Disease, 8th ed, vol 3. New York, McGraw-Hill, 2001, p 4181.
190. Bichet DG, Birnbaumer M, Lonergan M, et al: Nature and recurrence of AVPR2 mutations in X-linked nephrogenic diabetes insipidus. Am J Hum Genet 55:278, 1994.
191. Fujiwara TM, Morgan K, Bichet DG: Molecular analysis of X-linked nephrogenic diabetes insipidus. Eur J Endocrinol 134: 675, 1996.
192. Forssman H: On the mode of hereditary transmission in diabetes insipidus. Nord Med 16:3211, 1942.
193. Waring AG, Kajdi L, Tappan V: Congenital defect of water metabolism. Am J Dis Child 69:323, 1945.
194. Williams RM, Henry C: Nephrogenic diabetes insipidus transmitted by females and appearing during infancy in males. Ann Intern Med 27:84, 1947.
195. Crawford JD, Bode HH: Disorders of the posterior pituitary in children. In Gardner LI, (ed): Endocrine and Genetic Diseases of Childhood and Adolescence, 2nd ed. Philadelphia, WB Saunders, 1975, p 126.
196. van Lieburg AF, Knoers NVAM, Monnens LAH: Clinical presentation and follow-up of 30 patients with congenital nephrogenic diabetes insipidus. J Am Soc Nephrol 10:1958, 1999.
197. Hoekstra JA, van Lieburg AF, Monnens LA, et al: Cognitive and psychosocial functioning of patients with congenital nephrogenic diabetes insipidus. Am J Med Genet 61:81, 1996.
198. Niaudet P, Dechaux M, Trivin C, et al: Nephrogenic diabetes insipidus: Clinical and pathophysiological aspects. Adv Nephrol Necker Hosp 13:247, 1984.
199. van Lieburg AF, Verdijk MAJ, Schoute F, et al: Clinical phenotype of nephrogenic diabetes insipidus in females heterozygous for a vasopressin type 2 receptor mutation. Hum Genet 96: 70, 1995.
200. Nomura Y, Onigata K, Nagashima T, et al: Detection of skewed X-inactivation in two female carriers of vasopressin type 2 receptor gene mutation. J Clin Endocrinol Metab 82:3434, 1997.
201. Hobbs HH, Russell DW, Brown MS, et al: The LDL receptor locus in familial hypercholesterolemia: Mutational analysis of a membrane protein. Annu Rev Genet 24:133, 1990.
202. Schöneberg T, Yun J, Wenkert D, et al: Functional rescue of mutant $V_2$ vasopressin receptors causing nephrogenic diabetes insipidus by a coexpressed receptor polypeptide. EMBO J 15: 1283, 1996.
203. Schöneberg T, Sandig V, Wess J, et al: Reconstitution of mutant $V_2$ vasopressin receptors by adenovirus-mediated gene transfer. J Clin Invest 100:1547, 1997.
204. Oksche A, Schulein R, Rutz C, et al: Vasopressin $V_2$ receptor mutants that cause X-linked nephrogenic diabetes insipidus: Analysis of expression, processing, and function. Mol Pharmacol 50:820, 1996.
205. Tsukaguchi H, Matsubara H, Taketani S, et al: Binding-, intracellular transport–, and biosynthesis-defective mutants of vasopressin type 2 receptor in patients with X-linked nephrogenic diabetes insipidus. J Clin Invest 96:2043, 1995.
206. Wenkert D, Schoneberg T, Merendino JJ Jr, et al: Functional characterization of five $V_2$ vasopressin receptor gene mutations. Mol Cell Endocrinol 124:43, 1996.
207. Tamarappoo BK, Verkman AS: Defective aquaporin-2 trafficking in nephrogenic diabetes insipidus and correction by chemical chaperones. J Clin Invest 101:2257, 1998.
208. Kuznetsov G, Nigam SK: Folding of secretory and membrane proteins. N Engl J Med 339:1688, 1998.
209. Waheed A, Parkkila S, Zhou XY, et al: Hereditary hemochromatosis: Effects of C282Y and H63D mutations on association with beta$_2$-microglobulin, intracellular processing, and cell surface expression of the HFE protein in COS-7 cells. Proc Natl Acad Sci U S A 94:12384, 1997.
210. Kunchaparty S, Palcso M, Berkman J, et al: Defective processing and expression of thiazide-sensitive Na-Cl cotransporter as a cause of Gitelman's syndrome. Am J Physiol 277:F643, 1999.
211. Chillaron J, Estevez R, Samarzija I, et al: An intracellular trafficking defect in type I cystinuria rBAT mutants M467T and M467K. J Biol Chem 272:9543, 1997.
212. Carrell RW, Lomas DA: Conformational disease. Lancet 350: 134, 1997.
213. Bonnardeaux A, Bichet DG: Inherited disorders of the renal tubule. In Brenner BM (ed): The Kidney, 6th ed. Philadelphia, WB Saunders, 2000, p 1656.
214. Schulz A, Grosse R, Schultz G, et al: Structural implication for receptor oligomerization from functional reconstitution studies of mutant $V_2$ vasopressin receptors. J Biol Chem 275:2381, 2000.
215. Serradeil-Le Gal C: Nonpeptide antagonists for vasopressin receptors: Pharmacology of SR 121463A, a new potent and highly selective $V_2$ receptor antagonist. Adv Exp Med Biol 449: 427, 1998.
216. Chan PS, Coupet J, Park HC, et al: VPA-985 a nonpeptide orally active and selective vasopressin $V_2$ receptor antagonist. Adv Exp Med Biol 449:439, 1998.

217. Bernat A, Hoffmann P, Dumas A, et al: $V_2$ receptor antagonism of DDAVP-induced release of hemostasis factors in conscious dogs. J Pharmacol Exp Ther 282:597, 1997.
218. Morello JP, Salahpour A, Laperrière A, et al: Pharmacological chaperones rescue cell-surface expression and function of misfolded $V_2$ vasopressin receptor mutants. J Clin Invest 105:887, 2000.
219. Brenner B, Seligsohn U, Hochberg Z: Normal response of factor VIII and von Willebrand factor to 1-deamino-8-D-arginine vasopressin in nephrogenic diabetes insipidus. J Clin Endocrinol Metab 67:191, 1988.
220. Knoers N, Monnens LA: A variant of nephrogenic diabetes insipidus: $V_2$ receptor abnormality restricted to the kidney. Eur J Pediatr 150:370, 1991.
221. Langley JM, Balfe JW, Selander T, et al: Autosomal recessive inheritance of vasopressin-resistant diabetes insipidus. Am J Med Genet 38:90, 1991.
222. Lonergan M, Birnbaumer M, Arthus M-F, et al: Non-X-linked nephrogenic diabetes insipidus: Phenotype and genotype features. J Am Soc Nephrol 4:264A, 1993.
223. Deen PMT, Croes H, van Aubel RAMH, et al: Water channels encoded by mutant aquaporin-2 genes in nephrogenic diabetes insipidus are impaired in their cellular routing. J Clin Invest 95:2291, 1995.
224. Tamarappoo BK, Yang B, Verkman AS: Misfolding of mutant aquaporin-2 water channels in nephrogenic diabetes insipidus. J Biol Chem 274:34825, 1999.
225. van Os CH, Deen PM: Aquaporin-2 water channel mutations causing nephrogenic diabetes insipidus. Proc Assoc Am Physicians 110:395, 1998.
226. Mulders SM, Bichet DG, Rijss JPL, et al: An aquaporin-2 water channel mutant which causes autosomal dominant nephrogenic diabetes insipidus is retained in the Golgi complex. J Clin Invest 102:57, 1998.
227. Kamsteeg EJ, Wormhoudt TA, Rijss JP, et al: An impaired routing of wild-type aquaporin-2 after tetramerization with an aquaporin-2 mutant explains dominant nephrogenic diabetes insipidus. EMBO J 18:2394, 1999.
228. Boton R, Gaviria M, Batlle DC: Prevalence, pathogenesis, and treatment of renal dysfunction associated with chronic lithium therapy. Am J Kidney Dis 10:329, 1987.
229. Markowitz GS, Radhakrishnan J, Kambham N, et al: Lithium nephrotoxicity: A progressive combined glomerular and tubulointerstitial nephropathy. J Am Soc Nephrol 11:1439, 2000.
230. Christensen S, Kusano E, Yusufi AN, et al: Pathogenesis of nephrogenic diabetes insipidus due to chronic administration of lithium in rats. J Clin Invest 75:1869, 1985.
231. Cogan E, Svoboda M, Abramow M: Mechanisms of lithium-vasopressin interaction in rabbit cortical collecting tubule. Am J Physiol 252:F1080, 1987.
232. Goldberg H, Clayman P, Skorecki K: Mechanism of Li inhibition of vasopressin-sensitive adenylate cyclase in cultured renal epithelial cells. Am J Physiol 255:F995, 1988.
233. Kwon TH, Laursen UH, Marples D, et al: Altered expression of renal AQPs and Na(+) transporters in rats with lithium-induced NDI. Am J Physiol Renal Physiol 279:F552, 2000.
234. Marples D, Christensen S, Christensen EI, et al: Lithium-induced downregulation of aquaporin-2 water channel expression in rat kidney medulla. J Clin Invest 95:1838, 1995.
235. Marples D, Frokiaer J, Dorup J, et al: Hypokalemia-induced downregulation of aquaporin-2 water channel expression in rat kidney medulla and cortex. J Clin Invest 97:1960, 1996.
236. Amlal H, Krane CM, Chen Q, et al: Early polyuria and urinary concentrating defect in potassium deprivation. Am J Physiol Renal Physiol 279:F655, 2000.
237. Frokiaer J, Marples D, Knepper MA, et al: Bilateral ureteral obstruction downregulates expression of vasopressin-sensitive AQP-2 water channel in rat kidney. Am J Physiol 270:F657, 1996.
238. Sands JM, Flores FX, Kato A, et al: Vasopressin-elicited water and urea permeabilities are altered in IMCD in hypercalcemic rats. Am J Physiol 274:F978, 1998.
239. Batlle DC, von Riotte AB, Gaviria M, et al: Amelioration of polyuria by amiloride in patients receiving long-term lithium therapy. N Engl J Med 312:408, 1985.
240. Barlow ED, de Wardener HE: Compulsive water drinking. QJM 28:235, 1959.
241. Robertson GL: Dipsogenic diabetes insipidus: A newly recognized syndrome caused by a selective defect in the osmoregulation of thirst. Trans Assoc Am Physicians 100:241, 1987.
242. Amico JA: Diabetes insipidus and pregnancy. In Czernichow P, Robinson AG (eds): Frontiers of Hormone Research, vol 13, Diabetes Insipidus in Man. Basel, S. Karger, 1985, p 266.
243. Davison JM, Shiells EA, Philips PR, et al: Serial evaluation of vasopressin release and thirst in human pregnancy: Role of human chorionic gonadotrophin in the osmoregulatory changes of gestation. J Clin Invest 81:798, 1988.
244. Iwasaki Y, Oiso Y, Kondo K, et al: Aggravation of subclinical diabetes insipidus during pregnancy. N Engl J Med 324:522, 1991.
245. Forssman H: On hereditary diabetes insipidus, with special regard to a sex-linked form. Acta Med Scand 159:1, 1945.
246. Barron WM, Cohen LH, Ulland LA, et al: Transient vasopressin-resistant diabetes insipidus of pregnancy. N Engl J Med 310: 442, 1984.
247. Durr JA, Hoggard JG, Hunt JM, et al: Diabetes insipidus in pregnancy associated with abnormally high circulating vasopressinase activity. N Engl J Med 316:1070, 1987.
248. Ford SM Jr: Transient vasopressin-resistant diabetes insipidus of pregnancy. Obstet Gynecol 68:288, 1986.
249. Leaf A: Neurogenic diabetes insipidus. Kidney Int 15:572, 1979.
250. Robertson GL: Diagnosis of diabetes insipidus. In Czernichow P, Robinson AG (eds): Frontiers of Hormone Research, vol 13, Diabetes Insipidus in Man. Basel, Karger, 1985, p 176.
251. Boyd SD, Raz S, Ehrlich RM: Diabetes insipidus and nonobstructive dilatation of urinary tract. Urology 16:266, 1980.
252. Gautier B, Thieblot P, Steg A: Mégauretère, mégavessie et diabète inspide familial. Sem Hop 57:60, 1981.
253. Robertson GL: Diseases of the posterior pituitary. In Felig D, Baxter JD, Broadus AE, Frohman LA (eds): Endocrinology and Metabolism. New York, McGraw-Hill, 1981, p 251.
254. Bettinelli A, Ciarmatori S, Cesareo L, et al: Phenotypic variability in Bartter syndrome type I. Pediatr Nephrol 14:940, 2000.
255. Bichet DG: Nephrogenic diabetes insipidus. Semin Nephrol 14:349, 1994.
256. Robertson GL, Klein LA, Roth J, et al: Immunoassay of plasma vasopressin in man. Proc Natl Acad Sci U S A 66:1298, 1970.
257. Robertson GL, Mahr EA, Athar S, et al: Development and clinical application of a new method for the radioimmunoassay of arginine vasopressin in human plasma. J Clin Invest 52: 2340, 1973.
258. Bichet DG, Kortas C, Mettauer B, et al: Modulation of plasma and platelet vasopressin by cardiac function in patients with heart failure. Kidney Int 29:1188, 1986.
259. Bichet DG, Arthus M-F, Barjon JN, et al: Human platelet fraction arginine-vasopressin. J Clin Invest 79:881, 1987.
260. Davison JM, Gilmore EA, Durr J, et al: Altered osmotic thresholds for vasopressin secretion and thirst in human pregnancy. Am J Physiol 246:F105, 1984.
261. Vokes TP, Aycinena PR, Robertson GL: Effect of insulin on osmoregulation of vasopressin. Am J Physiol 252:E538, 1987.
262. Hartter E, Woloszczuk W: Radioimmunological determination of arginine vasopressin and human atrial natriuretic peptide after simultaneous extraction from plasma. J Clin Chem Clin Biochem 24:559, 1986.
263. LaRochelle FT Jr, North WG, Stern P: A new extraction of arginine vasopressin from blood: The use of octadecasilyl-silica. Pflugers Arch 387:79, 1980.
264. Ysewijn-Van Brussel KA, De Leenheer AP: Development and evaluation of a radioimmunoassay for Arg8-vasopressin, after extraction with Sep-Pak C18. Clin Chem 31:861, 1985.
265. Preibisz JJ, Sealey JE, Laragh JH, et al: Plasma and platelet vasopressin in essential hypertension and congestive heart failure. Hypertension 5:I129, 1983.
266. Seckl JR, Dunger DB, Bevan JS, et al: Vasopressin antagonist in early postoperative diabetes insipidus. Lancet 355:1353, 1990.
267. Maas AH, Siggaard-Andersen O, Weisberg HF, et al: Ion-selective electrodes for sodium and potassium: A new problem of what is measured and what should be reported. Clin Chem 31: 482, 1985.

268. Gennari FJ: Current concepts. Serum osmolality: Uses and limitations. N Engl J Med 310:102, 1984.
269. Knoers N, Monnens LA: Nephrogenic diabetes insipidus: Clinical symptoms, pathogenesis, genetics and treatment. Pediatr Nephrol 6:476, 1992.
270. Kirchlechner V, Koller DY, Seidl R, et al: Treatment of nephrogenic diabetes insipidus with hydrochlorothiazide and amiloride. Arch Dis Child 80:548, 1999.
271. Neifert MR: Prevention of breastfeeding tragedies. Pediatr Clin North Am 48:273, 2001.
272. Kennedy JR: Offer infants water. Pediatrics 105:686, 2000.
273. Antonarakis S, Nomenclature Working Group: Recommendations for a nomenclature system for human gene mutations. Hum Mutat 11:1, 1998.
274. Stern P, Valtin H: Verney was right, but . . . [editorial]. N Engl J Med 305:1581, 1981.
275. Berl T, Kumar S: Disorders of water metabolism. In Johnson RJ, Feehally J (eds): Comprehensive Clinical Nephrology. London, Mosby, 2000, p 9.1.
276. Carlotti AP, Bohn D, Mallie JP, et al: Tonicity balance, and not electrolyte-free water calculations, more accurately guides therapy for acute changes in natremia. Intensive Care Med 27: 921, 2001.
277. Mouillac B, Chini B, Balestre MN, et al: The binding site of neuropeptide vasopressin $V_{1a}$ receptor: Evidence for a major localization within transmembrane regions. J Biol Chem 270: 25771, 1995.
278. Vokes T, Robertson GL: Physiology of secretion of vasopressin. In Czernichow P, Robinson AG (eds): Diabetes Insipidus in Man. Basel, S. Karger, 1985, pp 127–155.
279. Zerbe RL, Robertson GL: Disorders of ADH. Med North Am 13:1570, 1984.
280. Pan Y, Metzenberg A, Das S, et al: Mutations in the $V_2$ vasopressin receptor gene are associated with X-linked nephrogenic diabetes insipidus. Nat Genet 2:103, 1992.
281. Rosenthal W, Seibold A, Antaramian A, et al: Molecular identification of the gene responsible for congenital nephrogenic diabetes insipidus. Nature 359:233, 1992.
282. van den Ouweland AM, Dreesen JC, Verdijk M, et al: Mutations in the vasopressin type 2 receptor gene (AVPR2) associated with nephrogenic diabetes insipidus. Nat Genet 2:99, 1992.
283. Holtzman EJ, Harris HWJ, Kolakowski LFJ, et al: Brief report: A molecular defect in the vasopressin $V_2$-receptor gene causing nephrogenic diabetes insipidus. N Engl J Med 328:1534, 1993.
284. Merendino JJJ, Speigel AM, Crawford JD, et al: Brief report: A mutation in the vasopressin $V_2$-receptor gene in a kindred with X-linked nephrogenic diabetes insipidus. N Engl J Med 328: 1538, 1993.
285. Tsukaguchi H, Matsubara H, Aritaki S, et al: Two novel mutations in the vasopressin $V_2$ receptor gene in unrelated Japanese kindreds with nephrogenic diabetes insipidus. Biochem Biophys Res Commun 197:1000, 1993.
286. Faa V, Ventruto ML, Loche S, et al: Mutations in the vasopressin $V_2$-receptor gene in three families of Italian descent with nephrogenic diabetes insipidus. Hum Mol Genet 3:1685, 1994.
287. Friedman E, Bale AE, Carson E, et al: Nephrogenic diabetes insipidus: An X chromosome–linked dominant inheritance pattern with a vasopressin type 2 receptor gene that is structurally normal. Proc Natl Acad Sci U S A 91:8457, 1994.
288. Holtzman EJ, Kolakowski LFJ, Geifman-Holtzman O, et al: Mutations in the vasopressin $V_2$ receptor gene in two families with nephrogenic diabetes insipidus. J Am Soc Nephrol 5: 169, 1994.
289. Knoers NV, van den Ouweland AM, Verdijk M, et al: Inheritance of mutations in the $V_2$ receptor gene in thirteen families with nephrogenic diabetes insipidus. Kidney Int 46:170, 1994.
290. Oksche A, Dickson J, Schülein R, et al: Two novel mutations in the vasopressin $V_2$ receptor gene in patients with congenital nephrogenic diabetes insipidus. Biophys Biochem Res Commun 205:552, 1994.
291. Pan Y, Wilson P, Gitschier J: The effect of eight $V_2$ vasopressin receptor mutations on stimulation of adenylyl cyclase and binding to vasopressin. J Biol Chem 269:31933, 1994.
292. Wenkert D, Merendino JJJ, Shenker A, et al: Novel mutations in the $V_2$ vasopressin receptor gene of patients with X-linked nephrogenic diabetes insipidus. Hum Mol Genet 3:1429, 1994.
293. Wildin RS, Antush MJ, Bennett RL, et al: Heterogeneous AVPR2 gene mutations in congenital nephrogenic diabetes insipidus. Am J Hum Genet 55:266, 1994.
294. Yuasa H, Ito M, Oiso Y, et al: Novel mutations in the $V_2$ vasopressin receptor gene in two pedigrees with congenital nephrogenic diabetes insipidus. J Clin Endocrinol Metab 79: 361, 1994.
295. Tsukaguchi H, Matsubara H, Inada M: Expression studies of two vasopressin $V_2$ receptor gene mutations, R202C and 804insG, in nephrogenic diabetes insipidus. Kidney Int 48: 554, 1995.
296. Jinnouchi H, Araki E, Miyamura N, et al: Analysis of vasopressin receptor type II (V2R) gene in three Japanese pedigrees with congenital nephrogenic diabetes insipidus: Identification of a family with complete deletion of the V2R gene. Eur J Endocrinol 134:689, 1996.
297. Oksche A, Moller A, Dickson J, et al: Two novel mutations in the aquaporin-2 and the vasopressin $V_2$ receptor genes in patients with congenital nephrogenic diabetes insipidus. Hum Genet 98:587, 1996.
298. Tajima T, Nakae J, Takekoshi Y, et al: Three novel AVPR2 mutations in three Japanese families with X-linked nephrogenic diabetes insipidus. Pediatr Res 39:522, 1996.
299. Yokoyama K, Yamauchi A, Izumi M, et al: A low-affinity vasopressin $V_2$-receptor gene in a kindred with X-linked nephrogenic diabetes insipidus. J Am Soc Nephrol 7:410, 1996.
300. Cheong HI, Park HW, Ha IS, et al: Six novel mutations in the vasopressin $V_2$ receptor gene causing nephrogenic diabetes insipidus. Nephron 75:431, 1997.
301. Sadeghi H, Robertson GL, Bichet DG, et al: Biochemical basis of partial NDI phenotypes. Mol Endocrinol 11:1806, 1997.
302. Vargas-Poussou R, Forestier L, Dautzenberg MD, et al: Mutations in the vasopressin $V_2$ receptor and aquaporin-2 genes in 12 families with congenital nephrogenic diabetes insipidus. J Am Soc Nephrol 8:1855, 1997.
303. Ala Y, Morin D, Mouillac B, et al: Functional studies of twelve mutant $V_2$ vasopressin receptors related to nephrogenic diabetes insipidus: Molecular basis of a mild clinical phenotype. J Am Soc Nephrol 9:1861, 1998.
304. Szalai C, Triga D, Czinner A: C112R, W323S, N317K mutations in the vasopressin $V_2$ receptor gene in patients with nephrogenic diabetes insipidus. Mutations in brief no. 165. Online. Hum Mutat 12:137, 1998.
305. Schöneberg T, Schulz A, Biebermann H, et al: $V_2$ vasopressin receptor dysfunction in nephrogenic diabetes insipidus caused by different molecular mechanisms. Hum Mutat 12:196, 1998.
306. Shoji Y, Takahashi T, Suzuki Y, et al: Mutational analyses of AVPR2 gene in three Japanese families with X-linked nephrogenic diabetes insipidus: Two recurrent mutations, R137H and delta V278, caused by the hypermutability at CpG dinucleotides. Hum Mutat Suppl 1:S278, 1998.
307. Wildin RS, Cogdell DE, Valadez V: AVPR2 variants and $V_2$ vasopressin receptor function in nephrogenic diabetes insipidus. Kidney Int 54:1909, 1998.
308. Kraulis PJ: MOLSCRIPT—a program to produce both detailed and schematic plots of proteins. J Appl Crystallogr 24:946, 1991.
309. van Lieburg AF, Verdijk MAJ, Knoers NVAM, et al: Patients with autosomal nephrogenic diabetes insipidus homozygous for mutations in the aquaporin 2 water-channel gene. Am J Hum Genet 55:648, 1994.
310. Canfield MC, Tamarappoo BK, Moses AM, et al: Identification and characterization of aquaporin-2 water channel mutations causing nephrogenic diabetes insipidus with partial vasopressin response. Hum Mol Genet 6:1865, 1997.
311. Hochberg Z, van Lieburg A, Even L, et al: Autosomal recessive nephrogenic diabetes insipidus caused by an aquaporin-2 mutation. J Clin Endocrinol Metab 82:686, 1997.
312. Goji K, Kuwahara M, Gu Y, et al: Novel mutations in aquaporin-2 gene in female siblings with nephrogenic diabetes insipidus: Evidence of disrupted water channel function. J Clin Endocrinol Metab 83:3205, 1998.
313. Kuwahara M: Aquaporin-2, a vasopressin-sensitive water channel, and nephrogenic diabetes insipidus. Int Med 37:215, 1998.
314. Cheng A, van Hoek AN, Yeager M, et al: Three-dimensional organization of a human water channel. Nature 387:627, 1997.

Section III

# Sodium

## Chapter 16

# Renin-Angiotensin-Aldosterone System

Roland C. Blantz, MD ▪ Francis B. Gabbai, MD

## INTEGRATIVE VIEW OF THE RENIN-ANGIOTENSIN-ALDOSTERONE SYSTEM

The renin-angiotensin-aldosterone system has been retained throughout evolutionary biology. The system supports multiple functions including maintenance of extracellular fluid volume and perfusion of various organs by maintenance of blood pressure despite perceived deficits in extracellular fluid volume. At the same time, the system maintains the kidney's capacity to generate and maintain the excretion of protons and potassium in the settings of extracellular volume deficits and lower rates of glomcrular filtration.

Various neurohumoral systems maintain defenses against the external environment, which include the renin-angiotensin system, the autonomic nervous system, endothelin, and various other vasoactive materials.[1] Interestingly, many of these vasoactive substances, both vasoconstrictors and vasodilators, exert systemic actions (maintenance of blood pressure and systemic hemodynamics) and actions at the cell level by which they regulate or stimulate cell proliferation and hypertrophy and participate in the generation of extracellular matrix and the scarring process.[2] We focus this discussion primarily on the functions that contribute to maintenance of extracellular fluid volume and blood pressure and, at the same time, prevent hyperkalemia and metabolic acidosis.

The renin-angiotensin-aldosterone system is reasonably complex and consists of the enzyme renin, which is located predominantly within the kidney but also within the systemic vasculature.[3] The substrate for this enzyme, angiotensinogen or renin substrate, is generated primarily in the liver but has also been demonstrated in both the juxtaglomerular apparatus and in renal tubular cells.[4] The enzyme, renin, generates the primary peptide, angiotensin I, which is then converted by angiotensin-converting enzyme (ACE) into the primary active material angiotensin II.[5]

Angiotensin II, which is then generated primarily in the kidney but also elsewhere, can act in a truly endocrine fashion to release aldosterone (a steroid hormone) from the glomerulosa of the adrenal cortex.[6] However, angiotensin also exerts numerous local effects. Aldosterone acts primarily within the kidney but also in other epithelial cells and, based on recent information, may also act on nonepithelial cells. A characteristic of this system is that the earliest documented functions for the systems were primarily endocrine; however, as time has passed, it is obvious that there are multiple local or paracrine effects for angiotensin II.[7] These effects are critical to organ function, particularly in the kidney.

### Renin and Its Regulation

Renin exists primarily in the juxtaglomerular apparatus adjacent to the glomerular capillary within juxtaglomerular cells and also within renal tubular cells.[3, 4] Renin activity appears to be modulated by two primary factors within the kidney. The first is a baroreceptor mechanism whereby reductions in arterial pressure at the preglomerular afferent arteriole lead to the release of renin.[8] The second mechanism, which involves reductions in delivery of NaCl to the macula densa, provides a second adjunctive mechanism whereby renin release is accomplished.[9] However, there are additional modulatory influences upon renin release in addition to the baroreceptor and macula densa systems. The prostaglandin system is important to the release of renin.[10, 11] The prostaglandins function to enhance renin release despite the fact that these substances generally function as antagonists of the hormone angiotensin II. Additionally, the adrenergic nervous system also plays a role in modulating the release of renin. Renal nerve stimulation enhances renin release primarily via β-adrenergic mechanisms.[12] It has been reported that $\alpha_2$-adrenergic systems inhibit renin release under certain circumstances.[13]

The substrate for the renin enzyme, angiotensinogen, is a large molecule and renin cleaves off a decapeptide, angiotensin I. In most circumstances, renin substrate is not rate limiting—at least not in the systemic circulation. It is more difficult to determine whether it might be rate limiting in certain other tissues (e.g., renal tubular cells) or within extrarenal and nonvascular cells (e.g., macrophage monocyte systems).[4, 14] An exception may be severe hepatic failure in which substrate generation may be partially rate limiting. It would be difficult to determine whether enough substrate is generated locally within the kidney. Another important modulator of renin activity and release is the concentration of angiotensin II.[15]

Angiotensin II suppresses renin synthesis via a calcium-dependent mechanism.[16]

ACE exists in multiple organs but primarily in lung and kidney and acts to rapidly convert angiotensin I to angiotensin II.[5] The regulatory influences on ACE are less well understood. It is likely to be a regulated enzyme, and certain mutations exhibit high rates of angiotensin II generation.[17] One of the angiotensin receptors, the angiotensin II receptor, may also downregulate ACE activity within the lung, kidney, and other sites.[18]

## Functions and Regulation of Angiotensin

### INTRARENAL VERSUS EXTRARENAL ANGIOTENSIN II CONCENTRATIONS

Angiotensin II generally circulates in the picomolar range or picograms per milliliter in the systemic circulation and extracellular fluid.[7] However, the kidney measurements of angiotensin II have suggested that much higher concentrations exist. Proximal tubular fluid samples have demonstrated values in the range of 10 to 20 nM.[19, 20] This angiotensin II may be generated by renal tubular cells, because glomerular filtration and access to the urinary space are not necessary to demonstrate high levels of angiotensin in proximal tubular fluid.[21] In the kidney, angiotensin II levels have been measured by highly specific radioimmunoassay. Rather high values for angiotensin II have been demonstrated, depending on the separation techniques, suggesting that much of the angiotensin II within the kidney may be bound to receptors or may already be in intracellular compartments as part of the process of receptor recycling.[22] Angiotensin II in the kidney has been estimated at 500 to 1500 pg on a normal to low salt intake. In support of high degrees of angiotensin II binding are the data that demonstrate that prolonged administration of losartan, a potent angiotensin II receptor blocker, decreases angiotensin II content in rats with low-salt diets to levels of approximately 250 pg, much less than 20% to 25% of the normal angiotensin II content on a low-NaCl diet.[23] Because the angiotensin II receptor blocker does not decrease the synthesis of angiotensin II, it is very likely that this reflects displacement of angiotensin II from receptors. As much as 75% of angiotensin II content may be bound to receptors or internalized within the cell at any given time,[24] suggesting that concentration of free angiotensin II in small compartments may be much lower.

Data from several laboratories have demonstrated very high proximal tubular luminal concentrations that decline fairly rapidly along the proximal tubule, which suggests that there are major gradients in angiotensin concentration from the lumen of the proximal tubule to the interstitial fluid and peritubular capillaries (10 to 100 pg/mL in plasma and 10 to 30 nM in early proximal tubular fluid).[19–21] These observations also imply certain distinct functions for the angiotensin II generated locally. The $K_D$ for these various receptor functions should be strikingly different.

### FUNCTION AND REGULATION OF ANGIOTENSIN RECEPTORS

Both angiotensin I and angiotensin II receptors have been cloned and have been found to be G protein–coupled seven transmembrane spanning polypeptides containing about 360 amino acids.[25, 26] Most of the biologic activities of angiotensin II have been documented as being mediated by the angiotensin receptor subtype type 1 (AT1). Angiotensin II receptors are expressed primarily during fetal life and also in and around the time of birth.[27] However, there have been reports that suggest that angiotensin II receptors may be expressed at the sites of vascular injury and that the receptors may mediate antiproliferative influences that counteract those of the AT1 receptor. Some of the vascular effects of angiotensin infusion may be mediated in part via actions of the angiotensin receptor type 2 (AT2). Regulation of both nitric oxide synthase and prostaglandins in the kidney may be mediated by the AT2 receptor.[28] Some of the beneficial effects of AT1 receptor blockade in clinical medicine may be mediated by the unopposed effect of angiotensin on AT2 receptors.

Clearly, AT1 receptors exist in abundance throughout the vasculature and within the kidney, within glomeruli, mesangial cells, and the vasculature, and also in renal tubules, both in the cortex and medulla.[29] Regulation of AT1 receptor expression is complex and is mediated over several time courses: (1) via G protein uncoupling, (2) with alterations in receptor recycling and trafficking, and (3) over longer periods via transcription of AT1 receptors. The primary regulators of the AT1 receptor number and affinity are the agonist concentration of angiotensin II, the NaCl content of the diet (which may be in major part mediated by the effects of angiotensin II), and via glucocorticoids and mineralocorticoids.

This regulation is highly cell type specific. Within the vasculature and the mesangial cell, increases in angiotensin II content and a low-salt diet are associated with downregulation of receptor number, producing decreased sensitivity to angiotensin infusion, in major part via decreased receptor expression.[30] However, in other cells, primarily proximal tubular cells, and cells within the adrenal cortex, increased angiotensin II concentration is paralleled by an increase in the number of AT1 receptors.[31, 32] On a low-salt diet, there is enhanced expression of AT1 receptors in the adrenal cortex and proximal tubule; on a high-salt diet, these receptors diminish in number compared with the parallel effects within mesangial and vascular smooth muscle cells. This peculiar difference in AT1 receptor expression may be absolutely critical to the normal response to variations in NaCl intake. The capacity to upregulate or downregulate appropriately in these diverse fashions may be critical to the complex renal and systemic responses to variations in NaCl intake.[33, 34]

The $K_D$ and transduction pathways utilized by the

AT1 receptor may differ significantly among cell types. For example, both the vasoconstrictor and the antinatriuretic effects of angiotensin II appear to occur in the range of $10^{-11}$ to $10^{-12}$ M, generating a positive effect on sodium reabsorption in the proximal tubule and vasoconstrictor effects within both the renal and systemic vasculature.[35, 36]

Many years ago, Harris and Young demonstrated that angiotensin II exerts a dose-dependent biphasic effect on proximal reabsorption.[37] These observations have been verified.[38] Concentrations of angiotensin II from $10^{-10}$ to $10^{-12}$ M perfused within peritubular capillaries stimulated sodium reabsorption, whereas perfusion with solutions at much higher concentrations ($10^{-7}$ M or higher) significantly inhibited proximal tubular reabsorption. These have been verified by in vivo studies, which have suggested that the AT1 receptor is tonically important to proximal reabsorption from the luminal side, implying that AT1 receptors stimulate proximal tubular reabsorption.[39, 40] Other in vivo microperfusion studies have suggested that there are significant luminal and antiluminal effects of angiotensin II, with luminal effects appearing to dominate and that the administration of higher concentrations of angiotensin II can be natriuretic.[41] Data from our laboratories have also indirectly suggested that nitric oxide might be a modulator of the effective concentration in which the natriuretic effects of angiotensin II may be mediated.[42] When L-NMMA is administered to rats, proximal tubular reabsorption decreases. This effect can be inhibited by co-administration of large doses of losartan, suggesting that losartan can inhibit both the stimulatory and inhibitory effects of angiotensin II and that the angiotensin II concentration mediating the inhibitory effect on proximal tubular reabsorption may be modified by other systems. Stimulatory effects of angiotensin II appear to be mediated partly by inhibition of adenyl cyclase, and the inhibitory pathway may depend on a calcium-signaling mechanism[43] that is similar to the one that mediates the vasoconstriction effects on smooth muscle at much lower angiotensin II concentrations.

Renal and systemic hemodynamic effects of angiotensin II are very important. Angiotensin II exerts a potent effect on both the afferent and efferent arterioles by slightly different mechanisms.[44] At lower angiotensin II infusion rates, the efferent arteriolar effect may dominate and act to increase the filtration fraction whereby the glomerular filtration rate (GFR) is somewhat better maintained than is renal blood flow. This increase in filtration fraction may also have a minor stimulatory effect on proximal tubular reabsorption by enhancing physical factors promoting proximal tubular reabsorption.

Contrary to prior observations, AII does have an afferent arteriolar effect that appears to be direct.[45] In addition, AII influences GFR by causing marked reductions in the glomerular ultrafiltration coefficient.[44] Although initial studies predicted that this effect might be mediated by angiotensin effects on mesangial contraction, it seems highly likely that the AII effect may in fact be mediated by effects on the glomerular visceral epithelial cell and on glomerular epithelial podocyte architecture.[46]

Angiotensin is also known to be a modulator of the function of the tubuloglomerular feedback (TGF) system.[47, 48] However, AII is definitely not a mediator of the system and may modulate by altering the balance between afferent and efferent arteriolar resistances, thereby influencing the contribution of the glomerular capillary hydrostatic pressure gradient. It is of interest that the two macula densa–based systems, the renin regulatory system and the TGF system, appear to counteract one another in the sense that reductions in distal delivery cause vasodilation of the afferent arteriole by TGF mechanisms, whereas reductions in distal delivery cause increased generation of renin and AII locally, which should lead to vasoconstriction.

## MODIFIERS AND ELEMENTS INTERACTING WITH AII

There are several influences that modify the actions of AII, especially within the renal vasculature. It is clear that renal nerve stimulation elicits an increase in AII generation. In the same manner there is synergism between AII and catecholamine release via exocytosis. Denervation, one would think, would diminish AII effects by removing that influence. In studies performed several years ago, the effects of infused AII were actually greater in kidneys that were denervated 5 to 7 days previously.[24] Denervation does not change the intrarenal content of AII,[49] but AII receptor number in denervated kidneys almost doubled and the sensitivity to increased AII is increased 5 to 7 days after denervation.[24] The specific mechanism that produces this effect is not specifically known. However, the β component of adrenergic activity does not appear to be the candidate system since β-adrenergic blockade did not change AII receptor number.[50]

Another candidate system with influence is the $\alpha_2$-adrenergic system. Administration of $\alpha_2$-adrenergic agonists enhances the effects of AII, and this relationship appears to be reciprocal and equally synergistic.[51] Interesting relationships exist in which $\alpha_2$-adrenergic stimulation diminishes renin activity,[13] and $\alpha_2$-adrenergic activity at effector cells, primarily mesangial and smooth cells, appears to enhance the effects of AII and vice versa. It is of interest that $\alpha_2$-adrenergic activity also modifies the effects of expression of blockers of nitric oxide synthase.[49]

Nitric oxide interacts with AII both at the level of renin and at the level of AII activity. L-NMMA, an inhibitor of NOS activity, elicits glomerular hemodynamic effects that are strikingly similar to those of AII, increased resistances of both afferent and efferent arterioles, an increase in the glomerular capillary hydrostatic pressure gradient, and a reduction in the glomerular ultrafiltration coefficient.[42, 45] These effects are totally eliminated by co-administration of losartan, the AT1 receptor blocker. Therefore, there are strong antagonistic interactions between NO and AII both at the level of glomerular hemodynamics and at the level of the proximal tubule, as previously mentioned.

Similar relationships exist between the renin-angiotensin system and the prostaglandin-cyclooxygenase system. Acute inhibition of cyclooxygenase 1 (COX-1) enhanced angiotensin II activity on glomerular hemodynamics, resulting in greater vasoconstriction and greater reductions in GFR.[52, 53] However, chronic administration of COX-1 inhibitors actually diminishes the activity of the renin-angiotensin system and can lead, as is discussed further, to diminished angiotensin II generation and aldosterone level.[53] The cyclooxygenase-prostaglandin system is thus similar in some respects to the relationship between $\alpha_2$-adrenergic activity and the synergism with angiotensin II and its influences on renin, the synthetic enzyme.

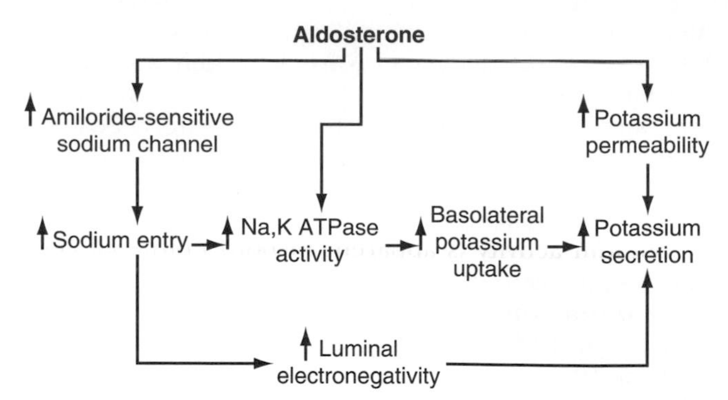


**FIGURE 16–1** ■ Effects of aldosterone on collecting tubular cells. Effects on potassium secretion.

### VASCULAR TRANSDUCTION PATHWAYS

Reduction in NaCl intake or, in a more exaggerated fashion, extracellular volume depletion, elicits an increase in activity of the renin-angiotensin system and higher levels of angiotensin II in the kidney and in the plasma. Very high levels of angiotensin II will elicit some reduction in GFR under volume-depleting circumstances,[54] but usually no changes in GFR are observed if the organism is placed only on a low-salt diet. However, throughout this range, angiotensin II exerts significant effects on proximal tubular reabsorption. It also elicits changes in aldosterone levels via its effect on the adrenal cortex. At the same time, adaptations in receptor number occur whereby low sodium intake elicits increases in angiotensin I receptor expression in the proximal tubule, possibly the distal tubule, and the adrenal cortex, thus enhancing the net tubular reabsorptive influence of the renin-angiotensin system.[31, 32] Concurrently, there is a general reduction in the number of AT1 receptors within the systemic vasculature, glomerular arterioles, and mesangial cells, making these structures less responsive to angiotensin II on a low-salt intake. The opposite general formulation occurs with the transition to a high-salt intake.[30] Therefore, a rapid transition to volume expansion seemingly may have a greater effect on the tubular reabsorptive influences of the renin-angiotensin system because the effects on the vasculature and the glomerulus will be buffered to an extent by reciprocal changes in the expression of AT1 receptors. It appears that this coordinated difference in receptor expression may be quite critical to the normal behavior of a transition from a low- to a high-salt intake. Abnormalities in angiotensin II receptor regulation could provide the basis of certain forms of salt-sensitive hypertension, acquired forms of hypertension in which there is abnormal regulation of the AT1 receptor in these various cell types.[33, 34]

## Aldosterone

Aldosterone secretion can be stimulated by angiotensin II at reasonably high plasma levels,[6] by elevated serum potassium,[55] and, in extreme cases, by an extremely low sodium concentration.[56] The elevated aldosterone levels in the plasma correlate best under normal physiologic circumstances with reductions in sodium delivery and tubular flow rate within the collecting duct. In a sense, this feedback system allows for continuous potassium and proton secretion during variations in NaCl intake and extracellular fluid volume status.

### RENAL AND OTHER EPITHELIAL EFFECTS

Aldosterone increases sodium reabsorption in the cortical collecting duct as an early event. Chronic tubular stimulation by aldosterone dramatically increases sodium reabsorption and especially potassium and proton secretion (Figs. 16–1 and 16–2).[57–59] Mineralocorticoids exert a reciprocal effect on sodium and potassium transport, but no fixed relationship exists between the sodium reabsorbed and the potassium secreted. The effects of aldosterone on either sodium reabsorption or potassium secretion can be separated by manipulations of method of administration, dietary pretreatment, and dose.[60] Prolonged treatment with mineralocorticoid produces only a temporary state of salt retention until the individual or animal "escapes" from the sodium-retaining effect, but increased potassium secretion tends to continue to a greater extent if placed on an increased sodium intake.[61] The mechanism of increased sodium reabsorption involves insertion of amiloride-sensitive sodium channels into the

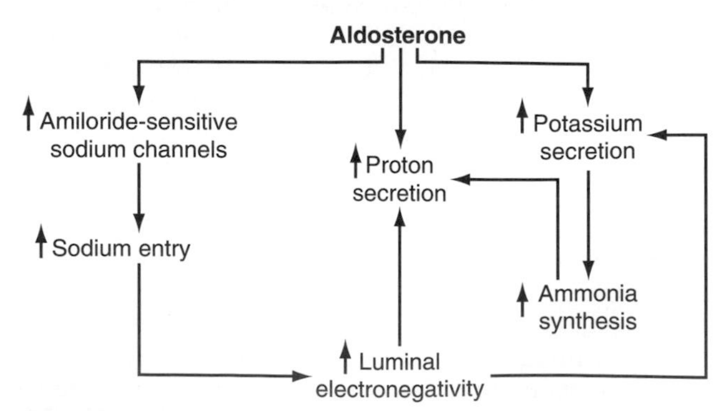


**FIGURE 16–2** ■ Effects of aldosterone on collecting tubular cells. Effects on proton secretion.

apical membrane.[62] Increased apical entry of sodium further stimulates $Na^+,K^+$ ATPase. Aldosterone also primarily increases $Na^+,K^+$ ATPase, leading to increased active basolateral potassium uptake.[63] After the insertion of apical epithelial sodium channels, the increased sodium entry activates $Na^+,K^+$ ATPase. The effect of aldosterone on $Na^+,K^+$ ATPase and intracellular sodium activity is apparent in both epithelial cells and vascular smooth muscle cells.

Aldosterone exerts a prolonged action to affect internal potassium homeostasis. After prolonged administration of mineralocorticoids, the animal is actually protected against potassium toxicity, but not as effectively as after chronic potassium loading. Administration of aldosterone at any given level of sodium delivery establishes the ability of the nephron segments to raise luminal potassium concentration. Mineralocorticoid deficiency is restricted primarily to the late distal tubule and collecting system.

The effects of aldosterone on sodium reabsorption and potassium secretion can be demonstrated in isolated cortical collecting tubules.[57] This effect increases with the duration of hormone treatment. Collecting ducts harvested from rabbits pretreated with mineralocorticoid secrete more potassium with a relatively low concentration of potassium in the bath and show exaggerated secretory responses when the concentration of potassium in the bath is increased. A high level of potassium excretion is achieved at lower plasma concentrations of potassium as aldosterone concentration is increased.[64] In this sense, aldosterone increases the gain of the relationship between tubular flow rate and sodium reabsorption and the amount of potassium secreted.

At any level of total body potassium, the plasma potassium concentration tends to be lower when aldosterone levels are high. The movement of potassium into the lumen occurs in response to the electronegativity in the lumen generated by sodium reabsorption, but at any given luminal electronegativity there is greater potassium secretion in the presence of aldosterone (see Fig. 16–1). When mineralocorticoids are withdrawn, there is a reduction in the electrical potential difference across both the luminal and the basolateral membrane of the cells, a significant decrease in intracellular potassium activity in distal tubular cells, and an apparent reduction in the permeability of the luminal membrane to potassium. With administration of mineralocorticoids, these changes are reversed. These results are most compatible with a dual action of aldosterone on apical potassium permeability and active uptake of potassium at the peritubular surface.[65]

Aldosterone administration produces the formation of aldosterone-induced proteins that result in the insertion of sodium channels into the apical membrane and increase activity of the basolateral pumps. These effects require 1 to 3 hours and are associated with increases in the apical conductance of sodium. Later responses involve increases in the conductance of the apical membrane for potassium and further activation of $Na^+,K^+$ ATPase.[66] Additional factors that modify potassium secretion and excretion over longer periods are associated with changes in the fine structure of specific cells in the late distal tubule and cortical collecting duct. These changes are associated with increased complexity of the basolateral surface of the principal cells, but not those intercalated cells.[67] This increased complexity is associated with increased $Na^+,K^+$ ATPase activity. It is important to note that other factors that are independent of aldosterone can also influence potassium secretion. These factors include the nature of the intraluminal anion, which in turn generates different levels of electronegativity within the lumen, and flow rate, which alters the potassium gradients. There is generally a reciprocal relationship between the urine flow rate and aldosterone levels.

For many years it was assumed that the effects of aldosterone within the collecting duct primarily related to sodium reabsorption and potassium secretion. However, it is quite clear that mineralocorticoids stimulate acidification and do so independent of aldosterone effects on volume status, potassium, and ammonia.[68, 69] Increased proton secretion may be simply the result of producing a more lumen-negative electrical potential as a result of increased sodium reabsorption (see Fig. 16–2).[70] There is also a more direct effect of mineralocorticoids on proton secretion.[71] Complete inhibition of sodium transport with ouabain, an inhibitor of $Na^+,K^+$ ATPase, did not prevent aldosterone-stimulated proton secretion. These effects were dependent upon transcription and were prevented by actinomycin D. Total proton secretion is increased by aldosterone, but the minimum urine pH is not reduced; thus, presumably proton permeability and the ability to maintain a high proton gradient are not greatly altered.[71] However, in humans under conditions of $Na_2SO_4$ infusion, spironolactone did increase the minimum urine pH from 4.8 to 5.2, which reflects a reduction in proton secretory activity. Clinical observations suggest that patients with hypoaldosteronism can lower their urine pH appropriately despite the presence of a secretory defect.[72] Hyperkalemia in these patients affects ammonia synthesis. In the presence of limited buffering of protons by ammonia, the patients are able to excrete an appropriately acid urine but with a reduced net acid excretion. The proton secretory effect of aldosterone can also be demonstrated in vitro. Proton secretion can be demonstrated even in a sodium-free medium.[73]

Therefore, there are three mechanisms whereby aldosterone administration leads to increased proton secretion. Mineralocorticoids directly stimulate proton secretion in the cortical and medullary collecting ducts by increasing activity of the proton pump and the chloride bicarbonate exchanger.[74] Second, aldosterone stimulates sodium entry and creates a more favorable negativity within the collecting duct lumen for proton secretion. Third, the more remote effect is that aldosterone stimulates potassium excretion and secretion. This action leads to potassium depletion and stimulates ammonia synthesis, which increases buffer production and luminal pH in the collecting duct and secondarily stimulates proton secretion and enhances net acid excretion.

## CONDITIONS ASSOCIATED WITH INCREASED RENIN-ANGIOTENSIN-ALDOSTERONE SYSTEM ACTIVITY

The overall effects of increased renin-angiotensin-aldosterone system activity on acid-base and electrolyte status cannot be fully predicted without knowing how concurrent renal function and volume status collectively contribute to NaCl and water delivery to sites in the distal tubule and collecting duct, where aldosterone and other factors affect sodium reabsorption and potassium and proton secretion. This is true whether all components of the renin-angiotensin-aldosterone system are increased or whether there are concurrent increases in aldosterone but defects in the action of aldosterone in the setting of increased renin-angiotensin activity.

In normal physiology, increased activity of the renin-angiotensin-aldosterone system correlates strongly with conditions of significant reductions in flow or delivery rates to the distal nephron.[75] The opposite is also the case. In fact, this normal physiologic relationship makes teleologic sense. Increased activity of renin and angiotensin components of this system in extreme forms will reduce load to the distal nephron by reducing plasma flow and GFR and also via effects on angiotensin receptors in the proximal tubule that enhance reabsorption within that segment. The net effect is that the delivery rate out of the proximal tubule and into the distal nephron is severely reduced. In order for normal dietary loads of protons and potassium to be secreted despite this reduction in distal delivery and flow rate, aldosterone is generated to increase the gain on this system, thus enhancing distal NaCl reabsorption and concurrently enhancing potassium and proton entry into the collecting duct. Not only is NaCl and water homeostasis maintained, but also this system permits appropriate secretion of potassium and protons over a wide range of volume delivery.

However, in many clinical conditions, hyperreninemia or increased activity of the renin-angiotensin system is not always associated with reductions in distal delivery or appropriately increased activity of aldosterone. These conditions result in various electrolyte and acid-base abnormalities that are rather predictable from an understanding of the normal physiology and the normal flow dependence of reabsorption and secretion.

### Increased Renin-Angiotensin-Aldosterone Activity Associated with Decreased Distal Delivery

Primary increases in renin-angiotensin activity are quite rare and must be considered to be confined to juxtaglomerular tumors. This conclusion then rele-

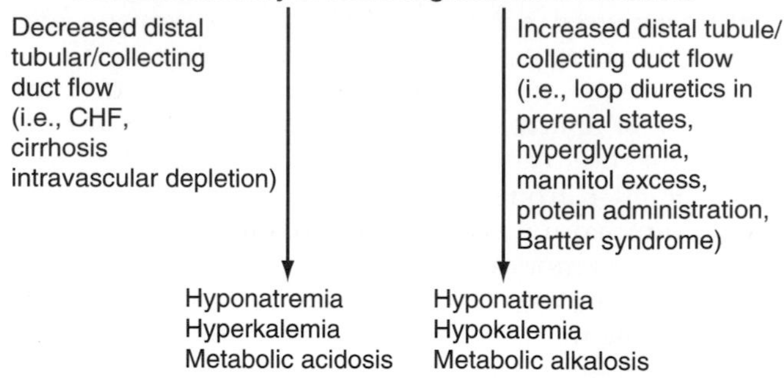


**FIGURE 16–3** ■ Electrolyte and acid-base disorders associated with increased renin-angiotensin-aldosterone activity.

gates most high renin-angiotensin conditions to secondary causes that are usually considered appropriate to the pathophysiologic conditions. In the untreated condition, prerenal states are associated with increased renin-angiotensin-aldosterone activity and reductions in distal tubular and collecting duct flow rate and delivery (Fig. 16–3).[76] These include the major clinical conditions of congestive heart failure, bilateral renal artery stenosis, plasma and extracellular volume depletion, cirrhosis, and intrarenal vascular obstructive diseases including vasculitis and malignant hypertension. In the untreated condition, the most common acid-base and electrolyte abnormalities that one might predict would be some degree of hyponatremia as a result of increased proximal tubular reabsorption and limitations of delivery of fluid to the diluting segment in a setting in which antidiuretic hormone is increased. In addition, if the prerenal condition is severe and the increase in angiotensin II, other vasoconstrictors, and factors that influence proximal reabsorption are great enough to override any of the beneficial effects of aldosterone, hyperkalemia and some degree of metabolic acidosis will occur, especially if there are major reductions in GFR. In some clinical conditions and in the absence of therapeutic interventions that may alter delivery to the distal nephron, hyponatremia, hyperkalemia, and metabolic acidosis are the conditions that one would predict as a consequence of the overall activity of the renin-angiotensin system.

### Increased Renin-Angiotensin-Aldosterone Activity Associated with Increases in Distal Tubular/Collecting Duct Flow or Delivery Rates

The conditions mentioned earlier are basically those characterized by secondary hyperreninemia and increased angiotensin II levels. The intrarenal generation of angiotensin II is usually increased, but systemic and intrarenal systems are compartmentalized and separate.[19–22] The most commonly encountered clinical condition in which increased renin-angiotensin and aldosterone levels are associated with increases in flow to the distal nephron are conditions in which therapy with loop diuretics is applied for the treatment of congestive heart failure, nephrotic syndrome, and cirrhosis (see Fig. 16–3). As mentioned earlier, hyponatremia can occur as a consequence of reduced delivery to the diluting segment in congestive heart failure but also occurs in other prerenal conditions. If one utilizes diuretics such as bumetanide, furosemide, and thiazides, the propensity to hyponatremia is enhanced greatly by reducing transport in those segments in the nephron in which dilution occurs. Hyponatremia can, therefore, be the consequence of both the initial prerenal condition and the additional effects of therapy with diuretics. However, most important, diuretic therapy applies a significant dissociation to the normal physiologic condition. Increased renin-angiotensin activity is usually associated with reductions in filtered load and enhanced proximal reabsorption. However, diuretic therapy increases delivery of fluid into the cortical distal tubule and the collecting duct as a normal consequence of the attempt to offload NaCl and $H_2O$. This increased flow rate maintains high rates of potassium and proton secretion in the presence of aldosterone, leading commonly to hypokalemic alkalosis.[77] Physicians can largely avoid many of those consequences of diuretic therapy by applying loop diuretics on a periodic basis, only once a day or even less, taking advantage of the fact that loop diuretics have a relatively short duration of action, and by allowing longer periods of time during the day for normal to reduced flow rates and lower rates of potassium and proton secretion. If there is significant azotemia or if the patient has chronic renal disease, diuretics might even be applied on an alternate-day basis in larger doses. Certainly, one should compulsively avoid dosing twice or three times a day with these short-acting agents if hyponatremia, hypokalemia, or alkalosis become problems, because this regimen maintains the kidney under the influence of diuretics and constantly produces normal to high flow rates in a setting of increased aldosterone activity.

Another increasingly common clinical problem that dissociates the renin-angiotensin-aldosterone system activity from expected flow rates into the distal nephron and collecting duct is the imposition of an osmotic diuresis sufficient to produce significant volume depletion.[78] The osmotic agents that are most likely to produce these conditions are hyperglycemia, as a consequence of uncontrolled diabetes, or the clinical administration of mannitol in the treatment of conditions such as high intracranial pressures.[79] More recently, an increasingly common cause of osmotic diuretic-induced volume depletion is overfeeding with protein and amino acid loads that generate large quantities of urea and obligate large flow rates to the distal nephron, inappropriately high urine volumes, volume depletion, and high aldosterone levels.[76] A common electrolyte disorder that occurs under these conditions is hypernatremia as a result of the large volumes of urine obligated for the excretion of urea. Occasionally, this clinical syndrome can occur not from protein overfeeding but from exaggerated catabolic conditions.[76] However, under these conditions of volume depletion, high angiotensin II, and high aldosterone, there can be significant losses of potassium and protons in the urine sufficient to produce modest degrees of hypokalemia and metabolic alkalosis. Increased angiotensin activity sufficient to lower GFR and enhance proximal reabsorption further allows for the maintenance of metabolic alkalosis,[80] because the filtered load of bicarbonate is decreased and angiotensin II is known to stimulate both apical sodium proton antiporter activity and basolateral exit of sodium bicarbonate from the proximal tubular cells, thus permitting high levels of serum bicarbonate and metabolic alkalosis.

A quite different clinical condition, which is not iatrogenic, is salt-losing nephropathy. In this condition, volume depletion commonly occurs and renin-angiotensin-aldosterone activity is increased. However, in these conditions, significant defects occur in NaCl reabsorption, primarily in the thick ascending limb of the loop of Henle, which allow for normal to elevated levels of delivery of NaCl and water into the distal tubule and collecting duct and result in high rates of potassium and proton secretion.[81, 82] Bartter's syndrome represents a specific example of this condition in which greater renin-angiotensin activity is associated with normal to low blood pressures, salt-wasting nephropathy, and significant hypokalemia and metabolic alkalosis.[83]

A more complex condition, which produces a contrast in function between the two kidneys, is that of one kidney renal artery stenosis. Under these conditions, the dogma states that the main renal artery stenosis or increased resistance in smaller vessels in the kidney generates increased renin-angiotensin activity, which then stimulates aldosterone secretion from the adrenal gland.[84] However, the other kidney, which does not have stenosis, responds to the elevated angiotensin II levels, systemic hypertension, and elevated systemic aldosterone levels. Under these circumstances, delivery of fluid into the distal tubule and collecting ducts is normal or increased, and aldosterone activity is increased. Gradients for protons and potassium secretion continue to be favorable at high flow rates under circumstances in which aldosterone has increased the number of transporters in these segments. For these reasons, hypokalemia and metabolic alkalosis may supervene in unilateral renal artery stenosis.

## ANGIOTENSIN II RECEPTOR MUTANTS OR ANGIOTENSIN-CONVERTING ENZYME MUTANTS

Although specific clinical conditions have not been well defined, there might be abnormalities in the angiotensin II receptor regulation or in the regulation of ACE whereby conditions of increased renin-angiotensin activity may be duplicated. If upregulation and downregulation of angiotensin II receptors in the proximal tubule and renal vasculature were not appropriate, one might find that there would be increased delivery of fluid out of the proximal tubule under circumstances in which angiotensin II had increased the aldosterone influence.[33, 34] Although these specific mutants have not been defined, it is possible that abnormal regulation of receptor expression in either tubule, adrenal, glomerulus, or vascular smooth muscle cells could result in some dissociation between filtered load, proximal reabsorption, and distal delivery in a setting of increased angiotensin-aldosterone activity. Speculation seems more likely when one considers the complexity and directional differences of receptor responses to large variations in NaCl intake and the fact that vascular smooth muscle cells and glomerular cells regulate angiotensin II receptors remarkably differently than does the proximal tubule and the adrenal.

### Increased Mineralocorticoid Activity/ Primary Aldosteronism

Mineralocorticoid excess states are not rare and do contribute to acid-base and electrolyte disorders. Although primary aldosteronism is not the most common form of hypertension, Cushing disease and various iatrogenic clinical conditions in which steroids produce mineralocorticoid effects can also influence overall renal function.

Aldosterone is primarily a hormone that influences sodium reabsorption. High aldosterone levels lead to volume expansion and increased GFR. Interestingly, primary aldosteronism is not associated with excess extracellular fluid or edema due to the "escape" phenomenon, which limits the effects of aldosterone on NaCl reabsorption.[85] Patients with primary aldosteronism or Cushing disease can encounter chronic renal insufficiency and progressive renal disease, which is only in part due to concomitant hypertension. A large amount of literature suggests that aldosterone exerts significant extrarenal influences beyond effects on the renal and colonic epithelium and salivary gland.[86, 87] Primary aldosteronism, a low renin form of hypertension, is not a benign form of hypertension, and recent data suggest that effects on renal function and the systemic vasculature are significant.[88, 89] There may also be detrimental cardiac effects of high aldosterone levels independent of the genesis of hypertension.

The symptoms of primary aldosteronism or mineralocorticoid excess are reasonably subtle. There are symptoms and signs that may characterize primary aldosteronism or other mineralocorticoid excess states that derive from obliteration of the normal diurnal variation in steroid levels and the consequences of exaggerated renal potassium wasting.[85] A symptom that occurs early in primary aldosteronism is nocturia, which may derive from the fact that the patients are volume expanded and that GFR increases at night under circumstances of constant and elevated levels of aldosterone. The second symptom is profound muscle weakness, which is related to the absolute level of potassium in the plasma and the total body potassium deficits.[90] Potassium deficits not only affect the muscle capacity to vasodilate in response to exercise but also affect the resting strength of muscles. In addition, earlier studies suggested that even myocardial cells may be adversely affected in terms of cardiac output reserve due to profound potassium depletion.[91, 92]

The pathophysiology of primary aldosterone is highly logical. There is total dissociation among the aldosterone influence in the collecting duct and the volume status of the patient, the GFR, and the delivery rate of fluid into the distal tubule and collecting duct. A high NaCl intake may have adverse consequences in patients with primary aldosteronism. A high NaCl intake may be the major determinant of the rate of potassium wasting rather than potassium intake. Spironolactone therapy in primary aldosteronism may be inadequate to prevent hypokalemia if the patient is on a high NaCl intake and has an elevated GFR.

## CONDITIONS ASSOCIATED WITH DECREASED RENIN-ANGIOTENSIN-ALDOSTERONE ACTIVITY

### Hyporeninemia or Low Renin-Angiotensin Activity

This section focuses on models in which either the renin-angiotensin activity response has been blunted or the normal physiologic increases do not occur in an appropriate manner. This discussion includes clinical syndromes that are part of the differential diagnosis of patients with hyperkalemia (Table 16–1).

A few decades ago, hyporeninemic hypoaldosteronism and variations on this theme were described.[93, 94] Initially, it was proposed that certain forms of renal disease, particularly renal disease associated with diabetes mellitus and certain forms of chronic interstitial disease, caused decreased renin-angiotensin system responses. However, more extensive analysis over the past few decades has suggested that kidney-generated models of hyporeninemic hypoaldosteronism (in the absence of severe chronic renal insufficiency) are not particularly common.

One must be careful in fully characterizing the true cause of these disorders. The major consequence of true hyporeninemic hypoaldosteronism is not salt wasting but rather a condition in which modest-to-severe hyperkalemia is associated with a modest metabolic acidosis. This suggests that the major impact of low renin-angiotensin activity is not hypotension and salt and volume deficits but rather abnormalities in the secretion of potassium and protons.[93] However, particularly in patients with diabetes mellitus, one must be careful to discern whether hyperkalemia is actually caused by a defect in the renin-angiotensin-aldosterone system and consequent renal effects or is a consequence of the nonrenal effects of inadequate insulin. Inadequate insulin therapy leads to low intracellular potassium and somewhat elevated extracellular fluid potassium, such that poor insulin control leads to total body potassium deficits despite the fact that hyperkalemia may be present.[95] Treatment of modest hyperkalemia in the diabetic patient with renal insufficiency with loop diuretics that increase distal delivery and

**TABLE 16–1.** The Patient with Hyperkalemic Renal Tubular Acidosis (Type IV Renal Tubular Acidosis)

| | Classification by Activity of Renin-Angiotensin-Aldosterone | | | |
|---|---|---|---|---|
| Renin-angiotensin | ↑ | ↑ | ↓ or normal | ↓ or normal |
| Aldosterone | ↑ | ↓ | Normal or ↓ | ↓ or normal |
| | • Congenital absence of receptors<br>• Distal tubular damage<br>• Interstitial disease<br>• Spironolactone<br>• Trimethoprim and amiloride | • Addison disease<br>• Adrenalectomy<br>• Heparin | • Acute GN<br>• Chloride shunt nephropathy | *Drugs*<br>• COX inhibitors<br>• CsA<br>• ACEI<br>• ARBs<br>*Renal Causes*<br>• Diabetic nephropathy<br>• Interstitial nephritis |

ACEI, angiotensin-converting enzyme inhibitor; ARB, angiotensin receptor blocker; CsA, cyclosporin A; GN, glomerulonephritis.

enhance potassium secretion could magnify the problem of total body potassium deficits in inadequately treated diabetes. Close monitoring of plasma potassium levels and proper administration of insulin, correction of hyperglycemia, and elimination of β-blocker therapy may be the best approach in the poorly controlled diabetic with modest hyperkalemia. In summary, one should be certain that hyporeninemic hypoaldosteronism is the primary cause for elevated potassium in the diabetic patient, especially if the hemoglobin A1C is elevated.

Extrarenal causes of hyperkalemia also exist. The patient with inadequate adrenal medullary function tends to have elevated potassium levels, especially after a potassium load, and in certain patients on β-blockers, hyperkalemia is not an uncommon finding.[96] This could relate to β-adrenergic effects on renin, but potassium translocation into cells is also a problem due to inadequate epinephrine and β-adrenergic responses, even in patients with an intact renin-angiotensin system. Administration of COX inhibitors and reduced prostaglandin generation can lead to a form of low renin-angiotensin activity.[97] Although prostaglandins are normally viewed as endogenous antagonists of angiotensin II activity, prostaglandins are necessary for normal renin responses. Therefore, if COX inhibitors are administered to certain patients over prolonged periods, a form of low renin-angiotensin activity can occur that is characterized by modest hyperkalemia and mild metabolic acidosis. The experiences with COX-2 inhibitors are less extensive, but one might expect that these agents also contribute to this form of low renin-angiotensin activity.

In many patients, cyclosporine administration produces not only hypertension and a tendency to prerenal conditions via renal vasoconstriction[98] but also commonly contributes to mild hyperkalemia and metabolic acidosis. Studies from various laboratories have presented different assessments of renin-angiotensin activity during cyclosporine administration, and some have purported that angiotensin II is critical to the renal vasoconstriction associated with cyclosporine toxicity.[99] However, studies in which angiotensin levels have actually been measured suggest that kidney angiotensin II content is decreased with this agent[100] and that nitric oxide and prostaglandin production are also reduced, which may provide the basis for this reduction in angiotensin II generation.[98] Functional studies in cyclosporine toxicity also suggest reduced angiotensin II influence on the kidney. The acid-base and electrolyte consequences of cyclosporine administration are hyperkalemia and metabolic acidosis.

Chronic renal insufficiency is not a true low renin-angiotensin condition, but one might expect that during advanced renal failure the responses to angiotensin II receptor blockers and ACE inhibitors may be somewhat exaggerated with regard to the impact on total potassium and proton secretion. In fact, renin-angiotensin activity is reasonably high with advancing renal failure such that kidneys with chronic renal insufficiency are highly dependent on aldosterone for normal potassium excretion and secretion.[101]

The last consideration in the differential diagnosis of hyporeninemic hypoaldosteronism might be considered functional hyporeninism. These conditions are moderately rare, and many cases are more theoretical in part. In this case, a renal process produces reductions in delivery and flow rates to the distal tubule and collecting duct that limit potassium and proton secretion. At the same time, inappropriate signals determining the activity of the renin-angiotensin system are perceived within the kidney and systemic vasculature.

A classic example is acute postinfectious glomerulonephritis.[102] This process limits glomerular filtration owing to vasoconstriction and major alterations in the glomerular ultrafiltration coefficient, which are based on immune-mediated events within the glomerular capillaries. This results in retention of NaCl and volume and the rapid development of hypertension. The hypertension develops suddenly over a short period of time. Both hypertension and fluid and NaCl accumulation functionally suppress the activity of the renin-angiotensin system. This reduction is really inappropriate when one considers that delivery rates of fluid to the distal nephron and GFR are reduced in all nephrons, and there is no absolute loss of nephron number. Under these circumstances, serum potassium may be remarkably increased, whereas the increases in creatinine and blood urea nitrogen are quite modest. Acute glomerulonephritis is a prerenal condition in which the baroreceptors dictating renin-angiotensin activity are provided with signals that the body is volume expanded. In this case, treatment should focus on increasing distal delivery. Diuretics such as furosemide and bumetanide are quite appropriate therapy to correct the salt and water retention and hypertension and to restore adequate potassium and proton secretion. Theoretically, any pathophysiologic condition characterized by accelerated proximal tubular reabsorption could lead to hyperkalemia and metabolic acidosis.

There is one major problem with all causes of hyporeninemic hypoaldosteronism. The renin-angiotensin activity is decreased and is the primary reason for the loss of normal angiotensin stimulation of aldosterone secretion. However, hyperkalemia is known to directly stimulate aldosterone secretion.[55] Older studies suggest that possibly the level at which serum potassium stimulates aldosterone output is sufficiently high that patients will experience a serum potassium of 5.5 to 6.5 mEq/L before significant increases in aldosterone occur. Alternatively, absolute angiotensin deficiency may alter some structural or cellular component within the adrenal glomerulosa that contributes to an inadequate aldosterone response to elevated serum potassium.

## Hypoaldosteronism with Normal Renin-Angiotensin Activity

Hypoaldosteronism has been simplified into two general categories: (1) inadequate secretion or functionally suppressed renin-angiotensin activity leading to low plasma aldosterone levels, and (2) conditions that simulate hypoaldosteronism in which serum aldosterone is normal or increased but no aldosterone effect is observed due to tubular damage or absence of receptors. This is a reasonable categorization of the clinical problem, but the differential diagnosis is actually rather broad. If defects are to be corrected, one has to consider all of the several possibilities that lead to the syndrome of chronic hyperkalemia with metabolic acidosis. Isolated underproduction of aldosterone is actually not common and could occur in an absolute sense only after adrenalectomy or in Addison disease, which is caused by destruction of the adrenal gland. However, in those circumstances, there is also a significant glucocorticoid deficiency, and the overall clinical picture differs. The isolated deficiency of aldosterone output despite normal renin-angiotensin activity is actually rare. One circumstance in a clinical setting that may simulate this condition is the administration of heparin, given in doses as low as 5000 U twice daily, which decreases aldosterone secretion and contributes to a condition associated with modest hyperkalemia.[103]

Conditions of aldosterone resistance or tubular aldosterone unresponsiveness, however, are fairly common. A frequently encountered clinical situation is that of distal tubular and collecting duct damage. The most common acquired condition is chronic obstructive uropathy, that has not been corrected by surgical therapy.[104, 105] One also encounters this syndrome in certain types of chronic interstitial diseases or after an episode of acute drug-induced interstitial nephritis. The latter condition usually resolves with time. Hyperkalemia can be attributed to relative unresponsiveness of the kidney to the elevated aldosterone levels in plasma. In this category must also be included the true absence of aldosterone receptors.[106, 107] Congenital or hereditary forms of this disorder are quite rare.

The general picture of distal tubular and collecting duct damage and aldosterone unresponsiveness is fairly classic. The patient often does badly during circumstances of extrarenal NaCl volume losses, and renal salt wasting is often associated with this disorder.[104, 105] If the latter is the case, the clinical picture may simulate Addison disease. Rather severe hyperkalemia and metabolic acidosis may occur under conditions of volume depletion. Under these circumstances, other organs continue responsive to aldosterone such as the salivary gland and the distal gastrointestinal tract. When one tests renal function with certain provocative tests such as $Na_2SO_4$ infusion, potassium excretory responses are relatively intact and driven by other factors such as the large electronegativity in the collecting duct lumen produced by the unreabsorbable sulfate anion. In addition, urinary pH decreases appropriately to low levels even in the absence of an aldosterone response (unpublished observations).

Various drugs, of course, produce diminished aldosterone responses, the most common of which are drugs that are designed for this purpose, such as spironolactone. However, other agents such as triamterene can emulate aldosterone antagonists and can produce significant hyperkalemia, especially with concurrent renal insufficiency. Another commonly used drug that can produce this condition is trimethoprim, which exhibits some amiloride-like effects and impairs potassium secretion.[108–110] This effect of trimethoprim produces mild elevations of serum potassium (1.1 mEq/L) in individuals with regular doses of this agent, and the severity of hyperkalemia depends to a certain extent on the simultaneous presence of reductions in GFR. Large doses of this agent used in patients with human immunodeficiency virus (HIV) infection may produce hyperkalemia with rather normal values of plasma creatinine.

There are other entities that one must consider in which both the adrenal response to aldosterone and the expression of aldosterone receptors are entirely normal, but the clinical outcome is hyperkalemia and metabolic acidosis. This clinical entity has been called variously "chloride shunt" nephropathy or Gordon syndrome.[111] The clinical picture is usually one of mild-to-moderate chronic hypertension associated with mild-to-moderate hyperkalemia and depressed bicarbonate concentration.[112] It has been proposed that this syndrome is produced by an abnormally elevated chloride permeability in the distal tubule in segments that express thiazide receptors. In these circumstances, sodium is reabsorbed; however, instead of generating an electronegative potential in the lumen of that segment, the elevated chloride permeability causes chloride reabsorption, thus "shunting" out the electrical potential in the lumen and causing abnormal NaCl retention leading to hypertension and reduction in $K^+$

and proton secretion. The important point is that a syndrome of modest hypertension, hyperkalemia, and metabolic acidosis can be treated effectively with long-acting thiazide diuretics, thus also successfully contributing to the treatment of hypertension. However, administration of loop diuretics such as furosemide and bumetanide are not successful despite the fact that they increase fluid delivery into the distal tubule and collecting duct. Apparently, the increase in tubular chloride permeability is of sufficient magnitude to negate the beneficial effects of loop diuretics on potassium and proton secretion.

Severe prerenal states obviously could produce a similar overall picture but usually in conditions in which massive volume losses or reductions in cardiac output have occurred.[76] Under these circumstances, all nephrons are being subjected to a reduction in renal blood flow and nephron GFR sufficient to greatly reduce delivery into the collecting duct. The elevated levels of renin-angiotensin-aldosterone activity under these circumstances do not sufficiently compensate for the marked prerenal condition, and hyperkalemia and metabolic acidosis ensue. In a sense, this is not an abnormality but just an extreme pathophysiologic response of nephron underperfusion, and angiotensin II and aldosterone secretion cannot completely compensate for the marked reductions in load to more distal portions in the nephron. The net effect of an inadequate renin-angiotensin-aldosterone system on acid-base, fluid, and electrolyte states is, therefore, modest hyperkalemia, particularly under circumstances of restricted NaCl or extrarenal losses and a modest metabolic acidosis associated with elevated chloride concentration. The anion gap in this case is usually normal, because no excess organic acids are generated.

## PHARMACOLOGIC MANIPULATIONS OF THE RENIN-ANGIOTENSIN-ALDOSTERONE SYSTEM

The availability of renin inhibitors, ACE inhibitors, angiotensin II receptor blockers, and aldosterone receptor blockers allows pharmacologic manipulation of the renin-angiotensin-aldosterone system at single or multiple steps along the system. With the exception of renin inhibitors and AT2 receptor blockers, all these agents are used extensively in our daily practices.

### Angiotensin-Converting Enzyme Inhibitors

ACE inhibitors have been commercially available for approximately 20 years. During the past 2 decades, these agents have proved to be excellent drugs in the management of systemic hypertension, congestive heart failure, proteinuria, and chronic renal failure.[113–117] A large number of them exist on the market, and they differ by the mechanism by which they inhibit the converting enzyme and their tissue solubility.[118] As implied by their name, these agents inhibit the ACE, and through this inhibition they reduce the amount of angiotensin II generated. Reductions in plasma as well as tissue angiotensin II have been proposed as a major mechanism to explain the antihypertensive, antiproteinuric, and renoprotective effects of ACE inhibitors.[119–122] Interestingly, not only does ACE cleave two amino acids from angiotensin I to generate angiotensin II, but this enzyme also is responsible for breaking down bradykinin into smaller peptides. The effects of ACE inhibitors on angiotensin II generation and bradykinin metabolism support a dual mechanism of action for these agents that may be important for understanding their antihypertensive and renoprotective effects.[123–127]

The use of ACE inhibitors in patients with essential hypertension has demonstrated that, at least during the first 3 months after initiation of therapy, plasma angiotensin II and aldosterone levels are significantly reduced.[119, 120] This reduction in plasma aldosterone levels leads to a state of "hypoaldosteronism," and as a consequence one observes increases in plasma potassium and under certain circumstances a type IV distal tubular acidosis.[128–130] The severity of the hyperkalemia and acidosis depends on the presence of aggregated factors or conditions. The presence of reduced GFR; concomitant use of other agents that decrease potassium excretion such as nonsteroidal anti-inflammatory drugs,[131, 132] potassium-sparing diuretics,[133] and heparin[133, 134]; and hyporeninemic hypoaldosteronism[135] can lead to severe hyperkalemia and non-gap metabolic acidosis in patients receiving ACE inhibitors. The development of hyperkalemia in patients receiving ACE inhibitors requires a few days and is clearly present usually within 1 week of initiation of treatment.[128] In the absence of aggregated factors or conditions, chronic administration of ACE inhibitors leads to minimal increases in plasma potassium. The effects of ACE inhibitors on angiotensin II and aldosterone can have great clinical benefits in conditions associated with hypokalemia, such as chronic administration of diuretics where the use of ACE reduces the need for potassium supplementation and the risk of hypokalemia.

### Angiotensin II Receptor Blockers

Angiotensin II type 1 (AT1) receptor blockers constitute a new class of agents capable of modifying the activity of the renin-angiotensin-aldosterone system. AT1 blockers bind to the angiotensin II type 1 receptor and through this mechanism prevent the effects of angiotensin II. AT1 receptors are widely distributed throughout the body, and this receptor is responsible for most of the well-known physiologic effects of angiotensin II including vasoconstriction, stimulation of aldosterone, and tubular sodium reabsorption.[136] AT1 blockers have proved very useful as antihypertensive agents, and some preliminary studies suggest a beneficial effect in the management of congestive heart failure and proteinuria.[137, 138] The renal protective effect of AT1 blockers has been demonstrated in experimental animals, but such protection in humans is awaiting the results of large clinical trials.[139–141]

The effects of AT1 blockers on plasma angiotensin II levels are quite opposite to those observed with ACE inhibitors. Due to the loss of the negative feedback effect of angiotensin II on renin secretion due to receptor blockade, AT1 blockers lead to rather striking increases in plasma angiotensin II levels. High levels of circulating angiotensin II produce no physiologic effects due to the AT1 receptor blockade.[136]

However, AT1 receptors are not the only type of angiotensin II receptor, and there is experimental evidence for AT2 and AT4 angiotensin II receptors.[142, 143] The role of AT2 and AT4 receptors has not been clearly defined, but there is increasing evidence of a role for AT2 receptors in renal morphogenesis in embryonic stages as well as endothelial proliferation after endothelial injury.[143] It is, therefore, possible that some of the beneficial effects observed with AT1 blockers may relate to the effects of stimulation of other angiotensin II receptors due to increased angiotensin II levels.

The effects of AT1 blockers on potassium excretion are very similar to the ones observed with ACE inhibitors.[136] Blockade of the AT1 receptor in aldosterone-producing cells reduces aldosterone secretion, generating "hypoaldosteronism" similar to that observed with ACE inhibitors. As mentioned earlier, in conditions of reduced renal function or in the presence of agents that suppress or limit aldosterone effects, the use of AT1 blockers can lead to hyperkalemia and metabolic acidosis. Otherwise, administration of AT1 blockers to patients with normal renal function is associated with mild increases in plasma potassium levels.

## Combination Angiotensin-Converting Enzyme Inhibitors and Angiotensin II Receptor Blockers

There is increasing clinical evidence for a synergistic effect of the combination of ACE inhibitors and AT1 blockers in proteinuria.[138, 144] Such synergism is likely to be a byproduct of the fact that: (1) AT1 blockers produce better long-standing inhibition of the angiotensin II effects, and (2) ACE inhibitors function through a dual mechanism of action, including increased bradykinin and vasodilatory factors (nitric oxide, prostaglandins). As a consequence of this potentially important synergism, it is likely that combination therapy with ACE inhibitors and AT1 will become more popular in our daily practice. Should we expect to see more hyperkalemia or acidosis in the setting of combination ACE inhibitors and AT1 blockers? Interestingly, evidence collected to date does not demonstrate an increased incidence of hyperkalemia in patients with combination therapy, but one should be cautious and not underestimate this possibility until larger numbers of patients with increased risk factors (e.g., decreased renal function) are treated.[138, 144]

## Aldosterone Receptor Blockers

Spironolactone, an aldosterone receptor blocker, has been commercially available for several decades. This agent reduces collecting tubule sodium reabsorption and exchange for potassium/hydrogen secretion, leading to natriuresis and reduced kaliuresis.[145, 146] The distal site of action makes spironolactone a very weak diuretic agent that is used mainly in conditions associated with increased aldosterone activity, including primary and secondary aldosteronism (e.g., congestive heart failure, cirrhosis associated with fluid retention).[113, 114] Administration of spironolactone in patients with primary or secondary aldosteronism corrects or prevents hypokalemia and metabolic alkalosis associated with excess aldosterone. In conditions not associated with primary or secondary aldosteronism, spironolactone is associated with mild increases in plasma potassium levels. Development of severe hyperkalemia and metabolic acidosis depends, as mentioned earlier, on the presence of associated conditions such as reduced GFR and increased potassium intake.

Results from recent clinical trials demonstrating a significant reduction in mortality in patients with congestive heart failure receiving a low dose of spironolactone have generated a great deal of interest and have led to increased use of spironolactone.[147] This increase in use of spironolactone, in combination with ACE inhibitors in the treatment of congestive heart failure, is likely to increase the number of patients with hyperkalemia and metabolic acidosis presenting for treatment in the emergency department. The beneficial effect of aldosterone blockade on mortality in the patient with congestive heart failure is stimulating the development of new aldosterone receptor blockers with reduced side-effect profiles (mainly gynecomastia), and it is very likely that some of these agents will become a very important tool in our therapeutic armamentarium.

# REFERENCES

1. Blantz RC, Thomson S, Gabbai FB: Interactions of angiotensin II with neurohumoral systems in normal and pathophysiological conditions. In Ulfendahl H, Aurell M (eds): Renin-Angiotensin: Proceedings of a Symposium Held at the Wenner-Gren Research Institute, vol 74. Stockholm, Portland Press, 1998, pp 57–65.
2. Wolf G: Vasoactive substances as regulators of renal growth [editorial]. Exp Nephrol 1:141, 1993.
3. Inagami T, Mizuno K, Naruse K, et al: Intracellular formation and release of angiotensin from juxtaglomerular cells. Kidney Int 38(suppl 30):S33, 1990.
4. Ingelfinger JR, Zuo WM, Fon EA, et al: In situ hybridization evidence for angiotensinogen messenger RNA in the rat proximal tubule: An hypothesis for the intrarenal renin angiotensin system. J Clin Invest 85:417, 1990.
5. Erdos EG: Angiotensin I–converting enzyme and the changes in our concepts through the years. Lewis K. Dahl Memorial Lecture. Hypertension 16:363, 1990.
6. Fredlund P, Saltman S, Catt KJ: Aldosterone production by isolated adrenal glomerulosa cells: Stimulation by physiological concentrations of angiotensin II. Endocrinology 97:1577, 1975.
7. Dzau VJ: Circulating versus local renin-angiotensin system in cardiovascular homeostasis. Circulation 77:1, 1988.

8. Davis JO: What signals the kidney to release renin? Circ Res 28:301, 1971.
9. Skøtt O, Briggs JP: Direct demonstration of macula densa-mediated renin secretion. Science 237:1618, 1987.
10. Larsson C, Weber P, Enggard E: Arachidonic acid increases and indomethacin decreases plasma renin activity in the rabbit. Eur J Pharmacol 28:391, 1974.
11. Freeman RH, Davis JO, Villarreal R: Role of renal prostaglandins in the control of renin release. Circ Res 54:1, 1984.
12. Berl T, Henrich WL, Erickson AL, et al: Prostaglandins in the beta-adrenergic and baroreceptor-mediated secretion of renin. Am J Physiol 236:F472, 1979.
13. Smythe DD, Umemura S, Yang E, et al: Inhibition of renin release by alpha-adrenoceptor stimulation in the isolated perfused rat kidney. Eur J Pharmacol 140:33, 1987.
14. Dzau VJ: Tissue renin-angiotensin system in myocardial hypertrophy and failure. Arch Intern Med 153:937, 1993.
15. Kurtz A, Pfeilschifter J, Hutter A, et al: Role of protein kinase C in inhibition of renin release caused by vasoconstrictors. Am J Physiol 250:C563, 1986.
16. Kurtz A, Penner R: Angiotensin II induces oscillations of intracellular calcium and blocks anomalous inward rectifying potassium current in mouse renal juxtaglomerular cells. Proc Natl Acad Sci U S A 86:3423, 1989.
17. Hunley TE, Julian BA, Phillips JQ III, et al: Angiotensin converting enzyme gene polymorphism: Potential silencer motif and impact on progression in IgA nephropathy. Kidney Int 49: 571, 1996.
18. Hunley TE, Tamura M, Stoneking BJ, et al: The angiotensin type II receptor tonically inhibits angiotensin-converting enzyme in AT2 null mutant mice. Kidney Int 57:570, 2000.
19. Seikaly MG, Arant BSJ, Seney FDJ: Endogenous angiotensin concentrations in specific intrarenal fluid compartments of the rat. J Clin Invest 86:1352, 1990.
20. Navar LG, Imig JD, Zou L, et al: Intrarenal production of angiotensin II. Semin Nephrol 17:412, 1997.
21. Braam B, Mitchell KD, Fox J, et al: Proximal tubular secretion of angiotensin II in rats. Am J Physiol 264:F891, 1993.
22. De Nicola L, Thomson SC, Wead LM, et al: Arginine feeding modifies cyclosporine nephrotoxicity in rats. Clin Invest 92: 1859, 1993.
23. Gabbai FB, Wead LM, Khang S, et al: Effect of combining an angiotensin converting enzyme inhibitor (ACEI) and angiotensin II (AII) receptor blocker (ARB) on plasma (AIIp) and kidney tissue (AIIk) AII levels in rats with salt depletion. J Am Soc Nephrol 11:618A, 2000.
24. Tucker BJ, Mundy CA, Maciejewski AR, et al: Changes in glomerular hemodynamic response to angiotensin II after subacute renal denervation in rats. J Clin Invest 78:680, 1986.
25. Goodfriend TL, Elliott ME, Catt KJ: Angiotensin receptors and their antagonists. N Engl J Med 334:1649, 1996.
26. Sasaki K, Yamano Y, Bardham S, et al: Cloning and expression of a complementary DNA encoding a bovine adrenal angiotensin II type 1 receptor. Nature 351:230, 1991.
27. Horiuchi M, Hayashida W, Kambe T, et al: Angiotensin type 2 receptor dephosphorylates Bcl–2 by activating mitogen-activated protein kinase phosphatase-1 and induces apoptosis. J Biol Chem 272:19022, 1997.
28. Siragy HM, Carey RM: The subtype-2 (AT2) angiotensin receptor regulates renal cyclic guanosine 3′,5′-monophosphate and AT1 receptor-mediated prostaglandin E2 production in conscious rats. J Clin Invest 97:1978, 1996.
29. Navar LG, Rosivall L: Contribution of the renin-angiotensin system to the control of intrarenal hemodynamics. Kidney Int 25:857, 1984.
30. Ruan X, Wagner C, Chatziantoniou C, et al: Regulation of angiotensin II receptor AT1 subtypes in renal afferent arterioles during chronic changes in sodium diet. J Clin Invest 99: 1072, 1997.
31. Cheng HF, Becker BN, Burns KD: Angiotensin II upregulates type-1 angiotensin II receptors in renal proximal tubule. J Clin Invest 95:2012, 1995.
32. Du Y, Guo DF, Inagami T, et al: Regulation of ANG II-receptor subtype and its gene expression in adrenal gland. Am J Physiol 271(2 Pt 2)H440, 1996.
33. Miller JA, Thai K, Scholey JW: Angiotensin II type I receptor gene polymorphism predicts response to losartan and angiotensin II. Kidney Int 56:2173, 1999.
34. Blantz RC: Why are some people more receptive to angiotensin II? Kidney Int 56:2316, 1999.
35. Hall JE: Control of sodium excretion by angiotensin II: Intrarenal mechanisms and blood pressure regulation. Am J Physiol 250:R960, 1986.
36. Cogan MG: Angiotensin II: A powerful controller of sodium transport in the early proximal tubule. Hypertension 15:451, 1990.
37. Harris PJ, Young JA: Dose-dependent stimulation and inhibition of proximal tubular sodium reabsorption by angiotensin II in the rat kidney. Pflugers Arch 367:295, 1977.
38. Schuster VL, Kokko JP, Jacobson HR: Angiotensin II directly stimulates sodium transport in rabbit proximal convoluted tubules. J Clin Invest 73:507, 1984.
39. Liu FY, Cogan MG: Angiotensin II stimulation of hydrogen ion secretion in the rat early proximal tubule: Modes of action, mechanism, and kinetics. J Clin Invest 82:601, 1988.
40. Quan A, Baum M: Endogenous production of angiotensin II modulates rat proximal tubule transport. J Clin Invest 97: 2878, 1996.
41. Geibel J, Giebisch G, Boron WF: Angiotensin II stimulates both $Na(^{+})$-$H^{+}$ exchange and $Na^{+}/HCO_3^{-}$ cotransport in the rabbit proximal tubule. Proc Natl Acad Sci U S A 87:7917, 1990.
42. De Nicola L, Blantz RC, Gabbai FB: Nitric oxide and angiotensin II: Glomerular and tubular interaction in the rat. J Clin Invest 89:1248, 1992.
43. Liu FY, Cogan MG: Angiotensin II stimulates early proximal bicarbonate absorption in the rat by decreasing cyclic adenosine monophosphate. J Clin Invest 84:83, 1989.
44. Blantz RC, Konnen KS, Tucker BJ: Angiotensin II effects upon the glomerular microcirculation and ultrafiltration coefficient of the rat. J Clin Invest 57:419, 1976.
45. Ito S, Arima S, Ren YL, et al: Endothelium-derived relaxing factor/nitric oxide modulates angiotensin II action in the isolated microperfused rabbit afferent but not efferent arteriole. J Clin Invest 91:2012, 1993.
46. Haley DP, Sarrafian M, Bulger RE, et al: Structural and functional correlates of effects of angiotensin-induced changes in rat glomerulus. Am J Physiol 1:272, 1987.
47. Persson AEG, Gushwa LC, Blantz RC: Feedback pressure flow responses in normal and angiotensin prostaglandin blocked rats. Am J Physiol 247:F925, 1984.
48. Braam B, Mitchell KD, Koomans HA, et al: Relevance of the tubuloglomerular feedback mechanism in pathophysiology. J Am Soc Nephrol 4:1257, 1993.
49. Gabbai FB, Thomson SC, Peterson O, et al: Glomerular and tubular interactions between renal adrenergic activity and nitric oxide. Am J Physiol 37:F1004, 1995.
50. Tucker BJ, Mundy CA, Blantz RC: Effects of $\beta_1$-adrenergic blockade on glomerular dynamics and angiotensin II response. Am J Physiol 26:F225, 1989.
51. Thomson SC, Gabbai FB, Tucker BJ, et al: Interaction between $\alpha_2$-adrenergic and angiotensin II systems in the control of glomerular hemodynamics as assessed by renal micropuncture in the rat. J Clin Invest 90:604, 1992.
52. Baylis C, Brenner BM: Modulation by prostaglandin synthesis inhibitors of the action of exogenous angiotensin II on glomerular ultrafiltration in the rat. Circ Res 43:889, 1978.
53. Tucker BJ, Blantz RC: Acute and subacute prostaglandin and angiotensin inhibition on glomerular and tubular dynamics in the rat. Am J Physiol 258:F1026, 1990.
54. Steiner RW, Tucker BJ, Blantz RC: Glomerular hemodynamics in rats with chronic sodium depletion: Effect of saralasin. J Clin Invest 64:503, 1979.
55. Boyd J, Mulrow PJ, Palmore WP, et al: Importance of potassium in the regulation of aldosterone production. Circ Res 32:39, 1973.
56. Dufau ML, Crawford JD, Kliman B: Effects of high sodium intake on the response of the rat adrenal to angiotensin II. Endocrinology 84:462, 1969.
57. Gross JB, Kokko JP: Effects of aldosterone and potassium-sparing diuretics on electrical potential differences across the distal nephron. J Clin Invest 59:82, 1977.

58. Doucet A, Katz AI: Mineralocorticoid receptors along the nephron: [$^3$H]aldosterone binding in rabbit tubules. Am J Physiol 241:F605, 1981.
59. Garg LC, Knepper MA, Burg MG: Mineralocorticoid effects on Na-K-ATPase in individual nephron segments. Am J Physiol 240:F536, 1981.
60. Bastl CP, Hayslett JP: The cellular action of aldosterone in target epithelia. Kidney Int 42:250, 1992.
61. Sansom S, Muto S, Giebisch G: Na-dependent effects of DOCA on cellular transport properties of CCDs from ADX rabbit. Am J Physiol 253:F753, 1987.
62. O'Neil RG: Aldosterone regulation of sodium and potassium transport in the cortical collecting duct. Semin Nephrol 10: 365, 1990.
63. Verry F: Transcriptional control of sodium transport in tight epithelia by adrenal steroids. J Membr Biol 244:93, 1995.
64. Young DB: Quantitative analysis of aldosterone's role in potassium regulation. Am J Physiol 255:F811, 1988.
65. Muto S, Giebisch G, Sansom S: An acute increase of peritubular K simulates K transport through cell pathways of CCT. Am J Physiol 255:F104, 1988.
66. Sansom SC, Muto S, Giebisch G: $Na^+$-dependent effects of DOCA on cellular transport properties of CCDs from ADX rabbits. Am J Physiol 253:F753, 1987.
67. Kaissling B, Stanton BA: Structure-function correlation in electrolyte transporting epithelia. In Seldin DW, Giebisch GH (eds): The Kidney: Physiology and Pathophysiology, 2nd ed. New York, Raven Press, 1992, p 779.
68. Hulter HN, Licht JH, Glynn RD, et al: Renal acidosis in mineralocorticoid deficiency is not dependent on NaCl depletion or hyperkalemia. Am J Physiol 236:F183, 1979.
69. Sebastian A, Schambelan M, Lindenfeld S, et al: Amelioration of metabolic acidosis with fludrocortisone therapy in hyporeninemic hypoaldosteronism. N Engl J Med 297:576, 1977.
70. Schwartz GJ, Burg MB: Mineralocorticoid effects on cation transport by cortical collecting tubules in vitro. Am J Physiol 235:F576, 1978.
71. Al-Awqati Q, Norby LH, Mueller A, Steinmetz PR: Characteristics of stimulation of H transport by aldosterone in turtle urinary bladder. J Clin Invest 58:351, 1976.
72. Hulter HN, Ilnicki LP, Harbottle JA, et al: Impaired renal H secretion and $NH_3$ production in mineralocorticoid-deficient glucocorticoid-replete dogs. Am J Physiol 232:F136, 1977.
73. Koeppen BM, Helman SI: Acidification of luminal fluid by the rabbit cortical collecting tubule perfused in vitro. Am J Physiol 242:F521, 1982.
74. Stone DK, Seldin DW, Kokko JP, et al: Mineralocorticoid modulation of rabbit medullary collecting duct acidification: A sodium independent effect. J Clin Invest 72:77, 1983.
75. Walser M: Phenomenological analysis of renal regulation of sodium and potassium balance. Kidney Int 27:837, 1985.
76. Blantz RC: Pathophysiology of pre-renal azotemia. Nephrology Forum. Kidney Int 53:512, 1997.
77. Siegel D, Hulley SB, Black, DM, et al: Diuretics, serum and intracellular electrolyte levels, and ventricular arrhythmias in hypertensive men. JAMA 267:1083, 1992.
78. Gennari FJ, Kassirer JP: Osmotic diuresis. N Engl J Med 291: 714, 1974.
79. Warren SE, Blantz RC: Mannitol. Arch Intern Med 141:493, 1981.
80. Cogan MG, Liu FY: Metabolic alkalosis in the rat: Evidence that reduced glomerular filtration rather than enhanced tubular bicarbonate reabsorption is responsible for maintaining the alkalotic state. J Clin Invest 71:1141, 1983.
81. Simon DB, Karet FE, Hamdan JM, et al: Bartter's syndrome, hypokalemic alkalosis with hypercalciuria, is caused by mutations in the Na-K-2Cl cotransporter NKCC2. Nat Genet 13: 183, 1996.
82. Simon DB, Karet FE, Rodriguez-Soriano J, et al: Genetic heterogeneity of Bartter's syndrome revealed by mutations in the $K^+$ channel, ROMK. Nat Genet 14:152, 1996.
83. Barter FC, Pronove P, Gill JR: Hyperplasia of the juxtaglomerular complex with hyperaldosteronism and hypokalemic alkalosis. Am J Med 33:811, 1962.
84. Simon N, Franklin SS, Bleifer KH, Maxwell MH: Clinical characteristics of renovascular hypertension. JAMA 220:1209, 1972.
85. Holland OB: Primary aldosteronism. Semin Nephrol 15:116, 1995.
86. Fromm M, Schulzke JD, Hegel U: Control of electrogenic $Na^+$ absorption in rat late distal colon by nanomolar aldosterone added in vitro. Am J Physiol 264:E68, 1993.
87. Duc C, Farman N, Canessa CM, et al: Cell-specific expression of epithelial sodium channel alpha, beta, and gamma subunits in aldosterone-responsive epithelia from the rat: Localization by in situ hybridization and immunocytochemistry. J Cell Biol 127:1907, 1994.
88. Ibrahim HN, Rosenberg ME, Greene EL, et al: Aldosterone is a major factor in the progression of renal disease. Kidney Int Suppl 63:S115, 1997.
89. Green EL, Kren S, Hostetter TH: Role of aldosterone in the remnant kidney model in the rat. J Clin Invest 98:1063, 1996.
90. Knochel JP: Rhabdomyolysis and effects of potassium deficiency on skeletal muscle structure and function. Cardiovasc Med 3:247, 1978.
91. Welt LG, Hollander W, Blythe WB: The consequences of potassium depletion. Ann Intern Med 11:213, 1960.
92. Hove EL, Herndon JF: Potassium deficiency in the rabbit as a cause of muscular dystrophy. J Nutr 55:363, 1955.
93. Schambelan M, Stockigt JR, Biglieri EG: Isolated hypoaldosteronism in adults: A renin-deficiency syndrome. N Engl J Med 287:573, 1972.
94. Perez GO, Lespier L, Jacobi J, et al: Hyporeninemia and hypoaldosteronism in diabetes mellitus. Arch Intern Med 137:852, 1977.
95. Goldfarb S, Strunk B, Singer I, Goldberg M: Paradoxical glucose-induced hyperkalemia: Combined aldosterone-insulin deficiency. Am J Med 59:744, 1975.
96. Bia MJ, Tyler KA, DeFronzo RA: Regulation of extrarenal potassium homeostasis by adrenal hormones in rats. Am J Physiol 242:F641, 1982.
97. Larsson C, Weber P, Anggard E: Arachidonic acid increases and indomethacin decreases plasma renin activity in the rabbit. Eur J Pharmacol 28:391, 1974.
98. Thomson SC, Tucker BJ, Gabbai FB, et al: Functional effects on glomerular hemodynamics of short-term chronic cyclosporine in male rats. J Clin Invest 83:960, 1989.
99. Kurtz A, Della Bruna R, Kuhn K: Cyclosporin A enhances renin secretion and production in isolated juxtaglomerular cells. Kidney Int 33:947, 1988.
100. De Nicola L, Thomson SC, Wead LM, et al: Arginine feeding modifies cyclosporine nephrotoxicity in rats. J Clin Invest 92: 1859, 1993.
101. Schrier RW, Regal EM: Influence of aldosterone on sodium, water and potassium metabolism in chronic renal disease. Kidney Int 1:156, 1972.
102. Don BR, Schambelan M: Hyperkalemia in acute glomerulonephritis due to transient hyporeninemic hypoaldosteronism. Kidney Int 38:1159, 1990.
103. Oster JR, Singer I, Fishman LM: Heparin-induced aldosterone suppression and hyperkalemia. Am J Med 98:575, 1995.
104. Battle DC, Arruda JA, Kurtzman NA: Hyperkalemic distal renal tubule acidosis associated with obstructed uropathy. N Engl J Med 304:373, 1981.
105. Pelleya R, Oster JR, Perez GO: Hyporeninemic hypoaldosteronism sodium wasting and mineralocorticoid-resistant hyperkalemia in two patients with obstructive uropathy. Am J Nephrol 3:223, 1983.
106. Bosson D, Kuhnle U, Mees N, et al: Generalized unresponsiveness to mineralocorticoid hormones: Familial recessive pseudohypoaldosteronism due to aldosterone-receptor deficiency. Acta Endocrinol Suppl (Copenh) 279:376, 1986.
107. Chang SS, Grunder S: Mutations in subunits of the epithelial sodium channel cause salt wasting with hyperkalemic acidosis, pseudohypoaldosteronism type 1. Nat Genet 12:248, 1996.
108. Greenberg S, Reiser IW, Chou S-Y, et al: Trimethoprim-sulfamethoxazole induces reversible hyperkalemia. Ann Intern Med 119:291, 1993.
109. Hsu I, Wordell CJ: Hyperkalemia and high-dose trimethoprim/sulfamethoxazole. Ann Pharmacother 29:427, 1995.
110. Perazella MA, Mahnensmith RL: Trimethoprim-sulfamethoxazole: Hyperkalemia is an important complication regardless of dose. Clin Nephrol 46:187, 1996.

111. Gordon RD: The syndrome of hypertension and hyperkalemia with normal GFR: A unique pathophysiological mechanism for hypertension? Clin Exp Pharmacol Physiol 13:329, 1986.
112. Klemm SA, Gordon RD, Tunny TJ, Thompson RE: The syndrome of hypertension and hyperkalemia with normal GFR (Gordon's syndrome): Is there increased proximal sodium reabsorption? Clin Invest Med 14:551, 1991.
113. Materson BJ, Preston RA: Angiotensin converting enzyme inhibitors in hypertension. Arch Intern Med 154:513, 1994.
114. Taal MW, Brenner BM: Renoprotective benefits of RAS inhibition: From ACEI to angiotensin II antagonists. Kidney Int 57: 1803, 2000.
115. Pahor M, Patsy BM, Alderman MH, et al: Therapeutic benefits of ACE inhibitors and other antihypertensive drugs in patients with type 2 diabetes. Diabetes Care 23:888, 2000.
116. Yusuf L, Lonn E, Bosch J, Gerstein H: Summary of randomized trials of angiotensin converting enzyme inhibitors. Clin Exp Hypertens 21:835, 1999.
117. Giatras I, Lau J, Levey AS: Effect of angiotensin-converting enzyme inhibitors on the progression of non-diabetic renal disease: A meta-analysis of randomized trials. Ann Intern Med 1127:337, 1997.
118. Nash DT: Comparative properties of angiotensin-converting enzyme inhibitors: Relations with inhibition of tissue angiotensin-converting enzyme and potential clinical implications. Am J Cardiol 69:26C, 1992.
119. Brunner HR, Waeber B, Nussberger J, et al: Long-term clinical experience with enalapril in essential hypertension. J Hypertens 1(suppl 1):103, 1983.
120. Ogihara T, Maruyama A, Hata T, et al: Hormonal responses to long-term converting enzyme inhibition in hypertensive patients. Clin Pharmacol Ther 30:328, 1981.
121. Garcia GE, Hammond TC, Wead LM, et al: Effect of angiotensin II on the renal response to amino acid in rats. Am J Kidney Dis 28:115, 1996.
122. Weir MR, Dzau VJ: The renin-angiotensin-aldosterone system: A specific target for hypertension management. Am J Hypertension 12:205S, 1999.
123. Swartz SL, Williams GH, Hollenberg NK, et al: Converting enzyme inhibition in essential hypertension: The hypotensive response does not reflect only reduced angiotensin II formation. Hypertension 1:106, 1979.
124. Biollaz J, Brunner HR, Gavras I, et al: Antihypertensive therapy with MK421: Angiotensin II–renin relationships to evaluate efficacy of converting enzyme blockade. J Cardiovasc Pharmacol 4:966, 1982.
125. Swartz SL: The role of prostaglandins in mediating the effects of angiotensin converting enzyme inhibitors and other antihypertensive drugs. Cardiovasc Drugs Ther 1:39, 1987.
126. Swartz SL, Williams GH, Hollenberg NK, et al: Captopril-induced changes in prostaglandin production. Relationship to vascular responses in man. J Clin Invest 65:1257, 1980.
127. Liu YH, Yang XP, Sharov VG, et al: Effects of angiotensin-converting enzyme inhibitors and angiotensin II type 1 receptor antagonists in rats with heart failure: Role of kinins and angiotensin II type 2 receptors. J Clin Invest 99:1926, 1997.
128. Reardon LS: Hyperkalemia in outpatients using angiotensin-converting enzyme inhibitors. Arch Intern Med 158:26, 1998.
129. Textor SC, Bravo EL, Fouad FM, Tarazi RC: Hyperkalemia in azotemic patients during angiotensin-converting inhibition and aldosterone reduction with captopril. Am J Med 73:719, 1982.
130. Keilani T, Danesh FR, Sclueter WA, et al: A subdepressor low dose of ramipril lowers urinary protein excretion without increasing plasma potassium. Am J Kidney Dis 33:450, 1999.
131. Zimran A, Kramer M, Plaskin M, Hershko C: Incidence of hyperkalaemia induced by indomethacin in a hospital population. BMJ 291:107, 1985.
132. Oates JA, Fitzgerald GA, Branch RA, et al: Clinical implications of prostaglandin and thromboxane A2 formation. N Engl J Med 319:761, 1988.
133. Rose BD (ed): Clinical Physiology of Acid-Base and Electrolyte Disorders, 4th ed. New York, McGraw-Hill, 1994, pp 834–843.
134. Oster JR, Singer I, Fishman LM: Heparin-induced aldosterone suppression and hyperkalemia. Am J Med 98:575, 1995.
135. DeFronzo RA: Hyperkalemia in hyporeninemic hypoaldosteronism. Kidney Int 17:118, 1980.
136. Messerli FH, Weber MA, Brunner HR: Angiotensin II receptor inhibition: A new therapeutic principle. Arch Intern Med 156: 1957, 1996.
137. Pitt B, Segal R, Martinez FA, et al: Randomized trial of losartan versus captopril in patients over 65 with heart failure (evaluation of losartan in the elderly study, ELITE). Lancet 349:747, 1997.
138. Russo D, Pisani A, Balletta MM, et al: Additive antiproteinuric effect of converting enzyme inhibitor and losartan in normotensive patients with IgA nephropathy. Am J Kidney Dis 33: 851, 1999.
139. Gandhi M, Meyer TW, Brooks DP: Effects of eprosartan on glomerular injury in rats with reduced renal mass. Pharmacology 59:89, 1999.
140. Lafayette RA, Mayer G, Park SK, Meyer TW: Angiotensin II receptor blockade limits glomerular injury in rats with reduced renal mass. J Clin Invest 90:766, 1992.
141. Remuzzi A, Perico NO, Sangalli F, et al: ACE inhibition and ANG II receptor blockade improve glomerular permselectivity in IgA nephropathy. Am J Physiol 276:F457, 1999.
142. Weber MA: Interrupting the renin angiotensin system: The role of angiotensin-converting enzyme inhibitors and angiotensin II receptor antagonists in the treatment of hypertension. Am J Hypertens 12:189S, 1999.
143. Unger T: The angiotensin type 2 receptor: Variations on an enigmatic theme. J Hypertens 17:1775, 1999.
144. Ruilope LM, Aldigier JC, Ponticelli C, et al: Safety of the combination of valsartan and benazepril in patients with chronic renal disease: European group for the investigation of valsartan in chronic renal disease. J Hypertens 18:89, 2000.
145. Rose BD: Diuretics. Kidney Int 39:336, 1991.
146. Hropot M, Fowler N, Kalmark B, Giebisch G: Tubular actions of diuretics: Distal effects on electrolyte transport and acidification. Kidney Int 28:477, 1985.
147. Pitt B, Zanned F, Remme WJ, et al: The effect of spironolactone on morbidity and mortality in patients with severe heart failure. Randomized aldactone evaluation study investigators. N Engl J Med 341:709, 1999.

CHAPTER 17

# Edematous Disorders

Robert J. Anderson, MD

Diuretics have been in widespread use for the treatment of edematous disorders and hypertension since oral agents became available in the late 1950s and early 1960s. The subsequent development of multiple agents acting at different nephron sites has enhanced the clinician's ability to effectively intervene to improve quality of life for patients with edematous disorders. In this chapter, a brief historical overview of diuretics is initially presented. Subsequently, clinical aspects of renal sodium handling and the principles of diuretic action are reviewed. Finally, clinical use of diuretics for the edematous disorders of congestive heart failure, hepatic cirrhosis, and nephrotic syndrome are discussed.

## HISTORICAL PERSPECTIVE

Although edematous disorders have been recognized for centuries, the "modern era" of diuretic treatment began in 1919, when injected mercury was found fortuitously to increase urine output.[1] Thirty years later, sulfonamide-based antibiotics were observed to cause metabolic acidosis and diuresis.[2] These agents were later classified as carbonic anhydrase inhibitors. In the 1950s, structural modifications of carbonic anhydrase inhibitors led to agents that cause natriuresis without bicarbonaturia—the "thiazide" diuretics.[3] In the early 1960s, further modifications of carbonic anhydrase inhibitors led to more potent natriuretic agents that were subsequently found to act in the loop of Henle. Also at about this time, potassium-sparing diuretics were identified.[4]

It was only later that the ion transporters on which diuretics act were identified (1970s and 1980s) and cloned (1990s). At present, a reasonably thorough understanding of diuretic action on the proximal tubule (carbonic anhydrase inhibitors), thick ascending limb of Henle (loop diuretics), distal convoluted tubule (thiazides and similar agents), and cortical collecting duct (potassium-sparing diuretics) is available.[5–11] During the past 2 decades, initially parenteral and now oral agents that inhibit the action of vasopressin to enhance water reabsorption at the collecting duct have been developed.[12] These agents, which induce a water diuresis and are called "aquaretics," are not yet available for routine clinical use.

## RENAL TUBULAR HANDLING OF SODIUM

A thorough discussion of the sites and mechanisms of renal tubular sodium and water handling can be found in Chapters 13 and 16. A brief overview of renal tubular sites and mechanisms of sodium reabsorption, relevant to diuretic action and edematous disorders, is presented in Figure 17–1 and Table 17–1. Clinical disorders characterized by generalized edema are associated with net positive sodium balance. Positive sodium balance occurs when intake exceeds output. The kidney is by far the most important regulator for elimination of sodium from the body.

Under normal circumstances, the kidney can be viewed as an avid, sodium-reabsorbing organ. In a normal individual with a glomerular filtration rate (GFR) of 100 mL/min, 6 L/hr or about 144 L/day of glomerular ultrafiltrate is formed. The concentration of sodium in glomerular filtrate is almost the same as that found in plasma. Thus, the filtered load of sodium (GFR × plasma concentration) is about 144 L/day × 140 mEq/L or about 20,160 mEq/day. The usual amount of sodium excreted by a healthy individual on a typical diet is about 150 to 200 mEq/day. This indicates that the nephron reabsorbs approximately 99% of the sodium it filters. This avid sodium reabsorption by the renal tubules, and the enhanced sodium reabsorption that occurs in patients with an edematous disorder, provides the substrate for diuretic action.

Almost all tubular sites within the nephron are involved in reabsorption of filtered sodium (see Fig. 17–1).[13] The proximal tubule reabsorbs 60% to 65%, the loop of Henle 25% to 30%, the distal tubule 5%, and the collecting duct 3% to 5%. The proximal tubule is a high-capacity system that reabsorbs the bulk of the filtered sodium. The collecting duct reabsorbs only a small amount of filtered sodium and represents an easily overwhelmed low-capacity system. However, the critical location of the collecting duct as the last

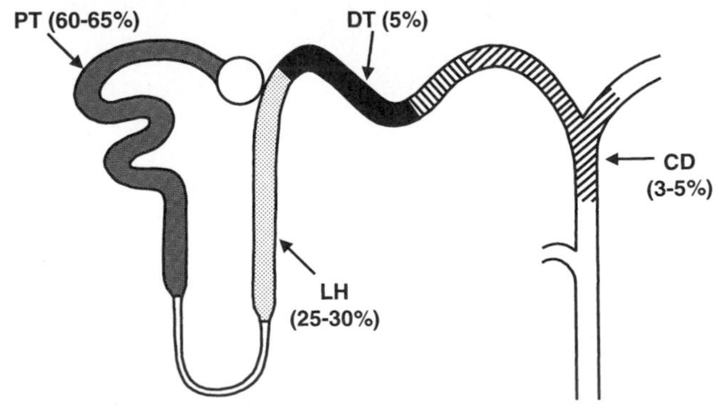


FIGURE 17–1 ■ Schematic representation demonstrating the sites of sodium reabsorption in the normal nephron. PT, proximal tubule; LH, loop of Henle; DT, distal tubule; CD, collecting duct.

**TABLE 17–1.** Nephron Site, Mechanism of Sodium Absorption, and Diuretic Agents Active at Each Site

| Nephron Site | $Na^+$ Transport | Transporter Characteristics | Diuretic Action |
|---|---|---|---|
| Proximal tubule | $Na^+$-$H^+$ exchanger | MW: 95 kDa<br>Structure: 12 transmembrane domains<br>Abbreviated: NHE3 | Carbonic anhydrase inhibitors impair function indirectly by preventing formation of $H^+$ |
| Thick ascending limb of Henle | $Na^+$-$K^+$-$2Cl^-$ cotransporter | MW: 120 kDa<br>Structure: 12 transmembrane domains | Loop diuretics directly inhibit $Na^+$-$K^+$-$2Cl^-$ transporter |
| Distal convoluted tubule | $Na^+$-$Cl^-$ cotransporter | MW: 110 kDa<br>Structure: 12 transmembrane domains | Thiazide diuretic and related agents directly inhibit cotransporter |
| Cortical collecting duct | Epithelial $Na^+$ channel | MW: 180 kDa (3 subunits of 60 kDa)<br>Structure: 3 subunits of 2 transmembrane domains each<br>Abbreviated: ENaC | Sodium channel blockers (amiloride, triamterene) directly inhibit $Na^+$ channel; spironolactone is a competitive inhibitor of the aldosterone receptor and may indirectly inhibit channel function by inhibiting $Na^+$,$K^+$ ATPase |

sodium-reabsorbing nephron segment renders the "fine tuning" of sodium reabsorption done by the collecting duct an important determinant of final urinary sodium concentration and overall sodium balance.

The mechanisms whereby the epithelial cells of the renal tubules reabsorb sodium can be visualized as a two-step process.[13] This process involves entry of sodium from the tubular fluid into the cell across the luminal or apical membrane with subsequent exit of sodium from the cell into the peritubular capillary across the basolateral membrane. The exit process involves the removal of sodium via the $Na^+$,$K^+$ ATPase pump. The action of the $Na^+$,$K^+$ ATPase pump removes three sodium ions in exchange for two potassium ions that are reabsorbed. This results in generation of an electrical potential that keeps the cell interior negative and results in a favorable gradient for sodium entry across the luminal cell membrane. This sodium exit process is the same in all nephron segments. The only currently used diuretic that may exert a clinically significant effect by acting, in part, by inhibiting $Na^+$,$K^+$ ATPase is the aldosterone antagonist—spironolactone. It is at the sodium entry step that renal epithelial cells exhibit specificity with regard to sodium reabsorption and thus nephron site specificity for diuretic action.

The sodium entry step is regulated in part by $Na^+$,$H^+$ exchange in the proximal tubule, a $Na^+$-$K^+$-$2Cl^-$ cotransporter in the thick ascending limb of Henle, a $Na^+$-$Cl^-$ cotransporter in the distal convoluted tubule, and an epithelial sodium channel (ENaC) in the principal cells of the cortical collecting duct.[13] The molecular weight and structure of each of these cell sodium entry participants is noted in Table 17–1 along with the diuretics that work at the corresponding site. Each of these transporters has now been cloned. Also, genetic mutations for each transporter, with the exception of the $Na^+$-$H^+$ exchanger, have been identified. The physiologic effects and resultant phenotype of these sodium transport mutations are discussed in Chapter 19. Additional sodium entry steps are involved in renal tubular epithelial cell sodium reabsorption (i.e., cotransporters in the proximal tubule in which sodium reabsorption is combined with reabsorption of sugars, amino acids, and other organic substances). To date, no diuretic agents acting through these pathways have been identified.

Knowledge of the nephron sites of sodium absorption and mechanisms of diuretic action has several important clinical implications. Reasonable evidence exists that most nephron sites participate in enhanced tubular sodium reabsorption that occurs in edematous disorders.[10] The clinical implication of this observation is that administration of a diuretic that acts solely at a proximal nephron site is unlikely to be effective, because enhanced sodium reabsorption at the remaining distal nephron sites may easily compensate for a diuretic-induced decreased proximal sodium reabsorption. Conversely, a diuretic agent that acts solely at a distal site may not be effective in edematous states, because markedly enhanced proximal tubular sodium reabsorption may result in little delivery of sodium to the distal site of diuretic action. A combination of diuretic agents that concomitantly block more than one nephron site of sodium reabsorption is, therefore, potentially more effective than a single agent.[14–18]

Diuretic agents such as the loop and thiazide diuretics and potassium-sparing diuretics exert their effect by preventing absorption of sodium from tubular fluid.[5–11] Thus, most diuretic agents must gain access to tubular fluid to be clinically effective. Because diuretics are generally protein bound, they are not extensively filtered. Most diuretics gain access to tubular fluid through tubular secretion by either organic anion (e.g., thiazides, loop diuretics) or cation (e.g., amiloride, triamterene) pathways of the proximal straight tubule.[19] Thus, either clinical conditions associated with impaired function of the proximal straight tubule (i.e., acute and chronic renal failure) or concomitant administration of drugs that compete for tubular secretion (i.e., nonsteroidal anti-inflammatory drugs [NSAIDs] and cimetidine) may be associated with relative diuretic resistance.[19]

Potential clinical complications can be anticipated by knowledge of the site and mechanism of diuretic action. For example, many edematous states are characterized by enhanced activity of the renin-angiotensin-aldosterone axis. Thus, a diuretic agent that acts proximal to the site of aldosterone-mediated sodium (reabsorption) for potassium (secretion) exchange in the distal nephron would result in enhanced natriuresis with marked hypokalemia. Also, because spironolactone blocks aldosterone action, aldosterone loss (which enhances potassium and hydrogen ion secretion in the distal nephron) could cause marked hyperkalemia and metabolic acidosis.[20] Finally, carbonic anhydrase inhibition, which ultimately causes diminished proximal tubular $Na^+$-$H^+$ exchange, would potentially result in $H^+$ retention and metabolic acidosis.[21]

## DETERMINANTS OF DIURETIC RESPONSE

### Pharmacokinetics

Several diuretic drug and patient variables interact to determine the natriuretic response to a given diuretic (Table 17–2) . Diuretic agents vary not only by nephron site and mechanism of action but also by structure (Fig. 17–2) and pharmacokinetic parameters (Table 17–3). With regard to structure, it is of clinical relevance with respect to possible allergic reactions to diuretics and cross-reactivity between diuretic agents that all commonly used diuretic agents contain a sulfur moiety except ethacrynic acid, amiloride, and triamterene.

The pharmacokinetic parameters that have clinical relevance include oral bioavailability, degree of protein binding, mechanisms of renal handling, plasma half-life, and site of metabolism.[6, 7, 19] Interindividual variation in bioavailability, which occurs with furosemide, could lead to apparent diuretic resistance. A high degree of bioavailability, which occurs with bumetanide and torsemide, means there is little need for dose titration when switching from an oral to an intravenous

**TABLE 17–2.** Determinants of Diuretic Response

| |
|---|
| **Host Variables** |
| Compliance |
| Sodium intake |
| Underlying health |
| Extracellular fluid volume status |
| Glomerular filtration rate |
| Activity of sodium-retaining mechanisms |
| Duration of diuretic use |
| Concomitant medication intake |
| **Diuretic Variables** |
| Agent |
| Dosage |
| Dose interval |
| Route of administration |
| Concomitant second diuretic administration |

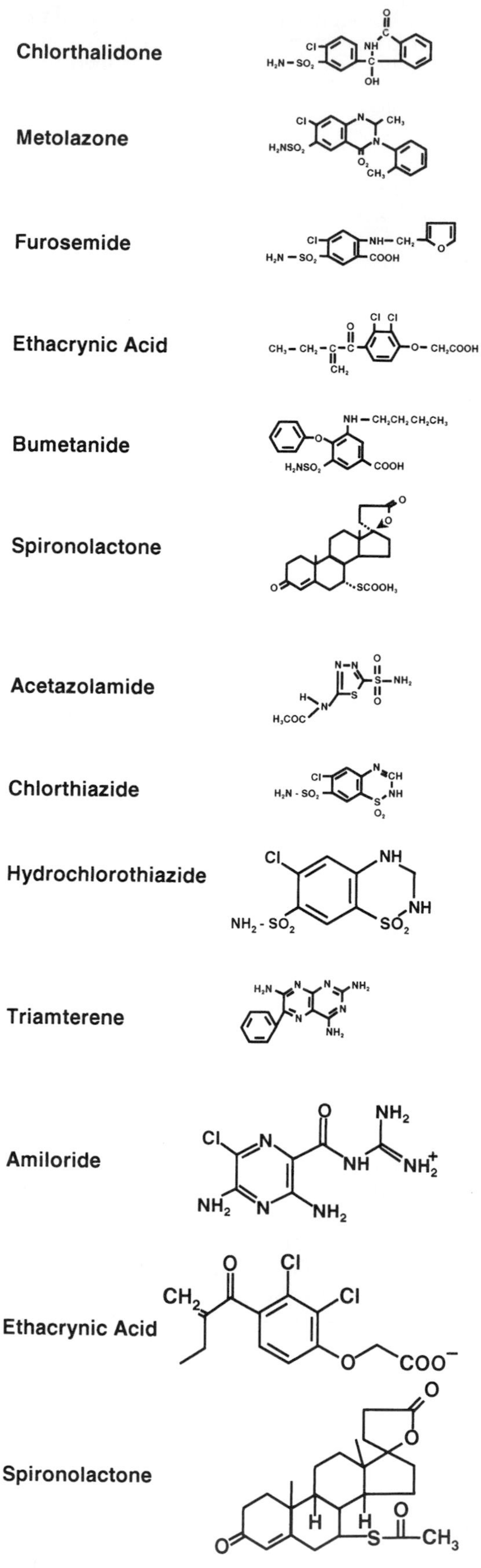

Chlorthalidone
Metolazone
Furosemide
Ethacrynic Acid
Bumetanide
Spironolactone
Acetazolamide
Chlorthiazide
Hydrochlorothiazide
Triamterene
Amiloride
Ethacrynic Acid
Spironolactone

**FIGURE 17–2** ■ Chemical structure of several commonly used diuretic agents.

**TABLE 17–3.** Selected Pharmacokinetic Parameters for Some Commonly Used Diuretics

| Diuretic | Oral Bioavailability (%) | Elimination Half-Life (hours) | | | |
|---|---|---|---|---|---|
| | | *Normal* | *Renal Failure* | *Heart Failure* | *Cirrhosis* |
| Thiazides | | | | | |
| Chlorothiazide | 30–50 | 1–2 | Unknown | Unknown | Unknown |
| Hydrochlorothiazide | 65–75 | 2–3 | Increased | Unknown | Unknown |
| Indapamide | 90–95 | 15–25 | Unknown | Unknown | Unknown |
| Chlorthalidone | 65 | 24–55 | Unknown | Unknown | Unknown |
| Loop | | | | | |
| Bumetanide | 80–100 | 1–2 | 2–3 | 2–3 | 2–3 |
| Furosemide | 10–100 | 1 | 1–2 | 1–2 | 2 |
| Torsemide | 80–100 | 3–4 | 4–5 | 6 | 8 |
| Distal | | | | | |
| Triamterene | 80–100 | 2–5 | Increased | Unknown | 2–5 |
| Spironolactone (active metabolites) | Unknown | >15 | Unknown | Unknown | Unknown |
| Amiloride | Unknown | 17–26 | 100 | Unknown | No change |

route. The plasma protein binding of diuretics, which is very high for thiazides, loop diuretics, and spironolactone, limits glomerular filtration. This protein binding confines loop and thiazide diuretics to the vascular space, where they are delivered to the secretory sites of the proximal tubule.

The plasma half-life of a diuretic is an important determinant of frequency of administration. Most thiazide and distal-acting diuretics have relatively long half-lives, such that once- or twice-daily administration is effective. The shorter half-life of loop diuretics, when combined with the phenomenon of postdiuretic-enhanced sodium reabsorption, may limit effectiveness, unless more frequent administration is used. The site of diuretic metabolism and the health of the organ involved in metabolism and elimination of diuretics can affect the plasma level and half-life.

With regard to pharmacokinetics, less information is available on thiazides than other agents.[6, 21] These agents have reasonably good bioavailability. Some thiazides are eliminated unchanged in the urine (e.g., chlorothiazide, hydrochlorothiazide, chlorthalidone, hydroflumethiazide, and trichlormethiazide). Other drugs undergo hepatic metabolism (e.g., indapamide, polythiazide, and bendroflumethiazide).[6, 19] Delivery of thiazide diuretics into tubular fluid occurs by the organic acid pathway.[6, 19] Members of the thiazide family differ from one another primarily in terms of half-life, which ranges from as short as 1 to 2 hours (e.g., chlorothiazide) to as long as 24 to 55 hours (e.g., chlorthalidone).[6, 21]

Some pharmacokinetic data are available with regard to the loop diuretics.[22–29] Oral bioavailability of the loop diuretic furosemide is highly variable (10% to 100%, average 50%), whereas the bioavailability of bumetanide and torsemide is excellent.[22, 25] Approximately 50% of furosemide is eliminated unchanged in the urine, whereas the remaining half is conjugated to glucuronic acid in the kidney.[22, 26] Thus, prolongation of the half-life of furosemide occurs with renal failure. By contrast, bumetanide and torsemide are significantly metabolized by the liver.[27–29] Thus, in liver disease, the plasma half-life of these agents is prolonged, and more drug may be present in renal tubular fluid. Little pharmacokinetic data are available for ethacrynic acid. Because of greater ototoxic potential than other loop diuretics, ethacrynic acid is rarely used at present.

The pharmacokinetics of distal-acting, potassium-sparing diuretics are complex.[30–34] Triamterene is converted to an active metabolite by the liver, and the metabolite is eliminated by the kidney.[32, 33] Amiloride is eliminated primarily by the kidney.[30, 31] Spironolactone is converted by the liver to numerous active metabolites.[34] Two other agents not commonly considered to be distal-acting diuretics—trimethoprim and pentamidine—have been found to inhibit sodium channel activity in distal nephron segments. Although any diuretic effect of these agents is minimal, they do have the potential to induce significant hyperkalemia.[36–40]

## Pharmacodynamics

### NORMAL FUNCTION

The relationship between diuretic delivery to its site of action and natriuretic response delineates the diuretic's pharmacodynamics. As noted previously, the delivery of a diuretic depends on dosage, selected pharmacokinetic parameters, and renal function. Several patient factors also influence the natriuretic response (see Table 17–2).

The relationship between diuretic delivery into renal tubular fluid and natriuresis is shown in Figure 17–3. Three aspects of this relationship are noteworthy. First, there is a threshold amount that must be delivered to achieve natriuresis. Dose titration to reach this threshold level in the urine is thus sometimes necessary, especially in states of apparent diuretic resistance. Second, there is a ceiling amount above which additional natriuresis does not occur. Administration of diuretic doses in excess of this ceiling amount poten-

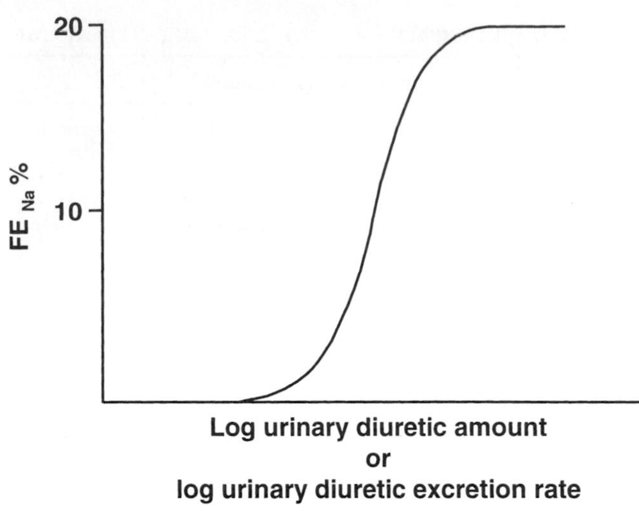


**FIGURE 17–3** ■ Pharmacodynamics of a loop diuretic. The relationship between the natriuretic response (on the vertical axis) and the amount of loop diuretic reaching its site of action (on the horizontal axis) is shown. (Adapted from Brater DC: Diuretic therapy. N Engl J Med 339:37, 1998.)

tially elevates plasma levels and could result in unwanted toxicity for no diuretic gain. Relative natriuretic potency and maximal effective doses, in the setting of normal renal function, for selected diuretics are depicted in Table 17–4. Maximum doses of loop diuretics that can be used to treat edematous disorders are in Table 17–5. Third, as will be discussed subsequently, pathologic conditions in the recipient of diuretics, such as the presence of renal failure or an edematous disorder as well as acute and chronic diuretic administration, may shift the relationship of diuretic delivery and natriuresis demonstrated in Figure 17–3 downward and to the right. There are likely several mechanisms that underlie this decrease in response (see later).

## RENAL FAILURE

The response to diuretics in the setting of renal insufficiency is impaired. This impairment is due both to limitations in renal sodium excretion and impaired diuretic pharmacokinetics. The relationship between the rate of diuretic excretion and the natriuretic response is normal in renal failure—at least for loop diuretics.[41, 42] The issue with renal insufficiency is getting sufficient diuretic to its site of action. In patients with a GFR of 15 mL/min, 10% to 20% as much loop diuretic is secreted into tubular fluid as in normal persons.[22, 26] Thus, higher doses of loop diuretics are required.

Renal insufficiency does not alter loop diuretic bioavailability.[24, 25, 35, 41–47] Thus, for well-absorbed agents such as bumetanide and torsemide, the oral and intravenous doses for patients with renal insufficiency, although significantly higher than for individuals with normal renal function, are equivalent. For furosemide, an agent with incomplete and variable oral absorption, the usual maximum oral dose for patients with moderate (160 to 320 mg) and severe (320 to 500 mg) renal failure is about twice the intravenous dose.

In patients with renal insufficiency in whom, despite large doses of intermittent loop diuretics, difficulty is experienced in achieving diuresis, a continuous infusion can be tried. Such a continuous infusion has been demonstrated to result in modest but significantly enhanced natriuresis over that which occurs with intermittent intravenous doses.[48, 49] A continuous infusion should be preceded by an intravenous bolus loading dose to achieve a significant plasma level. Suggested

**TABLE 17–4.** Relative Potency and Maximal Dosage in Normals of Commonly Used Diuretic Agents

| Agent | Relative Potency | Maximal Effective Dose in Normals |
|---|---|---|
| Furosemide | 2.00 | 40 |
| Bumetanide | 1.75 | 1 |
| Metolazone | 1.20 | 5 |
| Hydrochlorothiazide | 0.30 | 50 |
| Amiloride | 0.15 | 5 |
| Spironolactone | 0.15 | 50 |
| Triamterene | 0.10 | 50 |

**TABLE 17–5.** Maximal Intermittent Doses of Loop Diuretics in Patients with Edematous Disorders and Various Degrees of Renal Impairment

| Condition | Furosemide (mg) | | Bumetanide (mg) | | Torsemide (mg) | |
|---|---|---|---|---|---|---|
| | *Oral* | *IV* | *Oral* | *IV* | *Oral* | *IV* |
| Congestive Heart Failure | | | | | | |
| GFR >50 mL/min | 40–120 | 40–80 | 1–3 | 1–3 | 20–50 | 20–50 |
| GFR <50 mL/min | 40–240 | 160–240 | 2–10 | 2–10 | 50–100 | 50–100 |
| Cirrhosis | | | | | | |
| GFR >50 mL/min | 40–80 | 80–160 | 1–2 | 1–2 | 10–20 | 10–20 |
| GFR <50 mL/min | 80–160 | 160–240 | 2–8 | 2–8 | 20–100 | 20–100 |
| Nephrosis | | | | | | |
| GFR >50 mL/min | 40–120 | 80–120 | 1–3 | 1–3 | 20–50 | 20–50 |
| GFR <50 mL/min | 40–240 | 160–240 | 3–10 | 3–10 | 20–100 | 10–100 |

GFR, glomerular filtration rate; IV, intravenous.

**TABLE 17–6.** Intravenous Dosing of Loop Diuretics

| Diuretic | IV Loading Dose (mg) | Infusion Rate (mg/hr) | | |
|---|---|---|---|---|
| | | *GFR > 50* | *GFR = 25–50* | *GFR < 25* |
| Furosemide | 40 | 2–10 | 10–20 | 20–80 |
| Bumetanide | 1 | 0.2–0.5 | 0.5–1.0 | 1–4 |
| Torsemide | 20 | 1–5 | 5–10 | 10–50 |

GFR, glomerular filtration rate; IV, intravenous.

loading doses and infusion rates of three loop diuretics for patients with renal failure are listed in Table 17–6.

Another strategy to enhance loop-agent diuresis in patients with renal insufficiency is to add a thiazide diuretic.[6, 15, 16, 18, 50–54] Most thiazides are synergistic with loop diuretics. Higher than usual doses are, however, required with renal insufficiency.[52, 54] If hydrochlorothiazide is used, 50 to 100 mg/day is required with moderate and 100 to 200 mg/day is needed with more advanced renal failure.[6]

To summarize, in patients with renal insufficiency, titration to an effective dose is required. This effective dose is usually higher than in the presence of normal renal function. Once an effective dose is identified, the agent should be given as often as necessary to achieve the desired goal. If no diuresis occurs after a maximum dose has been given, then either intravenous dosing or the addition of a thiazide can be considered.

### DIURETIC TOLERANCE AND RESISTANCE

One aspect of diuretic pharmacodynamics that affects clinical response is the phenomenon of tolerance. Diuretic tolerance is viewed by many as composed of two components. The first is a short-term "braking phenomenon" that can occur after only a single dose.[55–58] This decreased diuretic effect after a single dose appears to be primarily an appropriate renal tubular enhanced sodium reabsorptive response to volume depletion, although a volume-independent component can also be identified.[55–58] Some of this braking phenomenon may be attributed to activation of the sympathetic nervous system and the renin-angiotensin-aldosterone system.[59–61] However, blockade of these systems, either alone or together, does not completely prevent the phenomenon.[59–61] Increased expression of distal convoluted tubular sodium-chloride cotransporter also occurs after short-term loop diuretic exposure.

Chronic loop diuretic administration leads to several adaptations in nephron sites distal to the loop of Henle. These adaptations, as determined from animal experiments, include increased sodium transport, increased Na-Cl cotransporter protein and message, increased $Na^+,K^+$ ATPase activity, and hypertrophy of distal convoluted tubules.[62–69] Some of these changes may be mediated by insulin-like growth factor 1.[66] Also, it has been postulated that loop diuretic–induced enhanced sodium delivery, and the increases in angiotensin II and aldosterone that can accompany diuretic use, lead to hyperfunction and hypertrophy of distal convoluted tubules.[62–69] In this regard, angiotensin-converting enzyme inhibitors (ACEIs) can prevent thickening but not hypertrophy of distal cells in the nephron.[69] Collectively, these observations reinforce clinical experiences demonstrating enhanced diuretic response when diuretics that act at distal nephron sites, such as the thiazide diuretics, are added to chronic loop diuretic regimens.[6, 15, 16, 18, 50–54, 70, 71]

Diuretic tolerance and renal insufficiency are two other factors that contribute to clinical resistance to diuretic agent–induced natriuresis.[70, 71] As will be discussed subsequently, intrinsic renal tubular resistance to any given concentration of diuretic agent also occurs in the edematous disorders.[70, 71] An overview of clinical strategies directed toward diuretic resistance is shown in Table 17–7.

## SPECIFIC DIURETIC AGENTS—THEIR EFFECTS AND SIDE EFFECTS

### Osmotic Diuretics

Osmotic diuretics are generally considered to be pharmacologically inert substances that are freely filtered at the glomerulus and are not reabsorbed by the tubules.[73] Thus, mannitol, sorbitol, sucrose, glucose, glycerin, urea, and contrast agents are all osmotic diuretics.[73] Clinically, only mannitol is widely used.[72, 73] Mannitol is a 6-carbon alcohol (molecular weight 182) prepared by the reduction of dextrose. After administration, mannitol remains in the extracellular fluid pool with a plasma half-life of 15 to 30 minutes in individuals with normal renal function. About 90% of an administered dose of mannitol is recovered in the urine within 24 hours. The precise mechanisms whereby mannitol exerts its diuretic effect remain debated.[72] In the proximal tubule, mannitol causes osmotic inhibition of water reabsorption. This inhibition of water reabsorption dilutes the tubular fluid sodium concentration and lowers the transtubular sodium concentration gradient, thus impairing sodium reabsorp-

**TABLE 17–7.** Management of Diuretic Resistance

- Optimize treatment of primary disorder.
- Consider dietary noncompliance.
  - Review the dietary history.
  - Measure 24-hour urinary sodium; if >100 mEq/L re-instruct on diet.
- Consider diuretic noncompliance.
- Review the history/records for interfering drugs.
  - NSAIDs
  - Vasodilators
  - Antihypertensive agents
- Double the oral dose of loop diuretic until therapeutic effect or maximal recommended dose is achieved.
- Increase frequency of administration or attempt intravenous route, especially if renal insufficiency is present.
- Add a distal-acting diuretic.
- Add a postassium-sparing diuretic.
- Consider other disease-specific fluid removal modalities.

NSAIDs, nonsteroidal anti-inflammatory drugs.

tion. Mannitol also increases medullary blood flow, decreasing medullary tonicity and the gradients for possible water and sodium reabsorption in the descending and ascending limbs of the loop of Henle, respectively. The net effect of mannitol in decreasing salt and water reabsorption in the proximal tubule and the limb of Henle is a high filtered load of these substances that exceeds the reabsorptive capacity of the distal tubule and collecting duct. In healthy men, the net effect of a large dose (100 g) of mannitol is an 8- to 10-mL/min urine flow containing 50 to 70 mEq/L of sodium.

Mannitol is not often currently used in therapy for generalized edematous states.[72, 73] On rare occasions, such as diuretic-resistant nephrosis, mannitol may be a helpful diuretic adjunct.[74] Clinical use of mannitol involves prophylactic administration to patients at high risk of acute renal failure, such as patients with pigmenturia (rhabdomyolysis, hemolysis).[73] Mannitol is also used to decrease cerebral edema and occasionally to induce an osmotic diuresis to facilitate drug or toxin removal (e.g., bromide, salicylate, barbiturates, or uric acid).[73]

The primary complications of mannitol relate to its osmotic effects. The increase in plasma osmolality induced by mannitol shifts water from the intracellular to the extracellular compartment. The consequence is expansion of extracellular fluid volume, hyponatremia, and loss of cell volume. When large doses of mannitol are given to patients who cannot eliminate it (i.e., patients with acute or chronic renal failure), congestive heart failure, pulmonary edema, and a hyperosmolar syndrome with hyponatremia and marked cerebral dysfunction can occur.[75–77] Administration of large doses of mannitol has been associated with the development of acute renal failure.[75–77] In these cases, the hyperosmolality induced by mannitol increases the osmotic pressure of glomerular capillary blood to such a level that net glomerular filtration pressure (i.e., glomerular hydrostatic pressure minus glomerular osmotic pressure) no longer exceeds tubular pressure.[75–77] As noted previously, the diuresis induced by mannitol can cause extracellular fluid volume depletion. Hyperkalemia may accompany infusion of mannitol.[78]

## Carbonic Anhydrase Inhibitors

Sulfanilamide, which is a carbonic anhydrase inhibitor, was the first orally available diuretic used to treat edema. Acetazolamide is the currently used prototypical carbonic anhydrase inhibitor.[2] Carbonic anhydrase, located both intracellularly and in the apical brush border of proximal tubular cells, catalyzes the hydration and dehydration of carbonic acid, thus regulating formation of $H^+$ for $Na^+$-$H^+$ exchange.[79, 80] Acutely, acetazolamide results in a modest alkaline diuresis with increased excretion of $Na^+$, $HCO_3^-$, and $K^+$. The diuresis is modest and self-limited, both because distal nephron segments increase sodium reabsorption and because the chronic diuretic action of acetazolamide is attenuated by the metabolic acidosis caused by bicarbonaturia. In addition, adverse effects such as abnormal taste (particularly with carbonated beverages), nausea, vomiting, paresthesia, encephalopathy, allergic reactions, liver function abnormalities, and bone marrow suppression occur occasionally, further limiting the clinical utility of these agents.[81–83] Interestingly, many of the adverse consequences of acetazolamide are more pronounced in patients with a greater degree of acidosis. Because of side effects and possible accumulation in the elderly, use of acetazolamide for diuresis is usually restricted to patients with metabolic alkalosis.[81–83] However, acetazolamide, when given to edematous patients treated with other diuretic agents, is clearly capable of augmenting diuresis.[14] Moreover, acetazolamide does not appear to induce a high frequency of hypokalemia.[83] Occasionally, acetazolamide is used to induce an alkaline diuresis to facilitate renal excretion of weak acids.

## Thiazide Diuretics

Commercially available agents in this class include hydroflumethiazide, chlorothiazide, methyclothiazide, hydrochlorothiazide, indapamide, metolazone, polythiazide, and chlorthalidone. These agents were introduced into clinical practice in the late 1950s and represented the first oral diuretics with reasonable potency and safety.[4, 84] As noted previously, these agents act by inhibiting the $Na^+$-$Cl^-$ cotransporter in the distal convoluted tubule. Thiazide diuretics generally result in modest natriuresis (two-fold increase in urine volume and sodium excretion in healthy individuals), transient magnesiuria, and a decrease in urinary excretion of calcium and uric acid.

The thiazide diuretics have been associated with the development of numerous fluid/electrolyte and metabolic complications.[84–96] Modest extracellular fluid volume depletion, metabolic alkalosis, and hypokalemia frequently occur in patients receiving thiazide diuretics. The average decrease in serum potassium is 0.1 to 0.5 mEq/L but can be higher in edematous patients with secondary aldosteronism, in magnesium-depleted patients, and in patients with limited potassium intake. Thiazide diuretics usually decrease renal excretion of calcium and increase serum calcium concentration. The hypercalcemia is usually modest and readily reversible unless another underlying factor causing hypercalcemia is present. Although the mechanism of hypercalcemia remains unclear, it is most likely to occur either when parathyroid hormone or vitamin D excess is present or when bone turnover is high. Thiazide diuretics produce an acute magnesium diuresis, and low serum and tissue magnesium levels occurred in several groups of patients receiving chronic thiazide therapy.[87]

Thiazide diuretics have been implicated in the development of hyponatremia.[89–96] Frail, elderly females are at highest risk for this complication. Some of the hyponatremia can be attributed to the fact that thiazide directly impairs renal tubular diluting mechanisms.[96] Mild extracellular fluid volume depletion with release of antidiuretic hormone can further impair renal water elimination after thiazide administration.[92] In some cases, marked hypokalemia is also present and restoration of plasma potassium concentration may correct some of the hyponatremia.[92] Hyponatremia can occur quickly (within hours) after the start of thiazide therapy and may be caused at least partly by an associated increase in fluid intake.[94] In such patients, a history of increased fluid intake usually exists, but the urinary concentration of monovalent cation (i.e., sodium and potassium) exceeds that of plasma. Balance studies have shown that most of the observed decrease in serum sodium is accounted for by the urinary loss of monovalent cation.[95] Such patients may develop symptomatic hyponatremia with resultant permanent brain damage.[95]

Other metabolic complications including hyperuricemia, carbohydrate intolerance, and lipid disorders have been associated with the use of thiazide agents.[4, 84–86] Thiazide-associated hyperuricemia is usually of modest magnitude (20% to 30% increase) and is probably caused by mild extracellular fluid volume depletion with decreased uric acid filtration and increased tubular reabsorption. The development of carbohydrate intolerance following chronic thiazide therapy is a concern. Most recent studies fail to find, however, that thiazide diuretics predispose to development of type 2 diabetes mellitus.[88] The effect of thiazides to marginally (4% to 14%) increase triglycerides, total cholesterol, very low density lipoproteins (VLDLs), and low-density lipoproteins (LDLs), while minimally affecting high-density lipoproteins (HDLs), is the source of considerable debate. These lipid changes are most marked in patients with lower levels at the start of therapy and are less evident with a longer duration of therapy. The mechanisms of these changes are unknown. Thiazide diuretics may also cause allergic responses (including allergic interstitial nephritis), gastrointestinal side effects, pancreatitis, liver function abnormalities, blood dyscrasias, and photosensitive dermatitis.

## Loop Diuretics

Commercially available agents in this class include furosemide, bumetanide, torsemide, and ethacrynic acid. These agents are the most potent diuretics currently available for clinical use and act by a $Na^+$-$K^+$-$2Cl^-$ cotransporter in the thick ascending limb of Henle. In normal men, a single dose of furosemide (40 mg) or ethacrynic acid (50 mg) usually results in a 10-fold increase in urine volume and sodium excretion for 2 to 4 hours.[6, 97] The loop diuretics generally produce moderate to marked natriuresis, even in patients with marked reductions in GFR.[6, 97, 98] Loop diuretics also substantially increase the fractional excretion of calcium and magnesium.[97] Acutely, loop diuretics increase uric acid excretion.[97] Subsequently, a decrease in uric acid excretion occurs, possibly because of extracellular fluid volume depletion and enhanced tubular reabsorption. Because of their potency, loop diuretics are often used to treat fluid-electrolyte (e.g., pulmonary edema and hypercalcemia) emergencies.[8] These agents are routinely used when either thiazide diuretics or potassium-sparing diuretics cause a suboptimal diuresis in edematous patients, or in patients with serum creatinine concentrations greater than 2 to 3 mg/dL.

The adverse consequences of loop diuretics include the potential for serious extracellular fluid volume depletion. Although furosemide may be a renal vasodilator, the volume depletion, if marked, can cause worsening of renal failure. Metabolic alkalosis, hypokalemia, and hypomagnesemia are also potential adverse consequences of loop diuretic therapy.[97] In contrast to thiazide diuretics (which impair urinary diluting capacity), the loop diuretics (which impair both urinary diluting and concentrating capacity) are rarely associated with the development of hyponatremia. In fact, loop diuretics may be helpful in therapy for some forms of hyponatremia.[99] In some patients with underlying hypoparathyroidism, loop diuretics may further decrease the serum calcium concentration.

One of the greatest concerns with furosemide therapy is ototoxicity.[48, 100–103] This toxicity, which may be permanent, usually occurs when large doses are given rapidly intravenously. Bumetanide is associated with less ototoxicity than furosemide. Furosemide, and perhaps to a lesser extent other diuretics, may increase urinary thiamine excretion, although the clinical consequences of this enhanced excretion are unknown.[104, 105] The loop diuretics may be associated with allergic reactions, including acute interstitial nephritis. Gastrointestinal side effects, liver function abnormalities, and blood dyscrasias have also been reported in conjunction with loop diuretic therapy.

## Potassium-Sparing Diuretics

Included in this grouping are spironolactone, amiloride, and triamterene. As noted previously, trimethoprim and pentamidine are other agents that may exert weak diuretic effects with hyperkalemia potential.[36–40] These agents act to inhibit the function of the apical sodium epithelial channel in the cortical collecting tubule. Amiloride, triamterene, and perhaps trimethoprim and pentamidine act to block the apical sodium channel, whereas spironolactone is an aldosterone antagonist.

In contrast to all other diuretics, these agents, by inhibiting distal tubular sodium uptake and potassium secretion, have the potential to increase serum potassium concentration. These agents are widely used as first-line therapy for patients with edematous disorders and are used in combination with either thiazide or loop diuretics to enhance diuresis while attenuating or preventing hypokalemia.

The predominant concern regarding these agents is the potential for development of significant hyperkalemia. Thus, these agents should be used with extreme caution in patients with either clinical conditions (e.g., renal failure, high potassium intake) or medications (e.g., potassium supplements, NSAIDs, β-blockers, angiotensin II–converting enzyme inhibitors, heparin) associated with hyperkalemia. Impaired net acid excretion occurs with these agents and may lead to acidosis.[20] Spironolactone can produce amenorrhea in women and painful gynecomastia in men. Triamterene can crystallize in urine and potentially cause renal stone formation.[106]

## CLINICAL USE OF DIURETICS TO TREAT EDEMATOUS DISORDERS

One suggested overview of the use of diuretic agents to treat edematous disorders is shown in Figure 17–4.[6] This overview provides a reasonable framework within which to discuss medical management of the edematous disorders.[6] An overview of the pathogenesis of edematous disorders is shown in Figure 17–5.

Before discussing diuretic therapy of each edematous disorder, a review of three potential adverse effects common to all diuretic agents is appropriate. By virtue of the fact that the purpose of diuretics is to induce natriuresis, extracellular volume contraction is a potential complication of all agents, especially if an actual or effective "underfilled" extracellular fluid volume state is present (see Fig. 17–5). Another concern with regard to diuretic use is electrolyte disturbances.[99] The potential occurrence of extracellular fluid volume depletion and electrolyte disturbances demands clinical and laboratory vigilance when diuretics are used to treat edematous disorders.

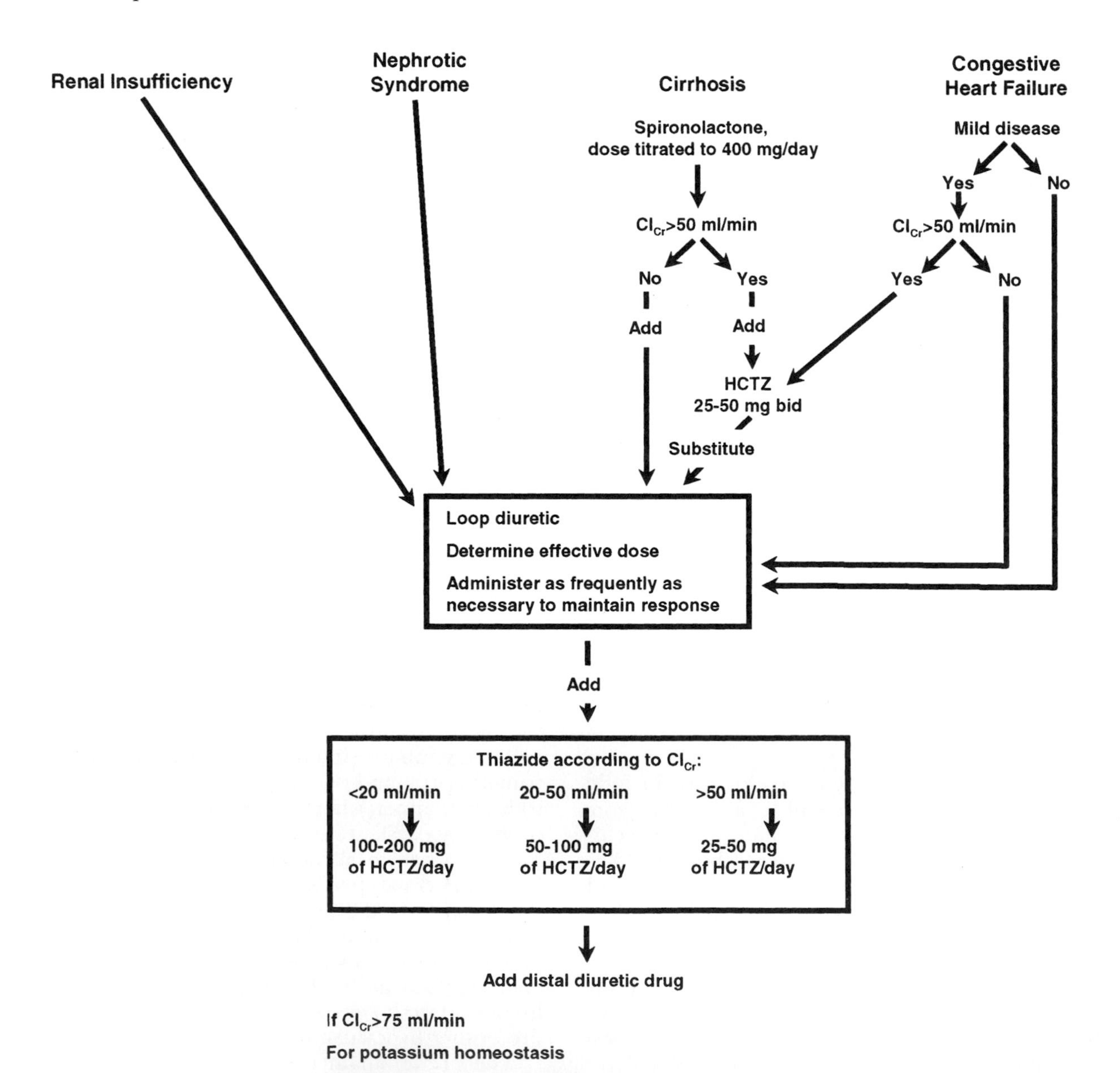


**FIGURE 17–4** ■ One suggested algorithm for diuretic use in patient with an edematous disorder. $Cl_{cr}$, creatinine clearance; HCTZ, hydrochlorothiazide; bid, twice daily. (From Brater DC: Diuretic therapy. N Engl J Med 339:37, 1998.)

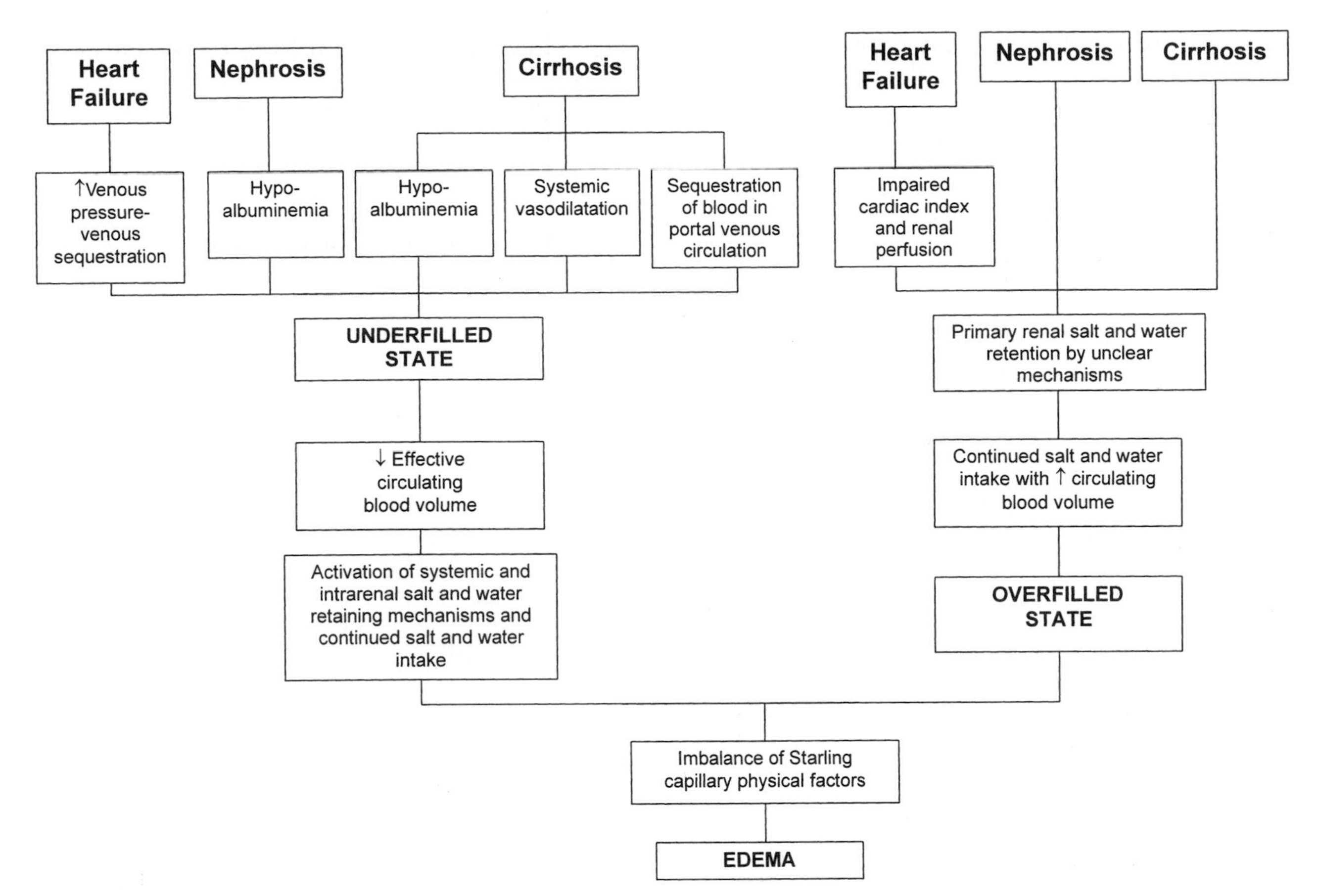


**FIGURE 17–5** ■ An overview of "overfilled" and "underfilled" theories of renal salt and water metabolism in edematous states.

Another recently emphasized concern regarding chronic diuretic use is the issue of relationship to renal cell carcinoma.[107, 108] To date, nine case control studies and three cohort studies of large numbers of patients revealed about a two-fold increased risk of renal cell carcinoma in patients treated with diuretics.[107, 108] This issue is likely more relevant to the setting of chronic diuretic use in nonedematous states such as hypertension where several years of therapy can be anticipated.

# CONGESTIVE HEART FAILURE

## Overview

The incidence and prevalence of congestive heart failure are increasing as populations age and as therapeutic interventions prolong survival. At present, congestive heart failure is the single most common medical discharge-from-hospital diagnosis in the United States.[109] It is estimated that 4.6 million Americans are currently being treated for heart failure and that 500,000 to 600,000 new cases are diagnosed each year.[110, 111] Heart failure is also the single most expensive health care item in the United States and accounts for an estimated $38 billion in direct costs of care and 1 million hospitalizations annually.[110, 111]

There are two major mechanisms of heart failure—failure of systolic function and failure of diastolic function.[112, 113] The most common causes of systolic dysfunction are coronary artery disease, hypertension, valvular disease, and several miscellaneous disorders of myocardium. Common causes of diastolic dysfunction include hypertensive heart disease, aortic stenosis, and heart disease occurring in the context of diabetes mellitus. The underlying cause of heart failure may be an important determinant of prognosis.[110] In general, prognosis is poor, with 1- and 5-year survival rates of about 75% and 35%, respectively.[114]

The mechanisms of renal salt and water retention in patients with heart failure are reasonably well understood.[10, 115–117] Cardiac pump failure often results in increased central venous pressure and transudation of fluid from the intravascular to the interstitial space. This loss of intravascular volume then results in neurohumoral activation with increased activity of the renin-angiotensin-aldosterone, vasopressin, and sympathetic systems.[10, 115–117] In addition to this long-held "backward failure" view of heart failure, "forward failure," with resultant decreases in renal perfusion, can also activate intrarenal and systemic mechanisms that activate various vasoconstrictor and antinatriuretic neuroendocrine systems. Collectively, systemic vasoconstriction and renal salt and water retention initially maintain systemic arterial pressure and cardiac output.[10, 115–117] Over time, renal salt and water retention and systemic vasoconstriction may become maladaptive, leading to pulmonary congestion and edema from positive salt and water balance and increased cardiac afterload from increased arterial pressure.[10, 115–117] These factors induce symptoms and potentially accelerate the worsening course of heart failure.

For many years, digitalis preparations and subsequently diuretic agents were the only available oral medical therapies to treat heart failure. Thus, from a historical perspective, diuretic therapy has traditionally been considered a mainstay of heart failure management. The occurrence of pedal and pulmonary edema in patients with heart failure often prompts the clinician to prescribe diuretics for this disorder. One survey of 1825 patients with congestive heart failure from nine European countries revealed that all patients were taking one or more diuretic agents.[118] This frequency of use of diuretics exceeded use of ACEIs (92%), digitalis preparations (64%), and β-adrenergic blocking agents (6%).

## Rationale for Therapy

The rationale for diuretic therapy for congestive heart failure is shown in Figure 17–6. At high left-ventricular filling pressures, congestive symptoms (e.g., cough, orthopnea, and nocturnal dyspnea), fine basilar rales, and hypoxemia are often present. If the filling pressure is chronically increased, then an associated increase in jugular venous pressure with pedal edema often occurs. Diuretics, by inducing negative sodium balance and reducing extracellular fluid volume, decrease left and right ventricular filling pressures, thus relieving congestive symptoms and edema. Diuretics have no known direct effect on the failing heart. In fact, in many cases, diuretic therapy either does not change or slightly decreases cardiac output in acute and chronic heart failure.[118–124] Occasionally, diuretic therapy reduces arterial pressure and peripheral vascular resistance.[125, 126] When this occurs, cardiac output can increase. Despite variable effects of diuretic therapy on cardiac output, exercise tolerance often increases.[118, 126–130]

When discussing the use of diuretic agents for treatment of congestive heart failure, it is important to review the overall goal of therapy.[131, 132] The short-term goal for patients with heart failure is to relieve symptoms and improve quality of life. It is this goal at which diuretic therapy is directed. The long-term goal of heart failure therapy is prolongation of life. To date, only one diuretic agent (spironolactone) has been demonstrated to prolong life in patients with heart failure.[133, 134] This prolongation of life appears to be independent of any true diuretic response in terms of diuresis with loss of weight. Diuretic treatment of congestive heart therapy is thus often viewed as "necessary but not sufficient" and should almost always be undertaken in the context of other pharmacologic treatments with proven survival benefits.[112, 131, 132] Such agents include ACEIs, combined afterload and preload reducers (hydralazine and isosorbide dinitrate), and β-blockers.[112, 131, 132] Digoxin does not appear to prolong life, although this drug does decrease deaths owing to worsening heart failure and hospitalization caused by heart failure.[135]

## Diuretic Pharmacokinetics and Pharmacodynamics

Studies have clarified the pharmacokinetics and pharmacodynamic aspects of diuretic use in patients with heart failure.[136–143] Generally, heart failure patients with normal renal function respond well to thiazide diuretic therapy. Most commonly, for unclear reasons, patients with heart failure are treated with loop diuret-

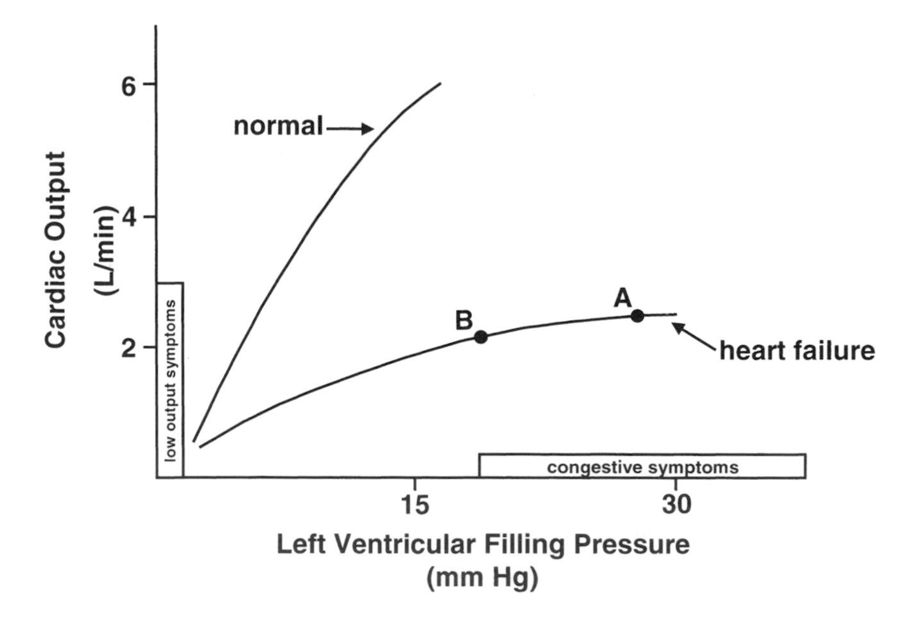


FIGURE 17–6 ■ Relationship between the left ventricular filling pressure (on the horizontal axis) and the cardiac index (on the vertical axis). Patients with heart failure usually have a flattening of the normal curve. Preload reduction with diuretic therapy can move a patient from point A to point B on the lower curve, thus reducing congestive symptoms and also reducing edema.

ics. With loop diuretics, patients with heart failure have delayed absorption and thus often have delayed natriuretic responses.[141] Although heart failure does not impair delivery of loop diuretics to their site of action, renal natriuretic responses to loop diuretics are decreased in patients with heart failure relative to normal contacts by a factor of two thirds to three quarters.[137, 138] The renal natriuretic response to loop diuretics declines as the severity of the heart failure increases and is not improved by the administration of dopamine.[137–142] Decreased renal tubular natriuretic responses to naturally occurring natriuretic peptides is also well documented in congestive heart failure.[10] There is evidence that a significant portion of impaired natriuretic response of the kidney to diuretics and peptides is caused by decreased delivery of tubular sodium to distal nephron sites.[10] Thus, if loop diuretics and dietary sodium restriction do not produce adequate diuresis, one therapeutic option is to add a thiazide diuretic such as hydrochlorothiazide or metolazone. Such dual diuretic therapy demands careful clinical observation, because a massive diuresis is occasionally observed.[143] Also, profound kaliuresis can occur. Thus, potassium and volume status must be closely observed if this type of regimen is selected.

In selected patients with heart failure, the addition of a distal potassium-sparing diuretic (e.g., spironolactone, amiloride, or triamterene) to either a thiazide or loop diuretic can increase natriuresis.[14–18, 71] Measurement of urinary concentration of sodium and potassium may help to predict diuretic response to addition of a potassium-sparing diuretic. If both urinary sodium and potassium are low, then a potassium-sparing diuretic will likely be ineffective because distal sodium delivery is presumably low. If the urinary sodium concentration is low and the urinary potassium concentration is high, then enhanced sodium-for-potassium distal nephron exchange can be presumed and a potassium-sparing diuretic will likely result in natriuresis.[17]

Because of comorbid conditions and perhaps other therapeutic agents such as ACEIs, many patients with congestive heart failure have some element of renal insufficiency. In patients with a creatinine clearance less than 50 mL/min, a diuretic response to a thiazide diuretic alone is unlikely and a loop diuretic will almost certainly be required.[6]

In patients with heart failure and renal insufficiency, although loop diuretic absorption remains constant, a marked decrease in secretion of the loop diuretic into tubular fluid occurs. Thus, a larger dose to obtain a reasonable diuretic effect must be given. When combined with the tubular insensitivity to loop diuretics that occurs with congestive heart failure, frequent, large doses of loop diuretics may need to be given.[42, 47, 48] In some settings in which a patient with heart failure and renal insufficiency appears refractory to a loop diuretic, intravenous administrations are often prescribed.[6] In this setting, continuous infusions appear to offer a slightly better natriuresis and diuresis than intermittent boluses.[48, 49]

## General Approach to Therapy

Once heart failure has been diagnosed, the clinician should consider whether treatable causes of cardiac dysfunction, such as unrecognized coronary artery occlusion or valve disease, are present. Occasionally, inflammatory and infiltrative processes are present. Also, a general medical review should be done, focusing on factors that can contribute to or worsen heart failure, such as anemia, altered thyroid hormone status, pulmonary emboli, sleep apnea, untreated hypertension, hypoxemic lung disease, cardiac arrhythmias, and sodium-retaining medications.

Diuretic therapy in patients with asymptomatic heart failure has not been extensively studied. In one study, 60 patients with a Q wave infarction and asymptomatic decreased ejection fraction (<45%) were randomized to furosemide (40 mg/day), captopril (75 mg/day), or a placebo and observed for 1 year.[144] Captopril decreased end-systolic volume and increased the ejection fraction. Both furosemide and placebo were associated with an opposite effect in which end-systolic volume was increased and ejection faction decreased.[118] Based on this study and other observations, diuretic therapy is limited to relieving symptoms in patients with heart failure and is not currently used for asymptomatic disease.

The traditional medical approach to treatment of symptomatic congestive heart failure has been to start therapy with a diuretic and then add an ACEI and digoxin as symptoms evolve.[112, 118, 131, 132, 145] Data extracted and pooled from two prospective randomized trials support this "triple therapy" approach.[146] The frequency of worsening heart failure was 5% in patients treated with diuretics, ACEIs, and digoxin and 39%, 43%, and 25% in patients treated with a diuretic alone, a diuretic and digoxin, and an ACEI plus a diuretic, respectively.[146] It is unclear exactly where, in the current pharmacologic armamentarium of heart failure treatment, spironolactone and a β-blocker should be added. In general, these agents are currently reserved for patients with New York Heart Association class III or IV heart failure who are already being treated with "triple therapy" (i.e., digoxin, ACEI, and diuretics). Some clinicians, however, are instituting spironolactone and β-blockers in cases of mild heart failure. Data that support this earlier use of spironolactone therapy are currently lacking. However, accumulating data suggest a benefit from use of β-blockers in NYHA class II disease.[147] Increasingly, a five-part regimen (diuretic, digoxin, ACEI, spironolactone and β-blockers) for advanced heart failure is common therapy. An overview of treatment of heart failure is in Table 17–8.

Because of their ability to reduce left ventricular filling pressure, diuretics have been used to treat both acute and chronic forms of heart failure. Once diuretics became available, their use was quickly incorporated into therapeutic pulmonary edema regimens. Initially, mercurial diuretics were used to treat pulmonary edema. In the late 1960s and early 1970s, loop diuretics became available and, because of their

**TABLE 17–8.** Overview of Treatment of Congestive Heart Failure (Ejection Fraction < 0.40) Based on Patient Symptoms as Categorized by New York Heart Association Class

| NYHA I | NYHA II or III | NYHA IV |
|---|---|---|
| • Titrate ACEI therapy; monitor blood pressure, sodium, potassium, and creatinine as clinically indicated<br>↓<br>(Some clinicians consider use of a low dose β-blocker therapy at this stage; there is very limited evidence for this therapy at present.) | • Titrate ACEI therapy<br>• Titrate diuretic therapy to alleviate congestive symptoms and edema<br>• For patients with stage III disease, spironolactone should be considered<br>• Consider the addition of digoxin if symptoms persist<br>• Consider slow titration of β-blockade | • Hospitalization for stabilization<br>• Acute diuretic therapy for congestive symptoms<br>• Titrate ACEI therapy<br>• Spironolactone therapy<br>• Consider digoxin<br>• Consider titration of β-blockade<br>• Consider ultrafiltration, intravenous inotropic therapy, or mechanical assist device therapy |

ACEI, angiotensin-converting enzyme inhibitor; NYHA, New York Heart Association.

greater potency and earlier onset of action, quickly became the diuretic agents of choice in therapy for acute pulmonary edema. However, a prospective comparison of a mercurial diuretic (mercaptomerin) and ethacrynic acid failed to demonstrate differences in the rate of clinical improvement in patients with acute pulmonary edema.[120] In this study, 2 mL of intramuscular mercaptomerin produced an average diuresis of 1240 mL within 6 hours of treatment, and all 18 patients improved. Two types of responses to ethacrynic acid were observed: 6 patients with minimal (290 mL in 6 hours) and 18 patients with marked (2510 mL in 6 hours) increases in urine output. The rate of clinical improvement in all patients was independent of the rapidity of diuresis.[120]

Early experience with the use of furosemide to treat myocardial infarction–associated pulmonary edema was reported by Kiely and associates.[121] In this study, 9 of 15 patients experienced diuresis after administration of 40 mg intravenous furosemide. In those responding, furosemide was associated with a decrease in pulmonary capillary wedge pressure and cardiac index and an increase in peripheral vascular resistance.[121] At the time this report was published, Dikshit and associates raised the possibility that furosemide exerts an extrarenal effect to lower left-ventricular filling pressure after myocardial infarction.[148] Left ventricular filling pressure decreased and venous capacitance increased after administration of furosemide; these changes occurred prior to onset of diuresis.[148] Together these observations suggest that intravenous furosemide potentially exerts a dual effect (early venodilatation, late diuresis) that causes decreased left ventricular filling pressures in acute pulmonary edema.

Subsequently, studies found that furosemide uniformly decreases left ventricular filling pressure.[123–135] However, the decrease in filling pressure is less than that produced by other direct venodilators, such as intravenous nitrate or nitroprusside. Moreover, when used in patients with acute pulmonary edema, furosemide can increase arterial pressure and peripheral vascular resistance and lower cardiac index.[123–135]

Diuretic agents as therapy for chronic congestive heart failure have been common clinical practice since the early 1960s. Studies demonstrate that many diuretic agents including mercurials, thiazides, loop diuretics, and potassium-sparing agents—alone or in combination—can reduce or eliminate edema, decrease congestive symptoms, and improve exercise tolerance and functional status.[14–18, 131, 132, 139, 143, 145, 148–151] Moreover, with careful clinical and biochemical monitoring, these improvements with diuretic therapy are generally not associated with a high risk of significant adverse effects.

To date, no diuretic agent has been proved superior to any other as therapy for heart failure.[140–142] As noted previously, relatively low-dose spironolactone therapy (25 to 50 mg/day) has been associated with significant reductions in morbidity and mortality among patients with severe heart failure when compared with standard therapy.[133, 134]

Several special circumstances regarding diuretic use in patients with heart failure merit discussion. First, use of diuretic agents in some types of heart disorders can be harmful. With right ventricular infarction, pericardial constriction and/or significant effusion and heart failure caused by marked diastolic dysfunction, diuretic-induced reduction of preload may greatly reduce cardiac index. Second, special attention must be given to the heart failure patient with concomitant hyponatremia. Thiazides should be avoided; a loop diuretic is the diuretic of choice. Alternatively, an angiotensin-converting enzyme inhibitor, particularly when used with a loop diuretic, may effectively restore plasma sodium concentration in hyponatremic patients with heart failure. Third, rigorous attention must be given to maintenance of normal potassium and magnesium levels when diuretic agents are used in patients with heart failure. Hypokalemia and hypomagnesemia following use of thiazides and loop diuretics can predispose to life-threatening ventricular arrhythmias, and life-threatening hyperkalemia can occur with use of potassium-sparing diuretics. Hyperkalemia is especially likely when potassium-sparing diuretics are used in patients with renal insufficiency or in those receiving concomitant therapy with ACEIs on NSAIDs. Fourth, it has become increasingly apparent that "diuretic resistance" is an ominous prognostic sign in patients with congestive heart failure.[152] In such resistant patients, sudden death is especially common. Fifth, recent studies clearly demonstrate the hazard of concurrent use of diuretics and NSAIDs in heart failure patients.[153] In one study of patients older than 55 years, use of an NSAID was associated with a two-fold increased risk of hospitalization for heart failure. This trend was especially severe in those with pre-existing serious congestive heart failure.[153] Finally, occasionally it is not possible to remove excess fluid via diuretics in patients with heart failure. In such settings, extracorporeal methods to remove excess fluid may need to be attempted.[154]

# CIRRHOSIS WITH ASCITES

## Overview

The association between advanced liver disease and sodium retention with ascites and edema formation has been recognized for hundreds of years. Most commonly, advanced cirrhosis with ascites occurs as a consequence of chronic alcoholism or chronic hepatitis B and C infections. Other less commonly encountered causes of cirrhosis include various forms of chronic active hepatitis, biliary cirrhosis, hemochromatosis, Wilson disease, $\alpha_1$-antitrypsin deficiency, and cardiac cirrhosis. All forms of hepatic cirrhosis can be complicated by portal hypertension and positive sodium balance with ascites and edema formation.

Two generalizations provide a reasonable framework for understanding the therapeutic approach to ascites treatment. First, ascites is the most common of the major complications of cirrhosis.[7, 10, 11, 156–163] Moreover, the development of ascites is an important landmark in the natural history of cirrhosis and per se represents an ominous prognostic marker. For example, almost 40% of cirrhotic patients followed for 5 years after the onset of ascites developed the hepatorenal syndrome.[164] Second, there is likely to be a continuum of enhanced renal tubular sodium reabsorptive abnormalities along the clinical spectrum of advancing cirrhosis with portal hypertension.[156–164] Initially, urinary sodium excretion is only modestly decreased, and negative sodium balance can be induced and maintained by modest restriction of sodium intake. As the disease progresses, neurohumoral and intrarenal physical factor influences result in enhanced sodium reabsorption, and there is evidence that this enhanced reabsorption occurs at each nephron site. If some sodium is delivered to the distal, aldosterone-sensitive nephron sites, spironolactone (or, alternatively, amiloride) will be an effective diuretic. As more intense proximal sodium reabsorption limits distal sodium delivery, then thiazides and loop diuretics must be added to spironolactone to induce and maintain a natriuresis. Still later, decreases in glomerular filtration, filtered load of sodium, and greatly enhanced tubular sodium reabsorption can induce a diuretic refractory state. At this point, either mechanical intervention (e.g., large-volume paracentesis, peritoneovenous shunt, portosystemic shunt) or liver transplantation is required.[7, 10, 11, 156–162]

## Rationale for Therapy

When discussing use of diuretic agents for cirrhotic ascites treatment, a review of the overall goals of therapy is important. To date, no diuretic regimen has been demonstrated to improve survival in patients with cirrhosis, ascites, and edema. Diuretics are used predominantly to relieve symptoms, improve quality of life, and as an adjunct to prevent spontaneous bacterial peritonitis that commonly complicates cirrhotic ascites.

In preascitic cirrhosis, moderate portal hypertension is present due to increased intrahepatic venous resistance. At this stage of illness, increases in cardiac index and total blood volume and decreases in total peripheral resistance are present but blood pressure remains normal. In preascitic cirrhosis, only modest abnormalities in renal sodium handling are present. These abnormalities consist of an inability to excrete sodium loads, failure to escape from mineralocorticoids, and enhanced renal tubular sodium reabsorption in the upright posture.[157, 163–167]

As cirrhosis progresses and ascites develops, increasingly severe portal hypertension occurs. Increases in cardiac index and total blood volume are present, and decreases in total peripheral resistance and mean arterial pressure are present.[156, 157, 163–167] In contrast to preascitic cirrhosis, activation of the renin-angiotensin and sympathetic nervous systems as well as increased nonosmotic release of vasopressin can be documented.[156, 157, 163–165, 168, 169] In animal models of cirrhosis and perhaps in patients, the peripheral vasodilation of advanced cirrhosis appears attributable, at least in part, to overproduction of nitric oxide.[163] In addition to renal sodium retention, renal capacity to excrete free water becomes impaired and intense renal vasoconstriction with declining GFR often occurs.[158, 164, 168, 169]

In the early stages of cirrhosis, modest sodium restriction may be sufficient to control edema and ascites. As the disease progresses, initially distally acting agents such as spironolactone, or, alternatively, amiloride, are effective. With still more progression, increasing dosage of distal agents plus addition of either thiazides or a loop diuretic becomes necessary. In some cases of refractory ascites, mechanical therapies (e.g., large-volume paracentesis, shunt procedures) become necessary.

For years, a debatable issue with regard to the pathophysiology of advanced cirrhosis was the status of the central blood volume (see Fig. 17–5).[10, 163, 170] Measurements of central blood volume are often diminished while peripheral blood volume is increased.[170, 171] Regardless of these static measurements, activation of the sympathetic nervous system and the renin-angiotensin system that is suppressible by volume expansion and/or other maneuvers that increase central blood volume (e.g., water immersion to the neck) support the contention that the blood volume responsible for activating cardiopulmonary and arterial receptors is diminished in hepatic cirrhosis.[10]

The status of the central blood volume in advanced cirrhosis has important clinical ramifications. If the central blood volume is normal or increased (the "overfilled state"), then careful diuresis should be readily attainable without risk of major complications in patients with cirrhosis, ascites, and edema. If central blood volume is low ("underfilled state") then patients with cirrhosis, edema, and ascites would be extremely difficult to diurese and complications related to extracellular fluid volume depletion might occur. Clinical studies suggest that patients with cirrhosis, ascites, and edema with normal renal function can usually be easily diuresed with minimal complications, thus resembling a normovolemic or "overfilled" state.[172] By contrast, diuresis in patients with cirrhosis and ascites but without edema and with renal failure is often associated with volume depletion. These patients physiologically resemble a central blood volume depletion or "underfilled" state.[172] These clinical observations are compatible with measurements of ascites fluid kinetics made about 30 years ago.[173] These studies found that mobilization of fluid from the ascitic fluid compartment was fixed and relatively limited to about 300 to 500 mL/day in the average patient.[173] Thus, if a diuresis of more than this amount occurs, fluid must be mobilized from either the interstitial space (edematous patients) or from the plasma volume (nonedematous patients).

The rationale for treating ascites and edema in cirrhosis is that ascites causes discomfort in many patients.[157–161] Also, ascites predisposes to spontaneous bacterial peritonitis. When severe, ascites can be associated with diminished vital capacity, decreased cardiac output, abdominal wall skin infections, and hernia formation.[157–161] Finally, in many patients, ascites is associated with anorexia, fatigue, and poor body image.

## Diuretic Pharmacokinetics and Pharmacodynamics

In patients with normal renal function, the concentration of loop diuretics in tubular fluid in cirrhosis is normal.[6, 174–176] Thus, any observed decrease in loop diuretic response in cirrhosis with ascites is not due to impaired delivery of the diuretic agent to its site of action. It follows that increasing the dosage of the diuretic will not increase natriuretic response as long as renal function remains normal. Although delivery of loop diuretic agents into tubular fluid is normal in cirrhosis, there is an 80% to 90% decrease in natriuretic response to a maximally effective dose of loop diuretic when cirrhotic patients are compared with controls.[172–174] Impaired natriuresis in response to atrial natriuretic peptide in patients with cirrhosis and ascites also occurs.[10, 177, 178]

The mechanism of this impaired relationship between loop diuretic excretion rate and natriuretic response is unknown. However, decreased delivery of sodium to the site of action of the diuretic as well as enhanced sodium reabsorption at sites distal to the action of the diuretic undoubtedly play a role in decreased diuresis.[10, 14] When lack of response to loop diuretics occurs in patients with cirrhotic ascites and well-maintained renal function, more frequent doses and the addition of diuretics that act at additional nephron sites may enhance natriuresis.[6, 14]

## General Approach to Therapy

The first principle of therapy in patients with ascites is to ascertain whether the ascites is indeed caused exclusively by portal hypertension. Thus, in almost all patients presenting with ascites, a diagnostic paracentesis is done initially to exclude infections and neoplastic, chylous, or other inflammatory causes of ascites. The clinician must also consider if factors contributing to worsening liver function are operative. Such factors include drugs and toxins (e.g., alcohol and acetaminophen), biliary tract obstruction, hepatitis, hepatoma, and other disorders.

In the stable cirrhotic patient whose condition does not respond to low sodium intake alone, several studies have compared the efficacy of various diuretic regimens.[157–161, 179, 180] Either spironolactone or amiloride alone or combinations of thiazide and loop diuretics and spironolactone and amiloride are effective in treating cirrhosis with ascites and edema (Table 17–9). In studies that have examined monotherapy, most patients respond to spironolactone therapy, and the diuretic response to adequate doses of spironolactone is more consistent than is the response to loop diuretics.[179, 180]

Many clinicians consider spironolactone to be the mainstay of therapy for cirrhotic ascites that is unresponsive to salt restriction and associated with normal renal function.[6] Almost always, spironolactone, or, in some cases, amiloride, is the initial diuretic agent of choice. The usual starting dose of spironolactone is 50 mg/day. The drug has a long half-life and, therefore, can be given once daily. An interval of 2 to 4 days is often required to attain a steady state and to ascertain if diuresis is occurring. If a suboptimal diuresis occurs, the dose can be titrated to 200 mg/day. If diuresis is not seen with spironolactone 200 mg/day, then either hydrochlorothiazide or furosemide therapy can be started and titrated upward depending on the rate of diuresis. Frequent daily doses of loop diuretics are often needed and are preferable to a single daily dose of furosemide. In patients with ascites and edema, the rate of diuresis can be up to 1 kg/day. In patients with ascites but without edema, a weight loss of less than 0.5 kg/day is the goal.

From a practical perspective, the urinary sodium level is thought by some to be an important indicator of diuretic use in cirrhotic ascites.[162, 182, 183] With a

**TABLE 17–9.** Approach to Treatment of Ascites due to Cirrhosis

1. Assess dietary sodium intake and restrict to 75–100 mEq/day.
2. Assess need for vigorous diuresis and risk factors for associated complications.
3. Start spironolactone at 50–100 mg/day if there is normal renal function and no hyperkalemia. Titrate to 200 mg/day.
4. Add either a loop diuretic or a thiazide diuretic, and titrate the dose and interval as necessary to obtain a response.
5. Consider large-volume paracentesis.

urinary sodium greater than 30 mEq/L, spironolactone therapy alone is usually effective. With urinary sodium between 10 and 30 mEq/L, some advocate combined spironolactone and furosemide treatment in a ratio of 100 mg to 40 mg.[162,183] If urinary sodium is less than 10 to 20 mEq/L, diuretic therapy is unlikely to be successful, and large-volume paracentesis should be considered.[162, 183]

Once ascites has been mobilized, diuretic therapy can usually be adjusted downward and, in most nonazotemic patients, 100 to 200 mg/day of spironolactone will keep the patient free of edema provided that sodium intake is limited to prevent a recurrence of positive sodium balance.

Approximately 10% to 20% of patients with advanced cirrhosis are found to be relatively resistant to diuretics, including combined spironolactone and furosemide.[181] Factors that predict likelihood of decreased diuretic response of cirrhotic patients with ascites include clinical features such as previous episodes of ascites, a history of gastrointestinal bleeding, the presence of pedal edema, and a large amount of ascites.[181] Laboratory features that often characterize "diuretic-resistant" cirrhotic ascites include the presence of elevated serum creatinine, hyponatremia, very low urinary sodium and potassium excretion, and marked increases in plasma renin activity and aldosterone.[162, 181–183] High renal vascular resistance, as determined by duplex Doppler ultrasonography, is also predictive of poor diuretic response in nonazotemic patients with ascites caused by cirrhosis.[181]

In patients with ascites resistant to diuretic therapy, several options are available. From a medical standpoint, whereas acetazolamide (administered orally) can enhance diuresis,[14] such therapy is rarely done. Diuresis can also be enhanced by intermittent intravenous albumin.[185, 186] Given the substantial expense of albumin in the United States (~$5 to $25/g), many clinicians would next consider large-volume or total paracentesis.

A series of controlled trials has demonstrated that large-volume paracentesis (4 to 5 L/day) is safe and effective for treating ascites complicating cirrhosis.[187–190] Initially, a randomized trial comparing repeated large-volume paracentesis (4 to 6 L/day) plus albumin infusion (40 g after paracentesis) with standard diuretic therapy was done on 117 relatively stable patients with cirrhosis and tense ascites.[187] Paracentesis was more effective (97% versus 73%) in eliminating ascites. The frequency of complications such as hyponatremia (5% versus 30%), impaired renal function (3% versus 27%), and encephalopathy (10% versus 29%) was lower in patients receiving paracentesis than in those receiving diuretics. Also, the cost and duration of hospitalization were less in patients treated with paracentesis. A second randomized trial examined the necessity of albumin infusion following repeated large-volume paracentesis.[188] In patients who did not receive albumin, a higher frequency of development of hyponatremia and renal impairment occurred. Albumin appears to be a more effective plasma volume expander than other proposed expanders such as dextran in this setting using plasma renin activity as a surrogate maker of effective circulating volume.[190] Large-volume paracentesis, with and without postparacentesis albumin infusion, is now used by many as not only therapy for diuretic-resistant ascites but also as the primary therapy for tense ascites.

Several comments are in order, however, when discussing the use of large-volume paracentesis for treating cirrhotic ascites. Up to 30% of the patients enrolled in some of these studies had never been treated with diuretics. The renal impairment caused by paracentesis without albumin was usually subtle, asymptomatic, and of unknown clinical relevance.[192] Finally, plasma volume expansion with albumin in this setting has not been demonstrated to improve survival. In a 1995 consensus report, albumin infusion after therapeutic paracentesis was regarded as inappropriate therapy.[191]

If total or large-volume paracentesis is done, then one study demonstrates need for diuretics immediately post procedure to prevent a recurrence of ascites.[193] In this study, 36 nonazotemic patients were randomized to either placebo or spironolactone following total paracentesis plus albumin infusion. Recurrence of ascites was almost uniform (93%) in the placebo group and uncommon (18%) in the treatment group.

Another modality used in therapy for refractory cirrhotic ascites is peritoneovenous shunting. An older study compared peritoneovenous shunting with medical therapy in 299 patients.[194] Although the group undergoing shunting had prompt relief of ascites, decreased length of initial hospital stay, and delayed recurrence of ascites, duration of survival and number of complications were comparable in the two groups.[194] Another study prospectively compared paracentesis plus albumin infusion with peritoneovenous shunting in patients with cirrhosis and refractory ascites.[195] Both treatments were equally effective in mobilizing ascites and in the frequency of development of complications, patient survival, and total time for hospitalization during follow-up.[195] The probability of shunt obstruction after 1 year was 40%. The high rate of complications and alternative therapies has rendered peritoneovenous shunting an uncommonly used modality at present.

Most recently, use of the transvenous route, approached percutaneously, to create a transvenous intrahepatic portosystemic shunt (TIPS) has been advocated to treat refractory ascites.[196, 197] In an observational study of 30 patients with refractory ascites due to cirrhosis, a TIPS procedure resulted in diuretic control of ascites in 26 patients. Refractory ascites recurred in eight following shunt stenosis. New onset or worsening hepatic encephalopathy occurred in 14 patients and was severe and disabling in 5. The 1-year and 2-year survival rates were 41% and 34%, respectively.[196] An overview of cirrhotic ascites therapy is shown in Table 17–9.

## Ascites Therapy—Complications

The primary complications of diuretic therapy in cirrhosis include hyponatremia, hyperkalemia, hypokalemia, azotemia, alkalemia, and encephalopathy. Hypokalemia can increase renal ammonia production, and, in concert with alkalemia, precipitate or worsen hepatic encephalopathy. Among other potential diuretic-induced complications, the development of azotemia is most feared because it is a common perception that diuretic-induced azotemia often precipitates an irreversible hepatorenal syndrome in patients with cirrhosis and ascites. More than 30 years ago, the clinical course of diuretic-induced azotemia was examined by Liebermann and Reynolds.[198] These investigators induced a 21-lb diuresis in 14 days in 43 patients with ascites and cirrhosis. This diuresis was associated with an average decrease in creatinine clearance from 70 to 60 mL/min. Five patients developed a marked decrease in creatinine clearance (77 to 30 mL/min). Creatinine clearance returned to pre-diuresis values, either spontaneously or with liberalization of sodium intake, in all patients. Although these observations suggest that diuretic-induced azotemia is usually reversible in the context of ascites treatment, most clinicians monitor renal failure closely and decrease or stop active diuresis if renal function declines.

## Ascites Special Considerations—Ascites Caused by Malignancy

Another difficult problem often encountered is management of ascites caused by malignancy. Ascites due to malignancy can be caused by peritoneal carcinomatosis, lymphatic occlusion with chylous ascites, or portal hypertension from massive hepatic metastases. Therapeutic options include paracenteses, intraperitoneal chemotherapy, diuretics, and peritoneovenous shunts.[199–205] In a large group of heterogeneous patients with malignancy-related ascites, diuretic therapy was of some benefit in approximately 35% of patients.[201] Studies by Pockros and associates indicate that responsiveness to diuretics is strongly dependent on the mechanism of malignancy-associated ascites.[202] Diuretic therapy of ascites that was either chylous or was caused by peritoneal carcinomatosis was not effective in mobilizing ascitic fluid and was associated with a high frequency of extracellular fluid volume depletion, azotemia, and symptomatic hypotension.[202] Diuretic therapy was efficacious, however, in mobilizing ascites caused by portal hypertension resulting from hepatic metastases.

In 42 retrospectively studied patients with ascites caused by cancer, peritoneovenous shunts were inserted. In two thirds of these patients, ascites was controlled.[201] Interestingly, shunt patency was not related to type of shunt, type of cancer, or any characteristic of the ascitic fluid.[201] Survival and quality of life were comparable in patients undergoing paracentesis and in those undergoing shunt therapy.

# NEPHROTIC SYNDROME WITH EDEMA

## Overview

Exact population prevalence and incidence data with regard to nephrotic syndrome are not available. However, one commonly encountered clinical entity, diabetes mellitus, is often complicated by the development of nephrotic syndrome. Moreover, nephrotic syndrome is often encountered in the referral practice of nephrology.

Although edema is a cardinal feature of nephrotic syndrome, it is important to acknowledge that nephrotic syndrome is heterogeneous with regard to cause, renal histopathology, associated renal function, and pathophysiology of sodium retention.[206, 207] One cause of nephrotic syndrome—minimal change disease—is characterized by well-maintained renal architecture and GFR. Renal albumin leak causes hypoalbuminemia, decreased effective arterial volume and renal perfusion, and renal sodium retention. This disorder may represent an "underfilled" state with regard to plasma volume. Affected patients can be contrasted with patients with nephrotic syndrome caused by diffuse proliferative glomerulonephritis with substantial renal impairment. In the latter group, volume expansion and hypertension are often present, and the patients have an "overfilled" plasma volume. The pathophysiology of renal sodium retention in these two groups of patients obviously differs. Clinical studies using plasma renin activity profiling support the contention that nephrotic patients can be divided into "underfilled" (i.e., minimal change disease) and "overfilled" (i.e., diffuse glomerulonephritis) categories with regard to plasma volume.[208–210]

As noted previously, diabetic glomerulopathy is one of the most common causes of nephrotic syndrome. This disorder is often associated with renal and cardiac insufficiency further complicating treatment. Thus, differences among nephrotic patients have important implications for appropriate diuretic therapy and potential complications from such treatment.

## Rationale for Therapy

The rationale for diuretic therapy of nephrotic syndrome is to improve patient comfort and well-being. There is no evidence that diuretic treatment of nephrotic syndrome improves morbidity or mortality.

The pathophysiology of edema formation in the nephrotic syndrome can best be visualized as occurring on at least a two-step level (see Fig. 18–5).[10, 115, 209, 210] The hypoalbuminemia that occurs as a result of urinary protein loss with inadequate hepatic synthesis to maintain normal levels of plasma albumin is widely believed to decrease colloid oncotic pressure, thus leading to extravasation of intravascular fluid into the interstitial space. Although this may occur, it requires a profound decrease in colloid oncotic pressure. Such a shift in intravascular volume would decrease effective circulating blood volume, thus activating systemic and intrarenal sodium-retaining mechanisms.

Blood volume studies in nephrotic patients have demonstrated variable results and are often normal.[10, 115, 209, 210] These static blood volume studies are often done in the maintenance phase of the disease, and the relationship of these volume measurements to effective organ perfusion remains unknown.

Because measurements of plasma volume are often normal in nephrotic syndrome, some feel primary renal sodium retention occurs with nephrosis and that this "intrarenal" mechanism of sodium retention is more important than systemic, neural, or humoral effectors. In studies in animal models of nephrotic syndrome, enhanced collecting duct sodium reabsorption has been found.[10, 209–211] Also, enhanced activity of cyclic GMP phosphodiesterase leading to decreased response to natriuretic peptides and increased activity of $Na^+,K^+$ ATPase have also been found.[10, 209–212] Collectively, these animal observations suggest that not only systemic but also primary intrarenal mechanisms can cause renal sodium retention in nephrosis. Regardless of the primary mechanism, avid renal tubular reabsorption of sodium occurs in nephrotic syndrome. If a positive sodium balance ensues, then diuretic therapy is often needed to treat the edema of nephrosis.

## Diuretic Pharmacokinetics and Pharmacodynamics

In most but not all patients with the nephrotic syndrome and normal GFR, renal tubular secretion of furosemide is normal.[160, 213–219] Despite the normal rate of excretion of diuretic into tubular fluid, diuretic response is diminished.[6, 14, 158, 209–217] The cause of this decreased renal tubular response may be related to intratubular binding of loop diuretic to albumin in tubular fluid with subsequent decreased amount of active, unbound drug.[215–219] Thus, doses two to three times normal may be necessary to achieve sufficient free drug to result in natriuresis. Some of the decreased response to loop diuretics also appears attributable to enhanced sodium reabsorption at distal nephron sites.[220] Not only is the natriuretic response to furosemide decreased in nephrotic syndrome, but also a decreased natriuretic response to atrial natriuretic peptide may occur.[211] Some of the resistance to atrial natriuretic peptide appears attributable to decreased cyclic GMP, which may be reversed by a cGMP phosphodiesterase inhibitor.[212]

The relative tubular resistance of nephrotic patients to loop diuretics and evidence for enhanced tubular sodium reabsorption at distal nephron sites suggests that combinations of higher-than-usual doses of loop diuretics and additional thiazide diuretics may be needed for some nephrotic patients.[221, 222]

## General Approach to Therapy

The first principle of therapy for nephrotic syndrome is directed toward the primary disease process. Many forms of nephrotic syndrome respond to corticosteroids or immunosuppressive agents.[206, 209] Also, angiotensin-converting enzyme inhibition can significantly reduce proteinuria in some patients with nephrotic syndrome.[223–226]

As with patients with cirrhosis and ascites, the state of the central blood volume in patients with nephrotic syndrome may have important therapeutic implications. If low, then diuretic therapy may result in worsened hypovolemia and azotemia. If high, then diuretic therapy should potentially be easily accomplished. Evidence does not support a "uniform" change of the central blood volume in patients with nephrosis. Thus, individualized therapy with clinical and, in some cases, biochemical monitoring is necessary with diuretic treatment of nephrotic syndrome.

Few prospective studies exist that compare efficacy and safety of various diuretic regimens in well-matched patients with nephrosis.[6, 160, 222, 227–234] In patients with well-maintained GFRs, thiazide diuretics with or without a distal-acting, potassium-sparing diuretic may produce a satisfactory diuresis. Most recent data show that loop diuretics are usually effective and safe when used in patients with nephrosis.[6, 161, 226–234] When loop diuretics are used, relatively high doses (to overcome binding to albumin in intratubular fluid) given at frequent intervals are often needed. Concomitant decreases in GFR make it necessary to increase the dosage further. Combination therapy with large doses of a loop diuretic and metolazone is often an effective combination in nephrotic syndrome that is relatively resistant to standard dosages of diuretics.[221, 222, 233] Occasionally, intravenous infusions are necessary. Other regimens that may be efficacious with relative diuretic resistance in nephrotic syndrome include coadministration of furosemide and mannitol.[74] Finally, limited experimental and clinical data suggest that in patients with severe nephrotic syndrome and diuretic resistance, administration of a mixture of albumin and a loop diuretic (30 mg furosemide mixed with 25 g of albumin) will enhance diuresis.[235]

Albumin infusions have been used as a therapeutic adjunct in attempted diuresis of patients with nephrosis for several years.[235–240] For example, 6 of 12 patients with nephrosis whose condition was either resistant to diuresis or who experienced complications on this regimen were given 300 mL of a 15% solution of salt-poor albumin, with a resultant safe diuresis and resolution of edema.[237] One study compared intravenous furosemide, with the same dose of furosemide plus 200 mL of 20% human albumin and 200 mL of 20% human albumin alone in nine nephrotic patients.[240] Furosemide alone produced a significantly greater diuresis than human albumin alone. The coadministration of furosemide and human albumin produced a modest but significant increased diuresis over that seen with furosemide alone. Infusions of albumin may be helpful adjuncts to diuretic agents in selected patients with diuretic-resistant nephrosis. Finally, "head-out" immersion in water up to the patient's neck can cause a diuresis of 0.5 to 2 kg in 4 hours in

**TABLE 17–10.** Approach to Treatment of Edema due to Nephrosis

1. Assess dietary sodium intake and restrict to 75–100 mEq/day.
2. Assess the need for vigorous diuresis and risk factors for associated complications.
3. Start with a loop diuretic and titrate dosage and interval to achieve and maintain an adequate response.
4. Add a thiazide diuretic on either an intermittent or daily basis.
5. Consider a potassium-sparing diuretic if either hypokalemia is present or the GFR is well maintained.
6. Consider an infusion of albumin.
7. Consider extracorporeal fluid removal.

GFR, glomerular filtration rate.

some patients with nephrosis. An overview of diuretic therapy for nephrosis is shown in Table 17–10.

## USE OF URINARY ELECTROLYTES TO GUIDE DIURETIC THERAPY

An alternative approach to the use of diuretic agents in various edematous states is to tailor an initial therapeutic plan based upon the pattern of measured urinary electrolyte excretion. Some limited clinical experience supports such an approach.[6, 14, 17, 71, 182, 183, 241] Collectively, several clinical observations support the following generalizations about urinary electrolytes and diuretic use in edematous states. First, the lower the urinary sodium excretion, the more difficult it is to achieve a diuretic-induced natriuresis. Thus, if a spot urinary sodium excretion is less than 10 to 20 mEq/L or a calculated fractional excretion of sodium is less than 0.2%, a diuretic-resistant state is highly likely. To achieve a clinically significant diuresis in such patients, generally large doses of loop diuretics are required combined with additional distal or proximally acting diuretics.[14, 17, 71, 182, 183, 241] Second, the urinary $Na^+$:$K^+$ ratio generally correlates well with plasma aldosterone and may serve as a useful guide to diuretic therapy of edematous states.[17, 182] Thus, a urinary $Na^+$:$K^+$ ratio greater than 1.0 generally is associated with a good response to loop or (depending on the GFR) thiazide diuretics, and little additional response to potassium-sparing diuretics would be anticipated to occur.[1, 7, 182] Conversely, a $Na^+$:$K^+$ ratio less than 1.0 portends a less good diuretic response to loop and thiazide diuretics and often a marked kaliuresis with these agents. In patients with a urinary $Na^+$:$K^+$ ratio less than 1.0, distal-acting, potassium-sparing diuretics such as spironolactone are often effective and additive to loop diuretics.

## CONCLUSION

Diuretic agent treatment of edematous disorders is usually done to improve quality of life. Use of diuretics based on an understanding of diuretic pharmacokinetic and pharmacodynamic parameters usually leads to an effective diuresis. One key to safe use of diuretics is tailoring the diuretic program to meet the needs of individual patients along with careful clinical and laboratory monitoring. Such individualized therapy and monitoring should lead to safe, effective therapy in most cases.

## REFERENCES


1. Vogl A: The discovery of the organic mercurial diuretics. Am Heart J 39:881, 1950.
2. Schwartz WB: The effect of sulfanilamide on salt and water excretion in congestive heart failure. N Engl J Med 240:173, 1949.
3. Novello FC, Sprague JM: Benzothiadiazine dioxides as novel diuretics. J Am Chem Soc 79:2028, 1950.
4. Rose BD: Diuretics. Kidney Int 39:336, 1991.
5. Greger R: New insights into the molecular mechanism of the action of diuretics. Nephrol Dial Transplant 14:536, 1999.
6. Brater DC: Diuretic therapy. N Engl J Med 339:37, 1998.
7. Antes LM, Fernandez PC: Principles of diuretic therapy. Dis Mon 44:254, 1998.
8. Antes LM: Use of diuretics in the acute care setting. Kidney Int 66(s):67, 1998.
9. Morrison RT: Edema and principles of diuretic use. Med Clin North Am 81:689, 1997.
10. Abraham WT, Schrier RW: Cardiac failure, liver disease and the nephrotic syndrome. In Schrier RW, Gottschalk CW (eds): Diseases of the Kidney, 6th ed. Boston, Little Brown, 1997, p 2353.
11. Ellison DA: Diuretic drugs and the treatment of edema: From clinic to bench and back again. Am J Kidney Dis 23:623, 1994.
12. Kityarkara C, Wilcox CS: Vasopressin $V_2$ antagonists: Panacea for hyponatremia? Curr Opin Nephrol Dial 6:461, 1997.
13. Reeves WB, Andreoli T: Tubular sodium transport. In Schrier RW, Gottschalk CW (eds): Diseases of the Kidney, 6th ed. Boston, Little Brown, 1997, p 127.
14. Knauf H, Mutschler E: Sequential nephron blockage breaks resistance to diuretics in edematous states. J Cardiovasc 29: 367, 1997.
15. Fliser D, Schroter M, Neubeck M, et al: Coadministration of thiazide diuretics increases the efficacy of loop diuretics even in patients with advanced renal failure. Kidney Int 46:482, 1994.
16. Dormans TP, Gerlay PG: Combination of high-dose furosemide and hydrochlorothiazide in the treatment of refractory congestive heart failure. Eur Heart J 17:1867, 1996.
17. Van Vliet AA, Donker AJ, Nauta JP, et al: Spironolactone in congestive heart failure refractory to high-dose loop diuretics and low-dose angiotensin-converting enzyme inhibitors. Am J Cardiol 71:214, 1993.
18. Ellison DH: The physiologic basis of diuretic synergism: Its role in treating diuretic resistance. Ann Intern Med 114:886, 1991.
19. Weiner IM: General pharmacologic aspects of diuretics. In Dirks JH, Sutton RA (eds): Diuretics. Philadelphia, WB Saunders, 1996, p 3.
20. Gabow PA, Moore S, Schrier RW: Spironolactone-induced hyperchloremic acidosis in cirrhosis. Ann Intern Med 90:338, 1979.
21. Epstein DL, Grant WM: Carbonic anhydrase inhibitor side effects. Arch Ophthalmol 95:1378, 1997.
22. Boxtel CJ, Holford NHG, Danhof M (eds): The In Vivo Study of Drug Action: Principles and Applications of Kinetic-Dynamic Modelling. Amsterdam, Elsevier Science, 1992, pp 253–275.
23. Schwartz S, Brater DC, Pound D, et al: Bioavailability, pharmacokinetics, and pharmacodynamics of torsemide in patients with cirrhosis. Clin Pharmacol Ther 54:90, 1993.
24. Gehr TWB, Rudy DW, Matzke D, et al: The pharmacokinetics of intravenous and oral torsemide in patients with chronic renal insufficiency. Clin Pharmacol Ther 56:31, 1994.
25. Vargo DL, Kramer WG, Black PK, et al: DC. Bioavailability, pharmacokinetics, and pharmacodynamics of torsemide and furosemide in patients with congestive heart failure. Clin Pharmacol Ther 57:601, 1995.

26. Beermann B: Aspects of pharmacokinetics of some diuretics. Acta Pharmacol Toxicol (Copenh) 54(suppl 1):17, 1984.
27. Brater DC, Leinfelder J, Anderson SA: Clinical pharmacology of torsemide, a new loop diuretic. Clin Pharmacol Ther 42: 187, 1987.
28. Davies DL, Lant AF, Millard NR, et al: Renal action, therapeutic use, and pharmacokinetics of the diuretic bumetanide. Clin Pharmacol Ther 15:141, 1974.
29. Brater DC, Chennavasin P, Day B, et al: Bumetanide and furosemide. Clin Pharmacol Ther 34:27, 1983.
30. Smith AJ, Smith RN: Kinetics and bioavailability of two formulations of amiloride in man. Br J Pharmacol 48:646, 1973.
31. Sahn H, Reuter K, Mutdcher E, et al: Pharmacokinetics of amiloride in renal and hepatitis disease. Eur J Clin Pharmacol 33:493, 1987.
32. Knauf H, Mohrke W, Mutschler E: Delayed elimination of triamterene and its active metabolite in chronic renal failure. Eur J Clin Pharmacol 24:453, 1983.
33. Villenevue JP, Rocheleau F, Raymond G: Triamterene kinetics and dynamics in cirrhosis. Clin Pharmacol Ther 35:831, 1984.
34. Ochs HR, Greenblatt DJ, Bordem G, et al: Spironolactone. Am Heart J 96:389, 1978.
35. Overdick HWPM, Hermens WAJJ, Matzke GR, et al: The pharmacokinetics of intravenous and oral torsemide in patients with chronic renal insufficiency. Clin Pharmacol Ther 56:31, 1994.
36. Kleyman TR, Roberts C, Ling BN: A mechanism for pentamidine-induced hyperkalemia: Inhibition of distal nephron sodium transport. Ann Intern Med 122:103, 1995.
37. Velazquez H, Perazella MA, Wright FS, et al: Renal mechanism of trimethoprim-induced hyperkalemia. Ann Intern Med 119: 296, 1993.
38. Schlanger LE, Kleyman TR, Ling BN: $K^+$-sparing diuretic actions of trimethoprim: Inhibition of $Na^+$ channels in A6 distal nephron cells. Kidney Int 45:1070, 1994.
39. Greenberg S, Reiser IW, Chou S-Y, et al: Trimethoprim-sulfamethoxazole induces reversible hyperkalemia. Ann Intern Med 119:291, 1993.
40. Perlmutter EP, Sweeney D, Herskovitz G, et al: Case report: Severe hyperkalemia in a geriatric patient receiving standard doses of trimethoprim-sulfamethoxazole. Am J Med Sci 311: 54, 1996.
41. Voelker JR, Cartwright-Brown D, Anderson S, et al: Comparison of loop diuretics in patients with chronic renal insufficiency. Kidney Int 32:522, 1987.
42. Van Olden RW, van Meyel JJM, Gerlag PGG: Sensitivity of residual nephrons to high dose furosemide described by diuretic efficiency. Eur J Clin Pharmacol 47:483, 1995.
43. Chaturvedi PR, O'Donnell JP, Nicholas JM, et al: Furosemide in congestive heart failure. Int J Clin Pharmacol Ther Toxicol 25:123, 1987.
44. Van Meyel JJM, Gerlag PG Smith P, et al: Absorption of high-dose furosemide (frusemide) in congestive heart failure. Clin Pharmacokinet 22:308, 1992.
45. Bailie GR, Grennan A, Waldek S: Bioavailability of bumetanide in grossly oedematous patients. Clin Pharmacokinet 12:440, 1987.
46. Brater DC, Day B, Burdette A, Anderson S: Bumetanide and furosemide in heart failure. Kidney Int 26:183, 1984.
47. Vasko MR, Cartwright DB, Knochel JP, et al: Furosemide absorption altered in decompensated congestive heart failure. Ann Intern Med 102:314, 1985.
48. Rudy DW, Voelker JR, Greene PK, et al: Loop diuretics for chronic renal insufficiency: A continuous infusion is more efficacious than bolus therapy. Ann Intern Med 115:360, 1991.
49. Lahan M, Regev A, Raanani P, et al: Intermittent administration of furosemide vs continuous infusion preceding a loading dose for congestive heart failure. Chest 102:725, 1992.
50. Sica DA, Gehr TW: Diuretic combinations in refractory oedema states: Pharmacokinetic-pharacodynamic relationships. Clin Pharmacokinet 30:229, 1996.
51. Epstein M, Leep BA, Hoffman DS, et al: Potentiation of furosemide by metolazone in refractory edema. Curr Ther Res 21: 656, 1997.
52. Olsen KH, Sigurd B: The supra-additive natriuretic effect of addition of quinethazone or bendroflumethiazide during long-term treatment with furosemide and spironolactone. Acta Med Scand 190:253, 1971.
53. Wollam GL, Tarazi RC, Bravo EL, et al: Diuretic potency of combined hydrochlorothazide and furosemide therapy in patients with azotemia. Am J Med 72:929, 1982.
54. Knauf H, Mutschler E: Diuretic effectiveness of hydrochlorothiazide and furosemide alone and in combination in chronic renal failure. J Cardiovasc Pharmacol 26:394, 1995.
55. Hammarlund MM, Odlind B, Paalzow LK: Acute tolerance to furosemide diuresis in humans: Pharmacokinetic-pharmacodynamic modeling. J Pharmacol Exp Ther 233:447, 1985.
56. Wakelkamp M, Alvan G, Gabrielsson J, et al: Pharmacodynamic modeling of furosemide tolerance after multiple intravenous administration. Clin Pharmacol Ther 60:75, 1996.
57. Almeshari K, Ahlstrom NG, Capraro FE, et al: A volume-independent component of postdiuretic sodium retention in humans. J Am Soc Nephrol 3:1878, 1993.
58. Wilcox CS, Mitch WE, Kelly RA, et al: Response of the kidney to furosemide. I: Effects of salt intake and renal compensation. J Lab Clin Med 102:450, 1983.
59. Kelly RA, Wilcox CS, Mitch WE, et al: Response of the kidney to furosemide. II: Effect of captopril on sodium balance. Kidney Int 24:233, 1983.
60. Wilcox CS, Guzman NJ, Mitch WE, et al: $Na^+$, $K^+$, and BP homeostasis in man during furosemide: Effects of prazosin and captopril. Kidney Int 31:135, 1987.
61. Petersen JS, Shalmi M, Abildgaard U, et al: Renal effects of $\alpha$-adrenoceptor blockage during furosemide diuresis in conscious rats. Pharmacol Toxicol 70:3, 1992.
62. Kaissling B, Stanton BA: Adaptation of distal tubule and collecting duct to increased sodium delivery. I: Ultrastructure. Am J Physiol 255:F1256, 1998.
63. Stanton BA, Kaissling B: Adaptation of distal tubule and collecting duct to increased Na delivery. II: $Na^+$ and $K^+$ transport. Am J Physiol 255:F1269, 1988.
64. Ellison DH, Velazquez H, Wright FS: Adaptation of the distal convoluted tubule of the rat: Structural and functional effects of diatary salt intake and chronic diuretic infusion. J Clin Invest 83:113, 1989.
65. Loon NR, Wilcox CS, Unwin RJ: Mechanism of impaired natriuretic response to furosemide during prolonged therapy. Kidney Int 36:682, 1989.
66. Kobayashi S, Clemmons DR, Nogami H, et al: Tubular hypertrophy due to work load induced by furosemide is associated with increases of IGF-1 and IGFBP-1. Kidney Int 47:818, 1995.
67. Scherger P, Wald H, Popopvitzer MM: Enhanced glomerular filtration and $Na^+$-$K^+$-ATPase with furosemide administration. Am J Physiol 252:F910, 1987.
68. Obermuller N, Bernstein PL, Udaquez H, et al: Expression of the thiazide-sensitive Na-Cl cotransporter in rat and human kidney. Am J Physiol 269:F900, 1995.
69. Beck FX, Olno A, Muller E, et al: Inhibition of angiotensin-converting enzyme modulates structural and functional adaptation to loop diuretic-induced diuresis. Kidney Int 52:36, 1997.
70. Suki WN: Diuretic resistance. Miner Electrolyte Metab 25:28, 1999.
71. Kramer BK, Duherfs G, Riegger GA: Diuretic treatment and diuretic resistance in heart failure. Am J Med 106:90, 1999.
72. Gennari FJ, Kassirer JP: Osmotic diuresis. N Engl J Med 291: 714, 1974.
73. Better OS, Rubenstein I, Winaver JM, et al: Mannitol revisited. Kidney Int 51:886, 1997.
74. Lewis MA, Arvan A: Mannitol and furosemide in the treatment of diuretic resistant edema in nephrotic syndrome. Arch Dis Child 80:184, 1999.
75. Powers SR, Boba A, Hostnik W, et al: Prevention of postoperative acute renal failure with mannitol in 100 cases. Surgery 55: 15, 1964.
76. Borges HF, Hocks J, Kjellstrand CM: Mannitol intoxication in patients with renal failure. Ann Intern Med 142:63, 1982.
77. Dorman HR, Sondheimer JN, Cadnapapornchai P: Mannitol-induced acute renal failure. Medicine 69:153, 1990.
78. Moreno M, Murphy C, Goldsmith C: Increase in serum potassium resulting from the administration of hypertonic mannitol and other solutions. J Lab Clin Med 73:291, 1969.

79. Priesig PA, Toto RD, Alpern RJ: Carbonic anhydrase inhibitors. Renal Physiol Biochem 10:136, 1987.
80. Dirks JH, Sutton RAL (eds): Diuretics. Philadelphia, WB Saunders, 1986.
81. Epstein DL, Grant WM: Carbonic anhydrase inhibitor side effects. Arch Ophthalmol 95:1378, 1977.
82. Chaperon DJ, Freebourne SF, Roddie RA: Influence of advanced age on the deposition of acetazolamide. Br J Clin Pharmacol 19:363, 1985.
83. Davis AR, Diggory P, Seward HC: Prevalence of chronic hypokalemia amongst elderly patients using acetazolamide and diuretics. Eye 9:381, 1995.
84. Fried TA, Kunau RT: Thiazide diuretics. In Dirkls JH, Sutton RAL (eds): Diuretics. Philadelphia, WB Saunders, 1986, p 66.
85. Freis ED: The efficacy and safety of diuretics in treating hypertension. Ann Intern Med 122:223, 1995.
86. Siegel D, Hulley SB, Black DM, et al: Diuretics serum and intracellular electrolyte levels, and ventricular arrhythmias in hypertensive men. JAMA 267:1083, 1992.
87. Martin BJ, Milligan K: Diuretic-associated hypomagnesemia in the elderly. Ann Intern Med 147:1768, 1987.
88. Gress TW, Nieto FJ, Shalar E, et al: Hypertension and antihypertensive therapy as risk factors for type 2 diabetes mellitus. N Engl J Med 342:905, 2000.
89. Spital A: Diuretic-induced hyponatremia. Am J Nephrol 19: 447, 1999.
90. Baglin A, Boulard JC, Hanslik T, et al: Metabolic adverse reactions to diuretics. Drug Safety 12:161, 1995.
91. Ruml LA, Gonzales G, Taylor R, et al: Effect of varying doses of potassium-magnesium citrate on thiazide-induced hypokalemia and magnesium loss. Am J Ther 6:45, 1999.
92. Fichman MP, Vorhers H, Kleeman CR, et al: Diuretic-induced hyponatremia. Ann Intern Med 75:853, 1971.
93. Ashouri OS: Severe diuretic-induced hyponatremia in the elderly. Arch Intern Med 146:1355, 1986.
94. Friedman E, Shadel M, Halkin H, et al: Thiazide-induced hyponatremia. Ann Intern Med 110:24, 1987.
95. Ashrof N, Locksley R, Arieff AI: Thiazide-induced hyponatremia associated with death or neurologic damage in outpatients. Am J Med 70:1163, 1981.
96. Szatalowicz VL, Miller PD, Lacher JW, et al: Comparative effects of diuretics on renal water excretion in hyponatremic edematous disorders. Clin Sci 62:235, 1982.
97. Quamme GA: Loop diuretics. In Dirks JH, Sutton RAL (eds): Diuretics. Philadelphia, WB Saunders, 1986, p 86.
98. Van Olden RW, Van Megel JJ, Gerlaz PG: Acute and long-term effects of therapy with high-dose furosemide in chronic hemodialysis. Am J Nephrol 12:351, 1992.
99. Schrier RW, Lehman D, Zacherle B, et al: Effect of furosemide on free water excretion in edematous patients with hyponatremia. Kidney Int 3:30, 1973.
100. Rybak LP: Ototoxicity of loop diuretics. Otolaryngol Clin North Am 26:829, 1993.
101. Dormans TP, van Mezel JJ, Gurlay PG, et al: Diuretic efficacy of high dose furosemide in severe heart failure: Bolus injection versus continuous infusion. J Am Coll Cardiol 28:376, 1996.
102. Gallagher KL, Jones JK: Furosemide-induced ototoxicity. Ann Intern Med 91:744, 1979.
103. Cooperman LB, Rubin IL: Toxicity of ethacrynic acid and furosemide. Am Heart J 85:831, 1973.
104. Rieck J, Halkin H, Almog S, et al: Urinary loss of thiamine is increased by low doses of furosemide in healthy volunteers. J Lab Clin Med 134:238, 1999.
105. Lubetsky A, Winauer J, Seligmann H, et al: Urinary thiamine excretion in the rat: Effects of furosemide, other diuretics and volume load. J Lab Clin Med 134:232, 1999.
106. Perazella MA: Crystal-induced acute renal failure. Am J Med 106:459, 1999.
107. Grossman E, Messenli FH, Goldbourt U: Does diuretic therapy increase the risk of renal cell carcinoma? Am J Cardiol 83: 1090, 1999.
108. Schnieder RT, Delles C: Renal cell carcinoma—should one restrict the use of diuretics? Nephrol Dial Transplant 14:1621, 1999.
109. Ghali JK, Cooper R, Ford E: Trends in hospitalization for heart failure. 1973–1986. Arch Intern Med 150:769, 1990.
110. Givertz MM: Underlying causes and survival in patients with heart failure. N Engl J Med 342:119, 2000.
111. 2000 Heart and Stroke Statistical Update. Dallas, American Heart Association, 1999.
112. Schrier RW, Abdallah JG, Weinberger HD, et al: Therapy of heart failure. Kidney Int 57:1418, 2000.
113. Gasch WH: Diagnosis and treatment of heart failure based on left ventricular systolic or diastolic dysfunction. JAMA 271: 1276, 1994.
114. Senni M, Triboillory CM, Rodeheffer RJ, et al: Congestive heart failure in the community: A study of all incident cases in Olmstead County, Minnesota in 1991. Circulation 98:2282, 1998.
115. Schrier RW: Pathogenesis of sodium and water retention in high output and low output cardiac failure, nephrotic syndrome, cirrhosis and pregnancy. N Engl J Med 319:1065, 1988.
116. Abraham WT, Part JD, Bristow MR: Neurohumoral receptors in the failing heart. In Poole-Wilson PA (ed): Heart Failure. Massie, Churchill Livingstone, 1997, p 127.
117. Schrier RW, Abraham WT: Hormones and hemodynamics in heart failure. N Engl J Med 341:577, 1999.
118. Van Veldhuisen DJ, Charlesworth A, Crijins HJ, et al: Differences in drug treatment of chronic heart failure between European countries. Eur Heart J 20:666, 1999.
119. Stampfer M, Epstein SE, Beiser GD, et al: Hemodynamic effects of diuresis at rest and during intense upright exercise in patients with impaired cardiac function. Circulation 37:900, 1968.
120. Lesch M, Caranasos GJ, Mulholland JR: Controlled study comparing ethacrynic acid to mercaptomerin in the treatment of acute pulmonary edema. N Engl J Med 279:115, 1968.
121. Kiely J, Kelly DT, Taylor DR, Pitt B: The role of furosemide in the treatment of left ventricular dysfunction associated with myocardial infarction. Circulation 48:581, 1973.
122. Nelson GI, Silke B, Forsythe DR, et al: Hemodynamic comparison of primary venous or arteriolar dilation and the subsequent effect of furosemide in left ventricular failure after acute myocardial infarction. Am J Cardiol 52:1036, 1983.
123. Nelson GI, Silke B, Ahuja RC, et al: Haemodynamic advantages of isosorbide dinitrate over furosemide in acute heart-failure following myocardial infarction. Lancet 1:730, 1983.
124. Franciosa JA, Silverstein SR: Hemodynamic effects of nitroprusside and furosemide in left ventricular failure. Clin Pharmacol Ther 32:62, 1982.
125. Ikram H, Chan W, Esponer EA, et al: Haemodynamic and hormone responses to acute and chronic furosemide therapy in congestive heart failure. Clin Sci 59:443, 1980.
126. Wilson JR, Reichek N, Dunkman WB, et al: Effect of diuresis on the performance of the failing left ventricle in man. Am J Med 70:235, 1981.
127. Dixon DW, Barwolf-Gohlke C, Gunnar RM: Comparative efficacy and safety of bumetanide and furosemide in long-term treatment of edema due to congestive heart failure. J Clin Pharmacol 21:680, 1981.
128. Konecke LL: Clinical trial of bumetanide versus furosemide in patients with congestive heart failure. J Clin Pharmacol 21: 688, 1981.
129. Viherkaski M, Huikko M, Vajoranta K: The effect of amiloride-hydrochlorothiazide combination versus furosemide plus supplementation in the treatment of edema of cardiac origin. Ann Clin Res 13:11, 1981.
130. Bayliss J, Norell M, Canepa-Anson R, et al: Untreated heart failure: Clinical and neuroendocrine effects of introducing diuretics. Br Heart J 57:17, 1987.
131. Freudenberg RS, Gottlieb SS, Robinson SW, et al: A four-part regimen for clinical heart failure. Hosp Pract 30:51, 1999.
132. Cohn JN: The management of chronic heart failure. N Engl J Med 335:490, 1996.
133. Pitt B, Zannad F, Remme WJ, et al: The effect of spironolactone on morbidity and mortality in patients with severe heart failure. N Engl J Med 341:709, 1999.
134. Weber KT: Aldosterone and spironolactone in heart failure. N Engl J Med 341:753, 1999.
135. Digitalis Investigation Group: The effect of digoxin on mortality and morbidity in patients with heart failure. N Engl J Med 336:525, 1997.

136. Anderson F, Mikkelsen E: Distribution, elimination and effect of furosemide in normal subjects and in patients with heart failure. Eur J Clin Pharmacol 12:15, 1977.
137. Greither A, Goldman S, Edelen JS, et al: Pharmacokinetics of furosemide in patients with congestive heart failure. Pharmacology 19:121, 1977.
138. Brater DC, Chennavasin P, Sewall R: Furosemide in patients with heart failure: Shift in dose-response curves. Clin Pharmacol Ther 28:182, 1986.
139. Perez J, Setar DS, Ogilvie RI: Kinetic disposition and diuretic effect of fursemide in acute pulmonary edema. Br J Clin Pharmacol 9:471, 1980.
140. Brater DC, Day B, Bardette A, et al: Bumetanide and furosemide in heart failure. Kidney Int 26:183, 1984.
141. Vasko MR, Cartwright DB, Knochel JP, et al: Furosemide absorption is altered in decompensated heart failure. Ann Intern Med 102:314, 1985.
142. Vargo DL, Brater DC, Rudy DW, et al: Dopamine does not enhance furosemide-induced natriuresis in patients with congestive heart failure. J Am Soc Nephrol 7:1032, 1996.
143. Oster JR, Epstein M, Smaller S: Combined therapy with thiazide-type and loop diuretic agents for resistant sodium retention. Ann Intern Med 99:405, 1983.
144. Sharpe N, Murphy J, Smith H, et al: Treatment of symptomless left ventricular dysfunction after myocardial infarction. Lancet 1:255, 1980.
145. Cody RJ: Diuretics in the management of congestive heart failure. Cardiologia 43:25, 1998.
146. Young JB, Gheorghiade M, Uretsky BF, et al: Superiority of "triple" drug therapy in heart failure: Insights from the PROVED and RADIANCE trials. J Am Coll Cardiol 32:686, 1998.
147. Abraham WT: Boblockers: The new standard of therapy for mild heart failure. Arch Intern Med 160:1237, 2000.
148. Dikshit K, Vyden JK, Forrester JS, et al: Renal and extrarenal hemodynamic effects of furosemide in congestive heart failure after myocardial infarction. N Engl J Med 228:1087, 1973.
149. Dormans TP, Gerlag PG, Russel FG, Smith P: Combination diuretic therapy in severe congestive heart failure. Drugs 55: 165, 1998.
150. Adams KF, Ellis ML, Williamson KM, Patterson JH: The AHCPR clinical practice guideline for heart failure revisited. Ann Pharmacol 31:1197, 1997.
151. Huonker M, Sarichter S, Schmidt-Trucksass A, et al: Effectiveness of digitoxin versus trichlormethiazide/amiloride in congestive heart failure, NYHA class II/III and sinus rhythm. Cardiovasc Drugs Ther 13:233, 1999.
152. Philbin EF, Cotto M, Rocco TA, et al: Association between diuretic use, clinical response, and death in heart failure. Am J Cardiol 80:519, 1997
153. Herrdink ER, Keufkens HG, Herinap RM, et al: NSAIDs associated with increased risk of congestive heart failure in elderly patients taking diuretics. Arch Intern Med 158:1108, 1998.
154. Agostini P, Marenzi G, Lauri G, et al: Sustained improvement in functional capacity after removal of body fluid with escalated ultrafiltration in chronic cardiac insufficiency: Failure of furosemide to provide the same result. Am J Med 96:191, 1994.
155. Marenzi GC, Lauri G, Guazzi M, et al: Ultrafiltration in moderate heart failure. Chest 108:94, 1995.
156. Gines P, Arroyo V, Rades J: Ascites and hepatorenal syndrome: Pathogenesis and treatment strategies. Ann Intern Med 1998; 43:99.
157. Palmer BF: Pathogenesis of ascites and renal salt retention in cirrhosis. J Invest Med 47:183, 1999.
158. Runyon BA: Management of adult patients with ascites caused by cirrhosis. Hepatology 27:264, 1998.
159. Bataller R, Arroyo V, Gines P: Management of ascites in cirrhosis. J Gastroenterol Hepatol 12:723, 1997.
160. Wilkinson SP: Treatment options for cirrhotic ascites. Eur J Gastroenterol Hepatol 10:1, 1998.
161. Brater DC: Use of diuretics in cirrhosis and nephrotic syndrome. Semin Nephrol 19:575, 1999.
162. Narayanan KV, Kamath PS: Managing the complications of cirrhosis. Mayo Clin Prac 75:501, 2000.
163. Martin P-Y, Gines P, Schrier RW: Nitric oxide as a mediator of hemodynamic abnormalities and sodium and water retention in cirrhosis. N Engl J Med 339:533, 1998.
164. Gines P: Incidence, predictive factors, and prognosis of the hepatorenal syndrome in cirrhosis with ascites. Gastroenterology 105:229, 1993.
165. Wood LJ, Massie D, McLean AJ, et al: Fluid retention in cirrhosis: Tubular site and relation to hepatic dysfunction. Hepatology 8:831, 1988.
166. LaVilla G, Salmeron JM, Arroyo V, et al: Mineralocorticoid escape in patients with compensated cirrhosis, and portal hypertension. Gastroenterology 102:2114, 1992.
167. Bernardi M, DiMarco C, Tevisani F, et al: Renal sodium retention during upright posture in preascitic cirrhosis. Gastroenterology 105:188, 1993.
168. Bichet DG, VanPatton VJ, Schrier RW: Potential role of increased sympathetic activity in impaired sodium and water excretion in cirrhosis. N Engl J Med 307:1552, 1982.
169. Bichet D, Szatolowicz V, Chamovitz C, et al: Role of vasopressin in abnormal water excretion in cirrhotic patients. Ann Intern Med 76:413, 1982.
170. Fernandez-Seara J, Prieto J, Queroga J, et al: Systemic and regional hemodynamics in patients with liver cirrhosis and ascites with and without functional renal failure. Gastroenterology 97:1304, 1987.
171. Wong F, Liu P, Tobe S, et al: Central blood volume in cirrhosis: Measurement with radionuclide angiography. Hepatology 19: 312, 1994.
172. Pockros PJ, Reynolds TB: Rapid diuresis in patients with ascites from chronic liver disease: The importance of pedal edema. Gastroenterology 90:1827, 1986.
173. Shear L, Chung S, Gabuzda GJ: Compartmentalization of ascites and edema in patients with hepatic cirrhosis. N Engl J Med 282:1391, 1970.
174. Fuller R, Happel C, Ingalls ST: Furosemide kinetics in patients with hepatic cirrhosis with ascites. Clin Pharmacol Ther 30: 461, 1981.
175. Villeneve JP, Veabeck RK, Wilkinson GR, et al: Furosemide kinetics and dynamics in patients with cirrhosis. Clin Pharmacol Ther 140:14, 1986.
176. Schwartz S, Brater DC, Pound D, et al: Bioavailability, pharmacokinetics and pharmacodynamics of torsemide in patients with cirrhosis. Clin Pharmacol Ther 54:90, 1993.
177. Gines P, Jiminez W, Arroyo V, et al: Atrial natriuretic factor in cirrhosis with ascites: Plasma levels, cardiac release and splanchnic extraction. Hepatology 8:636, 1988.
178. Carstons J, Grisein J, Jensen KT, et al: Renal effects of urodilatin infusion in patients with liver cirrhosis with and without ascites. J Am Soc Nephrol 9:1489, 1998.
179. Decios L, Gauthier A, Levy VG, et al: Comparison of six treatments of ascites in patients with liver cirrhosis: A clinical trial. Hepatogastroenterology 30:15, 1983.
180. Perez-Ayuso RM, Arroyo V, Planas R, et al: Randomized comparative study of efficacy of furosemide vs spironolactone in non-azotemic cirrhosis with ascites. Gastroenterology 84:961, 1988.
181. Ljubicic N, Kujundgic M, Banie M, et al: Predictive factors influencing the therapeutic response to diuretic treatment of ascites in nonazotemic cirrhosis patients. J Gastroenterol 33: 441, 1998.
182. Alexander WD, Branch RA, Levine DF, et al: The urinary sodium:potassium ratio and response to diuretics in resistant edema. Postgrad Med J 53:117, 1977.
183. Roberts LR, Kamath PS: Ascites and the hepatorenal syndrome: Pathophysiology and management. Mayo Clin Proc 71:874, 1996.
184. Chang SC, Chang HI, Chan FJ, et al: Therapeutic efficacy of diuretics and paracentesis on lung function in patients with non-alcoholic cirrhosis and tense ascites. J Hepatol 26:833, 1997.
185. Gentilini P, Casini-Raggi V, DiFiore G, et al: Albumin improves the response of diuretics in patients with cirrhosis and ascites: Results of a randomized, controlled trial. J Hepatol 30:639, 1999.
186. Blendis L, Wong F: Intravenous albumin with diuretics: Protein lessons to be learnt? J Hepatol 30:727, 1999.

187. Gines P, Arroyo V, Quintero E, et al: Comparison of paracentesis and diuretics in the treatment of cirrhosis with tense ascites: Results of randomized study. Gastroenterology 93:234, 1987.
188. Gines P, Tito LI, Arroyo V et al: Randomized comparative study of therapeutic paracentesis with and without intravenous albumin in cirrhosis. Gastroenterology 94:1493, 1988.
189. Lucas A, Garcia-Pagan JC, Bosch J, et al: Beneficial effects of intravenous albumin infusion on the hemodynamic and humoral changes after total paracentesis. Hepatology 22:753, 1997.
190. Forovzandeh B, Konicik F, Sheagren JN: Large-volume paracentesis in the treatment of cirrhotic patients with refractory ascites: The role of post paracentesis plasma volume expansion. J Clin Gastroenterol 22:207, 1996.
191. Vermeulen LC, Ratko TA, Erstand BL, et al: A paradigm for concensus: The University Hospital consortium guidelines for the use of albumin, nonprotein colloid and crystalloid solution. Arch Intern Med 155:373, 1995.
192. Peltekian KM, Wong F, Liu PP, et al: Cardiovascular, renal and neurohumoral responses to single large-volume paracentesis in patients with cirrhosis and diuretic-resistant ascites. Am J Gastroenterol 92:394, 1997.
193. Fernandez-Esparrach G, Guerara M, Sart P, et al: Diuretic requirements after therapeutic paracentesis in nonazotemic patients with cirrhosis. J Hepatol 26:614, 1997.
194. Stanley MM, Orchi S, Lee KK, et al: Peritoneovenous shunting as compared with medical treatment in patients with alcoholic cirrhosis and massive ascites. N Engl J Med 321:1632, 1989.
195. Gines P, Arroyo V, Vargas V, et al: Paracentesis with intravenous infusion of albumin as compared with peritoneovenous shunting in cirrhosis with refractory ascites. N Engl J Med 325: 829, 1991.
196. Martinet JD, Fenyves D, Legault L, et al: Treatment of refractory ascites using transjugular intrahepatic portosystemic shunt (TIPS): A caution. Dig Dis Sel 42:161, 1997.
197. Lebrec D, Giuily N, Hadengue A, et al: Transjugular intrahepatic portosystemic shunts: Comparison with paracentesis in patients with cirrhosis and ascites: A randomized trial. J Hepatol 25:135, 1996.
198. Lieberman FL, Reynolds TP: Renal failure with cirrhosis. Ann Intern Med 64:1221, 1966.
199. Greenway B, Johnson PA, Williams R: Control of malignant ascites with spironolactones. Br J Surg 1982;69:441
200. Pockros PJ, Esrason KT, Nguyen C, et al: Motilization of malignant ascites with diuretics is dependent on ascites fluid characteristics. Gastroenterology 103:1302, 1992.
201. Gough IR, Balderson GA: Malignant ascites: A comparison of peritoneovenous shunting and nonoperative management. Cancer 71:2377, 1993.
202. Roussel JG, Kroon BB, Hart GA: The Denver type shunt for peritoneovenous shunting of malignant ascites. Surg Gynecol Obstet 162:235, 1986.
203. Lee CW, Baciek G, Faught W: A survey of practice in management of malignant ascites. J Pain Symptom Manage 16:96, 1988.
204. Sonnerfeld T, Tyden G: Peritoneovenous shunts for malignant ascites. Acta Chir Scand 152:1171, 1986.
205. Wickremesekera SK. Stubbs RS: Peritoneovenous shunting for malignant ascites. N Engl Med J 110:33, 1997.
206. Orth SR, Ritz E: The nephrotic syndrome. N Engl J Med 1998; 338:1202.
207. Usberti M, Gazzotti RM, Pocisi C, et al: Considerations on the sodium retention in nephrotic syndrome. Am J Nephrol 15: 38, 1995.
208. Meltzer JI: Nephrotic syndrome: Vasoconstriction and hypervolemic types indicated by renin-sodium profiling. Ann Intern Med 71:688, 1979.
209. Glassock RJ: Management of intractable edema in nephrotic syndrome. Kidney Int 58(s):575, 1997.
210. Donkerwalcke RN, Vande Welle JG: Pathogenesis of edema formation in the nephrotic syndrome. Kidney Int 51:558, 1997.
211. Valentin JP, Qiu CG, Mildewing WP, et al: Cellular basis for blunted volume expansion natriuresis in experimental nephrotic syndrome. J Clin Invest 90:1302, 1992.
212. Valentin JP, Ying WZ, Sechi LA, et al: Phosphodiesterase inhibitors correct resistance to natriuretic peptides in rats with Hegmann nephritis. J Am Soc Nephrol 7:582, 1996.
213. Rane A, Villeneuve JP, Stone WJ, et al: Plasma binding and disposition of furosemide in the nephrotic syndrome and in uremia. Clin Pharmacol Ther 24:199, 1978.
214. Keller E, Hoppe-Seyler G, Schollmeyer P: Disposition and diuretic effect of furosemide in the nephrotic syndrome. Clin Pharmacol Ther 33:442, 1982.
215. Green TP, Mirkin BL: Resistance of proteinuric rats to furosemide: Urinary drug protein binding as a determinant of drug effect. Life Sci 26:623, 1980.
216. Green TP: Furosemide disposition in normal and proteinuric rats: Urinary drug-protein binding as a determinant of drug excretion. J Pharmacol Exp Ther 218:122, 1981.
217. Kirchner KA, Voelker JR, Brater DC: Intratubular albumin bunts the response of furosemide: A mechanism for diuretic resistance in the nephrotic syndrome. J Pharmacol Exp Ther 252:1097, 1990.
218. Herchner KA: Binding inhibitors restore furosemide potency in tubule fluid containing albumin. Kidney Int 40:418, 1991.
219. Herchner KA: Tubular resistance to furosemide contributes to the attenuated diuretic response in nephrotic rats. J Am Soc Nephrol 2:1201, 1992.
220. Grausz H, Lieberman R, Earley LE: Effect of plasma albumin on sodium reabsorption in patients with nephrotic syndrome. Kidney Int 1:47, 1972.
221. Nakahama H, Orita Y, Yamazaki M, et al: Pharmacokinetic and pharmacodynamic interactions between furosemide and hydrochlorothiazide in nephrotic patients. Nephrology 47: 223, 1988.
222. Harris A, Rado JP: Patterns of potassium wasting in response to stepwise combinations of diuretics in nephrotic syndrome. Int J Clin Pharmacol Ther 37:332, 1999.
223. Gansevoort RT, Hemmelder MH: Antiproteinuric effect of blood pressure–lowering agents: A meta-analyses of comparative results. Nephrol Dial Transplant 10:1963, 1995.
224. Hemmelder MH, de Zeewiv D, Gansevoort RT, et al: Blood pressure reduction initiates the antiproteinuric effect of ACE inhibition. Kidney Int 49:174, 1996.
225. Weidmann P, Baehlen LM, deCourten M: Effects of different antihypertensive drugs on human diabetic proteinuria. Nephrol Dial Transplant 8:582, 1993.
226. Ruggenenti P, Mosconi L, Vendramin G, et al: ACE inhibition improves glomerular size selectively in patients with idiopathic membranous nephropathy and persistent nephrotic syndrome. Am J Kidney Dis 35:381, 2000.
227. Lemieux G, Beauchemin M, Gaugoux A, et al: Treatment of nephrotic edema with bumetanide. Can Med Assoc 125:1111, 1981.
228. Lau K: Effectiveness of bumetanide in nephrotic syndrome: A double-blind crossover study with furosemide. J Clin Pharmacol 20:489, 1976.
229. Marone C, Reubi FC: Effect of a new diuretic (piretanide) compared with furosemide on renal diluting and concentrating mechanisms in patients with the nephrotic syndrome. Eur J Clin Pharmacol 17:165, 1980.
230. Keller E, Hoppe-Seyler G, Schollmeyer D: Disposition and diuretic effect of furosemide in the nephrotic syndrome. Clin Pharmacol Ther 12:442, 1982.
231. Smith DE, Hyneck ML, Berardi RR, et al: Urinary protein binding, kinetics and dynamics of furosemide in nephrotic patients. J Pharm Sci 74:603, 1985.
232. Shapiro MD, Hasbargen J, Henson J, et al: Role of aldosterone in the sodium retention of patients with nephrotic syndrome. Am J Nephrol 10:44, 1990.
233. Garin EH, Richard GA: Edema resistant to furosemide therapy in nephrotic syndrome: Treatment with furosemide and metolazone. Int J Pediatric Nephrol 2:181, 1981.
234. Sica DA, Gehr TW: Diuretic combinations in refractory edema states: Pharmacokinetic-pharmacodynamic relationships. Clin Pharmacokinet 30:229, 1996.
235. Inoue A, et al: Mechanisms of furosemide resistance in analbuminemic rats and hypoalbuminemic patients. Kidney Int 32: 198, 1987.
236. Luetscher JA, Hall AD, Kramer VL: Treatment of nephrosis with concentrated human serum albumin. J Clin Invest 29: 896, 1950.

237. Davidson AM, Lambrie AT, Verth AH, et al: Salt-poor human albumin in management of nephrotic syndrome. BMJ 1:481, 1974.
238. Koomans HA, Geers AB, Meriracker AH, et al: Effects of plasma volume expansion on renal salt handling in patients with the nephrotic syndrome. Am J Nephrol 4:227, 1984.
239. Dorhout Mees EJ: Does it make sense to administer albumin to the patient with nephrotic edema? Nephrol Dial Transplant 11:1221, 1996.
240. Fliser D, Zurbruggen I, Mulschler E, et al: Coadministration of albumin and furosemide in patients with the nephrotic syndrome. Kidney Int 55:629, 1999.
241. Arroyo V, Bosch J, Casamitjana R, et al: Use of piretanide, a new loop diuretic, in cirrhosis with ascites. Gut 21:855, 1980.

CHAPTER 18

# Salt-Wasting Disorders

David H. Ellison, MD

*Renal salt wasting* connotes inappropriate sodium and chloride losses in the urine. Because salt (used here to indicate sodium chloride [NaCl]) excretion is determined largely by the extracellular fluid (ECF) volume and mean arterial pressure, the term *renal salt wasting* indicates that renal salt excretion continues at an ECF volume at which renal salt excretion normally ceases. Yet renal salt wasting does not necessarily imply unrelenting renal salt losses. Recent experimental results have clarified the nature of renal salt wasting and emphasize that earlier definitions of the syndrome were often incomplete. For example, the diagnosis of renal salt wasting was thought to require persistent sodium and chloride losses in the face of symptomatic ECF volume depletion. Yet genetic disruption of several renal ion transport proteins, in either humans or experimental animals, leads to subtle salt-wasting disorders that are not associated with unremitting salt losses or even with easily perceptible ECF volume depletion. These are often of considerable clinical importance. To aid in understanding salt-wasting disorders, it is useful first to consider some aspects of normal salt homeostasis. Cellular and molecular details of salt transport physiology in the kidney are beyond the scope of this chapter.

## PHENOMENOLOGY OF NORMAL SALT HOMEOSTASIS

The rate at which kidneys excrete NaCl is related to the ECF volume and the blood pressure. Although the nature of the relation between ECF volume and urinary NaCl excretion has been debated, Walser argued that human urinary NaCl excretion, at steady state, is a *linear function* of the ECF volume.[1] When the ECF volume declines below a critical threshold value (called by some the set point), renal salt excretion ceases. The relation between salt excretion and ECF volume describes a "renal function curve," as shown in Figure 18–1*A*. Because this model describes steady-state conditions, it implies that urinary NaCl excretion is linearly related to dietary NaCl intake, as well as to ECF volume. This is an intuitively satisfying corollary. According to this model, the term *salt wasting* implies that the renal function curve is shifted downward (see Fig. 18–1*A*). Guyton demonstrated that renal salt excretion determines the mean arterial pressure.[2] According to a related but distinct analysis, the relation between mean arterial pressure and urinary salt excretion at steady state is also nearly linear through a wide range of dietary salt intake. This defines a different but closely related renal function curve.[2] According to *this* model, salt-wasting disorders are those in which urinary salt excretion persists at blood pressures below normal, or when the renal function curve is shifted downward.

These models are essentially phenomenologic and do not provide specific insight into physiologic control mechanisms. Both models, however, have been corroborated by experimental data and accurately describe renal salt homeostasis under many conditions. They also have interesting implications for understanding renal salt-wasting disorders. For example, the slope of the relation between ECF volume and renal salt excretion determines the speed with which an individual can adapt to a change in dietary intake (Fig. 18–2). The slope appears to be reduced by chronic renal failure and by aging.[3] This means that it takes longer for the kidney to adapt to a change in dietary NaCl intake when renal function is compromised or an individual is aged. Thus, if dietary salt intake is reduced suddenly, ECF volume will decline more slowly in older individuals and in individuals with chronic renal failure than in younger individuals with normal renal function. Salt wasting resulting from chronic renal failure is discussed later. Surprisingly, a reduced slope of the relation between ECF volume and dietary NaCl intake also predicts that the ECF volume will be elevated when the dietary NaCl intake is normal or high in such patients.[4] This is precisely the response observed when the dietary NaCl intake of individuals suffering from chronic renal failure is varied. When dietary salt intake is abundant, the blood pressure is usually elevated. When dietary salt intake is restricted suddenly, however, salt wasting ensues.

Another important implication of the relation between ECF volume (or mean arterial pressure) and renal salt excretion is that salt wasting may be present despite a preserved ability to reduce urinary salt excretion to negligible levels. A downward shift in the renal function curve (see Fig. 18–1) does not mean that urinary salt excretion cannot fall to negligible levels. Clinical and experimental examples of salt-wasting disorders in which urinary NaCl excretion is very low are discussed later. The observation indicates that the diagnosis of salt wasting relies on the ability to estimate the ECF volume precisely. Because such determinations are nearly always imprecise clinically, the diagnosis of subtle renal salt wasting may be difficult.

## CLINICAL SALT-WASTING SYNDROMES

Depending on their severity and the clinical setting, salt-wasting disorders may present as unrelenting poly-

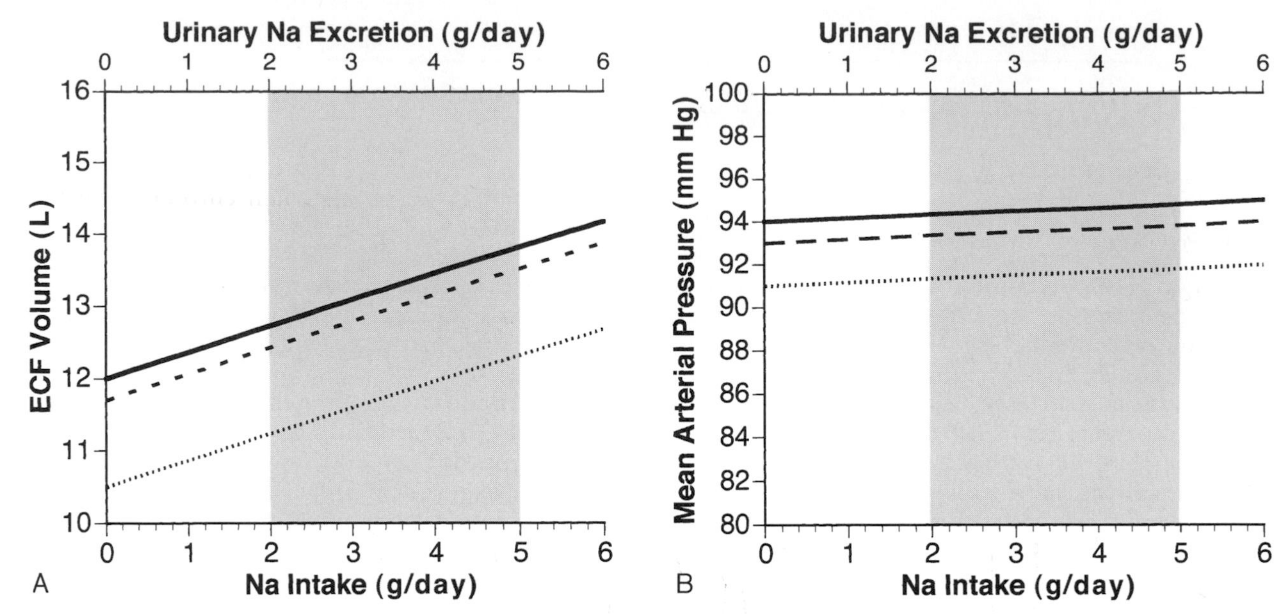


**FIGURE 18–1** ■ Renal function curves. *A,* The relationship is shown between extracellular fluid volume and dietary NaCl intake at steady state, as demonstrated by Walser.[1] Because steady state conditions apply, the data also describe the relationship between urinary NaCl excretion and extracellular fluid volume. The gray areas represent typical salt intakes. *B,* The relationship is shown between dietary NaCl intake and mean arterial blood pressure, as demonstrated by Guyton.[2] *A* and *B,* The *solid line* represents normal individuals. The *dashed line* indicates an individual with mild salt wasting. The *dotted line* depicts an individual with massive salt wasting. Note that an individual with mild salt wasting can reduce urinary salt excretion to very low levels with only a very modest reduction in extracellular fluid volume.

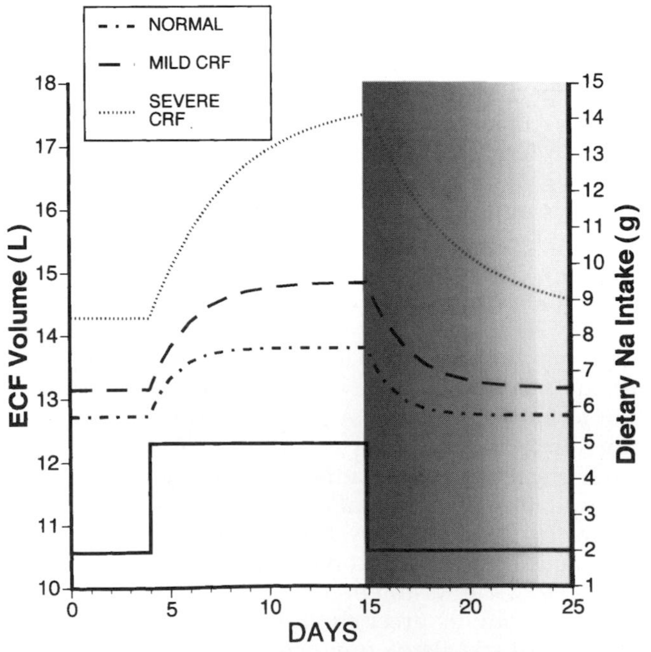


**FIGURE 18–2** ■ Effects of dietary salt intake on extracellular fluid volume in individuals with normal and abnormal renal function. Data extrapolated from Walser.[1] When dietary salt intake (indicated by the *solid line*) is reduced, urinary salt intake declines rapidly in normal individuals. The *shaded area* represents the period of negative salt balance. In patients with mild or severe chronic renal failure, there is a prolonged time necessary to achieve steady-state conditions when dietary NaCl intake is reduced (compare the shapes of the curves).

uria with extreme depletion of the ECF volume, leading rapidly to death, or as mild but troubling syndromes in which depletion of the ECF volume is nearly undetectable. Several clinical features, however, are typical of most salt-wasting disorders. These features include malaise, lassitude, fatigability, and salt craving. When mild, these symptoms can be subtle enough to cause diagnostic difficulty.

One classification of salt-wasting disorders is shown in Tables 18–1 and 18–2. According to this scheme, salt wasting can be classified as either inherited or acquired. A great deal of progress has been made during the past 10 years in understanding the physiologic basis of inherited salt-wasting disorders. Our understanding of acquired salt-wasting disorders is less complete.

## Acquired Salt-Wasting Disorders

### RENAL DISEASE

#### *Chronic Renal Failure*

**Physiologic Salt Wasting.** The phenomenon of salt wasting resulting from chronic renal failure was first described by Peters and colleagues.[5] Later, the term *salt-wasting nephritis* was proposed to characterize the minority of patients with chronic renal failure who lose large amounts of NaCl in their urine. The majority of patients with chronic renal failure have only a modest tendency to waste salt; they cannot reduce urinary NaCl excretion promptly during dietary salt restriction (see Fig. 18–2) but usually are volume replete when

**TABLE 18–1.** Acquired Salt-Wasting Disorders

- I. Renal
  - A. Chronic renal failure
    - 1. Physiologic
    - 2. Massive
      - a. Interstitial kidney disease
      - b. Other
  - B. Post–acute renal failure
  - C. Postobstructive
  - D. Renal tubular acidosis
- II. Extrarenal
  - A. Mineralocorticoid deficiency
    - 1. Addison disease
    - 2. Isolated hypoaldosteronism
    - 3. Hyporeninemic hypoaldosteronism
  - B. Natriuretic peptide mediated
    - 1. Cerebral salt wasting
    - 2. Syndrome of inappropriate antidiuretic hormone
- III. Drug induced
  - A. Solute diuresis
    - 1. Mannitol
    - 2. Urea
    - 3. Glucose
    - 4. Bicarbonate
  - B. Diuretics
    - 1. Proximal
    - 2. Loop
    - 3. Distal convoluted tubule
    - 4. Cortical collecting tubule

**TABLE 18–2.** Inherited Salt-Wasting Disorders

- I. Renal ion transport defects
  - A. Bartter syndrome
    - 1. Type I (*SLC12A1*; #600839)
    - 2. Type II (*KCNJ1*; #600359)
    - 3. Type III (*CLCNKB*; #602023)
    - 4. Type IV
  - B. Gitelman syndrome (*SLC12A3*; #263800)
  - C. Pseudohypoaldosteronism (PHA) type I
    - 1. PHA I*e* (*SCNN1*; #264350)
    - 2. PHA I*x*
- II. Mineralocorticoid receptor defects
  - A. PHA type I*mr* (*MLR*; #177735)
- III. Hypoaldosteronism
  - A. Adrenal hyperplasia
    - 1. Type I (*StAR*; #201710)
    - 2. Type II (*HSD3B2*; #20180)
    - 3. Type III (*CYP21*; #201910)
  - B. Aldosterone deficiency
    - 1. Type I (corticosterone methyl oxidase deficiency type I) (*CYP11B2*; #203400)
    - 2. Type II (corticosterone methyl oxidase deficiency type II) (*CYP11B2; #124080)*
- IV. Addison disease
  - A. X-linked (*NROB1*; #30020)
  - B. Recessive (*AIRE*; #240200)
- V. Inherited kidney disease
  - A. Juvenile nephronophthisis (NPH)
    - 1. NPH 1 (*NPH1*; #256100)
    - 2. NPH 2 (*NPH2*; #602088)
    - 3. NPH 3 (*NPH3*; #604387)
  - B. Medullary cystic kidney disease (MCKD)
    - 1. MCKD 1 (*MCKD1*; #174000)
    - 2. MCKD 2 (*MCKD2*; #603860)

Mendelian syndromes are followed by the gene symbol and by the Online Mendelian Inheritance in Man number (#).

consuming a typical diet. These patients do not usually manifest symptoms of salt wasting unless an intercurrent illness develops or dietary salt intake is reduced suddenly. Four theories have been advanced to explain this salt-wasting tendency.

*First,* natriuresis may result from an increased osmotic load per nephron. When chronic renal failure occurs, the osmotic load (600 to 1000 mOsm/day) is excreted by fewer functional nephrons. Thus, when the glomerular filtration rate declines from the normal 120 mL/min to 12 mL/min in a typical human, the number of osmoles excreted *per nephron* increases from 0.7 nmol/day to 7 nmol/day. This increased osmotic load should lead to an osmotic diuresis, thereby impairing renal salt conservation. Evidence in favor of an osmotic mechanism was obtained by Coleman and coworkers,[6] who compared the effects of a water diuresis in individuals with normal renal function and in those with chronic renal failure. In normal individuals consuming a salt-restricted diet, a water diuresis does not increase urinary salt excretion, because the urinary sodium concentration declines to very low levels. In contrast, in humans with chronic renal failure, the urinary sodium concentration does not decline to the same extent during a water diuresis; therefore, urinary sodium excretion rises along with urine volume. These workers showed that administering mannitol (an osmotic diuretic) to normal volunteers could mimic the situation in chronic renal failure; in this case, a water diuresis superimposed on a mannitol diuresis led to increments in urinary sodium excretion.[6]

The urinary osmoles that are believed to contribute to the salt-wasting tendency of chronic renal failure include urea, sodium sulfate, sodium phosphate, sodium urate, and sodium creatinine. Urea, which is the most important, is a "conditional" osmole in the urine. It is osmotically active only when the urinary electrolyte concentration is low,[7] as in the patients studied by Coleman ingesting a low-salt diet. In contrast, when urinary electrolyte concentrations are higher, urinary urea does not induce an osmotic diuresis.[7]

Despite the contribution of osmotic effects to the salt-wasting tendency of chronic renal failure, other factors probably play roles as well. None of these mechanisms is mutually exclusive, and several probably participate importantly. The *second* mechanism by which renal failure leads to salt wasting involves compensatory adaptations that occur in chronic renal disease. Chronic renal failure is usually viewed as resulting from a reduced number of functioning nephrons (the "intact nephron" hypothesis).[8] When the number of nephrons is reduced, the single-nephron glomerular filtration rate of the remaining nephrons increases. An increased single-nephron glomerular filtration rate increases sodium delivery to the proximal tubule. This increased sodium delivery leads to an increased sodium reabsorption along the nephron (the phenomenon of glomerulotubular balance).[9] Although glomerulotubular balance tends to return urinary salt excretion to normal when the single-nephron glomerular filtration rate increases, it does not do so completely, and some excess sodium may escape reabsorption.[10]

A *third* mechanism for salt wasting in chronic renal failure involves damage to the kidney tubules, leading to defective salt transport. This mechanism is probably most prominent when massive salt wasting (discussed later) results from tubulointerstitial or medullary cystic disease. In this case, salt wasting is often associated with hyperkalemia and hyponatremia, suggesting Addison disease, but these patients do not respond to exogenous mineralocorticoid hormones. Thus, severe damage to the renal medulla can lead to massive salt wasting owing to damage to the distal nephron.

A *fourth* mechanism involves adaptive changes in transport capacity. According to Danovitch and colleagues,[11] many cases of salt wasting associated with chronic renal failure are reversible if the dietary salt deprivation is imposed gradually. According to this scenario, the kidney must adapt to maintain salt excretion when renal failure develops gradually. This adaptation may result from mild ECF volume expansion, from hypertension, or from other undetermined factors. Regardless of its cause, the adaptation leads to decreased expression or activity of renal salt transporters. When dietary salt is restricted suddenly, the kidney cannot increase the density of salt transporters rapidly enough to compensate, and salt wasting ensues. Evidence in favor of this mechanism includes the description of a patient with Crohn disease who developed chronic renal failure owing to polycystic kidney disease. Because of ongoing NaCl losses via an ileostomy, the patient remained relatively volume contracted; in this setting, the urine sodium concentration remained less than 5 mM, indicating minimal salt wasting.[12] Experimental support for this theory was obtained by Kwon and colleagues,[13] who detected decreases in the expression of the $Na^+$-$H^+$ exchanger-3 (NHE-3), the apical sodium phosphate cotransporter (NaPi-II), and $Na^+,K^+$ ATPase in the cortex of kidneys from animals with chronic renal failure. Although these changes were not detected when transport protein density was examined per remnant nephron, they contrasted markedly with the behavior of sodium transport proteins that are expressed along the distal nephron. The total kidney expression of the thiazide- and bumetanide-sensitive transporters of the distal convoluted tubule and thick ascending limb, respectively, was *unchanged* by chronic renal failure (whereas proximal transporters were decreased). These workers concluded that the findings reflect an increased distal salt delivery resulting from a decrease in proximal salt reabsorption. This glomerulotubular "imbalance" may contribute to the salt-wasting tendency of chronic renal failure.[13]

**Massive Salt Wasting.** Massive salt wasting is a devastating complication of chronic renal disease that can lead to cardiovascular collapse and death (Fig. 18–3). In contrast to the mild salt wasting described earlier, patients with this disorder waste salt even when consuming a high-salt diet. Thorn and colleagues described two patients who presented with progressive volume depletion, hemoconcentration, lassitude, and eventually shock.[14] The patients were shown to have chronic renal failure and massive salt wasting. The adrenal glands were normal, and adrenal hormone replacement was not effective. The authors coined the term *salt-losing nephritis* to describe this syndrome. Enticknap found that chronic interstitial nephritis (also called chronic pyelonephritis), a disease primarily of the renal medulla, was responsible for most cases of massive salt wasting.[15] Many patients also demonstrate cystic changes in the renal medulla,[16] although inherited medullary cystic disease (described later) can present in a similar manner and might be confused with this entity clinically.

Patients typically present with weakness and tiredness, together with polyuria and nocturia. Hundreds of millimoles of NaCl may be lost in the urine daily.[17] The clinical presentation resembles that of Addison disease, with hyponatremia, hyperkalemia, hypotension, and lassitude. Many patients develop a hyperpig-

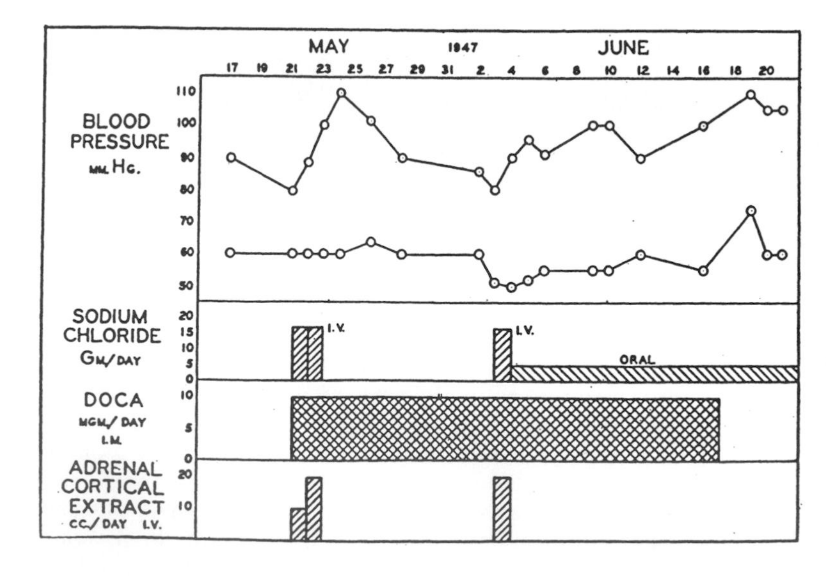


**FIGURE 18–3** ■ Salt-losing nephritis. Ineffectiveness of desoxycorticosterone acetate in oil on salt reabsorption and blood pressure in a patient with renal failure and salt wasting. (From Sawyer WH, Solez C: Salt-losing nephritis simulating adrenocortical insufficiency. N Engl J Med 240:210–215, 1949, with permission.)

mented appearance resembling that typical of Addison disease.[16] The blood urea nitrogen is elevated, often out of proportion to the creatinine, suggesting a prerenal component to the azotemia, but volume repletion does not correct the renal failure. Four criteria for the diagnosis of massive salt wasting associated with renal failure were described many years ago and remain valid.[18] They are (1) signs and symptoms consistent with ECF volume depletion; (2) low serum sodium and chloride levels on a normal salt intake, relieved by increasing dietary salt intake to 10 to 20 g/day; (3) unresponsiveness to exogenous fludrocortisone with normal rates of 17-ketosteroid excretion; and (4) evidence of renal disease with a low urinary specific gravity, elevated blood urea nitrogen and creatinine, and polyuria, all persistent on a high-salt diet. Although this disorder is well characterized, a relatively limited number of cases have been described in the literature, and the syndrome is encountered only rarely today.[16,19–29]

Many patients with massive salt wasting and renal failure have tubulointerstitial disease, as noted earlier, and often medullary calcifications. Among the disorders reported to lead to salt wasting are the milk-alkali syndrome and hyperparathyroidism.[30–33] Patients with the milk-alkali syndrome can develop profound ECF volume depletion owing to salt wasting, but renal salt wasting often improves following correction of the alkalosis and hypercalcemia. Thus, once the calcium and acid-base disorders are corrected, patients retain salt normally, falsely suggesting that depletion of the ECF volume does not result from renal salt wasting. Other interstitial renal conditions also lead to salt wasting on occasion. These include multiple myeloma,[34] analgesic nephropathy,[35] kidney transplantation,[36] and amyloidosis.[37] Many of these have been associated with nephrocalcinosis.

Obstructive uropathy can lead to a salt-losing tendency, as discussed later, but the syndrome occurs most commonly in children when acute pyelonephritis complicates the obstruction. In this case, the presentation is often confused with pseudohypoaldosteronism or adrenal hyperplasia (see later), two other salt-wasting diseases of infancy.[38, 39] In one series, 52 episodes of pyelonephritis were evaluated in 50 children.[40] A salt-losing syndrome was recognized in 17. All these children had severe urinary tract anomalies. Infants with pyelonephritis without urinary malformations did not manifest the salt-losing syndrome. It is important to seek this diagnosis in salt-wasting infants, because the renal dysfunction and salt wasting are reversible with appropriate treatment.

#### *Acute Tubular Necrosis*

Renal salt wasting has been observed during recovery from acute tubular necrosis, perhaps related to persistent tubular dysfunction. Although this phenomenon engendered a great deal of interest shortly after acute tubular necrosis was defined as a syndrome, it is now believed that most early reports reflected elimination of *excess* salt and water because of excessive solute and water administration during oliguria.[41] This was suggested because the magnitude of the salt loss correlates with the amount of salt retained during oliguria.[42] Another cause may be the osmotic effects of retained solutes, such as urea. Although most patients recovering from acute tubular necrosis do not develop profound salt wasting, this does not indicate that salt homeostasis is normal in this setting. Several groups have shown that experimental postischemic acute tubular necrosis decreases the expression of sodium transport proteins in the kidney (Fig. 18–4). Proximal injury leads to loss of normal polarization of cells and a redistribution of $Na^+,K^+$ ATPase to the apical membrane.[43, 44] Between 1 and 5 days after an ischemic insult, expression of $Na^+,K^+$ ATPase, NHE-3, NaPi-II, the apical $Na^+$-$K^+$-$2Cl^-$ cotransporter (NKCC2), and the thiazide-sensitive transporter (NCC) are all reduced.[45–48] These reductions in transport gene and protein expression are associated with increases in fractional sodium excretion, as well as activation of the tubuloglomerular feedback mechanism. They may contribute to a moderate tendency to waste salt during recovery from acute tubular necrosis.

Few authors provide specific recommendations for water and salt replacement during the recovery phase of oliguric acute tubular necrosis. Some continue to suggest that such patients may be at risk for ECF volume depletion owing to a tendency toward salt wasting.[49] Others suggest that this rarely occurs.[17, 50] Swann and Merrill, who originally observed that salt wasting after acute tubular necrosis most commonly reflects excessive salt and water administration, recommended that 75 mmol of NaCl be administered daily during recovery from acute tubular necrosis.[42]

#### *Postobstructive Salt Wasting*

Urine output is frequently high following relief of urinary tract obstruction. As discussed earlier with respect to acute tubular necrosis, much of the increased salt and water excretion following relief of urinary tract obstruction results from ECF volume expansion and from the osmotic effects of retained solutes.[51] Salt wasting to the point of cardiovascular collapse following relief of urinary tract obstruction is therefore unusual.[52, 53] Nevertheless, urinary tract obstruction can lead to salt wasting. In experimental models of obstruction, defects in proximal and distal sodium transport have been observed.[54] Salt wasting may be a greater problem in infants, especially when complicated by pyelonephritis. Terzi and colleagues studied infants undergoing surgical correction of congenital obstructive disease and found persistently elevated rates of urinary salt excretion.[55] Serum aldosterone concentrations were elevated both before and after surgery, indicating ECF volume depletion rather than expansion. Several infants required saline infusion to correct hyperkalemic volume depletion. When excessive volume losses are observed following relief of urinary tract obstruction, some authors advocate administration of half normal saline at 50% of the urine output.[56]

#### *Renal Tubular Acidosis*

Both proximal (type 2) and distal (type 1) renal tubular acidosis (RTA) may be associated with salt

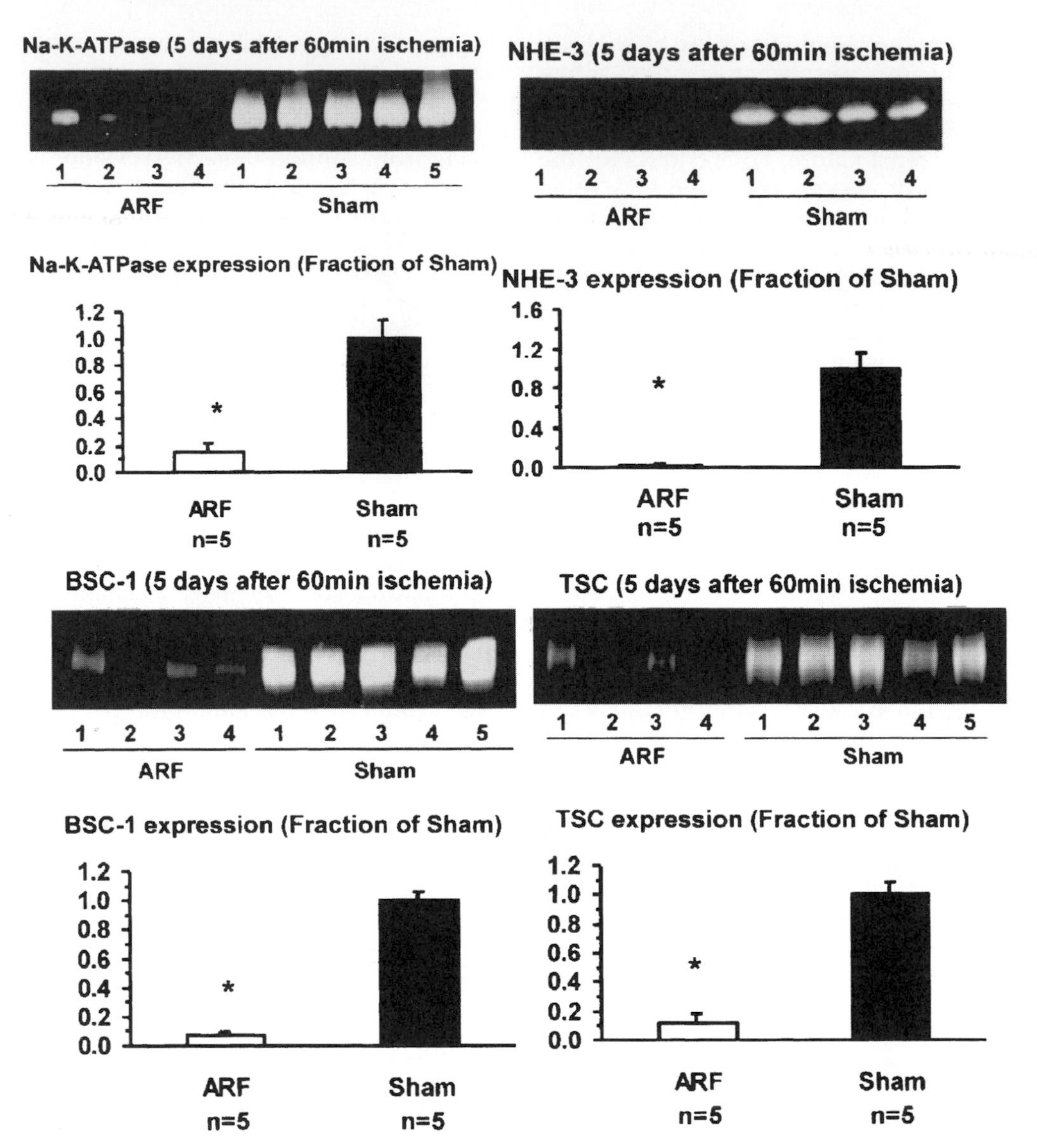


**FIGURE 18–4** ■ Effects of ischemia and reperfusion on expression of sodium transporters. Following ischemia, the expression of the Na/H exchanger (NHE3), the Na-phosphate cotransporter (NaPiII), the bumetanide-sensitive Na-K-2C cotransporter (BSC1 or NKCC2), and the thiazide-sensitive Na-Cl cotransporter (TSC or NCC) are all reduced compared with the control. (Adapted from Kwon et al[235] with permission.)

wasting. Type 4 RTA, although part of the spectrum of hyporeninemic hypoaldosteronism, does not usually present with salt wasting.

Proximal RTA is associated with losses of sodium and bicarbonate in the urine, owing to deficient proximal sodium bicarbonate ($NaHCO_3$) reabsorption. Increased distal $NaHCO_3$ delivery overwhelms the distal nephron's capacity for reabsorption, leading to increased sodium and bicarbonate excretion. Sodium wasting occurs only when the serum bicarbonate is normal, because sodium wasting is directly dependent on increased distal delivery.[57] Thus, patients who present with acidosis and a low urine pH generally do not waste sodium.[58] Although treatment of proximal RTA is difficult, because oral bicarbonate is rapidly excreted, sufficient correction of metabolic abnormalities by $NaHCO_3$ can be achieved to normalize growth.[59]

Distal (type 1) RTA is also associated with salt wasting. As with proximal RTA, the salt wasting is usually not severe enough to cause cardiovascular collapse,[60] but it can be demonstrated following sudden dietary salt restriction and may contribute to salt craving.[60] Correction of acidosis ameliorates salt wasting in many patients with distal RTA.[60] Some investigators, however, suggest that a defect in sodium reabsorption persists after correction of the acidosis.[61] This would be consistent with a more generalized disorder of distal nephron function. A mendelian dominant form of distal RTA was shown to result from mutations in the anion exchanger *AE1*.[62, 63] The mechanisms by which such mutations lead to salt wasting remain to be elucidated.

Treatment of salt wasting and acidosis in patients with type 1 RTA is relatively straightforward. Sodium bicarbonate can be administered (1 to 1.5 mmol/kg/day). Bicarbonate can be administered as sodium or potassium salt, because the salt wasting resolves following correction of the acidosis. Alternatively, Shohl solution can be used (1 mL of Shohl solution provides 1 mmol of bicarbonate). Shohl solution is often better tolerated than is $NaHCO_3$.

## EXTRARENAL DISEASE

### *Mineralocorticoid Deficiency*

Addison disease is adrenocortical insufficiency, but the disease can present with symptoms of glucocorticoid, mineralocorticoid, or androgen deficiency.[64] Patients with secondary or tertiary adrenal insufficiency usually have normal mineralocorticoid function and therefore do not waste salt (see later). In contrast, patients with primary Addison disease often develop salt wasting as the predominant manifestation. In this case, the disease has an insidious onset, leading to diagnosis only when an adrenal crisis occurs.[64, 65] Clinical findings, shown in Table 18–3, include malaise, lassitude, fatigability that is worsened by exertion, weakness, anorexia, and weight loss. Gastrointestinal symptoms—usually nausea, vomiting, abdominal pain, and constipation—are common. Hypoglycemia can occur after prolonged fasting, most commonly in infants and children. Hyperpigmentation is present in nearly all patients with primary adrenal insufficiency. It is caused in part by increased melanin in the skin, owing to the melanocyte-stimulating activity of plasma adrenocorticotropic hormone (ACTH). These symptoms are nonspecific and do not distinguish Addison disease from other syndromes associated with hyponatremia and weakness (see later).

**TABLE 18–3.** Clinical Manifestations of Adrenal Insufficiency

| Manifestation | Frequency (%) |
|---|---|
| **Symptom** | |
| Weakness, tiredness, fatigue | 100 |
| Anorexia | 100 |
| Gastrointestinal symptoms | 92 |
| Nausea | 86 |
| Vomiting | 75 |
| Constipation | 33 |
| Abdominal pain | 31 |
| Diarrhea | 16 |
| Salt craving | 16 |
| Postural dizziness | 12 |
| Muscle or joint pains | 6–13 |
| **Sign** | |
| Weight loss | 100 |
| Hyperpigmentation | 94 |
| Hypotension (systolic blood pressure <110 mmHg) | 88–94 |
| Vitiligo | 10–20 |
| Auricular calcification | 5 |
| **Laboratory Abnormality** | |
| Electrolyte disturbances | |
| Hyponatremia | 92 |
| Hyperkalemia | 88 |
| Hypercalcemia | 64 |
| Azotemia | 6 |
| Anemia | 55 |
| Eosinophilia | 40 |

Adrenal crisis can occur when a patient suffering from Addison disease has acute stress, or it can occur after bilateral adrenal infarction or hemorrhage. The most important manifestation of adrenal crisis is shock, although hypoglycemia can also occur. The major symptoms of an adrenal crisis result from mineralocorticoid deficiency and salt wasting, and the major clinical problem is hypotension. Thus, adrenal crisis can occur in patients who are receiving synthetic glucocorticoids if their mineralocorticoid requirements are not met.[66, 67] Adrenal crisis often presents as shock in a previously undiagnosed patient with primary adrenal insufficiency subjected to a major stress. It can also occur in a patient with known adrenal insufficiency who does not take more glucocorticoid during a bacterial infection or other major illness. Two other common symptoms are abdominal tenderness and fever. The cause is unknown, but in adrenal insufficiency associated with polyglandular autoimmune failure, it may be a manifestation of serositis.[68] Fever is usually caused by infection and should always be assumed to have an infectious cause, but it may be exaggerated by hypocortisolemia. The combination of abdominal pain and fever may lead to the incorrect diagnosis of an acute surgical abdomen, with potentially catastrophic surgical exploration. It is important to consider the possibility of acute adrenal crisis in critically ill patients, because a missed diagnosis may result in an unnecessary death.

Volume depletion in Addison disease results primarily from aldosterone deficiency.[65, 69] Cardiovascular symptoms include postural dizziness and syncope (see Table 18–3). In most patients the blood pressure is low, but some have only postural hypotension. In patients with preexisting hypertension, Addison disease may become manifest when blood pressure control improves. Eighty-five percent to 90% of patients develop hyponatremia; salt craving is common. Hyperkalemia occurs in 60% to 65% of patients.

The diagnosis of Addison disease may be straightforward.[64] Adrenal insufficiency is present if the serum cortisol is less than 3 μg/dL when measured between 8 and 9 AM. Conversely, it is excluded when the values are greater than 19 μg/dL, measured at the same time.[64] Patients whose values fall between 3 and 19 μg/dL need dynamic testing. Dynamic tests are summarized in Table 18–4.

Although it can be inherited as a mendelian trait (see later), Addison disease can also occur as an acquired disorder (Table 18–5). Tuberculosis was previously the most common cause, but autoimmune disease is now more common. Autoimmune adrenalitis may occur as an isolated disorder, but it is more commonly part of the inherited disorders known as polyglandular autoimmune syndromes types 1 and 2. Although infectious causes of Addison disease are less common than previously, they still occur, especially in patients with acquired immunodeficiency syndrome (AIDS).[70–73] Yet AIDS patients may develop orthostatic hypotension and hyperkalemia independent of Addison disease.[74, 75] Several drugs can also depress secretion of adrenal hormones (see Table 18–5).

**TABLE 18–4.** Hormonal Function Tests for Adrenal Insufficiency

| Reason for Test | Hormone Test | Normal Range | Interpretation of Result | Reference |
|---|---|---|---|---|
| Rule out adrenal insufficiency | Measurement of basal plasma cortisol between 8 and 9 AM | Plasma cortisol, 6–24 μg/dL | If plasma cortisol ≤3 μg/dL, adrenal insufficiency confirmed; if ≥19 μg/dL, adrenal insufficiency ruled out | 222 |
| | Conventional corticotropin test | Basal or postcorticotropin plasma cortisol, ≥20 μg/dL | Insufficient increase in plasma cortisol in most cases of adrenal insufficiency | 222, 223 |
| | Low-dose corticotropin test | Basal or postcorticotropin plasma cortisol, ≥18 μg/dL | Probably insufficient increase in plasma cortisol in all cases of adrenal insufficiency | 224, 225 |
| Primary adrenal insufficiency suspected | Conventional corticotropin test | Basal or postcorticotropin plasma cortisol, ≥20 μg/dL | No increase in plasma cortisol in primary adrenal insufficiency | 222 |
| | Measurement of basal plasma cortisol and corticotropin | Plasma cortisol, 6–24 μg/dL; plasma corticotropin, 5–45 pg/mL | Plasma cortisol low or in low-normal range, but plasma corticotropin always >100 pg/mL in primary adrenal insufficiency | 226, 227 |
| Secondary adrenal insufficiency suspected | Insulin-induced hypoglycemia | Plasma glucose, <40 mg/dL; plasma cortisol, ≥20 μg/dL | Little or no increase in plasma cortisol in secondary adrenal insufficiency | 222, 228 |
| | Short metyrapone test | Plasma 11-deoxycortisol at 8 hr, ≤7 μg/dL; plasma corticotropin, >150 pg/mL | Insufficient increase in plasma corticotropin (very sensitive) and 11-deoxycortisol in secondary adrenal insufficiency | 230, 231 |
| | Corticotropin-releasing hormone test | Depends on dose, time of administration, and species of origin (human, ovine) of corticotropin-releasing hormone | Insufficient increase in plasma corticotropin and cortisol in secondary adrenal insufficiency | 222, 232, 233 |
| | Low-dose corticotropin test | Basal or corticotropin-stimulated plasma cortisol, ≥18 μg/dL | Probably insufficient stimulation in all cases of secondary adrenal insufficiency | 224, 225 |
| Secondary adrenal insufficiency due to hypothalamic disease suspected | Insulin-induced hypoglycemia | Plasma glucose, <40 mg/dL; plasma cortisol, ≥20 μg/dL | Little or no increase in plasma cortisol in secondary adrenal insufficiency due to hypothalamic disease | 222, 228 |
| | Corticotropin-releasing hormone test on different day | Transient increase in plasma corticotropin and cortisol | Prolonged, exaggerated plasma corticotropin response; weak plasma cortisol response in hypothalamic disease | 222, 234 |

To convert values for cortisol to nanomoles per liter, multiply by 27.6; to convert values for corticotropin to picomoles per liter, multiply by 0.22; to convert values for 11-deoxycortisol to nanomoles per liter, multiply by 28.9; and to convert values for glucose to millimoles per liter, multiply by 0.055.

### *Syndrome of Inappropriate Antidiuretic Hormone and Cerebral Salt Wasting*

Hyponatremia is a common finding in hospitalized patients, especially those with diseases of the lung and central nervous system. Patients with the syndrome of inappropriate antidiuretic hormone secretion (SIADH) usually excrete large amounts of salt in the urine. Although this has been called salt wasting, it is usually associated with mild expansion of the ECF volume, as indicated by reductions in serum uric acid levels[76] and increases in atrial natriuretic peptide.[77] According to the criteria described earlier, therefore, SIADH does not qualify as a salt-wasting disorder. Instead, NaCl excretion is appropriate to the volume-expanded state, even though it seems inappropriate to the hyponatremia. Peters and coworkers suggested that patients with cerebral disease may manifest a true salt-losing tendency.[78] Although most cases of salt wasting associated with cerebral disease were subsequently ascribed to SIADH, interest in *cerebral salt wasting* has resurfaced.[79] Nelson and colleagues showed that 10 of 12 patients with intracranial disease who met the criteria for SIADH had decreased plasma volume.[80] Wijdicks and colleagues found that the ECF volume was decreased in a patient with ruptured intracranial aneurysm and natriuresis.[81] Other investigators have provided indications that salt wasting may occur despite contraction of the ECF volume.[79] Potential mediators of natriuresis in patients with intracranial disease include atrial natriuretic peptide and an endogenous ouabain-like factor.[79] Recently, most interest has centered on the role of brain natriuretic peptide. Circulat-

**TABLE 18–5.** Causes of Addison Disease

- Autoimmune adrenalitis
  - Isolated adrenal insufficiency
  - Polyglandular autoimmune syndrome type I
  - Polyglandular autoimmune syndrome type II
- Infectious adrenalitis
  - Tuberculosis
  - Disseminated fungal infection
    - Histoplasmosis
    - Paracoccidioidomycosis
  - HIV infection and AIDS
  - Syphilis
  - African trypanosomiasis
- Metastatic cancer
  - Primary lung, breast, stomach, and colon cancer or lymphoma
- Adrenal hemorrhage or infarction
- Drugs
  - Ketoconazole
  - Rifampin
  - Phenytoin
  - Barbiturates
  - Megestrol acetate
  - Other—aminoglutethimide, etomidate, metyrapone, suramin, mitotane
- Other
  - Adrenoleukodystrophy and adrenomyeloneuropathy
  - Congenital adrenal hypoplasia
  - Familial glucocorticoid deficiency
  - Familial glucocorticoid resistance
  - Defective cholesterol metabolism
    - Abetalipoproteinemia
    - Homozygous familial hypercholesterolemia

ing levels of this atrial natriuretic peptide–like hormone were found to be increased in 10 patients with cerebral salt wasting.[82]

The possibility that some patients with cerebral disease may have a salt-wasting disorder that is not SIADH has important therapeutic implications. Treatment of SIADH usually involves water restriction but not isotonic saline. Treatment of a volume-depleted state, however, demands normal saline. Damaraju and colleagues suggested that patients with central nervous system disease who fulfill the usual criteria for diagnosis of SIADH (hyponatremia, an "inappropriately" elevated urine sodium concentration, and clinical euvolemia) should receive central venous pressure monitoring.[83] If the central venous pressure is low, fluid and salt should be administered.

#### *Idiopathic Orthostatic Hypotension*

Idiopathic orthostatic hypotension results from dysfunction of the autonomic nervous system. Although the acute symptoms derive from an inadequate vascular response to standing, and therefore are not related directly to the kidney, renal salt wasting also occurs. This occurs because efferent renal nerves stimulate sodium retention directly.[84] Efferent renal nerves also stimulate renin secretion; plasma renin activity is frequently low in patients with orthostatic hypotension, and the response to upright posture may be blunted.[85–90] Some investigators have detected an excessive diurnal natriuretic response (increased salt excretion at night) in patients with orthostatic hypotension. This is believed to contribute to subtle ECF volume depletion.[91] Fludrocortisone, together with a high dietary NaCl intake, forms the cornerstone of treatment for this disorder.[92]

### SOLUTE DIURESIS

The most important cause of solute diuresis is glucose. When the glucose filtration rate exceeds 200 mg/min (corresponding to a serum concentration of 200 mg/dL), sodium-glucose cotransporters in the proximal tubule become saturated.[93] The resulting increase in luminal glucose reduces water reabsorption. Solute reabsorption is impaired as a result. The ECF volume is nearly always reduced in patients suffering from hyperglycemia associated with either diabetic ketoacidosis or nonketotic hyperosmolar coma. This results largely from the osmotic diuretic effects of hyperglycemia.

### DRUG-INDUCED SALT WASTING

The most important drug-induced cause of salt wasting is the administration of diuretic drugs. Of course, this is precisely the therapeutic effect of these agents, and except in cases of surreptitious ingestion, such salt wasting does not usually present diagnostic or therapeutic problems. As discussed earlier, tubulointerstitial nephritis can lead to profound salt wasting. Some cases have reportedly been caused by drug reactions.[94] Salt wasting and hypokalemia can develop during treatment with cisplatin,[95, 96] often in association with acute tubular necrosis. The patients reported by Hutchison and coworkers received a mean dose of 342 $mg/m^2$ before developing orthostatic hypotension.[95] Some of these patients also developed hyporeninemic hypoaldosteronism. Recently, transcriptional activity of the mineralocorticoid receptor was shown to be suppressed by cisplatin.[97] Other drugs that may cause salt wasting include amphotericin B, ifosfamide, trimethoprim, and gentamicin.[98, 99]

## Inherited Salt-Wasting Disorders

### RENAL ION TRANSPORT DEFECTS

#### *Bartter Syndrome*

Bartter and colleagues described several children who presented with failure to thrive.[100, 101] The patients were found to be hypokalemic and alkalotic and to have juxtaglomerular hyperplasia. Shortly thereafter, Gitelman and colleagues described a similar group of patients who had, in addition, severe magnesium wasting and hypocalciuria.[102] During the ensuing 20 years, Bartter syndrome was defined by the presence of hypokalemic metabolic alkalosis, a "normal" blood pressure (which differentiated it from the hypertensive alkaloses), hyperreninemia, and hyperaldosteronism. The syndrome was shown to be inherited as an autosomal recessive disease. Other features of the syndrome, such as an impaired vascular response to angiotensin

II, were subjects of intense interest but are now known to result from renal salt wasting. Bettinelli showed that patients with normotensive hypokalemic alkalosis generally fall into two categories—a hypocalciuric group and a normocalciuric group—commonly referred to as *Gitelman* and *Bartter* syndromes, respectively.[103] During the past 6 years, the molecular basis of Bartter and Gitelman syndromes has been elucidated. The molecular insights have greatly simplified and enhanced our understanding of the clinical features of these disorders. A contemporary classification of these disorders is presented in Table 18–2. A comparison of symptoms of Bartter and Gitelman syndromes is presented in Table 18–6.

Bartter syndrome is caused by defective salt transport by the thick ascending limb of the loop of Henle (Fig. 18–5). Based on the molecular defects leading to Bartter syndrome, Simon and colleagues proposed classifying the syndrome into three distinct subtypes, I, II, and III.[104–109] *Type I* disease is caused by mutations in the bumetanide-sensitive NKCC2. *Type II* disease is caused by mutations in the epithelial potassium channel, ROMK. *Type III* disease is caused by mutations in a kidney-specific chloride channel, CLCNKB. Although such a classification is based on the results of genetic analysis and is physiologically compelling, some phenotypic overlap between genetically distinct disorders does exist, as discussed later. Features that are specific to one particular subtype of Bartter syndrome are discussed later.

Most patients with Bartter syndrome have hypokalemic alkalosis and normotension. Rates of urinary sodium and chloride excretion are typically high,[110] and many patients report drinking pickle juice or canned soup to satisfy tremendous salt craving (for an interesting discussion of symptoms, see the Bartter syndrome Web site at http://www.zyworld.com/bartter/). Although many symptoms of Bartter syndrome result from renal salt wasting, some patients can reduce urinary NaCl excretion to very low levels upon challenge. In the initial report by Bartter and colleagues, it was observed that "when the sodium intake was lowered to 17 mEq a day, urinary sodium fell to intake values."[100] Thus, it is the excretion of sodium and chloride at rates equal to dietary intake in the presence of hypokalemic alkalosis that defines the presence of salt wasting rather than an absolute inability to reduce urinary NaCl excretion to very low levels.

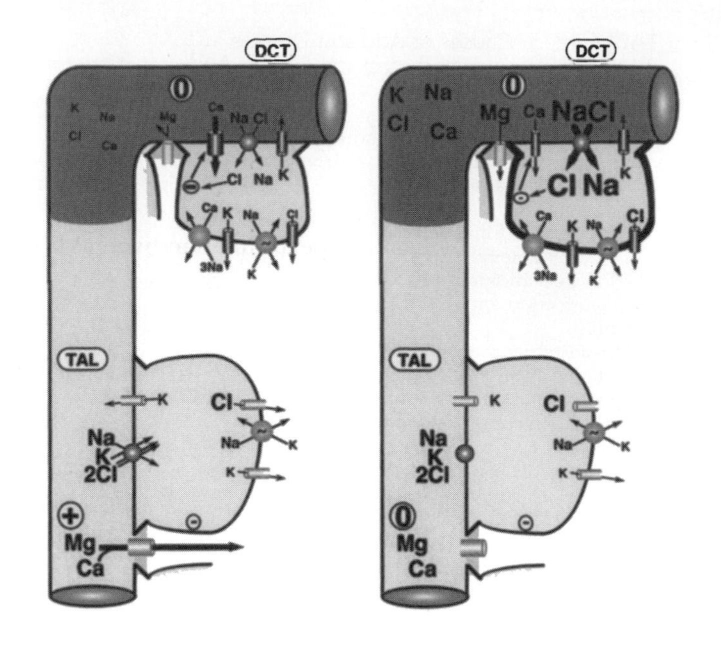


**FIGURE 18–5** ■ Pathogenesis of Bartter syndrome. *A,* A normal thick ascending limb (TAL) and distal convoluted tubule (DCT) are shown. A representative cell is shown in each segment. Note that the luminal voltage of the TAL is positive, and the DCT voltage is near to 0 mV. In the figure, calcium and magnesium are shown traversing the same paracellular pathway. In patients with Bartter syndrome *(B)* or during loop diuretic treatment, NaCl transport is inhibited along the TAL. This reduces the transepithelial voltage to almost zero, thus secondarily reducing magnesium and calcium absorption. It also increases distal delivery of Na, K, Cl, Ca, and Mg. This leads to hypertrophy of the DCT and increases in NaCl transport. This reduces Ca absorption, according to mechanisms described in the text. (From Ellison DH: Divalent cation transport by the distant nephron: Insights from Bartter's and Gitelman's syndromes. Am J Physiol Renal Physiol 279:F616–F625, 2000.)

Kidney biopsies are rarely performed on patients with Bartter syndrome, but when available, they typically show juxtaglomerular hyperplasia, with increases in the thickness of the afferent arteriole and increased abundance of macula densa cells.[100] Recent molecular-clinical correlations make it clear that Bartter syn-

**TABLE 18–6.** Symptoms and Signs of Bartter and Gitelman Syndrome

| | Gitelman Syndrome | Bartter Type I | Bartter Type II | Bartter Type III |
|---|---|---|---|---|
| Age at presentation | 22.5 yr (8 mo–65 yr) | Prenatal to neonatal | Prenatal to neonatal | Neonatal to childhood |
| Prematurity | Absent | Present | Present | Absent |
| Polyhydramnios | Absent | Present | Present | Absent |
| Potassium | 2.6 mM (1–3.5 mM) | Low | Normal to low (⇑ at birth) | Low |
| Bicarbonate | 30.7 mM (22–37.4 mM) | ⇑ | ⇑ (can be ⇓ at birth) | ⇑ |
| Urinary calcium-creatinine ratio | 0.088 (0.001–0.36 mol/mol) | ⇑ | ⇑ | ⇑ to ⇓ |
| Serum magnesium | 1.2 mg/dL (0.3–1.7 mg/dL) | Normal | Normal | ⇓ to normal |
| Tetany | 11.7% | Absent | Absent | Absent |
| Nephrocalcinosis | Absent | Present | Present | Absent |
| Chondrocalcinosis | Present | Absent | Absent | Absent |

drome represents several discrete phenotypes. These are discussed in the following paragraphs.

**Type I.** Many patients with type I disease are born prematurely, with polyhydramnios and birth weight less than 2 kg.[108, 111] Patients often present in the neonatal period with severe dehydration associated with marked hypokalemia and hyperreninemic hyperaldosteronism. Although this phenotype is most common, some patients have been reported without severe hypokalemia or alkalosis.[112] Isosthenuria is usually present. Hypercalciuria is a characteristic feature, and nephrocalcinosis may be detected by renal ultrasonography. Hypercalciuria results because defective salt reabsorption along the thick ascending limb reduces the magnitude of the lumen-positive voltage. It is this voltage that drives paracellular calcium transport in this segment (see Fig. 18–5).[113] Hypercalciuria is best documented using the molar calcium-creatinine ratio, measured after an overnight fast. Using this technique, a value greater than 0.5 (corresponding to greater than 0.18 mg/mg) may be considered elevated for children older than 5 years and for adults.[111]

Many patients with type I disease represent those previously identified as suffering from hyperprostaglandin E (antenatal Bartter) syndrome. In 1985, Seyberth and coworkers described five infants with hypokalemic metabolic alkalosis; a prenatal onset with polyhydramnios and premature labor; postnatal failure to thrive; episodes of fever, vomiting, diarrhea, and convulsions; and massive hypercalciuria.[114] Most of these findings could be corrected with nonsteroidal anti-inflammatory drugs.[114] Although clear molecular verification of hyperprostaglandin E syndrome as identical to type I Bartter syndrome has not been provided, it appears that many cases are caused by mutations in NKCC2. Evidence includes the observation that the response of patients with hyperprostaglandin E syndrome to furosemide is markedly impaired.[115] Further, NKCC2 knockout mice demonstrated elevated urinary prostaglandin $E_2$ excretion and could be rescued from lethality by treatment with indomethacin.[116]

**Type II.** Patients with mutations in ROMK have many phenotypic features in common with type I patients. These patients frequently result from pregnancies complicated by polyhydramnios, and they manifest nephrocalcinosis and hypercalciuria, as well as isosthenuria.[117] Many of these patients have excessive prostaglandin E secretion and require treatment with nonsteroidal anti-inflammatory drugs. Certain unique phenotypic features have recently emerged as highly characteristic of type II patients, however. Hypokalemia is less severe in type II patients, and many patients present during infancy with frank *hyperkalemia*.[109, 117] In fact, 14 of 20 patients with ROMK mutations were found to have transient hyperkalemia.[117] This has commonly led some infants with type II Bartter syndrome to be misdiagnosed as suffering from pseudohypoaldosteronism type I.[109, 117] As they grow out of infancy, hypokalemia begins to develop. Even then, however, potassium supplementation is less frequently required in this group than in type I patients.[117] These differences are believed to reflect the dual roles of ROMK in renal potassium transport (Fig. 18–6). ROMK mediates potassium recycling across the luminal membrane of thick ascending limb cells, where it is essential for normal sodium and chloride reabsorption.[118] Dysfunction of the protein at this site would be expected to lead to a phenotype that is similar to that induced by loop diuretics. ROMK, however, also plays an important role as a potassium secretory channel in the distal nephron.[119, 120] The absence of this channel greatly attenuates renal potassium wasting, because the majority of excreted potassium derives from that secreted along the connecting and collecting tubules.[121]

**Type III.** Patients with mutations of the renal chloride channel CLCNKB usually present with a phenotype that is intermediate between that described for antenatal Bartter (hyperprostaglandin E) syndrome and Gitelman syndrome. As such, these patients tend to present in infancy, but not at birth, and are infrequently the product of pregnancies complicated by polyhydramnios. Although polyuria is common, the urinary concentrating defect is less severe in these patients than in patients with types I and II. In addition, hypomagnesemia and hypocalciuria can be observed in such patients. Some patients with type III Bartter syndrome have a phenotype that is quite similar to Gitelman syndrome.[117, 122] In one study, three patients with type III Bartter syndrome presented early in life with failure to thrive and were found to be normomagnesemic, with elevated prostaglandin excretion. Later in life, however, hypomagnesemia (0.5 to 0.6 mM) developed in all, and the molar urinary calcium-creatinine ratio declined to subnormal values (0.06 to 0.1).[122]

The phenotype of type III Bartter syndrome fits well with recent molecular results concerning sites of CLCNKB expression and function (see Fig. 18–6).[123] CLCNKB is a member of the CLC family of chloride channels. These channels serve a variety of physiologic roles, but emerging data suggest that the predominant function of CLCNKB is similar to that of the rat channel CLC-K2. CLC-K2 is expressed at the basolateral surface of cells along the thick ascending limb, distal convoluted tubule, and connecting tubule.[123] This channel appears to form the predominant pathway for chloride to exit the cell, once it has been taken up via either the $Na^+$-$K^+$-$2Cl^-$ (in the thick ascending limb) or $Na^+$-$Cl^-$ (in the distal convoluted tubule) cotransporter. Thus, dysfunction of this gene product would be expected to *interfere with transport along both the thick ascending limb and the distal convoluted tubule.* The unique phenotype of this subset of patients appears to reflect the important role of basolateral chloride channels for NaCl transport along the thick ascending limb, leading to a Bartter syndrome phenotype, and along the distal convoluted tubule, leading to a Gitelman phenotype.

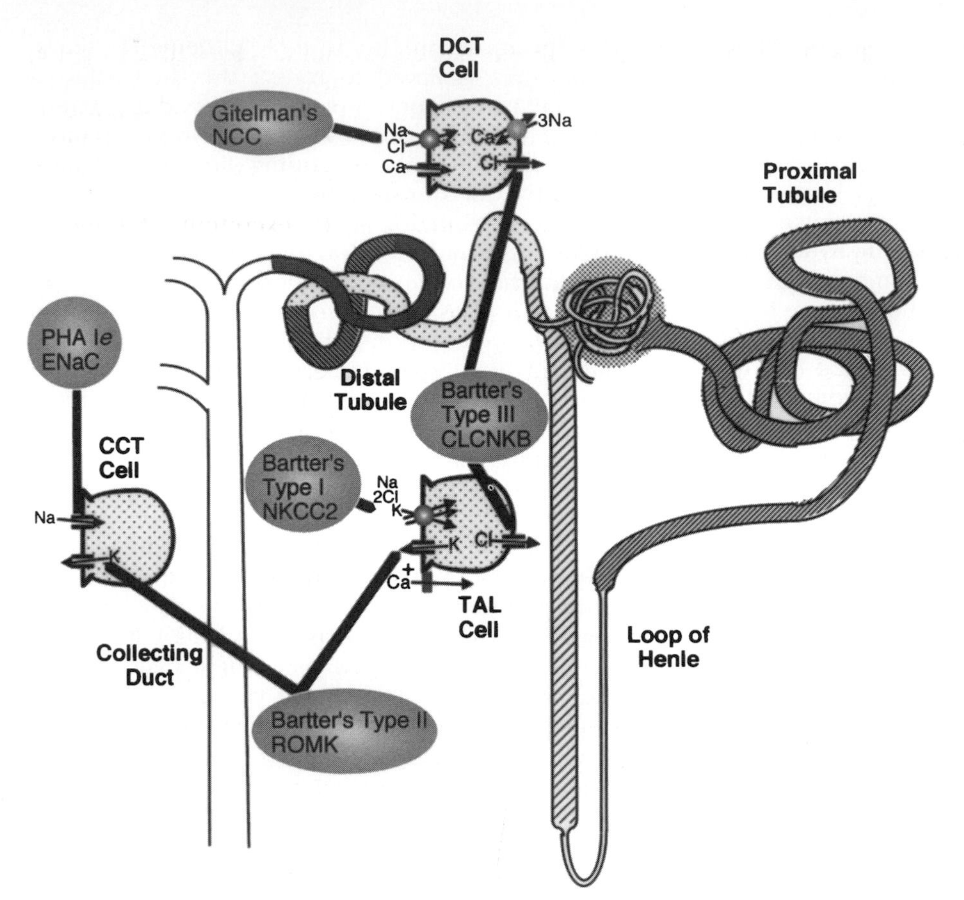


**FIGURE 18–6** ■ Sites and mechanisms of transport defects in Bartter and Gitelman syndromes. Note that type I Bartter syndrome and Gitelman syndrome affect transport pathways that are expressed exclusively in a single nephron segment. In contrast, Bartter syndrome type II involves mutation in the potassium channel ROMK, which is expressed in both the thick ascending limb and the cortical collecting tubule (CCT). Thus, the clinical phenotype of this disorder is intermediate between type I Bartter syndrome and pseudohypoaldosteronism. In contrast, type III Bartter syndrome affects a channel that is expressed along the thick ascending limb and distal convoluted tubule. This disorder manifests a phenotype that is intermediate between Bartter syndrome and Gitelman syndrome.

**Type IV.** Landau and colleagues described a variant of Bartter syndrome associated with sensorineural deafness.[124] This syndrome is typically associated with a characteristic triangular facies, with a drooping mouth and large eyes and pinnae.[124] The molecular pathogenesis of this syndrome has been linked to a novel gene expressed in the kidney.[125]

**Diagnosis.** The diagnosis of Bartter syndrome is suggested when an infant fails to thrive or grow normally and is found to have hypokalemic metabolic alkalosis. The urinary chloride concentration is typically above 20 mM in the presence of alkalosis; this is in contrast to patients who develop hypokalemic alkalosis after protracted vomiting, in whom the urinary chloride concentration is typically less than 20 mM. Many of these infants are the result of consanguineous marriage and are born prematurely after pregnancies complicated by polyhydramnios. In several series, amniotic fluid was shown to contain higher than normal concentrations of sodium (Bartter, ~135 mM; normal, 30 mM) and chloride.[126–131] Of therapeutic importance, the prostaglandin concentrations of amniotic fluid remain normal. The plasma renin activity and aldosterone concentration are typically elevated, but the blood pressure is normal.[132] The urinary calcium excretion, or the molar ratio of calcium to creatinine (see earlier), is often elevated. Nephrocalcinosis may be detected by ultrasonography.[133, 134]

Patients with Bartter syndrome demonstrate an impaired response to furosemide.[115] Furosemide treatment increased urine output by 7.5 mL/kg/hr in healthy control subjects but by only 4.4 mL/kg/hr in patients with Bartter syndrome. During the past 35 years, several clearance methods have been used to infer potential mechanisms of Bartter syndrome.[135] These have assessed tubule function during diuresis induced by intravenous hypotonic saline, by intravenous 5% dextrose in water, or by oral water loads. They have produced a confusing array of results, owing partly to previously unrecognized molecular heterogeneity and to limitations of the tests.[136, 137] The fractional distal solute reabsorption has been estimated as $C_{H_2O}/(C_{H_2O} + C_{Na})$. This value is typically reduced in patients with Bartter syndrome, reflecting the salt reabsorptive defects along the thick ascending limb.

As noted earlier, some patients develop hyperkalemia initially and are mistakenly diagnosed as pseudohypoaldosteronism type I.[109, 111]

**Treatment.** The treatment of Bartter syndrome is often difficult, but many patients can be managed effectively. Replacement of electrolyte losses is a central feature of all treatment regimens. In patients suffering from neonatal Bartter syndrome, fluid losses may surpass 500 mL/kg/day, with very large NaCl losses as well (up to 45 mmol/kg/day).[138] Many infants, especially those with type II disease, do not require potassium supplementation during the first weeks of life. After intravenous treatment has restored electrolyte balance, oral treatment with 1.5% NaCl/KCl can be given three or four times per day.[138]

The most important pharmaceutical agents for treating classic Bartter syndrome are the prostaglandin synthase inhibitors (nonsteroidal anti-inflammatory drugs). Indomethacin is the most widely used agent. Some patients respond dramatically, with decreases in salt wasting and metabolic alkalosis and improvements in urinary concentrating ability.[138] The issue of whether indomethacin should be administered during pregnancy remains unresolved. Some investigators suggest that indomethacin not be given to the mother of a Bartter syndrome fetus because amniotic fluid prostaglandin concentrations tend to be normal and the ductus arteriosus may remain patent.[127] Others, however, have reported that indomethacin, administered to the mother at 26 to 31 weeks of gestation, prevented progression of polyhydramnios without major side effects.[139] Similarly, whereas some investigators suggest that indomethacin is contraindicated in premature infants because of a high incidence of side effects, such as neonatal enterocolitis,[140] others have reported successful reduction of urinary electrolyte losses and improved growth once indomethacin was administered (at 0.8 mg/kg/day) to premature infants.[141] In one study of indomethacin use, 8% of infants developed major gastrointestinal complications, but the complications generally occurred in those with a gestational age of less than 29 weeks.[142] For older infants and children, indomethacin can be administered at 1.5 to 2.5 mg/kg/day in two to three divided doses.[127] Doses above 3 mg/kg/day are frequently nephrotoxic.[143]

Spironolactone can be useful in patients with Bartter syndrome, although this drug may increase calcium excretion.[127] This treatment, when combined with potassium supplementation, has been shown to improve appetite and growth.[127] Amiloride, captopril, and aspirin have also been used, but only limited results have been reported.

### *Gitelman Syndrome*

In 1966, Gitelman and colleagues described several patients with impaired conservation of potassium and magnesium. Of note, the three original patients were all adults; two were sisters, and all presented mild symptoms.[102] The report noted that "a generalized defect in tubular reabsorption seemed unlikely since *sodium conservation was unimpaired.*"[102] In a transcribed discussion accompanying this report, Bartter noted that patients with the syndrome of hypokalemic alkalosis and juxtaglomerular hyperplasia (Bartter syndrome) did not display marked hypomagnesemia, in contrast to Gitelman patients.[102] Despite these unique features, *Gitelman syndrome* was, for many years, lumped or confused with classic Bartter syndrome, until Bettinelli documented that Gitelman syndrome represents a clinically distinct entity.[103] The key factors permitting the distinction of Gitelman and Bartter syndromes are the rates of urinary calcium excretion and the serum magnesium concentration[103] (see Table 18–1). Simon and colleagues,[144] and later other groups,[145–148] showed that Gitelman syndrome is caused by mutations of a gene on human chromosome 16 (*SLC12A3* gene) encoding the thiazide-sensitive $Na^+$-$Cl^-$ cotransporter (NCC, NCCT, or TSC). Although the vast majority of patients with a Gitelman phenotype have mutations in the thiazide-sensitive $Na^+$-$Cl^-$ cotransporter, results suggest that some patients with type III Bartter syndrome manifest urine calcium excretion rates and serum magnesium concentrations that overlap those of Gitelman patients.[122]

Gitelman syndrome can present at any age (8 months to 65 years),[103, 149] and it does not usually cause prematurity or polyhydramnios. Frequently, the symptoms are mild, but up to 90% of patients report salt craving, 80% report nocturia, 82% report fatigue, 80% report dizziness, and 84% report cramps.[150] The overall frequency of symptoms is near 100%, much higher than previously believed.[150] Tetany is more common in Gitelman patients than in those with classic Bartter syndrome. This symptom, as well as many others, appears to be related to magnesium deficiency. Hypomagnesemia can cause muscle cramps, hyperreflexia, and tetany, even in the absence of hypocalcemia or alkalosis.[151] The serum magnesium concentration of Gitelman patients is frequently less than 0.5 mM (<1 mEq/L), although it can range from 0.12 to 0.7 mM.[149]

The fact that Gitelman syndrome is a salt-wasting disorder was not appreciated for many years, because the salt wasting is very mild.[102] When dietary NaCl intake is restricted, urinary NaCl excretion rapidly declines to very low values, recapitulating a normal response.[102] The existence of salt wasting, however, is suggested by the presence of a hypokalemic metabolic alkalosis and "normal" blood pressure in the setting of continued NaCl excretion (a "chloride-resistant" metabolic alkalosis). Although normal blood pressure was once considered to be a diagnostic criterion for Gitelman syndrome, more careful analysis, using genetically defined individuals, indicates that the blood pressure of affected patients is significantly lower than normal. When affected members of a large Amish kindred were compared with unaffected members, both the systolic and the diastolic pressures were 7.7 mm Hg lower ($P < 0.01$ and $P < 0.001$, respectively).[152] Thus, according to the scheme in Figure 18–1, Gitelman syndrome represents a disease in which the renal function curve is shifted downward, but only slightly. Dietary NaCl restriction can contract the ECF volume enough to reduce urinary NaCl excretion to zero, but the costs are metabolic abnormalities and systemic symptoms. Although ECF volume depletion is sufficient to cause the metabolic abnormalities, it is surprisingly difficult to document clinically.[153]

Gitelman syndrome is now known to be much more common than classic Bartter syndrome,[144, 154] and it is a common cause of unexplained hypokalemic alkalosis in the absence of hypertension.[154] Although the true frequency is unknown, most Gitelman patients are not the result of consanguineous marriage.[144] Some estimates suggest that at least 1% of Swedish and Italian populations are heterozygous for the disease.[144]

Gitelman syndrome is caused by loss-of-function mutations in the NCC. This hypothesis is supported by the Gitelman phenotype of an NCC knockout mouse[155] and by the confirmation that many Gitelman mutant NCC proteins are not functional when expressed in heterologous assay systems.[156] Many Gitelman mutations appear to generate misfolded proteins that are recognized by the quality-control mechanism of the endoplasmic reticulum and do not traffic to the plasma membrane normally.[156] Many phenotypic features result directly or indirectly from the salt-wasting phenotype. ECF volume depletion leads to hypotension[152]; it also stimulates aldosterone, which, coupled with enhanced sodium delivery to the connecting tubule and collecting duct, causes potassium wasting and alkalosis. The hypomagnesemia may contribute to the hypokalemia, because correction of hypomagnesemia reduces urinary potassium excretion in some Gitelman patients. The origin of other features, however, is not as obvious. Hypocalciuria is pathognomonic of Gitelman syndrome.[111] It is believed to result primarily from a reduction in sodium and chloride concentrations inside distal convoluted tubule cells. This hyperpolarizes the cells, activating an apical calcium entry pathway and stimulating basolateral calcium exit (Fig. 18–7).[157, 158] Recently, it was shown that chronic thiazide infusion increases expression of the calcium-binding protein calbindin D28K by distal convoluted tubule

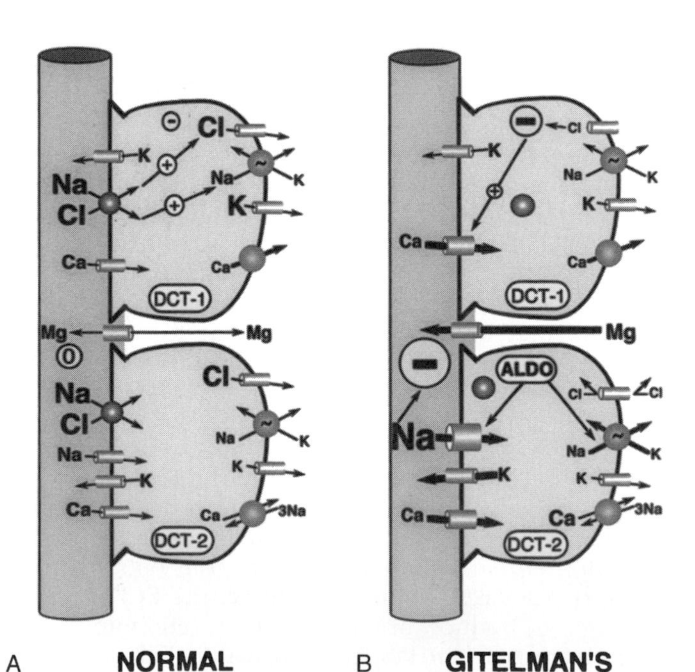


FIGURE 18–7 ■ Pathogenesis of Gitelman syndrome. *A*, The distal convoluted tubule (DCT) cells of the type 1 and 2 varieties are shown (see text for details). Under normal conditions, Na and Cl are absorbed electroneutrally by both cell types. When Gitelman syndrome occurs, the thiazide-sensitive Na-Cl transporter is misprocessed and does not appear at the plasma membrane. Cellular chloride concentrations decline, hyperpolarizing the cell. This activates the apical calcium channel, ECaC. In addition, the absence of electroneutral pathways for Na transport in this aldosterone-sensitive epithelium leads to an increase in the transepithelial voltage, which favors paracellular magnesium secretion via paracellin-1. Other secretory pathways for magnesium may also contribute. (From Ellison DH: Divalent cation transport by the distal nephron: Insights from Bartter's and Gitelman's syndromes. Am J Physiol Renal Physiol 279: F616–F625, 2000.)

cells.[159] This provides further support for the concept that distal convoluted tubule cells that lack the thiazide-sensitive $Na^+$-$Cl^-$ transporter move increased amounts of calcium, because this calcium-binding protein is believed to play a crucial role in transepithelial calcium shuttling.[113, 160]

The molar ratio of urinary calcium-creatinine is typically less than 0.1 (0.036 mg/mg) in Gitelman patients, although values can range from 0.0001 to 0.36.[149] The low rates of urinary calcium excretion that affect Gitelman patients, coupled with other abnormalities of calcium metabolism[161, 162] and with hypomagnesemia,[163] can lead to chondrocalcinosis (pseudogout, or calcium pyrophosphate deposit disease).[164–169] Hypomagnesemia has been proposed to contribute to calcium pyrophosphate deposition because magnesium acts as a cofactor in the conversion of pyrophosphate ($P_2O_7$) to inorganic phosphate ($PO_4$).[168, 170] Magnesium has also been shown to increase the solubility of calcium pyrophosphate crystals in vitro.[170]

The mechanisms by which magnesium wasting develops in Gitelman syndrome remain unclear.[157, 171] Some investigators suggest that high circulating aldosterone levels, together with transport deficiency in the distal convoluted tubule, *cause* magnesium wasting.[157] This is supported by the observation that spironolactone can reduce magnesium excretion in these patients.[169, 172] Other investigators suggest that high aldosterone levels *reduce* magnesium excretion in Gitelman patients.[171, 173] This issue requires further investigation.

**Treatment.** Many aspects of treatment for patients with Gitelman syndrome resemble those described earlier for Bartter syndrome. Specifically, the provision of adequate electrolyte replacement is essential. Recent reports, reflecting the current understanding of the pathogenesis of Gitelman syndrome, suggest that aggressive administration of salt effectively suppresses aldosterone secretion, increases serum potassium, and improves symptoms in Gitelman patients.[174] In this respect, Gitelman patients differ from Bartter patients in that hyperreninemia and hyperaldosteronism may be suppressible with adequate volume replacement. Kamel and colleagues showed that bicarbonaturia does not play a critical role in maintaining potassium wasting, but that hypomagnesemia does contribute importantly to urinary potassium losses in some patients.[175] Magnesium is usually given as $MgCl_2$, but recent reports show that potassium-magnesium citrate is an effective method to treat thiazide-induced magnesium and potassium losses.[176] The same treatment may be useful for patients with Gitelman syndrome. Spironolactone is frequently effective in reducing potassium and magnesium wasting.[167, 172] In contrast to patients with classic Bartter syndrome, patients suffering from Gitelman syndrome do not usually manifest increased rates of urinary prostaglandin $E_2$ excretion[177]; therefore, treatment with nonsteroidal anti-inflammatory drugs is usually not indicated.

## EPITHELIAL SODIUM CHANNEL DEFECTS (PSEUDOHYPOALDOSTERONISM TYPE I*e*)

The term *pseudohypoaldosteronism* (PHA) is used to describe two different syndromes. The first, PHA type

I, is a salt-wasting disorder characterized by hyperkalemia and acidosis. The second, PHA type II, is a salt-retaining disorder associated with hyperkalemia and hypertension. Only the first type is discussed here. PHA I is a rare syndrome that usually presents in neonates as failure to thrive. Salt wasting, hyperkalemic acidosis, and unresponsiveness to mineralocorticoid hormones are also present.[178–183] Hyponatremia frequently develops, and the renin and aldosterone concentrations in plasma are very high. Hypercalciuria may be present. Some patients are the products of pregnancies complicated by polyhydramnios.[184] Clinical studies initially identified two distinct clinical syndromes assigned the name PHA I.[185] Genetic studies later identified mutations in two different genes associated with PHA I: the epithelial sodium channel (ENaC), causing PHA I*e*,[186] and the mineralocorticoid receptor, causing PHA I*mr*.[187] Not all cases of PHA I have been found to be caused by mutations in either ENaC or the mineralocorticoid receptor.[187] One additional cause may be mutations in the potassium channel ROMK. Recall that type II Bartter syndrome (caused by dysfunction of ROMK) can also present as PHA.[188]

PHA I*e* is an autosomal recessive disorder caused by mutations in the α, β, or γ subunits of ENaC.[186, 189] Expression of a PHA I*e*–causing mutant ENaC in *Xenopus* oocytes generated currents that were significantly lower than currents in oocytes expressing wild-type ENaC,[186] confirming that the disease results from dysfunction of the sodium channel. One missense mutation (G37S) of the β subunit appears to identify a conserved glycine that is involved in channel gating.[190] Knockout mice have been generated to study the PHA phenotype. Disruption of the β subunit of ENaC leads to a PHA phenotype with salt wasting and high serum aldosterone.[191] In contrast, disruption of the α subunit leads to neonatal death from pulmonary congestion.[192] This may indicate a special role for α – ENaC in neonatal pulmonary function. Patients with PHA have been shown to have excess pulmonary water.[193] The severity of the phenotype in PHA I*e* indicates the important role that ENaC plays in maintaining ECF volume; it suggests that the relative impotence of amiloride as a diuretic is related primarily to its nature as a competitor for sodium at the channel pore.[186]

**Treatment.** PHA I*e* usually presents as a severe salt-wasting disorder requiring large amounts of NaCl replacement. Patients have required 50 mmol/kg/day. In addition to dietary potassium restriction, cation exchange resins are frequently used.[194, 195] As in Bartter syndrome, indomethacin has been reported to reduce polyuria and hypercalciuria in some patients,[196] although the possibility of exacerbating hyperkalemia must be considered. Hydrochlorothiazide (2 mg/kg/day) has been reported to improve hyperkalemia and hypercalciuria.[194]

## MINERALOCORTICOID RECEPTOR DEFECTS (PSEUDOHYPOALDOSTERONISM TYPE I*mr*)

PHA I*mr* is an autosomal dominant and sporadic disease caused by mutations in the mineralocorticoid receptor (MR).[187] The disease is milder than PHA I*e*, and it tends to remit spontaneously by puberty.[187] Most adults who harbor these mutations are asymptomatic, but spontaneous mutations also account for a fraction of the described cases. Some patients may show manifestations of salt wasting and hyperkalemia only following an insult, such as the development of pyelonephritis.[197] MR mutations that cause PHA I*mr* include frameshift mutations, premature stop codons, and splice site mutations.[187] These are believed to lead to partial loss of MR activity, compared with wild-type individuals who inherit two copies. The loss of one MR allele leads to salt wasting, and stimulation of the renin-angiotensin-aldosterone system is supported by the phenotype of an MR knockout mouse. Heterozygotes show significant increases in plasma renin concentration, plasma angiotensin II concentration, and plasma aldosterone concentration. These animals also demonstrate increases in urinary sodium concentration and in fractional salt excretion.[198] It has been suggested that the renin-angiotensin-aldosterone system is activated and necessary shortly after birth because the NaCl content of milk is low.[187, 199] As dietary NaCl intake increases during weaning, the need for two MR gene copies wanes. This may not be the only explanation for clinical improvement in PHA I*mr* patients. Serum sodium and potassium appear to improve gradually, reaching normal values only by 7 to 10 years of age.[200] This is well beyond the age of weaning, suggesting that non-nutritional factors may play a role in the improvement. Interestingly, some patients with the autosomal dominant form of PHA I respond to carbenoxolone (which inhibits the glucocorticoid metabolic enzyme 11β-hydroxysteroid dehydrogenase). This drug can stimulate salt retention and reduce activation of the renin-angiotensin-aldosterone system in these patients.[201]

**Treatment.** Treatment of PHA I*mr* usually involves replacement of electrolyte losses. Because of the mild and transient nature of this illness, treatment is usually successful in achieving normal growth and development.

## HYPOALDOSTERONISM

### *Adrenal Hyperplasia*

The biosynthetic pathways for adrenal corticosteroids are shown in Figure 18–8. Inherited deficiencies in several of the metabolic enzymes that catalyze conversion of the steroid precursors lead to syndromes characterized by adrenal hyperplasia. All these syndromes are examples of mixed hypo- and hyperadrenocorticism. When the synthesis of either aldosterone or cortisol is impaired, compensatory increases in angiotensin or ACTH occur. These increases may, in some cases, restore aldosterone and cortisol levels to normal, but at the expense of increased production of bioactive precursors. Many of these syndromes are associated with deficient aldosterone production and therefore lead to salt wasting. Crucial clinical and genetic features are reviewed briefly.

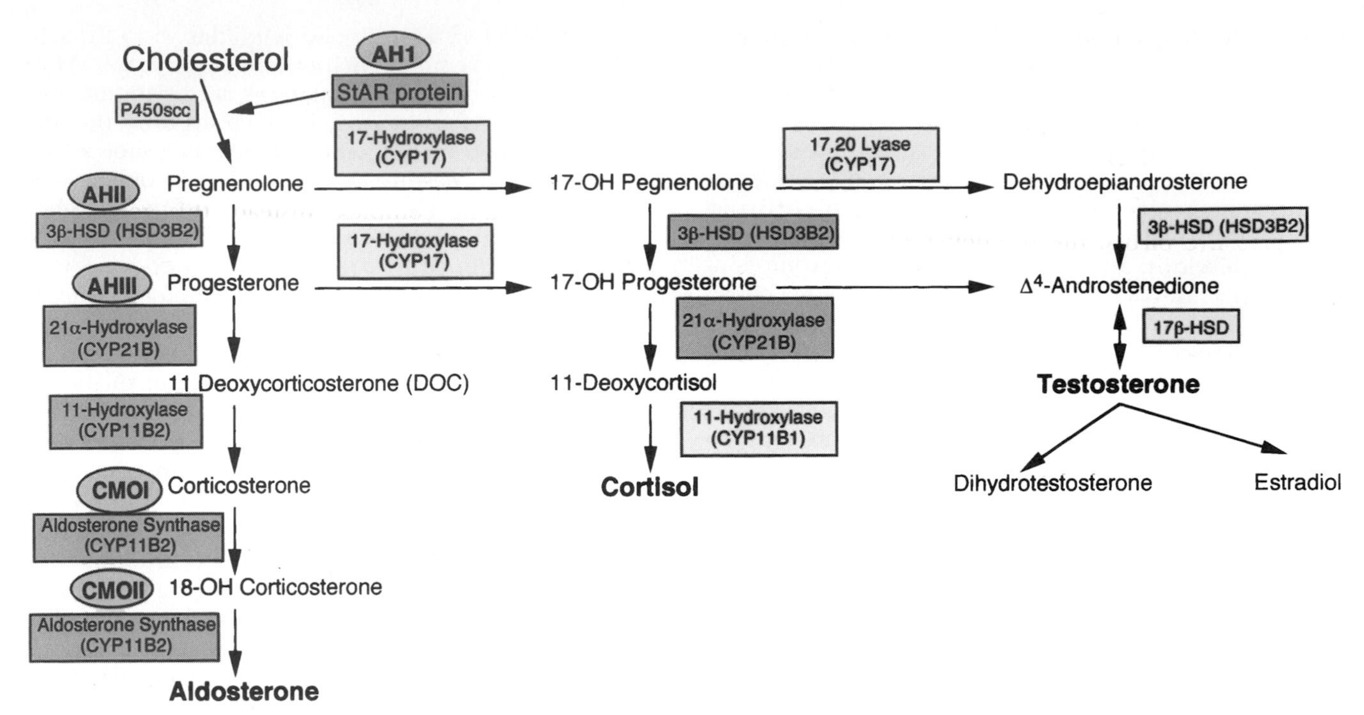


**FIGURE 18–8** ■ Pathways of steroid biosynthesis in the adrenal cortex and diseases resulting from enzyme deficiencies. Those disorders that lead to salt wasting are indicated by *shaded boxes*. The enzyme name is followed (in parentheses) by the gene symbol. The abbreviation for a resulting clinical syndrome is provided in the *shaded circle*. The syndromes are defined and described in the text; Adrenal hyperplasia type I (AHI), II (AHII), and III (AHIII), and corticosterone methyl oxidase deficiencies type I (CMOI) and II (CMOII).

**Adrenal Hyperplasia I (Lipoid Congenital Adrenal Hyperplasia).** This is the most severe form of adrenal hyperplasia because the synthesis of steroid hormones is almost completely deficient. Most genetic males are phenotypic females. Females may have normal genitalia, but both males and females may suffer from salt wasting, although the degree of salt wasting and hyperkalemia is variable.[202] Patients may die in infancy if mineralocorticoid and glucocorticoid replacement is not instituted. The first, rate-limiting step in steroidogenesis in the adrenal cortex (as well as the ovary, testis, and placenta) is cleavage of the cholesterol side chain to form pregnenolone. This reaction is catalyzed by a form of cytochrome P450, called P450scc (*CYP11A1* gene; see Fig. 18–8). Surprisingly, analysis of this gene in patients with adrenal hyperplasia I did not show abnormalities. Instead, these individuals carry mutations in the *StAR* gene (8p 11.2).[203] The *StAR* protein is necessary for P450scc to convert cholesterol to pregnenolone. Apparently, this protein shuttles cholesterol to the inner mitochondrial membrane, where it can be acted on by the P450 enzymes.[204] Several disease-causing mutants were shown to be incapable of promoting steroid biosynthesis when transfected into COS cells.[202] A late phase of the disease was proposed to result from the accumulation of cholesterol esters in the adrenal cortex, leading to salt wasting, hyponatremia, and hypovolemia.[202] Treatment of this disorder consists of steroid hormone replacement.

**Adrenal Hyperplasia II (3β-Hydroxysteroid Dehydrogenase Deficiency).** Male patients with adrenal hyperplasia II may present with hypospadias as well as pseudohermaphroditism. These patients can also present with adrenal crisis; salt wasting frequently leads to death.[205] Rheaume and coworkers described nonsense and frameshift mutations in the type II 3β-hydroxysteroid dehydrogenase gene in patients with this syndrome.[206]

**Adrenal Hyperplasia III (21α-Hydroxylase Deficiency).** This is a common disorder that can present with four relatively distinct phenotypes: salt wasting, simple virilizing, nonclassic, and late onset. The classic forms of the disorder present with ambiguity of the external genitalia in females, making diagnosis at birth relatively straightforward.[207] The phenotype of affected males is normal, requiring screening tests for neonatal diagnosis. Untreated patients develop progressive virilism and accelerated growth, but the adult stature is reduced because advanced bone age leads to premature epiphyseal closure.[208] Salt wasting is manifested by hyponatremia, hyperkalemia, high levels of plasma renin activity, and ECF volume depletion.[207] These features, together with deficiency in cortisol production, can lead to repeated adrenal crises, but as in other disorders of aldosterone production and action, salt wasting may abate as the affected individual ages.[209] Nonclassic adrenal hyperplasia presents in females with delayed menarche, secondary amenorrhea, hirsutism, infertility, and polycystic ovary disease.[207] Males may present with precocious puberty and acne.[207]

Diagnosis of classic adrenal hyperplasia III is made by demonstrating excess excretion of C19 steroid metabolites, including progesterone, 17-OH progesterone, androstenedione, and testosterone. The best method for diagnosis, however, is an ACTH stimulation test, in which the levels of 17-OH progesterone are determined before and 60 minutes after synthetic ACTH administration. Values are plotted on a logarithmic scale and compared with normative data.[207]

The incidence of classic adrenal hyperplasia III is 1 in 15,000 live births; the frequency of nonclassic disease may be as high as 1 in 100, making it the most common autosomal recessive disorder.[210] These phenotypic differences result from different mutations in the 21α-hydroxylase gene (*CYP21*). 21α-Hydroxylase mediates the conversion of progesterone to deoxycorticosterone, as well as the formation of 11-deoxycortisol from 17-OH progesterone (see Fig. 18–8). Deficiency or malfunction of this enzyme leads to inadequate aldosterone and cortisol synthesis and increased production of androgenic steroids. Increased production of androgenic steroids is driven by ACTH secretion, which is stimulated by the low cortisol levels. Approximately two thirds of patients with 21α-hydroxylase deficiency have low or undetectable aldosterone and cortisol levels and salt wasting,[211, 212] whereas the other third can maintain relatively normal aldosterone and cortisol levels, driven by high circulating ACTH levels.

The majority of cases of 21α-hydroxylase deficiency result from recombinations between the functional gene, *CYP21* (also called *CYP21B*), and a closely related pseudogene, *CYP21P* (or *CYP21A*).[213] These mutations either delete the functional gene or insert deleterious mutations. When these mutations completely abrogate gene function, aldosterone deficiency and salt wasting result. When the defect is milder, and increased substrate can maintain aldosterone within a reasonably normal range, androgenic effects tend to predominate.

**Treatment.** Prenatal diagnosis is recommended for families in which a previous member has been affected.[207, 214, 215] Dexamethasone (20 μg/kg/day in three divided doses) is administered orally to the mother beginning before the ninth week of gestation. Dexamethasone is begun before determining whether the fetus is affected or is male or female. Diagnosis can then be made by chorionic villus sampling at the eighth to tenth week or by amniocentesis during the second trimester. Treatment can be discontinued if the fetus is unaffected or is a male. Salt wasting in newborns responds well to exogenous mineralocorticoid hormones. Treatment of children is usually with fludrocortisone and a glucocorticoid. Some patients do not respond to cortisone acetate (probably because of low 11β-hydroxysteroid dehydrogenase activity). Thus, hydrocortisone is the recommended glucocorticoid.[216]

#### *Aldosterone Deficiency*

**Aldosterone Deficiency I (18-Hydroxylase Deficiency; Corticosterone Methyl Oxidase Deficiency Type I).** The final steps in aldosterone synthesis are mediated by multifunctional enzymes. One such enzyme (*CYP11B2* gene), which is expressed in the zona glomerulosa, appears to have 11-hydroxylase activity, 18-hydroxylase activity, and 18-hydroxysteroid dehydrogenase activity. Thus, the same protein mediates the final three steps in aldosterone synthesis (see Fig. 18–8). Another enzyme homologous with 11-hydroxylase activity (*CYP11B1* gene) was previously believed to be part of the same complex. Instead, this gene is expressed exclusively in the zona fasciculata and participates in glucocorticoid biosynthesis. Defects in the activity of *CYP11B1* lead to inadequate glucocorticoid production, stimulate ACTH secretion, and generate adrenal hyperplasia and hypertension (adrenal hyperplasia IV). In this case, hypertension results from excessive production of mineralocorticoids owing to the block in glucocorticoid synthesis. In contrast, defects in *CYP11B2* can lead to distinct syndromes, depending on the site of mutation. The activity of the *CYP11B2* gene product has been called corticosterone methyl oxidase. When the defect in enzyme activity is severe, corticosterone methyl oxidase deficiency type I occurs. These patients present as infants with failure to thrive, dehydration, vomiting, hyponatremia, and hyperkalemia. Serum aldosterone is undetectable; its immediate precursor, 18-hydroxycorticosterone, is low or normal.

Treatment of this disorder includes NaCl and the mineralocorticoid fludrocortisone.

**Aldosterone Deficiency II (18-Hydroxysteroid Dehydrogenase Deficiency; Corticosterone Methyl Oxidase Deficiency Type II).** This disorder is closely related to aldosterone deficiency I and results from a less severe mutation in the *CYP11B2* gene. This means that the steroid production block is less complete, and some aldosterone can be generated (see Fig. 18–8). This, however, is at the expense of greatly increased secretion of 18-hydroxycorticosterone. A high ratio of 18-hydroxycorticosterone to aldosterone suggests the diagnosis of corticosterone methyl oxidase deficiency type II. The clinical presentation is similar to that described earlier, but the symptoms are less severe.

## ADDISON DISEASE, X-LINKED

The *DAX1* gene (also called *NROB1*) encodes a protein that participates importantly in the regulation of adrenal development. The X-linked form of Addison disease results from a mutation in this gene.[217] The syndrome becomes apparent in infancy, when children may develop hypogonadotropic hypogonadism as well as adrenal hypoplasia. Aldosterone deficiency typically precedes cortisol deficiency, so that salt wasting is a common presentation.

## JUVENILE NEPHRONOPHTHISIS AND MEDULLARY CYSTIC KIDNEY DISEASE

Juvenile nephronophthisis (NPH) is an autosomal recessive kidney disease that is the most common genetic cause of end-stage renal disease in children.[218] This disorder belongs to a group of diseases that share common features, including their clinical symptoms, macroscopic pathology, and renal histology. Patients typically present as children with anemia, growth retardation, polyuria, and polydipsia. In the most common form of the disease, NPH 1 (*NPH1* gene), children become polydipsic around 6 years of age,[218] and end-stage renal disease invariably ensues. Two other forms of NPH have been described, encoded by distinct genes called *NPH2* and *NPH3*. Both cause similar symptoms, but patients with different forms of NPH develop end-stage renal disease at different ages; the median age is 13 years for NPH 1, 1 to 3 years for NPH 2, and 19 years for NPH 3.[218] The cysts occur primarily at the corticomedullary junction, and the kidneys remain normal in size; in contrast, cysts appear throughout the kidney in autosomal dominant polycystic kidney disease. The microscopic appearance of NPH kidneys is also characteristic. They show a triad of tubular basement membrane disintegration, tubular atrophy with cyst development, and interstitial cell infiltration with fibrosis.[218] The *NPH1* gene encodes a protein called nephrocystin, which contains an Src-homology 3 domain flanked by two glutamic acid–rich domains.[219] Hildebrandt and Otto showed that nephrocystin engages in protein-protein interactions that may be important for cell-cell interactions.[218]

Medullary cystic kidney diseases are dominantly inherited. They also lead to renal failure, but at a much later age. Two types have been described, associated with two loci termed *MCKD1* and *MCKD2*.[220] These lead to end-stage renal disease at median ages of 62 and 32 years, respectively. Polyuria is a characteristic feature of these disorders; salt wasting may occur, but it is usually less prominent than in PHA.[221]

### Acknowledgments

Work in the author's laboratory has been supported by grants from the National Institutes of Health (DK-51496 and P50 HL-5507), the Veterans Administration, and the American Heart Association.

## REFERENCES

1. Walser M: Phenomenological analysis of renal regulation of sodium and potassium balance. Kidney Int 27:837–841, 1985.
2. Guyton AC: Blood pressure control—special role of the kidneys and body fluids. Science 252:1813–1816, 1991.
3. Epstein M, Hollenberg NK: Age as a determinant of renal sodium conservation in normal man. J Lab Clin Med 87:411–417, 1976.
4. Ellison DH: Disorders of sodium balance. In Berl T (ed): Atlas of Diseases of the Kidney. Philadelphia, Blackwell Science, 1998, pp 2.1–2.22.
5. Peters JP, Wakeman AM, Lee C: Total acid-base equilibrium of plasma in health and disease. J Clin Invest 6:551–575, 1929.
6. Coleman AJ, Arias M, Carter NW: The mechanism of salt wasting in chronic renal disease. J Clin Invest 45:1116–1125, 1966.
7. Gowrishankar M, Lenga I, Cheung RY, et al: Minimum urine flow rate during water deprivation: Importance of the permeability of urea in the inner medulla. Kidney Int 53:159–166, 1998.
8. Bricker NS: On the pathogenesis of the uremic state: An exposition of the "trade-off hypothesis." N Engl J Med 286:1093–1099, 1972.
9. Palmer BF, Alpern RJ, Seldin DW: Physiology and pathophysiology of sodium retention. In Seldin DW, Giebisch G (eds): The Kidney: Physiology and Pathophysiology, 3rd ed. Philadelphia, Lippincott–Williams & Wilkins, 2000, pp 1473–1517.
10. Bricker NS, Klahr S, Rieselbach RE: The functional adaptation of the diseased kidney. I. Glomerular filtration rate. J Clin Invest 43:1915–1921, 1964.
11. Danovitch GM, Bourgoignie J, Bricker NS: Reversibility of the "salt-losing" tendency of chronic renal failure. N Engl J Med 296:14–19, 1977.
12. Danovitch GM, Jacobson E, Licht A: Absence of renal sodium adaptation in chronic renal failure. Am J Nephrol 1:173–176, 1981.
13. Kwon TH, Frokiaer J, Fernandez-Llama P, et al: Altered expression of Na transporters NHE-3, NaPi-II, Na-K-ATPase, BSC-1, and TSC in CRF rat kidneys. Am J Physiol 277:F257–F270, 1999.
14. Thorn GW, Koepf GF, Clinton M Jr: Renal failure simulating adrenocortical insufficiency. N Engl J Med 231:76–85, 1944.
15. Enticknap JB: The condition of the kidneys in salt-losing nephritis. Lancet 2:458–461, 1952.
16. Joiner CL, Thorne MG: Salt-losing nephritis. Lancet 2:454–458, 1952.
17. Toto RD, Seldin DW: Salt wastage. In Seldin DW, Giebisch G (eds): The Kidney: Physiology and Pathophysiology, 3rd ed. Philadelphia, Lippincott–Williams & Wilkins, 2000, pp 1519–1536.
18. Levere AH, Wesson LG Jr: Salt-losing nephritis: Review and report of a case. N Engl J Med 255:373–376, 1956.
19. Murphy FD, Settimi AL, Kozokoff NJ: Renal disease with the salt losing syndrome: A report of four cases of so-called "salt-losing nephritis." Ann Intern Med 38:1160–1176, 1953.
20. Nussbaum HE, Bernhard WG, Mattia VD: Chronic pyelonephritis simulating adrenocortical insufficiency. N Engl J Med 246: 289–293, 1952.
21. Sawyer WH, Solez C: Salt losing nephritis simulating adrenocortical insufficiency. N Engl J Med 240:210–215, 1949.
22. Miller WL: Dexamethasone treatment of congenital adrenal hyperplasia in utero: An experimental therapy of unproven safety. J Urol 162:537–540, 1999.
23. Bose HS, Whittal RM, Baldwin MA, Miller WL: The active form of the steroidogenic acute regulatory protein, StAR, appears to be a molten globule. Proc Natl Acad Sci U S A 96:7250–7255, 1999.
24. Stanbury SW, Mahler RF: Salt-wasting renal disease. QJM 28: 425–447, 1959.
25. Platt R: Sodium and potassium excretion in chronic renal failure. Clin Sci 9:367–377, 1950.
26. Nickel JF, Lowrance PB, Leifer E: Renal function, electrolyte excretion and body fluids in patients with chronic renal insufficiency before and after sodium deprivation. J Clin Invest 32: 68–79, 1953.
27. Petersen VP: Renal function and electrolyte metabolism in salt-losing nephritis. Acta Med Scand 154:187–199, 1956.
28. Better OS, Chaimowitz C, Gellei B, et al: Salt-losing nephropathy. J Pediatr 75:872–875, 1969.
29. Hughes JM: Salt-losing nephritis. Ann Intern Med 114:190–195, 1964.
30. Ansari A, Vennes JA: Chronic milk-alkali syndrome and salt-losing nephropathy. Minn Med 54:611–616, 1971.
31. Cheyne AI, Witehead TP: Thorn's syndrome following excessive ingestion of alkalies. Lancet 1:550–552, 1954.
32. Frank A, Greenspan G: Milk-alkali syndrome complicated by salt-losing nephritis. N Engl J Med 260:210–213, 1959.
33. Bell NH, Del Greco F, Colwell JA: Primary hyperparathyroidism and salt-wasting nephropathy. J Chronic Dis 28:601–607, 1975.
34. Kahn T, Levitt MF: Salt wasting in myeloma. Arch Intern Med 126:664–667, 1970.
35. Cove-Smith JR, Knapp MS: Sodium handling in analgesic nephropathy. Lancet 2:70–72, 1973.
36. Ferguson RK, Reed DM, Barber KG, et al: Sodium-losing nephropathy and nephrocalcinosis after transplantation. Am J Kidney Dis 5:206–210, 1985.
37. Conte G, Dal Canton A, Marcuccio F, et al: Polyuric prerenal

failure after reduction from high to normal dietary intake of sodium. Arch Intern Med 146:1814–1816, 1986.

38. Levin TL, Abramson SJ, Burbige KA, et al: Salt losing nephropathy simulating congenital adrenal hyperplasia in infants with obstructive uropathy and/or vesicoureteral reflux—value of ultrasonography in diagnosis. Pediatr Radiol 21:413–415, 1991.
39. Kuhnle U, Guariso G, Sonega M, et al: Transient pseudohypoaldosteronism in obstructive renal disease with transient reduction of lymphocytic aldosterone receptors: Results in two affected infants. Horm Res 39:152–155, 1993.
40. Melzi ML, Guez S, Sersale G, et al: Acute pyelonephritis as a cause of hyponatremia/hyperkalemia in young infants with urinary tract malformations. Pediatr Infect Dis J 14:56–59, 1995.
41. Loughridge LW, Milne MD, Shackman R: Clinical course of uncomplicated acute tubular necrosis. Lancet 1:351–355, 1960.
42. Swann RC, Merrill JP: The clinical course of acute renal failure. Medicine 1953.
43. Molitoris BA, Geerdes A, McIntosh JR: Dissociation and redistribution of $Na^+$,$K^{(+)}$-ATPase from its surface membrane actin cytoskeletal complex during cellular ATP depletion. J Clin Invest 88:462–469, 1991.
44. Spiegel DM, Wilson PD, Molitoris BA: Epithelial polarity following ischemia: A requirement for normal cell function. Am J Physiol 256:F430–F436, 1989.
45. Edelstein CL, Shi Y, Berkman J, Ellison DH: Renal ischemia decreases thiazide-sensitive Na-Cl cotransporter expression [abstract]. J Am Soc Nephrol 9:34A, 1998.
46. Kwon TH, Frokiaer J, Han JS, et al: Decreased abundance of major Na(+) transporters in kidneys of rats with ischemia-induced acute renal failure. Am J Physiol Renal Physiol 278: F925–F939, 2000.
47. Wang Z, Rabb H, Haq M, et al: A possible molecular basis of natriuresis during ischemic-reperfusion injury in the kidney. J Am Soc Nephrol 9:605–613, 1997.
48. Wang Z, Rabb H, Craig T, et al: Ischemic-reperfusion injury in the kidney: Overexpression of colonic $H^+$-$K^+$-ATPase and suppression of NHE-3. Kidney Int 51:1106–1115, 1997.
49. Kjellstrand CM, Berkseth RO, Klinkmann H: Treatment of acute renal failure. In Schrier RW (ed): Diseases of the Kidney, 4th ed. Boston, Little, Brown, 1988, pp 1501–1540.
50. Green J, Abassi Z, Winaver J, Skorecki KL: Acute renal failure: Clinical and pathophysiological aspects. In Seldin DW, Giebisch G (eds): The Kidney: Physiology and Pathophysiology, 3rd ed. Philadelphia, Lippincott–Williams & Wilkins, 2000, pp 2329–2374.
51. Maher JF, Schriener GF, Waters TJ: Osmotic diuresis due to retained urea after relief of urinary obstruction. N Engl J Med 268:1099–1104, 1963.
52. Muldowney FP, Duffy GJ, Kelly DG, et al: Sodium diuresis after relief of obstructive uropathy. N Engl J Med 274:1294–1298, 1966.
53. Falls WF, Stacy WK: Post obstructive diuresis. Am J Med 54: 404–412, 1973.
54. McDougal WS, Wright FS: Defect in proximal and distal sodium transport in post-obstructive diuresis. Kidney Int 2:304–317, 1972.
55. Terzi F, Assael BM, Claris-Appiani A, et al: Increased sodium requirement following early postnatal surgical correction of congenital uropathies in infants. Pediatr Nephrol 4:581–584, 1990.
56. Gillenwater JN: Hydronephrosis. In Gillenwater JN, Grayhack JT, Howards SS, Duckett JW (eds): Adult and Pediatric Urology, 3rd ed. St. Louis, Mosby, 1996, pp 973–998.
57. Rodriquez-Soriano J, Vallo A, Castillo G, Oliveros R: Renal handling of water and sodium in children with proximal and distal renal tubular acidosis. Nephron 25:193–198, 1980.
58. Sebastian A, McSherry E, Morris RCJ: On the mechanism of renal potassium wasting in renal tubular acidosis associated with the Fanconi syndrome (type 2 RTA). J Clin Invest 50: 231–243, 1971.
59. McSherry E: Renal tubular acidosis in childhood. Kidney Int 20:799–809, 1981.
60. Gill JR, Bell NH, Bartter FC: Impaired conservation of sodium and potassium in renal tubular acidosis and its correction by buffer anions. Clin Sci 33:577–592, 1967.
61. Sebastian A, McSherry E, Morris RCJ: Impaired renal conservation of sodium and chloride during sustained correction of systemic acidosis in patients with type 1, classic renal tubular acidosis. J Clin Invest 58:454–469, 1976.
62. Bruce LJ, Cope DL, Jones GK, et al: Familial distal renal tubular acidosis is associated with mutations in the red cell anion exchanger (band 3, AE1) gene. J Clin Invest 100:1693–1707, 1997.
63. Karet FE, Gainza FJ, Gyory AZ, et al: Mutations in the chloride-bicarbonate exchanger gene AE1 cause autosomal dominant but not autosomal recessive distal renal tubular acidosis. Proc Natl Acad Sci U S A 95:6337–6342, 1998.
64. Oelkers W: Adrenal insufficiency. N Engl J Med 335:1206–1212, 1996.
65. Harrop GA, Weinstein ASLJ: The diagnosis and treatment of Addison's disease. JAMA 100:1850–1855, 1933.
66. Jacobs TP, Whitlock RT, Edsall J, Holub DA: Addisonian crisis while taking high-dose glucocorticoids: An unusual presentation of primary adrenal failure in two patients with underlying inflammatory diseases. JAMA 260:2082–2084, 1988.
67. Cronin CC, Callaghan N, Kearney PJ, et al: Addison disease in patients treated with glucocorticoid therapy. Arch Intern Med 157:456–458, 1997.
68. Tucker WS, Niblack GD, McLean RH, et al: Serositis with autoimmune endocrinopathy: Clinical and immunogenetic features. Medicine (Baltimore) 66:138–147, 1987.
69. Brown JJ, Fraser R, Lever AF, et al: Renin, angiotensin, corticosteroids, and electrolyte balance in Addison's disease. QJM 37: 97–118, 1968.
70. Seel K, Guschmann M, van Landeghem F, Grosch-Worner I: Addison disease—an unusual clinical manifestation of CMV–end organ disease in pediatric AIDS. Eur J Med Res 5:247–250, 2000.
71. Strauss KW: Endocrine complications of the acquired immunodeficiency syndrome. Arch Intern Med 151:1441–1444, 1991.
72. Takasawa A, Morimoto I, Wake A, et al: Autopsy findings of Addison's disease caused by systemic cytomegalovirus infection in a patient with acquired immunodeficiency syndrome. Intern Med 34:533–536, 1995.
73. Wissner Greene L, Cole W, Greene JB, et al: Adrenal insufficiency as a complication of the acquired immunodeficiency syndrome. Ann Intern Med 101:497–498, 1984.
74. Cobbs R, Pepper BM, Rorres JG, Gruenspan HL: Adrenocortical insufficiency with normal serum cortisol levels and hyporeninemia in a patient with acquired immunodeficiency syndrome (AIDS). J Intern Med 230:179–181, 1991.
75. Perazella M: Electrolyte and acid-base disorders associated with AIDS: an etiologic review. J Gen Intern Med 3:232–236, 1994.
76. Beck LH: Hypouricemia in the syndrome of inappropriate secretion of antidiuretic hormone. N Engl J Med 301:528–530, 1979.
77. Cogan E, Debieve MF, Philipart I, et al: High plasma levels of atrial natriuretic factor in SIADH. N Engl J Med 314:1258–1259, 1986.
78. Peters JP, Welt LG, Sims EAH, et al: A salt wasting syndrome associated with cerebral disease. Trans Assoc Am Physicians 63: 57–64, 1950.
79. Harrigan MR: Cerebral salt wasting syndrome: A review. Neurosurgery 38:152–160, 1996.
80. Nelson PB, Seif SM, Maroon JC, Robinson AG: Hyponatremia in intracranial disease: Perhaps not the syndrome of inappropriate secretion of antidiuretic hormone (SIADH). J Neurosurg 55:938–941, 1981.
81. Wijdicks EF, Vermeulen M, ten Haaf JA, et al: Volume depletion and natriuresis in patients with a ruptured intracranial aneurysm. Ann Neurol 18:211–216, 1985.
82. Berendes E, Walter M, Cullen P, et al: Secretion of brain natriuretic peptide in patients with aneurysmal subarachnoid haemorrhage. Lancet 349:245–249, 1997.
83. Damaraju SC, Rajshekhar V, Chandy MJ: Validation study of a central venous pressure–based protocol for the management of neurosurgical patients with hyponatremia and natriuresis. Neurosurgery 40:312–316; discussion 316–317, 1997.
84. Kopp UC, DiBona GF: Neural control of volume homeostasis. In Brenner BM, Stein JH (eds): Body Fluid Homeostasis New York, Churchill Livingstone, 1987, pp 185–220.

85. Wilcox CS, Aminoff MJ: Blood pressure responses to noradrenaline and dopamine infusions in Parkinson's disease and the Shy-Drager syndrome. Br J Clin Pharmacol 3:207–214, 1976.
86. Wilcox CS, Aminoff MJ, Kurtz AB, Slater JD: Comparison of the renin response to dopamine and noradrenaline in normal subjects and patients with autonomic insufficiency. Clin Sci Mol Med 46:481–488, 1974.
87. Wilcox CS, Aminoff MJ, Penn W: Basis of nocturnal polyuria in patients with autonomic failure. J Neurol Neurosurg Psychiatry 37:677–684, 1974.
88. Wilcox CS, Aminoff MJ, Slater JD: Sodium homeostasis in patients with autonomic failure. Clin Sci Mol Med 53:321–328, 1977.
89. Wilcox CS, Puritz R, Lightman SL, et al: Plasma volume regulation in patients with progressive autonomic failure during changes in salt intake or posture. J Lab Clin Med 104:331–339, 1984.
90. Slaton PE Jr, Biglieri EG: Reduced aldosterone excretion in patients with autonomic insufficiency. J Clin Endocrinol Metab 27:37–45, 1967.
91. Pechere-Bertschi A, Nussberger J, Biollaz J, et al: Circadian variations of renal sodium handling in patients with orthostatic hypotension. Kidney Int 54:1276–1282, 1998.
92. Stumpf JL, Mitrzyk B: Management of orthostatic hypotension. Am J Hosp Pharm 51:648–660; quiz 697–698, 1994.
93. Gennari FJ, Kassirer JP: Osmotic diuresis. N Engl J Med 291: 714–720, 1974.
94. Cogan MC, Arieff AI: Sodium wasting, acidosis and hyperkalemia induced by methicillin interstitial nephritis: Evidence for selective distal tubular dysfunction. Am J Med 64:500–507, 1978.
95. Hutchison FN, Perez EA, Gandara DR, et al: Renal salt wasting in patients treated with cisplatin. Ann Intern Med 108:21–25, 1988.
96. Kurtzberg J, Dennis VW, Kinney TR: Cisplatinum-induced renal salt wasting. Med Pediatr Oncol 12:150–154, 1984.
97. Iida T, Makino Y, Okamoto K, et al: Functional modulation of the mineralocorticoid receptor by cis-diamminedichloroplatinum (II). Kidney Int 58:1450–1460, 2000.
98. Velázquez H, Perazella MA, Wright FS, Ellison DH: Renal mechanism of trimethoprim-induced hyperkalemia. Ann Intern Med 119:296–301, 1993.
99. Springate JE: Toxic nephropathies. Curr Opin Pediatr 9:166–169, 1997.
100. Bartter FC, Pronove P, Gill JR, MacCardle RC: Hyperplasia of the juxtaglomerular complex with hyperaldosteronism and hypokalemic alkalosis. Am J Med 33:811–828, 1962.
101. Pronove P, MacCardle RC, Bartter FC: Aldosteronism, hypokalemia, and a unique renal lesion in a five year old boy. Acta Endocrinol Suppl 51:167–168, 1960.
102. Gitelman HJ, Graham JB, Welt LG: A new familial disorder characterized by hypokalemia and hypomagnesemia. Trans Am Assoc Phys 79:221–235, 1966.
103. Bettinelli A: Use of calcium excretion values to distinguish two forms of primary renal tubular hypokalemic alkalosis: Bartter and Gitelman syndromes. J Pediatr 120:38–43, 1992.
104. Simon DB, Bindra RS, Mansfield TA, et al: Mutations in the chloride channel gene, CLCNKB, cause Bartter's syndrome type III. Nat Genet 17:171–178, 1997.
105. Simon DB, Lifton RP: Ion transporter mutations in Gitelman's and Bartter's syndromes. Curr Opin Nephrol Hypertens 7: 43–47, 1998.
106. Simon DB, Lifton RP: Mutations in Na(K)Cl transporters in Gitelman's and Bartter's syndromes. Curr Opin Cell Biol 10: 450–454, 1998.
107. Simon DB, Lifton RP: Mutations in renal ion transporters cause Gitelman's and Bartter's syndromes of inherited hypokalemic alkalosis. Adv Nephrol Necker Hosp 27:343–359, 1997.
108. Simon DB, Karet FE, Hamdan JM, et al: Bartter's syndrome: Hypokalaemic alkalosis with hypercalciuria is caused by mutations in the Na-K-2Cl cotransporter NKCC2. Nat Genet 13: 183–188, 1996.
109. Simon DB, Karet FE, Rodriquez-Soriano J, et al: Genetic heterogeneity of Bartter's syndrome revealed by mutations in the $K^+$ channel, ROMK. Nat Genet 14:152–156, 1996.
110. Schwartz ID, Alon US: Bartter syndrome revisited. J Nephrol 9:81–87, 1996.
111. Bettinelli A, Vezzoli G, Colussi G, et al: Genotype-phenotype correlations in normotensive patients with primary renal tubular hypokalemic metabolic alkalosis. J Nephrol 11:61–69, 1998.
112. Bettinelli A, Ciarmatori S, Cesareo L, et al: Phenotypic variability in Bartter syndrome type I. Pediatr Nephrol 14:940–945, 2000.
113. Friedman PA: Calcium transport in the kidney. Curr Opin Nephrol Hypertens 8:589–595, 1999.
114. Seyberth HW, Rascher W, Schweer H, et al: Congenital hypokalemia with hypercalciuria in preterm infants: A hyperprostaglandinuric tubular syndrome different from Bartter syndrome. J Pediatr 107:694–701, 1985.
115. Kockerling A, Reinalter SC, Seyberth HW: Impaired response to furosemide in hyperprostaglandin E syndrome: Evidence for a tubular defect in the loop of Henle. J Pediatr 129:519–528, 1996.
116. Takahashi N, Chernavvsky DR, Gomez RA, et al: Uncompensated polyuria in a mouse model of Bartter's syndrome. Proc Natl Acad Sci U S A 97:5434–5439, 2000.
117. Hess M, Jeck N, Klaus G, et al: Clinical presentation and treatment of genetic defined hypokalemic salt losing tubulopathies (Bartter-like syndromes) [abstract]. J Am Soc Nephrol 11: 407A, 2000.
118. Mount DB, Hoover RS, Hebert SC: The molecular physiology of electroneutral cation-chloride cotransport. J Membr Biol 158:177–186, 1997.
119. Xu JZ, Hall AE, Peterson LN, et al: Localization of the ROMK protein on the apical membranes of rat kidney nephron segments. Am J Physiol 273:F739–F748, 1997.
120. Mennitt PA, Wade JB, Ecelbarger CA, et al: Localization of ROMK channels in the rat kidney. J Am Soc Nephrol 8:1823–1830, 1997.
121. Malnic G, Muto S, Giebisch G: Regulation of potassium excretion. In Seldin DW, Giebisch G (eds): The Kidney: Physiology and Pathophysiology, 3rd ed. Philadelphia, Lippincott-Williams & Wilkins, 2000, pp 1575–1614.
122. Jeck N, Konrad M, Peters M, et al: Mutations in the chloride channel gene, CLCNKB, leading to a mixed Bartter-Gitelman phenotype. Pediatr Res 48:754–758, 2000.
123. Uchida S: In vivo role of CLC chloride channels in the kidney. Am J Physiol Renal Physiol 279:F802–F808, 2000.
124. Landau D, Shalev H, Ohaly M, Carmi R: Infantile variant of Bartter syndrome and sensorineural deafness: A new autosomal recessive disorder. Am J Med Genet 59:454–459, 1995.
125. Birkenhager R, Otto E, Schurmann MJ, et al: Mutation of BSND causes Bartter syndrome with sensorineural deafness and kidney failure. Nat Genet 29:310–314, 2001.
126. Massa G, Proesmans W, Devlieger H, et al: Electrolyte composition of the amniotic fluid in Bartter syndrome. Eur J Obstet Gynecol Reprod Biol 24:335–340, 1987.
127. Proesmans W: Bartter syndrome and its neonatal variant. Eur J Pediatr 156:669–679, 1997.
128. Proesmans W, Devlieger H, Van Assche A, et al: Bartter syndrome in two siblings—antenatal and neonatal observations. Int J Pediatr Nephrol 6:63–70, 1985.
129. Proesmans W, Massa G, Vandenberghe K, Van Assche A: Prenatal diagnosis of Bartter syndrome [letter]. Lancet 1:394, 1987.
130. Matsushita Y, Suzuki Y, Oya N, et al: Biochemical examination of mother's urine is useful for prenatal diagnosis of Bartter syndrome. Prenat Diagn 19:671–673, 1999.
131. Di Pietro A, Proverbio MR, Tammaro V, et al: [Fetal polyuria and decrease of electrolytes in amniotic fluid as principal markers of neonatal Bartter's syndrome]. Pediatr Med Chir 19: 267–268, 1997.
132. Kurtz I: Molecular pathogenesis of Bartter's and Gitelman's syndromes [clinical conference]. Kidney Int 54:1396–1410, 1998.
133. Al-Rasheed SA, Patel PJ, Kolawole TM, et al: Renal sonographic patterns in Bartter's syndrome. Pediatr Radiol 26:116–119, 1996.
134. Shultz PK, Strife JL, Strife CF, McDaniel JD: Hyperechoic renal medullary pyramids in infants and children. Radiology 181: 163–167, 1991; see comments.
135. Stein JH: The pathogenetic spectrum of Bartter's syndrome [clinical conference]. Kidney Int 28:85–93, 1985.

136. Bartoli E, Branca GF, Satta A, Faedda R: Sodium reabsorption by the Henle loop in humans. Nephron 46:288–300, 1987.
137. Bartoli E, Romano G, Favret G: Segmental reabsorption measured by micropuncture and clearance methods during hypertonic sodium infusion in the rat. Nephrol Dial Transplant 11: 1996–2003, 1996.
138. Amirlak I, Dawson KP: Bartter syndrome: An overview. QJM 93:207–215, 2000.
139. Konrad M, Leonhardt A, Hensen P, et al: Prenatal and postnatal management of hyperprostaglandin E syndrome after genetic diagnosis from amniocytes. Pediatrics 103:678–683, 1999.
140. Marlow N, Chiswick ML: Neonatal Bartter's syndrome, indomethacin and necrotising enterocolitis. Acta Paediatr Scand 71:1031–1032, 1982.
141. Mackie FE, Hodson EM, Roy LP, Knight JF: Neonatal Bartter syndrome—use of indomethacin in the newborn period and prevention of growth failure. Pediatr Nephrol 10:756–758, 1996.
142. Alpan G, Eyal F, Vinograd I, et al: Localized intestinal perforations after enteral administration of indomethacin in premature infants. J Pediatr 106:277–281, 1985.
143. Schachter AD, Arbus GS, Alexander RJ, Balfe JW: Non-steroidal anti-inflammatory drug–associated nephrotoxicity in Bartter syndrome. Pediatr Nephrol 12:775–777, 1998.
144. Simon DB, Nelson-Williams C, Bia MJ, et al: Gitelman's variant of Bartter's syndrome, inherited hypokalemic alkalosis, is caused by mutations in the thiazide-sensitive Na-Cl cotransporter. Nat Genet 12:24–30, 1996.
145. Lemmink HH, Knoers NV, Karolyi L, et al: Novel mutations in the thiazide-sensitive NaCl cotransporter gene in patients with Gitelman syndrome with predominant localization to the C-terminal domain. Kidney Int 54:720–730, 1998.
146. Lemmink HH, van den Heuvel LP, van Dijk HA, et al: Linkage of Gitelman syndrome to the thiazide-sensitive sodium-chloride cotransporter gene with identification of mutations in Dutch families. Pediatr Nephrol 10:403–407, 1996.
147. Pollak MR, Delaney VB, Graham RM, Hebert SC: Gitelman's syndrome (Bartter's variant) maps to the thiazide-sensitive cotransporter gene locus on chromosome 16q13 in a large kindred. J Am Soc Nephrol 7:2244–2248, 1996.
148. Karolyi L, Ziegler A, Pollak M, et al: Gitelman's syndrome is genetically distinct from other forms of Bartter's syndrome. Pediatr Nephrol 10:551–554, 1996.
149. Simon DB, Cruz DN, Lu Y, Lifton RP: Genotype-phenotype correlation of NCCT mutations and Gitelman's syndrome [abstract]. J Am Soc Nephrol 9:111A, 1998.
150. Cruz DN, Shaer AJ, Bia MJ, et al: Gitelman's syndrome revisited: An evaluation of symptoms and health-related quality of life. Kidney Int 59:710–717, 2001.
151. al-Ghamdi SM, Cameron EC, Sutton RA: Magnesium deficiency: Pathophysiologic and clinical overview. Am J Kidney Dis 24:737–752, 1994.
152. Cruz DN, Simon DB, Farhi A, Gill JLRP: Reduced blood pressure in Gitelman's syndrome: A study of a large extended kindred [abstract]. J Am Soc Nephrol 9:322A, 1998.
153. Garrick R, Ziyadeh FN, Jorkasky D, Goldfarb S: Bartter's syndrome: A unifying hypothesis. Am J Nephrol 5:379–384, 1985.
154. Gladziwa U, Schwarz R, Gitter AH, et al: Chronic hypokalaemia of adults: Gitelman's syndrome is frequent but classical Bartter's syndrome is rare. Nephrol Dial Transplant 10:1607–1613, 1995.
155. Schultheis PJ, Lorenz JN, Meneton P, et al: Phenotype resembling Gitelman's syndrome in mice lacking the apical $Na^+$-$Cl^-$ cotransporter of the distal convoluted tubule. J Biol Chem 273: 29150–29155, 1998.
156. Kunchaparty S, Palcso M, Berkman J, et al: Defective processing and expression of thiazide-sensitive Na-Cl cotransporter as a cause of Gitelman's syndrome. Am J Physiol 277:F643–F649, 1999.
157. Ellison DH: Divalent cation transport by the distal nephron: Insights from Bartter's and Gitelman's syndromes. Am J Physiol Renal Physiol 279:F616–F625, 2000.
158. Gesek FA, Friedman PA: Mechanism of calcium transport stimulated by chlorothiazide in mouse distal convoluted tubule cells. J Clin Invest 90:429–438, 1992.
159. Capasso G, Rizzo M, Ferrara D: Chronic administration of bendroflumethiazide up-regulates calbindin D28K mRNA expression and protein abundance along the rat distal tubule [abstract]. J Nephrol 13:450, 2000.
160. Sooy K, Kohut J, Christakos S: The role of calbindin and 1,25 dihydroxyvitamin D3 in the kidney. Curr Opin Nephrol Hypertens 9:341–347, 2000.
161. Bianchetti MG, Bettinelli A, Casez JP, et al: Evidence for disturbed regulation of calciotropic hormone metabolism in Gitelman syndrome. J Clin Endocrinol Metab 80:224–228, 1995.
162. Colussi G, Macaluso M, Brunati C, Minetti L: Calcium metabolism and calciotropic hormone levels in Gitelman's syndrome. Miner Electrolyte Metab 20:294–301, 1994.
163. Calo L, Punzi L, Semplicini A: Hypomagnesemia and chondrocalcinosis in Bartter's and Gitelman's syndrome: Review of the pathogenetic mechanisms. Am J Nephrol 20:347–350, 2000.
164. Cobeta-Garcia JC, Gascon A, Iglesias E, Estopinan V: Chondrocalcinosis and Gitelman's syndrome: A new association? [letter]. Ann Rheum Dis 57:748–749, 1998.
165. Fam AG: What is new about crystals other than monosodium urate? Curr Opin Rheumatol 12:228–234, 2000.
166. Gascon A, Cobeta-Garcia JC, Iglesias E: Hypomagnesemia and chondrocalcinosis in Gitelman syndrome [letter; comment]. Am J Med 107:301–302, 1999.
167. Hisakawa N, Yasuoka N, Itoh H, et al: A case of Gitelman's syndrome with chondrocalcinosis. Endocr J 45:261–267, 1998.
168. Punzi L, Calo L, Schiavon F, et al: Chondrocalcinosis is a feature of Gitelman's variant of Bartter's syndrome: A new look at the hypomagnesemia associated with calcium pyrophosphate dihydrate crystal deposition disease. Rev Rheum Engl Ed 65: 571–574, 1998.
169. de Heide LJ, Birkenhager JC: Bartter's syndrome, hypomagnesaemia and chondrocalcinosis. Neth J Med 39:148–152, 1991.
170. Smilde TJ, Haverman JF, Schipper P, et al: Familial hypokalemia/hypomagnesemia and chondrocalcinosis. J Rheumatol 21:1515–1519, 1994.
171. Cole DE, Quamme GA: Inherited disorders of renal magnesium handling. J Am Soc Nephrol 11:1937–1947, 2000.
172. Colussi G, Rombola G, De Ferrari ME, et al: Correction of hypokalemia with antialdosterone therapy in Gitelman's syndrome. Am J Nephrol 14:127–135, 1994.
173. Bettinelli A, Consonni D, Bianchetti MG, et al: Aldosterone influences serum magnesium in Gitelman syndrome. Nephron 86:236, 2000.
174. Kleta R, Frevel T, Cetinkaya I, et al: Physiological treatment of Gitelman's syndrome [abstract]. J Am Soc Nephrol 11:107A, 2000.
175. Kamel KS, Harvey E, Douek K, et al: Studies on the pathogenesis of hypokalemia in Gitelman's syndrome: Role of bicarbonaturia and hypomagnesemia. Am J Nephrol 18:42–49, 1998.
176. Pak CY: Correction of thiazide-induced hypomagnesemia by potassium-magnesium citrate from review of prior trials. Clin Nephrol 54:271–275, 2000.
177. Luthy C, Bettinelli A, Iselin S, et al: Normal prostaglandinuria E2 in Gitelman's syndrome, the hypocalciuric variant of Bartter's syndrome. Am J Kidney Dis 25:824–828, 1995.
178. Dillon MJ, Leonard JV, Buckler JM, et al: Pseudohypoaldosteronism. Arch Dis Child 55:427–434, 1980.
179. Savage MO, Jefferson IG, Dillon MJ, et al: Pseudohypoaldosteronism: Severe salt wasting in infancy caused by generalized mineralocorticoid unresponsiveness. J Pediatr 101:239–242, 1982.
180. Cheek DB, Perry JW: A salt-wasting syndrome in infancy. Arch Dis Child 97:252–256, 1958.
181. Donnell GN, Litman N, Roldan M: Pseudohypoadrenalocorticism. Am J Dis Child 97:813–828, 1959.
182. Popow C, Pollak A, Herkner K, et al: Familial pseudohypoaldosteronism. Acta Paediatr Scand 77:136–141, 1988.
183. Rosler A, Theodor R, Gazit E, et al: Salt wasting, raised plasma-renin activity, and normal or high plasma-aldosterone: A form of pseudohypoaldosteronism. Lancet 1:959–962, 1973.
184. Greenberg D, Abramson O, Phillip M: Fetal pseudohypoaldosteronism: Another cause of hydramnios. Acta Paediatr 84:582–584, 1995.
185. Hanukoglu A: Type I pseudohypoaldosteronism includes two

clinically and genetically distinct entities with either renal or multiple target organ defects. J Clin Endocrinol Metab 73: 936–944, 1991.
186. Chang SS, Grunder S, Hanukoglu A, et al: Mutations in subunits of the epithelial sodium channel cause salt wasting with hyperkalemic acidosis, pseudohypoaldosteronism type 1. Nat Genet 12:248–253, 1996.
187. Geller DS, Rodriguez-Soriano J, Vallo Boado A, et al: Mutations in the mineralocorticoid receptor gene cause autosomal dominant pseudohypoaldosteronism type I. Nat Genet 19:279–281, 1998.
188. Jeck N, Konrad M, Hess M, Seyberth HW: The diuretic- and Bartter-like salt-losing tubulopathies. Nephrol Dial Transplant 15(suppl 6):19–20, 2000.
189. Strautnieks SS, Thompson RJ, Gardiner RM, Chung E: A novel splice-site mutation in the gamma subunit of the epithelial sodium channel gene in three pseudohypoaldosteronism type 1 families. Nat Genet 13:248–250, 1996.
190. Grunder S, Firsov D, Chang SS, et al: A mutation causing pseudohypoaldosteronism type 1 identifies a conserved glycine that is involved in the gating of the epithelial sodium channel. EMBO J 16:899–907, 1997.
191. McDonald FJ, Yang B, Hrstka RF, et al: Disruption of the beta subunit of the epithelial $Na^+$ channel in mice: Hyperkalemia and neonatal death associated with a pseudohypoaldosteronism phenotype. Proc Natl Acad Sci U S A 96:1727–1731, 1999.
192. Hummler E, Barker P, Gatzy J, et al: Early death due to defective neonatal lung liquid clearance in alpha-ENaC–deficient mice. Nat Genet 12:325–328, 1996.
193. Kerem E, Bistritzer T, Hanukoglu A, et al: Pulmonary epithelial sodium-channel dysfunction and excess airway liquid in pseudohypoaldosteronism. N Engl J Med 341:156–162, 1999.
194. Stone RC, Vale P, Rosa FC: Effect of hydrochlorothiazide in pseudohypoaldosteronism with hypercalciuria and severe hyperkalemia. Pediatr Nephrol 10:501–503, 1996.
195. Mathew PM, Manasra KB, Hamdan JA: Indomethacin and cation-exchange resin in the management of pseudohypoaldosteronism. Clin Pediatr (Phila) 32:58–60, 1993.
196. Shalev H, Ohali M, Abramson O: Nephrocalcinosis in pseudohypoaldosteronism and the effect of indomethacin therapy. J Pediatr 125:246–248, 1994.
197. Bayer M, Kutilek S: A hereditary form of pseudohypoaldosteronism may be manifested in the course of pyelonephritis [letter]. Acta Paediatr 82:504, 1993.
198. Berger S, Bleich M, Schmid W, et al: Mineralocorticoid receptor knockout mice: Pathophysiology of $Na^+$ metabolism. Proc Natl Acad Sci U S A 95:9424–9429, 1998.
199. Koo WW, Gupta JM: Breast milk sodium. Arch Dis Child 57: 500–502, 1982.
200. Rosler A: The natural history of salt-wasting disorders of adrenal and renal origin. J Clin Endocrinol Metab 59:689–700, 1984.
201. Hanukoglu A, Joy O, Steinitz M, et al: Pseudohypoaldosteronism due to renal and multisystem resistance to mineralocorticoids respond differently to carbenoxolone. J Steroid Biochem Mol Biol 60:105–112, 1997.
202. Bose HS, Sugawara T, Strauss JF III, Miller WL: The pathophysiology and genetics of congenital lipoid adrenal hyperplasia: International Congenital Lipoid Adrenal Hyperplasia Consortium. N Engl J Med 335:1870–1878, 1996.
203. Bose HS, Sato S, Aisenberg J, et al: Mutations in the steroidogenic acute regulatory protein (StAR) in six patients with congenital lipoid adrenal hyperplasia. J Clin Endocrinol Metab 85: 3636–3639, 2000.
204. Lin D, Sugawara T, Strauss JF III, et al: Role of steroidogenic acute regulatory protein in adrenal and gonadal steroidogenesis. Science 267:1828–1831, 1995; see comments.
205. Cravioto MD, Ulloa-Aguirre A, Bermudez JA, et al: A new inherited variant of the 3 beta-hydroxysteroid dehydrogenase-isomerase deficiency syndrome: Evidence for the existence of two isoenzymes. J Clin Endocrinol Metab 63:360–367, 1986.
206. Rheaume E, Simard J, Morel Y, et al: Congenital adrenal hyperplasia due to point mutations in the type II 3 beta-hydroxysteroid dehydrogenase gene. Nat Genet 1:239–245, 1992.
207. New MI, Wilson RC: Steroid disorders in children: Congenital adrenal hyperplasia and apparent mineralocorticoid excess. Proc Natl Acad Sci U S A 96:12790–12797, 1999.
208. New MI, Gertner JM, Speiser PW, Del Balzo P: Growth and final height in classical and nonclassical 21-hydroxylase deficiency. J Endocrinol Invest 12:91–95, 1989.
209. Rosler A, Levine LS, Schneider B, et al: The interrelationship of sodium balance, plasma renin activity and ACTH in congenital adrenal hyperplasia. J Clin Endocrinol Metab 45:500–512, 1977.
210. Speiser PW, Dupont B, Rubinstein P, et al: High frequency of nonclassical steroid 21-hydroxylase deficiency. Am J Hum Genet 37:650–667, 1985.
211. New MI, Miller B, Peterson RE: Aldosterone excretion in normal children and in children with adrenal hyperplasia. J Clin Invest 45:412–428, 1966.
212. New MI, Seaman MP: Secretion rates of cortisol and aldosterone precursors in various forms of congenital adrenal hyperplasia. J Clin Endocrinol Metab 30:361–371, 1970.
213. White PC: Disorders of aldosterone biosynthesis and action. N Engl J Med 331:250–257, 1994.
214. Forest MG, Betuel H, Couillin P, Boue A: Prenatal diagnosis of congenital adrenal hyperplasia (CAH) due to 21-hydroxylase deficiency by steroid analysis in the amniotic fluid of mid-pregnancy: Comparison with HLA typing in 17 pregnancies at risk for CAH. Prenat Diagn 1:197–207, 1981.
215. Forest MG, Betuel H, David M: Prenatal treatment in congenital adrenal hyperplasia due to 21-hydroxylase deficiency: Update 88 of the French multicentric study. Endocr Res 15:277–301, 1989.
216. Nordenstrom A, Marcus C, Axelson M, et al: Failure of cortisone acetate treatment in congenital adrenal hyperplasia because of defective 11 beta-hydroxysteroid dehydrogenase reductase activity. J Clin Endocrinol Metab 84:1210–1213, 1999.
217. Zanaria E, Muscatelli F, Bardoni B, et al: An unusual member of the nuclear hormone receptor superfamily responsible for X-linked adrenal hypoplasia congenita. Nature 372:635–641, 1994.
218. Hildebrandt F, Otto E: Molecular genetics of nephronophthisis and medullary cystic kidney disease. J Am Soc Nephrol 11: 1753–1761, 2000.
219. Otto E, Kispert A, Schatzle S, et al: Nephrocystin: Gene expression and sequence conservation between human, mouse, and *Caenorhabditis elegans*. J Am Soc Nephrol 11:270–282, 2000.
220. Gardner KDJ: Evolution of clinical signs in adult-onset cystic disease of the renal medulla. Ann Intern Med 74:47–54, 1971.
221. Chagnac A, Zevin D, Weinstein T, et al: Combined tubular dysfunction in medullary cystic disease. Arch Intern Med 146: 1007–1009, 1986.
222. Grinspoon SK, Biller BM: Clinical review 62: Laboratory assessment of adrenal insufficiency. J Clin Endocrinol Metab 79: 923–931, 1994.
223. Oelkers W, Diederich S, Bahr V: Recent advances in diagnosis and therapy of Addison's disease. In Bhatt HR, James VHT, Besser GM, et al (eds): Advances in Thomas Addison's Diseases, vol 1. London, Thomas Addison Society, 1994, pp 69–80.
224. Tordjman K, Jaffe A, Grazas N, et al: The role of the low dose (1 microgram) adrenocorticotropin test in the evaluation of patients with pituitary diseases. J Clin Endocrinol Metab 80: 1301–1305, 1995.
225. Broide J, Soferman R, Kivity S, et al: Low-dose adrenocorticotropin test reveals impaired adrenal function in patients taking inhaled corticosteroids. J Clin Endocrinol Metab 80:1243–1246, 1995.
226. Blevins LS, Shankroff J, Moser HW, Ladenson PW: Elevated plasma adrenocorticotropin concentration as evidence of limited adrenocortical reserve in patients with adrenomyeloneuropathy. J Clin Endocrinol Metab 78:261–265, 1994.
227. Oelkers W, Diederich S, Bahr V: Diagnosis and therapy surveillance in Addison's disease: Rapid adrenocorticotropin (ACTH) test and measurement of plasma ACTH, renin activity, and aldosterone. J Clin Endocrinol Metab 75:259–264, 1992.
228. Pavord SR, Girach A, Price DE, et al: A retrospective audit of the combined pituitary function test, using the insulin stress test, TRH and GnRH in a district laboratory. Clin Endocrinol (Oxf) 36:135–139, 1992.
229. Fiad TM, Kirby JM, Cunningham SK, McKenna TJ: The over-

night single-dose metyrapone test is a simple and reliable index of the hypothalamic-pituitary-adrenal axis. Clin Endocrinol (Oxf) 40:603–609, 1994.
230. Oelkers W: Dose-response aspects in the clinical assessment of the hypothalamo-pituitary-adrenal axis, and the low-dose adrenocorticotropin test. Eur J Endocrinol 135:27–33, 1996.
231. Steiner H, Bahr V, Exner P, Oelkers PW: Pituitary function tests: Comparison of ACTH and 11-deoxy-cortisol responses in the metyrapone test and with the insulin hypoglycemia test. Exp Clin Endocrinol 102:33–38, 1994.
232. Schlaghecke R, Kornely E, Santen RT, Ridderskamp P: The effect of long-term glucocorticoid therapy on pituitary-adrenal responses to exogenous corticotropin-releasing hormone. N Engl J Med 326:226–230, 1992.
233. Trainer PJ, Faria M, Newell-Price J, et al: A comparison of the effects of human and ovine corticotropin-releasing hormone on the pituitary-adrenal axis. J Clin Endocrinol Metab 80: 412–417, 1995.
234. Orth DN: Corticotropin-releasing hormone in humans. Endocr Rev 13:164–191, 1992.
235. Kwon TH, Frokiaer J, Fernandez-Llama P, et al: Reduced abundance of aquaporins in rats with bilateral ischemia-induced acute renal failure: Prevention by alpha-MSH. Am J Physiol 277:F413–F427, 1999.

CHAPTER 19

# Genetic Disorders of Renal Apical $Na^+$ Transporters

Pierre Meneton, PhD ▪ Young S. Oh, PhD ▪ David G. Warnock, MD

Genetic studies and gene targeting techniques suggest that the genes encoding renal apical $Na^+$ transport proteins play an essential role in the control of extracellular fluid volume and blood pressure. Significant advancements in the understanding of the role of these genes in mendelian forms of extracellular volume homeostatic disorders have been achieved in recent years. Of even greater importance will be definition of the various factors that regulate the expression and activity of the $Na^+$ transport systems. These regulatory pathways and the responses to environmental factors such as dietary salt and stress may play a central role in determining the appearance, severity, and complexity of the clinical phenotypes that result from genetic disorders of the renal apical $Na^+$ transporters.

Blood pressure level depends on both peripheral vascular resistance, which is continuously controlled by the arterioles to adjust blood flow to the metabolic needs of each tissue[1] and cardiac output, which is determined primarily by extracellular fluid volume. The kidneys play a critical role in the control of extracellular fluid volume by matching urinary $Na^+$ and water output to dietary intake.[2] The functions of the kidneys, heart, and blood vessels are tightly integrated by multiple regulatory systems acting by neuronal, endocrine or paracrine pathways.[3]

From a genetic viewpoint, we are beginning to gain significant insights into the identity of the genes conferring to these organs the ability to control blood pressure. Using linkage studies and positional cloning in humans, a dozen genes responsible for monogenic forms of hypertension and hypotension or associated to essential hypertension have been identified at this time (Fig. 19–1). Remarkably, all of these genes are either mediating or involved in the regulation of renal $Na^+$ transport.[4] Gene targeting experiments in the mouse also furnish striking evidence for the importance of renal $Na^+$ handling in blood pressure control. Among the approximately 2000 genes modified to date by homologous recombination, approximately 30 genes, including the genes described as being involved in blood pressure control in humans, are shown to trigger a chronic change of blood pressure in adult mice when they are inactivated or activated.[5] Most of these genes encode for components of neuronal, hormonal, or paracrine systems that are known to participate in the regulation of renal $Na^+$ reabsorption.[6] In addition, it appears that blood pressure level is not determined by the preponderant action of a few genes but rather by a large number of genes, each having only a relatively small effect. Thus, the currently available genetic data strongly reinforce the concept that regulation of extracellular fluid volume by the kidneys is the major blood pressure control mechanism in the long-term and emphasize the crucial role of tubular $Na^+$ transport in this process.[2]

The reabsorption of $Na^+$ along the nephron follows a general rule; that is, $Na^+$ entry across the apical membrane is the primary determinant of intracellular $Na^+$ concentration in the epithelial cells. In turn, intracellular $Na^+$ concentration directly controls the activity of the $Na^+,K^+$-ATPase responsible for $Na^+$ extrusion across the basolateral membrane.[7] Thus, apical $Na^+$ entry is limiting for transepithelial $Na^+$ and fluid transport, and any change in the quantity and/or activity of the proteins mediating this entry should affect the reabsorption rate. Various genetic disorders have been described which result from mutations of renal tubular transport proteins.[8] Four major apical $Na^+$ transport

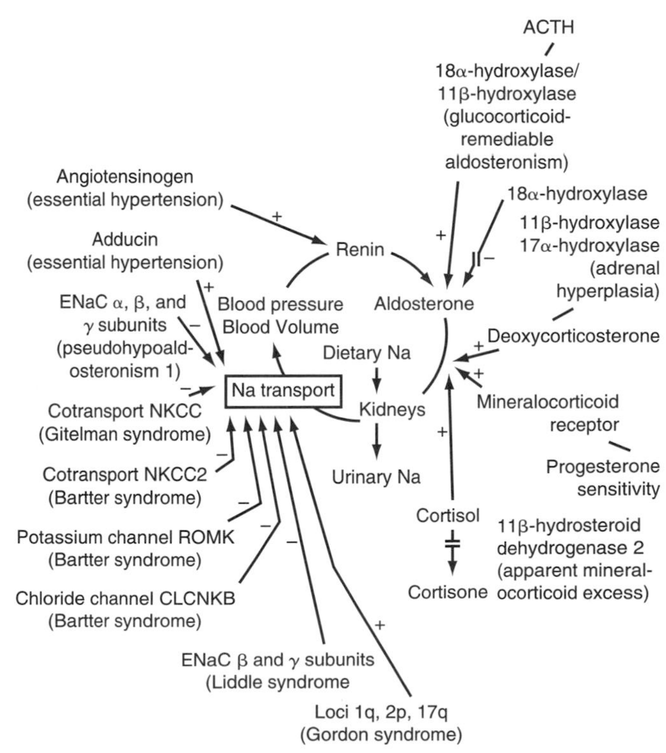


**FIGURE 19–1** ▪ Mutations and polymorphisms altering blood pressure in humans. All the genes are involved directly or indirectly in the control of renal Na reabsorption. The mutations have been found in monogenic human diseases that cause disorders of blood pressure regulation. (From Meneton P, Warnock DG: Involvement of renal apical Na transport systems in the control of blood pressure. Am J Kidney Dis 37:S39–S47, 2001.)

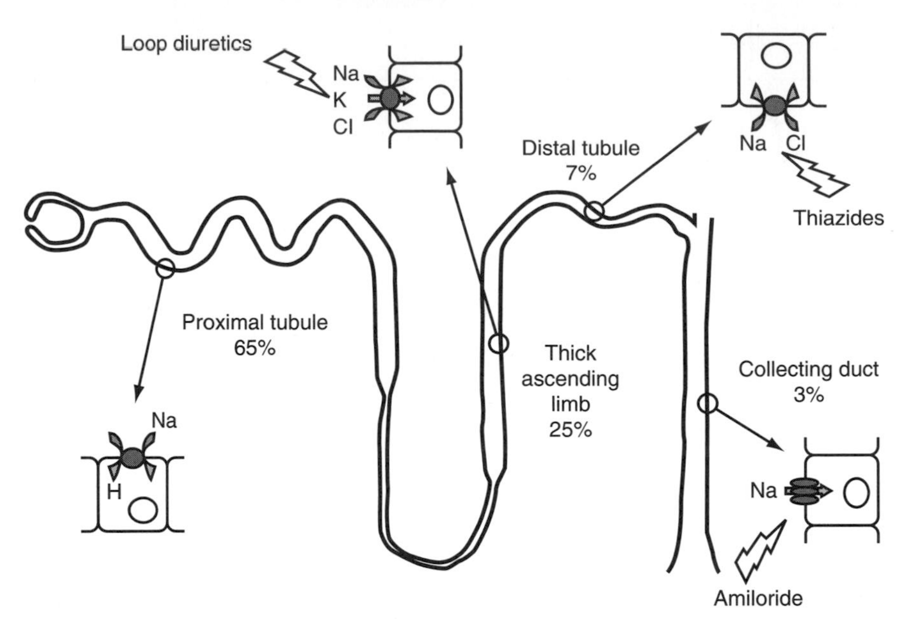


FIGURE 19–2 ■ Main apical Na$^+$ transport systems expressed along the nephron. The reabsorbed fraction of filtered Na load and specific inhibitors used as diuretics are indicated for each transport system. (From Meneton P, Oh YS, Warnock DG: Genetic renal tubular disorders of renal ion channels and transporters. Semin Nephrol 21:81–93, 2001.)

systems are present along the nephron,[9] each being expressed in a specific segment as shown in Figure 19–2. The Na$^+$-H$^+$ exchanger-3 (NHE-3) mediates bulk reabsorption of filtered $NaHCO_3$ in the proximal convoluted tubule while the furosemide-sensitive Na$^+$-K$^+$-2Cl$^-$ cotransporter 2 (NKCC2), located in the thick ascending limb of the loop of Henle, reabsorbs much of the remaining luminal NaCl. The remaining few percent of the filtered Na$^+$ are reabsorbed by the thiazide-sensitive Na$^+$-Cl$^-$ cotransporter (NCC) in the distal convoluted tubule and by the amiloride-sensitive epithelial Na$^+$ channel (ENaC) in the connecting tubule and collecting duct. Our aim is to review the data gathered on the pathophysiologic roles of these apical Na$^+$ transport systems using linkage and cohort studies in humans and gene targeting techniques in mice. Gene targeting techniques have produced mouse strains in which each of the genes encoding the apical Na$^+$ transport systems has been separately inactivated so that the effects of these mutations on fluid homeostasis and blood pressure can be investigated. The integration of these genes into the physiology and the development of the organism can be addressed in these mouse models by analyzing the compensatory phenomena. The observed phenotype in the adult (e.g., hypertension) is the result of the effect of the primary mutation and all of the compensatory processes that have taken place throughout the fetal, neonatal, and postnatal development of the organism in reaction to the primary mutation.

## Na$^+$-H$^+$ EXCHANGER-3

Most of the filtered Na$^+$ load is reabsorbed in the proximal convoluted tubule and NHE-3 has been shown to be responsible for up to 60% of the Na$^+$ reabsorption in this segment.[10] Therefore, one would predict that NHE-3 exerts a major influence on overall fluid and electrolyte balance and blood pressure. In the absence of functional mutations described in humans, the only available model for studying the role of NHE-3 in vivo are the NHE-3–deficient mice generated by gene targeting.[11]

On a normal-salt diet, NHE-3–deficient mice present marked disturbances such as low blood pressure, hyperkalemic metabolic acidosis, and hyperactivity of the renin-angiotensin-aldosterone system. The sharp reduction of fluid reabsorption in the proximal convoluted tubule of these mice overloads downstream segments of the nephron, which develop compensatory responses in order to limit Na$^+$ and water wasting in the urine. Thus, ENaC activity is found to be upregulated in the connecting tubule and collecting duct due to the highly elevated plasma aldosterone level. Increased Na$^+$ reabsorption in the loop of Henle, presumably mediated by NKCC2, is also demonstrated in these mice.[12] However, the main renal compensatory mechanism seems to be the decrease in single-nephron glomerular filtration rate, which is mediated in part by the activation of the tubuloglomerular feedback.[12] Owing to these various adaptive processes, distal delivery of fluid to the distal nephron is similar between NHE-3–deficient mice and wild-type mice. In fact, NHE-3–deficient mice excrete even less Na$^+$ and water daily in the urine than wild-type mice. Despite these adaptations, NHE-3–deficient mice have decreased blood pressure when fed a normal salt diet and are unable to survive on a low-salt diet.

In contrast to the NCC and NKCC2 transporters for which there are renal-specific isoforms, NHE-3 is also strongly expressed along the intestine where the exchanger normally mediates Na$^+$ and water reabsorption in cooperation with the apical $Cl^-$-$HCO_3^-$ exchanger.[13] It is, therefore, not surprising to observe in NHE-3–deficient mice, in addition to the renal phenotype, absorptive intestinal defects resulting in diarrhea and marked increase (two to fivefold) in the content volume of the distal segments of the intestine. As a consequence, several compensatory mechanisms occur in the distal colon to limit fluid wasting in the feces. For example, mRNAs encoding ENaC β- and γ-subunits are upregulated and transepithelial amiloride-sensitive Na current is sharply increased as expected from the very high plasma aldosterone level. The massive induction of the colonic $H^+$,$K^+$-ATPase mRNA seems to be related to the recovery of $K^+$, which is abnormally secreted into the lumen due to the increased electrogenic $Na^+$ reabsorption. However, despite these compensatory phenomena, adult NHE-3–deficient mice at steady state lose $Na^+$ and water in the feces compared with wild-type mice.

Given the phenotype of NHE-3–deficient mice, it is obvious that linkage and mutations in the NHE-3 gene should be investigated in several human disorders ranging from hypertension to hyperkalemic metabolic acidosis and diarrhea. Type II (proximal) renal tubular acidosis, in the absence of the Fanconi syndrome, could be also explained by NHE-3 dysfunction even though hypokalemia rather than hyperkalemia is usually seen in these patients.

## LOOP DIURETIC–SENSITIVE $Na^+$-$K^+$-$2Cl^-$ COTRANSPORTER (NKCC2)

Patients diagnosed with Bartter syndrome can present at an early age with severe urinary $Na^+$ wasting associated with extracellular fluid volume depletion, hypokalemic metabolic alkalosis, increased urinary $Ca^+$ excretion, and normal or low blood pressure despite a hyper-activation of the renin-angiotensin-aldosterone system.[14] Mutations in the gene encoding NKCC2[15–17] as well as in the genes encoding chloride channel CLCNKB[18] and potassium channel ROMK[19–24] have been found in patients with Bartter syndrome. As for the two other genes, the NKCC2 mutations (nonconservative amino acid changes, frameshifts, or truncations) are thought to result in a loss of function of the protein which normally reabsorbs about 30% of the filtered $Na^+$ load along the thick ascending limb of the loop of Henle and plays an essential role in the establishment of the corticopapillary interstitial osmotic gradient necessary for urine concentration.[25]

In confirmation of this hypothesis, NKCC2-deficient mice generated by gene targeting have many similarities to patients with Bartter syndrome.[26] These mice display signs of dehydration (increased hematocrit) as early as 1 day after birth. They subsequently failed to thrive and usually die before weaning. At 7 days, they exhibit hyperkalemic metabolic acidosis, hydronephrosis, and upregulation of the renin-angiotensin system as observed in some human perinatal Bartter syndrome.[27, 28] When treated with prostaglandin synthesis inhibitor indomethacin, NKCC2-deficient mice can survive to the adult stage but exhibit severe polyuria and hydronephrosis, hypokalemic metabolic alkalosis, and hypercalciuria. In addition, they have a low blood pressure when fed a normal-salt diet and are unable to survive on a low-salt diet (Nobuyuki Takahashi, personal communication). All these features are typical of Bartter syndrome, even though their extent clearly differs from the human phenotype.[29] Hydronephrosis is very severe in Bartter mice but is only observed occasionally in patients with Bartter syndrome. On the other hand, hypokalemia is very mild in Bartter mice, whereas patients with Bartter syndrome have usually profound hypokalemia. Despite these phenotypic differences between the two species, which appear to be quantitative rather than qualitative, NKCC2-deficient mice represent an interesting animal model of Bartter syndrome to investigate the mechanisms by which the mutation provokes the phenotype. For example, it is not obvious why the loss of function of NKCC2 leads to a hyperkalemic metabolic acidosis in the perinatal period and to hypokalemic metabolic alkalosis in adulthood. The understanding of the very high phenotypic heterogeneity of the syndrome in humans,[30] which is likely related to the influence of the individual genetic background, should also be greatly facilitated by the exploration of the phenotype of these mice in different genetic inbred backgrounds.

## THIAZIDE-SENSITIVE $Na^+$-$Cl^-$ COTRANSPORTER

Gitelman syndrome is an autosomal recessive disorder characterized by hypokalemic metabolic alkalosis, hypomagnesemia, and hypocalciuria with normal or low blood pressure and some evidence of salt wasting and hypovolemia.[31] Complete linkage of the syndrome to the locus encoding NCC has been demonstrated in several affected families, and more than 80 different mutations in the NCC gene have been found in patients diagnosed with the syndrome.[19, 32–39] Most of these mutations are nonconservative amino acid changes or deletions likely to be associated with loss of function of NCC. For example, a mutation deleting the carboxy-terminal 54 amino acids has been shown in an in vitro expression system to lead to misfolding and premature degradation of the protein in the endoplasmic reticulum.[40] At least 10 other mutations have been shown to prevent the delivery of NCC to the plasma membrane by misfolding-induced degradation of the protein in the endoplasmic reticulum.[41]

An NCC-deficient mouse strain with a phenotype similar to Gitelman syndrome has been generated by homologous recombination.[11] These mice exhibit low rates of urinary $Ca^{2+}$ excretion and low plasma magnesium concentrations together with some evidence of $Na^+$ wasting (slight overactivation of the renin-angiotensin system and low blood pressure under dietary $Na^+$ depletion). In contrast to the human syndrome, the NCC-deficient mice do not manifest hypokalemia or alkalosis. This discrepancy may be explained by some difference in species but may also be related to a recruitment bias of patients with Gitelman syndrome. Hypokalemia and alkalosis are among the inclusion criteria used to diagnose Gitelman syndrome, and it is not surprising to find both of these features in all patients. It may well be that in other people, mutations in the NCC gene provoke only hypomagnesemia and hypocalciuria without hypokalemic alkalosis due to the different genetic background of the individuals. This should be settled in the future by searching for subsets of patients without hypokalemic alkalosis, by carefully phenotyping extended pedigrees, and by looking at the phenotype of NCC-deficient mice in different genetic inbred backgrounds.

Immunologic and morphologic studies show that a large part of the distal convoluted tubule is completely missing in the NCC-deficient mice, so that the cortical thick ascending limb is almost directly in continuity with the connecting tubule (Jan Loffing, Personal communication). Given that NCC normally reabsorbs about 7% of the filtered Na load along the distal convoluted tubule, the loss of function of the transporter induces an increased $Na^+$ delivery to the connecting tubule and collecting duct. As an expected compensatory phenomenon, the amount of ENaC is upregulated in the apical membrane of principal cells along the connecting tubule (Jan Loffing, Personal communication). This adaptation is not observed in the collecting duct, suggesting that the increased ENaC-mediated $Na^+$ reabsorption in the connecting tubule is sufficient for compensating NCC inactivation when the mice are fed a normal-salt diet. If minimal $K^+$ and $H^+$ secretion occurs in the connecting tubule, this could explain why the NCC-deficient mice do not develop hypokalemia and metabolic alkalosis. These adaptations in the connecting tubule are efficient enough to allow the mice to survive indefinitely on a low-salt diet, and they probably also explain why the renin-angiotensin-aldosterone system is not strongly activated in NCC-deficient mice.

Concerning the mechanisms of the hypocalciuria; if reduced urinary $Ca^+$ excretion is due to increased tubular $Ca^+$ reabsorption,[42] this cannot be occurring in the upstream part of the distal convoluted tubule because it is virtually absent in NCC-deficient mice. The other sites where tubular $Ca^+$ reabsorption could be increased are the downstream part of the distal convoluted tubule where $Ca^+$ transport systems are heavily expressed and the thick ascending limb, which shows signs of a global adaptation with a twofold increase in the amount of apical NKCC2 cotransporter (Jan Loffing, Personal communication). If, in addition, the pericellular permeability for divalent cations favors $Ca^+$ over $Mg^+$, then the clinical phenotype would include enhanced $Ca^+$ reabsorption in the thick ascending limb and hypocalciuria, with renal $Mg^+$ wasting and hypomagnesemia. The possibility that divalent cation permeabilities could be differentially affected during hypertrophy is supported by the description of differentially selective divalent cation permeation pathways mediated by paracellins.[43]

## EPITHELIAL $Na^+$ CHANNEL (ENaC) AND THE DEG/ENaC SUPERFAMILY

The low-conductance ENaC present in the apical membranes of many $Na^+$-absorptive epithelia, such as the renal tubules, distal colon, sweat ducts, and lungs, is specifically inhibited by the diuretic drug amiloride.[44, 45] ENaC is well suited for participating in the maintenance of $Na^+$ homeostasis, blood volume, and blood pressure by providing an apical entry pathway for $Na^+$ ions to permit rapid vectorial transport of $Na^+$ from the luminal to the interstitial compartment in these epithelia (Fig. 19–3). The participation of ENaC in the control of blood pressure has been demonstrated effectively in the last several years with the description of gain or loss of function mutations in both humans and mice. In that sense, ENaC can be

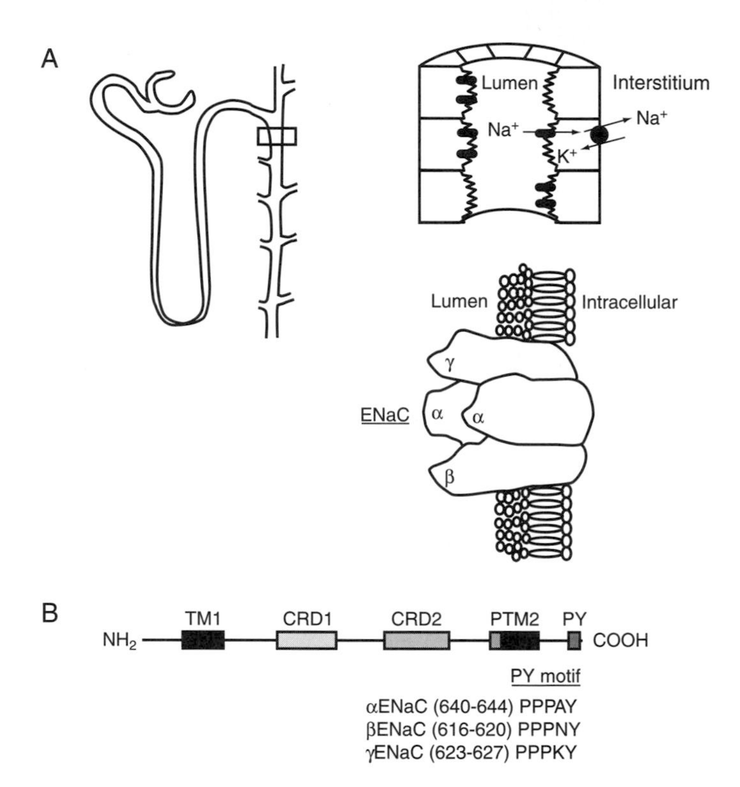


**FIGURE 19–3** ■ *A*, Schematic illustration showing the localization of epithelial $Na^+$ channels (ENaCs) in the collecting duct of the kidney. ENaC is expressed in the principal cells of the collecting duct, and its presence is polarized at the apical membrane in the cell. $Na^+$ enters the cell passively through ENaC following its electrochemical concentration gradient which is set across the apical membrane. $Na^+$ leaves the cell by way of $Na^+/K^+$ ATPase localized in the basolateral membrane. The subunit stoichiometry of the ENaC complex has been suggested either to be 4 subunits (2α, 1β, and 1γ)[56, 57] or 9 subunits (3α, 3β, and 3γ).[58, 59] In this figure, a model of the heterotetrameric architecture of ENaC is shown. *B*, The three ENaC subunits (α, β, and γ) have a common structure, containing two transmembrane domains (TMs) with a large extracellular loop (~65% of total amino acids) and two short cytoplasmic amino and carboxy termini. In the extracellular region, there are two conserved cystein-rich domains (CRDs), which seem to play an important role in channel assembly and targeting.[94] In each ENaC subunit, the pore-forming region (P) is localized just before TM2,[108] and the PY motif (PPPXY; X denotes any amino acid) is localized in the carboxy terminus. Numbers in parentheses correspond to the amino acid positions of the PY motif in each human ENaC subunit. The PY motif is shown to regulate channel density in the plasma membrane by interacting with the WW domains of Nedd4 protein.[86, 109] The PY motif in αENaC has also been suggested to interact with the SH3 domain of α-spectrin for proper targeting of the ENaC complex to the apical membranes.[110] (From Oh Y, Warnock DG: Disorders of the epithelial $Na^+$ channel in Liddle's syndrome and autosomal recessive pseudohypoaldosteronism, type 1. Exp Nephrol 8:320–325, 2000.)

used as a paradigm of what could be done with the other apical $Na^+$ transport systems.

Three subunits of ENaC have been cloned, α, β, and γ, which are homologous to each other, having about 35% amino acid identity over the entire length of coding regions.[46] ENaC shares significant sequence similarity with the nematode *Caenorhabditis elegans* degenerin (DEG) genes, such as *mec-4, mec-10,* and *deg-1,* which are involved in sensory touch transduction and, when mutated, neuronal degeneration.[47] Therefore, it has been proposed that ENaC subunits and the *mec-4, mec-10,* and *deg-1* proteins all belong to the same gene family (DEG/ENaC superfamily) that encodes cation channels involved in the control of the cellular and extracellular volume.[48] Other members of the DEG/ENaC superfamily include the ENaC δ subunit cloned from the rat and human brain,[49] mammalian degenerin (MDEG) or brain $Na^+$ channels (BNaCs),[50] the acid-sensing ionic channel (ASIC),[51] and a FRMFamide-activated $Na^+$ channel (FaNaC) cloned from the nervous system of the snail *Helix aspersa.*[52] The DEG/ENaC superfamily contains similar sequences and the same predicted structure—intracellular N- and C-termini, two hydrophobic membrane-spanning regions, and a large extracellular loop. This topology has been experimentally demonstrated for the ENaC α subunit[46, 53, 54] and MEC-4.[47, 55]

## FUNCTIONAL STUDIES OF ENaC

Functional expression studies have demonstrated that the three ENaC subunits form a heteromultimeric, constitutively active channel when coexpressed in *Xenopus* oocytes as well as in mammalian cells. The stoichiometry of the functional ENaC complex is not yet established, and it has been suggested to be either a tetramer[56, 57] or nanomer.[58, 59] The α-ENaC alone can produce an amiloride-sensitive $Na^+$ current in *Xenopus* oocytes, but the amplitude of the $Na^+$ current is small.[60–62] Nevertheless, the critical role of α-ENaC in forming a functional $Na^+$ channel in vivo was demonstrated by knocking out α-ENaC gene in mice, which then died within 40 hours of birth due to the failure of lung liquid clearance.[63] It is known that ENaC plays a critical role in clearing lung liquid during birth.[64] The role of α-ENaC for proper subunit assembly and targeting of the assembled channel complex to the apical membrane of epithelial cells has been described.[65–67] Several naturally occurring splice variants of human α-ENaC have been identified,[68, 69] but their physiologic significance remains to be characterized.

Two other ENaC subunits (β and γ) can potentiate the amiloride-sensitive current by more than 20-fold when all three subunits are coexpressed together in *Xenopus* oocytes.[61, 62] Interestingly, neither the ENaC β nor γ subunit alone could readily generate significant amiloride-sensitive currents, which is consistent with an unique role of the α subunit in forming and delivering of the assembled channel complex to the membrane. Moreover, coexpression of α and β subunits (or α and γ subunits) generated a small (three to fivefold) or no potentiation in current,[61, 62] suggesting that maximal ENaC activity can only be obtained when all three subunits are coexpressed together. Bonny and associates[65] have described a truncated α-ENaC that lacks the critical pore-forming (P) region (see Fig. 19–3) but is still capable with extended in vitro incubation of delivering a functional amiloride-sensitive channel, presumably composed of truncated α-ENaC and wild-type β and γ subunits, to the surface membrane in oocytes. The findings reported by Bonny and associates suggest that the truncated α-ENaC, which retains the N-terminus and the extracellular cysteine-rich domain, may contain a sorting signal that promotes the assembly and intracellular trafficking of the assembled ENaC complexes to the cell membrane.

Although ENaCs of different species are highly homologous to each other, there are some minor functional differences between different species. For example, Chraibi and Horisberger[70] have reported that human and *Xenopus* ENaCs (but not rat ENaCs) can be activated by glibenclamide, an inhibitor of sulfonylurea receptor and cystic fibrosis conductance regulator, in the oocyte expression system. The amiloride-sensitivity current obtained with α plus β subunits of each species is also quite different. Rat α-ENaC plus β-ENaC showed 5% to 30% of the amiloride-sensitive current compared with wild-type α plus β and γ subunits.[71] In contrast, extremely low amiloride-sensitive currents were observed with human α plus β-ENaC subunits after expression in the oocyte system.[62] Moreover, it appears that human ENaC can be activated by a membrane-permeable cyclic adenosine monophosphate (cAMP) analog, 8-CPT-cAMP, whereas the effect on rat ENaC activity is transient and can be easily missed, especially in the flow-through perfusion system (Tamba and associates, unpublished data). These findings emphasize the necessity of using human ENaCs when investigating the structure-function relationship of human disease-related ENaC mutations in the heterologous expression system.

In vivo, the localization and synthesis of ENaC subunits are tightly controlled by environmental factors such as dietary salt intake. For example in the mouse, feeding a high (3%)- or low (0.05%)-salt diet for 3 weeks influences strongly the distribution pattern of ENaC in the late portion of the distal convoluted tubule down to the medullary collecting duct.[72] On a high-salt diet with suppressed plasma aldosterone levels, the α subunit is undetectable, whereas the β and γ subunits are present in intracellular membranous dispersed sites but not in the apical plasma membrane. On a low-salt diet with elevated plasma aldosterone levels, all three subunits are displayed in the subapical cytoplasm and apical plasma membrane. The extent of the apical labeling for the β and γ subunits decreases from the connecting tubule to the medullary collecting duct, whereas the opposite is true for the cytoplasmic staining, indicating the existence of an adaptive gradient along this portion of the nephron. Thus, the regulation of ENaC activity in the kidneys involves both translocation of pre-existing β and γ subunits between intracellular sites and the apical plasma membrane as well as de novo synthesis of new α subunits.

## PSEUDOALDOSTERONISM

Liddle syndrome represents a rare form of low-renin, volume-expanded, salt-sensitive hypertension. It was first described by Liddle and associates in 1963[73] in a large kindred from Alabama. Liddle's original publication is a classical description of clinical investigation. They did not find any beneficial effect of spironolactone, a mineralocorticoid antagonist, but triamterene (an ENaC blocker) did correct the hypertension, renal $K^+$ wasting, and hypokalemia as long as the subjects restricted their dietary salt intake; salt restriction is necessary because low $Na^+$ in the filtered fluid in the kidney can enhance the inhibitory effect of triamterene on ENaC activity. Liddle and associates[73] correctly interpreted these findings as indicating an intrinsic renal defect in the regulation of salt absorption rather than the effects of some unidentified mineralocorticoid other than aldosterone on the distal tubules. In 1994, the autosomal dominant inheritance of this syndrome was demonstrated by Botero-Velez and associates,[74] and subsequently ENaC mutations associated with the original Liddle's kindred as well as with four other families were demonstrated by Shimkets and associates using genetic linkage analysis.[75] Several other ENaC mutations associated with Liddle syndrome have been identified since then.[76–84] Interestingly, all of the identified mutations of Liddle syndrome reside in the carboxy terminus of the β- or γ-ENaC subunits, respectively, either deleting or modifying the functionally important PY motif (see Fig. 19–3). Deletion or modification of the PY motif in Liddle syndrome results in increased channel number (as well as increased open probability of the single ion channel) in expression systems.[85–87] Constitutive activation of ENaC activity in Liddle syndrome would explain the pathophysiology of this rare form of low-renin hypertension. Unregulated, continuing $Na^+$ reabsorption across the connecting and collecting tubules of the kidney would result in volume expansion, suppression of plasma renin activity and aldosterone secretion, and consequent hypertension (Fig. 19–4). As such, this phenotype has been referred to as pseudoaldosteronism.[73]

A second form of pseudoaldosteronism has been described; this form results from a mutation in the hormone-binding domain of the mineralocorticoid receptor.[88] Although the phenotype of this disorder (pseudoaldosteronism, type 2) strongly resembles Liddle syndrome (pseudoaldosteronism, type 1) with hypertension and suppressed peripheral renin activity and aldosterone secretion (see Fig. 19–4), there is also an especially severe presentation during pregnancy.[88] A serine to leucine mutation in the hormone-binding domain changes the affinity of the receptor for a number of steroids. Progesterone in particular has an exceptionally high affinity for the receptor, thus accounting for the especially severe presentation during pregnancy. Spironolactone is also an agonist for the mutated receptor; therefore, spironolactone is ineffective in pseudoaldosteronism, type 1,[73] and is contraindicated in pseudoaldosteronism, type 2.[88] It appears that the mutated receptor has constitutively activated basal activity or may be responding to other endogenous steroids (e.g., 19-norprogesterone or 17-OH progesterone) to account for the clinical phenotype in males and nonpregnant females.[88]

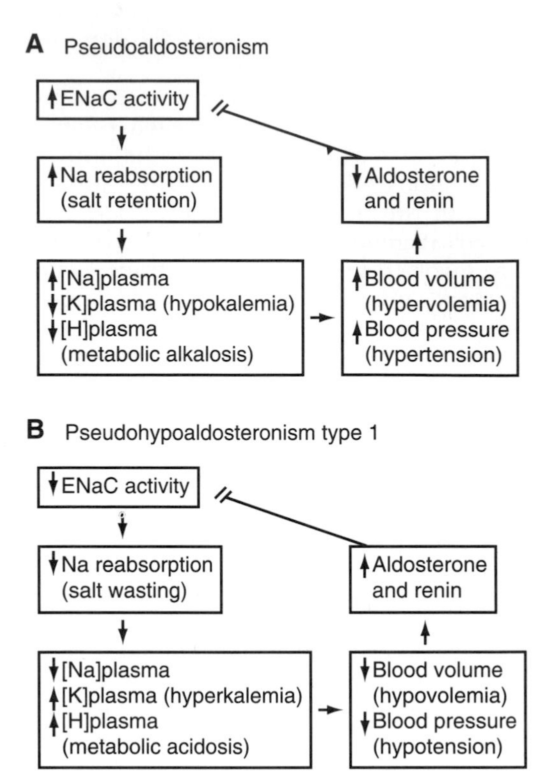


**FIGURE 19–4** ■ Possible pathways that are involved in pseudoaldosteronism *(A)* and autosomal recessive PHA-1 *(B)*. In both cases, the "dysregulation" of ENaC activity (enhanced channel activity in pseudoaldosteronism or reduced channel activity in PHA-1) underlies the pathophysiology. In pseudoaldosteronism, gain of function mutations in ENaC, per se (type 1), or in the mineralocorticoid receptor (type 2) are the cause of the enhanced ENaC activity. (From Oh Y, Warnock DG: Disorders of the epithelial $Na^+$ channel in Liddle's syndrome and autosomal recessive pseudohypoaldosteronism, type 1. Exp Nephrol 8:320–325, 2000.)

Recently, the truncation of the ENaC β subunit found in the original Liddle pedigree was reproduced in the mouse using gene targeting and Cre/loxP techniques.[89] Under a normal-salt diet, these mice have a blood pressure that does not differ from that of wild-type mice, despite evidence of chronic hypervolemia such as increased $Na^+$ reabsorption in the distal colon and low plasma aldosterone. Under high-salt diet, the mice develop hypokalemic metabolic alkalosis, high blood pressure and cardiac hypertrophy, thus reproducing to a large extent the human syndrome. These mice furnish a useful animal model of Liddle syndrome to investigate the relationships between renal

Na+ reabsorption, dietary salt intake, and blood pressure.

## PSEUDOHYPOALDOSTERONISM TYPE 1

Genetic linkage analysis has also demonstrated an association of ENaC gene mutations with autosomal recessive pseudohypoaldosteronism type 1 (PHA-1), an inherited human disorder characterized by salt wasting, hyperkalemic acidosis, and unresponsiveness to mineralocorticoids.[90–92] Premature truncations of α-ENaC occurring before the first transmembrane domain (I68fr) or before the second transmembrane domain (R508x) have been found (Fig. 19–5). Expression of these mutants in *Xenopus* oocytes generated no appreciable level of amiloride-sensitive current,[92] which is consistent with the pathophysiology ("loss-of-channel function") of PHA-1. In γ-ENaC, splice-site mutations occurring immediately after the first transmembrane domain (K106sp) have been found, which result in either a premature truncation or substitution of three conserved amino acids of 106 to 108KYS by an asparagine.[90] Kerem and associates[93] have reported several PHA-1 mutations causing premature truncation of α- or β-ENaC by point mutation or frameshift (see Fig. 19–5). The functional consequences of these mutations have not been reported, but it seems likely that they will generate reduced ENaC activity.

Two single amino acid point mutations have been found in PHA-1 (see Fig. 19–5). One mutation occurs at the extracellular region of α-ENaC (C133Y), which replaces cysteine to tyrosine.[91] In each ENaC subunit, there are two cysteine-rich domains (CRDs) at the extracellular region (see Fig. 19–5). Firsov and associates[94] have performed mutational analysis of CRDs in rat ENaC and have found that certain cysteines in CRD1 and CRD2, respectively, are involved in forming a disulfide bridge within each domain. It appears that C133 may form a disulfide bridge with a cysteine in CRD1. Mutation of the C133-equivalent cysteine in rat α-ENaC (C158S) produced significantly reduced amiloride-sensitive currents in oocytes.[94] Interestingly, this loss-of-function mutation in C158S showed further reduced currents after incubating oocytes at a higher temperature (i.e., 30°C; standard incubation temperature for oocytes is 19°C), suggesting an involvement of the temperature-sensitive ENaC delivery mechanism to the membrane and/or structural stabilization of ENaCs associated with the cysteine mutation. The critical role of CRD in ENaC function is also consistent with the expression study of a human α-ENaC splice variant, hα-ENaC + 22.[68] In hα-ENaC + 22, an additional 22 amino acids are inserted in frame in CRD2, and negligible levels of amiloride-sensitive currents are produced after expression of this splice variant together with wild-type human ENaC β and γ subunits in oocytes. Another point mutation in PHA-1 has been found in β-ENaC, replacing a conserved glycine with a serine (G37S) in the cytoplasmic amino terminus.[92] Functional expression of this mutation in *Xenopus* oocytes showed an ENaC activity that was reduced to about 40% of the activity of wild-type channels. Grunder and associates[91] have provided evidence that this amino acid may be critically involved in channel gating (i.e., regulation of channel open probability). Reduced ENaC activity in PHA-1 would result in reduced Na+ reabsorption in the kidneys, colon, and sweat glands and cause salt wasting, volume reduction, high plasma K+ level, elevated plasma renin activity and aldosterone level, and consequent hypotension. PHA-1 shows mineralocorticoid resistance at the target organ level due to the "dysregulation" of ENaC activity (see Fig. 19–4).

A mouse model for PHA-1 has been generated by disrupting the gene encoding the β subunit.[89] On a

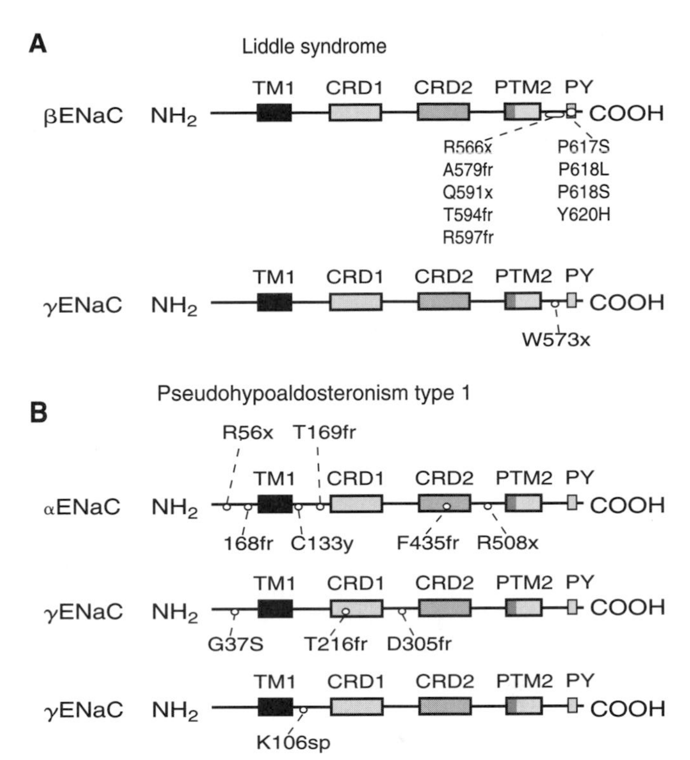


**FIGURE 19–5** ■ ENaC mutations identified in Liddle syndrome *(A)* and autosomal recessive pseudohypoaldosteronism type 1 (PHA-1) *(B)*. Liddle syndrome, an autosomal dominant form of low-renin hypertension, is caused by gain-of-function mutations in the carboxy terminus of the β- or γ-ENaC subunits that constitutively activate ENaC function. In contrast, loss-of-function mutations in the α-, β-, and γ-ENaC subunits have been found in autosomal recessive PHA-1.[91, 92, 112] The mutated amino acids in Liddle's syndrome or PHA-1 have been numbered according to human ENaC sequences. "x" denotes a truncated protein caused by new stop codon that is generated by point mutation. "fr" denotes a frame shift mutation. "sp" denotes splice-site mutation. In Liddle's syndrome, R566x is described by Shimkets et al[75] and Melander et al[84]; A579fr by Jeunemaitre et al[83]; Q589x by Shimkets et al[75]; T594fr by Shimkets et al[75]; R597fr by Shimkets et al,[75] Jackson et al,[82] and Inoue et al[81]; P617S by Inoue et al[80]; P618L by Hansson et al[79] and Uehara et al[76]; P618S by Uehara et al[76]; Y620H by Tamura et al[77]; W573x by Hansson et al,[78] respectively. In PHA-1, R56x is described by I68fr[92, 93] by Chang et al[92]; C133Y by Grunder et al[91]; T169fr by Kerem et al[93]; F435fr by Kerem et al[93]; R508x by Chang et al[92] and Kerem et al[93]; G37S by Chang et al[92]; T216fr and D305fr[92, 93] by K106sp by Strautnieks et al,[90] respectively. (From Oh Y, Warnock DG: Disorders of the epithelial Na+ channel in Liddle's syndrome and autosomal recessive pseudohypoaldosteronism, type 1. Exp Nephrol 8:320–325, 2000.)

normal-salt intake, β subunit–deficient mice exhibit elevated plasma aldosterone level and compensated metabolic acidosis compared with wild-type mice, but no change in blood pressure. When fed a low-salt diet, these mice develop features of an acute PHA-1 with weight loss, salt wasting in the urine, hyperkalemia, and decreased blood pressure, and they are unable to survive more than a few weeks after the dietary switch. This mouse model should be very useful in understanding human PHA-1, which is a very heterogeneous clinical syndrome that usually involves multiple organ systems (respiratory tract in particular) in addition to the kidneys.[95]

## ENaC AND ESSENTIAL HYPERTENSION

As well as its involvement in monogenic forms of blood pressure disorders, it is important to explore whether ENaC plays a role in the more common forms of hypertension such as low-renin hypertension, salt-sensitive hypertension, and even multifactorial polygenic essential hypertension. Despite numerous screening efforts of various ethnic populations, it appears that Liddle syndrome is a rare cause of human hypertension. Although activating mutations of ENaC subunits appear to be uncommon in essential hypertension, there may be polymorphisms in these genes, which may affect the regulation of ENaC activity. It is important to characterize such polymorphisms, especially in defined patients with low renin hypertension and relatively low levels of aldosterone secretion. In a comprehensive survey undertaken with the HYPERGENE data set of hypertensive families, sequence analysis of the last exon in the β-ENaC subunit was carried out in 532 hypertensive probands, and complete β subunit sequencing was performed in 101 probands who had low renin hypertension.[96] Missense mutations were identified in seven unrelated individuals; three probands of African ancestry had mutations that changed threonine to methionine at position 594 (T594M) with an overall incidence of 6% in the hypertensive probands of African ancestry. A G442V β subunit variant was identified in 19 probands; all except one was of African ancestry and eight of the probands were from the low renin subset. There was a low incidence of the G442V in whites, but it was found in 34.8% of the low renin hypertensive probands of African ancestry. Are there functional consequences of such polymorphisms, which could plausibly explain the hypertensive phenotype in these individuals? Unfortunately, the *Xenopus* oocyte expression system used to document the gain of function effect of the original mutation described in Liddle syndrome[97] did not demonstrate any significant effect of the T594M or G442V mutations on ENaC activity.[96] Hypersensitivity of the T594M mutation to cAMP had been identified in studies of the amiloride-sensitive $Na^+$ channel activity in B lymphocytes from affected individuals.[98] Although human B lymphocytes express an amiloride-sensitive $Na^+$ channel with a relevant regulatory repertoire,[99] and the causal truncating mutation of the β subunit was identified at the mRNA level in lymphocytes of the original Liddle pedigree,[100] the identification of the B lymphocyte amiloride-sensitive channel as ENaC has not yet been accomplished. Mindful of this proviso, it was then demonstrated that the T594M β subunit mutation could abolish a modulating effect of protein kinase C on the cAMP response in B lymphocytes.[101] The incidence of the T594M mutation was limited to African Americans in the original report with an incidence of the heterozygous mutation in African-American hypertensive subjects of 5.6%,[98] similar to that later found in the HYPERGENE data set.[96] Although the loss of a regulatory protein kinase C site on the β subunit was provocative, and hypersensitivity to cAMP could explain blood pressure variation related to environmental stresses,[102] the original population of African-American patients was relatively small and not fully defined with respect to plasma renin and aldosterone and dietary salt intake.[98] A larger scale case-control study was carried out on 206 hypertensive subjects referred to a central hypertension clinic in London, and 142 normotensive controls selected from the local general practice roles in the same area.[103] Despite the fact that most of the subjects were first-generation immigrants of African ancestry, so that detailed family histories were not readily available, there was a striking increase (fourfold) in the incidence of the heterozygous T594M mutation in the hypertensive patients compared with controls. Surprisingly, most of the normotensive and hypertensive subjects with the T594 mutation were females. This gender difference was not evident in previous studies on the incidence of the T594M variant in blacks[96, 98] and may have reflected some sort of selection bias in defining the hypertensive subjects in this case-control study.[104] Because direct measurements of ENaC activity in the collecting tubule cannot be easily obtained in humans, a surrogate marker is needed to estimate the effects of mutations on ENaC activity. In the original Liddle pedigree, it was reported that overnight urinary potassium excretion was high and urinary aldosterone excretion was low in affected individuals, giving very low urinary aldosterone-potassium ratios, consistent with the physiologic effect of an increased ENaC activity at the potassium secretory site in the collecting tubule.[74] This approach was used to estimate the intrinsic level of ENaC activity in a thorough study of ENaC polymorphisms, blood pressure, and renin-angiotensin-aldosterone system in a group of young white and African-American subjects.[105] In overnight urine samples collected from 249 white and 181 black subjects, the urinary aldosterone-$K^+$ ratio was significantly lower in blacks than in whites. In addition, four of five ENaC polymorphisms were found to be much more common in blacks than in whites. G442V in the β subunit was present in 16% of the blacks and in only one white and was associated with indices of greater $Na^+$ retention and potentially greater ENaC activity: lower plasma aldosterone concentration, lower urinary aldosterone excretion rate, higher $K^+$ excretion, and lower urinary aldosterone-$K^+$ ratio. Based on these findings, it was suggested that

ENaC activity is higher in blacks than in whites and that this activity could contribute to racial differences in $Na^+$ retention and subsequent risk of developing low renin hypertension.[105] In a second adult cohort of 126 black and 161 white normotensive subjects and 232 black and 188 white hypertensive subjects, G442V in the β subunit was not significantly associated with hypertension, but plasma renin and aldosterone levels were not available for comparison. On the other hand, a variant (T663A), which was twice as common in whites than in blacks was associated with normal blood pressure both in blacks and whites.

## CONCLUSIONS

Our understanding of epithelial $Na^+$ transport defects has greatly expanded in the last several years with the convergence of genetic linkage and mutation search efforts in clinically well characterized human pedigrees and the use of gene targeting techniques in the mouse. The overall data largely confirm that primary mutations in the apical $Na^+$ transport proteins can produce chronic and dramatic changes in blood pressure in accordance with the views of Guyton on the regulation of body fluid volumes and blood pressure by the kidneys.[2] Mutations in these $Na^+$ transport systems have been linked to several mendelian forms of human hypertension or hypotension that are relatively rare in the population.[25] It will be important to determine if variants of the genes encoding the apical $Na^+$ transport systems, as well as the genes encoding the numerous natriuretic and antinatriuretic regulatory systems that exert their effects via the $Na^+$ transport systems, contribute to the more common forms of systemic blood pressure disorders, in particular essential human hypertension.

The development of gene targeting techniques in the mouse has made it possible to assess directly in vivo the roles of the apical $Na^+$ transport proteins in the control of extracellular fluid volume and blood pressure.[26] These genetically modified mouse models have already proved to be very useful in deciphering the mechanisms linking the primary epithelial $Na^+$ transport defect to the overall phenotype. By comparing the consequences of the individual inactivation of the four main apical $Na^+$ transport systems expressed along the nephron, one can gain meaningful insights into how these different transport systems are functionally integrated in renal and whole body physiology. For example, the currently accepted dogma that regulation of $Na^+$ balance occurs primarily in the collecting duct should be tempered with a more refined understanding of the contribution of the more proximal segments of the nephron.[106] A primary $Na^+$ reabsorption defect in the collecting duct does not seem to have a more significant impact on fluid homeostasis and blood pressure than a reabsorption defect in the thick ascending limb of the loop of Henle or proximal convoluted tubule, at least in the mouse. Clearly, the most detrimental mutation is the inactivation of NKCC2, which affects directly the countercurrent urine concentrating mechanism and triggers profound disorganization of the renal tissue. Inactivation of NHE-3 demonstrates that the proximal convoluted tubule has also a crucial role in the control of fluid homeostasis and blood pressure. Part of the overall effect of NHE-3 inactivation may also be related to the absorptive defects in the intestine where the exchanger normally mediates $Na^+$ reabsorption. Given the relatively small contribution of the intestine to the $Na^+$ balance compared with the renal contribution, normal kidneys should easily correct any intestinal reabsorption defect in order to maintain fluid homeostasis. However, in NHE-3–deficient mice, the mutation alters both renal and intestinal function and it is possible that the kidneys, which must compensate for their own dysfunction, cannot compensate properly for the intestinal defects. The same phenomenon may occur in ENaC-deficient mice, because the channel is expressed in the colon.

Further investigations on the role of apical $Na^+$ transport systems should include interbreeding of mutant mouse strains to assess additive or synergistic relationships existing between the segments of the nephron concerning their ability to affect $Na^+$ balance and blood pressure. Tissue-specific gene inactivation should also help to clarify the importance of fecal $Na^+$ and water wasting in overall fluid homeostasis in the cases where the genes are expressed in both the intestine and the kidneys.[89] In addition, attention needs to be paid to the possibility that there may be segment-specific regulatory processes that determine the functional expression of the same apical transporter (e.g., ENaC, NHE-3) at different sites in the distal tubule and intestine.

### ACKNOWLEDGMENTS

We would like to thank Gary E. Shull, François Alhenc-Gelas, and Brigitte Kaissling for the work conducted in their laboratories, part of the presented work was supported by NIH grants DK-50594, HL-41496, DK-39626, DK-48816 (PM), DK19407, DK53161 (DGW), and NS-34877 (YO) and by INSERM.

## REFERENCES

1. Guyton AC: Dominant role of the kidneys and accessory role of whole-body autoregulation in the pathogenesis of hypertension. Am J Hypertens 2:575–585, 1989.
2. Guyton AC: Blood pressure control: Special role of the kidneys and body fluids. Science 252:1813–1816, 1991.
3. Cowley AW Jr: Long-term control of arterial blood pressure. Physiol Rev 72:231–300, 1992.
4. Lifton RP: Molecular genetics of human blood pressure variation. Science 272:676–680, 1996.
5. Meneton P, Warnock DG: Involvement of renal apical Na transport systems in the control of blood pressure. Am J Kidney Dis 37:S39–S47, 2001.
6. Knox FG, Granger JP: Control of sodium excretion: An integrative approach. In Windhager EE (ed): Handbook of Physiology—Renal Physiology. Oxford, Oxford University Press, 1992, pp 927–967.

7. Stanton BA, Kaissling B: Regulation of renal ion transport and cell growth by sodium. Am J Physiol 257:F1–F10, 1989.
8. Scheinman SJ, Guay-Woodford LM, Thakker RV, et al: Genetic disorders of renal electrolyte transport. N Engl J Med 340: 1177–1187, 1999.
9. Reeves WB, Andreoli TE: Tubular sodium transport. In Schrier RW, Gottschalk CW (eds): Diseases of the Kidney, Vol 1. Boston, Little Brown, 1993, pp 139–179.
10. Wang T, Yang CL, Abbiati T, et al: Mechanism of proximal tubule bicarbonate absorption in NHE3 null mice. Am J Physiol 277:F298–F302, 1999.
11. Schultheis PJ, Clarke LL, Meneton P, et al: Renal and intestinal absorptive defects in mice lacking the NHE3 $Na^+/H^+$ exchanger. Nat Genet 19:282–285, 1998.
12. Lorenz JN, Schultheis PJ, Traynor T, et al: Micropuncture analysis of single-nephron function in NHE3-deficient mice. Am J Physiol 277:F447–F453, 1999.
13. Shull GE, Miller ML, Schultheis PJ: VIII. Absorption and secretion of ions in the gastrointestinal tract. Am J Physiol Gastrointest Liver Physiol 278:G185–G190, 2000.
14. Bartter FC, Pronove P, Gill J, et al: Hyperplasia of the juxtaglomerular complex with hyperaldosteronism and hypokalemic alkalosis: A new syndrome. Am J Med 33:811–828, 1962.
15. Simon DB, Karet FE, Hamdan JM, et al: Bartter syndrome, hypokalaemic alkalosis with hypercalciuria, is caused by mutations in the Na-K-2Cl cotransporter NKCC2. Nat Genet 13: 183–188, 1996.
16. Kurtz CL, Karolyi L, Seyberth HW, et al: A common NKCC2 mutation in Costa Rican Bartter's syndrome patients: Evidence for a founder effect. J Am Soc Nephrol 8:1706–1711, 1997.
17. Vargas-Poussou R, Feldmann D, Vollmer M, et al: Novel molecular variants of the Na-K-2Cl cotransporter gene are responsible for antenatal Bartter syndrome. Am J Hum Genet 62:1332–1340, 1998.
18. Simon DB, Bindra RS, Mansfield TA, et al: Mutations in the chloride channel gene, CLCNKB, cause Bartter's syndrome type III. Nat Genet 17:171–178, 1997.
19. Simon DB, Karet FE, Rodriguez-Soriano J, et al: Genetic heterogeneity of Bartter's syndrome revealed by mutations in the $K^+$ channel, ROMK. Nat Genet 14:152–156, 1996.
20. Flagg TP, Tate M, Merot J, et al: A mutation linked with Bartter's syndrome locks Kir 1.1a (ROMK1) channels in a closed state. J Gen Physiol 114:685–700, 1999.
21. Feldmann D, Alessandri JL, Deschenes G: Large deletion of the 5' end of the ROMK1 gene causes antenatal Bartter syndrome. J Am Soc Nephrol 9:2357–2359, 1998.
22. Schwalbe RA, Bianchi L, Accili EA, et al: Functional consequences of ROMK mutants linked to antenatal Bartter's syndrome and implications for treatment. Hum Mol Genet 7: 975–980, 1998.
23. Vollmer M, Koehrer M, Topaloglu R, et al: Two novel mutations of the gene for Kir 1.1 (ROMK) in neonatal Bartter syndrome. Pediatr Nephrol 12:69–71, 1998.
24. Derst C, Konrad M, Kockerling A, et al: Mutations in the ROMK gene in antenatal Bartter syndrome are associated with impaired K+ channel function. Biochem Biophys Res Commun 230:641–645, 1997.
25. Delpire E, Kaplan MR, Plotkin MD, et al: The Na-(K)-Cl cotransporter family in the mammalian kidney: Molecular identification and function(s). Nephrol Dial Transplant 11:1967–1973, 1996.
26. Takahashi N, Chernavvsky DR, Gomez RA, et al: Uncompensated polyuria in a mouse model of Bartter's syndrome. Proc Natl Acad Sci U S A 97:5434–5439, 2000.
27. Rodriguez-Soriano J, Vallo A, Oliveros R: Bartter's syndrome presenting with features resembling renal tubular acidosis. Improvement of renal tubular defects by indomethacin. Helv Paediatr Acta 33:141–151, 1978.
28. Ammenti A, Montali S: "Neonatal variant" of Bartter syndrome presenting with acidosis. Pediatr Nephrol 10:79–80, 1996.
29. Schwartz ID, Alon US: Bartter syndrome revisited. J Nephrol 9:81–87, 1996.
30. Kurtz I: Molecular pathogenesis of Bartter's and Gitelman's syndromes [clinical conference]. Kidney Int 54:1396–1410, 1998.
31. Gitelman HJ, Graham JB, Welt LG: A new familial disorder characterized by hypokalemia and hypomagnesemia. Trans Assoc Am Physicians 79:221–235, 1966.
32. Lemmink HH, Knoers NV, Karolyi L, et al: Novel mutations in the thiazide-sensitive NaCl cotransporter gene in patients with Gitelman syndrome with predominant localization to the C-terminal domain. Kidney Int 54:720–730, 1998.
33. Mastroianni N, Bettinelli A, Bianchetti M, et al: Novel molecular variants of the Na-Cl cotransporter gene are responsible for Gitelman syndrome. Am J Hum Genet 59:1019–1026, 1996.
34. Takeuchi K, Kure S, Kato T, et al: Association of a mutation in thiazide-sensitive Na-Cl cotransporter with familial Gitelman's syndrome. J Clin Endocrinol Metab 81:4496–3399, 1996.
35. Takeuchi K, Kato T, Taniyama Y, et al: Three cases of Gitelman's syndrome possibly caused by different mutations in the thiazide-sensitive Na-Cl cotransporter. Intern Med 36:582–585, 1997.
36. Abuladze N, Yanagawa N, Lee I, et al: Peripheral blood mononuclear cells express mutated NCCT mRNA in Gitelman's syndrome: evidence for abnormal thiazide-sensitive NaCl cotransport. J Am Soc Nephrol 9:819–826, 1998.
37. Lemmink HH, van den Heuvel LP, van Dijk HA, et al: Linkage of Gitelman syndrome to the thiazide-sensitive sodium-chloride cotransporter gene with identification of mutations in Dutch families. Pediatr Nephrol 10:403–407, 1996.
38. Monkawa T, Kurihara I, Kobayashi K, et al: Novel mutations in thiazide-sensitive Na-Cl cotransporter gene of patients with Gitelman's syndrome. J Am Soc Nephrol 11:65–70, 2000.
39. Yahata K, Tanaka I, Kotani M, et al: Identification of a novel R642C mutation in Na/Cl cotransporter with Gitelman's syndrome. Am J Kidney Dis 34:845–853, 1999.
40. Kunchaparty S, Palcso M, Berkman J, et al: Defective processing and expression of thiazide-sensitive Na-Cl cotransporter as a cause of Gitelman's syndrome. Am J Physiol 277:F643–F649, 1999.
41. Reilly RF, Ellison DH: Mammalian distal tubule: Physiology, pathophysiology, and molecular anatomy. Physiol Rev 80:277–313, 2000.
42. Friedman PA: Codependence of renal calcium and sodium transport. Annu Rev Physiol 60:179–97, 1998.
43. Simon DB, Lu Y, Choate KA, et al: Paracellin-1, a renal tight junction protein required for paracellular $Mg^{2+}$ resorption. Science 285:103–106, 1999.
44. Benos DJ, Cunnigham S, Baker RR, et al: Molecular characteristics of amiloride sensitive sodium chanels. Rev Physiol Biochem Pharmacol 120:31–113, 1992.
45. Garty H, Palmer LG: Epithelial sodium channels: Function, structure, and regulation. Physiol Rev 77:359–396, 1997.
46. Canessa CM, Merillat A-M, Rossier BC: Membrane topology of the epithelial sodium channel in intact cells. Am J Physiol 267: C1682–C1690, 1994.
47. Hong K, Driscoll M: A transmembrane domain of the putative channel subunit MEC-4 influences mechanotransduction and neurodegeneration in *C. elegans.* Nature 367:470–473, 1994.
48. Chalfie M, Driscoll M, Huang M: Degenerin similarities. Nature 361:504, 1993.
49. Waldmann R, Champigny G, Lazdunski M: Functional degenerin-containing chimeras identify residues essential for amiloride-sensitive $Na^+$ channel function. J Biol Chem 270:11735–11737, 1995.
50. Corey DP, Garcia-Anoveros J: Mechanosensation and the DEG/ENaC ion channels. Science 273:323–324, 1996.
51. Waldmann R, Champigny G, Bassilana F, et al: A proton-gated cation channel involved in acid-sensing. Nature 386:173–176, 1997.
52. Lingueglia E, Champigny G, Lazdunski M, et al: Cloning of the amiloride-sensitive FMRFamide peptide-gated sodium channel. Nature 378:730–733, 1995.
53. Renard S, Lingueglia E, Voilley N, et al: Biochemical analysis of the membrane topology of the amiloride-sensitive $Na^+$ channel. J Biol Chem 269:12981–12986, 1994.
54. Snyder PM, McDonald FJ, Stokes JB, et al: Membrane topology of the amiloride-sensitive epithelial sodium channel. J Biol Chem 269:24379–24383, 1994.
55. Garcia-Anoveros J, Ma C, Chalfie M: Regulation of *Caenorhab-*

*ditis elegans* degenerin proteins by a putative extracellular domain. Curr Biol 5:441–448, 1995.
56. Kosari F, Sheng S, Li J, et al: Subunit stoichiometry of the epithelial sodium channel. J Biol Chem 273:13469–13474, 1998.
57. Firsov D, Gautschi I, Merillat AM, et al: The heterotetrameric architecture of the epithelial sodium channel (ENaC). EMBO J 17:344–352, 1998.
58. Eskandari S, Snyder PM, Kreman M, et al: Number of subunits comprising the epithelial sodium channel. J Biol Chem 274: 27281–27286, 1999.
59. Snyder PM, Cheng C, Prince LS, et al: Electrophysiological and biochemical evidence that DEG/ENaC cation channels are composed of nine subunits. J Biol Chem 273:681–684, 1998.
60. Canessa CM, Horisberger J-D, Rossier BC: Epithelial sodium channel related to proteins involved in neurodegeneration. Nature 361:467–470, 1993.
61. Canessa CM, Schild L, Buell G, et al: Amiloride-sensitive epithelial $Na^+$ channel is made of three homologous subunits. Nature 367:463–467, 1994.
62. McDonald FJ, Price MP, Snyder PM, et al: Cloning and expression of the β- and γ-subunits of the human epithelial sodium channel. Am J Physiol 268:C1157–C1163, 1995.
63. Hummler E, Barker P, Gatzy J, et al: Early death due to defective neonatal lung liquid clearance in αENaC-deficient mice. Nat Genet 12:325–328, 1996.
64. Matalon S: Mechanisms and regulation of ion transport in adult mammalian alveolar type II pneumocytes. Am J Physiol 261:C727–C738, 1991.
65. Bonny O, Chraibi A, Loffing J, et al: Functional expression of a pseudohypoaldosteronism type I mutated epithelial $Na^+$ channel deleting the pore-forming region of its α subunit. J Clin Invest 104:967–974, 1999.
66. Masilamani S, Kim G-H, Mitchell C, et al: Aldosterone-mediated regulation of ENaC α, β, and γ subunit proteins in rat kidney. J Clin Invest 104:R19–R23, 1999.
67. Oh YS, Saxena S, Warnock DG: αENaC: Leading the charge. J Clin Invest 104:849–850, 1999.
68. Tucker JK, Tamba K, Lee Y-J, et al: Cloning and functional studies of splice variants of the α-subunit of the amiloride-sensitive $Na^+$ channel. Am J Physiol 274:C1081–C1089, 1998.
69. Thomas C, Auerbach S, Stokes JB, et al: 5' Heterogeneity in epithelial sodium channel α-subunit mRNA leads to distinct $NH_2$-terminal variant proteins. Am J Physiol 274:C1312–C1323, 1998.
70. Chraibi A, Horisberger J-D: Stimulation of epithelial sodium channel activity by the sulfonylurea gilbenclamide. J Pharmacol Exp Ther 290:341–347, 1999.
71. McNicholas CM, Canessa CM: Diversity of channels generated by different combinations of epithelial sodium channel subunits. J Gen Physiol 109:681–692, 1997.
72. Loffing J, Pietri L, Aregger F, et al: Differential subcellular localization of ENaC subunits in mouse kidney in response to high- and low-Na diets. Am J Physiol (Renal Physiol) 279: F252–F258, 2000.
73. Liddle GW, Bledsoe T, Coppage WSJ: A familial renal disorder simulating primary aldosteronism but with negligible aldosterone secretion. Trans Assoc Am Physicians 76:199–213, 1963.
74. Botero-Velez M, Curtis JJ, Warnock DG: Brief report: Liddle's syndrome revisited: A disorder of sodium reabsorption in the distal tubule. N Engl J Med 330:178–181, 1994.
75. Shimkets RA, Warnock DG, Bositis CM, et al: Liddle's syndrome: Heritable human hypertension caused by mutations in the beta subunit of the epithelial sodium channel. Cell 79: 407–414, 1994.
76. Uehara Y, Sasaquri M, Kinoshita A, et al: Genetic analysis of the epithelial sodium channel in Liddle's syndrome. J Hypertens 16:1131–1135, 1998.
77. Tamura H, Schild L, Enomoto N, et al: Liddle disease caused by a missense mutation of beta subunit of the epithelial sodium channel gene. J Clin Invest 97:1780–1784, 1996.
78. Hansson JH, Nelson-Williams C, Suzuki H, et al: Hypertension caused by a truncated epithelial sodium channel γ subunit: Genetic heterogeneity of Liddle syndrome. Nat Genet 11:76–82, 1995.
79. Hansson JH, Schild L, Lu Y, et al: A de novo missense mutation of the beta subunit of the epithelial sodium channel causes hypertension and Liddle syndrome, identifying a proline-rich segment critical for regulation of channel activity. Proc Natl Acad Sci U S A 92:11495–11499, 1995.
80. Inoue J, Iwaoka T, Tokunaga H, et al: A family with Liddle's syndrome caused by a new missense mutation in the β subunit of the epithelial sodium channel. J Clin Endocrinol Metab 83: 2210–2213, 1998.
81. Inoue T, Okauchi Y, Matsuzaki Y, et al: Identification of a single cytosine base insertion mutation at Arg 597 of the β subunit of the human epithelial sodium channel in a family with Liddle's disease. Eur J Endocrinol 138:691–697, 1998.
82. Jackson SN, Williams B, Houtman P, et al: The diagnosis of Liddle syndrome by identification of a mutation in the β subunit of the epithelial sodium channel. J Med Genet 35:510–512, 1998.
83. Jeunemaitre X, Bassilana F, Persu A, et al: Genotype-phenotype analysis of a newly discovered family with Liddle's syndrome. J Hypertens 15:1091–1100, 1997.
84. Melander O, Orho M, Fagerudd J, et al: Mutations and variants of the epithelial sodium channel gene in Liddle's syndrome and primary hypertension. Hypertension 31:1118–1124, 1998.
85. Firsov D, Schild L, Gautschi I, et al: Cell surface expression of the epithelial Na channel and a mutant causing Liddle syndrome: A quantitative approach. Proc Natl Acad Sci U S A 93: 15370–15375, 1996.
86. Staub O, Dho S, Henry PC, et al: WW domains of Nedd4 bind to the proline-rich PY motifs in the epithelial $Na^+$ channel deleted in Liddle's syndrome. EMBO J 15:2371–2380, 1996.
87. Snyder PM, Price MP, McDonald FJ, et al: Mechanism by which Liddle's syndrome mutations increase activity of a human epithelial $Na^+$ channel. Cell 83:969–978, 1995.
88. Geller DS, Farhi A, Pinkerton N, et al: Activating mineralocorticoid receptor mutation in hypertension exacerbated by pregnancy. Science 289:119–123, 2000.
89. Pradervand S, Wang Q, Burnier M, et al: A mouse model for Liddle's syndrome. J Am Soc Nephrol 10:2527–2533, 1999.
90. Strautnieks SS, Thompson RJ, Gardiner RM, et al: A novel splice-site mutation in the gamma subunit of the epithelial sodium channel gene in three pseudohypoaldosteronism type 1 families. Nat Genet 13:248–250, 1996.
91. Grunder S, Chang SS, Lifton R, et al: PHA-1: a novel thermosensitive mutation in the ectodomain of αENaC. J Am Soc Nephrol 9:35A, 1998.
92. Chang SS, Grunder S, Hanukoglu A, et al: Mutations in subunits of the epithelial sodium channel cause salt wasting with hyperkalaemic acidosis, pseudohypoaldosteronism type 1. Nat Genet 12:248–253, 1996.
93. Kerem E, Bistritzer T, Hanukoglu A, et al: Pulmonary epithelial sodium-channel dysfunction and excess airway liquid in pseudohypoaldosteronism. N Engl J Med 341:156–162, 1999.
94. Firsov D, Robert-Nicoud M, Gruender S, et al: Mutational analysis of cystein-rich domains of the epithelial sodium channel (ENaC). J Biol Chem 274:2743–2749, 1999.
95. Hanukoglu A, Bistritzer T, Rakover Y, et al: Pseudohypoaldosteronism with increased sweat and saliva electrolyte values and frequent lower respiratory tract infections mimicking cystic fibrosis. J Pediatr 125:752–755, 1994.
96. Persu A, Barbry P, Bassilana F, et al: Genetic analysis of the beta subunit of the epithelial $Na^+$ channel in essential hypertension. Hypertension 32:129–137, 1998.
97. Schild L, Canessa CM, Shimkets RA, et al: A mutation in the epithelial sodium channel causing Liddle disease increases channel activity in the Xenopus laevis oocyte expression system. Proc Natl Acad Sci U S A 92:5699–5703, 1995.
98. Su YR, Rutkowski MP, Klanke CA, et al: A novel variant of the beta-subunit of the amiloride-sensitive sodium channel in African Americans. J Am Soc Nephrol 7:2543–2549, 1996.
99. Bubien JK, Jope RS, Warnock DG: G-proteins modulate amiloride-sensitive sodium channels. J Biol Chem 269:17780–17783, 1994.
100. Oh Y, Warnock DG: Expression of the amiloride-sensitive sodium channel beta subunit gene in human B lymphocytes. J Am Soc Nephrol 8:126–129, 1997.

101. Cui Y, Su YR, Rutkowski M, et al: Loss of protein kinase C inhibition in the beta-T594M variant of the amiloride-sensitive $Na^+$ channel. Proc Natl Acad Sci U S A 94:9962–9966, 1997.
102. Warnock DG: Polymorphism in the beta subunit and $Na^+$ transport [editorial]. J Am Soc Nephrol 7:2490–2494, 1996.
103. Baker EH, Dong YB, Sagnella GA, et al: Association of hypertension with T594M mutation in beta subunit of epithelial sodium channels in black people resident in London. Lancet 351:1388–1392, 1998.
104. Warnock DG: T594M mutation in the ENaC beta subunit and low-renin hypertension in blacks. Am J Kidney Dis 34:579–587, 1999.
105. Ambrosius WT, Bloem LJ, Zhou L, et al: Genetic variants in the epithelial sodium channel in relation to aldosterone and potassium excretion and risk for hypertension. Hypertension 34:631–637, 1999.
106. Hummler E: Reversal of convention: From man to experimental animal in elucidating the function of the renal amiloride-sensitive sodium channel. Exp Nephrol 6:265–271, 1998.
107. Meneton P, Oh YS, Warnock DG: Genetic renal tubular disorders of renal ion channels and transporters. Semin Nephrol 21:81–93, 2001.
108. Schild L, Schneeberger E, Gautschi I, et al: Identification of amino acid residues in the α, β, and γ? subunits of the epithelial sodium channel (ENaC) involved in amiloride block and ion permeation. J Gen Physiol 109:15–26, 1997.
109. Goulet CC, Volk KA, Adams CM, et al: Inhibition of the epithelial $Na^+$ channel by interaction of Nedd4 with a PY motif deleted in Liddle's syndrome. J Biol Chem 273:30012–30017, 1998.
110. Rotin D, Bar-Sagi D, O'Brodovich H, et al: An SH3 binding region in the epithelial $Na^+$ channel (αrENaC) mediates its localization at the apical membrane. EMBO J 13:4440–4450, 1994.
111. Oh Y, Warnock DG: Disorders of the epithelial $Na^+$ channel in Liddle's syndrome and autosomal recessive pseudohypoaldosteronism, type 1. Exp Nephrol 8:320–325, 2000.
112. Strautnieks SS, Thompson RJ, Hanukoglu A, et al: Localisation of pseudohypoaldosteronism genes to chromosome 16p12.2–13.11 and 12p13.1-pter by homozygosity mapping. Hum Mol Genet 5:293–299, 1996.

CHAPTER 20

# Electrolyte Abnormalities in the Intensive Care Unit

Kevin W. Finkel, MD

Critical illness causes major stress on all regulatory functions of the body including those responsible for maintaining normal electrolyte balance. In addition, many of the therapies directed at sustaining vital organ function directly or indirectly affect these regulatory systems. Hence, electrolyte abnormalities in the critically ill patient are both common and complex. In this chapter, electrolyte disorders are approached as they specifically apply to clinical scenarios commonly encountered in the intensive care unit (ICU). It assumes a rudimentary understanding of the principles involved in evaluating electrolyte disorders detailed in other chapters of this text.

## APPROACH TO THE CRITICALLY ILL PATIENT

Traditionally, the evaluation of an electrolyte disorder in a patient is approached as a relatively isolated problem. By use of physical examination and key blood and urine tests, it is often possible to identify a single defect in a regulatory system to explain the abnormal finding. For example, in a patient with hyponatremia, the evaluation is usually focused on determining the mechanism of persistent free water retention in the face of ongoing serum hypotonicity. The sequence involves identifying any signs of true or effective volume depletion and verifying normal renal, adrenal, and thyroid function before making a diagnosis of the syndrome of inappropriate antidiuretic hormone secretion (SIADH). In the critically ill patient such an approach is often too simplistic, and it is prudent to assume that multiple factors are involved. The stress of critical illness or trauma, positive-pressure ventilation, sepsis, acute renal failure, multiple organ dysfunction syndrome (MODS), and administration of vasoactive medications all perturb the neuroendocrine systems that control serum electrolyte balance. Evaluation is further complicated by the infusion of a variety of intravenous electrolyte solutions and hyperalimentation. Critical illness also alters the laboratory results commonly used to diagnose the cause of an abnormality. Therefore, electrolyte disturbances in the ICU are multifactorial in etiology and require an understanding of the effects of critical illness and its treatment on electrolyte homeostasis.

## NEUROENDOCRINE RESPONSES TO CRITICAL ILLNESS

### Thyroid Gland

Normal functioning of the thyroid gland is crucial to regulation of water excretion and serum tonicity. Deficiency of the hormone impairs the kidneys' ability to excrete a free water load and can lead to hypotonic hyponatremia.[1] The mechanism for this observation is not established. It may be that hyponatremia associated with hypothyroidism is caused by both decreased delivery of filtrate to the diluting segment and persistent antidiuretic hormone (ADH) secretion. Hypothyroidism is associated with reduced glomerular filtration rate (GFR) and renal plasma flow.[2] It has also been shown in hypothyroidism that ADH levels remain elevated despite water loading.[3]

Abnormalities in thyroid function tests are common in critically ill patients and are referred to as euthyroid sick syndrome.[4] Three general patterns of disturbance have been described: (1) low $T_3$ syndrome; (2) low $T_3$ and low $T_4$ syndrome; and (3) low thyroid-stimulating hormone (TSH) syndrome. Such patients are considered clinically euthyroid. It is not clear if euthyroid sick syndrome is an adaptive response, decreasing metabolic demand during stress, or a maladaptive one adversely affecting patient outcome.

Given the frequency of euthyroid sick syndrome in the ICU, there is the potential to misdiagnose a patient as having hypothyroidism and erroneously attribute the hyponatremia to it. Conversely, it may be incorrect to assume that euthyroid sick syndrome does not contribute in some way to impaired water excretion by the kidneys.

### Adrenal Gland

The adrenal cortex produces cortisol and aldosterone, whereas the adrenal medulla synthesizes the catecholamines norepinephrine and epinephrine. Because these substances can affect electrolyte balance, disturbances of adrenal function in the critically ill patient will complicate the evaluation of electrolyte abnormalities in the ICU.

#### CORTISOL

Cortisol is the major glucocorticoid produced by the adrenal cortex during stressful conditions. Like thyroid hormone, it plays a permissive role in normal water metabolism. Low cortisol levels impair the kidneys' ability to excrete a free water load and can result in hyponatremia.[5] Hypocortisolism leads to hypotension resistant to volume expansion and vasopressor administration. The resultant renal hypoperfusion promotes the retention of free water.

In the critically ill patient, cortisol levels are usually

elevated. However, several patients have been described who develop transient hypoadrenalism with unexplained hypotension and inappropriately normal cortisol levels as a result of stress.[6] In such patients, there may be impaired free water excretion despite a "normal" cortisol level.

#### ALDOSTERONE

Aldosterone secretion is stimulated by angiotensin II and catecholamines released in response to true or effective volume depletion. Its release is also directly triggered by hyperkalemia. Excessive aldosterone production produces hypernatremia and hypokalemia, whereas a deficiency causes hyponatremia and hyperkalemia.

There are numerous factors in the critically ill patient that affect aldosterone levels and cause electrolyte disturbances. Positive-pressure ventilation, severe hypoalbuminemia, congestive heart failure (CHF), and administration of diuretics raise circulating aldosterone levels. Critically ill patients are also at risk for the development of adrenal failure. Adrenal necrosis is caused by hypotension, disseminated intravascular coagulation (DIC), sepsis (Waterhouse-Friderichsen syndrome), or heparin administration, leading to hyponatremia and hyperkalemia. Several medications used in the ICU can impair aldosterone secretion or action such as angiotensin-converting enzyme inhibitors (ACEIs), angiotensin II receptor blockers (ARBs), spironolactone, and heparin.

Some critically ill patients develop a dissociation between renin and aldosterone secretion, so-called *hyperreninemic hypoaldosteronism.*[7] This condition is associated with an increased severity of illness and mortality rate. Although hyperkalemia has not been reported, this defect is likely to contribute to impaired potassium secretion by the kidneys. Hyperreninemic hypoaldosteronism develops in 20% of ICU patients.

#### CATECHOLAMINES

Adrenal catecholamines are well-recognized stress hormones and are released in response to various stimuli present in the critically ill patient. They redirect blood flow away from the kidneys, which impairs free water excretion and renal potassium handling. Catecholamines stimulate aldosterone release, thus altering sodium and potassium excretion by the kidneys. Through effects on the cellular $Na^+$-$K^+$ ATPase, catecholamines can change serum potassium levels by affecting transcellular shifting.

### Posterior Pituitary Gland

#### ANTIDIURETIC HORMONE

ADH secretion is stimulated by the physiologic stimuli of hypertonicity and decreased effective arterial blood volume (EABV). ADH release is quite sensitive to changes in serum osmolality. The suppressive effect of serum hypotonicity is overridden in the face of concurrent volume depletion. In this situation, the body "sacrifices" serum tonicity to conserve water. There are several other causes of ADH release in critically ill patients despite serum hypotonicity. These include pain, head injury, positive-pressure ventilation, use of narcotics, and administration of epinephrine.

## HYPONATREMIA

### Clinical Features

Hyponatremia is common in the critically ill patient.[8] It results from a complex interplay between the underlying disease state, neurohumoral activation, and intravenous administration of medications and electrolyte solutions. Traditionally, hyponatremia is classified as acute or chronic; however, in clinical practice, such a differentiation is difficult. Furthermore, there is evidence that neither the duration nor the magnitude of hyponatremia correlates with brain damage.[9] Symptoms of hyponatremia range from increased thirst and muscle cramping to obtundation, seizure, or coma. In many patients in the ICU, symptoms are masked by drug-induced sedation.

Patients with hyponatremia who are otherwise stable have no or only minor symptoms. They report increased thirst, muscle cramping, and anorexia. In more severe cases, clouding of the sensorium and respiratory muscle fatigue develop. More ominous is the development of neurologic signs. In patients who develop hyponatremic encephalopathy, the mortality rate may be as high as 20%.[9] Symptoms include headache, nausea, and vomiting. Severe manifestations such as grand mal seizures, obtundation, and respiratory arrest are less frequent. Typically, these manifestations are seen in subsets of patients, such as prepubertal children and postoperative women (see later).

In ICU patients, ADH levels are usually elevated despite the presence of hyponatremia and low serum tonicity. Most often, the persistence of circulating ADH is the result of a volume-mediated release of ADH. There are numerous conditions in critically ill patients that cause continued ADH release (Table 20–1).

Evaluation of hyponatremia in the ICU, which is covered in detail in Chapter 14, is summarized in Figure 20–1.

### Treatment of Hyponatremia

Guidelines for treatment of hyponatremia depend on its cause, severity, and the presence or absence of symptoms.

**Hypovolemic Hyponatremia.** Patients have deficits in both total body salt and water. Resuscitation with intravenous saline will correct the volume depletion and terminate the volume-mediated release of ADH.

**Hypervolemic Hyponatremia.** These patients are total body salt and water overloaded. Because the volume is maldistributed owing to poor cardiac function, por-

**TABLE 20–1.** Persistent Antidiuretic Hormone Release in Patients in the Intensive Care Unit

| |
|---|
| **True Volume Depletion** |
| Hemorrhage |
| Diarrhea |
| Nasogastric suction/vomiting |
| Pancreatitis |
| Rhabdomyolysis |
| Addisonian crisis |
| Diuretics |
| Osmotic diuresis |
| **Effective Volume Depletion** |
| Congestive heart failure |
| Cirrhosis/hepatorenal syndrome |
| Severe nephrotic syndrome |
| Positive-pressure ventilation |
| Systemic inflammatory response syndrome |

tal hypertension, or severe third spacing, the kidneys are hypoperfused and salt and water retention persist. Treatment consists of fluid restriction and administration of diuretics. In the case of heart failure, afterload reduction and inotropic support are also helpful. These therapies are often ineffective because they fail to reverse the underlying pathophysiology. In the ICU, control of anasarca and correction of the hyponatremia may only be achieved by application of slow continuous ultrafiltration modalities.

**Euvolemic Hyponatremia.** In the ICU, euvolemic hyponatremia is usually caused by SIADH. When mild, it can be simply treated by restriction of free water intake. This requires appropriate adjustment of the sodium content of diluent solutions used for drug administration. When hyponatremia is severe (<110 mEq/L), more aggressive therapy is indicated. Close attention to the rate of correction is necessary to avoid the potential of precipitating cerebral demyelination and permanent neurologic damage. The risk of such an occurrence is greatest in patients with severe chronic hyponatremia in which cerebral adaptation to the hyponatremia has returned brain volume toward normal. Although the results of various clinical and animal studies are conflicting, it is prudent to strive toward correcting the hyponatremia by 0.5 mEq/L/hr or 12 mEq/L/day.[10] This is achieved by calculating the sodium deficit and by administration of saline or hypertonic saline with a loop diuretic, the latter of which will increase free water loss. Once the sodium concentration has reached a safe level, water restriction can be instituted.

In the case of severe neurologic manifestations such as seizures, emergency treatment should be instituted with hypertonic saline infused at a rate of 1 to 2 mL/kg/hr for 2 to 4 hours until symptoms resolve.[11] Even with this aggressive approach, the overall goal is to raise the sodium concentration by no more than 12 to 15 mEq/L in the first 24 hours or to a concentration of 120 to 125 mEq/L.

## ICU Scenarios

### POSTOPERATIVE HYPONATREMIA

Postoperative hyponatremia is an uncommon and potentially lethal condition. It results from a combination of nonosmotic stimulation of ADH release in the postoperative state and the infusion of hypotonic fluid. Although it can occur in any postoperative patient, it is much more common in women and is related to the phase of the menstrual cycle.[9] Patients with postoperative hyponatremia typically have nonspecific complaints of headache, nausea, and vomiting. Although these symptoms are common to many postoperative patients, if a patient has been receiving hypotonic intravenous fluids (including lactated Ringer solution), a serum sodium level should be measured. If

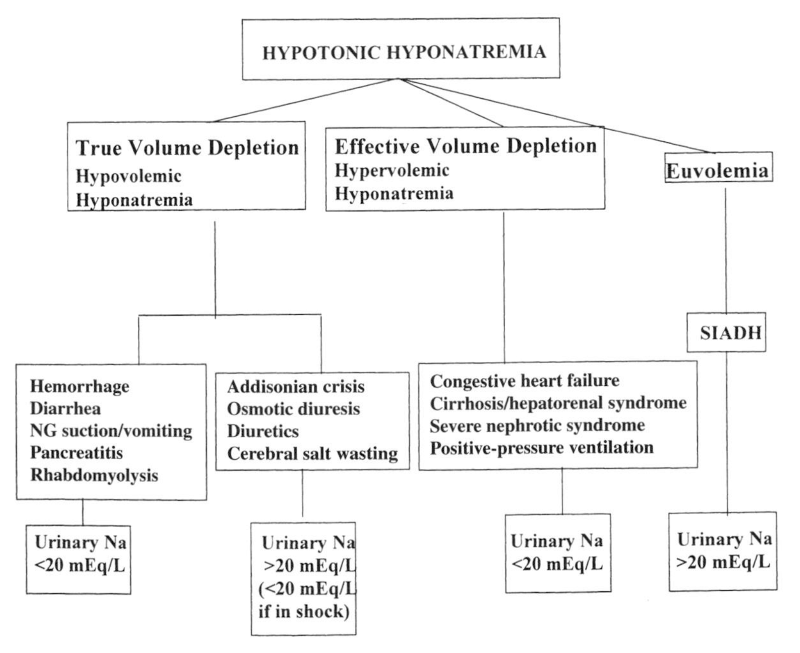


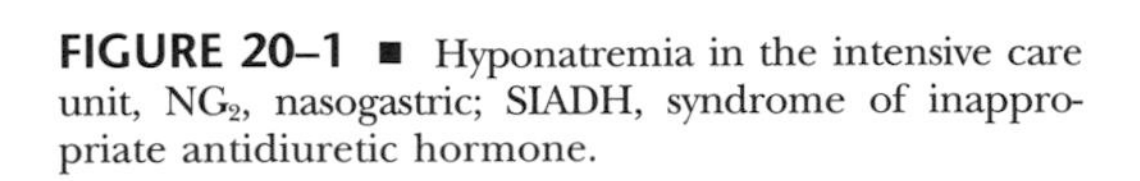
**FIGURE 20–1** ■ Hyponatremia in the intensive care unit, $NG_2$, nasogastric; SIADH, syndrome of inappropriate antidiuretic hormone.

the serum sodium concentration is low, early treatment can be initiated before an anoxic-hypoxic insult, such as seizure or respiratory arrest, results.

Since the 1930s, there have been several hundred reported cases of postoperative hyponatremia. The occurrence of death or permanent neurologic damage is more common in prepubertal children and menstruant women. Among patients who die of hyponatremic encephalopathy, three general neuropathologic patterns have been described.[12] In patients who died within 48 hours of respiratory arrest, there is cerebral edema, often with evidence of herniation. In patients who die several days after respiratory arrest, multiple cerebral infarcts with diffuse demyelinating lesions are found. Finally, in some patients who developed central diabetes insipidus, pituitary necrosis in addition to demyelinating lesions is evident.

The pathogenesis of the lesions seen in hyponatremia includes hypoxia, brain herniation, and rapid correction of hyponatremia. The demyelinating lesions seen after rapid correction of hyponatremia are often referred to as central pontine myelinolysis (CPM). However, numerous clinical conditions not associated with hyponatremia, such as increased intracranial pressure, radiotherapy, or cerebral hemorrhage, show lesions that resemble CPM.[13, 14] Furthermore, animal studies on rapid correction of hyponatremia have failed to consistently show lesions in the pons. When CPM has been specifically sought by detailed examination of the pons in humans with hyponatremia, it is generally absent.[15]

Therapy should first be directed at prevention. In the subset of patients at risk for hyponatremic encephalopathy, hypotonic fluid administration should be avoided. Once patients develop seizures or respiratory arrest, therapy may not effect a positive outcome. In general, it is neither necessary nor wise to raise the sodium level to normal levels. Hypertonic saline can be administered to raise the sodium level by 1 to 2 mEq/L/hr until symptoms abate. In an emergency situation, hypertonic saline is given at a rate of 1 to 2 mL/kg/hr. Frequent monitoring of serum and urine electrolytes is mandatory. Overall, the goal is to raise the serum sodium concentration by no more than 12 to 15 mEq/L in 24 hours.

## SYNDROME OF INAPPROPRIATE ANTIDIURETIC HORMONE SECRETION

Most patients with hyponatremia have impaired urinary free water excretion from the presence of circulating ADH despite serum hypotonicity. This ADH effect is demonstrated by the laboratory finding of an inappropriately concentrated urine in the face of severe hyponatremia. The work-up of such patients is directed at determining whether the persistent ADH secretion is stimulated by the physiologic trigger of true or effective volume depletion.[16] The clinical examination and determination of central venous pressures and urinary sodium concentrations are used to determine a patient's volume status. Clinical conditions such as CHF and nephrotic syndrome are classic examples in which ADH release is maintained by effective volume depletion despite low serum osmolality. When volume mediated release of ADH is not operative (a clinically euvolemic patient with a urinary sodium concentration >20 mEq/L), then ADH release is considered "inappropriate" and the diagnosis of SIADH is established.

**TABLE 20–2.** Syndrome of Inappropriate Diuretic Hormone Secretion in the Intensive Care Unit

| |
|---|
| **CNS Lesions** |
| Infection |
| Traumatic brain injury |
| Subarachnoid or subdural hemorrhage |
| **Pulmonary Disease** |
| Pneumonia |
| Tuberculosis |
| Pneumothorax |
| **Malignancy** |
| Brain |
| Lung |
| Gastrointestinal |

CNS, central nervous system.

The potential causes of SIADH are exhaustive, but some predominate in the critical care setting (Table 20–2). In summary, SIADH is characterized by the following findings: (1) hypotonic hyponatremia, (2) inappropriately concentrated urine (Uosm >100 mOsm/kg), (3) euvolemia, (4) urinary sodium greater than 20 mEq/L, and (5) normal adrenal, thyroid, and renal function. Another laboratory abnormality found in SIADH is hypouricemia, the result of enhanced urinary excretion of uric acid.[17]

Asymptomatic hyponatremia is treated by restricting water intake. However, as with postoperative hyponatremia, more vigorous therapy with hypertonic saline is indicated when symptoms are present because irreversible neurologic damage and death can occur.

## CEREBRAL SALT WASTING

Cerebral salt wasting (CSW) is an uncommonly recognized complication of cerebral injury that mimics many of the laboratory findings of SIADH. Because the two disorders occur in similar clinical scenarios but require different therapies, it is essential to differentiate between them.

CSW results in hyponatremia and natriuresis, which are often associated with a worsening of the patient's neurologic status.[18] The basic feature of CSW is hypovolemia compared with SIADH in which mild fluid overload or hypervolemia prevails. When hyponatremia with natriuresis in a neurosurgical patient is attributed to SIADH, fluid restriction is often initiated. However, several authors have found that fluid restriction in such patients may be harmful, because most of these patients are hypovolemic.[19]

The laboratory features of CSW include hyponatremia, concentrated urine, and elevated urinary sodium concentration. Despite the presence of volume depletion, serum uric acid levels are often low, again adding to the confusion with the diagnosis of SIADH. Correction of hyponatremia in SIADH normalizes serum urate levels, whereas in CSW serum urate levels remain persistently low.[20]

The mechanism by which intracranial disease leads to renal salt wasting is not understood, although several candidate mediators have been suggested by experimental data. These include elevated levels of brain natriuretic peptide, brain ouabain-like compound, bradykinin, oxytocin, adrenocorticotropic hormone (ACTH), α-melanocyte stimulation hormone (MSH), parathyroid hormone (PTH), and calcitonin.

Because most patients with CSW seem to meet the laboratory criteria for SIADH, a thorough evaluation is necessary to distinguish between the two disorders. Signs of volume depletion such as orthostatic hypotension, dry mucous membranes, absence of perspiration, and tachycardia should be sought. An accurate assessment of weight loss should be made. Invasive measurements such as central venous pressure and pulmonary artery occlusion pressure are low. Elevations in hematocrit, blood urea nitrogen (BUN) to creatinine ratio, and protein concentration suggest dehydration and the presence of CSW.

Treatment of CSW consists of volume replacement and maintenance of a positive sodium balance. This goal can be achieved by the administration of intravenous saline or hypertonic saline, or oral salt, depending on the severity of the hyponatremia and the patient's clinical status. Some argue that administration of hypertonic saline may cause volume expansion and increased urinary loss, thus oral administration is preferred.[21] Others suggest that prevention of volume depletion by decreasing urinary sodium loss with the mineralocorticoid fludrocortisone is more appropriate.[22] Others have used a combination of urea and saline.[23] Urea induces a mild osmotic diuresis that increases water loss, whereas the supplemental salt restores sodium deficits. In general, however, volume expansion and salt supplementation remain the primary therapy for CSW.

## MECHANICAL VENTILATION

Many patients in the ICU are intubated for respiratory failure. Often it goes unappreciated the effect positive-pressure ventilation has on the neuroendocrine systems that control electrolyte balance. Positive intrathoracic pressure impairs cardiac filling, leading to renal hypoperfusion. This results in elevated circulating levels of renin, angiotensin, aldosterone, catecholamines, and ADH. Therefore, mechanical ventilation may cause a volume-mediated release of ADH and perpetuate hyponatremia.[24]

## CIRRHOSIS

Patients with cirrhosis of the liver and portal hypertension are often hyponatremic. They have persistently elevated ADH levels, despite serum hypotonicity, attributed to the peripheral vasodilatation theory. In this scenario, effective EABV is enlarged, particularly in the splanchnic circulation.[25] Studies suggest that the vasodilatation is mediated by increased nitric oxide levels.[26] This underfilling stimulates the kidneys and other neurohumoral systems to retain salt and water despite the ensuing ascites and edema.

Treatment is unsatisfactory short of an orthotopic liver transplant. Diuretics are not only ineffective because of the profound sodium retentive state but can also further aggravate the decreased EABV and precipitate the hepatorenal syndrome. Slow continuous ultrafiltration or dialysis is effective in controlling symptoms but futile if a liver transplant is unavailable.

## CONGESTIVE HEART FAILURE

Patients with CHF are often hyponatremic. Heart failure decreases EABV, which activates baroreceptors and raises ADH levels. The presence of hyponatremia upon hospital presentation in a patient with CHF is associated with an increased mortality rate.[27]

## SYSTEMIC INFLAMMATORY RESPONSE SYNDROME

Systemic inflammatory response syndrome (SIRS) develops most commonly in patients with sepsis or trauma. Its pathogenesis remains poorly understood, although several cytokine pathways involving tumor necrosis factor (TNF), nitric oxide, and various interleukins are thought to play a role. SIRS causes a massive capillary leak leading to organ dysfunction, acute respiratory distress syndrome, and anasarca. Patients require massive quantities of intravenous fluids to maintain adequate tissue perfusion even with the use of numerous vasopressor drugs. ADH levels remain elevated owing to the decreased EABV, and hyponatremia can develop.

Currently, there is no known effective therapy for this disorder. Diuretic administration is ill-advised in patients with decreased EABV. Blocking antibodies to various cytokines have proved to be ineffective.[28] Enthusiasm for lowering cytokine levels with continuous dialysis is not justified by properly conducted clinical trials.[29] Slow continuous ultrafiltration or dialysis to help regulate electrolyte and fluid balance appears to be most appropriate, although there is no proven benefit on long-term outcome.

## PSEUDOHYPONATREMIA/SEVERE HYPERGLYCEMIA

Pseudohyponatremia is defined as the presence of hyponatremia in the face of normal or elevated serum osmolality. In the ICU, pseudohyponatremia is most commonly seen with severe hyperglycemia associated with diabetic ketoacidosis or nonketotic, hyperosmolar syndrome. In these cases, glucose induces a shift of water from the intra- to extracellular space. Therapy is directed at resuscitation of the volume depletion from osmotic diuresis and insulin administration. Traditionally, the correction factor that is used is a 1.6 mEq/L decrease in sodium concentration for every 100 mg/dL increase in glucose concentration.[30] However, one report refutes this practice. It found that in cases of severe hyperglycemia, a correction factor of 2.4 mEq/L per 100 mg/dL increase in glucose concentration provided a better approximation of the change in sodium concentration.[31]

# HYPERNATREMIA

## Clinical Features

Hypernatremia is also a common electrolyte disorder in ICU patients.[32] Although hypernatremia can result from the use of hypertonic fluids (e.g., sodium bicarbonate, trisodium citrate, or intravenous hyperalimentation), it is typically caused by a relative lack of free water, rendering the body fluids hyperosmolar.

Normally, hypernatremia stimulates the thirst mechanism and renal water conservation by stimulating the release of ADH. The importance of the thirst mechanism to maintain normonatremia is demonstrated in the clinical scenario of diabetes insipidus. In patients with intact thirst mechanism and adequate access to free water, serum sodium levels remain normal despite massive urine output.

Several factors contribute to the development of hypernatremia in the ICU. Many patients are mechanically ventilated and have some impairment of mental functioning. They are incapable of compensating for any free water loss associated with their underlying disease or its treatment. In the ICU, it is also likely that the kidneys' ability to conserve free water is impaired. This state exists at the same time that large quantities of intravenous medications and electrolyte solutions are being administered.

The elderly, who comprise a substantial proportion of ICU patients, are particularly likely to develop hypernatremia.[33] They commonly develop a diminution in their thirst mechanism. In addition, many older patients cannot maximally concentrate their urine and conserve free water during stress. Causes of hypernatremia in the ICU are listed in Table 20–3.

**TABLE 20–3.** Hypernatremia in the Intensive Care Unit

| |
|---|
| **Diabetes Insipidus** |
| *Neurogenic* |
| Neurosurgery |
| Pituitary apoplexy |
| *Nephrogenic* |
| Hypercalcemia |
| Hypokalemia |
| **Impaired Urinary Concentrating Ability** |
| Renal failure |
| Elderly |
| Osmotic diuresis |
| Loop diuretics |
| **Increased Free Water Loss** |
| Fever |
| Burns/Stevens-Johnson syndrome/GVH disease |
| Intestinal decontamination with lactulose |
| **Hypertonic Solution Administration** |
| Enteral tube feedings |
| Sodium bicarbonate |

GVH, graft versus host.

The development of symptoms from hypernatremia are related to its degree, and more important, the rapidity of onset.[34] Neurologic symptoms are the result of transcellular shifts of water out of brain cells. Early symptoms include lethargy and weakness, which can progress to muscular rigidity, seizures, and coma. A rapid decrease in brain water content can cause intracranial hemorrhage from rupture of cerebral veins.[35] These symptoms are often masked in critically ill patients by underlying medical conditions, intubation, and numerous medications.

## Treatment of Hypernatremia

Therapy for hypernatremia is directed at correcting any concurrent volume depletion and replacing the calculated free water deficit. When treating hypernatremic patients without overt signs of volume depletion, administration of water by mouth or intravenously as 5% dextrose in water is usually sufficient. Patients with evidence of volume depletion require both salt and water resuscitation. Regardless of the severity of hypernatremia, isotonic saline remains the initial treatment of choice in volume-contracted hypernatremic patients. Because isotonic saline is relatively hypotonic to plasma in such patients, it will initially repair both the sodium and water deficits. The potential complication of vigorous treatment of hypernatremia is cerebral edema. Thus, fluids should be administered with a plan to correct the hypernatremia over a period of 48 to 72 hours.[36] This can be accomplished by the administration of hypotonic fluids at a rate calculated to decrease the serum sodium by 0.5 to 1 mEq/L/hr. After calculating the free water deficit, one half is provided over the first 24 hours and the remaining deficit is corrected during the next 2 days. At the same time, appropriate fluids must be given for any ongoing fluid losses. The reader is referred to Chapter 15 for more complete details.

## ICU Scenarios

### NEUROGENIC DIABETES INSIPIDUS

Neurogenic (central) diabetes insipidus results from the lack of ADH secretion by the brain. Although various causes exist, in the ICU, surgical injury to the pituitary stalk is a noteworthy example.

Patients who experience damage to the pituitary stalk may have a classically described triphasic clinical syndrome of initial diabetes insipidus, followed by transient ADH excess, before permanent diabetes insipidus results.[37] After injury, patients develop polyuria with a maximally dilute urine and the development of hypernatremia. Later, owing to the release of previously stored ADH, urine output falls; the urine becomes concentrated; and hypernatremia can develop if the composition of intravenous fluids is not appropriately adjusted. Once the stores of ADH are exhausted, permanent diabetes insipidus emerges. As discussed earlier, such patients require adequate access to free water or infusion of hypotonic fluids to maintain normonatremia.

#### BURN PATIENTS

Unrecognized loss of water through excessive insensible fluid loss is common in patients with extensive thermal injuries. These deficits are often difficult to quantify so that adequate replacement is not achieved. Similar circumstances exist in patients with drug-induced Stevens-Johnson syndrome and dermal graft-versus-host disease (GVHD).

#### ENTERAL TUBE FEEDINGS

Critically ill patients are hypercatabolic and often have a negative nitrogen balance. In order to avoid the complications of starvation in these patients, nutrition in the form of hypertonic enteral feeding formulations is administered. Without proper attention to the composition of intravenous fluids, patients can rapidly develop the tube feeding syndrome of hypernatremia, azotemia, and dehydration.[38] Two factors cause this syndrome. Most tube feedings, when used in full strength, are hypertonic and result in hypernatremia if sufficient quantities of free water are not supplied. In addition, the protein in the diet may be converted to excess urea by the hypercatabolic patient, thus causing an osmotic diuresis that impairs the kidneys' ability to conserve free water. In order to avoid the development of hypernatremia, newer enteral feeding solutions have been developed that are isotonic. Another method employed is to dilute the feeding solution with water. Nevertheless, it is imperative to pay close attention to net fluid balance and serum sodium values in critically ill patients to avoid this pitfall.

#### DIURETICS

Diuretic use is common in patients in the ICU. Loop diuretics such as furosemide, by interfering with the countercurrent mechanism of the loop of Henle, impair the kidneys' ability to concentrate urine. These patients cannot conserve free water, and will develop hypernatremia if adequate quantities of free water are not supplied.

#### OSMOTIC DIURESIS

Osmotic diuresis results from the presence of a nonreabsorbed, osmotically active agent in the urinary space. Its presence increases urinary flow with a resultant wash-out of the renal medulla and impaired renal concentrating ability. Patients are, therefore, unable to conserve water and are at risk of developing hypernatremia. Although mannitol or carbonic anhydrase inhibitors are typical osmotic diuretics, in the critically ill patient, it is the osmotic agent urea that is often the culprit. The classic scenario is an ICU patient receiving increased protein loads from either intravenous or enteral hyperalimentation in an attempt to compensate for a hypercatabolic state. These patients often develop high BUN levels. The increased renal filtration and excretion of urea results in an osmotic diuresis and the increased propensity to develop hypernatremia.[39]

#### NEPHROGENIC DIABETES INSIPIDUS: HYPERCALCEMIA/HYPOKALEMIA

Hypercalcemia or hypokalemia may develop in critically ill patients and contribute to the development of hypernatremia by causing nephrogenic diabetes insipidus. The mechanism by which hypercalcemia causes diabetes insipidus is incompletely understood, although calcium deposition in the renal medulla with tubulointerstitial injury may play an important role.[40] In addition, the $Ca^{2+}$-sensing receptor (CaSR) has been localized in the thick ascending loop of Henle and the collecting duct. The interaction of calcium with this receptor may inhibit ADH stimulated cyclic adenosine monophosphate (cAMP) accumulation.[41]

In hypokalemia-induced polyuria, distal nephron responsiveness to ADH is diminished in part by a reduction in cAMP generation.[42] Hypokalemia may also interfere with the countercurrent multiplier in the loop of Henle.[43]

## HYPERKALEMIA

### Clinical Features

Hyperkalemia in the ICU is particularly important because of the adverse effects on the cardiac conduction system. Simplistically, the causes of hyperkalemia can be categorized as increased input, decreased renal excretion, or shifting from the intracellular to extracellular space (Table 20–4).

The symptoms of hyperkalemia depend on the degree of elevation and rapidity of onset. Patients may experience paresthesias, weakness, and if severe, flaccid paralysis. The most ominous complication is cardiac conduction system defects. The initial electrocardiogram (ECG) change is "tenting" or peaking of T waves. As the serum potassium level rises, there is prolongation of the PR interval and widening of the QRS complex. In severe cases, the P wave disappears and the QRS complex merges with the T wave, resulting in the classic sine wave pattern. Ventricular fibrillation or asystole can result.

### Treatment of Hyperkalemia

Treatment of hyperkalemia is covered in detail in Chapter 23, and is summarized in Figure 20–2. If the

**TABLE 20–4.** Hyperkalemia in the Intensive Care Unit

| |
|---|
| **Increased Input** |
| Inappropriate dialysis solution |
| Inappropriate total parenteral nutrition |
| **Decreased Output** |
| Renal failure |
| Urinary tract obstruction |
| Decreased distal sodium delivery |
| Hypoadrenalism |
| Drugs |
| **Transcellular Shifts** |
| Rhabdomyolysis |
| Tumor lysis syndrome |
| Tissue necrosis |
| Hyperosmolality |
| Insulin deficiency |

serum potassium level is elevated, an ECG tracing should be obtained immediately. It is foolhardy to repeat the serum level to "rule out" hemolysis first before obtaining the ECG tracing. Any ECG abnormality consistent with hyperkalemia demands immediate intravenous administration of calcium. It does not affect serum potassium level but antagonizes potassium's effect on cardiac cell membranes.[44]

The ultimate therapy of hyperkalemia is removal of potassium from the body by either dialysis or the ion-exchange resin Kayexalate, but more immediate results are achieved by temporarily shifting potassium into the intracellular compartment. This intracellular shifting of potassium is done with administration of intravenous insulin (along with glucose to avoid hypoglycemia) and inhaled β-agonists. Although routine administration of sodium bicarbonate has been used in the past, several recent studies question its overall effectiveness in treating hyperkalemia.[45] The use of bicarbonate should probably be reserved for therapy of hyperkalemia associated with severe metabolic acidosis. It is critical to remember that these maneuvers are transient. Without removing potassium from the body, hyperkalemia will recur after the effects of the drug wear off.

Increased renal excretion of potassium is produced with a brisk saline diuresis and administration of loop diuretics. However, in most circumstances in the ICU, renal function is inadequate to achieve significant potassium loss. Kayexalate, given as a retention enema, can significantly decrease serum potassium levels in 1 to 2 hours.[46] Because it exchanges sodium ions for potassium, caution should be exercised in patients with decompensated CHF. Intestinal necrosis has been reported with the use of rectal Kayexalate and has been attributed to the sorbitol added to the solution.[47] Hemodialysis is the most effective method of removing potassium from the body. Although peritoneal dialysis and continuous forms of dialysis are also effective, they are less useful in emergency situations. It must be emphasized that hemodialysis is not the treatment of first choice. The inherent time delay for initiation of dialysis (e.g., calling in a dialysis nurse from home, insertion of a dialysis catheter) mandates that previously described methods for lowering serum potassium levels take precedence.

## ICU Scenarios

### POTASSIUM CONTAINING INTRAVENOUS SOLUTIONS

Increased input alone is rarely a cause of hyperkalemia. A rise in serum potassium levels stimulates adrenal secretion of aldosterone, which increases renal potassium excretion. In addition, hyperkalemia, as has been shown in adrenalectomized dogs, directly increases renal potassium loss. Therefore, without impairment in either adrenal or renal function, hyperkalemia from increased input rarely causes significant hyperkalemia. Most often, hyperkalemia from increased input is the result of inappropriately prescribed intravenous or enteral nutrition in the face of impaired renal function.

### RENAL FAILURE

Renal failure is the prototypical disorder that causes hyperkalemia. However, potassium retention from re-

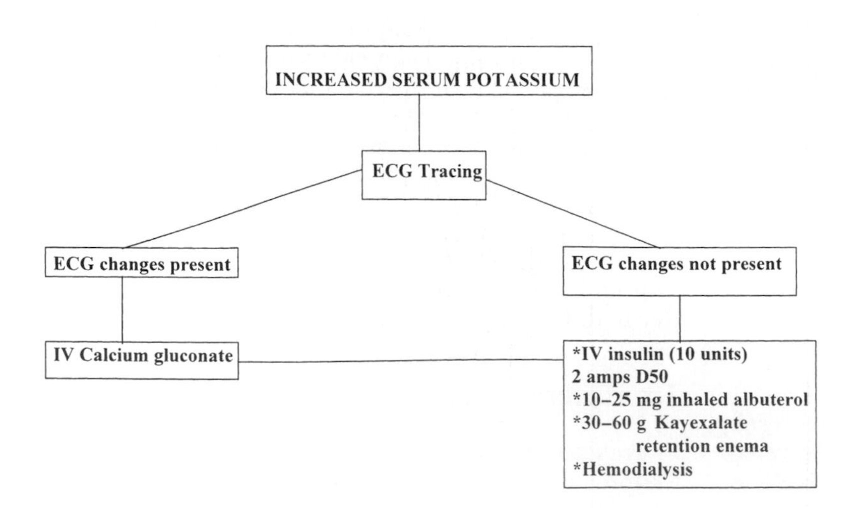


**FIGURE 20–2** ■ Emergency treatment of hyperkalemia. ECG, electrocardiogram; IV, intravenous.

nal insufficiency is seen only when the GFR falls below 15 mL/min.[48] Therefore, in patients with mild renal impairment who experience hyperkalemia, another mechanism is usually operative.

## IMPAIRED DISTAL SODIUM DELIVERY

Renal potassium excretion is dependent on adequate sodium delivery to the distal nephron. In the collecting duct, sodium reabsorption from the urinary space creates a negative electrogenic gradient that favors potassium secretion. When sodium delivery is impaired, this negative potential is dissipated and potassium retention results.[49] This mechanism is referred to as a voltage defect.

Many ICU patients have true or effective volume depletion from previous diuretic use, aggressive ultrafiltration, positive-pressure ventilation, severe hypoalbuminemia, CHF, sepsis, pancreatitis, or rhabdomyolysis. These disease states enhance proximal reabsorption of sodium and impair distal flow. In some patients, administration of intravenous saline can correct the problem. However, in disease states such as severe third-spacing or CHF, this therapy is rarely successful and usually only worsens anasarca or pulmonary edema.

## DRUGS

*Trimethoprim,* a component of the antibiotic Bactrim, is used in high doses to treat pneumocystis pneumonia in patients with acquired immunodeficiency syndrome (AIDS) and can cause hyperkalemia. Analogous to the mechanism of decreased distal sodium delivery, trimethoprim causes a voltage defect by blocking the apical sodium channel in the distal nephron and dissipates the electrogenic potential that favors potassium secretion.[50]

ACEIs, by decreasing angiotensin II stimulation of aldosterone secretion, can result in decreased renal excretion of potassium.

Cyclosporine, which is used to prevent rejection in transplant recipients and to treat various renal and rheumatologic conditions, can cause hyperkalemia, although the mechanism is incompletely understood. It may involve blocking of the apical potassium channels or inhibiting the basolateral $Na^+/K^+$ ATPase.[51, 52]

Finally, *spironolactone,* by directly antagonizing the action of aldosterone in the kidney, can cause hyperkalemia. Although spironolactone is used most commonly to treat ascites in patients with cirrhosis of the liver, studies have shown that it may prolong survival when given to patients with symptomatic CHF.[53] Hyperkalemia may become commonplace in the ICU when spironolactone and ACEIs are used together for treating severe CHF.

### *Heparin*

Heparin has varied uses in the ICU and can cause hyperkalemia. Prophylaxis for deep venous thrombosis, treatment of pulmonary embolism, deep venous thrombosis or DIC, and anticoagulation for continuous dialysis are just some of its indications. The mechanism by which heparin causes hyperkalemia remains unclear, although it appears to affect the adrenal gland. It has been reported that heparin administration decreases the density of angiotensin II receptors in the adrenal gland.[54] It is important to note that hyperkalemia from heparin does not require intravenous administration, because it has been reported after subcutaneous use.

## HYPERRENINEMIC HYPOALDOSTERONISM

In some critically ill patients, a dissociation between renin and aldosterone secretion develops. Its presence is associated with an increased severity of illness and mortality rate.[7] It is estimated that hyperreninemic hypoaldosteronism occurs in up to 20% of patients in the ICU. Although rarely an isolated cause of hyperkalemia, it contributes to the propensity of critically ill patients to develop hyperkalemia.

## ADRENAL INSUFFICIENCY

Patients in the ICU are at risk for developing adrenal failure. Adrenal gland necrosis from sepsis (Waterhouse-Friderichsen syndrome), hypotension, or heparin administration may occur in ICU patients. Although these patients develop hypotension, hyponatremia, hyperkalemia, and metabolic acidosis, the diagnosis can be easily missed because many other explanations for these findings are present in critically ill patients. When in doubt, a corticotropin stimulation test should be performed.

## DIABETIC KETOACIDOSIS

Patients with diabetic ketoacidosis (DKA) universally have depleted total body potassium stores from osmotic diuresis but typically are hyperkalemic on presentation.[55] The pathogenesis of this paradox is multifactorial. Hyperglycemia raises serum osmolality, which draws out intracellular water and potassium ions. At the same time, the insulin deficiency favors the movement of potassium out of the cells. Finally, most patients admitted with DKA are volume depleted from osmotic diuresis and vomiting. The resultant decreased distal sodium delivery impairs renal potassium secretion.

During the initial phases of DKA, patients lose a substantial quantity of potassium in their urine owing to excessive urine flow from hyperglycemia-induced osmotic diuresis. Elevated serum aldosterone levels from the ensuing volume depletion add to the renal potassium loss. Only in the later stages of DKA, usually upon presentation to the emergency center or ICU, when severe volume depletion is present, will hyperkalemia be manifest.

Treatment is directed at restoration of normal intravascular volume with infusion of saline and administration of insulin. Once adequate urine flow is established and the serum potassium is less than 5.5 mEq/L, potassium must be added to the intravenous fluids to avoid precipitating frank hypokalemia.

### RHABDOMYOLYSIS/TUMOR LYSIS SYNDROME/TISSUE NECROSIS

These disorders share the same mechanism for producing hyperkalemia, namely, release of intracellular potassium from cellular disruption. Although treatment follows the general guidelines discussed earlier, it can be very difficult to control the potassium levels in these patients. Revascularization of an ischemic limb or administration of chemotherapy to an acute leukemia patient with a white blood cell count greater than 100,000/mm$^3$ can result in fatal hyperkalemia. In these patients, immediate postoperative dialysis or prophylactic dialysis is commonly utilized at our institution.

### URINARY TRACT OBSTRUCTION

Hyperkalemia with hyperchloremic metabolic acidosis can develop in patients with urinary tract obstruction, independent of any change in the GFR. Three mechanisms have been found to explain these findings: (1) aldosterone deficiency secondary to decreased renal production of renin, (2) a defect in distal nephron sodium reabsorption that decreases the intraluminal negative potential difference and diminishes potassium secretion (voltage defect), and (3) a combination of these two defects.[56] Obstructive uropathy should be considered in any patient with unexplained renal disease and hyperkalemic, hyperchloremic metabolic acidosis.

# HYPOKALEMIA

## Clinical Features

The differential diagnosis of hypokalemia mirrors that of hyperkalemia: decreased input, increased output, and transcellular shifts (Table 20–5).

**TABLE 20–5.** Hypokalemia in the Intensive Care Unit

| |
|---|
| **Decreased Input** |
| NPO state |
| Inappropriate fluid/dialysis prescription |
| **Increased Loss** |
| NG suction/vomiting |
| Diarrhea |
| Diuretics |
| Postobstructive diuresis |
| Post-ATN diuresis |
| Amphotericin B |
| Hypomagnesemia |
| Urinary nonreabsorbed anions |
| **Transcellular Shifts** |
| Epinephrine |
| $\beta_2$-Agonists |
| Insulin |
| Refeeding syndrome |

ATN, acute tubular necrosis; NG, nasogastric; NPO, nothing by mouth.

Symptoms of hypokalemia include muscular weakness, cramping, and pain, which can progress to paralysis. These signs are usually not apparent in critically ill patients. Cardiac rhythm disturbances may also occur. Findings on ECG include flattening of the T wave and the appearance of a U wave. Atrial and ventricular extrasystoles can appear. Ventricular tachycardia and fibrillation are rare in otherwise normal patients. However, this is not the case in ICU patients who may be receiving digoxin, epinephrine, dobutamine, or dopamine or those who have underlying cardiac disease. Therefore, hypokalemia should be treated aggressively in such patients.

## Treatment of Hypokalemia

Because potassium is an intracellular cation, relatively small decrements in serum levels can represent large absolute deficits in total body potassium stores. For example, a serum potassium level below 3 mEq/L can represent a deficit of 100 to 300 mEq, whereas a value below 2 mEq/L may require replacement of up to 800 mEq over several days.[57]

In most cases, when the oral route cannot be used, or there are symptoms of hypokalemia, potassium is administered intravenously. When cardiac toxicity is present, 5 to 10 mEq of potassium can be given over 15 to 20 minutes. This dose is repeated as necessary. Continuous monitoring of the ECG and frequent measurement of the serum potassium levels are necessary. In severe cases, as much as 40 to 80 mEq/hr of potassium via a central venous catheter during continuous ECG monitoring has been utilized.[58]

## ICU Scenarios

### POSTOBSTRUCTIVE DIURESIS/POST-ACUTE TUBULAR NECROSIS DIURESIS

Approximately 15% of patients who develop acute renal failure have obstruction of the urinary tract. Relief of obstruction usually reverses the renal failure and is accompanied by a brisk increase in urine output—the so-called postobstructive diuresis. The increased urine output is usually considered "appropriate" because of the prior accumulation of water and solutes. However, the tubular reabsorption rate is still greatly reduced; therefore, a patient may excrete large volumes of an isosthenuric urine. In such patients, hypokalemia, hypomagnesemia, hypernatremia, and volume depletion can occur. A similar syndrome can develop in patients who experience polyuria after recovery from acute tubular necrosis (ATN).

Although intravenous fluids are often administered to match urine output during a postobstructive diuresis, this can lead to a perpetuation of the polyuria because the sodium in the fluid is another solute that requires excretion. Physicians may "wean" the postobstructive patient by providing fluids in a 1:2 or 1:3 ratio to the urine output. In the ICU, more prudent treatment is to avoid volume depletion and supplement patients with appropriate intravenous fluids as directed by frequent assessment of the clinical status, central venous pressure, and electrolyte levels.

#### HYPOMAGNESEMIA

Hypomagnesemia is a common condition in ICU patients. It is typically seen in states of nutritional deprivation or after administration of diuretics. Hypomagnesemia results in increased renal potassium loss, although the mechanism is unclear.[59] Enhanced secretion of aldosterone and direct cellular effects on the loop of Henle have been implicated. In general, correction of hypokalemia requires restoration of magnesium balance. Administration of potassium alone is insufficient, because it is excreted in the urine.

#### AMPHOTERICIN B

Amphotericin B is administered to critically ill patients with life-threatening fungal infections. By interacting with membrane sterols, it increases membrane permeability and causes increased urinary potassium loss.[60] Amphotericin B can also cause a type 1 renal tubular acidosis with hypokalemia.[61]

#### NASOGASTRIC SUCTION/VOMITING

Initially, loss of gastric fluids raises the serum bicarbonate level above the reabsorption threshold of the kidneys and bicarbonaturia develops.[62] Loss of this urinary anion obligates renal potassium excretion. This effect is transient. Ongoing gastric fluid loss eventually causes volume depletion that increases proximal bicarbonate reabsorption and stops the renal potassium wasting. Hypokalemia is maintained by continued loss of potassium in gastric fluids and volume depletion. A reasonable treatment approach is to match nasogastric output with intravenous half-normal saline with 20 mEq/L of potassium.

#### URINARY NONREABSORBED ANIONS

Delivery of sodium with a nonreabsorable anion other than chloride to the distal nephron increases renal potassium loss.[63] In the ICU, this commonly results from infusion of large volumes of sodium bicarbonate to patients with either tumor lysis syndrome or rhabdomyolysis in order to alkalinize the urine. In these settings, a lumen-negative potential favoring potassium secretion is created by sodium reabsorption, which cannot be dissipated by chloride reabsorption. This effect of nonreabsorbed anions is most prominent when there is concurrent volume depletion.

#### DIABETIC KETOACIDOSIS

Total potassium stores are depleted in patients with diabetic ketoacidosis (DKA) despite the presence of hyperkalemia on presentation. During the hyperglycemia-induced osmotic diuresis, massive amounts of potassium are lost in the urine. This deficit is masked by the hyperkalemia produced by insulin deficiency, hyperosmolality, and decreased sodium delivery to the distal nephron.

## HYPOCALCEMIA

### Clinical Features

Ionized hypocalcemia is common in ICU patients, although its cause often remains obscure (Table 20–6). Critically ill patients with hypocalcemia appear to have a higher mortality rate, longer ICU stay, and a higher incidence of bacteremia.[64]

In ICU patients, ionized calcium levels should always be measured rather than total calcium values. Hypoalbuminemia is common in critically ill patients and lowers total calcium levels without a fall in ionized values. It is wise in such sick patients to measure ionized calcium values rather than relying on a "correction factor" for the low albumin concentration. This edict is especially true in patients receiving citrate for regional anticoagulation on continuous dialysis.

Hypocalcemia affects neurologic, cardiovascular, and muscular functions. Early signs include circumoral numbness and limb paresthesias, which can progress to spasms, tetany, or seizures. Trousseau and Chvostek signs may be present. Cardiac involvement can manifest as prolongation of the QT interval, hypotension, heart block, or ventricular fibrillation.

### Treatment of Hypocalcemia

Although treatment of hypocalcemia is directed at the underlying cause, acute symptomatic hypocalcemia must be considered a medical emergency in a critically ill patient. Usually it requires intravenous administration of a calcium preparation. Caution must be exercised when concurrent hyperphosphatemia is present. In this case, calcium administration may precipitate metastatic calcification in tissues. Also, concurrent hypomagnesemia (as discussed later) must be corrected or the administered calcium will fail to raise serum calcium levels. If metabolic acidosis is present, hypocalcemia must be corrected before administering bicarbonate to avoid precipitating tetany or seizures.

**TABLE 20–6.** Hypocalcemia in the Intensive Care Unit

| |
|---|
| Sepsis/SIRS |
| Acute pancreatitis |
| Rhabdomyolysis |
| Tumor lysis syndrome |
| Acute hyperphosphatemia |
| Renal failure |
| Hypomagnesemia |
| Citrate administration |
| Alkali administration |

SIRS, systemic inflammatory response syndrome.

When hypocalcemia is severe or symptomatic, calcium gluconate may be given as 10 mL of a 10% solution intravenously over 5 to 10 minutes.[65] This agent should never be given through any line containing a bicarbonate-based solution, because it will cause precipitation. For more prolonged treatment, 50 mL of calcium gluconate in 500 mL of 5% dextrose in water can be infused over 8 hours. In the face of severe hyperphosphatemia, hemodialysis is necessary.

## ICU Scenarios

### SEPSIS/SYSTEMIC INFLAMMATORY RESPONSE SYNDROME

Low serum calcium can be found in 50% to 70% of patients with sepsis or SIRS without evidence of conditions otherwise associated with hypocalcemia, such as renal failure or rhabdomyolysis.[64] Although the mechanism or mechanisms have not been firmly established, data suggest that hypocalcemia may result directly from the inflammatory response in these patients. In a study of ICU patients with sepsis, the development of hypocalcemia correlated with the rise of the inflammatory mediators tumor necrosis factor-α (TNF-α), interleukin-6 (IL-6), C-reactive protein, and procalcitonin.[66] Although it had been previously suggested that the hypocalcemia of sepsis results from PTH resistance in the kidney and bone, in these patients, serum PTH levels were elevated, and urinary calcium levels were low. Markers of bone turnover were also elevated. Thus, there was no evidence for PTH resistance. How the inflammatory response induces hypocalcemia is unknown, but in human subjects and in septic shock models, intracellular calcium accumulation has been demonstrated.[67]

### ACUTE PANCREATITIS

Severe acute pancreatitis is a multisystemic disease that reflects the ability of the pancreas to produce a variety of vasoactive peptides, hormones, and enzymes. In approximately 25% of patients, severe hypocalcemia develops and is associated with decreased survival rates.[68]

The pathogenesis of hypocalcemia in acute pancreatitis is incompletely understood.[69, 70] Some studies have suggested an impairment in PTH release by the parathyroid gland. Other studies have implicated imbalances of calcitonin and glucagon, binding of calcium by free fatty acid–albumin complexes, and intracellular translocation of calcium. Finally, the theory of intraperitoneal saponification of calcium by fatty acids in areas of fat necrosis is still favored by some investigators.

### RHABDOMYOLYSIS

Rhabdomyolysis denotes an acute or subacute event that leads to necrosis of striated muscle. It is associated with numerous electrolyte disorders, including altered calcium metabolism.

Hypocalcemia develops in the initial phase of rhabdomyolysis and has been attributed to the deposition of calcium salts in necrotic muscle.[71] Muscle necrosis releases large amounts of organic and inorganic phosphate into the circulation, elevating the calcium-phosphate product with subsequent deposition of calcium salts into tissues and muscles. The hypocalcemia may be compounded by a fall in plasma levels of 1,25-dihydroxyvitamin D owing to hyperphosphatemia and renal failure. In later stages, up to 30% of patients with rhabdomyolysis and renal failure develop hypercalcemia. The etiology of this rebound hypercalcemia is multifactorial and includes release of calcium from damaged tissues, persistently elevated PTH levels, and increased 1,25-dihydroxyvitamin D synthesis with recovery of renal function.[72, 73]

### SODIUM PHOSPHATE ENEMAS

Any cause of acute hyperphosphatemia can produce hypocalcemia secondary to the formation of calcium-phosphate complexes. Patients with renal failure and an inability to excrete phosphate are particularly susceptible to this occurrence. Enemas such as Fleet (sodium phosphate) contain large quantities of phosphate. When given to patients with renal failure, there have been several reports of life-threatening hypocalcemia from acute hyperphosphatemia.[74]

### HYPOMAGNESEMIA

Hypocalcemia in ICU patients can be caused by hypomagnesemia. Hypomagnesemia impairs both the release of PTH and the action of PTH on the skeleton.[75] It is usually resistant to calcium repletion until the low magnesium level is corrected.

### CITRATE ADMINISTRATION/CONTINUOUS RENAL REPLACEMENT THERAPIES

Citrate chelates ionized calcium in the blood and can result in hypocalcemia. Although this can occur with massive blood transfusions, the more common etiology is the use of citrate for regional anticoagulation in continuous renal replacement therapies (CRRTs).

In CRRT, citrate is administered in a prefilter mode, chelating calcium and rendering blood anticoagulated. Calcium is infused through a central line so that the patient's serum calcium level remains normal and the blood can coagulate appropriately. Errors in prescription can easily result in hypocalcemia.

Hypocalcemia can also be seen in patients with liver failure who are unable to metabolize circulating calcium citrate complexes and appropriately release free calcium into the circulation.[76]

### ALKALI ADMINISTRATION

Sodium bicarbonate may be administered to patients in the ICU for metabolic acidosis. Calcium and protons compete for binding sites on serum proteins, particularly albumin. When bicarbonate is infused, there is the potential to precipitate acute symptomatic hypocalcemia. This is especially true in patients who already have low serum calcium levels. In these cases, it is important to correct the calcium deficit before administering bicarbonate.

#### TUMOR LYSIS SYNDROME/RENAL FAILURE

In these disorders, high serum phosphorus chelates circulating calcium and produces hypocalcemia. Lowering the phosphorus level will correct the calcium disorder. Administration of calcium in these patients can raise the calcium-phosphorus level and cause calcium precipitation into tissues. In the ICU, correction of a patient's hyperphosphatemia usually requires dialysis.

## HYPERCALCEMIA

### Clinical Features

Hypercalcemia is seen less often in critically ill patients than other electrolyte disturbances. Although the list of disorders that cause hypercalcemia is extensive, some are more commonly seen in the ICU (Table 20–7).

The clinical presentation of hypercalcemia correlates with the rapidity of the rise and absolute elevation of serum calcium. As with hypocalcemia, neurologic abnormalities predominate. Patients may develop lethargy, confusion, weakness, and headache. Stupor and coma may ensue. Hypercalcemia shortens the QT interval, broadens the T wave, and produces a first-degree atrioventicular block. Hypercalcemia can also lead to numerous renal abnormalities. Polyuria is caused by hypercalcemia-induced ADH resistance and nephrogenic diabetes insipidus. Acute renal failure results from dehydration, renal vasoconstriction, and nephrocalcinosis.

### Treatment of Hypercalcemia

Treatment of hypercalcemia is directed at the underlying disorder. However, in symptomatic patients, or when serum calcium levels exceed 13 mg/dL, acute therapy is warranted. The mainstay of treatment is the induction of a saline diuresis in patients with relatively normal renal and cardiac function. Infusion of intravenous saline at rates of 200 to 250 mL/hr are typical. Loop diuretics, which have a calciuric effect, can be added once any volume depletion has been corrected. Use of thiazide diuretics is avoided, because they decrease renal calcium excretion. In patients with renal or heart failure, removal of calcium is best achieved by hemodialysis using a low calcium dialysate bath. In most cases, severe hypercalcemia results from an underlying malignancy so that the aforementioned measures are only temporizing. Concomitant measures aimed at reducing bone resorption should be initiated.

Calcitonin inhibits osteoclastic bone formation and enhances renal calcium excretion.[77] Calcitonin has the advantage of rapid onset, which begins within 2 hours of administration. However, because its effect on serum calcium levels is both modest and transient, it should not be given as a single agent. Instead, it is used as an adjunct to bisphosphonates for rapid calcium reduction while waiting for the latter agent to take effect. Bisphosphonates are the principal agents used to treat hypercalcemia caused by increased osteoclastic bone resorption.[78] Pamidronate is the drug of choice for treating hypercalcemia, and causes calcium levels to return to normal, usually within 1 week. Plicamycin and gallium nitrate are other agents that lower serum calcium levels when hypercalcemia is the result of increased bone resorption. However, because of their side effect profile and the efficacy of bisphosphonates, these agents are used infrequently. Finally, glucocorticoids may be a useful agent in treating hypercalcemia associated with hematologic malignancies such as multiple myeloma and lymphoma. Treatment of severe hypercalcemia in malignancy is outlined in Figure 20–3.

**TABLE 20–7.** Hypercalcemia in the Intensive Care Unit

| |
|---|
| **Malignancy** |
| Solid tumors |
| Multiple myeloma |
| Hematopoietic cancers |
| **Rhabdomyolysis** |
| Trauma |
| Toxic/metabolic |
| Ischemic |
| **Immobilization** |

### ICU Scenarios

#### MALIGNANCY

Hypercalcemia is one of the skeletal complications of malignancies, but the reported prevalence is highly variable. More than half of the patients with malignancy associated hypercalcemia have lung or breast carcinoma. Less common malignancies such as multiple myeloma, head and neck cancers, and renal cell carcinoma have a higher incidence of hypercalcemia.

Although direct invasion and destruction of bone may result in malignancy associated hypercalcemia, more often it is caused by secretion of a calcemic factor by malignant cells.[79] Many tumors produce PTH-related peptide (PTHrP) in which the first 8 of 13 amino acids are identical to PTH. Other tumors produce transforming growth factor-α (TGF-α), interleukin-1 (IL-1), or cytokines such as lymphotoxin that promote bone resorption, or hormones such as 1,25 dihydroxy-vitamin D that promote intestinal calcium absorption, leading to hypercalcemia.

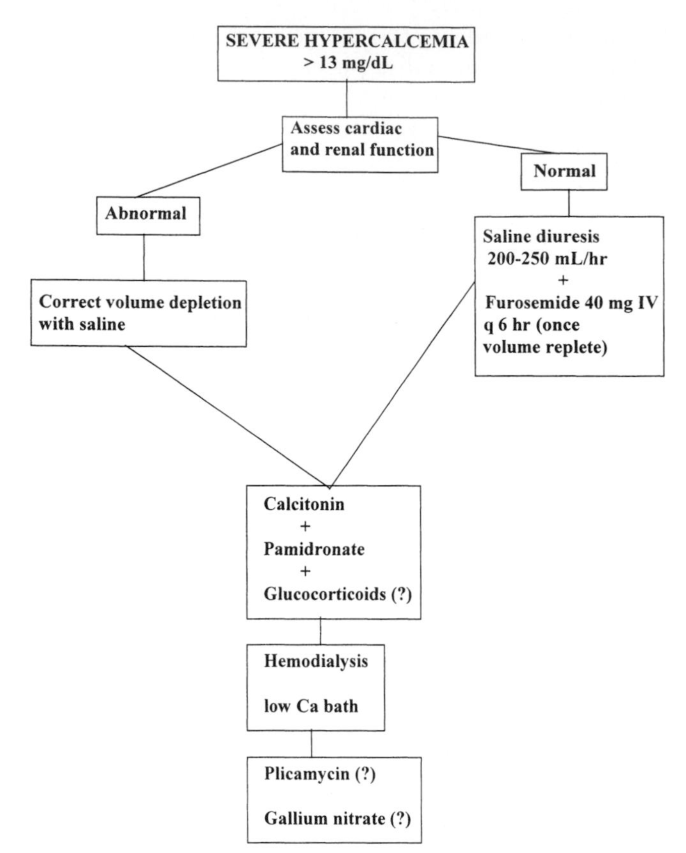


**FIGURE 20–3** ■ Treatment of malignant hypercalcemia.

### RHABDOMYOLYSIS

In the late stages of rhabdomyolysis, with the recovery of renal function, 30% of patients can develop hypercalcemia. It results from the release of calcium from injured tissues and elevated PTH and 1,25-dihydroxyvitamin D levels.

### IMMOBILIZATION

Similar to weightlessness in space travel, immobilization leads to a rapid increase in bone resorption for poorly understood reasons.[80] Although a rare cause of hypercalcemia, it is not surprising that it would play a role in the ICU, where patients are immobilized for prolonged periods of time. Although the rise in serum calcium is usually modest, in the face of impaired renal function, it can become severe and difficult to control. This disorder is most often seen in younger patients who sustain a traumatic injury, particularly to the spinal cord. Although treatment with saline usually suffices, the addition of bisphosphonate is occasionally necessary.[81]

# HYPERPHOSPHATEMIA

## Clinical Features

Hyperphosphatemia in the ICU is typically caused by retention of phosphate during acute renal failure or by release from intracellular stores owing to massive tissue breakdown (Table 20–8).

The clinical symptoms of patients with hyperphosphatemia, such as tetany and seizures, are caused by the subsequent fall in serum calcium levels. The formation of calcium-phosphate complexes result in ectopic calcification, especially in previously injured tissues.

## Treatment of Hyperphosphatemia

Treatment of hyperphosphatemia is directed at increasing renal excretion and decreasing intestinal absorption of phosphate. If renal function is normal, extracellular fluid volume expansion with saline can lower renal phosphate reabsorption. However, in patients with acute renal failure, hemodialysis is the treatment of choice. Similarly, in disorders such as rhabdomyolysis and tumor lysis syndrome, enhancing renal clearance with saline is often insufficient in controlling serum levels, and acute hemodialysis is necessary. Phosphate binders may be added to decrease intestinal absorption of phosphate. However, many patients in the ICU are not being fed or are receiving intravenous hyperalimentation, thus this treatment is of little use.

## ICU Scenarios

### ACUTE RENAL FAILURE

In acute renal failure, hyperphosphatemia develops from decreased renal excretion. Symptoms are due to the subsequent hypocalcemia. If the symptoms are mild and the patient is eating, hyperphosphatemia can be controlled by oral administration of phosphate binders with meals, such as calcium carbonate or calcium acetate. In severe cases, hemodialysis is necessary.

### TUMOR LYSIS SYNDROME/ RHABDOMYOLYSIS

Cellular disruption releases large quantities of phosphate into the serum and causes hypocalcemia. If renal function is normal, a saline diuresis can be attempted, but in the ICU, hemodialysis is usually necessary.

# HYPOPHOSPHATEMIA

## Clinical Features

Whereas mild hypophosphatemia is generally asymptomatic, severe hypophosphatemia (<1 mg/dL)

**TABLE 20–8.** Hyperphosphatemia in the Intensive Care Unit

| | |
|---|---|
| Acute renal failure | Hypercatabolic state |
| Rhabdomyolysis | Hyperthermia |
| Tumor lysis syndrome | |

**TABLE 20–9.** Hypophosphatemia in the Intensive Care Unit

| | |
|---|---|
| Refeeding syndrome | Respiratory alkalosis |
| Diabetic ketoacidosis | Chronic alcoholism |

is associated with various clinical symptoms and can result in death. Hypophosphatemia is caused by decreased intake, increased excretion, or a shift from the extracellular to the intracellular space (Table 20–9).

Patients with severe hypophosphatemia may develop neurologic dysfunction characterized by weakness, paresthesias, confusion, seizures, and coma. Hematologic effects include hemolytic anemia and impaired leukocyte and platelet function. Hypophosphatemia is associated with muscle edema and rhabdomyolysis. Decreased cardiac output and respiratory muscle paralysis can occur and result in death.

## Treatment of Hypophosphatemia

Treatment of hypophosphatemia, if not severe, is best accomplished by oral administration. Milk is an excellent source of phosphate. In patients unable to receive oral supplements, or in severe symptomatic hypophosphatemia, intravenous therapy is indicated. In this case, 2 mg/kg of phosphorus is infused over 6 hours. Levels should be checked frequently during replacement. If necessary, 1 g of phosphorus in 1 L of fluid may be infused over 8 to 12 hours.[65]

## ICU Scenarios

### REFEEDING SYNDROME

Severe hypophosphatemia and its associated complications in patients receiving intravenous hyperalimentation after massive weight loss has been termed the refeeding syndrome.[82] In this syndrome, depletion of potassium, magnesium, and vitamins also develops.

In the starved individual, the catabolism of fat and protein leads to a loss of lean muscle mass. Although phosphate stores are depleted, serum levels generally remain normal due to adjustments in renal excretion rates. When carbohydrates become available during refeeding, insulin release is stimulated. Carbohydrate repletion and insulin release together enhance cellular uptake of phosphorus and stimulate protein synthesis. Profound extracellular hypophosphatemia results. By a similar mechanism, refeeding syndrome causes severe hypokalemia and hypomagnesemia.

This syndrome may be unappreciated in the critical care setting, although patients in the ICU are clearly at risk (Table 20–10). In patients at risk, routine administration of vitamins, slow advancement of calories, and frequent electrolyte monitoring are necessary precautions.

**TABLE 20–10.** Patients at Risk for Refeeding Syndrome

| | |
|---|---|
| Chronic alcoholism | Nursing home resident |
| Prolonged intravenous hydration | Anorexia nervosa |
| Unfed patient with sepsis/stress | Recent massive weight loss |

### DIABETIC KETOACIDOSIS

In severe DKA, there is excessive urinary loss of phosphate due to hyperglycemia-induced osmotic diuresis. With the initiation of insulin therapy, phosphorus is shifted to the intracellular space. When patients first present, if hypophosphatemia is already present, aggressive replenishment is necessary.

### RESPIRATORY ALKALOSIS

Respiratory alkalosis is common in ICU patients and can result from overbreathing on a ventilator, too rapid a ventilator rate, sepsis, liver failure, or salicylate intoxication. The alkalosis results in an intracellular shifting of phosphate.[83]

### ALCOHOLISM

Many chronic abusers of alcohol are hypophosphatemic from poor nutrition. In addition, alcohol impairs renal phosphorus reabsorption. Even if the serum phosphorus level is normal, these patients should be considered at high risk for the development of refeeding syndrome when prescribing nutritional supplementation.

# HYPERMAGNESEMIA

## Clinical Features

Hypermagnesemia is relatively uncommon because patients with normal renal function are generally able to easily excrete a magnesium load. Hypermagnesemia is typically seen in ICU patients with renal failure who receive magnesium-containing laxatives or antacids. Severe hypermagnesemia (>5 mg/dL) may present with nausea, vomiting, flushing, and sedation. Deep tendon reflexes disappear, and hypotension and bradycardia develop. Muscle weakness can progress to frank paralysis and precipitate respiratory arrest. ECG changes include prolongation of the PR, QRS, and QT intervals. Coma and cardiac arrest may occur.

## Treatment of Hypermagnesemia

Treatment starts with removing any exogenous source of magnesium. For patients with renal failure, hemodialysis with a low magnesium bath may be required. In acute, life-threatening situations, rapid infusions of intravenous calcium result in a transient reduction of symptoms.

**TABLE 20–11.** Hypomagnesemia in the Intensive Care Unit

| | |
|---|---|
| Diuretics | Amphotericin B toxicity |
| Starvation | Postobstructive diuresis |
| Diarrhea | Post-ATN diuresis |
| Aminoglycoside toxicity | Chronic alcoholism |

ATN, acute tubular necrosis.

# HYPOMAGNESEMIA

## Clinical Features

Hypomagnesemia is a relatively common electrolyte disorder in hospitalized patients, especially in the ICU (Table 20–11).

Neuromuscular hyperexcitability is often observed in patients with magnesium deficiency. Patients may develop tremors, spasticity, ataxia, nystagmus, or seizures. Chvostek and Trousseau signs may be present. An ECG shows prolongation of the PR and QT intervals, and atrial and ventricular arrhythmias can develop. Finally, hypomagnesemia can cause hypokalemia and hypocalcemia, which are both refractory to treatment until the magnesium deficit is corrected.

## Treatment of Hypomagnesemia

Mild hypomagnesemia can be treated with oral supplementation, although this often causes diarrhea. Severe hypomagnesemia may be treated with parenteral preparations. Two grams of $MgSO_4$ will provide 16.2 mEq of magnesium and should be administered slowly every 8 hours until the deficit is corrected. In emergency situations, 1 to 2 g can be given rapidly over 5 to 10 minutes. In patients with normal renal function, approximately half of an intravenous dose will be excreted in the urine despite the presence of hypomagnesemia, thus therapy may need to be continued for several days. On the other hand, patients with renal failure require a lower dose with frequent monitoring of serum levels and reflexes.

# SUMMARY

Electrolyte disorders in the ICU are both common and complex. Critical illness causes disturbances in the neurohumoral systems that maintain normal electrolyte homeostasis. The wide variety of disease states and their respective therapies encountered in the ICU often result in numerous electrolyte disorders with multiple pathogenic mechanisms. Frequent monitoring and vigilance by the critical care nephrologist are necessary to evaluate and manage these complicated disorders.

The following clinical vignettes should give the reader an appreciation of the complexity of electrolyte abnormalities in the ICU.

## Rhabdomyolysis

Rhabdomyolysis has multiple causes and results in several electrolyte disorders. Owing to the release of intracellular contents, patients develop severe hyperkalemia and hyperphosphatemia. The hyperphosphatemia then chelates circulating calcium and causes hypocalcemia. The calcium-phosphate complexes deposit in necrotic tissue and contribute to hypocalcemia. In addition, patients may develop acute renal failure from myoglobinuria. The renal failure worsens the hyperphosphatemia and hypocalcemia. During the recovery phase of rhabdomyolysis with renal failure, patients can develop rebound hypercalcemia.

The damaged muscles in rhabdomyolysis accumulate large quantities of fluid, resulting in decreased extracellular fluid volume and elevated ADH levels. Patients treated with hypotonic intravenous fluids may develop hyponatremia.

Finally, treatment of rhabdomyolysis usually includes administration of sodium bicarbonate to alkalinize the urine. The sodium bicarbonate infusion can result in hypernatremia and precipitate tetany or seizures by worsening hypocalcemia.

## Citrate Anticoagulation for Continuous Renal Replacement Therapy

Citrate is used for regional anticoagulation in CRRT. Because it binds calcium, if inadequate calcium is infused through a central line, hypocalcemia can result. As mentioned earlier, some patients with liver failure are unable to metabolize citrate-calcium complexes and develop hypocalcemia.

In addition, citrate contains large quantities of sodium, thus there is a potential risk of developing hypernatremia. In order to avoid hypernatremia, the sodium concentration in the dialysate is usually lowered to 110 to 120 mEq/L.

Citrate is converted by the liver into bicarbonate causing a metabolic alkalosis. Hydrochloric acid in 5% dextrose in water is then administered and can lead to hyponatremia.

## Acute Renal Failure

Acute renal failure is the epitome of a disorder encountered in the ICU in which multiple, simultaneous electrolyte disorders occur. Hyperkalemia, hyperphosphatemia, and hypocalcemia are common. Hypermagnesemia may be seen if magnesium-containing antacids or laxatives are given. Life-threatening hyperphosphatemia is possible if sodium phosphate enemas are prescribed. If bicarbonate is given for metabolic acidosis, hypocalcemia will worsen and seizures can develop. Finally, because urinary dilution and concentration are impaired, hyponatremia or hypernatremia may develop depending on the type of intravenous fluids and electrolyte solutions administered.

## Diabetic Ketoacidosis

Multiple electrolyte disorders develop in patients with DKA. Hyponatremia is common caused by the shift of water to the extracellular space by hyperglycemia (pseudohyponatremia). Despite the decrease in total body potassium stores from prior osmotic diuresis, hyperkalemia is usually present because of hyperosmolality, insulin deficiency, and decreased sodium delivery to the distal nephron. Patients are also phosphate depleted from osmotic diuresis despite relatively normal serum levels. With the initiation of therapy with insulin and fluid resuscitation, severe hypokalemia and hypophosphatemia can develop.

ACKNOWLEDGMENTS

The author would like to acknowledge Dr. Pamela Bailey for her expert review of this manuscript and Ms. Patricia Carpenter for her excellent secretarial skills.

## REFERENCES

1. Weiss NM, Robertson GL: Water metabolism in endocrine disorders. Semin Nephrol 4:303, 1987.
2. DeRubertis FR, Michelis MF, Bloom ME, et al: Impaired water excretion in myxedema. Am J Med 51:41, 1971.
3. Skowsky WR, Kikuchi TA: The role of vasopressin in the impaired water excretion of myxedema. Am J Med 64:613, 1978.
4. Wartofsky L, Burman KD: Alterations in thyroid function in patients with systemic illness: The "euthyroid sick syndrome." Endocr Rev 3:164, 1982.
5. Linas SL, Berl T, Robertson GL, et al: Role of vasopressin in the impaired water excretion of glucocorticoid deficiency. Kidney Int 18:58, 1980.
6. Kidess AI, Caplan RH, Reynerston RH, et al: Transient corticotropin deficiency in critical illness. Mayo Clin Proc 68:435, 1993.
7. Zipser RD, Davenport MW, Martin KL, et al: Hyperreninemic hypoaldosteronism in the critically ill: A new entity. J Clin Endocrinol Metab 53:867, 1981.
8. Devita MV, Gardenswartz MH, Koneclay A, et al: Incidence and etiology of hyponatremia in an intensive care unit. Clin Nephrol 34:163, 1990.
9. Ayus JC, Wheeler JM, Arieff AI: Postoperative hyponatremic encephalopathy in menstruant women. Ann Intern Med 117: 891, 1992.
10. Sterns RH: The management of symptomatic hyponatremia. Semin Nephrol 10:503, 1990.
11. Lauriat SM, Berl T: The hyponatremic patient: Practical focus on therapy. J Am Soc Nephrol 8:1599, 1997.
12. Arieff AI: Acid-base, electrolyte, and metabolic abnormalities. In Parrillo JE, Bone RC (eds): Critical Care Medicine. St. Louis, CV Mosby, 1995, pp 1071–1105.
13. Miller GM, Baker HL, Okazaki H, et al: Central pontine myelinolysis and its imitators: MR findings. Radiology 168:795, 1988.
14. Wolman L: Ischemic lesions in the brain-stem associated with raised intracranial pressure. Brain 76:364, 1953.
15. Tieri R, Arieff AI, Kucharczyk W, et al: Hyponatremic encephalopathy: Is central pontine myelinolysis a component? Am J Med 92:513, 1992.
16. Gines P, Abraham WT, Schrier RW: Vasopressin in pathophysiological states. Semin Nephrol 4:384, 1994.
17. Shichiri M, Shinoda T, Kijima Y, et al: Renal handling of urate in the syndrome of inappropriate secretion of antidiuretic hormone. Arch Intern Med 145:2045, 1985.
18. Harrigon MR: Cerebral salt wasting: A review. Neurosurgery 38: 152, 1996.
19. Nelson PB, Seif SM, Maroon JC, et al: Hyponatremia in intracranial disease: Perhaps not the syndrome of inappropriate secretion of antidiuretic hormone (SIADH). J Neurosurg 55:938, 1982.
20. Maesaka JK, Gupta S, Fishbane S: Cerebral salt-wasting syndrome: Does it exist? Nephron 82:100, 1999.
21. Ishiguro S, Kimura A, Munemoto S, et al: Hyponatremia due to excess natriuresis. No Shinkei Geka 16:707, 1988.
22. Ishikawa S, Saito T, Kaneko K: Hyponatremia responsive to fludrocortisone acetate in elderly patients after head injury. Ann Intern Med 106:187, 1987.
23. Reeder RF, Harbaugh RE: Administration of intravenous urea and normal saline for the treatment of hyponatremia in neurosurgical patients. J Neurosurg 70:201, 1989.
24. Kaczmarczyk G: Pulmonary-renal axis during positive-pressure ventilation. New Horiz 2:512, 1994.
25. Epstein M: Hepatorenal syndrome: Emerging perspectives of pathophysiology and therapy. J Am Soc Nephrol 4:1735, 1994.
26. Martin P-Y, Gines P, Schrier RW: Nitric oxide as a mediator of hemodynamic abnormalities and sodium and water retention in cirrhosis. N Engl J Med 339:533, 1998.
27. Lee W, Packer M: Prognostic importance of serum sodium concentration and its modification by converting enzyme inhibitors. Circulation 73:257, 1986.
28. Fisher CJ, Agasti JM, Opal SM: Treatment of septic shock with the tumor necrosis factor receptor: Fc fusion protein. N Engl J Med 334:1697, 1996.
29. Van Bommel EFH: Should continuous renal replacement therapy be used for 'non-renal' indications in critically ill patients with shock? Resuscitation 33:257, 1997.
30. Katz MA: Hyperglycemia-induced hyponatremia: Calculation of expected serum sodium depression. N Engl J Med 289:843, 1973.
31. Hillier TA, Abbott RD, Barrett EJ: Hyponatremia: Evaluating the correction factor for hyperglycemia. Am J Med 106:399, 1999.
32. Polderman KH, Schrender WO, Strack RJ, et al: Hypernatremia in the intensive care unit: An indicator of quality of care? Crit Care Med 27:1105, 1999.
33. Synder NA, Feigal DW, Arieff AI: Hypernatremia in elderly patients: A heterogeneous, morbid, and iatrogenic entity. Ann Intern Med 107:309, 1987.
34. Ross EJ, Christie SBM: Hypernatremia. Medicine 48:441, 1969.
35. Arieff AI, Guisado R: Effects on the central nervous system of hypernatremic and hyponatremic states. Kidney Int 10:104, 1976.
36. Tonicity. In Kaissirer JP, Hricik DE, Cohen JJ: Repairing Body Fluids: Principles and Practice. Philadelphia, WB Saunders, 1989, pp 27–45.
37. Randall RV, Clar EC, Dodge HW Jr, et al: Polyuria after operation for tumors in the region of the hypophysis and hypothalamus. J Clin Endocrinol Metab 20:1614, 1960.
38. Bowman M, Eisenberg P, Katz B, et al: Effect of tube-feeding osmolality on serum sodium levels. Crit Care Nurse 9:22, 1989.
39. Gault MH, Doyle M, Cohen WM, et al: Hypernatremia, azotemia, and dehydration due to high-protein tube feeding. Ann Intern Med 68:778, 1968.
40. Rosen S, Greenfeld Z, Bernheim J, et al: Hypercalcemic nephropathy: Chronic disease with prominent medullary inner stripe injury. Kidney Int 37:1067, 1990.
41. Herbert SC, Brown EM, Harris HW: Role of the Ca(2+)-sensing receptor in divalent mineral ion homeostasis. J Exp Biol 200: 295, 1997.
42. Jim K, Summer SN, Berl T: The cyclic AMP system in the inner medullary collecting duct of the potassium depleted rat. Kidney Int 26:384, 1984.
43. Luke RG, Wright FS, Fowler N, et al: Effects of potassium depletion on renal tubular chloride transport in the rat. Kidney Int 14:414, 1978.
44. Schwartz AB: Potassium-related cardiac arrhythmias and their treatment. Angiology 29:194, 1978.
45. Allon M, Shanklin N: Effect of bicarbonate administration on plasma potassium in dialysis patients: Interactions with insulin and albuterol. Am J Kidney Dis 28:508, 1996.
46. Weiner ID, Wingo CS: Hyperkalemia: A potential silent killer. J Am Soc Nephrol 9:1535, 1998.

47. Lithemoe KD, Romolo JL, Hamilton SR, et al: Intestinal necrosis due to sodium polystyrene (Kayexalate) in sorbitol enemas: Clinical and experimental support for the hypothesis. Surgery 101:267, 1987.
48. Bourgoignie JJ, Kaplan M, Pincus J, et al: Renal handling of potassium in dogs with chronic renal insufficiency. Kidney Int 20:482, 1981.
49. Wingo CS, Weiner ID: Disorders of potassium balance. In Brenner BM (ed): The Kidney, 6th ed. Philadelphia, WB Saunders, 2000, pp 998–1035.
50. Velazquez H, Perazella MA, Wright FS, et al: Renal mechanism of trimethoprim-induced hyperkalemia. Ann Intern Med 119: 296, 1993.
51. Tumlin JA, Sands JM: Nephron segment-specific inhibition of $Na^+/K^+$-ATPase activity by cyclosporin A. Kidney Int 43:246, 1993.
52. Ling BN, Eaton DC: Cyclosporin A inhibits apical secretory $K^+$ channels in rabbit cortical collecting tubule principal cells. Kidney Int 44:974, 1993.
53. Pitt B, Zannad F, Remme WJ, et al: The effect of spironolactone on morbidity and mortality in patients with severe heart failure. N Engl J Med 341:709, 1999.
54. Oster JR, Singer I, Fishman LM: Heparin-induced aldosterone suppression and hyperkalemia. Am J Med 98:575, 1995.
55. Adrogue HJ, Lederer ED, Suki WN, et al: Determinants of plasma potassium levels in diabetic ketoacidosis. Ann Intern Med 106:615, 1987.
56. Battle DC, Arruda JA, Kurtzman NA: Hyperkalemic distal renal tubular acidosis associated with obstructive uropathy. N Engl J Med 304:373, 1980.
57. Weiner ID, Wingo CS: Hypokalemia: Consequences, causes, and correction. J Am Soc Nephrol 8:1179, 1997.
58. Pullen H, Doig A, Lambie AT: Intensive intravenous potassium replacement therapy. Lancet 2:809, 1967.
59. Whang R, Whong DD, Ryan MP: Refractory potassium repletion: A consequence of magnesium deficiency. Arch Intern Med 152: 40, 1992.
60. Cheng J-T, Witty RT, Robinson RR, et al: Amphotericin B nephrotoxicity: Increased renal resistance and tubular permeability. Kidney Int 22:626, 1982.
61. Douglas JB, Healy JK: Nephrotoxic effects of amphotericin B, including renal tubular acidosis. Am J Med 46:154, 1979.
62. Kassirer JP, Schwartz WB: The response of normal man to selective depletion of hydrochloric acid: Factors in the genesis of persistent gastric alkaloses. Am J Med 40:10, 1966.
63. Carlisle EJ, Donnelly SM, Ethier JH, et al: Modulation of the secretion of potassium by accompanying anions in humans. Kidney Int 39:1206, 1991.
64. Desai TK, Carlson RW, Gehab MA: Prevalence and clinical implications of hypocalcemia in acutely ill patients in a medical intensive care setting. Am J Med 84:209, 1988.
65. Monk RD, Bushinsky DA: Treatment of calcium, phosphorous and magnesium disorders. In Brady RH, Wilcox CS (eds): Therapy in Nephrology and Hypertension: A Companion to Brenner and Rector's The Kidney. Philadelphia, WB Saunders, 1999, pp 303–315.
66. Lind L, Carlstedt F, Rastad J, et al: Hypocalcemia and parathyroid hormone secretion in critically ill patients. Crit Care Med 28:93, 2000.
67. Zaloga GP, Washburn D, Black KW, et al: Human sepsis increases lymphocyte intracellular calcium. Crit Care Med 21:196, 1993.
68. Ranson JH-C: Risk factors in acute pancreatitis. Hosp Pract 20: 69, 1985.
69. Agarwal N, Pitchumoni CS: Acute pancreatitis: A multisystem disease. Gastroenterologist 1:115, 1993.
70. Pitchumoni CS, Agarwal N, Jain NK: Systemic complications of acute pancreatitis. Am J Gastroenterol 83:597, 1988.
71. Alkmal M, Goldstein DA, Tefler N, et al: Resolution of muscle calcification in rhabdomyolysis and acute renal failure. Ann Intern Med 89:928, 1978.
72. Llach F, Felsenfeld AJ, Haussler MR: The pathophysiology of altered calcium metabolism in rhabdomyolysis-induced acute renal failure. N Engl J Med 305:117, 1981.
73. Meneghini LF, Oster JR, Camacho JR, et al: Hypercalcemia in association with acute renal failure and rhabdomyolysis. Miner Electrolyte Metab 19:1, 1993.
74. Korzets A, Dicker D, Chaimoff C, et al: Life-threatening hyperphosphatemia and hypocalcemic tetany following the use of Fleet enemas. J Am Geriatr Soc 40:620, 1992.
75. Agus ZS: Hypomagnesemia. J Am Soc Nephrol 10:1616, 1999.
76. Meier-Kriesche H-U, Finkel KW, Gitomer JJ, et al: Unexpected severe hypocalcemia during continuous venovenous hemodialysis with regional citrate anticoagulation. Am J Kidney Dis 33: E8, 1999.
77. Hosking DJ, Gilson D: Comparison of the renal and skeletal actions of calcitonin in the treatment of severe hypercalcemia of malignancy. Q J Med NS 53:359, 1984.
78. Adami S, Rossini M: Hypercalcemia of malignancy: Pathophysiology and treatment. Bone 13:551, 1992.
79. Mosekilde L, Eriksen EF, Charles P: Hypercalcemia of malignancy: Pathophysiology, diagnosis and treatment. Crit Rev Oncol/Hematol 11:1, 1991.
80. Stewert AF, Adler M, Beyers CM, et al: Calcium homeostasis in immobilization: An example of resorptive hypercalciuria. N Engl J Med 306:1136, 1982.
81. Tamion F, Bonmarchand F, Girault C, et al: Intravenous pamidronate sodium therapy in immobilization-related hypercalcemia [letter]. Clin Nephrol 43:138, 1995.
82. Solomon SM, Kirby DF: The refeeding syndrome: A review. JPEN 14:90, 1990.
83. Agarwal R, Knochel J: Hypophosphatemia and hyperphosphatemia. In Brenner BM (ed): The Kidney, 6th ed. Philadelphia, WB Saunders, 2000, pp 1071–1125.

# Section IV
# *Potassium*

## CHAPTER 21

# Regulation of Renal Potassium Transport

Ruth A. Schwalbe, PhD ▪ I. David Weiner, MD ▪ Charles S. Wingo, MD

## PRINCIPLES OF POTASSIUM TRANSPORT AND REGULATION

Potassium is the major intracellular cation and is vital for normal cellular function. Most cells exhibit substantial K conductance that maintains membrane potential and regulates electrical excitability and transepithelial transport. K uptake is an energetically unfavorable process and requires active transport primarily by $Na^+,K^+$ ATPase or in certain cells cotransport with Na and Cl ions via the $Na^+$-$2Cl^-$-$K^+$ cotransporter.[1] The vast majority of K is contained within the intracellular fluid, and only a small component (~2%) is in the extracellular fluid.[2] The concentration of K in the extracellular fluid is tightly regulated by factors that determine the distribution of K between the intra- and extracellular compartments, referred to as extrarenal or internal potassium balance, and by the excretion of potassium, primarily by the kidney.

Extrarenal or cellular K homeostasis is important in preventing acute shifts of K, and hormones that affect this process by stimulating cellular K uptake include insulin, β-catecholamines, and aldosterone. Long-term K homeostasis is regulated by the kidney, which accounts for 90% of the excretion of K intake.[1] The colon has a more limited capacity to secrete K but may adapt during chronic renal failure to a limited degree.

### Internal (Cellular) K Balance

Although the kidney is the major organ that regulates the elimination of potassium from the body, acute administration of potassium, particularly if given intravenously and at high rates, can overwhelm the capacity of the kidney to maintain extracellular potassium concentrations within safe limits. Under such circumstances, extrarenal mechanisms primarily in skeletal and vascular smooth muscle, and to a lesser extent liver, red blood cells, and bone, defend the individual against potentially lethal increases in serum potassium concentration.

Figure 21–1 illustrates the importance of this extrarenal, or cellular (internal), mechanism of potassium homeostasis. The infusion of 0.75 mEq/kg KCl to healthy, young subjects resulted in a 0.9 mEq/L rise in plasma potassium concentration.[3] During the ensuing 6 hours, approximately 40% of this potassium load was excreted in the urine, and there were negligible other apparent losses of potassium. Thus, approximately 30 mEq of K were retained by the individual, which

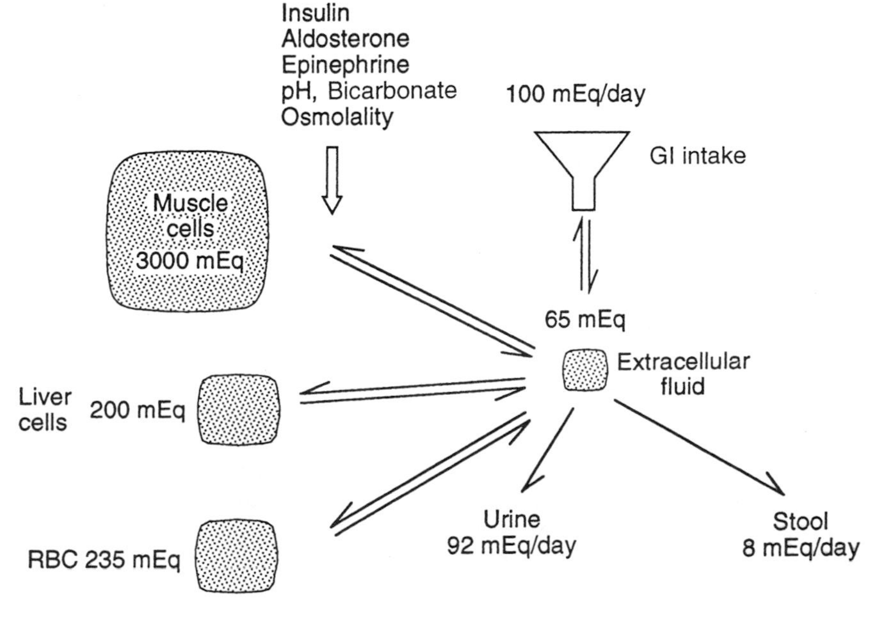


**FIGURE 21–1** ▪ Cellular (internal) potassium homeostasis and the distribution of K between intra- and extracellular fluid. (Adapted from Black DAK: Potassium metabolism. In Maxwell MH, Kleeman CR: Clinical Disorders of Fluid and Electrolyte Metabolism. New York, McGraw-Hill, 1962, p 121.)

amounted to approximately 60% of the original K load that was administered. If all this potassium remained in the extracellular space, plasma potassium concentration would have risen by more than 3 mEq/L, to levels that would be potentially life threatening. However, the actual increment in plasma potassium was less than 1 mEq/L (see Fig. 21–1). This stabilization of serum plasma potassium concentration reflects the intrinsic properties of most cells to actively translocate potassium from the extracellular fluid to the intracellular compartment. Similar K loads can occur with large meals or with heavy exercise. The primary enzyme responsible for this action is the ubiquitous Na,K pump or $Na^+$,$K^+$ ATPase. As noted later, the regulation of internal potassium homeostasis is largely dictated by the activity of this ion motive ATPase, which is regulated by three hormonal systems (discussed later).

### POTASSIUM TOLERANCE

For more than half a century, chronic administration of a large potassium load results in the adaptation of the individual so that infusions of potassium that would otherwise be lethal can be tolerated with impunity.[4, 5] This adaptation has been referred to as potassium tolerance and is caused both by renal adaptation as well as by extrarenal adaptation.[6, 7] However, the extrarenal adaptation appears to be more important acutely in stabilization of plasma potassium concentration, whereas the renal mechanisms serve to enhance the rapid elimination of potassium once a potassium surfeit has been achieved.[7, 8]

In addition to the extrarenal defense against hyperkalemia and hypokalemia, the kidney, and to a lesser extent the colon, respond to preserve potassium homeostasis.[9] Thus, internal or cellular defense mechanisms operate in concert with external (primarily renal) mechanisms for preserving the stability of plasma potassium concentration. When animals are chronically adapted to a high potassium diet, both internal and external mechanisms of potassium homeostasis are stimulated. This results in a more rapid uptake of potassium by tissues, reflecting internal homeostasis, and a more rapid elimination of potassium load, reflecting external potassium homeostasis. The mechanisms that regulate internal potassium homeostasis are not identical to those of external potassium homeostasis, although at least one hormone, aldosterone, clearly affects both systems.

## External K Balance

External K balance is normally regulated primarily by the kidney, which is responsible for approximately 90% of K elimination.[9–11] The majority of the remainder of K is excreted in the stool by active colonic secretion of potassium.[12, 13] In most cases, the amount of K elimination by perspiration is insignificant, but in extremely hot climates, K loss in sweat can be important.

### RENAL K EXCRETION

Under normal circumstances, when renal function is well preserved and with a normal K intake, the amount of K excreted reflects only a fraction (~20%) of the filtered load of K. From such observations, it was proposed that K excretion was regulated by selective reabsorption of filtered K. Some early studies, however, suggested that K could be actually secreted under certain circumstances. Studies by Berliner and coworkers[14] established that the majority of K that is excreted enters the urine by a process of active tubular K secretion and that this process was dependent on the delivery or reabsorption of Na within "distal tubular segments."[10] These clearance studies were largely confirmed and extended by more specific techniques (see later). In addition, alterations in systemic acid-base balance have marked effects on the rates of K elimination, with alkalinization frequently associated with enhanced kaliuresis. Acidosis, however, at least acutely, decreased K excretion.

Studies by Giebisch and coworkers extended these observations and identified the distal convolution, now known to be a heterogenous structure (see later), as a major site of distal tubule K secretion.[11, 15] Further studies also demonstrated that the majority of the effects of changes in acid-base balance occurred within or distal to the early distal convoluted tubule.[16] Additional micropuncture studies by Jamison and colleagues demonstrated that K underwent recycling in the renal medulla.[17–19] For example, in studies from K-loaded animals, it was noted that the fractional delivery of K to the thin descending limb of juxtamedullary nephrons frequently exceeded the filtered load of K, which clearly indicates net K secretion between the glomerulus and the site of sampling. Because K-sparing diuretics (e.g., amiloride) decreased K delivery into the thin descending limb, the authors inferred that the source of K that entered the thin descending limb originated in K that was secreted from the distal nephron and cortical collecting duct (CCD).[17] Thus, a fraction of K is reabsorbed in the medullary collecting duct into the medullary interstitium and thence into the thin descending limb. Additional microperfusion studies of isolated collecting ducts further supported this pathway of K transport, because decreasing K intake enhanced the K absorptive flux and suggested that this medullary K reabsorption was a regulated process.[20] The mechanism for both active tubular secretion and active tubular reabsorption in the collecting duct is discussed later.

Additional work by Giebisch and colleagues demonstrated that despite large changes in dietary K content, most (~90%) of the filtered load of K is reabsorbed prior to the early distal convoluted tubule.[11, 21, 22] In contrast to the lack of changes observed in more proximal segments, dietary K loading and dietary K restriction greatly altered transport within the distal convolution and more distal sites. With K loading, fractional delivery of K increased progressively along the distal convolution, indicating net K secretion. During K depletion, however, little change in the fractional delivery of K occurred, and there was a striking reduction in fractional delivery between the late distal convoluted tubule and the final urine, suggesting reabsorption along the collecting duct. Although heterogenous handling of K by superficial and juxtamedullary nephrons could also explain these findings, direct evidence for active K reabsorption in the medullary collecting duct supports the former interpretation.[23]

#### COLONIC K EXCRETION

The colon also participates in K elimination and, similar to the collecting duct, has the capacity to actively secrete as well as actively reabsorb potassium. Active K secretion exhibits many of the characteristics observed in the collecting duct; however, significant rates of K secretion remain in the absence of mucosal Na, presumably because of an active $Na^+$-$2Cl^-$-$K^+$ cotransporter at the basolateral membrane that allows Na recycling across the basolateral membrane and active K secretion.[12] The mechanism of K absorption is similar to that characterized in the collecting duct and appears to be caused by an active $H^+$-K-ATPase.[24] Studies in knockout animals have demonstrated significant impairment in K absorptive flux during K deprivation in the colon due to $HK\alpha_2$ gene products.[25]

#### OTHER K EXCRETION

Normally, K elimination from sources other than the kidney or colon are negligible; however, Knochel has demonstrated that, with strenuous exertion and under extremely hot conditions, loss in sweat can amount to approximately 200 mEq.[26] In the presence of enteric fistulas or other gastrointestinal diseases, external losses of K can also be substantial.

# SEGMENTAL ANALYSIS OF POTASSIUM TRANSPORT ALONG THE NEPHRON AND COLLECTING DUCT

## Overview of Renal Potassium Handling

#### RENAL HANDLING OF POTASSIUM

Potassium is freely filtered at the glomerulus. Under normal circumstances, approximately 15% to 30% of the filtered load of K is excreted, depending on dietary intake and the individual's degree of renal function.[27] Initially, K excretion was thought to be regulated by the rate of reabsorption of filtered K. Extensive studies have now confirmed, however, that urinary K excretion is largely due to secretion of K in the collecting duct, which is highly regulated.[27] This segment also possesses the capacity for active K absorption.[28]

Thus, K is regulated in a complex fashion. K filtered at the glomerulus is largely reabsorbed (~90%) in the proximal tubule and loop of Henle, regardless of dietary K intake. K is actively secreted in the initial CCD (iCCD) and CCD under normal conditions.[29, 30] Under normal conditions, the majority of this distally secreted potassium is excreted, although a component is reabsorbed to enter the medullary interstitium and to be secreted in the descending loop of Henle.[17] This reabsorption of distally secreted K helps to explain why K recycling occurs. Under conditions of K deprivation, however, active K absorption occurs both in the cortical and medullary collecting ducts. The mechanisms that are responsible for these transport events are discussed later.

## Glomerular Filtration

K is freely filtered at the glomerulus with minimal alterations owing to the Donnan equilibrium. Sampling in micropuncture studies reveals that the ultrafiltrate K concentration is approximately equal to the plasma K concentration.

## Proximal Tubule

**Proximal Tubule K Transport.** Potassium filtered at the glomerulus is reabsorbed largely in proportion to fluid and volume reabsorption along the proximal tubule; thus, approximately 60% of filtered K load is reabsorbed along the proximal tubule iso-osmotically in proportion to fluid reabsorption.[11, 15, 22] Micropuncture studies demonstrate that the tubular fluid to plasma K concentration [$(TF/P)_K$] changes little along the length of the proximal tubule, which indicates that K absorption is proportionate to fluid reabsorption.[15] The mechanism of K absorption in the early portion of the proximal tubule is illustrated in Figure 21–2. Three factors favor an increase in $(TF/P)_K$. First, in the early proximal tubule, transepithelial voltage ($V_T$) is lumen-negative and favors passive paracellular K secretion. Second, the apical membrane of the proximal

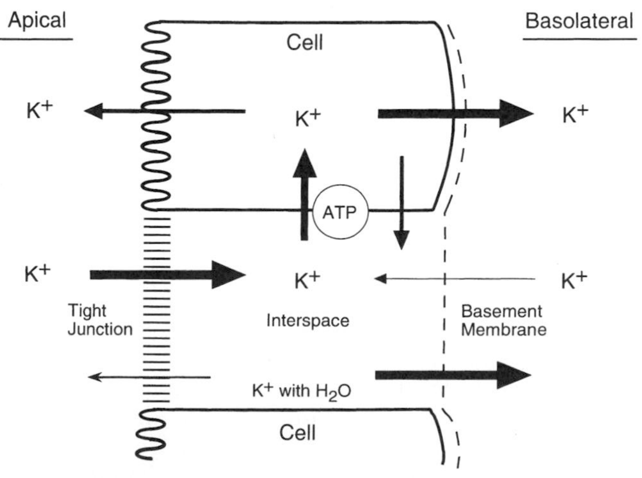


**FIGURE 21–2** ■ Mechanism of K transport by the proximal tubule. (From Giebisch G, Malnic G, Berliner RW: Control of renal potassium excretion. In Brenner BM [ed]: The Kidney. Philadelphia, WB Saunders, 2000, p 428.)

tubule contains a low density of apical K channels that allows transcellular K secretion. Third, the continued reabsorption of fluid leads to an increase of luminal fluid K concentration in the absence of K transport.

Measurements of intracellular potassium ion activity in the proximal tubule indicate that potassium remains above the electrochemically equilibrium compared with the potassium in the extracellular fluid. Thus, potassium absorption must occur either by active apical absorption or by passive paracellular potassium absorption. An analysis of the known transport mechanisms in the proximal tubule by Weinstein[31, 32] suggests that movement of potassium across the epithelium against an electrochemical gradient can occur by means of active potassium uptake via laterally located $Na^+,K^+$ ATPase. A salient feature of this model is active potassium absorption into the lateral intercellular space, which allows paracellular potassium absorption by entrainment (solvent drag) and passive diffusion. This model requires that diffusion of potassium from the plasma to the intercellular space be actively absorbed across the lateral plasma membrane and exit by passive diffusion through K channels at the basal plasma membrane. According to this model, potassium movement is both paracellular and transcellular. In support of passive paracellular potassium movement in the proximal tubule, Barfuss and Schafer observed more rapid egress of the potassium marker rubidium from the luminal space than from proximal tubule cells.[33] Osmotic diuretics that retard fluid reabsorption in the proximal tubule also significantly decrease proximal tubule potassium reabsorption. These observations are consistent with the notion that a significant amount of potassium movement is by entrainment.

## Loop of Henle

Micropuncture studies reveal that approximately 20% to 30% of the filtered load of potassium is reabsorbed within the loop of Henle. Fluid that exits the proximal tubule undergoes water abstraction in the descending loop of Henle; if this volume flux is not accompanied by commensurate potassium removal, a significant increase in luminal potassium concentration results that could favor passive potassium exit. Studies by Johnson and associates provide evidence for a concentration gradient favoring movement of sodium from the thin loop of Henle.[34] However, the thin descending limb of Henle, where the majority of water abstraction occurs, exhibits a relatively low potassium permeability, which would suggest that the high $(TF/P)_K$ resulted mainly from water abstraction. If the rise in the $(TF/P)_K$ is based solely on water abstraction, then maneuvers that affect distal potassium secretion should have little effect to alter the rise in $(TF/P)_K$, unless they have commensurate effects on interstitial solute concentration that could secondarily affect the rate of water abstraction. However, benzolamide, a carbonic anhydrase inhibitor that inhibits reabsorption of sodium and bicarbonate in the proximal tubule, also affects potassium excretion and results in a highly significant increase in the filtered load of potassium to the thin descending limb of juxtamedullary nephrons.[35] Similarly, administration of the high potassium diet results in a striking increase in the fraction of filtered potassium at the end of juxtamedullary descending limb. This increase appears to be principally a result of enhanced potassium secretion, because the administration of amiloride results in a sharp reduction in the delivery of potassium to the end thin descending limb.[36, 37] These observations indicate that potassium undergoes recycling in the kidney with a portion of potassium secreted in the collecting duct being reabsorbed into the medullary interstitium in the medullary collecting duct and then secreted into thin descending limbs of the juxtamedullary nephrons.

The mechanism for potassium entry into the luminal fluid of the thin descending limb has not been studied extensively. However, a ouabain-sensitive active potassium secretory mechanism has been reported in the rabbit proximal tubule.[38] Although the rates of potassium secretion were modest, the magnitude of potassium secretion could be greatly increased by a modest (5 mmol) bath-to-lumen potassium gradient. In the absence of a potassium gradient, the basolateral addition of ouabain largely inhibited the secretion of potassium. Luminal 1 mM amiloride also inhibited secretion. These observations indicate that a component of potassium secretion in the pars recta is active, transcellular, and dependent on basolateral $Na^+,K^+$ ATPase. Whether a component of potassium secretion occurs passively and paracellularly remains to be defined.

**Thick Ascending Limb.** The transport mechanisms of the thick ascending limb have been studied extensively. The basic transport mechanisms are similar in both the cortical and medullary thick ascending limb (mTALH), although in some species antidiuretic hormone stimulates solute transport in the mTALH, and $CO_2/HCO_3^-$ stimulates solute absorption in the cortical thick ascending limb. The basic function of this segment is to effect sodium chloride absorption in the absence of appreciable water flux serving to dilute the luminal fluid. When studied in vitro in the absence of ion gradients, only small rates of either potassium absorption or secretion have been observed.[39] However, modest ion gradients result in appreciable potassium flux, but, as noted by Stokes,[39] the medullary thick ascending limb of Henle (mTALH) exhibits significant rectification indicating that a significant component of this flux is transcellular.

The mechanism of potassium transport in the TALH is shown in Figure 21–3. K absorption is mediated by a secondary active transport via the $Na^+$-$2Cl^-$-$K^+$ cotransporter. This electroneutral transport of K is driven by sodium and chloride concentration gradients from the lumen to the cell. The majority of potassium that is absorbed at the apical membrane recycles by an apical K channel. The apical membrane is largely K selective with a transference number for potassium of 0.9 to 1.0.[40] Chloride that is reabsorbed via the apical $Na^+$-$2Cl^-$-$K^+$ cotransporter exits the basolateral membrane both conductively through a chlo-

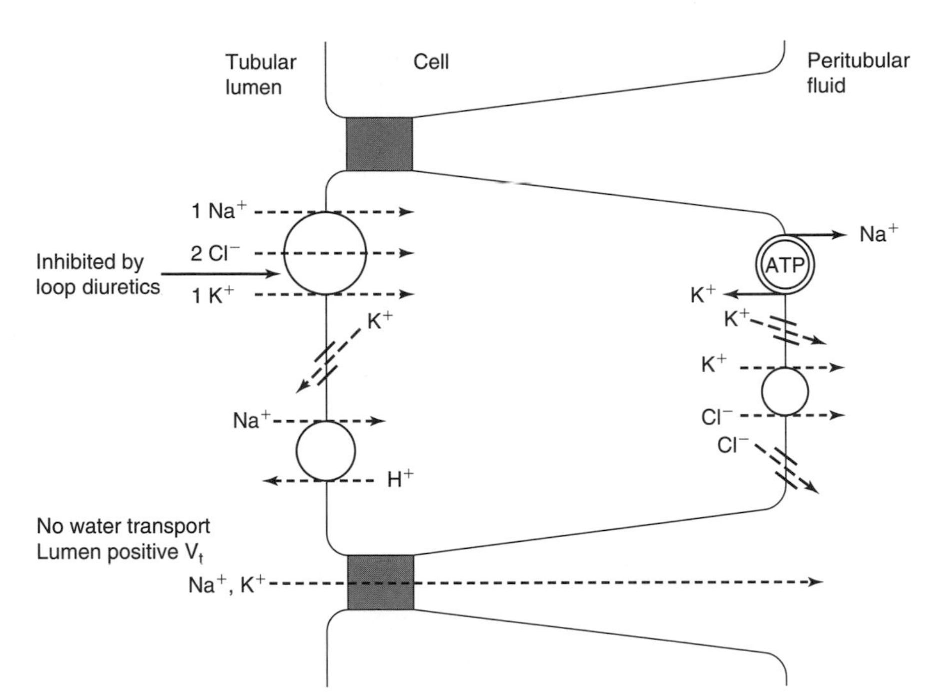


**FIGURE 21–3** ■ Mechanism of K transport by the thick ascending limb of Henle. (Adapted from Valtin H, Schafer JA: Renal Function. Boston, Little Brown, 1995, p 244.)

ride channel and electroneutrally through a KCl cotransporter. Sodium is reabsorbed both transcellularly and paracellularly, driven by the lumen-positive voltage and the cation selectivity of the paracellular pathway. In particular, the coupling between K transport and sodium chloride absorption is illustrated by the work of Hebert and colleagues,[41] which demonstrates that in the mTALH vasopressin enhances sodium chloride absorption in the absence of water flux by increasing the apical K conductance and the activity of the $Na^+$-$2Cl^-$-$K^+$ cotransporter, which appear to be functionally coupled. In additional studies, these workers have identified that the mode of operation of transport is also altered by vasopressin from a potassium-independent NaCl absorptive mechanism to a potassium-dependent NaCl absorptive mechanism that serves to transport sodium chloride more efficiently by increasing the efficiency of paracellular voltage-mediated sodium absorption as potassium is recycled at the apical membrane.

Two K channels have been identified at the apical membrane of the thick ascending limb with intermediate and low conductances.[42] Both exhibit high open probability and are sensitive to external Ba, cytosolic adenosine triphosphate (ATP) (mM), and acidic pH. One represents an intermediate conductance K channel, approximately 72 pS, which is inhibited by millimoles of cytosolic ATP, cytosolic acidification, $Ba^{2+}$, and quinidine. The second is a low-conductance K channel with a unitary conductance of ~30 pS. It has an open probability of 0.8 in cell-attached patches, does not display voltage dependence, but is inhibited by 2 mmol ATP in inside-out patches. This channel is also inhibited by 250 μm glyburide. In contrast, the 72-pS K channel is not inhibited by this concentration of glyburide. The small conductance K channel is stimulated by maneuvers that increase protein kinase A activity, such as the addition of cAMP congeners or 50 to 100 pM vasopressin to cell-attached patches. These apical K channels are activated by vasopressin and by the protein kinase A catalytic subunit when examined in inside-out patches. The apical K channels are also pH sensitive, stimulated by cytoplasmic alkalinization, and inhibited by acidification. The effects of pH on apical K channel activity, as well as $Na^+$-$2Cl^-$-$K^+$ cotransport activity, may partly explain why acidosis inhibits transport in the TALH.[43]

**KCl Exit**. Studies by Greger and Schlatter[44] provided evidence that in the rabbit, cTALH K exit exhibited properties that were most consistent with electroneutral KCl cotransport as the mechanism of K and Cl extrusion basolaterally. They observed that an increase in peritubular K concentration depolarizes the basolateral membrane. This effect could be abolished by 3 mM Ba in the peritubular fluid, but the rate of depolarization was slower than expected for a channel. Ba alone produced the same depolarization as that produced by Ba plus a K concentration step change. Moreover, the effect of Ba was not accompanied by a change in transepithelial resistance or the fractional resistance of the basolateral membrane. These facts indicate that Ba was not effecting a basolateral conductance. The authors concluded that K exit at the basolateral membrane was electroneutral and that Cl leaves the cell both electroneutrally and by Cl conductance. Other evidence by Oberleithner and associates indicates that nonconductive Cl exit occurs across the basolateral membrane.[45]

## Distal Convolution

**Distal Convoluted Tubule.** The distal convoluted tubule (DCT) is a morphologically and physiologically distinct subsegment of the distal convolution that consists of the DCT, connecting segment, and the iCCD.

Only limited information is available for this segment in the rabbit, because of the difficulty of dissection and the short length of this segment. However, the DCT of the rabbit possesses discrete borders between the cTALH and the connecting segment, which allows for precise identification. This segment possesses a lumen-negative voltage and secretes potassium.[46] The studies in the rat by in vivo microperfusion of the early distal convolution by Stanton and associates[30, 47] and by Wright and coworkers[48–51] demonstrate that this segment possesses substantially smaller rates of potassium secretion than does the late distal convolution, which includes the connecting segment and iCCD. The DCT does not respond to changes in mineralocorticoid status and, based on adenylate cyclase activity or fluid transport, does not respond to vasopressin.[52]

### MOLECULAR MECHANISMS OF K TRANSPORT

Molecular genetic studies have identified genes responsible for mendelian, or single gene, forms of inherited hypokalemic tubulopathies, which previously were grouped under the term Bartter syndrome. These syndromes are differentiated into at least three subtypes: (1) the Gitelman variant of Bartter syndrome (GS); (2) the antenatal variant of Bartter syndrome (HPS/aBS); and (3) the classic Bartter syndrome (cBS). Common characteristics of these syndromes are hypokalemic metabolic alkalosis and salt wasting. Bartter and colleagues proposed that Cl reabsorption was defective in the thick ascending limb of the loop of Henle.[53] In addition, microperfusion and molecular biology studies helped to identify candidate genes that may be responsible for these syndromes. Interestingly, the symptoms of GS are similar to chronic administration of thiazides, which was known to inhibit the NaCl cotransporter in the apical membrane of the distal convoluted tubule.[54] Molecular genetic studies confirmed that mutations in the NaCl cotransporter gene (*SLC12A3*) cause GS.[55–57] Mutations have also been identified, in individuals affected by antenatal Bartter syndrome, in two candidate genes—$Na^+$-$2Cl^-$-$K^+$ cotransporter (*SLC12A1*)[58–60] and renal outer medullary K channel (ROMK) (*KCNJ1*),[61–63] whose roles were proposed to be involved in salt reabsorption in the TALH. Identification of these mutations provides strong molecular evidence for the role of the $Na^+$-$2Cl^-$-$K^+$ cotransporter as a mediator and ROMK as a modulator of renal salt reabsorption. In addition, mutations of the basolateral chloride channel (*CLCNKB*) have been identified as a cause of classic Bartter syndrome, supporting the role of this channel in Cl reabsorption in the thick ascending limb.[64, 65]

**Connecting Segment and Initial Cortical Collecting Duct.** The connecting segment is an anatomically discrete segment in the rabbit nephron. In the rat, this represents a transition region between the DCT and the iCCD. In the rabbit, the $V_T$ of this segment is affected by amiloride, but neither sodium nor chloride transport is affected by furosemide. However, thiazide diuretics inhibit sodium and chloride transport in this segment in the rabbit.[66]

The iCCD represents the major site within the distal convolution for potassium secretion.[30, 47] The transport characteristics of this segment have been most fully characterized by in vivo microperfusion. Transepithelial voltage is significantly more lumen negative when compared with more proximal portions of the distal convolution, and rates of potassium secretion are commensurately greater. Both the flow and delivery of sodium appear to stimulate potassium secretion. However, the luminal flow rate appears to be quantitatively of greater importance.[50, 67–69] The flow dependence of the distal convolution and the iCCD indicates a substantial apical K permeability.[70] Dietary K content clearly affects potassium secretion in this segment, with large rates of potassium secretion in K-loaded animals. However, during potassium depletion, secretion of potassium is virtually abolished and there is a tendency toward absorption of potassium.[71]

## Collecting Duct

**Collecting Duct K Transport.** The collecting duct is comprised of three discrete regions: the CCD, the outer medullary collecting duct (OMCD), and the inner medullary collecting duct (IMCD). The OMCD can be further subdivided into the OMCD from the outer stripe and the OMCD from the inner stripe. The IMCD consists of three regions: the $IMCD_1$, $IMCD_2$, and $IMCD_3$. Each of these segments exhibits distinct transport characteristics, as discussed later.

**Potassium Secretion in the CCD.** The CD consists of two cell types: principal cells and intercalated cells. In the CCD and the $OMCD_o$, two types of intercalated cells, type A and type B, can be distinguished based on ultrastructural criteria.[72] Type A intercalated cells have an extensive apical tubulovesicular membrane compartment and prominent surface microprojections, whereas type B intercalated cells are characterized by a well-developed vesicular compartment and short sparse surface microprojections. The principal cells are involved in K secretion, whereas intercalated cells appear to be responsible for K absorption during K deprivation. The mechanisms of K transport in the CCD are illustrated in Figure 21–4. K secretion depends on the basolateral $Na^+$,$K^+$ ATPase and requires Na absorption at the apical membrane via an amiloride-sensitive Na channel for turnover of the $Na^+$,$K^+$ ATPase and basolateral K uptake. K exits apically both conductively and via secretion with Cl. The apical membrane of the CCD possesses several K channels that could be in part responsible for K secretion. Initially, a large conductance (Ca activated) K channel was identified at the apical membrane of the CCD and was proposed as a candidate K channel for K secretion.[73, 74] However, the pharmacologic profile of this channel and its single channel characteristics, which include a small open probability, suggest that it does not participate in K secretion under resting conditions. More recently, a small conductance K channel with a high open probability and external Ba sensitivity has been identified at the CCD apical mem-

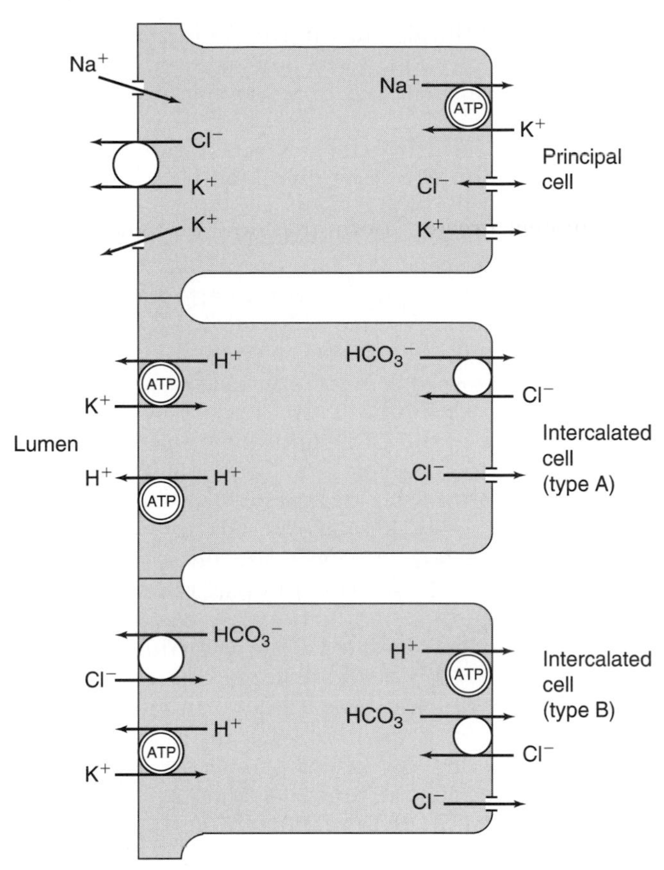


**FIGURE 21–4** ■ Mechanism of K transport in the different cell types of the cortical collecting duct. (From Wingo CS, Weiner ID: Ion transport by the renal tubule. In Jamison RL, Wilkinson R [eds]: Nephrology. London, Chapman & Hall, 1997, p 50.)

brane.[75–79] It is largely voltage insensitive and is not activated by changes in cytosolic Ca; it appears to be a plausible candidate for a K channel responsible for K secretion.

**KCl Secretion.** The nature of Cl transport with K is more complex. Cl transport occurs in part passively via the paracellular pathway and is driven via electrogenic Na absorption and the resultant lumen-negative voltage. However, under appropriate circumstances, the CCD can actively secrete Cl.[80] The precise mechanism for this KCl secretion is not fully established but represents either KCl cotransport or parallel conductive channels.[81, 82] As noted previously, evidence in the rat iCCD supports the assertion that K secretion occurs by an apical cotransporter.[48–51] During K loading, a component of K secretion occurs coupled to Cl,[83] and the coupled secretion of K with Cl helps to explain why conditions associated with a low luminal Cl concentration promote K wasting.[48, 50, 51]

**Potassium Absorption in the CCD.** As illustrated in Figure 21–5, the intercalated cells of the CCD possess a mechanism of K absorption coupled to proton secretion and mediated via an $H^+,K^+$ ATPase.[84] Luminal K is absorbed against its electrochemical gradient via this primary active P-type proton pump in exchange for cytosolic protons. During K restriction K exits basolaterally via a Ba-sensitive pathway, whereas during K repletion K is recycled across the apical membrane. In both situations, acute increases in $P_{CO_2}$ stimulate $H^+,K^+$ ATPase activity.[85–87]

**Potassium Transport in the $OMCD_i$.** The $OMCD_i$ possesses limited capacity to secrete K during K loading but is a major site of K reclamation during K deprivation.[88] Studies in the rat demonstrate intense hypertrophy of the cells of the $OMCD_i$ in response to K depletion.[89, 90] The mechanism of K absorption in the $OMCD_i$ is similar to that present in the type A intercalated cell of the CCD (see Fig. 21–5). At present, little is known about the regulation of this transport process.

**Potassium Transport in the IMCD.** When animals are fed a normal K diet, little net K transport occurs in the IMCD,[91] but with severe K loading this segment can contribute substantially to K excretion.[92] On the other hand, during severe K depletion the rat IMCD reabsorbs most (~90%) of the K delivered to this segment.[91] Thus, the IMCD, similar to the CCD, possesses the capacity for bidirectional K transport. Although under normal dietary intake it contributes little to changes in K excretory rates, this segment may be viewed as an additional site that adapts to more extreme changes in dietary K content. As with the more proximal CD segments, K absorption probably involves the action of an apical $H^+,K^+$ ATPase and a basolateral K channel, because this segment possesses $H^+,K^+$ ATPase activity[84] and has been shown to exhibit a K conductance at the basolateral membrane.[93] The mechanism of K secretion is not well characterized but may reflect the activity of a nonselective cation channel that has been identified at the apical membrane of the IMCD.[94]

# REGULATION OF POTASSIUM EXCRETION

## Potassium Recycling

A fraction of potassium that is secreted in the distal nephron is reabsorbed in the OMCD into the medul-

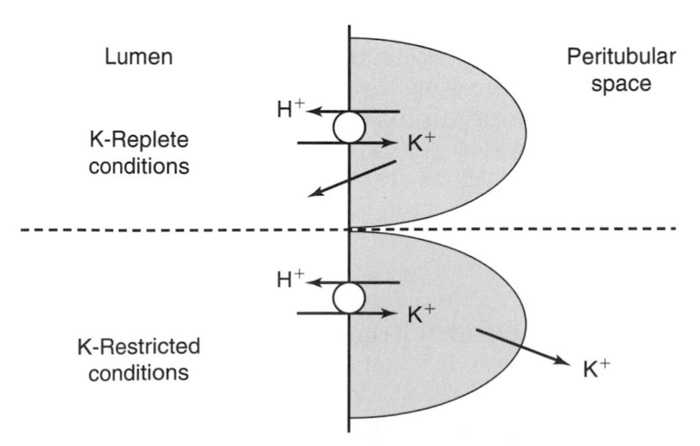


**FIGURE 21–5** ■ Mechanism of intercalated cell K transport under K-replete and K-restricted conditions. (From Zhou X, Lynch IJ, Xia SL, Wingo CS: Activation of $H^+,K^+$ ATPase by $CO_2$ requires a basolateral $Ba^{+2}$-sensitive pathway during K restriction. Am J Physiol 279:F158, 2000.)

lary interstitium. This results in an increase in interstitial K concentration within the outer medulla and may favor secretory movement of K into the thin descending limb.

### Circadian Rhythm of K Excretion: Sensors and Effectors (CNS and Hepatic)

There is a characteristic daily variation in K excretion that follows a circadian pattern. In humans, K excretion typically increases during the waking hours and reaches a maximum in the early afternoon. Although this pattern lags behind a typical oscillation in plasma cortisol, which also exhibits a circadian rhythm, studies in adrenalectomized animals demonstrate that the adrenal glands are not essential to the establishment of this cyclical rate of urinary K excretion.[95] In fact, Moore-Ede has noted that the circadian variations in K excretion are some of the most stable of circadian rhythms and take more than 1 week to shift after adjustment to a new time zone.[96] Other experiments have determined that this circadian rhythm is independent of feeding, drinking, or activity in laboratory animals (squirrel monkeys). Studies in humans on constant bed rest and provided with identical meals every 3 hours throughout the day and night, demonstrated that this characteristic circadian pattern persisted.[97]

This circadian fluctuation in K excretion is associated with alterations in the ability to defend against a K load and impairment in K homeostatic mechanisms. Notably, infusion of the same 37 mEq of KCl results in a significantly higher plasma K concentration when infused at night when compared with mid-day, and urinary K excretion is attenuated when infused during the nighttime infusion, indicating an impaired homeostatic response at night compared with daytime.[98] Moore-Ede found electrocardiographic evidence of this impaired nocturnal homeostatic ability with T waves in V5 of the electrocardiogram being elevated by 18% during a midday infusion but by 52% by nighttime infusion.[98]

The rhythmic nature of this K excretion has led to the proposal that oscillators in the central nervous system (CNS), possibly the hypothalamus, determine a circadian rhythm in renal excretion of K.[99] Other studies have supported peripheral K-sensitive receptors located in the liver or the hepatic portal circulation, which initiates a reflux increase in K excretion via vagal afferents that is lost with hypophysectomy.[99]

### Cellular Mechanisms for Renal K Adaptation

On a cellular level, the factors that are known as proximate signals that regulate the stimulation of K secretion and reabsorption are only partially understood. Although aldosterone markedly increases K secretion in the distal convolution and CCD when administered chronically, this hormone has only modest effect on K excretion when administered acutely, in part because of offsetting flow-dependent effects (see next).

The mechanism by which K intake modulates urinary K excretion is in part mediated by alterations in the activity of the apical and basolateral K channels (see Fig. 21–5). During K loading, K secretion is augmented by activity of the basolateral $Na^+,K^+$ ATPase, and an increased apical permeability that, in part, reflects increased presence of functional K channels at the apical membrane. Moreover, in the K-replete state, it has been shown that respiratory acidosis (increased ambient $P_{CO_2}$) stimulates the activity of the apical $H^+,K^+$ ATPase in the CCD, and this process occurs by a barium-sensitive mechanism, presumably related to apical recycling of K via this pump.[86]

In contrast, when K intake is reduced, the basolateral $Na^+,K^+$ ATPase activity is also decreased,[100] as is apical K permeability,[101] which in part reflects a reduction in the number of functional K channels at the apical membrane. Commensurate with this reduction in K intake, there is a decrease in net secretory capacity by the CCD,[102] which in part is due to an enhancement in K absorption, presumably via intercalated cells. Studies examining the effect of changes in ambient $P_{CO_2}$ on $H^+,K^+$ ATPase function demonstrate that under K depletion, increasing ambient $P_{CO_2}$ in perfused tubules is associated with augmented net acid secretion that is insensitive to luminal but inhibited by basolateral barium.[87] Taken together, the observations suggest that K depletion reduces the apical permeability to K of both principal and intercalated cells and the development of K exit pathways in intercalated cells, which can mediate net K absorption as shown in Figure 21–5.

## KNOWN FACTORS THAT AFFECT OR REGULATE K SECRETION AND/OR EXCRETION

### Potassium Intake: Potassium Loading/Deprivation

Analysis of K excretion must take into account the fact that net K secretion is a vectorial function of secretion and reabsorption. Increased excretion occurs with either increases in secretory flux or decreases in reabsorptive flux. Conversely, reduction in luminal K excretion may be synergistically effected by reducing K secretion and enhancing K absorption.

Thus, K excretion may be increased by inhibiting K reabsorption in more proximal segments and also by increasing distal luminal Na delivery, which increases CCD K secretion. Loop diuretics can also inhibit K secretion within the distal nephron or collecting duct[51, 103] by inhibiting KCl cotransporters that contribute to K secretory flux. This observation may explain why loop diuretics have somewhat less of a tendency to be kaliuretic than thiazide diuretics, even though they are more potent natriuretic agents. Diuretics can also inhibit K secretion within the distal nephron or collecting duct.[51, 103] This observation may explain why loop diuretics have somewhat less of a tendency to be kaliuretic than thiazide diuretics, even though they are more potent natriuretic agents.

When K intake is habitually increased, the ability to excrete a K load is greatly augmented. This renal mechanism preserves K homeostasis, although extrarenal mechanisms contribute to the stability of plasma K concentration with abrupt changes in K intake or loading. Intake of high levels of K leads to a state of K tolerance. The ability to survive otherwise lethal loads of K is partly owing to enhanced renal excretion, although extrarenal mechanisms, as noted earlier, also contribute.[4–6] Studies in laboratory animals have demonstrated that the renal mechanism for enhanced kaliuresis in response to K loading is caused by enhanced distal tubular K secretion, which occurs within the distal convolution and CCD. Part of the mechanism for this enhanced excretion is enhanced K uptake from peritubular fluid, suggesting enhanced activity of the Na,K pump. This increase in $Na^+$,$K^+$ ATPase activity, induced by K loading, occurs by aldosterone-dependent and aldosterone-independent mechanisms.[101, 104, 105] Because aldosterone is also known to stimulate $Na^+$,$K^+$ ATPase activity in the CCD, these pathways act cooperatively to enhance net K secretory capacity.

In addition to enhanced $Na^+$,$K^+$ ATPase activity, K loading greatly increases the apical membrane K permeability. Thus, the adaptation to a high K diet stimulates basolateral $Na^+$,$K^+$ ATPase and peritubular K uptake as well as increases an apical K permeability. The fundamental mechanism for these adaptive responses is aldosterone independent, but this mechanism is further stimulated by aldosterone. Other hormones have also been implicated in K homeostasis, including glucagon that is released after a protein meal and shown to increase urinary K excretion.[106, 107]

## Adaptive Changes to Potassium Deprivation and Potassium Loading

Studies by Fourman demonstrated that healthy individuals had the capacity to excrete urine with K values less than plasma, suggesting an active reabsorptive process.[108]

Based on substantial literature, this adaptation to K deficiency involves inhibition of active K secretion and stimulation of active tubular K absorptive mechanisms.[28, 109] This increase in K absorption occurs at least in part by intercalated cells of the collecting duct, although other cell types may also participate in this process. Structural studies demonstrate that K depletion results in striking morphologic changes of the intercalated cells, particularly in the OMCD.[90, 110]

The decrease in K excretion that accompanies K deprivation also results in alteration in the kaliuretic response to aldosterone.[111] Similar to K loading, the fundamental response to K depletion does not require a functioning adrenal cortex because this decrease in K excretion occurs even in adrenalectomized animals. These changes may reflect alterations in $H^+$,$K^+$ ATPase activity that have been shown to be, in part, independent of plasma aldosterone.[112]

Although decreases in K secretion undoubtedly contribute to this K conservation,[113] the laboratory studies demonstrate that an active K absorptive process is also responsible for this K conservation. This occurs throughout the entire collecting duct, but the most prominent morphologic changes occur in the outer medullary collecting duct, a site of high-capacity distal nephron proton secretion that contains an abundance of intercalated cells.

## Distal Luminal Na Delivery and Distal Nephron Luminal Flow Rate

### DIURETICS/CARBONIC ANHYDRASE

Nearly all diuretics have substantial effects on renal potassium excretion, which in large part are due to their effects on distal luminal Na delivery and luminal flow rate (see later). With the exception of potassium-sparing diuretics, these agents substantially increase renal K excretion, but the magnitude of the kaliuresis is not merely proportional to their natiuretic potential. Such observations suggest that these agents have additional, direct effects on net K transport. When factored for their natiuretic potential, carbonic anhydrase inhibitors, given acutely, produce a substantial kaliuretic response. The magnitude of the kaliuresis observed with thiazide diuretics, which is substantial, may reflect the combined effects of their natiuretic action and their ability to inhibit carbonic anhydrase.

### LUMINAL Na DELIVERY AND DISTAL NEPHRON LUMINAL FLOW RATE

The delivery of Na to the distal nephron and distal nephron luminal flow rate are major determinants of renal K excretion (Fig. 21–6[29, 69]). These two factors are codependent because increasing Na delivery is almost invariably associated with a greater luminal flow rate within the distal nephron. Thus, from a clinical perspective, these two factors are considered together. Nevertheless, where they have been studied and controlled separately, as in the rat distal convolution perfused in vivo, luminal flow rate appears to be a more important determinant of K secretion in this segment.[67] In contrast, in the perfused tubule, reduction in luminal Na concentration below approximately 10 to 15 mmol results in a precipitous reduction in K secretion.[29]

Certain agents, termed K-sparing diuretics, have their major action to reduce Na conductance of the apical membrane of the collecting duct. Two of the agents, amiloride and triamterene, directly inhibit Na channels, and other agents such as trimethoprim and pentamidine, when used in high doses, also act to block this same amiloride Na channel and, therefore, inhibit K secretion. Spironolactone, which antagonizes

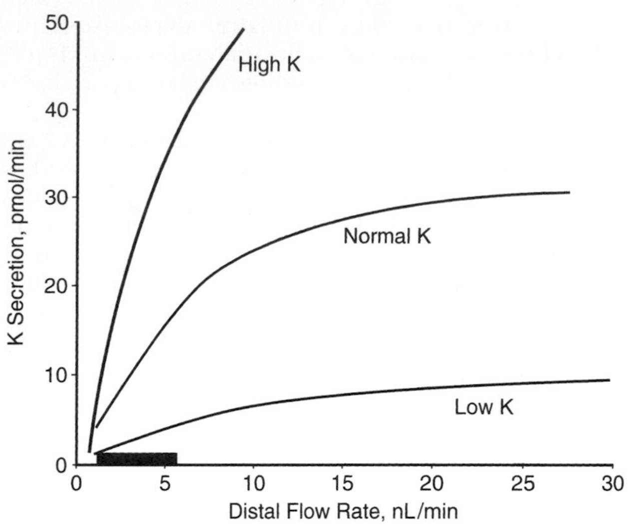


**FIGURE 21–6** ■ Effect of luminal flow rate on the rate of net K secretion in animals adapted to a low, normal, and high K diet. (From Malnic G, Berliner RW, Giebisch G: Flow dependence of $K^+$ secretion in cortical distal tubules of the rat. Am J Physiol 256: F932, 1989.)

the action of aldosterone, also reduces K secretion. Because aldosterone increases Na conductance within the collecting duct, antagonism of this action will reduce Na conductance and decrease the driving force for K secretion.

Osmotic diuretics such as mannitol, and to a lesser degree urea, inhibit volume reabsorption in the proximal tubule, which increases delivery to the loop of Henle and distal nephron. Other agents, such as the high-ceiling or loop diuretics, furosemide and bumetinide and related analogs are potent inhibitors of the $Na^+$-$2Cl^-$-$K^+$ cotransporter in the thick ascending limb. Inhibition of this transporter leads to marked increases in the distal nephron and collecting duct Na delivery and luminal flow. As such, these diuretics are kaliuretic primarily owing to their indirect effects. Inhibition of K absorption by the $Na^+$-$2Cl^-$-$K^+$ cotransporter is associated with a commensurate reduction in K secretion by the apical ROMK channel; however, a component of the kaliuresis reflects decreased K absorption on the $Na^+$-$2Cl^-$-$K^+$ cotransporter in the loop of Henle. Thiazide diuretics, which are also kaliuretic, when factored for their effect on Na excretion exhibit a more intense kaliuretic response. However, most thiazide diuretics also inhibit carbonic anhydrase activity, which may contribute to their acute kaliuretic response.

## Luminal Anion Composition/ Transepithelial Voltage

Additional factors that influence K excretion include the luminal anion composition and transepithelial voltage. Although distinct, these factors are frequently influenced by the same maneuvers, such as the infusion of impermeant anions including sulfate, phosphate, and ferrocyanide.[15, 114] Where these factors have been studied separately, such as in micropuncture and microperfusion studies, the evidence suggests that luminal anion composition is the predominant factor. Specifically, alterations in the luminal Cl composition in the distal convolution or CCD result in only small changes in transepithelial voltage that are not sufficient to account for the changes in the rate of net K secretory flux.[68, 115, 116] This effect of luminal anion composition appears to be caused by a decrease in Cl concentration in the tubular fluid in both the late distal nephron[48, 49, 51] and the CCD[116] and has been attributed to the stimulation of KCl cotransport in these segments, which is increased upon reduction in luminal Cl concentration and the gradient for KCl secretion.[50]

The most frequently observed clinical condition that is associated with an enhanced kaliuresis related to alterations in distal anion composition is Cl-depletion metabolic alkalosis. Under these conditions, K depletion can be substantial and is largely attributable to renal K wasting.[117–119] The simplest model of this form of metabolic alkalosis is that induced either by vomiting or nasogastric suction. Under these conditions, the selective removal of hydrochloric acid, particularly under conditions where NaCl intake is reduced, can yield a substantial metabolic alkalosis, and renal K wasting also occurs. The induction of metabolic alkalosis is associated with a renal kaliuretic response as well as a bicarbonaturic response, which can result in substantial K depletion. In this form of metabolic alkalosis, the K depletion is the consequence, not the cause, of the metabolic alkalosis, and reduction in luminal Cl composition appears to be a major contributor to this kaliuretic response.

## Acid-Base Balance/Ammonium Effects

It has been appreciated for many years that acid-base balance exerts large effects on renal K excretion.[16, 120] Clearance experiments demonstrate that acute systemic metabolic alkalosis induced by sodium bicarbonate infusion increases renal K excretion for all plasma K concentrations measured and that metabolic acidosis induced by hydrochloric acid infusion suppresses renal K excretion throughout the measurable range of plasma K (Fig. 21–7). Micropuncture experiments demonstrated that these effects of changes in systemic acid-base balance affect K excretion by altering the rates of tubular transport within the distal nephron and collecting duct. Metabolic alkalosis induced by Na bicarbonate infusion stimulates distal tubular K secretion, and metabolic acidosis inhibits K secretion in the distal convolution and CCD.[16] However, changes in acid-base balance induced by changes in $P_{CO_2}$ produce smaller effects on K excretion than do metabolic changes or carbonic anhydrase inhibition. The effects of metabolic changes in systemic acid-base balance may be in part due to changes in luminal pH, because in the perfused rabbit CCD reduction in luminal pH depresses tubular K secretion consistent with the effect of acidosis to reduce apical K conductance in the CCD. These findings are consistent with the observed effects of pH on individual ROMK channels, which are known to be present in this segment

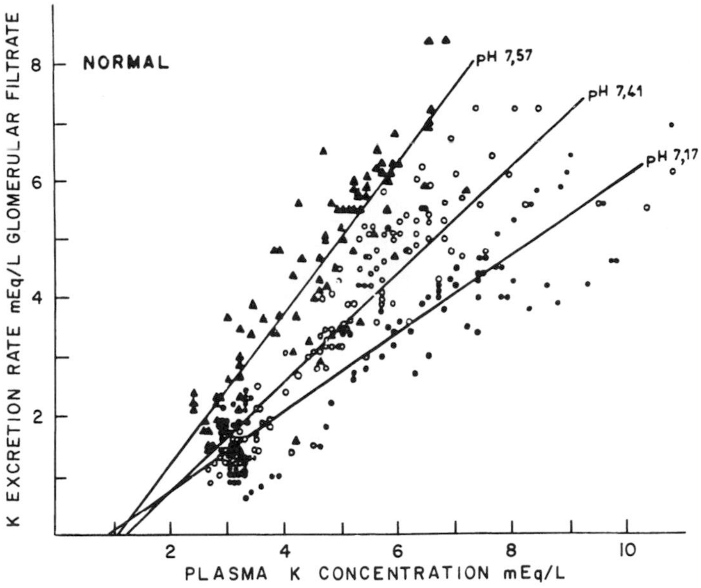

**FIGURE 21–7** ■ Effect of acid-base balance on net K excretion. (From Toussaint C, Vereerstraeten P: Effects of blood pH changes on potassium excretion in the dog. Am J Physiol 202: 768–772, 1962.)

of the nephron. Additional studies demonstrate that reduction in peritubular bicarbonate concentration also reduces net K secretion—an effect that has been largely attributed to a decrease in apical K conductance.[121] When luminal K and luminal flow rate are controlled by in vivo microperfusion, metabolic alkalosis stimulates distal nephron K secretion, whereas metabolic acidosis inhibits K secretion.[122]

The mechanism by which acute changes in acid-base perturbations affect renal K excretion includes both direct and indirect effects on tubular transport mechanisms. These direct and indirect effects may have opposing actions so that the precise clinical conditions will dictate the resultant effect on K excretion. For example, metabolic acidosis is known to inhibit transport in the thick ascending limb of Henle,[43] which will increase luminal Na delivery to the distal nephron and collecting duct and thus increase distal K secretion. On the other hand, metabolic acidosis decreases tubular K secretion.[122]

Other factors, as noted earlier, affect net K secretion and include alterations in luminal anion composition (see earlier) and changes in ambient $P_{CO_2}$. Changes in luminal Cl concentration frequently attend changes in metabolic acid-base disturbances, which may be due to an alteration in KCl secretion by the principal cells of the CCD. Although changes in ambient $P_{CO_2}$ stimulate K-absorptive flux under low K-restricted conditions, changes in $P_{CO_2}$ do not have appreciable effects on net K flux under K replete conditions, suggesting that substantial K recycling occurs under K replete circumstances. The observations suggest that alterations in the apical and basolateral K permeabilities are important determinants of net absorptive flux and are dictated by dietary K conditioning or some factor related to such conditioning. Additional studies have shown that chronic metabolic acidosis induces enhanced ammoniagenesis and that ammonium excretion, in part, serves to defend against K depletion that is a consequence of chronic metabolic acidosis.[123]

## Hormones

### MINERALOCORTICOIDS

Aldosterone is the most potent mineralocorticoid yet identified and exerts major effects on transport within the collecting duct as well as in vascular smooth muscle. This hormone exerts its effects through both genomic and nongenomic mechanisms of action. However, most of the renal effects appear to be mediated by de novo protein synthesis and via transcriptionally active mechanisms mediated by the mineralocorticoid receptor. This action requires approximately 1 to 2 hours before an effect on transport can be observed. Such observations have been observed both in clearance experiments and in microperfusion studies.[124] A consistent antinatriuresis and an enhanced Na reabsorption within the collecting duct is observed after aldosterone administration. The antinatriuresis is associated with an antidiuresis and a reduction in urine flow rate.[124, 125] Recent patch clamp studies demonstrate that one of the earliest transport effects of aldosterone is to enhance amiloride-sensitive Na channel activity in the collecting duct before changes in the activity of K channels.[126] Nevertheless, aldosterone exerts significant effects on extrarenal as well as renal mechanisms of K homeostasis. This is in part a consequence of its effect to enhance sodium reabsorption within the collecting duct and partly because of its effects on acid-base balance.

Chronic mineralocorticoid stimulation results in dramatically enhanced Na reabsorption and K secretory capacity of the CCD. Although aldosterone-independent mechanisms also participate in the effects of K loading on Na and K transport in the collecting duct, maximal rates of Na reabsorption and K secretion require mineralocorticoid action. In tubules from animals chronically treated with potent mineralocorticoid 11-desoxycorticosterone (DOCA), increasing bath K concentration is associated with more robust rates

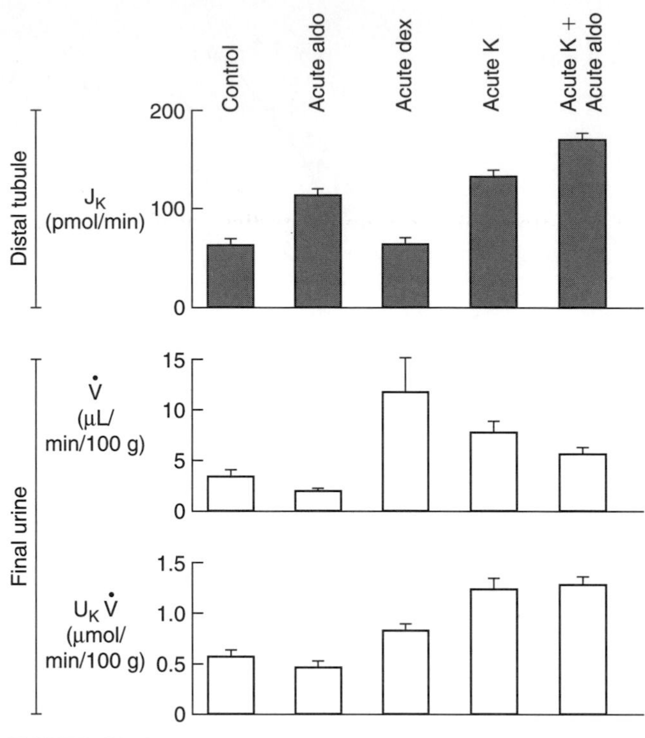


**FIGURE 21–8** ■ Effect of aldosterone and dexamethasone on distal nephron K secretion, urine flow rate and urinary K excretion (From Field MJ, Stanton B, Giebisch G: Differential acute effects of aldosterone, dexamethasone and hyperkalemia on distal tubular potassium secretion in the rat kidney. J Clin Invest 74:1792, 1984.)

of net K secretion.[127] This enhancement in transport is associated with an enhancement in the lumen-negative voltage and enhanced electrogenic Na reabsorption and K secretion.

The interaction of luminal flow rates and direct tubular transport effects of aldosterone on K secretion is illustrated in Figure 21–8.[125] In these free-flow micropuncture studies, aldosterone administration was associated with a significant increase in K secretion within the distal tubule; however, the flow rate was actually reduced after aldosterone administration and urinary K excretion remained unchanged. Acute K administration also augmented K secretion in the distal tubule to a comparable degree. However, this increase was associated with a modest increase in urine flow rate and consequently an increase in urinary K excretion. The addition of aldosterone to the same K load resulted in only modest increases in distal tubule K secretion, but this was associated with an attendant reduction in urine flow rates. Consequently, urine K excretion with aldosterone plus K administration was no greater than comparable experiments with the same K load.[125]

In addition to its potent effect on Na and K transport primarily in the distal convolution and CCD, aldosterone exerts substantial effects on proton secretion primarily via $H^+$ ATPase and possibly also by $H^+,K^+$ ATPase, primarily in the medullary collecting duct. These observations suggest that aldosterone may also augment K reabsorption, via direct or indirect mechanisms, as well as K secretion. Such observations are in keeping with previous studies that noted that the action of aldosterone is substantially modified by the pre-existing dietary treatment. Specifically, K depletion reduces the kaliuretic action of aldosterone on urinary K excretion. In addition to these renal mechanisms of action, aldosterone exerts significant effects on extrarenal K homeostasis.[8] In part, this mineralocorticoid-dependent mechanism helps to stabilize serum K concentrations. Chronic steady-state experiments demonstrate that aldosterone serves to enhance renal K clearance by augmenting the rate of K secretion as well as the redistribution of K intracellularly for any given plasma K concentration.[128] These observations are entirely consistent with the known action of aldosterone to enhance $Na^+,K^+$ ATPase activity in the CCD, colon, and nontransporting epithelial tissue.

## GLUCOCORTICOIDS

Glucocorticoids are known to be kaliuretic,[129, 130] although the mechanism by which their kaliuretic action occurs is not entirely established. The effect of mineralocorticoid or glucocorticoid antagonism was studied in healthy human subjects, who were administered either a mineralocorticoid antagonist or a glucocorticoid antagonist prior to a KCl load, during a maximum water diuresis.[131] Clearance studies were extended for 5 hours after the K load, and the effect of antagonism of the glucocorticoid or mineralocorticoid receptors was compared with that of the control group that received only the KCl load. KCl increased both K excretion and Na excretion. Canrenoate, the active metabolite of spironolactone, increased the rate of Na excretion but had no effect on K excretion. However, this agent blunted the kaliuresis after the KCl load. The glucocorticoid antagonist RU486 did not influence excretion of the KCl load or affect renal Na handling, although antagonism of the glucocorticoid effect was supported by its effect on plasma cortisol. Such data would suggest that in healthy subjects, mineralocorticoid activity but not glucocorticoid activity is involved in the elimination of an oral K load during the water diuresis.[131]

The effects of glucocorticoids on K excretion have been studied under multiple different physiologic and experimental conditions, and the differences in the interpretation of these results should take cognizance of different physiologic conditions and methods of analysis. For example, studies in adrenalectomized animals or in individuals with hypophysectomy, in which glucocorticoid function is compromised, provide results different from those of studies in which glucocorticoid receptor antagonism is studied in normal, healthy human subjects. Likewise, the studies during water diuresis, in which vasopressin levels are suppressed but distal nephron flow rate is augmented, provide a different physiologic model than that in which individuals are studied during hydropenia, which is associated with low distal nephron flow rates and high plasma vasopressin concentrations. Other differences that should be noted are the response to an oral versus an intravenous K load because studies have suggested a sensing mechanism in the portal circulation (see earlier). Finally, the coadministered anion may influence the kaliuretic response.[132]

Glucocorticoids are known to have diverse effects both on the immune system and on metabolism, including gluconeogenesis, protein metabolism and degradation, ureagenesis, and ammoniagenesis. Glucocorticoids also have a substantial effect on the glomerular filtration rate (GFR), which influences fluid and solute delivery to the distal nephron. Part of the kaliuretic effect of glucocorticoids, when administered chronically, may reflect their effects on muscle catabolism and tissue breakdown with the ensuing liberation of an endogenous K load. Nevertheless, additional studies demonstrate that glucocorticoids enhance K excretion by their effects on distal luminal flow rates mediated in part by changes in GFR,[133] which influences fluid delivery to the distal convolution. When examined by in vivo microperfusion, glucocorticoids have a substantial effect on urine flow rate and a modest effect on K excretion with very little effect on net tubular K excretion.[125] However, other studies have found that glucocorticoids increase K excretion[129, 130] and have direct effects on net K secretion.[124]

### STEROID RECEPTOR SPECIFICITY AND 11β-OH STEROID DEHYDROGENASE

Studies have identified that the enzyme 11β-hydroxysteroid dehydrogenase type II is an important enzyme in the protection of the mineralocorticoid receptor from occupancy by glucocorticoids.[134] Rare conditions associated with defects in this enzyme are associated with early onset of severe hypertension that mimics hyperaldosteronism.[135] Specifically, children with the syndrome of apparent mineralocorticoid excess are afflicted with hypokalemia and metabolic alkalosis and severe hypertension often manifesting in the first few years of life, leading to severe cardiovascular consequences.

Clinically, certain drugs are known to inhibit this enzyme, including carbenoxolone, which is associated with a mineralocorticoid-like effect, and glycyrrhetinic acid. Certain candies, most notably candies with natural licorice flavoring that contain large quantities of glycyrrhetinic acid, may mimic primary hyperaldosteronism, except that aldosterone levels are suppressed.[136]

### VASOPRESSIN

As previously noted, one of the important factors that determines renal K excretion is flow within the distal nephron. However, the induction of the water diuresis is not associated with a kaliuresis that would be anticipated if flow-dependent effects were the sole determinant of renal K excretion. The resolution of this paradox is explained partly by the effects of vasopressin on distal nephron and collecting duct K secretion.[137] Vasopressin significantly augments K secretion in the CCD; however, the urine flow rate is substantially reduced because of the antinatriuretic effect of vasopressin. Thus, increases in vasopressin action, which results in fluid reabsorption of the collecting duct, occur without major alterations in renal K excretion because the direct effects of vasopressin on renal tubular K secretory rates are opposed by alterations in luminal flow rate.[137]

Other hormones may also affect renal K excretion. In free-flow micropuncture studies, perfusion with a glomerular ultrafiltrate results in substantially higher rates of K secretion in a flow-dependent manner than does perfusion with artificial tubular fluid of the same ionic composition. This observation suggests that some substance in either plasma and filtered at the glomerulus or secreted into the luminal fluid effectively increases net K secretion. Interestingly, vasopressin receptors have been identified at the luminal membrane of the collecting duct. Whether these or receptors for other hormones are involved in regulating K excretion awaits further studies.

## REFERENCES


1. Stanton BA, Giebisch G: Renal potassium transport. In Windhager EE (ed): Handbook of Physiology-Renal Physiology. New York, Oxford University Press, 1992, pp 813–874.
2. Brown RS: Extrarenal potassium homeostasis. Kidney Int 30: 116–127, 1986.
3. DeFronzo RA, Sherwin RS, Dillingham M, et al: Influence of basal insulin and glucagon secretion on potassium and sodium metabolism: Studies with somatostatin in normal dogs and in normal and diabetic human beings. J Clin Invest 61:472–479, 1978.
4. Thatcher TS, Radike AW: Tolerance to potassium intoxication in the albino rat. Am J Physiol 151:138–146, 1947.
5. Truszkowski R, Duszynska J: Protection of mice against potassium poisoning by corticoadrenal hormones. Endocrinology 27:117–124, 1940.
6. Schwartz WB: Potassium and the kidney. N Engl J Med 253: 601–603, 1955.
7. Stanton BA, Giebisch G: Renal potassium transport. In Windhager EE (ed): Handbook of Physiology-Renal Physiology. New York, Oxford University Press, 1992, pp 813–874.
8. Alexander EA, Levinsky NG: An extrarenal mechanism of potassium adaptation. J Clin Invest 47:740–748, 1968.
9. Hayslett JP, Binder HJ: Mechanism of potassium adaptation. Am J Physiol 243:F103–F112, 1982.
10. Berliner RW, Kennedy TJ, Hilton JG: Renal mechanisms for excretion of potassium. Am J Physiol 162:348–367, 1950.
11. Malnic G, Klose RM, Giebisch G: Microperfusion study of distal tubular potassium and sodium transfer in the rat kidney. Am J Physiol 211:548–559, 1966.
12. Foster ES, Hayslett JP, Binder HJ: Mechanism of active potassium absorption and secretion in the rat colon. Am J Physiol 246:G611–G617, 1984.
13. Sweiry JH, Binder HJ: Characterization of aldosterone-induced potassium secretion in rat distal colon. J Clin Invest 83:844–851, 1989.
14. Berliner RW, Kennedy TJ, Hilton JG: Renal mechanisms for excretion of potassium. Am J Physiol 162:348–367, 1950.
15. Malnic G, Klose RM, Giebisch G: Micropuncture study of distal tubular potassium and sodium transport in the rat nephron. Am J Physiol 211:529–547, 1966.
16. Malnic G, DeMello Aires M, Giebisch G: Potassium transport across renal distal tubules during acid-base disturbances. Am J Physiol 221:1192–1208, 1971.
17. Arrascue JF, Dobyan DC, Jamison RL: Potassium recycling in the renal medulla: Effects of acute potassium chloride administration to rats fed a potassium-free diet. Kidney Int 20:348–352, 1981.

18. Dobyan DC, Lacey FB, Jamison RL: Suppression of potassium-recycling in the renal medulla by short-term potassium deprivation. Kidney Int 16:701–709, 1979.
19. Roy DR, Blouch KL, Jamison RL: Effects of acute acid-base disturbances on $K^+$ delivery to the juxtamedullary end-descending limb. Am J Physiol 243:F188–F196, 1982.
20. Wingo CS: Potassium transport by the medullary collecting tubule of rabbit: Effects of variation in K intake. Am J Physiol 253:F1136–F1141, 1987.
21. Giebisch G, Malnic GL: Studies on the mechanism of tubular acidification. Physiologist 19:511–524, 1976.
22. Malnic G, Klose RM, Giebisch G: Micropuncture study of renal potassium excretion in the rat. Am J Physiol 206:674–686, 1964.
23. Wingo CS: Active proton secretion and potassium absorption in the rabbit outer medullary collecting duct—functional evidence for proton-potassium activated adenosine triphosphatase. J Clin Invest 84:361–365, 1989.
24. Sangan P, Rajendran VM, Mann AS, et al: Regulation of colonic H-K-ATPase in large intestine and kidney by dietary Na depletion and dietary K depletion. Am J Physiol 272:C685–C696, 1997.
25. Meneton P, Schultheis PJ, Greeb J, et al: Increased sensitivity to $K^+$ deprivation in colonic H,K,ATPase-deficient mice. J Clin Invest 101:536–542, 1998.
26. Knochel JP, Dotin LN, Hamburger RJ: Pathophysiology of intense physical conditioning in a hot climate. I. J Clin Invest 51: 242–255, 1972.
27. Wingo CS, Armitage FE: Potassium transport in the kidney: Regulation and physiological relevance of $H^+$,$K^+$-ATPase. Semin Nephrol 13:213–224, 1993.
28. Wingo CS, Cain BD: The renal H-K-ATPase: Physiological significance and role in potassium homeostasis. Annu Rev Physiol 55:323–347, 1993.
29. Stokes JB: Potassium secretion by cortical collecting tubule: Relation to sodium absorption, luminal sodium concentration, and transepithelial voltage. Am J Physiol 241:F395–F402, 1981.
30. Stanton BA, Biemesderfer D, Wade JB, Giebisch G: Structural and functional study of the rat distal nephron: Effects of potassium adaptation and depletion. Kidney Int 19:36–48, 1981.
31. Weinstein AM: A mathematical model of the rat proximal tubule. Am J Physiol 250:F860–F873, 1986.
32. Weinstein AM: Modeling the proximal tubule: Complications of the paracellular pathway. Am J Physiol 254:F297–F305, 1988.
33. Barfuss DW, Schafer JA: Rate of formation and composition of absorbate from proximal nephron segments. Am J Physiol 247: F117–F129, 1984.
34. Johnston TA, Battilana CA, Lacey FB, Jamison RL: Evidence of concentration gradient favoring outward movement of sodium from the thin loop of Henle. J Clin Invest 59:234–240, 1977.
35. Jamison RL, Lacey FB, Pennell JP, Sanjana VM: Potassium secretion by the descending limb or pars recta of the juxtamedullary nephron in vivo. Kidney Int 9:323–332, 1976.
36. Battilana CA, Dobyan DC, Lacey FB, et al: Effect of chronic potassium loading on potassium secretion by the pars recta or descending limb of the juxtamedullary nephron in the rat. J Clin Invest 62:1093–1103, 1978.
37. Jamison RL, Lacey FB, Pennell JP, Sanjana VM: Potassium secretion by the descending limb or pars recta of the juxtamedullary nephron in vivo. Kidney Int 9:323–332, 1976.
38. Wasserstein AG, Agus ZS: Potassium secretion in the rabbit proximal straight tubule. Am J Physiol 245:F167–F174, 1983.
39. Stokes JB: Consequences of potassium recycling in the renal medulla. Effects of ion transport by the medullary thick ascending limb of the loop of Henle. J Clin Invest 70:219–229, 1982.
40. Greger R, Schlatter E: Properties of the lumen membrane of the cortical thick ascending limb of Henle's loop of rabbit kidney. Pflugers Arch 396:315–324, 1983.
41. Sun A, Grossman EB, Lombardi M, Hebert SC: Vasopressin alters the mechanism of apical Cl-entry from $Na^+Cl^-$ to $Na^+K^+Cl^-$ cotransport in mouse medullary thick ascending limb. J Membr Biol 120:83–94, 1991.
42. Wang WH: Two types of $K^+$ channel in thick ascending limb of rat kidney. Am J Physiol 267:F599–F605, 1994.
43. Wingo CS: Effect of acidosis on chloride transport in the cortical thick ascending limb of Henle. J Clin Invest 78:1324–1330, 1986.
44. Greger R, Schlatter E: Properties of the basolateral membrane of the cortical thick ascending limb of Henle's loop of rabbit kidney. Pflugers Arch 396:325–334, 1983.
45. Oberleithner H, Ritter M, Lang F, Guggino W: Anthracene-9-carboxylic acid inhibits renal chloride reabsorption. Pflugers Arch 398:172–174, 1983.
46. Gross JB, Imai M, Kokko JP: A functional comparison of the cortical collecting tubule and the distal convoluted tubule. J Clin Invest 55:1284–1294, 1975.
47. Stanton BA, Giebisch GH: Potassium transport by the renal distal tubule: Effects of potassium loading. Am J Physiol 243: F487–F493, 1982.
48. Ellison DH, Velazquez H, Wright FS: Stimulation of distal potassium secretion by low luminal chloride in the presence of barium. Am J Physiol 248:F638–F649, 1985.
49. Ellison DH, Velazquez H, Wright FS: Unidirectional potassium fluxes in renal distal tubule: Effects of chloride and barium. Am J Physiol 250:F885–F894, 1986.
50. Velazquez H, Wright FS, Good DW: Luminal influences on potassium secretion: Chloride replacement with sulfate. Am J Physiol 242:F46–F55, 1982.
51. Velazquez H, Ellison DH, Wright FS: Chloride-dependent potassium secretion in early and late renal distal tubules. Am J Physiol 253:F555–F562, 1987.
52. Woodhall PB, Tisher CC: Response of the distal tubule and cortical collecting duct to vasopressin in the rat. J Clin Invest 52:3095–3108, 1973.
53. Gullner H-G, Gill JR Jr, Bartter FC, et al: A familial disorder with hypokalemic alkalosis, hyperreninemia, aldosteronism, high urinary prostaglandins and normal blood pressure that is Bartter's syndrome. Trans Assoc Am Physicians 92:175–188, 1979.
54. Sutton RA, Mavichak V, Halabe A, Wilkins GE: Bartter's syndrome: Evidence suggesting a distal tubular defect in a hypocalciuric variant of the syndrome. Miner Electrolyte Metab 18: 43–51, 1992.
55. Simon DB, Nelson-Williams C, Bia MJ, et al: Gitelman's variant of Bartter's syndrome, inherited hypokalaemic alkalosis, is caused by mutations in the thiazide-sensitive Na-Cl cotransporter. Nat Genet 12:24–30, 1996.
56. Lemmink HH, Knoers NV, Karolyi L, et al: Novel mutations in the thiazide-sensitive NaCl cotransporter gene in patients with Gitelman syndrome with predominant localization to the C-terminal domain. Kidney Int 54:720–730, 1998.
57. Lemmink HH, van den Heuvel LP, van Dijk HA, et al: Linkage of Gitelman syndrome to the thiazide-sensitive sodium-chloride cotransporter gene with identification of mutations in Dutch families. Pediatr Nephrol 10:403–407, 1996.
58. Kurtz CL, Karolyi L, Seyberth HW, et al: A common NKCC2 mutation in Costa Rican Bartter's syndrome patients: Evidence for a founder effect. J Am Soc Nephrol 8:1706–1711, 1997.
59. Simon DB, Karet FE, Hamdan JM, et al: Bartter's syndrome, hypokalaemic alkalosis with hypercalciuria, is caused by mutations in the Na-K-2Cl cotransporter NKCC2. Nat Genet 13: 183–188, 1996.
60. Vargas-Poussou R, Feldmann D, Vollmer M, et al: Novel molecular variants of the Na-K-2Cl cotransporter gene are responsible for antenatal Bartter syndrome. Am J Hum Genet 62:1332–1340, 1998.
61. Karolyi L, Konrad M, Kockerling A, et al: Mutations in the gene encoding the inwardly-rectifying renal potassium channel, ROMK, cause the antenatal variant of Bartter syndrome: Evidence for genetic heterogeneity. International Collaborative Study Group for Bartter-like syndromes [published erratum appears in Hum Mol Genet 6(4):650, 1997]. Hum Mol Genet 6:17–26, 1997.
62. Simon DB, Karet FE, Rodriguez-Soriano J, et al: Genetic heterogeneity of Bartter's syndrome revealed by mutations in the $K^+$ channel, ROMK. Nat Genet 14:152–156, 1996.
63. Vollmer M, Koehrer M, Topaloglu R, et al: Two novel mutations of the gene for Kir 1.1 (ROMK) in neonatal Bartter syndrome. Pediatr Nephrol 12:69–71, 1998.
64. Konrad M, Vollmer M, Lemmink HH, et al: Mutations in the

chloride channel gene CLCNKB as a cause of classic Bartter syndrome. J Am Soc Nephrol 11:1449–1459, 2000.
65. Simon DB, Bindra RS, Mansfield TA, et al: Mutations in the chloride channel gene, CLCNKB, cause Bartter's syndrome type III. Nat Genet 17:171–178, 1997.
66. Shimizu T, Yoshitomi K, Nakamura M, Imai M: Site and mechanism of action of trichlormethiazide in rabbit distal nephron segments perfused in vitro. J Clin Invest 82:721–730, 1988.
67. Good DW, Wright FS: Luminal influences on potassium secretion: Sodium concentration and luminal flow rate. Am J Physiol 236:F192–F205, 1979.
68. Good DW, Wright FS: Luminal influences on potassium secretion: Transepithelial voltage. Am J Physiol 239:F289–F298, 1980.
69. Good DW, Velazquez H, Wright FS: Luminal influences on potassium secretion: Low sodium concentration. Am J Physiol 246:F609–F619, 1984.
70. Wright FS, Giebisch G: Renal potassium transport: Contributions of individual nephron segments and populations. Am J Physiol 235:F515–F527, 1978.
71. Malnic G, Klose RM, Giebisch G: Micropuncture study of renal potassium excretion in the rat. Am J Physiol 206:674–686, 1964.
72. Verlander JW, Madsen KM, Tisher CC: Effect of acute respiratory acidosis on two populations of intercalated cells in the rat cortical collecting duct. Am J Physiol 253:F1142–F1156, 1987.
73. Frindt G, Palmer LG: Ca-activated K channels in apical membrane of mammalian CCT, and their role in K secretion. Am J Physiol 252:F458–F467, 1987.
74. Hunter M, Lopes AG, Boulpaep E, Giebisch G: Regulation of single potassium ion channels from apical membrane of rabbit collecting tubule. Am J Physiol 251:F725–F733, 1986.
75. Kubokawa M, Wang W, McNicholas CM, Giebisch G: Role of $Ca^{2+}$/CaMK II in $Ca^{2+}$-induced $K^+$ channel inhibition in rat CCD principal cell. Am J Physiol 268:F211–F219, 1995.
76. Wang W, Giebisch G: Protein kinase a(PKA) and protein kinase c(PKC) modulate the apical small-conductance $K^+$ channel of rat cortical collecting duct (CCD). J Am Soc Nephrol 1: 694, 1990.
77. Wang W, Giebisch G: Dual effect of adenosine triphosphate on the apical small conductance $K^+$ channel of the rat cortical collecting duct. J Gen Physiol 98:35–61, 1991.
78. Wang W, Sackin H, Giebisch G: Renal potassium channels and their regulation. Annu Rev Physiol 54:81–96, 1992.
79. Ling BN, Eaton DC: Cyclosporin A inhibits apical secretory $K^+$ channels in rabbit cortical collecting tubule principal cells. Kidney Int 44:974–984, 1993.
80. Wingo CS: Potassium secretion by the cortical collecting tubule: Effects of ouabain and Cl gradients. Am J Physiol 256: F306–F313, 1989.
81. Ling BN, Kokko KE, Eaton DC: Prostaglandin $E_2$ activates clusters of apical $Cl^-$ channels in principal cells via a cyclic adenosine monophosphate-dependent pathway. J Clin Invest 93:829–837, 1994.
82. Wingo CS: Reversible Cl dependent K flux across the rabbit cortical collecting tubule. Am J Physiol 256:F697–F704, 1989.
83. Wingo CS: Active and passive chloride transport by the rabbit cortical collecting duct. Am J Physiol 258:F1388–F1393, 1990.
84. Wingo CS, Smolka AJ: Function and structure of H,K-ATPase in the kidney. Am J Physiol 269:F1–F16, 1995.
85. Wingo CS, Zhou X, Smolka A, et al: The renal H-K-ATPase: Function and expression. In Hirst BH (ed): Molecular and Cellular Mechanisms of $H^+$ Transport. Berlin, Springer-Verlag, 1994, pp 153–161.
86. Zhou X, Wingo CS: Stimulation of total $CO_2$ flux by 10% $CO_2$ in rabbit CCD: Role of an apical Sch-28080- and Ba-sensitive mechanism. Am J Physiol 267:F114–F120, 1994.
87. Zhou X, Lynch IJ, Xia SL, Wingo CS: Activation of $H^+$-$K^+$-ATPase by $CO_2$ requires a basolateral $Ba^{2+}$-sensitive pathway during K restriction. Am J Physiol 279:F153–F160, 2000.
88. Wingo CS, Cain BD: The renal H-K-ATPase: Physiological significance and role in potassium homeostasis. Annu Rev Physiol 55:323–347, 1993.
89. Elger M, Bankir L, Kriz W: Morphometric analysis of kidney hypertrophy in rats after chronic potassium depletion. Am J Physiol 262:F656–F667, 1992.
90. Hansen GT, Tisher CC, Robinson RR: Response of the collecting duct to disturbances of acid base and potassium balance. Kidney Int 17:326–337, 1980.
91. Backman KA, Hayslett JP: Role of the medullary collecting duct in potassium conservation. Pflugers Arch 396:297–300, 1983.
92. Schon DA, Backman KA, Hayslett JP: Role of the medullary collecting duct in potassium excretion in potassium-adapted animals. Kidney Int 20:655–662, 1981.
93. Stanton BA: Characterization of apical and basolateral membrane conductances of rat inner medullary collecting duct. Am J Physiol 256:F862–F868, 1989.
94. Light DB, Schwiebert EM, Karlson KH, Stanton BA: Atrial natriuretic peptide inhibits a cation channel in renal inner medullary collecting duct cells. Science 243:383–385, 1989.
95. Rabinowitz L, Berlin R, Yamauchi H: Plasma potassium and diurnal cyclic potassium excretion in the rat. Am J Physiol 253: F1178–F1181, 1987.
96. Moore-Ede MC: Physiology of the circadian timing system: Predictive versus reactive homeostasis. Am J Physiol 250:R735–R752, 1986.
97. Moore-Ede MC, Brennan MF, Ball MR: Circadian variation of intercompartmental potassium fluxes in man. J Appl Physiol 38:163–170, 1975.
98. Moore-Ede MC, Meguid MM, Fitzpatrick GF, et al: Circadian variation in response to potassium infusion. Clin Pharmacol Ther 23:218–227, 1978.
99. Rabinowitz L, Aizman RI: The central nervous system in potassium homeostasis. Front Neurol 14:1–26, 1993.
100. Mujais SK: Renal memory after potassium adaptation: Role of $Na^+$-$K^+$-ATPase. Am J Physiol 254:F840–F850, 1988.
101. Muto S, Sansom S, Giebisch G: Effects of a high potassium diet on electrical properties of cortical collecting ducts from adrenalectomized rabbits. J Clin Invest 81:376–380, 1988.
102. Wingo CS: Active and passive chloride transport by the rabbit cortical collecting duct. Am J Physiol 258:F1388–F1393, 1990.
103. Velazquez H, Wright FS: Effects of diuretic drugs on Na, Cl, and K transport by rat renal distal tubule. Am J Physiol 250: F1013–F1023, 1986.
104. Mujais SK, Chekal MA, Hayslett JP, Katz AI: Regulation of renal $Na^+$-$K^+$-ATPase in the rat: Role of increased potassium transport. Am J Physiol 251:F199–F207, 1986.
105. Fujii Y, Mujais SK, Katz AI: Renal potassium adaptation: Role of the $Na^+$-$K^+$ pump in rat cortical collecting tubules. Am J Physiol 256:F279–F284, 1989.
106. Ahloulay M, Dechaux M, Laborde K, Bankir L: Influence of glucagon on GFR and on urea and electrolyte excretion: Direct and indirect effects. Am J Physiol 269:F225–F235, 1995.
107. Lang F, Ottl I, Haussinger D, et al: Renal hemodynamic response to intravenous and oral amino acids in animals. Semin Nephrol 15:415–418, 1995.
108. Fourman P: The ability of the normal kidney to conserve potassium. Lancet 1:1042–1044, 1952.
109. Mujais SK, Katz AI: Potassium deficiency. In Seldin DW, Giebisch G (eds): The Kidney Physiology and Pathophysiology. New York, Raven Press, 1992, pp 2249–2278.
110. Stetson DL, Wade JB, Giebisch G: Morphologic alterations in the rat medullary collecting duct following potassium depletion. Kidney Int 17:45–56, 1980.
111. Ornt DB, Radke KJ, Scandling JD: Effect of aldosterone on renal potassium conservation in the rat. Am J Physiol 270: E1003–E1008, 1996.
112. Eiam-Ong S, Kurtzman NA, Sabatini S: Regulation of collecting tubule adenosine triphosphatases by aldosterone and potassium. J Clin Invest 91:2385–2392, 1993.
113. Linas SL, Peterson LN, Anderson RJ, et al: Mechanism of renal potassium conservation in the rat. Kidney Int 15:601–611, 1979.
114. Berliner RW, Kennedy TJ, Hilton JG: Renal clearance of ferrocyanide in the dog. Am J Physiol 160:325–329, 1950.
115. Malnic G, Giebisch G: Some electrical properties of distal tubular epithelium in the rat. Am J Physiol 223:797–808, 1972.
116. Wingo CS: Potassium secretion by the cortical collecting tubule: Effects of ouabain and Cl gradients. Am J Physiol 256: F306–F313, 1989.
117. Bleich HL, Tannen RL, Schwartz WB: The induction of metabolic alkalosis by correction of potassium deficiency. J Clin Invest 45:573–579, 1966.

118. Kassirer JP, Schwartz WB: Correction of metabolic alkalosis in man without repair of potassium deficiency. Am J Med 40: 19–26, 1966.
119. Schwartz WB, van Ypersele de Strihou C, Kassirer JP: Role of anions in metabolic alkalosis and potassium deficiency. N Engl J Med 279:630–639, 1968.
120. Toussaint C, Vereerstraeten P: Effects of blood pH changes on potassium excretion in the dog. Am J Physiol 202:768–772, 1962.
121. Tabei K, Muto S, Furuya H, et al: Potassium secretion is inhibited by metabolic acidosis in rabbit cortical collecting ducts in vitro. Am J Physiol 268:F490–F495, 1995.
122. Stanton BA, Giebisch G: Effects of pH on potassium transport by renal distal tubule. Am J Physiol 242:F544–F551, 1982.
123. Tannen RL, Terrien T: Potassium-sparing effect of enhanced renal ammonia production. Am J Physiol 228:699–705, 1975.
124. Wingo CS, Kokko JP, Jacobson HR: Effects of in vitro aldosterone on the rabbit cortical collecting tubule. Kidney Int 28: 51–57, 1985.
125. Field MJ, Stanton BA, Giebisch GH: Differential acute effects of aldosterone, dexamethasone, and hyperkalemia on distal tubular potassium secretion in the rat kidney. J Clin Invest 74: 1792–1802, 1984.
126. Palmer LG, Frindt G: Aldosterone and potassium secretion by the cortical collecting duct. Kidney Int 57:1324–1328, 2000.
127. Muto S, Giebisch G, Sansom S: An acute increase of peritubular K stimulates K transport through cell pathways of CCT. Am J Physiol 255:F108–F114, 1988.
128. Young DB, Jackson TE: Effects of aldosterone on potassium distribution. Am J Physiol 243:R526–R530, 1982.
129. Bia MJ, Tyler K, DeFronzo RA: The effect of dexamethasone on renal electrolyte excretion in the adrenalectomized rat. Endocrinology 111:882–888, 1982.
130. Bia MJ, Tyler K, DeFronzo R: The effect of dexamethasone on renal potassium excretion and acute potassium tolerance. Endocrinology 113:1690–1696, 1983.
131. Vanburen M, Boer P, Kuomas HA: Effects of acute mineralocorticoid and glucocorticoid receptor blockade on the excretion of an acute potassium load in healthy humans. J Clin Endocrinol Metab 77:902–909, 1993.
132. Morris RCJ, Schmidlin O, Tanaka M, et al: Differing effects of supplemental KCl and $KHCO_3$: Pathophysiological and clinical implications. Semin Nephrol 19:487–493, 1999.
133. Baylis C, Brenner BM: Mechanism of the glucocorticoid-induced increase in glomerular filtration rate. Am J Physiol 234:F166–F170, 1978.
134. Funder JW, Pearce PT, Smith R, Smith AI: Mineralocorticoid action: Target tissue specificity is enzyme, not receptor, mediated. Science 242:583–585, 1988.
135. New MI, Levine LS, Biglieri EG, et al: Evidence for an unidentified steroid in a child with apparent mineralocorticoid hypertension. J Clin Endocrinol Metab 44:924–933, 1977.
136. Blachley JD, Knochel JP: Tobacco chewer's hypokalemia: Licorice revisited. N Engl J Med 302:784–785, 1980.
137. Field MJ, Stanton BA, Giebisch GH: Influence of ADH on renal potassium handling: A micropuncture and microperfusion study. Kidney Int 25:502–511, 1984.

CHAPTER 22

# Hypokalemia

Bruce C. Kone, MD

Hypokalemia, which is defined as a serum $K^+$ concentration of less than 3.5 mEq/L, is a commonly encountered clinical condition arising from diverse etiologies. The decrement in extracellular $K^+$ concentration hyperpolarizes the resting transmembrane potential and reduces the excitability of nerve and contractile cells. Although mild hypokalemia is typically well tolerated in otherwise healthy individuals, severe hypokalemia can result in cardiac arrhythmias, paralysis, and even death. Moreover, hypokalemia is associated with increased morbidity and mortality in patients with cardiovascular disease. Consequently, early recognition, etiologic discrimination, and treatment of hypokalemia are warranted. The goal of this chapter is to offer a practical review of the clinical consequences, diagnostic features, and appropriate therapies of hypokalemia.

## PHYSIOLOGY OF $K^+$ BALANCE

The total body $K^+$ content in humans is estimated to be approximately 50 mEq/kg body weight. Approximately 98% of $K^+$ is distributed in the intracellular compartment and is the result of active $K^+$ uptake by the $Na^+$-$K^+$-adenosine triphosphatase (ATPase) in the cell membrane. The remaining 2% of $K^+$ is located in the extracellular pool.[1,2] $K^+$ intake based on a typical Western diet averages 70 mEq/day. Under normal conditions, excretion balances intake, with renal mechanisms accounting for 90% of excreted $K^+$. The remaining 10% of $K^+$ excretion occurs principally in the stool. With $K^+$ deficiency, a portion of intracellular $K^+$ redistributes to the extracellular fluid to maintain the transmembrane electrochemical gradient. Consequently, small decrements in serum $K^+$ concentration may reflect large deficits in intracellular $K^+$ content. In general, the serum $K^+$ concentration decreases by approximately 0.3 mEq/L for each 100 mEq decrement in total body $K^+$ content below 3.5 mEq/L, although this response is highly variable.[2] Thus, a serum $K^+$ level less than 3 mEq/L typically represents a total body $K^+$ deficit of approximately 100 to 300 mEq, whereas a level less than 2 mEq/L may represent a deficit of 500 to 700 mEq in total body $K^+$ (Table 22–1).

**TABLE 22–1.** Approximation of Total Body $K^+$ Deficit

| Serum [$K^+$] (mEq/L) | $K^+$ Deficit (mEq/70 kg body wt) |
|---|---|
| 3.5 | 125–250 |
| 3.0 | 150–400 |
| 2.5 | 300–600 |
| 2.0 | 500–750 |

Adapted from data presented in Sterns RH, Cox M, Feig PU, Singer I: Internal potassium balance and the control of the plasma potassium concentration. Medicine 60:339–354, 1981.

The daily minimum requirement for $K^+$ is 40 to 50 mEq. $K^+$ intake varies considerably according to the individual's general medical status, age, type of diet consumed, and race. Adolescents may consume larger amounts of K, whereas elderly individuals may have more restricted K intake. Vegetarians who consume large amounts of K-rich vegetables and fruits may consume up to 275 mEq/day of $K^+$.[3] Urban white populations generally consume more $K^+$ than do their African-American counterparts.[4] Normal individuals on a typical Western diet absorb about 90% of intake and excrete an equivalent amount of $K^+$ in the urine. $K^+$ is freely filtered at the glomerulus. Approximately 85% of filtered $K^+$ is reabsorbed by the proximal tubule and the medullary thick ascending limb of the loop of Henle. The principal cells of the cortical collecting duct secrete excess $K^+$. During states of $K^+$ deficiency, the outer and inner medullary collecting ducts reabsorb $K^+$ to reclaim the filtered $K^+$.

Normal fecal $K^+$ excretion averages about 9 mEq/day.[5] The bulk of intestinal $K^+$ absorption in $K^+$-replete individuals occurs in the small intestine, whereas the colon contributes little to net $K^+$ absorption and secretion under basal conditions. $K^+$ is absorbed or secreted mainly by passive mechanisms; the rectum and perhaps the sigmoid colon have the capacity to secrete actively $K^+$, but the quantitative and physiologic significance of this active secretion is uncertain. Hyperaldosteronism, whether primary or secondary, increases fecal $K^+$ excretion by about 3 mEq/day in subjects with normal intestinal tracts. In situ microperfusion studies have demonstrated net $K^+$ reabsorption along the distal tubule in chronically hypokalemic rats.[3] Based on in vitro microperfusion studies in animals, the intercalated cells in the cortical and outer[4] medullary collecting duct appear to be the principal sites of $K^+$ reabsorption. Animal studies also suggest that the distal colon actively reabsorbs $K^+$ during chronic hypokalemia. Studies in mice with targeted deletion of the $H^+$-$K^+$-ATPase $\alpha_2$ gene indicate that this gene contributes significantly to active $K^+$ absorption in the distal colon during $K^+$ depletion.[6]

## CLINICAL FEATURES OF HYPOKALEMIA

Most patients with mild hypokalemia are asymptomatic and present without remarkable signs. In other asymptomatic patients, hypokalemia may manifest only as associated or incidental electrochemical and biochemical abnormalities. Symptomatic patients may present with potentially life-threatening features. In general, the incidence of symptoms appears to correlate directly with both the magnitude and the rate of decline in serum $K^+$ concentration. However, in many cases this correlation is weak. The most prominent clinical findings are detailed later and are also found in Table 22–2.

**Cardiovascular Effects.** Hypokalemia may be associated with electrocardiogram (ECG) changes. As the serum $[K^+]$ decreases, ST segment depression, reduced amplitude of the T wave, and prominent U waves are initially observed. With more severe decrements in serum $[K^+]$, the P wave amplitude increases and the QRS interval becomes prolonged.[7] However, these responses are variable, so that patients with ECG changes attributable to hypokalemia should be monitored closely. Cardiac arrhythmias, including atrial tachycardia with or without atrioventricular block, atrioventricular dissociation, premature ventricular contractions, torsades de pointes, ventricular tachycardia, and ventricular fibrillation[5, 6] represent a potentially fatal complication of hypokalemia. Accordingly, for all patients with severe hypokalemia (serum $[K^+]$, 2.5 mEq/L), an ECG should be obtained.

**TABLE 22–2.** Clinical Consequences of Hypokalemia

| |
|---|
| **Cardiac** |
| ECG changes (flat or inverted T waves, prominent U waves, ST segment depression) |
| Arrhythmias (atrial tachycardia with or without atrioventricular block, atrioventricular dissociation, premature ventricular contractions, ventricular tachycardia, and ventricular fibrillation) |
| **Neurologic/Neuromuscular** |
| Muscle weakness |
| Cramps |
| Myalgias |
| Rhabdomyolysis |
| Paralysis |
| Decreased deep tendon reflexes |
| Paresthesias |
| Worsening of hepatic encephalopathy |
| **Gastrointestinal** |
| Nausea, vomiting |
| Constipation |
| Paralytic ileus |
| **Pulmonary** |
| Respiratory failure from respiratory muscle paralysis |
| **Endocrine** |
| Hyperglycemia |
| Carbohydrate intolerance |
| **Renal** |
| Increased $HCO_3^-$ reabsorption in the proximal tubule |
| Increased $H^+$ secretion in the cortical collecting duct |
| Decreased urinary citrate excretion |
| Increased ammoniagenesis in the proximal tubule |
| Impaired urinary concentrating ability |
| Nephrogenic diabetes insipidus |
| Renal cystic disease, interstitial scarring, and renal insufficiency[24] |

ECG, electrocardiogram.

Patients with ischemic heart disease, congestive heart failure, or left ventricular hypertrophy appear to be at greatest risk for dysrhythmias related to hypokalemia. Notably, hypokalemia promotes the occurrence of digoxin-related arrhythmias. The Multicenter Study of Perioperative Ischemia Research Group reported that in patients undergoing elective coronary artery bypass grafting, perioperative arrhythmia and the need for cardiopulmonary resuscitation (CPR) increased as preoperative serum $K^+$ level decreased below 3.5 mmol/L.[7]

Hypokalemia has also been theorized to underlie the reduced benefit on cardiovascular events in hypertensive patients receiving thiazide diuretics.[8] Initial studies suggested that this occurred only with higher doses (50 to 100 mg) of thiazides. However, recent evidence from the Systolic Hypertension in the Elderly Program (SHEP), a 5-year randomized, placebo-controlled clinical trial of chlorthalidone-based treatment of isolated systolic hypertension in the elderly, found that this effect also extends to elderly patients on low-dose thiazides. In this study, approximately 7% of participants developed hypokalemia on low-dose thiazide therapy. The participants who had hypokalemia after 1 year of treatment with a low-dose diuretic failed to achieve the reduction in cardiovascular events experienced by those who did not have hypokalemia.[8] Accordingly, the dose of thiazide diuretic in patients should be maintained at the lowest effective dose, and the serum $K^+$ concentration should be monitored. $K^+$ repletion and the addition of a $K^+$-sparing diuretic may be indicated if hypokalemia supervenes.

The relationship between $K^+$ intake and the risk of cardiovascular and renovascular events has been the subject of intense scrutiny. Several observational studies have suggested a link between low $K^+$ intake and the risk of hypertension and stroke.[9, 10] In the case of stroke, the putative protective effects of $K^+$ seem to be most prominent in African-American and hypertensive males.[11] $K^+$ supplementation may suppress or abolish salt sensitivity in hypertensive patients, particularly blacks, in whom salt sensitivity may occur when dietary $K^+$ is only marginally deficient.[12] One pooled analysis of 33 randomized, controlled trials concluded that $K^+$ supplementation might be beneficial for normalizing blood pressure.[13] Consequently, the consensus of several study groups and health councils[14] has suggested that the daily dietary intake of $K^+$ should be at least 60 mEq. It should be emphasized, however, that no direct *causal* relationship between dietary K intake and increased cardiovascular or renovascular risk has yet been convincingly established.[15]

**Neurologic/Neuromuscular Effects.** The initial manifestation of $K^+$ depletion may be generalized muscle weakness, cramps, or myalgias. Worsening of the symptoms with exercise may occur. Hypokalemic myopathy tends to affect the lower extremities more than the upper extremities. Muscle necrosis and rhabdomyolysis may occur when serum $[K^+]$ is less than 2.5 mEq/L.[16] Severe hypokalemia (serum $[K^+] < 2$ mEq/L) can cause decreased deep tendon reflexes, paresthesias, and, rarely, paralysis, eventually involving the respiratory muscles. Respiratory paralysis, which is a rare but potentially fatal complication of severe hypokalemia, warrants emergent $K^+$ replacement.

**Metabolic and Hormonal Effects.** Hypokalemia is associated with impaired insulin secretion by the pancreatic beta cells and decreased peripheral glucose utilization.[17] This leads to carbohydrate intolerance and hyperglycemia, which is particularly problematic in diabetic patients. This complication may also be encountered in diuretic-induced hypokalemia.[17] Studies in female mice suggest that hypokalemia may suppress circulating progesterone levels, the preovulatory surge of gonadotropins, and the secondary surge of follicle-stimulating hormone at estrus.[18] Comparable studies in women have not been performed.

**Gastrointestinal and Hepatic Effects.** Nausea, vomiting, constipation, and paralytic ileus may occur with hypokalemia. Ileus typically occurs only with severe hypokalemia (serum $[K^+]$ of $<2.5$ mEq/L). Hypokalemia also promotes or aggravates hepatic encephalopathy by increasing renal ammoniagenesis and systemic ammonia levels.[19]

**Renal and Electrolyte Effects.** Hypokalemia is associated with increased $HCO_3^-$ reabsorption in the proximal tubule[20] and $H^+$ secretion in the cortical collecting duct, which promotes the evolution of metabolic alkalosis. Urinary citrate excretion may also be reduced. These effects are generally mild unless accompanied by sodium depletion.[21] Hypokalemia also results in increased ammoniagenesis[22] in the proximal tubule and impaired urinary concentrating ability. Patients with hypokalemia may develop both increased thirst and a mild nephrogenic diabetes insipidus.[23] In addition, patients with chronic hypokalemia may develop renal cystic disease, interstitial scarring, and renal insufficiency,[24] which may be related to increased ammoniagenesis.[25]

## ETIOLOGIES AND DIAGNOSTIC APPROACH

Hypokalemia usually reflects total body $K^+$ deficiency. Less commonly, hypokalemia results from transcellular $K^+$ redistribution with normal total body $K^+$ stores. The differential diagnosis of hypokalemia includes pseudohypokalemia, in vivo cellular $K^+$ redistribution, inadequate $K^+$ intake, excessive cutaneous or gastrointestinal $K^+$ losses, and renal $K^+$ wasting (Tables 22–3 and 22–4). Figure 22–1 presents a decision tree designed to establish the underlying etiology of hypokalemia. Accordingly, the history should be directed at determining the blood collection and transport procedure; the duration and timing of hypokalemia; the presence of hypokalemia-related symptoms; details of medications and diet; history of hypertension or gastrointestinal or renal disease; and a family history of

**TABLE 22–3.** Differential Diagnosis of Hypokalemia

| Normal Total Body $K^+$ | Decreased Total Body $K^+$ |
|---|---|
| Transcellular $K^+$ shifts | Inadequate $K^+$ intake |
| In vitro (pseudohypokalemia) | Nonrenal $K^+$ losses (gastrointestinal skin) |
| In vivo | Renal $K^+$ losses |

**TABLE 22–4.** Causes of Hypokalemia Associated with Depleted $K^+$ Stores

**Inadequate $K^+$ Intake**

Inadequate diet
Iatrogenic

**Excessive Sweating**

**Excessive GI Losses**

Vomiting, bulemia
Nasogastric suction
Biliary drainage
Diarrhea
- Infectious
- Tumor
- Watery diarrhea, hypokalemia, and achlorhydria syndrome
- Villous adenoma
- Laxative abuse
- Congenital chloride diarrhea
- Malabsorption syndromes

Enteric fistula
Clay ingestion
$K^+$ binding resin therapy
Uterosigmoid anastomosis

**Renal Losses**

Intrinisic renal disease
- Interstitial nephritides
- Diuretic (recovery) phase of acute tubular necrosis
- Postobstructive diuresis
- Classical distal RTA
- Alkali treatment of proximal RTA

Associated acid-base or electrolyte disorders
- Correction phase of metabolic disorders
- Hypomagnesemia

Drugs
- Diuretics
- Amphotericin B
- Penicillin and penicillin derivatives
- Aminoglycosides
- Cisplatin
- Ifosfamide
- Fludrocortisone
- High-dose glucocorticoids
- Gossypol
- Carbenoxolonc

Lysozymuria in acute leukemias
Mineralocorticoid excess
- Primary hyperaldosteronism
  - Bilateral adrenal hyperplasia
  - Adrenal adenoma
  - Adrenal carcinoma
  - Familial hyperaldosteronism
  - Idiopathic aldosteronism
- Primary hyperreninism
  - Malignant hypertension
  - Renal artery stenosis
  - Renin-producing tumors
- Primary excess of glucocorticoids exerting mineralocorticoid effects
  - Congenital adrenal hyperplasia (11β- or 17α-hydroxylase deficiency)
  - Cushing syndrome
  - Ectopic adrenocorticotropin syndrome

Disorders mimicking primary mineralocorticoid excess
- Liddle syndrome
- Apparent mineralocorticoid excess (11β-hydroxysteroid dehydrogenase type II deficiency)
- Bartter syndrome
- Gitelman syndrome

GI, gastrointestinal; RTA, renal tubular acidosis.

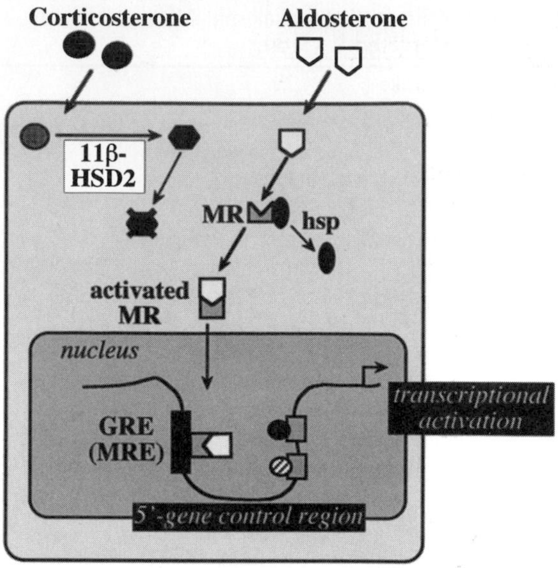

**FIGURE 22–1** ■ Diagnostic approach to defining the etiology of hypokalemia. (Modified from Weiner ID, Wingo CS: Hypokalemia—consequences, causes, and correction. J Am Soc Nephrol 8:1179–1188, 1977.)

hypertension, early stroke, or spontaneous hypokalemia.

**Transcellular $K^+$ Redistribution.** Cellular uptake of $K^+$ by blood in vitro can result in *pseudohypokalemia,* which occurs in three principal settings (Table 22–5). If blood specimens from leukemic patients with total leukocyte counts over 100,000/μL are kept at room temperature for prolonged periods, $K^+$ uptake by the leukocytes lowers the serum $K^+$ concentration in the test tube.[26, 27] Similarly, if blood samples obtained from patients who have been recently administered intravenous insulin are stored at room temperature, continued cellular uptake of $K^+$ may occur (Table 22–6). Delayed transit of venous blood samples during periods of high ambient temperature has also been reported to produce spurious hypokalemia.[27] Rapid separation of the plasma and storage at 4°C limit these in vitro problems.

Transcellular $K^+$ redistribution and hypokalemia in vivo occur by several mechanisms and in varied clinical settings. In these cases, total body $K^+$ is normal. $\beta_2$-Agonists (whether given for asthma or as tocolytic therapy in preterm labor[28]), theophylline, stress-induced catecholamine release, dobutamine, dopamine, aldosterone, and excessive insulin promote increased $Na^+$-$K^+$-ATPase activity, net cellular $K^+$ uptake, and hypokalemia. The effect of insulin on cellular $K^+$

**TABLE 22–5.** Causes of Pseudohypokalemia

- Blood specimens containing total leukocyte counts >100,000/μL kept at room temperature for prolonged periods
- Blood specimens from patients recently administered insulin that were stored at room temperature for prolonged periods
- Delayed transit of blood samples during periods of high ambient temperature

**TABLE 22–6.** Factors Promoting Increased Cellular $K^+$ Uptake

| |
|---|
| Insulin |
| Aldosterone |
| Extracellular alkalosis (minor effect) |
| Stress-induced catecholamine release membrane potential (depolarization) |
| $\beta_2$-Agonists |
| Dobutamine, dopamine |
| Theophylline |
| Barium intoxication |
| Chloroquine, hydroxychloroquine intoxication |
| Hypothermia |
| Acute anabolic states |
| Total parenteral nutrition in malnourished patients |
| Treatment of pernicious anemia |
| Rapidly growing leukemias and lymphomas |

redistribution must be considered when administering intravenous KCl solutions to replace $K^+$ deficits, because infusions of dextrose-containing solutions may actually aggravate hypokalemia. Competitive blockade of $K^+$ channels during barium[29–31] and hydroxychloroquine[32] poisoning stimulates net cellular $K^+$ uptake by unopposed operation of the $Na^+$-$K^+$-ATPase. Metabolic alkalosis or alkalemia promotes net $K^+$ uptake in exchange for the buffering effects of net $H^+$ efflux. In contrast, acute and chronic respiratory alkalosis have only minor effects on intracellular-extracellular $K^+$ balance and serum [$K^+$]. Although *intense exercise* may result in transient hyperkalemia, a rapid decrease in plasma $K^+$ concentration (often to 3 mEq/L or less), which may be maintained for prolonged periods, has been observed after cessation of intense exercise.[33] *Hypothermia* has also been reported to promote net cellular $K^+$ uptake and hypokalemia.[34] This effect is reversed with rewarming, and therapy with $K^+$ supplements during hypothermia may lead to hyperkalemia on rewarming.

Because $K^+$ is the principal intracellular cation, acute anabolic or cell proliferative states can result in severe hypokalemia. Malnourished patients treated with enteral or parenteral nutrition—the "refeeding" syndrome—commonly develop hypokalemia. Acute leukemias, aggressive lymphomas, or the cell proliferative response to treatment of severe pernicious anemia[35] may also lead to hypokalemia (see Table 22–3).

The *hypokalemic periodic paralyses* represent additional disorders that promote intracellular redistribution of extracellular $K^+$ and hypokalemia (Table 22–7). *Primary hypokalemic periodic paralysis* is a relatively uncommon illness that may occur sporadically or more commonly as an inherited disease. The familial disease is inherited in an autosomal dominant manner with reduced penetrance in women, and in some kindreds results from point mutations of the dihydropyridine-sensitive receptor $\alpha_1$ subunit gene (CACNA1S[36]) and an apparently defective ATP-sensitive $K^+$ channel (KATP[37]) in the sarcolemma of skeletal muscle. The dihydropyridine receptor functions as an L-type $Ca^{2+}$ channel that is critical for excitation-contraction coupling. One family has been described who has the

**TABLE 22–7.** Clinical Features of Primary Hypokalemic Periodic Paralysis

| | |
|---|---|
| Occurrence | • Sporadic<br>• Autosomal dominant (two thirds of cases) with reduced penetrance in women |
| Age of presentation | • Childhood to the third decade of life |
| Clinical presentation | • Episodes of hypokalemia and muscle weakness/paralysis<br>• Proximal muscles affected more than distal ones<br>• Normal serum [$K^+$] and strength between attacks (chronic muscle weakness may occur over time) |
| Precipitating factors | • Carbohydrate ingestion<br>• Emotional stress<br>• Overexertion |
| Molecular basis | • Mutations in ion channels of the skeletal muscle sarcolemma<br>Dihydropyridine-sensitive receptor $\alpha_1$ subunit gene (CACNA1S)[36]<br>$\alpha_1$ sodium channel gene (SCN4A)[38]<br>ATP-sensitive $K^+$ channel (KATP)[37] |
| Treatment | Acute: KCl administration<br>Preventive: low $Na^+$, low carbohydrate diet, carbonic anhydrase inhibitors, KC1 supplements |

disease on the basis of a point mutation in the skeletal muscle $\alpha_1$ sodium channel gene (SCN4A[38]). The disease typically manifests in childhood through the third decade of life as episodes of weakness in the face of mental alertness and normal strength between attacks. Serum [$K^+$] during an attack may fall below 2 mEq/L but generally falls to levels that would not typically be associated with muscle paralysis. In primary hypokalemic periodic paralysis, serum [$K^+$] is normal between attacks. Hypokalemia documented between paralytic episodes suggests secondary rather than primary hypokalemic paralysis. During the attack, proximal muscles are affected more than distal ones, with limb involvement being more common than bulbar. Attacks typically follow a carbohydrate meal, exercise, or sleep and may last a few hours or longer than 1 day. Preventive therapy consists of a low-sodium, low-carbohydrate diet; avoidance of the cold and overexertion; and supplemental KCl. Acetazolamide and, more recently, dichlorphenamide,[39] both potent carbonic anhydrase inhibitors, are also effective in reducing the frequency of episodic weakness in this disorder. Acute therapy typically consists of oral or intravenous KCl, depending on the severity of the weakness.

*Thyrotoxic periodic paralysis* is an unusual disorder that typically occurs among Asian and Latin-American men in the third decade of life, which often presents dramatically with severe hypokalemia and muscle paralysis. Precipitating factors for hypokalemia include exercise, carbohydrate ingestion, and alcohol consumption. In addition to hypokalemia, hypophosphatemia and mild hypomagnesemia are often present.[40] Graves disease represents the most common underlying disorder. Because signs and symptoms of hyperthyroidism may be subtle or absent on initial presentation, patients presenting with hypokalemic periodic paralysis and a negative family history should be screened for hyperthyroidism. KCl replacement and β-blockers may abbreviate the duration of a paralytic attack, but treatment of the underlying hyperthyroidism represents definitive therapy. Rebound hyperkalemia is a potential hazard of $K^+$ administration and occurred in 42% of 24 episodes reported in one series.[40]

**Inadequate $K^+$ Intake.** Chronic dietary $K^+$ deficiency as a primary cause of hypokalemia is relatively uncommon. Hypokalemia from inadequate dietary intake may occur in severe protein-calorie malnutrition, anorexia nervosa, and inadequate nutritional supplementation of severely catabolic patients. More frequently, however, low $K^+$ intake predisposes patients to hypokalemia when concurrent $K^+$ losses are occurring. Chronic ingestion of certain types of clay may also contribute to inadequate net $K^+$ intake. The clay functions as a $K^+$ binder and prevents adequate $K^+$ absorption from the gastrointestinal tract.[41]

**Excessive $K^+$ Losses.** Hypokalemia results most commonly from excessive cutaneous, gastrointestinal, or urinary $K^+$ losses. In addition, extracorporeal therapy may be associated with excessive net $K^+$ losses. When the prescription for dialysate [$K^+$] is too low in hemodialysis and peritoneal dialysis patients, hypokalemia may ensue. Hypokalemia may also complicate peripheral blood stem cell collection performed for allogeneic or autologous transplantation.[42]

**Renal Versus Nonrenal $K^+$ Losses.** To discriminate excessive renal from extrarenal $K^+$ losses as a cause for hypokalemia, a 24-hour urine collection for $K^+$ and $Na^+$ content should be performed. Urinary $K^+$ losses of more than 20 mEq/24 hr in the presence of adequate urinary $Na^+$ excretion (>100 mEq/24 hr) is indicative of excessive renal $K^+$ losses. Renal $Na^+$ excretion is measured, because distal nephron $Na^+$ delivery is rate limiting for $K^+$ secretion. If distal nephron $Na^+$ delivery is reduced, as approximated by the urinary $Na^+$ excretion, renal $K^+$ excretion may also be limited and thus mask excessive renal $K^+$ losses. In contrast, extrarenal $K^+$ wasting is expected when urinary $K^+$ excretion is less than 20 mEq/24 hr in the presence of adequate urinary $Na^+$ excretion. The fractional excretion of $K^+$ has also been used as a discriminating tool. In one study, the mean fractional excretion of $K^+$ in normokalemic subjects was found to be 8%. Patients with hypokalemia resulting from extrarenal $K^+$ losses exhibited a mean fractional excretion of $K^+$ of 2.8%, whereas those in whom renal $K^+$ loss was the main etiologic factor had mean values of 15%.[43]

The transtubular $K^+$ gradient (TTKG) has been proposed to provide a semiquantitative urinary index of the activity of the $K^+$ secretory process in the kidney. This equation describes the ratio of the urinary to venous $K^+$ concentrations after adjusting the urine $K^+$ concentration for medullary water abstraction:

$$\frac{[K^+]\ \text{urine}/[K^+]\ \text{venous blood}}{\text{urine osmolality}/\text{plasma osmolality}}$$

The use of TTKG is restricted to situations in which the urine is not hypotonic and distal nephron sodium delivery is adequate for normal $K^+$ secretion.[44] In a study of hypokalemia resulting from renal $K^+$ wasting (mineralocorticoid excess or diuretics) in humans, the TTKG was higher than 10, whereas the TTKG was less than 2 in conditions of hypokalemia owing to extrarenal $K^+$ losses.[45]

**Cutaneous Losses.** Excessive sweating, typically from intense exertion in hot climates (e.g., marathon runners), promotes excessive $K^+$ losses that may result in hypokalemia.[46] This is a relatively uncommon event, because sweat contains only approximately 5 mEq/L of $K^+$ and cutaneous losses of greater than 10 L would be required to deplete total body $K^+$ stores.

**Gastrointestinal Losses.** Excessive vomiting and nasogastric suction promote hypokalemia both by direct loss of $K^+$ in the gastric contents and by the consequent renal $K^+$ losses associated with metabolic alkalosis. Furthermore, if volume depletion ensues, secondary hyperaldosteronism aggravates renal and colonic $K^+$ losses. Hypokalemia often occurs in lower-weight bulimic or anorectic/bulimic patients and may also be a complication of hyperemesis gravidum.[47, 48]

Diarrheal states, intestinal fistulas, laxative abuse, and the use of oral cation exchange resins promote excessive fecal $K^+$ losses. In patients with cholera, for example, daily stool losses of $K^+$ may be substantial. Similarly, watery diarrhea, hypokalemia, and achlorhydria (WDHA) syndrome, an unusual paraneoplastic condition caused by excess vasoactive intestinal polypeptide (VIP) secreted by certain tumors,[49] may develop profound hypokalemia. Oral sodium phosphate administered as a bowel preparation for endoscopy may be complicated by hypokalemia.[50] In hypokalemia related to excessive stool losses, the presence of a nonanion gap metabolic acidosis with normal urinary acidification (as judged by urine pH and the urinary anion gap) often points to these disorders. If diarrhea is associated with severe volume depletion, however, high anion gap metabolic acidosis, owing to lactic acidemia, may evolve as well. In diarrheal states, the intestinal $K^+$ absorptive mechanisms are generally not disturbed, but fecal $K^+$ losses are increased by unabsorbed anions (which obligate $K^+$), by electrochemical gradients driven by active $Cl^-$ secretion, and by secondary hyperaldosteronism. In chronic diarrheal states, total body $K^+$ can be reduced by two mechanisms: loss of muscle mass because of malnutrition and reduced net absorption of $K^+$; only the latter causes hypokalemia. In cases of voluminous diarrhea accompanied by severe metabolic acidosis and volume depletion, distal nephron $Na^+$ delivery may be limited and promote excessive urinary $K^+$ excretion.

**Renal Losses.** Renal $K^+$ wasting represents the most common cause of hypokalemia. Primary increases in mineralocorticoids, distal $Na^+$ delivery, or reabsorption of $Na^+$ in the presence of a nonreabsorbable anion are the principal mechanisms for renal excessive $K^+$ losses. In general, assessment of the blood pressure and effective arterial blood volume aid in the discrimination of a primary increase in mineralocorticoids from a primary increase in distal $Na^+$ delivery.

**Drugs.** Diuretics, particularly the loop diuretics and thiazides, generate renal $K^+$ wasting and commonly produce hypokalemia. Careful monitoring of volume status and serum $K^+$ concentration, dosage adjustment, and replacement of electrolyte losses help to mitigate this complication. Some penicillin derivatives, such as ticarcillin and carbenicillin, generate nonreabsorbable anions that obligate excessive renal $K^+$ losses. Toluene intoxication may also present with hypokalemia.

Renal $K^+$ wasting and hypokalemia are common complications of amphotericin B therapy. Amphotericin B diluted in a lipid emulsion seems to be associated with a smaller number of acute adverse events and fewer cases of hypokalemia than does amphotericin B diluted in 5% dextrose.[51] A review of the published clinical data suggests that amiloride may be effective in preventing amphotericin B–related hypokalemia and hypomagnesemia. In patients treated with amphotericin B who have preserved glomerular filtration rate (GFR) and are at high risk for adverse events resulting from these electrolyte disorders, amiloride therapy should be considered.[52, 53]

Therapy with cisplatin,[54] ifosfamide,[55] or aminoglycosides[56] is also commonly complicated by renal $K^+$ wasting and hypokalemia. In these cases, coincident renal $Mg^2$ wasting and hypomagnesemia may occur and aggravate the hypokalemia and replacement of $K^+$ stores.[57] Chinese herbal medicines and teas also promote hypokalemia in some patients.[58] Sirolimus, which is used as therapy in the prophylaxis of acute renal transplant rejection, may also induce hypokalemia.[59]

**Intrinsic Renal Disease.** The interstitial nephritides, the diuretic phase of acute tubular necrosis, postobstructive diuresis, salt-wasting nephropathies, and lysozymuria in leukemic patients may promote excessive renal $K^+$ losses and hypokalemia. Both proximal and distal renal tubular acidoses commonly present with hypokalemia in addition to their hyperchloremic metabolic acidosis.

**Hypomagnesemia.** Magnesium depletion inhibits net $Na^+$ absorption by the thick ascending limb of Henle and often results in renal $K^+$ wasting[60, 61] and hypokalemia. Hypomagnesemia is often associated with hypokalemic metabolic alkalosis and with hypocalcemia. Hypokalemia and hypomagnesemia are commonly encountered in malnourished alcoholics and in patients receiving cisplatin.[57] Restoration of magnesium levels is essential for effective $K^+$ repletion in concurrent hypokalemia.

**Metabolic Acidosis.** Metabolic acidosis inhibits proximal tubular NaCl absorption.[62] If severe, this can limit distal $Na^+$ delivery and promote renal $K^+$ wasting. In cases of voluminous diarrhea accompanied by severe metabolic acidosis and volume depletion, urinary $K^+$ excretion may exceed 20 mEq/day and erroneously suggest mineralocorticoid excess as the primary cause of hypokalemia.

## Disorders of Mineralocorticoid Excess

**Primary Aldosteronism.** Patients with autonomous production of aldosterone classically present with hypertension, hypokalemia, elevated aldosterone levels, and suppressed plasma renin levels, but these features may be normal in some cases or early in the course of the disease. Primary aldosteronism is generally caused by aldosterone-producing adenomas (Conn syndrome), which are typically unilateral or bilateral idiopathic adrenal hyperplasia, adrenal carcinomas, familial disorders, or occur in sporadic cases. A simple and direct diagnostic test for primary aldosteronism has not yet been developed. The most commonly used screening test in patients with spontaneous hypokalemia in whom primary aldosteronism is suspected measures the random and ambulatory plasma aldosterone (PA) concentrations to plasma renin activity (PRA) (ng/mL/hr). A positive screen is demonstrated when the plasma aldosterone–plasma renin activity ratio is greater than 20 ng/dL, the plasma aldosterone concentration is greater than 15 ng/dL, and the plasma renin activity is less than 2.0. A plasma aldosterone concentration–plasma renin activity ratio higher than 20 alone is not diagnostic of primary aldosteronism. Primary aldosteronism is distinguished from volume contraction by demonstrating inappropriate aldosterone secretion with either the intravenous saline suppression test or measurement of 24-hour urinary aldosterone while on a high-sodium diet and after $K^+$ stores have been repleted. If imaging reveals normal-appearing adrenals or ambiguous findings, adrenal venous sampling or noriodocholesterol scintigraphy helps to solve these clinical dilemmas. Evaluation of the glucocorticoid status of the patient should also be performed.

Patients with *aldosterone-producing adenoma* are usually treated with unilateral adrenalectomy, and patients with idiopathic hyperplasia are treated medically. The subtype evaluation may require one or more tests, the first of which is imaging the adrenals with computed tomography (CT). Magnetic resonance imaging is also gaining favor in the diagnosis of these lesions.[63] When CT reveals a solitary unilateral macroadenoma (>1 cm) and normal contralateral adrenal morphology in a patient with primary aldosteronism, unilateral transperitoneal laparoscopic adrenalectomy has become the treatment of choice in many centers.[64]

Familial hyperaldosteronism is an unusual autosomal disorder that presents with hypokalemia and hypertension beginning in childhood and occurs as two subtypes. In familial hyperaldosteronism type I (FH-I, also called *glucocorticoid-suppressible hyperaldosteronism*), the underlying genetic defect is a chimeric gene in which regulatory elements of the 11β-hydroxylase gene are fused to the coding region of the aldosterone synthase gene[65, 66] (Table 22–8). The chimeric gene product escapes negative feedback control of aldosterone section, resulting in constitutive aldosterone secretion. Hypokalemia may occur, although many patients have, paradoxically, normal serum [$K^+$] values.[67] Patients with this disorder also exhibit early onset of hemorrhagic stroke and ruptured intracranial aneurysms.[68] Women with FH-I who exhibit chronic hypertension appear to be susceptible to exacerbations of hypertension during pregnancy.[53]

**Familial Hyperaldosteronism Type II (FH-II).** This type is characterized by aldosterone hypersecretion due to adrenocortical hyperplasia or an aldosterone-producing adenoma that is not suppressible by glucocorticoids. Linkage analysis of one large kindred demonstrated that the *CYP11B2* gene is not responsible for FH-II in this family.[69]

**Idiopathic Primary Aldosteronism.** In unusual cases, evidence of primary hyperaldosteronism may occur without evidence of affected family members or adrenal pathology. Genetic linkage studies in patients with this disorder demonstrated polymorphisms in the *CYP11B2* gene encoding aldosterone synthase.[70] These data suggest that dysregulation of aldosterone synthesis may contribute to or increase susceptibility to the disease.

All of these disorders of primary aldosteronism must be distinguished from cases of a primary increase in renin production. Many patients presenting with malignant hypertension exhibit hypokalemia. Many patients with renal artery stenosis and consequent hyperreninemia have hypokalemia.[71] More rarely, a renin-secreting tumor may be responsible for refractory hypertension (in a young patient), hyperreninism, and hypokalemia.[72, 73]

**Bartter Syndrome.** Bartter syndrome represents a group of autosomal recessive tubulopathies characterized by hypokalemia with renal $K^+$ and salt wasting, hypochloremia, metabolic alkalosis, and normal or low blood pressure despite hyperreninemia and secondary hyperaldosteronism (see Table 22–8). Three subclasses of the disease have been identified. *Antenatal Bartter syndrome* (also called hyperprostaglandin E syndrome) is a severe form that often presents with maternal polyhydramnios, prematurity, postnatal polyuria and dehydration, and hyposthenuria. Hypercalciuria with normal serum magnesium concentrations and nephrocalcinosis are typically evident. Defective $Na^+$ reabsorption resulting from mutations in the (*SLC12A1*) gene encoding the bumetanide-sensitive Na-K-2Cl cotransporter NKCC2 or the *KCNJ1* gene[69, 74] encoding the inwardly rectifying $K^+$ channel ROMK residing in the thick ascending limb of the loop of Henle gives rise to this syndrome. ROMK functions to recycle $K^+$ entering cells of the thick limb back into the lumenal fluid facilitating sodium reabsorption by the Na-K-2Cl cotransporter. *Classical Bartter syndrome* often presents in infancy with dehydration and is associated with hypomagnesemia in approximately 25% of cases and normal or increased calciuria. This form appears to be related to loss-of-function mutations in the *CLCNKB* gene encoding the voltage-gated chloride channel CLC-Kb in the thick ascending limb of Henle,[75, 76] impairing chloride reabsorption. No subclassification of Bartter syndrome fits all cases, because patients may present with overlapping features of the forms, or, rarely, with diabetes mellitus[77] or sensorineural deafness[78, 79]. Patients with *Gitelman syndrome* additionally exhibit renal magnesium wasting and hypocalciuria (see Table 22–8). Patients with Gitelman syndrome are often recognized by chance or present in childhood or adolescence with muscular weakness, constipation,

**TABLE 22–8.** Genomic Disorders Producing Hypokalemia

| Clinical Disorder | Clinical Presentation | ↑ BP | Renin Aldosterone | Genomic Defect | Plasma $[Mg^{2+}]$ |
|---|---|---|---|---|---|
| Bartter syndrome | • Infancy<br>• Failure to thrive, dehydration, unexpected laboratory finding<br>• Hypokalemic metabolic alkalosis<br>• Hypercalciuria | No | ↑ Renin<br>↑ Aldosterone | Loss of function mutations in<br>• CLCNKB (gene encoding a voltage-gated $Cl^-$ channel in mTAL)<br>• SLC12A3 (gene encoding the bumetanide-sensitive Na-K-2Cl cotransporter of mTAL)<br>• KCNJ1 (gene encoding inwardly-rectifying $K^+$ channel in mTAL) | Low |
| Gitelman syndrome | • Childhood or adolescence<br>• Constipation, muscle weakness, tetanies, unexpected lab finding<br>• Hypokalemic metabolic alkalosis<br>• Hypocalciuria | No | ↑ Renin<br>↑ Aldosterone | • Loss-of-function mutation in SLC12A3 (gene encoding the bumetanide-sensitive Na-K-2Cl cotransporter of mTAL) | Low |
| Liddle syndrome | • Childhood or adolescence<br>• Hypokalemic metabolic alkalosis<br>• Family history of hypertension and hypokalemia | Yes | ↓ Renin<br>Normal/near-normal aldosterone | Constitutive activating mutations of SCNN1B, and SCNN1G (genes encoding the β and γ subunits of the epithelial $Na^+$ channel) | Normal |
| AME | • Children<br>• Hypokalemic metabolic alkalosis<br>• Increased incidence of CVA<br>• Increased urine cortisone-cortisol | Yes | ↓ Renin<br>↓ Aldosterone | Loss of function mutation in HSD11B2 (gene encoding 11β-HSD2 gene) | Normal |
| CAH | • Children<br>• Hypokalemic metabolic alkalosis<br>• 11β-Hydroxylase deficiency: virilization<br>• 17α-Hydroxylase deficiency: hypogonadism, male pseudohermaphrodism | Yes | ↓ Renin<br>↓ Aldosterone | Loss of function mutations in<br>• CYP11B1 (gene encoding 11β-hydroxylase)<br>• CYP17 (gene encoding 17α-hydroxylase) | Normal |
| FH-I (GRA) | • Hypokalemia in some patients<br>• DEX-suppressed aldosterone release<br>• ↑ Cortisol C-18 oxidation metabolites | Yes | ↓ Renin<br>↓ Aldosterone | Chimera between regulatory elements of the gene encoding 11β-HSD2 and the coding sequence of aldosterone synthase | Normal |

AME, apparent mineralocorticoid excess; BP, blood pressure; CAH, congenital adrenal hyperplasia; CVA, cerebrovascular accident; DEX, dexamethasone; 11β-HSD2, 11β-hydroxysteroid dehydrogenase type II; GRA, glucocorticoid remediable aldosteronism; MTAL, medullary thick ascending limb of Henle's loop.

or tetanies resulting from hypokalemia and hypomagnesemia. The disease has been linked to mutations in the *SLC12A3* gene encoding the thiazide-sensitive Na-Cl cotransporter NCCT in the distal convoluted tubule.[80–83]

## Disorders Mimicking Aldosterone Excess

**Liddle Syndrome.** Patients with this rare autosomal dominant form of salt-sensitive hypertension typically present with clinical and biochemical findings consistent with hyperaldosteronism yet have normal or minor elevations in plasma aldosterone levels (see Table 22–8). Mutations in the β and γ subunits of the epithelial sodium channel (ENaC[84, 85]) responsible for $Na^+$ transport in the cortical collecting duct appear to promote constitutive activation of the channel, resulting in enhanced sodium reabsorption, secondarily increased $K^+$ and $H^+$ secretion, and the evolution of hypokalemic metabolic alkalosis with volume expansion and hypertension. These patients exhibit no beneficial response to SV-9055, an inhibitor of aldosterone secretion, or to spironolactone, a mineralocorticoid receptor antagonist. Amiloride and triamterene, inhibitors of the epithelial sodium channel, normalize blood pressure and serum $K^+$ levels of these patients.[86]

**Apparent Mineralocorticoid Excess.** In vitro, cortisol and aldosterone have a similar affinity for the mineralocorticoid receptor. The 11β-hydroxysteroid dehydrogenase type II enzyme catalyzes the interconversion of cortisol to its inactive 11-oxo-metabolite cortisone (Fig. 22–2). This interconversion is in part responsible for the in vivo specificity of the mineralocorticoid receptor. A defect of the 11β-hydroxysteroid dehydrogenase type II enzyme leads to hypertension, hypokalemia, and low renin levels despite subnormal or normal levels of aldosterone and other known mineralocorticoids ("pseudohyperaldosteronism"). A rare hyperten-

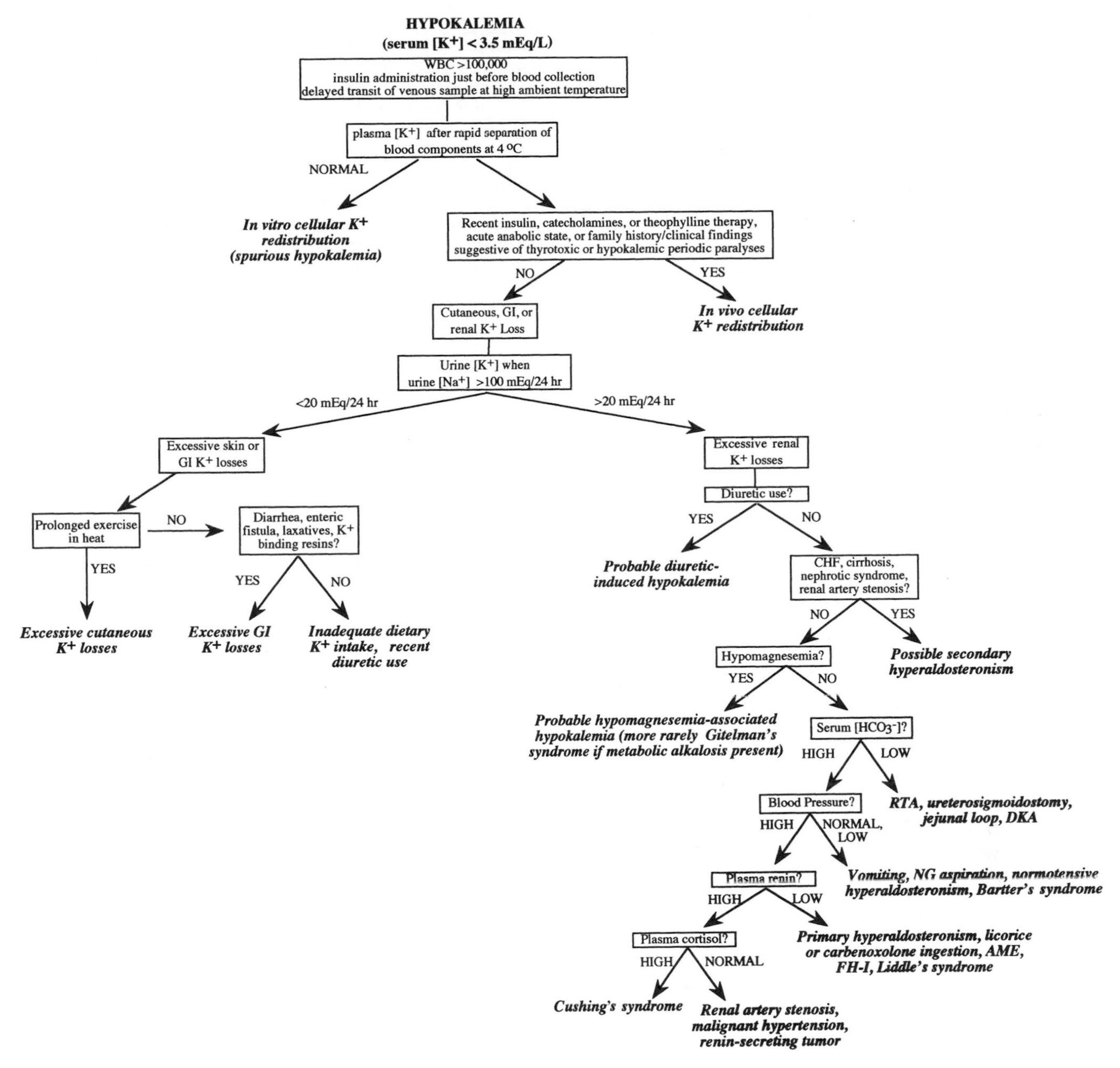


**FIGURE 22–2** ■ Effects of aldosterone on target gene transcription. Aldosterone mediates its effects through binding to nuclear mineralocorticoid receptors (MR). In the absence of hormone, latent MR is present in the cytoplasm in a complex comprised of hsp90 and other stress family proteins. Binding of aldosterone to the MR induces a conformational change in the receptor that promotes dissociation of the ligand-activated receptors from the inhibitory complex and rapid export of the hormone-receptor complex to the nucleus, where it binds to glucocorticoid response elements (GRE). The selective effect of aldosterone on target epithelia relates principally to 11β-hydroxysteroid dehydrogenase II (11β-HSD2) activity. 11β-HSD2 converts corticosterone and cortisol into 11-dehydrocorticosterone and cortisone, respectively, which have little affinity for the MR. Aldosterone, an enzyme-resistant steroid, therefore binds to MR relatively free from competing ligand.

sive syndrome, called the *apparent mineralocorticoid excess syndrome,* results from mutations in the 11β-hydroxysteroid dehydrogenase type II gene (see Table 23–8). The biochemical marker of this disorder is an increased ratio of tetrahydrocortisol plus allotetrahydrocortisol/tetrahydrocortisone in the urine. These patients experience early onset of hypertension and are at increased risk for cerebrovascular events. Dexamethasone is used to treat these patients but often fails to control blood pressure over the long term. A few cases of a second form of apparent mineralocorticoid excess, called type II, have been described that differ from the classic form in that the urinary tetrahydrocortisol plus allotetrahydrocortisol/tetrahydrocortisone is normal. Additional variants of the 11β-hydroxysteroid dehydrogenase type II gene may contribute to the enhanced blood pressure response to salt in humans.[87]

Acquired forms of apparent mineralocorticoid excess result from treatment with gossypol, which was developed as a male infertility drug [88] and is now being tested for antitumor activity in patients with recurrent gliomas,[89] or excessive ingestion of carbenoloxone or licorice, all of which inhibit the activity of the 11β-hydroxysteroid dehydrogenase type II gene. Carbenoxolone inhibits the reverse 11-oxoreductase reaction leading to somewhat different abnormalities of urinary cortisol/cortisone. The aldosterone-like effects of licorice have traditionally been attributed to glycyrrhizic acid, but its biochemical substrate has remained elusive. It is now known that glycyrrhetenic acid,[90, 91] the hydrolytic metabolite of glycerrhizic acid, is the active component of licorice. Glycyrrhetenic acid inhibits the peripheral metabolism of cortisol, leading to relative cortisol excess. Because cortisol binds with the same affinity as aldosterone to the mineralocorticoid receptor, a hypermineralocorticoid condition occurs.

**Other Disorders of Steroid Metabolism Promoting Renal $K^+$ Wasting.** *Congenital adrenal hyperplasia* is a rare congenital abnormality resulting from the absence of 11β-hydroxylase or 17α-hydroxylase[92] (see Table 22–8). These enzymatic disturbances result in sustained secretion of corticotropin-releasing hormone and, consequently, high levels of 11-deoxycorticosterone. 11-Deoxycorticosterone escapes metabolism by 11β-hydroxysteroid dehydrogenase II and consequently exerts potent mineralocorticoid action. Patients with 11β-hydroxylase deficiency manifest virilization, whereas those with 17α-hydroxylase deficiency typically present with absence of sex hormones.[93] Similarly, patients with severe *Cushing syndrome* or *ectopic adrenocorticotropin syndrome*[94] may have levels of circulating cortisol that exceed the capacity of 11β-hydroxysteroid dehydrogenase II to metabolize it. The excess cortisol, by virtue of its ability to bind to the mineralocorticoid receptor, exerts mineralocorticoid effects and promotes hypokalemia.

## THERAPY

**Goals of Therapy.** Therapy of hypokalemia is aimed at preventing life-threatening complications, reducing ongoing $K^+$ losses, correcting the total body $K^+$ deficit, and correcting the underlying disorder. When considering the rate and means by which $K^+$ is replaced, the benefits of correcting depleted $K^+$ stores should be carefully weighed against the risk of hyperkalemia from overcorrection and its attendant adverse effects (Table 22–9). The severity and pace of decline of hypokalemia should be judged, because a sudden or rapid fall in the serum [$K^+$] below 2.5 mEq/L carries the risk of dangerous arrhythmias and requires immediate $K^+$ replacement therapy. In general, the oral/enteral route should be used if possible, because it does not produce sudden large increases in plasma $K^+$ concentrations. It is important that renal function is assessed and judged to be adequate for the $K^+$ to be administered.

**Oral Therapy.** If the serum $K^+$ is in the range of 3 to 3.4 mEq/L and the patient is asymptomatic, oral or enteral therapy may suffice.

In general, 40 mEq of KCl elixir can be given; the serum $K^+$ is measured 4 hours later; and the dose can be repeated if needed.

**TABLE 22–9.** Principles of Therapy for Hypokalemia

Assess the risk-benefit ratio for therapy
- Severity and pace of decline of hypokalemia
- Presence of hypokalemia-associated signs or symptoms
- Presence of life-threatening conditions associated with hypokalemia (e.g., cardiac arrhythmias, acute MI, digitalis intoxication, severe muscle weakness or paralysis, respiratory failure)
- Assess adequacy of renal function: current BUN, creatinine, and urine output

Determine urgency and appropriate route of administration
- Enteral route is preferred

IV administration only if:
- Enteral access not available or contraindicated *or*
- Urgent repletion is warranted by associated conditions

Special situations
- If hypokalemic acidosis, treat hypokalemia before correcting acidosis
- If hypovolemic and hypokalemic with $Cl^-$-responsive metabolic alkalosis and hypovolemia, avoid overly vigorous volume expansion

BUN, blood urea nitrogen; IV, intravenous; MI myocardial infarction.

If this route cannot be used, a maximum KCl concentration of 20 mEq/100 mL can be administered via a central or peripheral intravenous line at a maximum rate of 10 mEq/hr. At these infusion rates, ECG monitoring is generally not needed and peripheral veins are not damaged.

Intravenous $K^+$ replacement therapy should generally be restricted to cases in which the enteral route cannot be used (e.g., lack of enteral access, enteral use contraindicated) or the patient is experiencing hypokalemia-associated signs or symptoms. Before ordering intravenous $K^+$ replacement, the degree of hypokalemia, the presence of hypokalemia-associated signs or symptoms, and the availability of ECG monitoring should be considered. It is important that all sources of $K^+$—the KCl prescribed as replacement therapy together with the KCl or potassium phosphate in total parenteral nutrition or maintenance intravenous fluids—be included in the calculation of the maximum intravenous infusion rate. Intravenous KCl is usually used unless concomitant hypophosphatemia (recovery from a catabolic state, diabetic ketoacidosis being treated with insulin) is present, in which case $K^+$ phosphate is sometimes used. When $K^+$ phosphate (3 mmol phosphate/mL and 4.4 mEq $K^+$/mL) is used, it should generally be infused at a rate of less than 50 mmol over 8 hours to avoid the risk of metastatic calcification and hypocalcemia. In a study of critically ill patients in a surgical ICU with hypophosphatemia, it was concluded that 15 mmol $K^+$ phosphate given IV over 3 hours to patients with mild-to-moderate hypophosphatemia (serum phosphate concentration of 1.27 to 2.48 mg/dL) was both safe and effective, whereas administration of 30 mmol $K^+$ phosphate to severely hypophosphatemic (serum phosphate concentration of 1.24 mg/dL or less) patients was safe but often required repeated doses to achieve normalization of phosphate levels.[95] $K^+$ phosphate can be used in patients with coincident hypokalemia and hypophosphatemia, such as patients with diabetic ketoacidosis receiving insulin or those in the acute recovery phase from a catabolic disorder.

In the setting of metabolic acidosis (e.g., diabetic ketoacidosis), it is preferable to correct the $K^+$ deficit with KCl to safer levels before administering phosphate or $HCO_3^-$. Similarly, glucose should not be given concomitantly with $K^+$ for treatment of severe hypokalemia unless warranted by hypoglycemia, because it will promote insulin release and cellular uptake of $K^+$ and thus worsen the hypokalemia. Therefore, KCl should be mixed in normal saline or half-normal saline when given for treatment of hypokalemia. In addition, volume repletion in patients presenting with $Cl^-$-responsive metabolic alkalosis and severe hypokalemia should be approached cautiously until the hypokalemia is corrected. Bicarbonaturia associated with volume expansion in this setting may aggravate renal $K^+$ wasting and worsen hypokalemia.

Urgent replacement is often required when hypokalemia-related ECG abnormalities, acute myocardial infarction, respiratory failure from respiratory muscle paralysis, digitalis intoxication, marked muscle weakness or tetany, or hepatic coma is present. Initial therapy should be directed toward rapidly restoring serum $K^+$ levels so that the life-threatening potential is mitigated. Repletion of the deficit of total body $K^+$ can then be more cautiously approached. For severe hypokalemia (typically serum $K^+$ <2.5 mEq/L) with acute hypokalemia-associated symptoms, KCl at a concentration of up to 40 mEq/L can be infused at a maximum rate of 20 mEq/hr via a peripheral or central vein with close monitoring of the ECG and the neuromuscular examination, preferably in an ICU setting. If cardiac dysrhythmia, respiratory failure from muscle paralysis, or severe hepatic encephalopathy related to severe hypokalemia is present, maximum infusion rates of 40 to 60 mEq $K^+$/hr can be given via a central vein with ECG monitoring in an ICU. In all cases, serum $K^+$ levels should be monitored frequently (at least every 2 to 4 hours depending on the response) to avoid hyperkalemia. Once the complicating disorder associated with hypokalemia is effectively treated by rapid therapy, repletion of total $K^+$ stores can be more cautiously approached.

**Chronic Therapy.** Microencapsulated and sustained-release forms of KCl tend to produce fewer gastrointestinal disturbances than do wax-matrix tablets or liquid preparations. Although wax-matrix preparations are generally well tolerated, they have been associated with gastric ulcerations. Oral replacement therapy includes K-rich foods, and KCl preparations in liquid, microencapsulated, and wax-matrix preparations. A banana contains approximately 6 mEq of $K^+$. Salt substitutes that contain several $K^+$ salts (Table 22–10) are available for correction of $K^+$ losses: $K^+$ chloride, $K^+$ phosphate, $K^+$ bicarbonate, and $K^+$ magnesium citrate. $K^+$ chloride is typically given for patients with hypokalemia, particularly when it is complicated by metabolic acidosis. $K^+$ phosphate can be used in patients with coincident hypokalemia and hypophosphatemia, such as patients with diabetic ketoacidosis receiving insulin or those in the acute recovery phase from a catabolic disorder. Some caution must be used in these situations, because symptomatic hypocalcemia has been reported in children with diabetic ketoacidosis treated with intravenous $K^+$ phosphate.[96] In these cases, an initial correction of the serum $K^+$ concentration with $K^+$ chloride followed by repletion of phosphate should be considered. KMg Citrate 4 tablets per day (24 mEq $K^+$, 12 mEq magnesium, and 36 mEq citrate per day) were effective in treating thiazide-induced hypokalemia. Four tablets are needed to correct thiazide-induced hypokalemia and to increase urinary pH and citrate sufficiently to prevent stones. Higher dosages are probably required to prevent magnesium loss and adverse symptoms of thiazide therapy.[97]

**TABLE 22–10.** Dietary Sources for $K^+$ Supplementation

| >10 mg $K^+$/g | >5 mg $K^+$/g | >2.5 mg $K^+$/g |
|---|---|---|
| Dried figs | Dried dates, prunes | Fruits |
| Seaweed | Nuts | Bananas |
| Molasses | Lima beans | Oranges |
| | Wheat germ | Cantaloupe |
| | Bran | Mangos |
| | Avocados | Kiwis |
| | | Vegetables |
| | | Tomatoes |
| | | Spinach |
| | | Broccoli |
| | | Beets |
| | | Carrots |
| | | Cauliflower |
| | | Potatoes |
| | | Winter squash |
| | | Meats |
| | | Beef |
| | | Pork |
| | | Veal |
| | | Lamb |

Modified from Gennari FJ: Hypokalemia. N Engl J Med 339:451–458, 1998.

Oral replacement therapy includes dietary sources, including salt substitutes (14 mEq $K^+$/g) and liquid, microencapsulated, and wax-matrix preparations of KCl. Replacement doses should be 40 to 120 mEq/day in divided doses, depending on the patient's weight and level of hypokalemia. Microencapsulated and sustained-release forms of KCl tend to produce fewer gastrointestinal disturbances than do wax-matrix tablets or liquid preparations.


## Acknowledgments

Work in the author's laboratory is sponsored in part by National Institutes of Health grants DK47981, DK-50745, and GM-20529 and an Established Investigatorship from the American Heart Association. The author acknowledges his past and current colleagues in the Division of Renal Diseases and Hypertension at The University of Texas Medical School at Houston for their helpful insights.

## REFERENCES


1. Higham PD, Adams PC, Murray A, Campbell RW: Plasma potassium, serum magnesium and ventricular fibrillation: A prospective study. Q J Med 86:609–617, 1993.
2. Holland OB, Nixon JV, Kuhnert L: Diuretic-induced ventricular ectopic activity. Am J Med 70:762–768, 1981.
3. Ophir O, Peer G, Gilad J, et al: Low blood pressure in vegetarians: The possible role of potassium. Am J Clin Nutr 37:755–762, 1983.
4. Adrogue HJ, Wesson DE: Role of dietary factors in the hypertension of African Americans. Semin Nephrol 16:94–101, 1996.
5. Agarwal R, Afzalpurkar R, Fordtran JS: Pathophysiology of potassium absorption and secretion by the human intestine. Gastroenterology 107:548–571, 1994.
6. Meneton P, Schultheis PJ, Greeb J, et al: Increased sensitivity to $K^+$ deprivation in colonic H,K-ATPase-deficient mice. J Clin Invest 101:536–542, 1998.
7. Surawicz B: Relationship between electrocardiogram and electrolytes. Am Heart J 73:814–834, 1967.
8. Franse LV, Pahor M, Di Bari M, et al: Hypokalemia associated with diuretic use and cardiovascular events in the Systolic Hypertension in the Elderly Program. Hypertension 35:1025–1030, 2000.
9. Iso H, Stampfer MJ, Manson JE, et al: Prospective study of calcium, potassium, and magnesium intake and risk of stroke in women. Stroke 30:1772–1779, 1999.
10. Ascherio A, Rimm EB, Hernan MA, et al: Intake of potassium, magnesium, calcium, and fiber and risk of stroke among US men. Circulation 98:1198–1204, 1998.
11. Fang J, Madhavan S, Alderman MH. Dietary potassium intake and stroke mortality. Stroke 31:1532–1537, 2000.
12. Morris RC Jr, Schmidlin O, Tanaka M, et al: Differing effects of supplemental KCl and $KHCO_3$: Pathophysiological and clinical implications. Semin Nephrol 19:487–493, 1999.
13. Whelton PK, He J, Cutler JA, et al: Effects of oral potassium on blood pressure: Meta-analysis of randomized controlled clinical trials. JAMA 277:1624–1632, 1997.
14. Burgess E, Lewanczuk R, Bolli P, et al: Lifestyle modifications to prevent and control hypertension. 6. Recommendations on potassium, magnesium and calcium. Canadian Hypertension Society, Canadian Coalition for High Blood Pressure Prevention and Control, Laboratory Centre for Disease Control at Health Canada, Heart and Stroke Foundation of Canada. CMAJ 160: S35–S45, 1999.
15. He J, Whelton PK: What is the role of dietary sodium and potassium in hypertension and target organ injury? Am J Med Sci 317:152–159, 1999.
16. Singhal PC, Abramovici M, Venkatesan J, Mattana J: Hypokalemia and rhabdomyolysis. Miner Electrolyte Metab 17:335–339, 1991.
17. Wilcox CS: Metabolic and adverse effects of diuretics. Semin Nephrol 19:557–568, 1999.
18. Tejada F, Cremades A, Aviles M, et al: Hypokalemia alters sex hormone and gonadotropin levels: Evidence that FSH may be required for luteinization. Am J Physiol 275:E1037–E1045, 1998.
19. Gabuzda GJ: Ammonium metabolism and hepatic coma. Gastroenterology 53:806–810, 1967.
20. Soleimani M, Bergman JA, Hosford MA, McKinney TD: Potassium depletion increases luminal $Na^+/H^+$ exchange and basolateral $Na^+:CO_3^-:HCO_3^-$ cotransport in rat renal cortex. J Clin Invest 86:1076–1083, 1990.
21. Hernandez RE, Schambelan M, Cogan MG, et al: Dietary NaCl determines severity of potassium depletion-induced metabolic alkalosis. Kidney Int 31:1356–1367, 1987.
22. Tannen RL, McGill J: Influence of potassium on renal ammonia production. Am J Physiol 231:1178–1184, 1976.
23. Berl T, Linas SL, Aisenbrey GA, Anderson RJ: On the mechanism of polyuria in potassium depletion: The role of polydipsia. J Clin Invest 60:620–625, 1977.
24. Torres VE, Young WF Jr, Offord KP, Hattery RR: Association of hypokalemia, aldosteronism, and renal cysts. N Engl J Med 322: 345–351, 1990.
25. Tolins JP, Hostetter MK, Hostetter TH: Hypokalemic nephropathy in the rat: Role of ammonia in chronic tubular injury. J Clin Invest 79:1447–1458, 1987.
26. Naparstek Y, Gutman A: Case report: Spurious hypokalemia in myeloproliferative disorders. Am J Med Sci 288:175–177, 1984.
27. Masters PW, Lawson N, Marenah CB, Maile LJ: High ambient temperature: A spurious cause of hypokalaemia. BMJ 312:1652–1653, 1996.
28. Braden GL, von Oeyen PT, Germain MJ, et al: Ritodrine- and terbutaline-induced hypokalemia in preterm labor: Mechanisms and consequences. Kidney Int 51:1867–1875, 1997.
29. Deng JF, Jan IS, Cheng HS: The essential role of a poison center in handling an outbreak of barium carbonate poisoning. Vet Hum Toxicol 33:173–175, 1991.
30. Sigue G, Gamble L, Pelitere M, et al: From profound hypokalemia to life-threatening hyperkalemia: A case of barium sulfide poisoning. Arch Intern Med 160:548–551, 2000.
31. Zschiesche W, Schaller KH, Weltle D: Exposure to soluble barium compounds: An interventional study in arc welders. Int Arch Occup Environ Health 64:13–23, 1992.
32. Jordan P, Brookes JG, Nikolic G, Le Couteur DG: Hydroxychloroquine overdose: Toxicokinetics and management. J Toxicol Clin Toxicol 37:861–864, 1999.
33. Lindinger MI: Potassium regulation during exercise and recovery in humans: Implications for skeletal and cardiac muscle. J Mol Cell Cardiol 27:1011–1022, 1995.
34. Zydlewski AW, Hasbargen JA: Hypothermia-induced hypokalemia. Mil Med 163:719–721, 1998.
35. Lawson DH, Murray RM, Parker JL, Hay G. Hypokalaemia in megaloblastic anemias. Lancet 2:588–590, 1970.
36. Ptacek LJ, Tawil R, Griggs RC, et al: Dihydropyridine receptor mutations cause hypokalemic periodic paralysis. Cell 77:863–868, 1994.
37. Tricarico D, Servidei S, Tonali P, et al: Impairment of skeletal muscle adenosine triphosphate-sensitive $K^+$ channels in patients with hypokalemic periodic paralysis. J Clin Invest 103:675–682, 1999.
38. Bulman DE, Scoggan KA, van Oene MD, et al: A novel sodium channel mutation in a family with hypokalemic periodic paralysis. Neurology 53:1932–1936, 1999.
39. Tawil R, McDermott MP, Brown R Jr, et al: Randomized trials of dichlorphenamide in the periodic paralyses. Working Group on Periodic Paralysis. Ann Neurol 47:46–53, 2000.
40. Manoukian MA, Foote JA, Crapo LM: Clinical and metabolic features of thyrotoxic periodic paralysis in 24 episodes. Arch Intern Med 159:601–606, 1999.
41. Severance HW Jr, Holt T, Patrone NA, Chapman L: Profound muscle weakness and hypokalemia due to clay ingestion. South Med J 81:272–274, 1988.
42. Perseghin P, Confalonieri G, Buscemi F, et al: Electrolyte monitoring in patients undergoing peripheral blood stem cell collection. J Clin Apheresis 14:14–17, 1999.
43. Elisaf M, Siamopoulos KC. Fractional excretion of potassium in normal subjects and in patients with hypokalaemia. Postgrad Med J 71:211–212, 1995.
44. West ML, Marsden PA, Richardson RM, et al: New clinical approach to evaluate disorders of potassium excretion. Miner Electrolyte Metab 12:234–238, 1986.
45. Ethier JH, Kamel KS, Magner PO, et al: The transtubular potassium concentration in patients with hypokalemia and hyperkalemia. Am J Kidney Dis 15:309–315, 1990.
46. Knochel JP: Exertional rhabdomyolysis. N Engl J Med 287:927–929, 1972.
47. Greenfeld D, Mickley D, Quinlan DM, Roloff P: Hypokalemia in outpatients with eating disorders. Am J Psychiatry 152:60–63, 1995.
48. Fukada Y, Ohta S, Mizuno K, Hoshi K: Rhabdomyolysis secondary to hyperemesis gravidarum. Acta Obstet Gynecol Scand 78: 71, 1999.
49. Grier JF: WDHA (watery diarrhea, hypokalemia, achlorhydria) syndrome: Clinical features, diagnosis, and treatment. South Med J 88:22–24, 1995.
50. Hill AG, Teo W, Still A, et al: Cellular potassium depletion predisposes to hypokalaemia after oral sodium phosphate. Aust N Z J Surg 68:856–858, 1998.
51. Nucci M, Loureiro M, Silveira F, et al: Comparison of the toxicity

of amphotericin B in 5% dextrose with that of amphotericin B in fat emulsion in a randomized trial with cancer patients. Antimicrob Agents Chemother 43:1445–1448, 1999.
52. Wazny LD, Brophy DF: Amiloride for the prevention of amphotericin B-induced hypokalemia and hypomagnesemia. Ann Pharmacother 34:94–97, 2000.
53. Wyckoff JA, Seely EW, Hurwitz S, et al: Glucocorticoid-remediable aldosteronism and pregnancy. Hypertension 35:668–672, 2000.
54. Milionis HJ, Bourantas CL, Siamopoulos KC, Elisaf MS: Acid-base and electrolyte abnormalities in patients with acute leukemia. Am J Hematol 62:201–207, 1999.
55. Jones DP, Chesney RW: Renal toxicity of cancer chemotherapeutic agents in children: Ifosfamide and cisplatin. Curr Opin Pediatr 7:208–213, 1995.
56. Goodhart GL, Handelsman S: Gentamicin and hypokalemia. Ann Intern Med 103:645–646, 1985.
57. Rodriguez M, Solanki DL, Whang R: Refractory potassium repletion due to cisplatin-induced magnesium depletion. Arch Intern Med 149:2592–2594, 1989.
58. Lee CT, Wu MS, Lu K, Hsu KT: Renal tubular acidosis, hypokalemic paralysis, rhabdomyolysis, and acute renal failure—a rare presentation of Chinese herbal nephropathy. Ren Fail 21:227–230, 1999.
59. Groth CG, Backman L, Morales JM, et al: Sirolimus (rapamycin)-based therapy in human renal transplantation: Similar efficacy and different toxicity compared with cyclosporine. Sirolimus European Renal Transplant Study Group. Transplantation 67: 1036–1042, 1999.
60. Shils ME: Experimental production of magnesium deficiency in man. Ann N Y Acad Sci 162:847–855, 1969.
61. Whang R: Magnesium deficiency: Pathogenesis, prevalence, and clinical implications. Am J Med 82:24–29, 1987.
62. Wang T, Egbert AL Jr, Aronson PS, Giebisch G: Effect of metabolic acidosis on NaCl transport in the proximal tubule. Am J Physiol 274:F1015–F1019, 1998.
63. Sohaib SA, Peppercorn PD, Allan C, et al: Primary hyperaldosteronism (Conn syndrome): MR imaging findings. Radiology 214: 527–531, 2000.
64. Shen WT, Lim RC, Siperstein AE, et al: Laparoscopic vs open adrenalectomy for the treatment of primary hyperaldosteronism. Arch Surg 134:628–632, 1999.
65. Dluhy RG, Lifton RP: Glucocorticoid-remediable aldosteronism. J Clin Endocrinol Metab 84:4341–4344, 1999.
66. Lifton RP, Dluhy RG, Powers M, et al: A chimaeric 11 β-hydroxylase/aldosterone synthase gene causes glucocorticoid-remediable aldosteronism and human hypertension. Nature 355:262–265, 1992.
67. Litchfield WR, Coolidge C, Silva P, et al: Impaired potassium-stimulated aldosterone production: A possible explanation for normokalemic glucocorticoid-remediable aldosteronism. J Clin Endocrinol Metab 82:1507–1510, 1997.
68. Litchfield WR, Anderson BF, Weiss RJ, et al: Intracranial aneurysm and hemorrhagic stroke in glucocorticoid-remediable aldosteronism. Hypertension 31:445–450, 1998.
69. Flagg TP, Tate M, Merot J, Welling PA: A mutation linked with Bartter's syndrome locks Kir 1.1a (ROMK1) channels in a closed state. J Gen Physiol 114:685–700, 1999.
70. Mulatero P, Schiavone D, Fallo F, et al: CYP11B2 gene polymorphisms in idiopathic hyperaldosteronism. Hypertension 35:694–698, 2000.
71. Bunchman TE, Sinaiko AR: Renovascular hypertension presenting with hypokalemic metabolic alkalosis. Pediatr Nephrol 4:169–170, 1990.
72. Haab F, Duclos JM, Guyenne T, et al: Renin secreting tumors: Diagnosis, conservative surgical approach and long-term results. J Urol 153:1781–1784, 1995.
73. Corvol P, Pinet F, Plouin PF, et al: Renin-secreting tumors. Endocrinol Metab Clin North Am 23:255–270, 1994.
74. Simon DB, Lifton RP: The molecular basis of inherited hypokalemic alkalosis: Bartter's and Gitelman's syndromes. Am J Physiol 271:F961–F966, 1996.
75. Simon DB, Bindra RS, Mansfield TA, et al: Mutations in the chloride channel gene, CLCNKB, cause Bartter's syndrome type III. Nat Genet 17:171–178, 1997.
76. Konrad M, Vollmer M, Lemmink HH, et al: Mutations in the chloride channel gene CLCNKB as a cause of classic Bartter syndrome. J Am Soc Nephrol 11:1449–1459, 2000.
77. Venkat Raman G, Albano JD, Millar JG, Lee HA: Bartter's syndrome and diabetes mellitus. J Intern Med 228:525–531, 1990.
78. Brennan TM, Landau D, Shalev H, et al: Linkage of infantile Bartter syndrome with sensorineural deafness to chromosome 1p. Am J Hum Genet 62:355–361, 1998.
79. Landau D, Shalev H, Ohaly M, Carmi R: Infantile variant of Bartter syndrome and sensorineural deafness: A new autosomal recessive disorder. Am J Med Genet 59:454–459, 1995.
80. Simon DB, Nelson-Williams C, Bia MJ, et al: Gitelman's variant of Bartter's syndrome, inherited hypokalemic alkalosis, is caused by mutations in the thiazide-sensitive Na-Cl cotransporter. Nat Genet 12:24–30, 1996.
81. Monkawa T, Kurihara I, Kobayashi K, et al: Novel mutations in thiazide-sensitive Na-Cl cotransporter gene of patients with Gitelman's syndrome. J Am Soc Nephrol 11:65–70, 2000.
82. Lemmink HH, Knoers NV, Karolyi L, et al: Novel mutations in the thiazide-sensitive NaCl cotransporter gene in patients with Gitelman syndrome with predominant localization to the C-terminal domain. Kidney Int 54:720–730, 1998.
83. Bhandari S: The pathophysiological and molecular basis of Bartter's and Gitelman's syndromes. Postgrad Med J 75:391–396, 1999.
84. Tamura H, Schild L, Enomoto N, et al: Liddle disease caused by a missense mutation of beta subunit of the epithelial sodium channel gene. J Clin Invest 97:1780–1784, 1996.
85. Hansson JH, Nelson-Williams C, Suzuki H, et al: Hypertension caused by a truncated epithelial sodium channel gamma subunit: genetic heterogeneity of Liddle syndrome. Nat Genet 11: 76–82, 1995.
86. Warnock DG: Liddle syndrome: An autosomal dominant form of human hypertension. Kidney Int 53:18–24, 1998.
87. Ferrari P, Krozowski Z: Role of the 11beta-hydroxysteroid dehydrogenase type 2 in blood pressure regulation. Kidney Int 57: 1374–1381, 2000.
88. Song D, Lorenzo B, Reidenberg MM: Inhibition of 11 beta-hydroxysteroid dehydrogenase by gossypol and bioflavonoids. J Lab Clin Med 120:792–797, 1992.
89. Bushunow P, Reidenberg MM, Wasenko J, et al: Gossypol treatment of recurrent adult malignant gliomas. J Neurooncol 43: 79–86, 1999.
90. Heilmann P, Heide J, Hundertmark S, Schoneshofer M: Administration of glycyrrhetinic acid: Significant correlation between serum levels and the cortisol/cortisone-ratio in serum and urine. Exp Clin Endocrinol Diabetes 107:370–378, 1999.
91. Kato H, Kanaoka M, Yano S, Kobayashi M: 3-Monoglucuronyl-glycyrrhetinic acid is a major metabolite that causes licorice-induced pseudoaldosteronism. J Clin Endocrinol Metab 80: 1929–1933, 1995.
92. White PC, New MI, Dupont B: Congenital adrenal hyperplasia. (1). N Engl J Med 316:1519–1524, 1987.
93. Kater CE, Biglieri EG: Disorders of steroid 17 alpha-hydroxylase deficiency. Endocrinol Metab Clin North Am 23:341–357, 1994.
94. Ulick S, Wang JZ, Blumenfeld JD, Pickering TG: Cortisol inactivation overload: A mechanism of mineralocorticoid hypertension in the ectopic adrenocorticotropin syndrome. J Clin Endocrinol Metab 74:963–967, 1992.
95. Perreault MM, Ostrop NJ, Tierney MG: Efficacy and safety of intravenous phosphate replacement in critically ill patients. Ann Pharmacother 31:683–688, 1997.
96. Zipf WB, Bacon GE, Spencer ML, et al: Hypocalcemia, hypomagnesemia, and transient hypoparathyroidism during therapy with potassium phosphate in diabetic ketoacidosis. Diabetes Care 2: 265–268, 1979.
97. Ruml LA, Gonzalez G, Taylor R, et al: Effect of varying doses of potassium-magnesium citrate on thiazide-induced hypokalemia and magnesium loss. Am J Ther 6:45–50, 1999.

CHAPTER 23

# Hyperkalemia

I. David Weiner, MD ▪ Charles S. Wingo, MD

Hyperkalemia is a common, silent, and potentially lethal clinical condition. It occurs in both outpatients and inpatients. In large part, this is because many medicines that treat common diseases can cause hyperkalemia. If hyperkalemia is not recognized, it can lead to either paralysis or death from cardiac arrest. Fortunately, the pathophysiology of hyperkalemia is relatively well understood, and the treatment is straightforward. Clinical management requires excluding pseudohyperkalemia, assessing the urgency for treatment, and instituting appropriate therapy. Long-term treatment requires identifying the cause and preventing recurrence.

## CLINICAL PRESENTATION

Hyperkalemia can cause adverse effects that range from subtle and difficult to detect to life-threatening. The majority of these effects are related to the influence of potassium on cellular membrane potential or voltage.

The primary determinant of membrane potential in most cells is the ratio of intracellular to extracellular potassium concentrations.[1,2] Under normal conditions, intracellular potassium concentration averages 120 mEq/L, whereas extracellular potassium concentration is approximately 4 mEq/L. Accordingly, a quantitatively small change in extracellular potassium concentration can result in large changes in the intracellular to extracellular potassium ratio, and thus large changes in resting membrane potential. For example, an increase in extracellular potassium concentration from 4 to 6 mEq/L reflects an increase in plasma potassium content of only about 10 mEq (assuming a normal plasma volume of 5 L). Yet this apparently small change in plasma potassium decreases the transmembrane potassium ratio from approximately 30:1 to 20:1. Substantial changes in resting membrane potential ensue, with secondary effects on a number of cellular processes.

The most prominent effect of hyperkalemia is on the myocardium.[3–6] A lower resting membrane potential decreases myocardial cell conduction velocity and increases the rate of repolarization. Decreasing the conduction velocity also leads to an increase in the PR interval and in the width of the QRS complex on the electrocardiogram (ECG). The greater repolarization rate leads to an increased height of the T waves, also known as peaked T waves. A slowed conduction velocity, especially in the presence of peaked T waves, increases the likelihood of ventricular fibrillation, leading to sudden death.

A rough correlation between the ECG findings and the degree of hyperkalemia is often observed, but progression from mild to severe hyperkalemia may be unpredictable. Mild hyperkalemia, 5.5 to 6 mEq/L, is more frequently associated with a balanced increase in the height of the T waves, otherwise known as tenting. More severe hyperkalemia is associated with delayed conduction through the His-Purkinje system and the ventricular myocardium, resulting in an increased PR interval and a longer QRS interval, followed by progressive flattening and eventual absence of P waves. Under extreme conditions, the QRS complex widens sufficiently that it merges with the T wave, resulting in a sine wave pattern. However, the correlation of absolute potassium levels with ECG findings is difficult and depends on a number of factors, including patient sensitivity and the rapidity of hyperkalemia development. Unfortunately, the progression of hyperkalemia from benign to lethal arrhythmias is unpredictable, and any hyperkalemia-induced ECG findings should be considered a medical emergency. Treatment methods are described later.

Hyperkalemia affects cells throughout the body. Skeletal muscles are particularly sensitive to hyperkalemia, resulting in increased weakness and fatigue. This is related in part to the importance of membrane potential for normal contraction of skeletal muscles. Hyperkalemia, particularly if acute, can lead to generalized weakness, which may proceed to paralysis.[7–9] If the hyperkalemia affects respiratory muscles, it can result in severe respiratory depression.[10]

## PATHOPHYSIOLOGY

Serum potassium concentration reflects the balance among potassium intake, potassium excretion, and transcellular potassium shifts. Abnormalities in any of these factors can lead to hyperkalemia. Figure 23–1 summarizes potassium distribution and movement in the body.

### Dietary Intake

Under normal conditions, dietary potassium intake is about 100 mEq/day. Net gastrointestinal tract absorption is generally 90%.[11] Approximately 10% of dietary potassium is excreted in the stool. Changes in gastrointestinal absorption do not result in hyperkalemia.

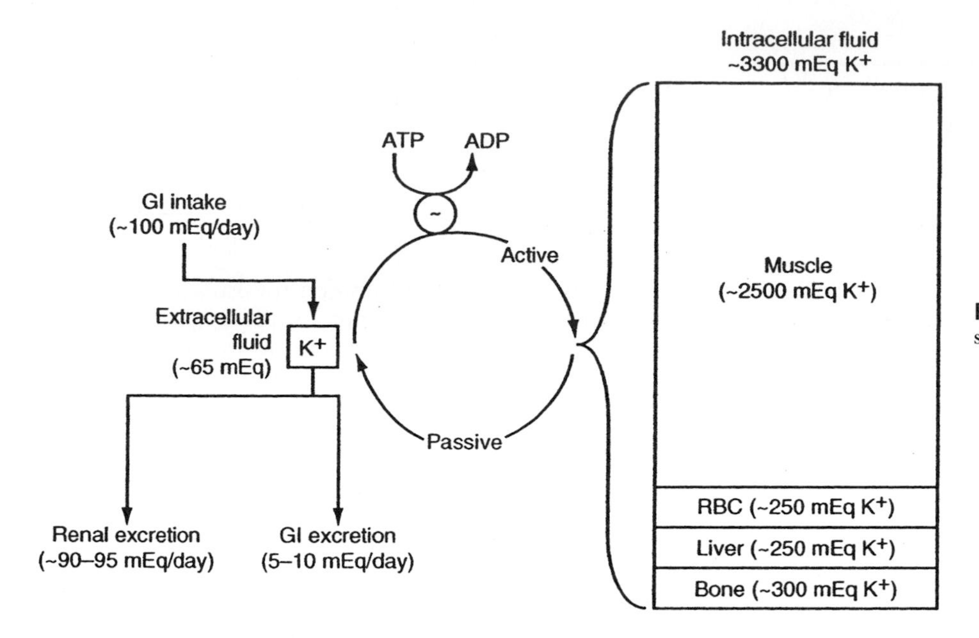


FIGURE 23–1 ■ Summary of potassium intake and excretion mechanisms.

## Renal Potassium Metabolism

Under normal conditions, about 90% of dietary potassium is eliminated via the kidneys, and the great majority of the physiologic response to altered potassium balance is through renal potassium elimination. The colon is responsible for the majority of the remaining potassium excretion.

Sweat contains small amounts of potassium. Under unusual conditions, potassium excretion through sweat can reach clinically significant magnitudes and cause hypokalemia. However, under basal conditions, sweat potassium losses are sufficiently low that decreases do not cause hyperkalemia. Potassium excretion through sweat does not increase appreciably in response to hyperkalemia. Accordingly, sweat potassium excretion does not contribute to potassium homeostasis.

Under normal conditions, the kidney can excrete large quantities of potassium. Ingesting 400 mEq of potassium chloride (KCl) increases serum potassium by less than 1 mEq/L if renal function is normal and potassium excretion mechanisms are intact.[12] This remarkably small increase reflects an increase in renal potassium excretion that parallels changes in potassium intake.

Renal potassium excretion reflects the net balance of glomerular filtration, tubular reabsorption, and tubular secretion. Potassium is freely filtered by the glomerulus, with luminal potassium concentrations equaling serum levels. The majority of filtered potassium is reabsorbed in the proximal tubule and the loop of Henle, with only 10% to 15% of filtered potassium being delivered to the distal tubule.[13, 14] The amount delivered to the distal tubule is relatively constant, even in the presence of hypokalemia or hyperkalemia.[15, 16]

The predominant regulation of renal potassium excretion occurs in the collecting duct.[17, 18] Figure 23–2 summarizes the major potassium transport mechanisms in the collecting duct. At least two cell populations are present in the collecting duct—the principal cell and the intercalated cell—and they appear to have fundamentally different roles in potassium homeostasis.[19, 20] The principal cell is generally modeled to secrete potassium, whereas the intercalated cell reabsorbs potassium.[19, 20]

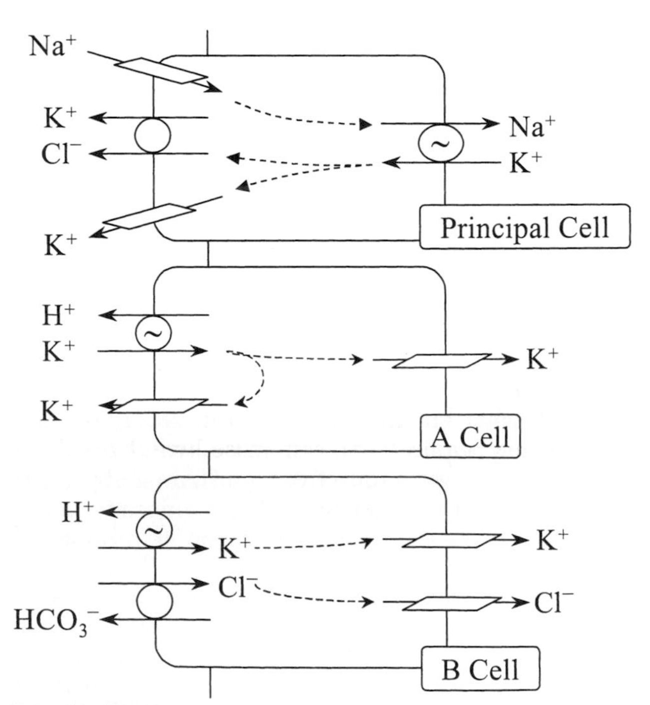


FIGURE 23–2 ■ Summary of potassium transport in the collecting duct. The principal cell secretes potassium via an apical potassium channel in series with basolateral $Na^+$, $K^+$ ATPase. An apical KCl cotransporter may also be present in the principal cell. The A-type intercalated cell (A cell) and the B-type intercalated cell (B cell) both reabsorb potassium via an apical $H^+$, $K^+$ ATPase in series with a peritubular barium-sensitive mechanism, most likely a potassium channel. An apical barium-sensitive transporter, probably a potassium channel, allows potassium recycling when necessary.

In the principal cell, a basolateral $Na^+$, $K^+$ ATPase transports potassium against its electrochemical gradient from the peritubular space into the cytoplasm.[21] Under most circumstances, cellular potassium is secreted into the luminal fluid, down its electrochemical gradient, via an apical potassium channel.[22, 23] To a large extent, the driving force for potassium secretion is regulated by luminal electronegativity generated by active sodium reabsorption through an apical sodium channel. An apical KCl cotransport mechanism, or parallel potassium and chloride transporters, may also contribute to potassium secretion.[24, 25]

Several factors regulate principal cell potassium secretion. Increased urine flow rates and luminal sodium delivery stimulate renal potassium secretion.[26] Oliguria is insufficient to yield hyperkalemia unless renal insufficiency is also present, but prerenal azotemia, as well as obstruction, frequently leads to hyperkalemia.

The mineralocorticoid aldosterone, by binding to the mineralocorticoid receptor, stimulates cortical collecting duct potassium secretion.[27–29] This occurs through stimulation of apical sodium channels, with an increase in both the number of sodium channels and their open probability,[30] and through stimulation of $Na^+$, $K^+$ ATPase. The increased sodium reabsorption makes the lumen more electronegative, which increases the electrochemical driving gradient for potassium secretion via the apical potassium channel.[31]

A second factor that increases potassium secretion is hyperkalemia. Although hyperkalemia stimulates aldosterone production, hyperkalemia also stimulates potassium secretion through mechanisms that are independent of aldosterone.[32, 33] Aldosterone-independent hyperkalemia-stimulated potassium secretion occurs through increases in the density of principal cell apical potassium channels.[34, 35] Gene transcription and translation are not necessary, suggesting that hyperkalemia activates quiescent potassium channels.[31] Hyperkalemia also increases basolateral $Na^+$, $K^+$ ATPase activity, further increasing the principal cells' ability to secrete potassium.[36]

Arachidonic acid metabolites are intracellular signaling molecules that stimulate collecting duct potassium secretion.[37] Inhibition of arachidonic acid production, through the use of nonsteroidal anti-inflammatory medications, can cause hyperkalemia by preventing normal stimulation of principal cell–mediated potassium secretion.[38–40]

## Potassium Reabsorption

In addition to secreting potassium, the collecting duct reabsorbs potassium.[41] Collecting duct intercalated cells possess an apical $H^+$, $K^+$ ATPase ion pump.[42–45] This transporter uses adenosine triphosphate (ATP) as an energy source for proton secretion and potassium reabsorption.[17, 46] Potassium that enters can recycle across the apical membrane via a barium-sensitive transporter, most likely a potassium channel, or can exit across the basolateral membrane, also via a barium-sensitive transport.[47] Net potassium reabsorption is determined by a variety of factors, including apical $H^+$, $K^+$ ATPase activity and the relative permeability of the apical and basolateral barium-sensitive transporters to potassium exit. $H^+$, $K^+$ ATPase–mediated potassium reabsorption appears to be stimulated by a wide variety of factors, including chronic metabolic acidosis,[43] acute respiratory acidosis,[47] and chronic respiratory acidosis.[48] Interestingly, aldosterone does not appear to regulate $H^+$, $K^+$ ATPase–mediated potassium reabsorption,[49] consistent with its role in protecting against hyperkalemia.

## Colon Potassium Secretion

The colon also secretes small amounts of potassium, actuated by chronic aldosterone stimulation and by hyperkalemia. The other mechanisms through which this occurs are not well defined. Some regulation of colonic potassium secretion occurs, particularly in renal insufficiency, although the absolute amounts of potassium secretion remain low.

## Transcellular Potassium Shifts

The great majority of potassium, more than 98% under most conditions, is present in the intracellular fluid compartment. The intracellular and extracellular compartments are not static; there is continuous movement of potassium from one compartment to the other. Potassium is concentrated in the intracellular fluid by a plasma membrane $Na^+$, $K^+$ ATPase that is present in almost all cells. An $Na^+$-$K^+$-$2Cl^-$ cotransporter also contributes to cellular potassium uptake in some cells. Simultaneously, potassium exits cells via a family of potassium channels. The relative rates of potassium uptake and exit determine the absolute amount of intracellular and extracellular potassium. Small changes in the relative rates of potassium transport by these processes can rapidly result in large changes in plasma potassium concentrations.

Several factors can cause transcellular potassium shifts. These include aldosterone, alterations in aldosterone synthesis, acidosis, insulin, β-adrenergic agonists, and exercise. Each of these is discussed in greater detail later. Because 98% of total body potassium is intracellular, relatively small changes in transcellular potassium shifts can have substantial and significant effects on serum potassium concentrations.

### ALDOSTERONE

Aldosterone induces substantial changes in transcellular potassium shifts, enabling it to play a major role in protection against hyperkalemia, even in the absence of its effects on renal potassium excretion. In particular, aldosterone decreases the percentage of total body potassium that is present as plasma potassium, indicating an increase in intracellular amount.[50] Aldosterone may increase intracellular potassium by stimulating $Na^+$, $K^+$ ATPase in both epithelial cells and vascular smooth muscle.[51, 52]

### INSULIN

Insulin induces rapid cellular potassium uptake.[53, 54] This effect occurs within minutes of insulin administration and is dose dependent.[55] Insulin's effect on potassium uptake is independent of its effect on glucose transport[56, 57] and is due to stimulation of $Na^+$, $K^+$ ATPase. Insulin stimulates potassium uptake predominantly in skeletal muscles,[58] but also in adipose tissues[59] and in hepatocytes.[60] Hepatic potassium uptake predominates during the initial hour of insulin-induced potassium uptake, whereas skeletal muscle potassium uptake predominates after the first hour.[61]

### β-ADRENERGIC AGONISTS

β-Adrenergic agonists stimulate transcellular potassium uptake, thereby reducing plasma potassium levels,[62] via $\beta_2$-receptor activation.[63] Activation of this receptor stimulates cellular cyclic adenosine monophosphate (cAMP) production, which leads to activation of $Na^+$, $K^+$ ATPase in both skeletal muscle cells and adipocytes.[64, 65]

β-Adrenergic–stimulated potassium uptake has a potentially important physiologic role in two common conditions. First, cellular uptake of a potassium load is much more efficient when the potassium is given via the gastrointestinal tract as compared with intravenous administration. Oral potassium intake is associated with stimulation of the sympathetic nervous system.[66] This may serve to stimulate, via activation of $\beta_2$-adrenergic receptors, cellular potassium uptake. Teleologically, this may serve to protect against otherwise lethal oral potassium loads.

A second important role for β-adrenergic agonist–mediated stimulation of potassium uptake is in response to exercise. Exercise stimulates skeletal muscle potassium release; increases in plasma potassium can easily exceed 1 mEq/L.[67] Exercise-related stimulation of the sympathetic nervous system serves to minimize the resulting hyperkalemia by stimulating cellular potassium uptake.[67] $\beta_2$-Adrenergic antagonists increase the degree of hyperkalemia that occurs following vigorous exercise, possibly resulting in substantial degrees of hyperkalemia.[67]

### α-ADRENERGIC RECEPTOR ACTIVATION

α-Adrenergic receptor activation causes cellular potassium losses that oppose those of β-adrenergic receptor activation.[68, 69] In humans, $\alpha_1$-adrenergic receptors appear to mediate the majority of this effect.[70] The cellular potassium losses seem to reflect activation of calcium-activated potassium channels,[71, 72] resulting in an increased rate of cellular potassium exit. At least part of this effect reflects activation of hepatic potassium exit.[71]

### HYPEROSMOLALITY

Increases in extracellular osmolality induce shifts of potassium from the intracellular to the extracellular compartment.[73] Presumably, this occurs because hyperosmolality causes cell shrinkage, an increase in intracellular potassium concentration, and a resultant stimulation of potassium extrusion. Even small increases in osmolality, 10 mOsm/kg, can cause detectable, 0.4 mEq/L, increases in plasma potassium.[74] More substantial increases can occur in response to hyperglycemia; the standard 100-g oral glucose tolerance can increase plasma potassium levels by as much as 1.8 mEq/L in susceptible diabetic patients.[75] Hyperosmolality caused by "ineffective osmoles," such as urea, that rapidly cross plasma membranes and therefore do not alter cell size, does not appear to stimulate cellular potassium loss and does not cause hyperkalemia.

# SPECIFIC CAUSES AND EVALUATION

The evaluation of hyperkalemia is a multistep process. First, one should verify that hyperkalemia is not an artifact of the in vitro measurement process. If so, this is termed *pseudohyperkalemia.* Second, one should determine the severity of the hyperkalemia. Finally, one should identify the underlying causes.

## Pseudohyperkalemia

The plasma potassium level may be artificially high when measured and may not reflect the actual potassium level, a condition known as pseudohyperkalemia. Potassium levels are typically measured in blood that has been allowed to clot and is then centrifuged to obtain the plasma. Potassium release from any of the cellular elements of blood can artificially elevate the plasma potassium level.

The diagnosis of pseudohyperkalemia should be considered whenever hyperkalemia and hemolysis, leukocytosis, or thrombocytosis coexist. It should also be considered whenever hyperkalemia occurs in the absence of other identifiable causes or in the absence of appropriate ECG changes. Identifying the presence of pseudohyperkalemia is critical to avoid the complications caused by treating pseudohyperkalemia and thereby inducing actual hypokalemia. This condition can be diagnosed by simultaneously measuring plasma (unclotted blood, obtained using a heparinized syringe) and serum (clotted) potassium levels. If plasma and serum potassium levels differ by more than 0.3 mEq/L, pseudohyperkalemia should be diagnosed, and further clinical decisions should be guided by the plasma, not the serum, potassium concentration.

### HEMOLYSIS

The most common cause of pseudohyperkalemia is hemolysis. This condition is easily identified in the laboratory by the pink tinge to the plasma, resulting from the release of hemoglobin from damaged red blood cells. Centrifuging the specimen before the clot has completely formed predisposes the red blood cells to membrane damage, leading to potassium leakage. In addition, an excessively tight tourniquet surrounding an exercising extremity (e.g., an opening and closing hand) can increase plasma potassium by more than 2 mEq/L.[76]

### THROMBOCYTOSIS

Platelets are the second most common cellular element in plasma, following erythrocytes. At normal platelet concentrations, potassium release from platelets during the clotting process does not measurably alter serum potassium values. However, when thrombocytosis is present, pseudohyperkalemia frequently occurs. The degree of pseudohyperkalemia correlates with the platelet count; as many as 34% of patients with platelet counts between 500 and 1000 $\times$ $10^9$/L exhibit pseudohyperkalemia.[77]

An underlying myeloproliferative condition is not necessary. Reactive thrombocytosis is sufficient to cause pseudohyperkalemia. This condition should be suspected whenever the platelet count is greater than 500 $\times$ $10^9$/L.

### LEUKOCYTOSIS

Potassium release from cells other than red blood cells can cause pseudohyperkalemia. Severe leukocytosis, greater than 70,000/$cm^3$, can lead to pseudohyperkalemia.[78–80] This is independent of the method and timing used to centrifuge the specimen and appears to be related to increased potassium release from the increased number of leukocytes.

### FAMILIAL PSEUDOHYPERKALEMIA

Occasional families have abnormal red blood cell membrane permeability, which leads to excessive potassium leakage and pseudohyperkalemia.[81–83] Specific causes of red blood cell fragility include hereditary spherocytosis[84] and abnormalities in the erythrocyte membrane (hereditary stomatocytosis).[85, 86] In most cases the defect causes an abnormally high rate of erythrocyte potassium loss that occurs at room temperature but not at 37°C.[85]

### OTHER CAUSES

There are rare reports of pseudohyperkalemia from other causes, such as rheumatoid arthritis[87] and infectious mononucleosis.[88] The underlying causes in these cases are unknown, but its occurrence reinforces the possibility that pseudohyperkalemia may be seen in a wide variety of conditions.

## True Hyperkalemia

Several classification methods have been developed for the evaluation of "true" hyperkalemia. We recommend one that is based on the mechanisms that govern potassium homeostasis and that uses common clinical principles. In this schema, hyperkalemia can result from excess intake, inadequate renal excretion, or redistribution between the intra- and extracellular fluid compartments. A careful history and physical examination should be sufficient to differentiate most cases.

### EXCESS POTASSIUM INTAKE

Excessive potassium ingestion is an infrequent cause of hyperkalemia in the absence of other contributing factors. If renal potassium excretion is unimpaired, the normal kidney can excrete hundreds of milliequivalents of potassium daily.[12] However, if renal potassium excretion is impaired, whether through drugs, renal insufficiency, or other causes, then excess potassium intake can produce hyperkalemia.

**Dietary Intake.** The primary means of potassium intake is through the diet.[89] Essentially all foods contain potassium, but the relative amounts of potassium differ greatly in different food groups. Fruits and vegetables tend to contain the highest concentrations of potassium. Table 23–1 lists a number of common high-potassium foods and their potassium content. Consultation with a trained dietitian may be helpful in assessing dietary potassium intake.

Commonly overlooked dietary potassium sources are salt substitutes; KCl is the primary constituent of many salt substitutes. Typical salt substitutes contain 10 to 13 mEq potassium per gram, or 283 mEq per tablespoon.[90]

Other dietary sources are oral and enteral nutritional supplements. Many of these products contain 40 mEq/L KCl or more. Table 23–2 summarizes the potassium content of a number of enteral food sources. When given continuously as an enteral nutritional support, the administration of 100 mL/hr of such products can result in a potassium intake of 100

**TABLE 23–1.** Potassium Content of Selected Foods

| Food | Portion Size | Approximate Potassium Content (mEq) |
|---|---|---|
| Almonds, dry roasted | 4 oz | 20 |
| Artichoke, boiled | 1, medium | 25 |
| Avocado | 1, medium | 40 |
| Banana | 1, medium | 11 |
| Beans, lima | 1 cup | 14 |
| Cantaloupe, cut up | 1 cup | 12 |
| Chocolate bar | 1.5 oz | 4 |
| Figs, dried | 10 | 30 |
| Fish, fillet, cooked | 6 oz | 15 |
| French fries | Medium fast-food portion | 15–20 |
| Grapefruit juice | 8 oz | 40 |
| Hamburger, cooked | 7 oz | 15 |
| Milk | 8 oz | 40 |
| Orange juice | 8 oz | 12 |
| Potato, baked | 7 oz | 20 |
| Raisins | ⅔ cup | 18 |
| Tomato paste | ½ cup | 30 |

**TABLE 23–2.** Potassium Content of Enteral Nutrition Supplements

| | Calories/mL | Potassium (mEq/L) | Sodium (mEq/L) | Osmolality (mOsm/kg) |
|---|---|---|---|---|
| Ensure | 1.06 | 40 | 37 | 470 |
| Ensure Plus | 1.50 | 54 | 49 | 690 |
| Glucerna | 1.00 | 40 | 40 | 375 |
| Osmolite | 1.06 | 26 | 27 | 300 |
| Pulmocare | 1.50 | 49 | 57 | 490 |
| Suplena | 2.00 | 29 | 34 | 615 |
| Ultracal | 1.06 | 41 | 41 | 310 |
| Vivonex T.E.N. | 1.00 | 20 | 20 | 630 |

mEq/day. Patients with renal failure receiving total nutritional support through enteral nutritional supplements frequently develop hyperkalemia.

Potassium is also an essential component of intravenous hyperalimentation fluids. The usually recommended potassium concentrations for hyperalimentation fluids may be excessive for patients with renal insufficiency; close monitoring and frequent reevaluations are necessary for this patient population.

**Medications.** A second major source of potassium is medications. The most obvious medication sources are potassium supplements, such as KCl. These are frequently administered to patients receiving diuretics who may also be taking other medications that predispose to hyperkalemia. In view of the evidence that potassium supplementation decreases blood pressure[91,92] and may improve mineral balance and skeletal calcium metabolism in postmenopausal women,[93] potassium may be prescribed more often for conditions other than hypokalemia in the future. As many as 4% of patients receiving KCl supplements develop hyperkalemia.[94]

Many pharmacies routinely place labels on prescriptions for diuretics, especially loop diuretics, that encourage patients to increase their fruit and vegetable intake in an attempt to prevent the development of hypokalemia. However, for patients with renal insufficiency, diuretic-induced hypokalemia is less of a concern than is hyperkalemia resulting from dietary potassium intake.

Similarly, fruits and vegetables decrease the incidence of ischemic strokes,[95] possibly through their potassium content. Increased use of fruit and vegetable intake as a medical therapy may lead to an increased incidence of hyperkalemia.

Other commonly used potassium-containing medications are penicillin and citrate salts. Penicillin G is supplied as a potassium salt, containing 1.7 mEq of potassium per 1 million U. High-dose penicillin G administration, such as for penicillin-sensitive pneumococcal meningitis, can involve a substantial potassium load and can be fatal.[96] If necessary, sodium penicillin G is available; it does not contain potassium. Although the oral formulation of penicillin, Pen-Vee K, contains potassium, the potassium present in usual doses is insufficient to be clinically important.

Citrate can be supplied as a sodium salt, a potassium salt, or a sodium-potassium salt. Table 23–3 summarizes the potassium content of various citrate preparations. Because certain citrate preparations can provide large amounts of potassium, significant hyperkalemia may develop if one does not monitor serum potassium levels and pay close attention to the type of citrate preparation.

**TABLE 23–3.** Potassium Content of Various Citrate Preparations

| | Potassium (mEq/mL) | Sodium (mEq/mL) | Citrate/ Citric Acid (mEq/mL) |
|---|---|---|---|
| Polycitra-K | 2 | — | 2 |
| Bicitra (Shohl solution) | — | 1 | 1 |
| Polycitra | 1 | 1 | 2 |

## INADEQUATE RENAL POTASSIUM EXCRETION

Chronic hyperkalemia is almost impossible to produce unless renal potassium secretion is impaired. Because the kidney regulates potassium excretion primarily via collecting duct–mediated potassium secretion, factors that affect potassium excretion can be classified into those due to reduced nephron mass (number of functioning collecting ducts) and those due to inhibition of active potassium secretion.

**Reduced Nephron Mass (Renal Insufficiency).** The primary mechanism by which the kidney excretes the daily load of ingested potassium is through active potassium secretion in the collecting duct. Accordingly, in the presence of renal insufficiency, when there is a decreased number of functional collecting ducts, the maximal rate of potassium secretion is decreased, and there is an increased incidence of hyperkalemia.

***Acute Renal Failure.*** In oliguric acute renal failure, the serum potassium level can rise as much as 0.4 mEq/L/day, and if renal failure is complicated by trauma, burns, infection, or other catabolic states, it may increase by 0.7 mEq/L/day or more.[97] When acute tubular necrosis or acute interstitial nephritis causes the acute renal failure, there may be sufficient damage to the collecting duct to blunt the normal increase in potassium secretion, thereby resulting in hyperkalemia. Additionally, ischemic renal failure may impair potassium secretion by suppressing the expression of mRNA for proteins that play an important role in collecting duct potassium secretion—namely, the renal outer medullary collecting duct potassium channel (ROMK) and its regulatory protein, channel-inducing factor (CHIF).[98]

The incidence of hyperkalemia appears to be lower in nonoliguric acute renal failure than in oliguric acute renal failure.[97] In part, this may reflect the observation that nonoliguric acute renal failure indicates a less severe renal injury. It may also reflect a continued ability to excrete potassium, albeit at reduced rates, in nonoliguric acute renal failure, whereas in oliguric acute renal failure, the loss of urine output indicates a loss of renal potassium excretion. This is predictable, because the distal nephron flow rate is a primary determinant of renal potassium excretion.

***Chronic Renal Insufficiency.*** The incidence of hyperkalemia appears to be lower in chronic renal insufficiency than in acute renal insufficiency of equal magnitude. In part, this reflects time for adaptation of collecting duct potassium secretion and increased rates of per nephron potassium secretion.[99, 100] As a result, hyperkalemia is said to be unusual in chronic renal disease unless the glomerular filtration rate is less than 15 mL/min.[99, 101] However, because medications that interfere with normal potassium homeostasis, such as angiotensin-converting enzyme inhibitors (ACEIs), angiotensin receptor antagonists, and aldosterone receptor antagonists (spironolactone), are more frequently used in patients with chronic renal insufficiency, it is likely that the incidence of hyperkalemia will rise. Moreover, the kidney's capacity to further increase potassium excretion in response to acute potassium loads is limited in patients with chronic renal insufficiency.[100, 102]

**Inhibition of Collecting Duct Potassium Secretion.** The great majority of hyperkalemia cases involve impaired collecting duct potassium secretion. Although acute hyperkalemia can occur in response to either acute potassium loads or redistribution, chronic hyperkalemia almost always involves at least a component of impaired renal potassium excretion. Because the collecting duct mediates the great majority of the kidney's regulated potassium transport, almost all cases of chronic hyperkalemia involve abnormal collecting duct potassium transport. Indeed, in the presence of normal renal function and normal tubular function, it is almost impossible to generate chronic hyperkalemia through dietary potassium intake.

Medications are probably the most common causes of impaired collecting duct potassium secretion.[103] A large number of medications inhibit this secretion, and many have multiple effects. Because of the central role that aldosterone plays in potassium homeostasis, through its effects on both collecting duct potassium secretion and transcellular potassium shifts, medications that alter aldosterone metabolism are among the most likely to cause hyperkalemia. Additionally, many of these medications have multiple effects on potassium metabolism that are independent of their effects on aldosterone metabolism.

***β-Adrenergic Antagonists.*** β-Adrenergic antagonists have multiple effects that contribute to the increase in serum potassium levels. First, β-adrenergic antagonists inhibit renin release by the macula densa.[104, 105] Plasma renin activity decreases, resulting in decreased aldosterone production. The $\beta_1$-adrenergic receptor appears to regulate renin release to a greater extent than the $\beta_2$-adrenergic receptor.[106] Indeed, β-receptor antagonist–induced decreases in plasma renin activity may play a role in the antihypertensive effect of this class of drugs.[107–109]

β-Adrenergic antagonists also alter transcellular potassium shifts. Early studies showed that β-adrenergic antagonists increased potassium levels predominantly through a shift from the intracellular to the extracellular space, not through changes in renal excretion.[110] β-Adrenergic antagonists also impair cellular uptake of a potassium load, resulting in greater increments in serum potassium levels.[111]

The combination of these effects—inhibition of renin production, stimulation of transcellular potassium shifts, and impaired tolerance of potassium loads—enables β-adrenergic antagonists to cause hyperkalemia. Patients with either chronic renal insufficiency or diabetes mellitus appear to be at the greatest risk of β-adrenergic antagonist–induced hyperkalemia.

***Angiotensin-Converting Enzyme Inhibitors.*** ACEIs have assumed a key role in current medical therapy because of their multiple beneficial effects. These include controlling hypertension,[112] decreasing mortality in patients with myocardial infarction or congestive heart failure,[113–115] and slowing the progression of chronic renal disease.[116, 117] However, the incidence of hyperkalemia in patients receiving ACEI therapy ranges from 1.2% to 11%.[118, 119] In large part, this is because ACEIs decrease peripheral conversion of angiotensin I to angiotensin II, thereby decreasing angiotensin II–mediated stimulation of adrenal aldosterone production.[120] In addition, ACEIs inhibit potassium-stimulated aldosterone production.[121] This dual effect of ACEIs on aldosterone production leads to hyperkalemia in susceptible individuals. Risk factors for hyperkalemia include underlying renal insufficiency, diabetes mellitus, congestive heart failure, use of long-acting ACEIs, and treatment with other medications that increase potassium levels.[118] A high dietary potassium intake, especially dried fruit, can also increase the risk of hyperkalemia. Because of the clear benefit of ACEIs on clinical outcome in many conditions, one may wish to consider using kaliuretic diuretics, such as thiazide or loop diuretics, to increase urinary potassium excretion in the treatment of ACEI-induced hyperkalemia[118] before discontinuing ACEI therapy.

***Angiotensin Receptor Blockers.*** Angiotensin receptor blockers inhibit the angiotensin II type 1 receptor, which is the receptor for the majority of the effects of angiotensin II in adults, including stimulation of adrenal gland aldosterone synthesis. Relatively few studies have reported the incidence of hyperkalemia with angiotensin receptor blockers; however, the incidence of hyperkalemia appears to be either similar to or slightly less than that observed with ACEIs.[122] Furthermore, early experience suggests that the incidence of hyperkalemia in individuals with renal insufficiency is low.[123] Whether combination therapy with both ACEIs and angiotensin receptor blockers will potentiate the effects of these medications on potassium levels remains to be seen.

***Heparin.*** Heparin can contribute to hyperkalemia by decreasing aldosterone levels.[124–126] Heparin inhibits the adrenal enzyme aldosterone synthase, which is the rate-limiting enzyme for adrenal aldosterone production.[124–126] This effect is specific for the adrenal zona glomerulosa; accordingly, glucocorticoid production is not altered.[126] The effect is dose dependent and may occur with heparin doses as low as 10,000 U/day (5000 U twice a day).[127] Clinically significant changes in potassium levels are generally not seen for 3 to 4 days after initiation of therapy and may require 3 to 4 days to reverse.[126, 128] Low-molecular-weight heparin may inhibit aldosterone synthesis,[129] although some studies suggest that the effect is less marked than with conventional heparin.[130, 131]

***Aldosterone Receptor Antagonists.*** Spironolactone is an effective medication that decreases mortality in chronic congestive heart failure[132, 133] and is also used for the treatment of primary hyperaldosteronism.[134] Because increasing evidence suggests that aldosterone causes detrimental effects that are independent ofitseffects on renal sodium and potassium transport—including inhibition of parasympathetic activity, induction of myocardial and vascular fibrosis, and vascular damage and impairment of arterial compliance[132, 135, 136]—it is likely that spironolactone or other aldosterone receptor antagonists will be used frequently in the future. However, spironolactone can cause hyperkalemia both by inhibiting mineralocorticoid-stimulated renal potassium excretion and by altering transcellular potassium shifts.[137, 138] The incidence of hyperkalemia is dose dependent, with detectable effects even at doses of 25 mg/day.[139] Figure 23–3 summarizes the incidence of hyperkalemia in individuals with congestive heart failure treated with spironolactone.[139]

Risk factors for spironolactone-induced hyperkalemia include the use of long-acting ACEIs, ACEI dose, and baseline elevation of serum creatinine or potassium levels.[139] However, if spironolactone is used at low doses, such as 25 mg/day, the incidence of severe hyperkalemia (>6 mEq/L) is low (about 2%).[132] At higher doses, the risk of severe hyperkalemia increases. In many cases of spironolactone-induced hyperkalemia, the potassium level can be safely decreased with diuretics or reevaluation of dietary potassium intake. Rare cases may necessitate the discontinuation of this medication.

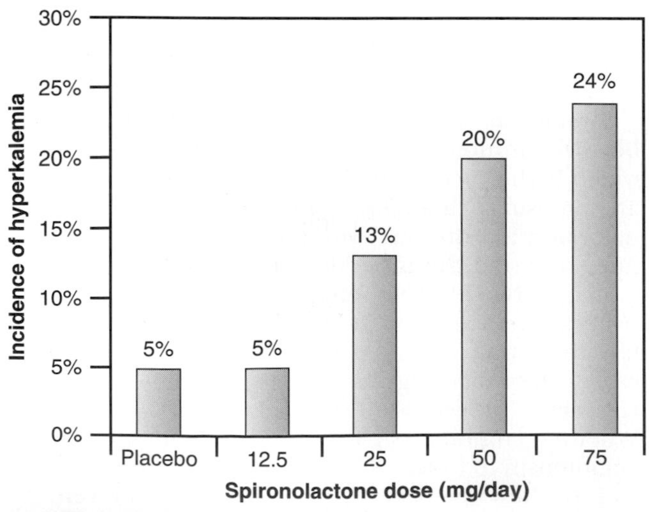


**FIGURE 23–3** ■ Incidence of hyperkalemia in response to spironolactone therapy for New York Heart Association class II to IV congestive heart failure. Hyperkalemia was defined as $[K^+] \geq 5.5$ mEq/L. (Data from Am J Cardiol 78:902–907, 1996.)

***Nonsteroidal Anti-inflammatory Drugs.*** Arachidonic acid metabolites play an important role in collecting duct potassium secretion; they are necessary for normal renin release and aldosterone synthesis,[140–142] and they regulate collecting duct sodium and potassium transport.[142] Because nonsteroidal anti-inflammatory drugs (NSAIDs) reduce arachidonic acid metabolite production, they can exert multifactorial effects on potassium metabolism. Clinically significant hyperkalemia can occur in the absence of underlying renal insufficiency.[103, 141, 143] In most cases, the hyperkalemia responds to discontinuation of the NSAID.

***Potassium-Sparing Diuretics.*** Potassium-sparing diuretics are specifically used to minimize or inhibit collecting duct potassium secretion. Accordingly, it is not surprising that they can cause hyperkalemia. As discussed earlier, collecting duct sodium reabsorption increases potassium secretion by increasing luminal electronegativity, thereby increasing the electrochemical gradient for potassium secretion. Several drugs in common use inhibit sodium reabsorption by blocking the principal cell apical sodium channel. The potassium-sparing diuretics amiloride and triamterene are specific inhibitors of this sodium channel.[144] Use of each has caused life-threatening hyperkalemia.[145, 146] The major risk factors for potassium-sparing diuretic–induced hyperkalemia are age greater than 60 years and concomitant diabetes mellitus.[147]

***Antibiotics.*** The antibiotics trimethoprim and pentamidine have been found to block the principal cell apical sodium channel,[148–150] leading to hyperkalemia.[151–153] High-dose trimethoprim, frequently used with sulfamethoxazole to treat *Pneumocystis carinii* pneumonia, routinely causes a mild increase in serum potassium, averaging 1.1 mEq/L,[154] and occasionally results in severe hyperkalemia.[154–157] Those with renal insufficiency and the elderly may develop hyperkalemia even on conventional doses of sulfamethoxazole-trimethoprim.[158, 159]

***Digoxin.*** Digoxin can cause hyperkalemia in predisposed patients, such as those with end-stage renal disease, even in the absence of toxic ingestion.[160] This may relate to both impaired renal excretion and impaired extrarenal cellular uptake of potassium. In particular, digoxin inhibits basolateral $Na^+$, $K^+$ ATPase in a wide variety of cells, including the collecting duct principal cell. In nonrenal cells, inhibiting $Na^+$, $K^+$ ATPase decreases cellular potassium uptake, thereby increasing the proportion in the extracellular fluid and increasing plasma potassium concentrations. In the collecting duct, inhibiting $Na^+$, $K^+$ ATPase inhibits sodium reabsorption and potassium secretion.[161, 162] Some poisoning deaths have been attributed to bufadienolides, a class of naturally occurring compounds with digoxin-like effects.[163]

***Cyclosporine and Tacrolimus.*** These potent immunosuppressive agents have become a mainstay of organ transplantation. However, hyperkalemia is a common electrolyte abnormality affecting patients receiving these medications.[164–166] As many as 73% of simultaneous kidney-pancreas transplant recipients and 44% of kidney transplant recipients develop hyperkalemia,[166] which tends to occur early after transplantation and then decreases in incidence and severity.[165] Hyperkalemia can also occur among patients taking these medications following other types of transplants[167] or when cyclosporine or tacrolimus is used for treatment of autoimmune disease. In part, cyclosporine and tacrolimus cause hyperkalemia by inhibiting potassium secretion.[168] This occurs through dual effects whereby these medications inhibit both apical potassium channels[169] and collecting duct $Na^+$, $K^+$ ATPase.[170] In addition, cyclosporine suppresses plasma renin activity and induces tubular insensitivity to aldosterone, both of which contribute to impaired potassium excretion.[171] Finally, cyclosporine may cause acute transcellular potassium shifts that contribute to hyperkalemia; the mechanism of these shifts is unknown.[172] The hyperkalemia is associated with hypertension and sodium retention. As a result, loop diuretics tend to be effective in this condition.

## REDISTRIBUTION

The vast majority of total body potassium is located in the intracellular fluid compartment; even small changes in the distribution between intra- and extracellular compartments can result in marked hyperkalemia. Several common clinical conditions are known to cause redistribution. These include acidosis, extracellular hyperosmolality due to "effective osmoles," and diabetes mellitus.

**Acidosis.** Metabolic acidosis due to mineral acids, such as hydrochloric acid or ammonium chloride, is commonly associated with hyperkalemia. In contrast, metabolic acidosis due to organic acids, such as β-hydroxybutyric acid or lactic acid, is an infrequent cause of hyperkalemia.[173, 174] The contrasting effects of organic and mineral acids on plasma potassium are attributed to differences in cellular potassium release. Hydrochloric acid, but not lactic acid and β-hydroxybutyric acid, causes cellular potassium release. Mineral acids are largely dissociated and cause intracellular acidification by electrogenic proton uptake, which results in membrane depolarization and a more favorable gradient for conductive potassium exit. In contrast, organic acids are incompletely dissociated and relatively permeable in the undissociated state across cell membranes. This results in cellular uptake with subsequent dissociation to protons and the weak base.[175, 176] Because this acid uptake step predominantly involves diffusion of a neutral molecule, membrane potential is largely unaffected, which minimizes conductive cellular potassium exit.

In practice, the factors that determine whether hyperkalemia occurs in response to acidosis are much more complicated than just the nature of the acid load. A potassium-reabsorbing $H^+$, $K^+$ ATPase is present in the apical membrane of collecting duct intercalated cells and contributes to a significant component of acid secretion and potassium reabsorption.[17, 46] Stimulation of $H^+$, $K^+$ ATPase by acidosis increases potassium reabsorption across the apical membrane.[42, 43, 45] This increases net potassium reabsorption and can contribute to the development of hyperkalemia. One factor known to regulate potassium exit mechanisms at the apical and basolateral membranes is prior potassium intake. Increased dietary potassium loads increase potassium recycling across the apical membrane, thereby decreasing net potassium reabsorption, whereas dietary potassium restriction enhances potassium exit basolaterally and potassium reabsorption.[47,177]

Acidosis inhibits potassium secretion in addition to stimulating potassium reabsorption. Both metabolic and respiratory acidosis cause intracellular acidosis, and intracellular acidosis decreases the open probability of collecting duct apical potassium channels,[34, 178] which should decrease potassium secretion. Chronic acidosis stimulates ammoniagenesis, and increased extracellular ammonia levels inhibit collecting duct potassium secretion. This effect may be due to ammonia-mediated inhibition of sodium reabsorption[179] and the resulting gradient for potassium secretion, or it may reflect direct regulation of the apical potassium channel by ammonium.[180]

**Hyperosmolality.** Another cause of redistribution-induced hyperkalemia is hyperosmolality. Increases in extracellular osmolality, when caused by "effective osmoles," can increase the extracellular potassium concentration by 1 to 2 mEq/L or more.[73, 181–183] Mannitol is the most commonly administered exogenous osmole, whereas hyperglycemia, in the absence of sufficient insulin or insulin responsiveness, is the most common endogenous osmole responsible for hyperosmolality. The increase in extracellular osmolality, when caused by effective osmoles, is attributed to cell shrinkage, which increases intracellular potassium concentration and stimulates potassium exit. "Ineffective osmoles" are those that rapidly cross plasma membranes (e.g., urea or glucose in the presence of sufficient insulin), do not lead to cell shrinkage, and do not lead to hyperkalemia. The hyperkalemia associated with diabetic ketoacidosis, in part, reflects the significant increase in extracellular osmolality that occurs in response to the hyperglycemia and lack of insulin.

**Diabetes Mellitus.** Diabetes mellitus is one of the most common causes of hyperkalemia. It is either a primary factor or a contributing factor in almost 40% of individuals with sustained hyperkalemia,[103] and almost 4% of outpatient diabetic patients have significant hyperkalemia.[184] As ACEIs become more widely used in diabetic patients for the prevention of ischemic heart disease,[185] for the treatment of congestive heart failure, and for their renoprotective effect in diabetic nephropathy, the incidence of diabetes-associated hyperkalemia will likely increase.

Diabetes contributes to hyperkalemia through several mechanisms. First, insulin deficiency or resistance leads to decreased insulin-stimulated potassium uptake. This results in transcellular potassium changes such that plasma potassium levels increase. Second, diabetes mellitus frequently results in hyporeninemia and hypoaldosteronism.[186] The hypoaldosteronism contributes to hyperkalemia through the absence of aldosterone's effect on both transcellular potassium shifts and collecting duct potassium secretion. This syndrome can be differentiated from primary hypoaldosteronism by the absence of hypotension.[186] Instead, the majority of patients exhibit hypertension, probably related to sodium retention. Some evidence suggests that the suppressed renin and aldosterone levels in this condition are due to atrial natriuretic peptide release in response to sodium retention and volume overload.[187] Third, hyperglycemia leads to hyperosmolarity. In the absence of insulin or in the presence of insulin resistance, this hyperosmolarity leads to cellular potassium loss and subsequent hyperkalemia. Finally, diabetes frequently leads to renal insufficiency, thereby impairing renal potassium excretion. The net effect is that diabetes mellitus is frequently either the cause of or a contributing factor in the development of hyperkalemia.[103]

**Human Immunodeficiency Virus Infection.** Potassium disorders are frequent in individuals infected with human immunodeficiency virus (HIV).[151, 188] A large number of these cases are precipitated only after initiation of medications that inhibit urinary potassium secretion. Both trimethoprim and pentamidine, important components of the therapy for *Pneumocystis carinii* pneumonia, cause hyperkalemia.[152–155] An unexpected finding was that each has renal effects identical to those of the potassium-sparing diuretic amiloride—inhibition of the collecting duct apical sodium channel, thereby inhibiting potassium secretion.[148, 150] However, HIV-infected patients appear to be more susceptible to the hyperkalemia-inducing effects of trimethoprim and pentamidine than are non–HIV-infected individuals. In some cases, the hyperkalemia appears to precede changes in urinary potassium excretion.[153] This may reflect an underlying state of hyporeninemic hypoaldosteronism.[189, 190] In addition, HIV-infected individuals appear to have a poorly defined systemic derangement in transmembrane potassium transport.[191] As a result of these multiple predisposing factors, HIV-infected individuals are at increased risk of hyperkalemia, especially when they are being treated with either trimethoprim or pentamidine for *P. carinii* pneumonia.

**Hypothermia.** Hyperkalemia is a common complication of hypothermia, whether accidental or related to a therapeutic strategy.[192, 193] The hyperkalemia may reflect cellular potassium loss from either cellular death or hypothermia-induced inhibition of $Na^+$, $K^+$ ATPase–mediated cellular potassium uptake. Hyperkalemia may also occur after rewarming of hypothermic patients, especially if potassium was used to treat hypokalemia that existed while the patient was hypothermic.[194] Whereas some studies have suggested that hypothermia-induced hyperkalemia is an adverse prognostic sign,[192] other studies have not found hyperkalemia to be predictive of outcome.[195] Until more information becomes available, aggressive treatment of hypothermic patients should be attempted, regardless of serum potassium levels. Hemodialysis, if needed, may be included in the therapy of these patients.

**Rhabdomyolysis.** Acute skeletal muscle death, rhabdomyolysis, frequently causes hyperkalemia.[196] The hyperkalemia results from both myocyte injury, with resultant leakage of intracellular potassium and the development of metabolic acidosis, and the coincident acute renal failure.[196] Because the hyperkalemia may predate the development of acute renal failure, cellular potassium loss appears to be the primary mechanism of early hyperkalemia in rhabdomyolysis. Because cellular potassium losses may be massive, early, aggressive treatment with hemodialysis may be necessary.

**Tumor Lysis Syndrome.** Chemotherapy-based treatment of large, rapidly growing tumors can produce life-threatening hyperkalemia.[197] The primary mechanism is cytoplasmic potassium release; however, coexisting acute renal failure may contribute to the hyperkalemia.[198, 199] Tumor lysis syndrome–related hyperkalemia is a particular concern when treating acute leukemia or Burkitt lymphoma,[197–199] but it can occur during the treatment of other tumors, including chronic lymphocytic leukemia, lymphosarcoma, breast cancer, and small cell lung cancer.[200–202] Prophylactic treatment with aggressive hydration and alkalinization of the urine substantially decreases the likelihood of tumor lysis–induced hyperkalemia. General recognition of the risk associated with tumor lysis syndrome and the effectiveness of prophylaxis probably explain the low occurrence rate of this condition.[203]

**Neuroleptic Malignant Syndrome.** Neuroleptic malignant syndrome is characterized by fever, muscle rigidity, and neurologic changes after treatment with neuroleptic agents such as haloperidol. These symptoms may progress to rhabdomyolysis and acute renal failure. This syndrome is similar in its fluid and electrolyte complications to rhabdomyolysis,[204] but the associated autonomic dysfunction may contribute to the hyperkalemia. Accordingly, the therapy is similar,[204] except that treatment with dantrolene sodium or bromocriptine may be beneficial.[204, 205]

**Malignant Hyperthermia.** Malignant hyperthermia is a hypermetabolic state after anesthesia with suxamethonium or volatile halogenated anesthetic agents. It may also be triggered in susceptible individuals by infections or by severe exercise in hot conditions. The hyperkalemia appears to result from massive increases in intracellular calcium in skeletal muscle cells, leading to cellular death and loss of intracellular potassium into the extracellular fluid. Dantrolene is effective therapy.[206] However, hemodialysis may be needed to treat the hyperkalemia or renal failure.

**Medications.** Drugs may interfere with the hormonal systems that regulate the distribution of potassium between the intra- and extracellular fluid compartments. The major hormones that regulate potassium distribution are insulin, aldosterone, and β-adrenergic agonists. The normal response to increased potassium intake is increased aldosterone synthesis, and increased aldosterone can increase the intracellular potassium content. Inhibition of aldosterone production or action can lead to significant hyperkalemia, due at least in part to decreased cellular potassium uptake. Many drugs in common use affect aldosterone synthesis or action. Aldosterone synthesis is regulated in large part by renin-stimulated angiotensin II production. Inhibitors of renin secretion, such as β-adrenergic antagonists, atrial natriuretic peptide analogues, ACEIs, and angiotensin II receptor antagonists, inhibit angiotensin II–mediated stimulation of adrenal aldosterone synthesis. Heparin inhibits adrenal aldosterone synthase, thereby inhibiting aldosterone production. Spironolactone, a mineralocorticoid receptor antagonist, inhibits aldosterone action at the cellular level. Drugs from any of these classes can cause hyperkalemia, in part through alterations in the cellular distribution of potassium.

**α-Adrenergic Receptor Agonists.** α-Receptor activation can increase basal potassium levels,[72] magnify the rise in serum potassium following a potassium load, and prolong the duration of potassium load–induced hyperkalemia.[69] α-Adrenergic receptor activation also worsens exercise-induced hyperkalemia.[67]

### OTHER CAUSES

Many causes of hyperkalemia are not easily categorized. Examples include obstructive uropathy, adrenal insufficiency, and pseudohypoaldosteronism.

**Obstructive Uropathy.** Obstructive uropathy leads to hyperkalemia frequently, but the mechanism is incompletely understood.[207, 208] The hyperkalemia may occur either in association with metabolic acidosis or separately. These patients have a degree of mineralocorticoid resistance; whether this is a receptor deficiency or is related to the interstitial nephritis that occurs is unclear.[207, 208] Many patients with obstructive uropathy–induced hyperkalemia remain hyperkalemic for up to several weeks following treatment of the obstruction.

**Adrenal Insufficiency.** Primary adrenal insufficiency, leading to hypoaldosteronism, is an unusual cause of hyperkalemia. It should be considered in patients presenting with hyponatremia, hypotension, and hyperkalemia. Acute adrenal insufficiency has a particularly high mortality, especially if unrecognized.[209] Hypoaldosteronism lead to alterations in both potassium distribution and renal potassium secretion; the accompanying sodium and volume depletion leads to decreased sodium reabsorption in the collecting duct, which secondarily decreases potassium secretion. As a result, life-threatening hyperkalemia may develop. In rare cases, selective hypoaldosteronism, in the absence of glucocorticoid deficiency, occurs.[209]

**Pseudohypoaldosteronism.** Pseudohypoaldosteronism is a rare, inherited disease characterized by renal sodium wasting, hyperkalemia, and metabolic acidosis in the presence of normal or even elevated plasma aldosterone levels. If medications that interfere with the response to aldosterone are not being used by the patient, pseudohypoaldosteronism should be considered. Molecular biology studies have shown that mutations in the genes for either the mineralocorticoid receptor[210] or the principal cell sodium channel subunits[211, 212] can cause pseudohypoaldosteronism.

**Gordon Syndrome.** In 1986, Gordon described a series of patients with hypertension, hyperkalemia, and normal glomerular filtration rate. Both plasma renin activity and aldosterone levels were suppressed, although they responded normally to volume depletion.[213] Patients typically present during adolescence or young adulthood with severe hypertension, short stature, intellectual impairment, and muscle weakness. This condition is known as either Gordon syndrome or pseudohypoaldosteronism type II. The cause may be either an increase in proximal tubule sodium reabsorption[214] or a defect in vasodilator prostaglandin metabolism.[215]

**Hyperkalemic Periodic Paralysis.** Hyperkalemic periodic paralysis is an autosomal dominant disorder characterized by episodic weakness, lasting minutes to days, in association with mild hyperkalemia.[216, 217] The underlying abnormality appears to be a defect in the normal voltage-dependent inactivation of skeletal muscle sodium channels. As a result of this defect, hyperkalemia-induced depolarization persists and inactivates normal sodium channels, which are then unable to generate an action potential.[216, 217]

## GERIATRIC MEDICINE

The geriatric population is one of the fastest growing populations in industrialized countries. It is also a population with high rates of hypertension, diabetes mellitus, coronary artery disease, congestive heart failure, and renal insufficiency—all conditions that predispose to the use of medications that interfere with transcellular potassium homeostasis and with renal potassium handling. In addition, advancing age is usually accompanied by a decline in glomerular filtration rate and by a decrease in the kidney's ability to compensate for electrolyte abnormalities.[218, 219] Aging also results in decreases in plasma renin activity and aldosterone levels.[220] The net effect is an increased susceptibility to hyperkalemia.[218, 221, 222] Close monitoring of elderly patients who take medications that interfere with potassium homeostasis is warranted.

## THERAPY

Therapies for hyperkalemia can be divided into those that minimize the cardiac effects of hyperkalemia; those that induce potassium uptake by cells, resulting in a decrease in plasma potassium; and those that remove potassium from the body.

### Blockage of Cardiac Effects

Intravenous calcium administration specifically antagonizes the effects of hyperkalemia on the myocardial conduction system and on myocardial repolarization.[223] Calcium is the most rapid way to treat hyperkalemia and is effective even in normocalcemic patients. Calcium can be administered as either calcium gluconate or calcium chloride and should be given intravenously. Effects can be documented on the ECG within 1 to 3 minutes, and they last for 30 to 60 minutes. A second dose can be given if no effect is seen within 5 to 10 minutes. Because of the rapid onset of its effect, intravenous calcium administration should be the initial treatment for individuals with ECG abnormalities related to hyperkalemia.

Several precautions should be observed with intravenous calcium. First, it should not be administered in solutions containing sodium bicarbonate, because calcium carbonate precipitation can occur. Second, hypercalcemia that occurs during rapid calcium infusion can potentiate the myocardial toxicity of digitalis. Hyperkalemic patients taking digoxin should be given calcium in a slow infusion over 20 to 30 minutes to avoid hypercalcemia.

### Increased Cellular Potassium Uptake

The second fastest way to treat hyperkalemia is to alter potassium distribution by increasing cellular uptake with either insulin or $\beta_2$-adrenergic agonist administration. Insulin rapidly stimulates cellular potassium uptake by extrarenal cells, primarily hepatocytes and myocytes.[56, 224] Insulin, 10 U, should be administered intravenously to ensure rapid and consistent bioavailability. It begins to affect serum potassium levels within 10 to 20 minutes and lasts for 4 to 6 hours.[224] Glucose is generally coadministered to avoid hypoglycemia but should not be given to hyperglycemic individuals. Glucose-induced hyperglycemia can lead to further increases in the potassium concentration due to hyperosmolality-induced potassium redistribution.

A second effective treatment for hyperkalemia is β-agonist administration. Intravenous albuterol, 0.5 mg, rapidly stimulates potassium uptake and can decrease serum potassium by about 1 mEq/L[225]; however, it is not approved for intravenous use in the United States. Nebulized $\beta_2$-agonists can be used. Albuterol administered by nebulizer at a dose of 10 or 20 mg decreases serum potassium by 0.62 or 0.98 mEq/L, respectively, with a rapid onset of action and maximal effect at 90 to 120 minutes.[226] The primary limitations of $\beta_2$-agonist therapy are tachycardia when given intravenously[225] and lack of response in 20% to 33% of patients when given by nebulizer.[226, 227] In addition, albuterol may decrease potassium removal during subsequent hemodialysis.[228] A frequent mistake when administering nebulized albuterol is underdosage; the dose required is two to eight times that usually given by nebulizer and 50 to 100 times the dose administered by metered-dose inhalers.[229] In severe hyperkalemia, combined therapy with insulin and albuterol may be more effective than either alone.[230]

Bicarbonate administration is probably less effective than either β-agonist or insulin administration. Studies have shown that the changes in serum potassium with intravenous bicarbonate are small and inconsistent.[231–233] Moreover, the associated sodium load may worsen hypertension and contribute to the development of acute congestive heart failure. At present, we do not recommend the routine use of sodium bicarbonate for hyperkalemia. In patients with hyperkalemia, metabolic acidosis, and volume depletion, rehydration with 5% dextrose solutions with the addition of 150 mEq/L sodium bicarbonate (3 amps of sodium bicarbonate in 1 L D-5-W) may be a preferable intravenous solution for rehydration than normal saline solutions.

### Potassium Removal

The definitive treatment for hyperkalemia is removal of potassium from the affected individual. Table 23–4 summarizes the available options for potassium removal.

In selected cases, renal potassium elimination may be adequate for treatment of hyperkalemia. With chronic, mild hyperkalemia, stimulation of renal potassium excretion with either loop or thiazide diuretics may suffice. Acute hyperkalemia should generally not be treated with diuretics because the rate of potassium excretion is inadequate. Most patients with hyperkalemia have underlying renal insufficiency as a contributing factor,[234] limiting the effectiveness of diuretics. If a rapidly reversible cause of renal failure is identified, such as obstructive uropathy, treatment of the underlying condition with close observation of the potassium level in association with continuous ECG observation may be adequate.

A second mode of potassium elimination is with the resin sodium polystyrene sulfonate. This resin exchanges sodium for potassium in the gastrointestinal tract, thereby allowing potassium elimination. In general, 1 g of sodium polystyrene sulfonate removes 0.5 to 1 mEq of potassium in exchange for 2 to 3 mEq of sodium. It can be administered either orally or per rectum as a retention enema. The rate of potassium removal is relatively slow, requiring approximately 4

**TABLE 23–4.** Potassium Treatment Options

| Mechanism | Therapy | Dose | Onset | Duration |
|---|---|---|---|---|
| Antagonize membrane effects | Calcium | Calcium gluconate, 10% solution, 10 mL IV over 10 min | 1–3 min | 30–60 min |
| Cellular potassium uptake | Insulin | Regular insulin, 10 U IV, with dextrose, 50%, 50 mL if plasma glucose < 250 mg/dL | 10–20 min | 4–6 hr |
| | $\beta_2$-adrenergic agonist | Nebulized albuterol, 10 mg | 30 min | 2–4 hr |
| Potassium removal | Sodium polystyrene sulfonate | Kayexalate, 60 g PO, in 20% sorbitol; or Kayexalate, 60 g per retention enema, without sorbitol | 1–2 hr | 4–6 hr |
| | Hemodialysis | — | Immediate | Until dialysis completed |

hours for full effect. When given orally, sodium polystyrene sulfonate is generally administered with 20% sorbitol to avoid constipation. If sodium polystyrene sulfonate is given as an enema, avoiding the use of sorbitol may be prudent; several case reports suggest an association between rectal administration with 20% sorbitol and subsequent colonic perforation.[235–237] Animal models suggest that the sorbitol is responsible for the colonic perforation, possibly due to mucosal dehydration related to fluid loss into the colon lumen.[236]

Dialysis should be considered the primary method of potassium removal when renal function is absent and hyperkalemia is persistent or severe. Hemodialysis is the most rapid method of potassium removal. If a potassium-free dialysate is used, serum potassium may decrease as much as 1.2 to 1.5 mEq/hr[98] and should be monitored closely.[231] The more severe the hyperkalemia, the more rapid the reduction in plasma potassium should be.[238] However, care should be used with 0 or 1 mEq/L potassium dialysate fluids to avoid precipitating hypokalemia. If a very low potassium dialysate is used, the serum potassium should be rechecked after 2 hours from either a peripheral site or the arterial side of the extracorporeal circulation. Peritoneal dialysis, chronic arteriovenous hemodialysis, and chronic venovenous hemodialysis are effective in chronic hyperkalemia, but they do not remove potassium quickly enough to be recommended for use in acute, severe hyperkalemia.

Although dialysis is the most rapid method of treating most cases of hyperkalemia, other modes of treatment should not be delayed while waiting to institute dialysis. In many cases, dialysis may be delayed for several hours if the dialysis unit is closed at the time; it can be delayed even longer if vascular access is not present and must be obtained before beginning dialysis. Thus, although dialysis removes more potassium than either restoration of renal function in obstructive uropathy or administration of sodium polystyrene sulfonate, the time required to institute hemodialytic therapy is often longer, and hyperkalemia may proceed to life-threatening levels if therapy with other techniques is not instituted in the meantime.

Specific therapies may be quite valuable in certain causes of hyperkalemia. For example, digoxin-specific Fab fragments are beneficial in many cases of digitalis toxicity.[239, 240] Patients with acute urinary tract obstruction and subsequent hyperkalemia may be effectively treated with relief of the urinary tract obstruction. Because the rate of potassium excretion in the latter condition may be variable, frequent measurement of plasma potassium is necessary.

### ACKNOWLEDGMENTS

The authors appreciate the secretarial assistance of Gina Cowsert. This work was supported in part by funds from NIH grants DK-45788 (to IDW) and DK-49750 (to CSW), Merit Review Grants from the Department of Veterans Affairs (to IDW and to CSW), and a Grant-in-Aid from the Florida Affiliate of the American Heart Association (to IDW).

## REFERENCES

1. Hodgkin AL, Horowicz P: The influence of potassium and chloride ions on the membrane potential of single muscle fibres. J Physiol 148:127–160, 1959.
2. Wingo CS, Weiner ID: Disorders of potassium balance. In Brenner BM (ed): The Kidney. Philadelphia, WB Saunders, 1998.
3. Browning JJ, Channer KS: Hyperkalaemic cardiac arrhythmia caused by potassium citrate mixture. BMJ 283:1366, 1981.
4. Surawicz B: Ventricular fibrillation. J Am Coll Cardiol 5:43B–54B, 1985.
5. Weizenberg A, Class RN, Surawicz B: Effects of hyperkalemia on the electrocardiogram of patients receiving digitalis. Am J Cardiol 55:968–973, 1985.
6. Ettinger PO, Regan TJ, Oldewurtel HA, et al: Ventricular conduction delay and arrhythmias during regional hyperkalemia in the dog: Electrical and myocardial ion alterations. Circ Res 33:521–531, 1973.
7. Rado JP, Marosi J, Szende L, et al: Hyperkalemic changes during spironolactone therapy for cirrhosis and ascites, with special reference to hyperkalemic intermittent paralysis. J Am Geriatr Soc 16:874–886, 1968.
8. Herman E, Rado J: Fatal hyperkalemic paralysis associated with spironolactone: Observation on a patient with severe renal disease and refractory edema. Arch Neurol 15:74–77, 1966.
9. Werner H: Observations of a case of tetraplegia in potassium intoxication. Med Klin 60:1278–1279, 1965.
10. Freeman SJ, Fale AD: Muscular paralysis and ventilatory failure caused by hyperkalaemia. Br J Anaesth 70:226–227, 1993.
11. Agarwal R, Afzalpurkar R, Fordtran JS: Pathophysiology of

potassium absorption and secretion by the human intestine. Gastroenterology 107:548–571, 1994.
12. Rabelink TJ, Koomans HA, Hene RJ, et al: Early and late adjustment to potassium loading in humans. Kidney Int 38: 942–947, 1990.
13. Malnic G, Klose RM, Giebisch G: Micropuncture study of distal tubular potassium and sodium transport in the rat nephron. Am J Physiol 211:529–547, 1966.
14. Schultze RG: Recent advances in the physiology and pathophysiology of potassium excretion. Arch Intern Med 131:885–897, 1973.
15. Brenner BM, Berliner RW: The transport of potassium. In Orloff J, Berliner RW (eds): Handbook of Physiology, Section 8: Renal Physiology. Washington, DC, American Physiological Society. 1973, pp 497–519.
16. Hierholzer K: Secretion of potassium and acidification in collecting ducts of mammalian kidney. Am J Physiol 201:318–324, 1961.
17. Wingo CS, Armitage FE: Potassium transport in the kidney: Regulation and physiological relevance of $H^+$-$K^+$-ATPase. Semin Nephrol 13:212–224, 1993.
18. Stanton BA, Giebisch G: Renal potassium transport. In Windhager EE (ed): Handbook of Physiology, Section 8: Renal Physiology. New York, Oxford University Press. 1992, pp 813–874.
19. Stanton BA: Renal potassium transport: Morphological and functional adaptations. Am J Physiol 257:R989–R997, 1989.
20. Madsen KM, Verlander JW, Tisher CC: Relationship between structure and function in distal tubule and collecting duct. J Electron Microsc Tech 9:187–208, 1988.
21. Ridderstrale Y, Kashgarian M, Koeppen BM, et al: Morphological heterogeneity of the rabbit collecting duct. Kidney Int 34: 655–670, 1988.
22. Koeppen BM, Biagi BA, Giebisch GH: Intracellular microelectrode characterization of the rabbit cortical collecting duct. Am J Physiol 244:F35–F47, 1983.
23. Ling BN, Hinton CF, Eaton DC: Potassium permeable channels in primary cultures of rabbit cortical collecting tubule. Kidney Int 40:441–452, 1991.
24. Wingo CS: Potassium secretion by the cortical collecting tubule: Effect of Cl gradients and ouabain. Am J Physiol 256: F306–F313, 1989.
25. Ellison DH, Velazquez H, Wright FS: Stimulation of distal potassium secretion by low luminal chloride in the presence of barium. Am J Physiol 248:F638–F649, 1985.
26. Malnic G, Berliner RW, Giebisch G: Flow dependence of $K^+$ secretion in cortical distal tubules of the rat. Am J Physiol 256: F932–F941, 1989.
27. Muto S, Giebisch G, Sansom S: Effects of adrenalectomy on CCD: Evidence for differential response of two cell types. Am J Physiol 253:F742–F752, 1987.
28. Muto S, Sansom S, Giebisch G: Effects of a high potassium diet on electrical properties of cortical collecting ducts from adrenalectomized rabbits. J Clin Invest 81:376–380, 1988.
29. O'Neil RG: Aldosterone regulation of sodium and potassium transport in the cortical collecting duct. Semin Nephrol 10: 365–374, 1990.
30. Garty H, Palmer LG: Epithelial sodium channels: Function, structure, and regulation. Physiol Rev 77:359–396, 1997.
31. Palmer LG, Frindt G: Aldosterone and potassium secretion by the cortical collecting duct. Kidney Int 57:1324–1328, 2000.
32. Wingo CS, Seldin DW, Kokko JP, et al: Dietary modulation of active potassium secretion in the cortical collecting tubule of adrenalectomized rabbits. J Clin Invest 70:579–586, 1982.
33. Stanton B, Pan L, Deetjen H, et al: Independent effects of aldosterone and potassium on induction of potassium adaptation in rat kidney. J Clin Invest 79:198–206, 1987.
34. Wang W, Schwab A, Giebisch G: The regulation of the small conductance $K^+$ channel in the apical membrane of rat cortical collecting tubule. Am J Physiol 259:F494–F502, 1990.
35. Palmer LG, Antonian L, Frindt G: Regulation of apical K and Na channels and Na/K pumps in rat cortical collecting tubule by dietary K. J Gen Physiol 104:693–710, 1994.
36. Hayslett JP, Binder HJ: Mechanism of potassium adaptation. Am J Physiol 243:F103–F112, 1982.
37. Sternheim W, Dalakos TG, Streeten DH, et al: Action of L-epinephrine on the renin-aldosterone system and on urinary electrolyte excretion in man. Metabolism 31:979–984, 1982.
38. Haragsim L, Dalal R, Bagga H, et al: Ketorolac-induced acute renal failure and hyperkalemia: Report of three cases. Am J Kidney Dis 24:578–580, 1994.
39. Murray MD, Brater DC: Renal toxicity of the nonsteroidal anti-inflammatory drugs. Annu Rev Pharmacol Toxicol 33:435–465, 1993.
40. Pirson Y, van Ypersele DS: Renal side effects of nonsteroidal antiinflammatory drugs: Clinical relevance. Am J Kidney Dis 8: 338–344, 1986.
41. Wingo CS: Potassium transport by medullary collecting tubule of rabbit: Effects of variation in K intake. Am J Physiol 253: F1136–F1141, 1987.
42. Milton AE, Weiner ID: Intracellular pH regulation in the rabbit cortical collecting duct A-type intercalated cell. Am J Physiol 273:F340–F347, 1997.
43. Silver RB, Mennitt PA, Satlin LM: Stimulation of apical H-K-ATPase in intercalated cells of cortical collecting duct with chronic metabolic acidosis. Am J Physiol 270:F539–F547, 1996.
44. Wingo CS, Madsen KM, Smolka A, et al: H-K-ATPase immunoreactivity in cortical and outer medullary collecting duct. Kidney Int 38:985–990, 1990.
45. Weiner ID, Milton AE: $H^+$-$K^+$-ATPase in rabbit cortical collecting duct B-type intercalated cell. Am J Physiol 270:F518–F530, 1996.
46. Wingo CS, Cain BD: The renal H-K-ATPase: Physiological significance and role in potassium homeostasis. Annu Rev Physiol 55:323–347, 1993.
47. Zhou X, Wingo CS: Stimulation of total $CO_2$ flux by 10% $CO_2$ in rabbit CCD: Role of an apical Sch-28080– and Ba-sensitive mechanism. Am J Physiol 267:F114–F120, 1994.
48. Eiam Ong S, Laski ME, Kurtzman NA, et al: Effect of respiratory acidosis and respiratory alkalosis on renal transport enzymes. Am J Physiol 267:F390–F399, 1994.
49. Garg LC: Respective roles of H-ATPase and H-K-ATPase in ion transport in the kidney. J Am Soc Nephrol 2:949–960, 1991.
50. Young DB, Jackson TE: Effects of aldosterone on potassium distribution. Am J Physiol 243:R526–R530, 1982.
51. Muto S, Nemoto J, Ohtaka A, et al: Differential regulation of $Na^+$-$K^+$-ATPase gene expression by corticosteroids in vascular smooth muscle cells. Am J Physiol 270:C731–C739, 1996.
52. Friedman SM: Evidence for an enhanced transmembrane sodium ($Na^+$) gradient induced by aldosterone in the incubated rat tail artery. Hypertension 4:230–237, 1982.
53. Harrop G, Benedict E: The role of phosphate and potassium in carbohydrate metabolism following insulin administration. Proc Soc Exp Biol Med 20:430–431, 1923.
54. Briggs A, Koechig I: Some changes in the composition of blood due to the injection of insulin. J Biol Chem 58:721–730, 1924.
55. Bia MJ, DeFronzo RA: Extrarenal potassium homeostasis. Am J Physiol 240:F257–F268, 1981.
56. Andres R, Baltazan MA, Cader G: Effect of insulin on carbohydrate metabolism and on potassium in the forearm of man. J Clin Invest 41:108–112, 1962.
57. Zierler K, Rabinowitz D: Effect of very small concentrations of insulin on forearm metabolism: Persistence of its action on potassium and free fatty acids without its effect on glucose. J Clin Invest 43:950–962, 1964.
58. Lytton J, Lin JC, Guidotti G: Identification of two molecular forms of ($Na^+$,$K^+$)-ATPase in rat adipocytes: Relation to insulin stimulation of the enzyme. J Biol Chem 260:1177–1184, 1985.
59. Lytton J: Insulin affects the sodium affinity of the rat adipocyte ($Na^+$,$K^+$)-ATPase. J Biol Chem 260:10075–10080, 1985.
60. Fehlmann M, Freychet P: Insulin and glucagon stimulation of ($Na^+$-$K^+$)-ATPase transport activity in isolated rat hepatocytes. J Biol Chem 256:7449–7453, 1981.
61. DeFronzo RA, Felig P, Ferrannini E, et al: Effect of graded doses of insulin on splanchnic and peripheral potassium metabolism in man. Am J Physiol 238:E421–E427, 1980.
62. Powell WJ Jr, Skinner NS: Effect of catecholamines on ionic balance and vascular resistance in skeletal muscle. Am J Cardiol 18:73–82, 1966.
63. Bia MJ, Lu D, Tyler K, et al: Beta adrenergic control of extrarenal potassium disposal: A beta-2 mediated phenomenon. Nephron 43:117–122, 1986.

64. Clausen T, Everts ME: Regulation of the Na,K-pump in skeletal muscle. Kidney Int 35:1–13, 1989.
65. Insel PA: Identification and regulation of adrenergic receptors in target cells. Am J Physiol 247:E53–E58, 1984.
66. Landsberg L, Young J: Fasting, feeding, and regulation of the sympathetic nervous system. N Engl J Med 298:1295–1301, 1978.
67. Williams ME, Gervino EV, Rosa RM, et al: Catecholamine modulation of rapid potassium shifts during exercise. N Engl J Med 312:823–827, 1985.
68. Brown RS: Extrarenal potassium homeostasis. Kidney Int 30: 116–127, 1986.
69. Williams ME, Rosa RM, Silva P, et al: Impairment of extrarenal potassium disposal by alpha-adrenergic stimulation. N Engl J Med 311:145–149, 1984.
70. Ensinger H, Dirks B, Altemeyer KH, et al: The role of alpha 1-adrenoceptors in adrenaline-induced hyperkalaemia. Br J Anaesth 65:786–790, 1990.
71. Koumi S, Sato R, Horikawa T, et al: Characterization of the calcium-sensitive voltage-gated delayed rectifier potassium channel in isolated guinea pig hepatocytes. J Gen Physiol 104: 147–171, 1994.
72. Reverte M, Garcia-Barrado MJ, Moratinos J: Role of alpha-adrenoceptors in control of plasma potassium in conscious rabbits. J Auton Pharmacol 11:305–313, 1991.
73. Makoff DL, Da Silva JA, Rosenbaum BJ: On the mechanism of hyperkalaemia due to hyperosmotic expansion with saline or mannitol. Clin Sci 41:383–393, 1971.
74. Moreno M, Murphy C, Goldsmith C: Increase in serum potassium resulting from the administration of hypertonic mannitol and other solutions. J Lab Clin Med 73:291–298, 1969.
75. Nicolis GL, Kahn T, Sanchez A, et al: Glucose-induced hyperkalemia in diabetic subjects. Arch Intern Med 141:49–53, 1981.
76. Skinner SL, Adelaide MB: A cause of erroneous potassium levels. Lancet 1:478–482, 1961.
77. Graber M, Subramani K, Corish D, et al: Thrombocytosis elevates serum potassium. Am J Kidney Dis 12:116–120, 1988.
78. Bellevue R, Dosik H, Spergel G, et al: Pseudohyperkalemia and extreme leukocytosis. J Lab Clin Med 85:660–664, 1975.
79. Bronson WR, DeVita VT, Carbone PP, et al: Pseudohyperkalemia due to release of potassium from white blood cells during clotting. N Engl J Med 274:369–375, 1966.
80. Lichtman MA, Rowe JM: Hyperleukocytic leukemias: Rheological, clinical, and therapeutic considerations. Blood 60:279–283, 1982.
81. Dagher G, Vantyghem MC, Doise B, et al: Altered erythrocyte cation permeability in familial pseudohyperkalaemia. Clin Sci 77:213–216, 1989.
82. Stewart GW, Corrall RJ, Fyffe JA, et al: Familial pseudohyperkalaemia: A new syndrome. Lancet 2:175–177, 1979.
83. James DR, Stansbie D: Familial pseudohyperkalaemia: Inhibition of erythrocyte $K^+$ efflux at 4 degrees C by quinine. Clin Sci 73:557–560, 1987.
84. Alani FS, Dyer T, Hindle E, et al: Pseudohyperkalaemia associated with hereditary spherocytosis in four members of a family. Postgrad Med J 70:749–751, 1994.
85. Iolascon A, Stewart GW, Ajetunmobi JF, et al: Familial pseudohyperkalemia maps to the same locus as dehydrated hereditary stomatocytosis (hereditary xerocytosis). Blood 93:3120–3123, 1999.
86. Carella M, Stewart GW, Ajetunmobi JF, et al: Genetic heterogeneity of hereditary stomatocytosis syndromes showing pseudohyperkalemia. Haematologica 84:862–863, 1999.
87. Ralston SH, Lough M, Sturrock RD: Rheumatoid arthritis: An unrecognized cause of pseudohyperkalaemia. BMJ 297:523–524, 1988.
88. Ho-Yen DO, Pennington CR: Pseudohyperkalaemia and infectious mononucleosis. Postgrad Med J 56:435–436, 1980.
89. Smith JD, Bia M, DeFronzo RA: Clinical disorders of potassium metabolism. In Arieff AI, DeFronzo RA (eds): Fluid, Electrolyte and Acid-Base Disorders. New York, Churchill Livingstone, 1985, pp 413–509.
90. Sopko JA, Freeman RM: Salt substitutes as a source of potassium. JAMA 238:608–610, 1977.
91. Smith SR, Klotman PE, Svetkey LP: Potassium chloride lowers blood pressure and causes natriuresis in older patients with hypertension. J Am Soc Nephrol 2:1302–1309, 1992.
92. Whelton PK, He J, Cutler JA, et al: Effects of oral potassium on blood pressure: Meta-analysis of randomized controlled clinical trials. JAMA 277:1624–1632, 1997.
93. Sebastian A, Harris ST, Ottaway JH, et al: Improved mineral balance and skeletal metabolism in postmenopausal women treated with potassium bicarbonate. N Engl J Med 330:1776–1781, 1994.
94. Lawson DH: Adverse reactions to potassium chloride. QJM 43: 433–440, 1974.
95. Joshipura KJ, Ascherio A, Manson JE, et al: Fruit and vegetable intake in relation to risk of ischemic stroke. JAMA 282:1233–1239, 1999.
96. Tullett GL: Sudden death occurring during "massive-dose" potassium penicillin G therapy: An argument implicating potassium intoxication. Wis Med J 69:216–217, 1970.
97. Bluemle LW, Webster GD, Elkinton JR: Acute tubular necrosis: Analysis of one hundred cases with respect to mortality, complications, and treatment with and without dialysis. Ann Intern Med 104:180–185, 1959.
98. Rabb H, Wang Z, Postler G, et al: Possible molecular basis for changes in potassium handling in acute renal failure. Am J Kidney Dis 35:871–877, 2000.
99. Gonick HC, Kleeman CR, Rubini ME, et al: Functional impairment in chronic renal disease. 3. Studies of potassium excretion. Am J Med Sci 261:281–290, 1971.
100. Bourgoignie JJ, Kaplan M, Pincus J, et al: Renal handling of potassium in dogs with chronic renal insufficiency. Kidney Int 20:482–490, 1981.
101. Kahn T, Kaji DM, Nicolis G, et al: Factors related to potassium transport in chronic stable renal disease in man. Clin Sci Mol Med 54:661–666, 1978.
102. Winkler AW, Hoff HE, Smith PK: The toxicity of orally administered potassium salts in renal insufficiency. J Clin Invest 20: 119–127, 1941.
103. Rimmer JM, Horn JF, Gennari FJ: Hyperkalemia as a complication of drug therapy. Arch Intern Med 147:867–869, 1987.
104. Lammintausta R, Syvalahti E, Iisalo E, et al: Selective and non-selective beta-blockade in renin release. Acta Pharmacol Toxicol (Copenh) 41:489–496, 1977.
105. Holmer SR, Kaissling B, Putnik K, et al: Beta-adrenergic stimulation of renin expression in vivo. J Hypertens 15:1471–1479, 1997.
106. Weber F, Brodde OE, Anlauf M, et al: Subclassification of human beta-adrenergic receptors mediating renin release. Clin Exp Hypertens [A] 5:225–238, 1983.
107. Moore SB, Goodwin FJ: Effect of beta-adrenergic blockade on plasma-renin activity and intractable hypertension in patients receiving regular dialysis treatment. Lancet 2:67–70, 1976.
108. Blumenfeld JD, Sealey JE, Mann SJ, et al: Beta-adrenergic receptor blockade as a therapeutic approach for suppressing the renin-angiotensin-aldosterone system in normotensive and hypertensive subjects. Am J Hypertens 12:451–459, 1999.
109. Holmer SR, Hense HW, Danser AH, et al: Beta adrenergic blockers lower renin in patients treated with ACE inhibitors and diuretics. Heart 80:45–48, 1998.
110. Pedersen G, Pedersen A, Pedersen EB: Effect of propranolol on total exchangeable body potassium and total exchangeable body sodium in essential hypertension. Scand J Clin Lab Invest 39:167–170, 1979.
111. DeFronzo RA, Bia M, Birkhead G: Epinephrine and potassium homeostasis. Kidney Int 20:83–91, 1981.
112. The sixth report of the joint national committee on prevention, detection, evaluation, and treatment of high blood pressure. Arch Intern Med 157:2413–2446, 1997.
113. Garg R, Yusuf S: Overview of randomized trials of angiotensin-converting enzyme inhibitors on mortality and morbidity in patients with heart failure. Collaborative Group on ACE Inhibitor Trials. JAMA 273:1450–1456, 1995.
114. Effect of enalapril on survival in patients with reduced left ventricular ejection fractions and congestive heart failure. The SOLVD Investigators. N Engl J Med 325:293–302, 1991.
115. Kober L, Torp-Pedersen C, Carlsen JE, et al: A clinical trial of the angiotensin-converting-enzyme inhibitor trandolapril in

patients with left ventricular dysfunction after myocardial infarction. Trandolapril Cardiac Evaluation (TRACE) Study Group. N Engl J Med 333:1670–1676, 1995.
116. Ruggenenti P, Perna A, Gherardi G, et al: Renoprotective properties of ACE-inhibition in non-diabetic nephropathies with non-nephrotic proteinuria. Lancet 354:359–364, 1999.
117. Navis G, de Zeeuw D, de Jong PE: ACE-inhibitors: Panacea for progressive renal disease. Lancet 349:1852–1853, 1997.
118. Reardon LC, Macpherson DS: Hyperkalemia in outpatients using angiotensin-converting enzyme inhibitors: How much should we worry? Arch Intern Med 158:26–32, 1998.
119. Kostis JB, Shelton B, Gosselin G, et al: Adverse effects of enalapril in the Studies of Left Ventricular Dysfunction (SOLVD). SOLVD Investigators. Am Heart J 131:350–355, 1996.
120. Gupta P, Franco-Saenz R, Mulrow PJ: Locally generated angiotensin II in the adrenal gland regulates basal, corticotropin-, and potassium-stimulated aldosterone secretion. Hypertension 25:443–448, 1995.
121. Pratt JH: Role of angiotensin II in potassium-mediated stimulation of aldosterone secretion in the dog. J Clin Invest 70: 667–672, 1982.
122. Pitt B, Segal R, Martinez FA, et al: Randomised trial of losartan versus captopril in patients over 65 with heart failure (Evaluation of Losartan in the Elderly Study, ELITE). Lancet 349: 747–752, 1997.
123. Toto R, Shultz P, Raij L, et al: Efficacy and tolerability of losartan in hypertensive patients with renal impairment. Collaborative Group. Hypertension 31:684–691, 1998.
124. Bailey RE, Ford HC: The effect of heparin on sodium conservation and on the plasma concentration, the metabolic clearance and the secretion and excretion rates of aldosterone in normal subjects. Acta Endocrinol (Copenh) 60:249–264, 1969.
125. Majoor CL: Aldosterone suppression by heparin. N Engl J Med 279:1172–1173, 1968.
126. Oster JR, Singer I, Fishman LM: Heparin-induced aldosterone suppression and hyperkalemia. Am J Med 98:575–586, 1995.
127. Sherman RA, Ruddy MC: Suppression of aldosterone production by low-dose heparin. Am J Nephrol 6:165–168, 1986.
128. Edes TE: Heparin-induced hyperkalemia. Postgrad Med 87: 104–106, 1990.
129. Cailleux N, Moore N, Levesque H, et al: A low molecular weight heparin decreases plasma aldosterone in patients with primary hyperaldosteronism. Eur J Clin Pharmacol 43:185–187, 1992.
130. Marcelli JM, Lalau JD, Abourachid H, et al: Unlike heparin, low-molecular weight heparin does not suppress aldosterone production. Horm Metab Res 21:402, 1989.
131. Hottelart C, Achard JM, Moriniere P, et al: Heparin-induced hyperkalemia in chronic hemodialysis patients: Comparison of low molecular weight and unfractionated heparin. Artif Organs 22:614–617, 1998.
132. Pitt B, Zannad F, Remme WJ, et al: The effect of spironolactone on morbidity and mortality in patients with severe heart failure. Randomized Aldactone Evaluation Study Investigators. N Engl J Med 341:709–717, 1999.
133. Richards AM, Nicholls MG: Aldosterone antagonism in heart failure. Lancet 354:789–790, 1999.
134. Holland OB: Primary aldosteronism. Semin Nephrol 15:116–125, 1995.
135. MacFadyen RJ, Barr CS, Struthers AD: Aldosterone blockade reduces vascular collagen turnover, improves heart rate variability and reduces early morning rise in heart rate in heart failure patients. Cardiovasc Res 35:30–34, 1997.
136. Duprez DA, De Buyzere ML, Rietzschel ER, et al: Inverse relationship between aldosterone and large artery compliance in chronically treated heart failure patients. Eur Heart J 19:1371–1376, 1998.
137. McGeown MG: Spironolactone and hyperkalaemia in patients with impaired renal failure. Lancet 2:1207, 1987.
138. Morton AR, Crook SA: Hyperkalaemia and spironolactone. Lancet 2:1525, 1987.
139. Effectiveness of spironolactone added to an angiotensin-converting enzyme inhibitor and a loop diuretic for severe chronic congestive heart failure (the Randomized Aldactone Evaluation Study). Am J Cardiol 78:902–907, 1996.
140. Saruta T, Kaplan NM: Adrenocortical steroidogenesis: The effects of prostaglandins. J Clin Invest 51:2246–2251, 1972.
141. Tan SY, Shapiro R, Franco R, et al: Indomethacin-induced prostaglandin inhibition with hyperkalemia: A reversible cause of hyporeninemic hypoaldosteronism. Ann Intern Med 90:783–785, 1979.
142. Houston MC: Nonsteroidal anti-inflammatory drugs and antihypertensives. Am J Med 90:42S–47S, 1991.
143. Ponce SP, Jennings AE, Madias NE, et al: Drug-induced hyperkalemia. Medicine (Baltimore) 64:357–370, 1985.
144. Busch AE, Suessbrich H, Kunzelmann K, et al: Blockade of epithelial $Na^+$ channels by triamterenes—underlying mechanisms and molecular basis. Pflugers Arch 432:760–766, 1996.
145. Chiu TF, Bullard MJ, Chen JC, et al: Rapid life-threatening hyperkalemia after addition of amiloride HCl/hydrochlorothiazide to angiotensin-converting enzyme inhibitor therapy. Ann Emerg Med 30:612–615, 1997.
146. Cohen AB: Hyperkalemic effects of triamterene. Ann Intern Med 65:521–527, 1966.
147. Hollenberg NK, Mickiewicz C: Hyperkalemia in diabetes mellitus: Effect of a triamterene-hydrochlorothiazide combination. Arch Intern Med 149:1327–1330, 1989.
148. Kleyman TR, Roberts C, Ling BN: A mechanism for pentamidine-induced hyperkalemia: Inhibition of distal nephron sodium transport. Ann Intern Med 122:103–106, 1995.
149. Velazquez H, Perazella MA, Wright FS, et al: Renal mechanism of trimethoprim-induced hyperkalemia. Ann Intern Med 119: 296–301, 1993.
150. Schlanger LE, Kleyman TR, Ling BN: $K^+$-sparing diuretic actions of trimethoprim: Inhibition of $Na^+$ channels in A6 distal nephron cells. Kidney Int 45:1070–1076, 1994.
151. O'Brien JG, Dong BJ, Coleman RL, et al: A 5-year retrospective review of adverse drug reactions and their risk factors in human immunodeficiency virus–infected patients. Clin Infect Dis 24: 854–859, 1997.
152. Briceland LL, Bailie GR: Pentamidine-associated nephrotoxicity and hyperkalemia in patients with AIDS. DICP 25:1171–1174, 1991.
153. Lachaal M, Venuto RC: Nephrotoxicity and hyperkalemia in patients with acquired immunodeficiency syndrome treated with pentamidine. Am J Med 87:260–263, 1989.
154. Greenberg S, Reiser IW, Chou S-Y, et al: Trimethoprim-sulfamethoxazole induces reversible hyperkalemia. Ann Intern Med 119:291–295, 1993.
155. Greenberg S, Reiser IW, Chou SY: Hyperkalemia with high-dose trimethoprim-sulfamethoxazole therapy. Am J Kidney Dis 22:603–606, 1993.
156. Hsu I, Wordell CJ: Hyperkalemia and high-dose trimethoprim/sulfamethoxazole. Ann Pharmacother 29:427–429, 1995.
157. Marinella MA: Trimethoprim-induced hyperkalemia: An analysis of reported cases. Gerontology 45:209–212, 1999.
158. Perazella MA, Mahnensmith RL: Trimethoprim-sulfamethoxazole: Hyperkalemia is an important complication regardless of dose. Clin Nephrol 46:187–192, 1996.
159. Perlmutter EP, Sweeney D, Herskovits G, et al: Case report: Severe hyperkalemia in a geriatric patient receiving standard doses of trimethoprim-sulfamethoxazole. Am J Med Sci 311: 84–85, 1996.
160. Papadakis MA, Wexman MP, Fraser C, et al: Hyperkalemia complicating digoxin toxicity in a patient with renal failure. Am J Kidney Dis 5:64–66, 1985.
161. Reza MJ, Kovick RB, Shine KI, et al: Massive intravenous digoxin overdosage. N Engl J Med 291:777–778, 1974.
162. Citrin D, Stevenson IH, O'Malley K: Massive digoxin overdose: Observations on hyperkalaemia and plasma digoxin levels. Scott Med J 17:275–277, 1972.
163. Deaths associated with a purported aphrodisiac—New York City, February 1993–May 1995. MMWR Morb Mortal Wkly Rep 44:853–855, 861, 1995.
164. Adu D, Turney J, Michael J, et al: Hyperkalaemia in cyclosporin-treated renal allograft recipients. Lancet 2:370–372, 1983.
165. Foley RJ, Hamner RW, Weinman EJ: Serum potassium concentrations in cyclosporine- and azathioprine-treated renal transplant patients. Nephron 40:280–285, 1985.
166. Kaplan B, Wang Z, Abecassis MM, et al: Frequency of hyperka-

lemia in recipients of simultaneous pancreas and kidney transplants with bladder drainage. Transplantation 62:1174–1175, 1996.
167. Fleming DR, Ouseph R, Herrington J: Hyperkalemia associated with cyclosporine (CsA) use in bone marrow transplantation. Bone Marrow Transplant 19:289–291, 1997.
168. Kamel KS, Ethier JH, Quaggin S, et al: Studies to determine the basis for hyperkalemia in recipients of a renal transplant who are treated with cyclosporine. J Am Soc Nephrol 2:1279–1284, 1992.
169. Ling BN, Eaton DC: Cyclosporin A inhibits apical secretory $K^+$ channels in rabbit cortical collecting tubule principal cells. Kidney Int 44:974–984, 1993.
170. Tumlin JA, Sands JM: Nephron segment-specific inhibition of $Na^+/K^+$-ATPase activity by cyclosporin A. Kidney Int 43:246–251, 1993.
171. Bantle JP, Nath KA, Sutherland DE, et al: Effects of cyclosporine on the renin-angiotensin-aldosterone system and potassium excretion in renal transplant recipients. Arch Intern Med 145: 505–508, 1985.
172. Pei Y, Richardson R, Greenwood C, et al: Extrarenal effect of cyclosporine A on potassium homeostasis in renal transplant recipients. Am J Kidney Dis 22:314–319, 1993.
173. Perez GO, Oster JR, Vaamonde CA: Serum potassium concentration in acidemic states. Nephron 27:233–243, 1981.
174. Oster JR, Perez GO, Vaamonde CA: Relationship between blood pH and potassium and phosphorus during acute metabolic acidosis. Am J Physiol 235:F345–F351, 1978.
175. Rogers TA: Tissue buffering in rat diaphragm. Am J Physiol 191:363–369, 1957.
176. Rogers TA, Wachenfeld AE: Effect of physiologic acids on electrolytes in rat diaphragm. Am J Physiol 193:628, 1958.
177. Zhou X, Lynch IJ, Xia SL, Wingo CS: Activation of $H^+$-$K^+$-ATPase by $CO_2$ requires a basolateral $Ba^{2+}$-sensitive pathway during K restriction. Am J Physiol Renal 279:F153–F160, 2000.
178. Choe H, Zhou H, Palmer LG, et al: A conserved cytoplasmic region of ROMK modulates pH sensitivity, conductance, and gating. Am J Physiol 42:F516–F529, 1997.
179. Hamm LL, Gillespie C, Klahr S: $NH_4Cl$ inhibition of transport in the rabbit cortical collecting tubule. Am J Physiol 248:F631–F637, 1985.
180. Schlatter E, Haxelmans S, Hirsch J, et al: pH Dependence of $K^+$ conductances of rat cortical collecting duct principal cells. Pflugers Arch 428:631–640, 1994.
181. Makoff DL, Silva JA, Rosenbaum BJ, et al: Hypertonic expansion: Acid-base and electrolyte changes. Am J Physiol 218: 1201–1207, 1970.
182. Goldfarb S, Strunk B, Singer I, et al: Paradoxical glucose-induced hyperkalemia: Combined aldosterone-insulin deficiency. Am J Med 59:744–750, 1975.
183. Viberti GC: Glucose-induced hyperkalaemia: A hazard for diabetics? Lancet 1:690–691, 1978.
184. Jarman PR, Kehely AM, Mather HM: Hyperkalaemia in diabetes: Prevalence and associations. Postgrad Med J 71:551–552, 1995.
185. Yusuf S, Sleight P, Pogue J, et al: Effects of an angiotensin-converting-enzyme inhibitor, ramipril, on cardiovascular events in high-risk patients. The Heart Outcomes Prevention Evaluation Study Investigators. N Engl J Med 342:145–153, 2000.
186. DeFronzo RA: Hyperkalemia and hyporeninemic hypoaldosteronism. Kidney Int 17:118–134, 1980.
187. Chan R, Sealey JE, Michelis MF, et al: Renin-aldosterone system can respond to furosemide in patients with hyperkalemic hyporeninism. J Lab Clin Med 132:229–235, 1998.
188. Perazella MA, Brown E: Electrolyte and acid-base disorders associated with AIDS: An etiologic review. J Gen Intern Med 9: 232–236, 1994.
189. Cobbs R, Pepper GM, Torres JG, et al: Adrenocortical insufficiency with normal serum cortisol levels and hyporeninaemia in a patient with acquired immunodeficiency syndrome (AIDS). J Intern Med 230:179–181, 1991.
190. Etzel JV, Brocavich JM, Torre M: Endocrine complications associated with human immunodeficiency virus infection. Clin Pharm 11:705–713, 1992.
191. Caramelo C, Bello E, Ruiz E, et al: Hyperkalemia in patients infected with the human immunodeficiency virus: Involvement of a systemic mechanism. Kidney Int 56:198–205, 1999.
192. Schaller MD, Fischer AP, Perret CH: Hyperkalemia: A prognostic factor during acute severe hypothermia. JAMA 264:1842–1845, 1990.
193. Hauty MG, Esrig BC, Hill JG, et al: Prognostic factors in severe accidental hypothermia: Experience from the Mt. Hood tragedy. J Trauma 27:1107–1112, 1987.
194. Zydlewski AW, Hasbargen JA: Hypothermia-induced hypokalemia. Mil Med 163:719–721, 1998.
195. Mair P, Kornberger E, Furtwaengler W, et al: Prognostic markers in patients with severe accidental hypothermia and cardiocirculatory arrest. Resuscitation 27:47–54, 1994.
196. Abassi ZA, Hoffman A, Better OS: Acute renal failure complicating muscle crush injury. Semin Nephrol 18:558–565, 1998.
197. Arrambide K, Toto RD: Tumor lysis syndrome. Semin Nephrol 13:273–280, 1993.
198. Jones DP, Mahmoud H, Chesney RW: Tumor lysis syndrome: Pathogenesis and management. Pediatr Nephrol 9:206–212, 1995.
199. Cunningham SG: Fluid and electrolyte disturbances associated with cancer and its treatment. Nurs Clin North Am 17:579–593, 1982.
200. Barton JC: Tumor lysis syndrome in nonhematopoietic neoplasms. Cancer 64:738–740, 1989.
201. Kalemkerian GP, Darwish B, Varterasian ML: Tumor lysis syndrome in small cell carcinoma and other solid tumors. Am J Med 103:363–367, 1997.
202. Van Der Klooster JM, Van Der Wiel HE, Van Saase JL, et al: Asystole during combination chemotherapy for non-Hodgkin's lymphoma: The acute tumor lysis syndrome. Neth J Med 56: 147–152, 2000.
203. Tsokos GC, Balow JE, Spiegel RJ, et al: Renal and metabolic complications of undifferentiated and lymphoblastic lymphomas. Medicine (Baltimore) 60:218–229, 1981.
204. Becker BN, Ismail N: The neuroleptic malignant syndrome and acute renal failure. J Am Soc Nephrol 4:1406–1412, 1994.
205. Kurien T, Rajeev KK, Abraham OC, et al: Management of neuroleptic malignant syndrome—a series of eight cases. J Assoc Physicians India 41:91–93, 1993.
206. Denborough M: Malignant hyperthermia. Lancet 352:1131–1136, 1998.
207. Batlle DC, Arruda JA, Kurtzman NA: Hyperkalemic distal renal tubule acidosis associated with obstructed uropathy. N Engl J Med 304:373–380, 1981.
208. Pelleya R, Oster JR, Perez GO: Hyporeninemic hypoaldosteronism, sodium wasting and mineralocorticoid-resistant hyperkalemia in two patients with obstructive uropathy. Am J Nephrol 3:223–227, 1983.
209. Werbel SS, Ober KP: Acute adrenal insufficiency. Endocrinol Metab Clin North Am 22:303–328, 1993.
210. Geller DS, Rodriguez-Soriano J, Vallo BA, et al: Mutations in the mineralocorticoid receptor gene cause autosomal dominant pseudohypoaldosteronism type I. Nat Genet 19:279–281, 1998.
211. Chang SS, Grunder S, Hanukoglu A, et al: Mutations in subunits of the epithelial sodium channel cause salt wasting with hyperkalaemic acidosis, pseudohypoaldosteronism type 1. Nat Genet 12:248–253, 1996.
212. Grunder S, Firsov D, Chang SS, et al: A mutation causing pseudohypoaldosteronism type 1 identifies a conserved glycine that is involved in the gating of the epithelial sodium channel. EMBO J 16:899–907, 1997.
213. Gordon RD: The syndrome of hypertension and hyperkalaemia with normal GFR: A unique pathophysiological mechanism for hypertension? Clin Exp Pharmacol Physiol 13:329–333, 1986.
214. Klemm SA, Gordon RD, Tunny TJ, et al: The syndrome of hypertension and hyperkalemia with normal GFR (Gordon's syndrome): Is there increased proximal sodium reabsorption? Clin Invest Med 14:551–558, 1991.
215. Klemm SA, Hornych A, Tunny TJ, et al: The syndrome of hypertension and hyperkalaemia with normal glomerular filtration rate: Is there a deficiency in vasodilator prostaglandins? Clin Exp Pharmacol Physiol 18:309–313, 1991.
216. Cannon SC: Spectrum of sodium channel disturbances in the

nondystrophic myotonias and periodic paralyses. Kidney Int 57:772–779, 2000.
217. Cannon SC, Brown J, Corey DP: A sodium channel defect in hyperkalemic periodic paralysis: Potassium-induced failure of inactivation. Neuron 6:619–626, 1991.
218. Biswas K, Mulkerrin EC: Potassium homeostasis in the elderly. QJM 90:487–492, 1997.
219. Beck LH: Changes in renal function with aging. Clin Geriatr Med 14:199–209, 1998.
220. Noth RH, Lassman MN, Tan SY, et al: Age and the renin-aldosterone system. Arch Intern Med 137:1414–1417, 1977.
221. Michelis MF: Hyperkalemia in the elderly. Am J Kidney Dis 16: 296–299, 1990.
222. Perazella MA, Mahnensmith RL: Hyperkalemia in the elderly: Drugs exacerbate impaired potassium homeostasis. J Gen Intern Med 12:646–656, 1997.
223. Schwartz AB: Potassium-related cardiac arrhythmias and their treatment. Angiology 29:194–205, 1978.
224. Clausen T, Hansen O: Active Na-K transport and the rate of ouabain binding: The effect of insulin and other stimuli on skeletal muscle and adipocytes. J Physiol (Lond) 270:415–430, 1977.
225. Montoliu J, Lens XM, Revert L: Potassium-lowering effect of albuterol for hyperkalemia in renal failure. Arch Intern Med 147:713–717, 1987.
226. Allon M, Dunlay R, Copkney C: Nebulized albuterol for acute hyperkalemia in patients on hemodialysis. Ann Intern Med 110:426–429, 1989.
227. Liou HH, Chiang SS, Wu SC, et al: Hypokalemic effects of intravenous infusion or nebulization of salbutamol in patients with chronic renal failure: Comparative study. Am J Kidney Dis 23:266–271, 1994.
228. Allon M, Shanklin N: Effect of albuterol treatment on subsequent dialytic potassium removal. Am J Kidney Dis 26:607–613, 1995.
229. Greenberg A: Hyperkalemia: Treatment options. Semin Nephrol 18:46–57, 1998.
230. Allon M, Copkney C: Albuterol and insulin for treatment of hyperkalemia in hemodialysis patients. Kidney Int 38:869–872, 1990.
231. Blumberg A, Weidmann P, Shaw S, et al: Effect of various therapeutic approaches on plasma potassium and major regulating factors in terminal renal failure. Am J Med 85:507–512, 1988.
232. Allon M, Shanklin N: Effect of bicarbonate administration on plasma potassium in dialysis patients: Interactions with insulin and albuterol. Am J Kidney Dis 28:508–514, 1996.
233. Kim HJ: Combined effect of bicarbonate and insulin with glucose in acute therapy of hyperkalemia in end-stage renal disease patients. Nephron 72:476–482, 1996.
234. Acker CG, Johnson JP, Palevsky PM, et al: Hyperkalemia in hospitalized patients: Causes, adequacy of treatment, and results of an attempt to improve physician compliance with published therapy guidelines. Arch Intern Med 158:917–924, 1998.
235. Gerstman BB, Kirkman R, Platt R: Intestinal necrosis associated with postoperative orally administered sodium polystyrene sulfonate in sorbitol. Am J Kidney Dis 20:159–161, 1992.
236. Lillemoe KD, Romolo JL, Hamilton SR, et al: Intestinal necrosis due to sodium polystyrene (Kayexalate) in sorbitol enemas: Clinical and experimental support for the hypothesis. Surgery 101:267–272, 1987.
237. Rashid A, Hamilton SR: Necrosis of the gastrointestinal tract in uremic patients as a result of sodium polystyrene sulfonate (Kayexalate) in sorbitol: An underrecognized condition. Am J Surg Pathol 21:60–69, 1997.
238. Feig PU, Shook A, Stearns RH: Effect of potassium removal during hemodialysis on the plasma potassium concentration. Nephron 27:25–30, 1981.
239. Marchlinski FE, Hook BG, Callans DJ: Which cardiac disturbances should be treated with digoxin immune Fab (ovine) antibody? Am J Emerg Med 9:24–28, 1991.
240. Smith TW, Butler VPJ, Haber E, et al: Treatment of life-threatening digitalis intoxication with digoxin-specific Fab antibody fragments: Experience in 26 cases. N Engl J Med 307:1357–1362, 1982.

CHAPTER 24

# Aldosterone Deficiency and Resistance

Amit Mitra, MD ■ Daniel Batlle, MD

Hyperkalemia with varying degrees of metabolic acidosis develops in syndromes in which the primary disturbance is deficiency of aldosterone, resistance to the action of aldosterone, or a more diffuse tubular derangement of electrolyte transport causing a form of hyperkalemic distal renal tubular acidosis (dRTA). These syndromes span from pure genetic defects at the level of one transporter (mutations in the epithelial renal sodium channel or the mineralocorticoid receptor in pseudohypoaldosteronism type I) to overlapping syndromes associated with chronic renal disease in which "relative" aldosterone deficiency may coexist with "relative" tubular resistance or with hyperkalemic dRTA. Notwithstanding this overlap, two pathogenic types of hyperkalemic metabolic acidosis are frequently encountered in adults with underlying chronic renal disease.[1–17] One type, which corresponds to the animal model of selective aldosterone deficiency (SAD) created experimentally by adrenalectomy and glucocorticoid replacement, is manifested in humans by low plasma and urinary aldosterone levels, reduced ammonium excretion, and preserved ability to lower urine pH below 5.5.[1–22] This is also referred to as type IV RTA.[2, 18] In the other type of hyperkalemic metabolic acidosis, ammonium excretion is also reduced and there is a tubular defect in distal hydrogen ion ($H^+$) secretion, as evidenced by the finding that urine pH cannot be lowered below 5.5 not only during acidemia but also after stimulation of sodium-dependent distal $H^+$ secretion by the administration of either sodium sulfate or a loop diuretic such as furosemide or bumetanide.[6–14] The term *hyperkalemic dRTA* is used to designate the latter syndrome, regardless of whether plasma aldosterone levels are normal, low, or elevated.[6–8, 11–14]

This chapter is organized in sections describing the various hyperkalemic syndromes caused by mineralocorticoid deficiency and mineralocorticoid resistance. The iatrogenic causes of hyperkalemia are also described. An overlap is unavoidable at times, because mineralocorticoid deficiency and resistance may coexist at the clinical level. As an introduction to the syndromes of mineralocorticoid deficiency and resistance, we briefly review the pathways of aldosterone biosynthesis and the regulatory mechanisms of its secretion.

## ALDOSTERONE SYNTHESIS AND SECRETION

Aldosterone is synthesized in the zona glomerulosa of the adrenal cortex, as summarized in Figure 24–1.[23] The first three steps of aldosterone and cortisol biosynthesis are identical, but the final step in the synthesis of the two steroids differs. Cortisol biosynthesis involves a 17 (α)-hydroxylation step by 17 α-hydroxylase in the zona fasciculata. Aldosterone biosynthesis, by contrast, requires the presence of aldosterone synthase, an enzyme normally present in the zona glomerulosa.[23]

The main regulator of aldosterone biosynthesis is angiotensin II (Fig. 24–2). This hormone binds to a G protein–coupled membrane receptor on the surface of cells in the zona glomerulosa, activating phospholipase C, which hydrolyzes phosphatidylinositol biphosphate, producing inositol triphosphate and diacylglycerol. These substances raise intracellular calcium concentrations and rapidly activate aldosterone biosynthesis through their effects on steroidogenic enzymes.[23]

All the components of the renin-angiotensin system are expressed in the adrenal cortex, and convincing evidence has accumulated demonstrating that the local renin-angiotensin system in the adrenal gland acts as a paracrine-autocrine system, regulating aldosterone secretion in response to physiologic stimuli. It is therefore likely that the source of angiotensin II that drives aldosterone synthesis is not only angiotensin II from the systemic circulation but also locally formed angiotensin II within the adrenal gland.[24]

The effect of dietary sodium and volume status on aldosterone production is regulated by the renin-angiotensin system via the control of renin secretion by the kidney. In the renal juxtaglomerular apparatus, renin is formed by virtue of stimulation of receptors in the wall of the afferent arteriole that respond to a decrease in intravascular volume. Renin is a proteolytic enzyme that cleaves angiotensinogen to produce a decapeptide, angiotensin I. Angiotensin I is then converted to angiotensin II, mainly in the lungs by the action of a converting enzyme that then stimulates aldosterone production. Aldosterone production increases markedly in subjects in whom sodium intake is restricted, primarily as a result of stimulation of renal renin. Under conditions of severe sodium restriction (≤25 mEq/24 hr), aldosterone levels may increase to a value fivefold that seen in normal subjects on a diet with normal sodium intake (100 to 200 mEq/24 hr). Conversely, the administration of large amounts of salt, either orally or intravenously, markedly decreases plasma aldosterone levels.[15]

A low-sodium diet has also been shown to increase adrenal renin and renin mRNA concentrations in the zona glomerulosa of the adrenal capsule, where aldosterone is synthesized; a high-sodium diet has the opposite effect.[25, 26] Importantly, these changes in dietary

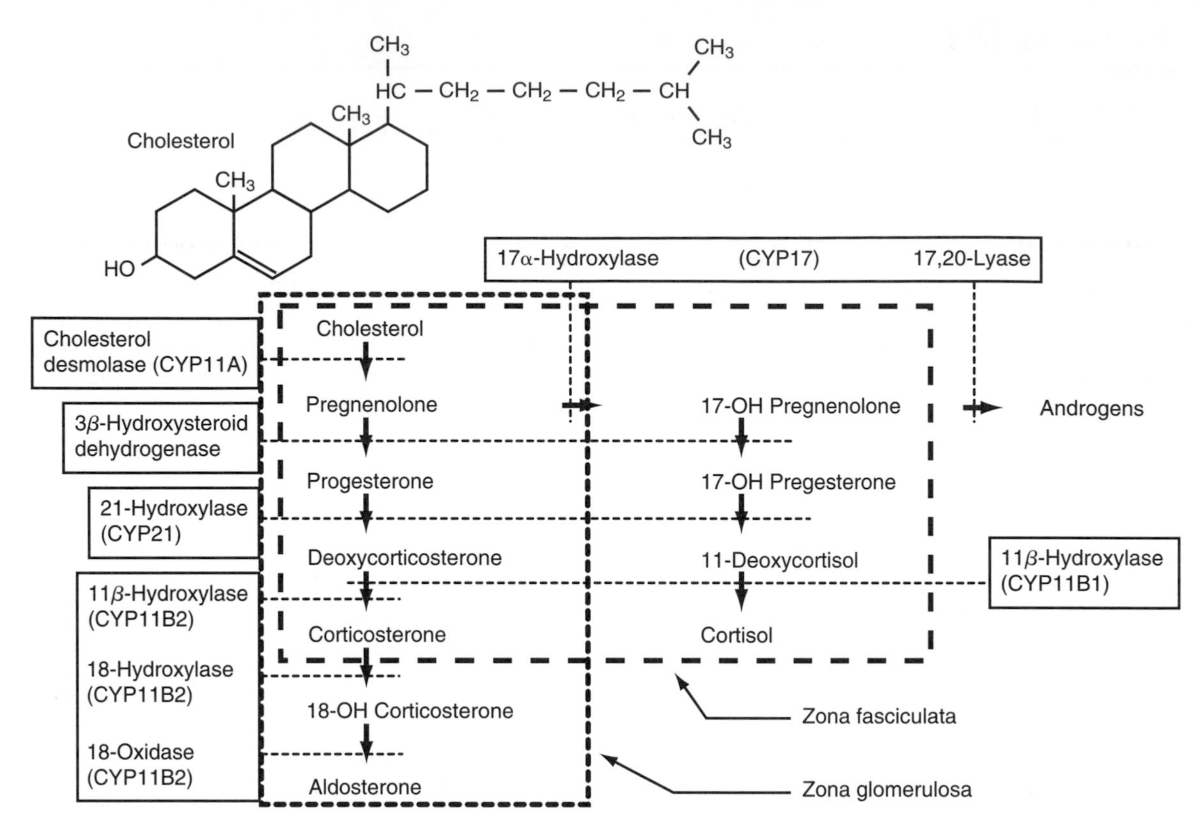


**FIGURE 24–1** ■ Pathway of aldosterone biosynthesis. The *CYP11B2* gene encodes one single P450 enzyme, aldosterone synthase, which catalyzes the last three reactions leading to aldosterone synthesis. (From White PC: Mechanisms of disease: Disorders of aldosterone biosynthesis and action. N Engl J Med 331:250–258, 1994.)

sodium intake have no effect on renin or renin mRNA in the decapsular portions of the adrenal gland that do not produce aldosterone (zona fasciculata-reticularis). Further evidence of the adrenal renin-angiotensin system's impact on aldosterone is the finding that in the rat, aldosterone secretion correlates more closely with adrenal renin activity than with plasma renin activity.[25–27]

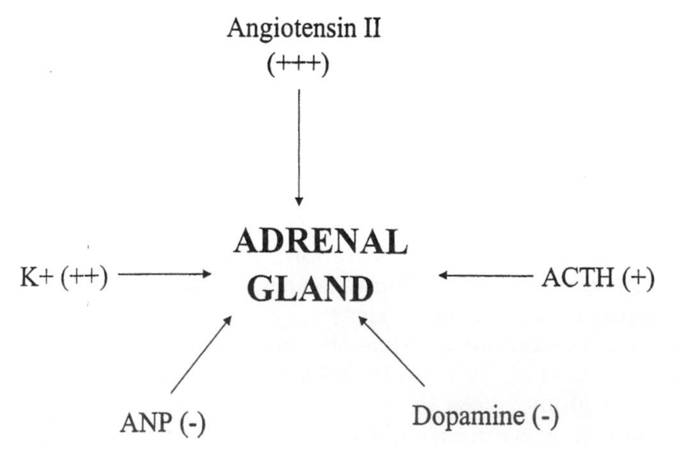


**FIGURE 24–2** ■ Factors affecting adrenal aldosterone release.

The second major regulator of aldosterone release is provided by the level of plasma potassium (see Fig. 24–2). Hyperkalemia results in an increase in plasma aldosterone, whereas hypokalemia results in decreased plasma aldosterone.[28] The mechanism by which potassium regulates aldosterone secretion remains unclear, although it may involve depolarization of the cell membrane with a consequent influx of calcium through voltage-gated channels.[23] Interestingly, a high-potassium diet or bilateral nephrectomy has been shown to dissociate plasma renin activity from adrenal renin.[25] A high-potassium diet decreased plasma renin activity, but it increased adrenal capsular renin, and this was associated with an increase in aldosterone secretion.[25] After bilateral nephrectomy, plasma renin activity was virtually nonexistent, but adrenal capsular renin and aldosterone secretion increased in response to an increase in plasma potassium.[25, 26] Therefore, the local adrenal renin-angiotensin system seems to play an important role in regulating aldosterone secretion in response to physiologic and pathophysiologic stimulus.[24]

Relatively minor regulators of aldosterone production in humans are adrenocorticotropic hormone (ACTH) and the natriuretic peptides (see Fig. 24–2). ACTH administration results in an approximately twofold increase in plasma aldosterone levels, although this effect is short-lived. Natriuretic peptides, such as atrial natriuretic peptide (ANP), suppress aldosterone release. Another stimulus for aldosterone release may be hyponatremia. Although low plasma sodium levels have been shown experimentally to stimulate aldosterone secretion, such an effect has not been convincingly demonstrated in clinical studies.[15]

## MINERALOCORTICOID DEFICIENCY SYNDROMES

These syndromes can be conveniently classified according to whether there is a combined deficiency of both mineralocorticoids and glucocorticoids or an isolated mineralocorticoid deficiency (Table 24–1). The syndromes characterized by combined deficiencies of mineralocorticoid and glucocorticoid hormones are associated with a high plasma renin activity and are easily diagnosed by the finding of a low plasma cortisol level. The rare syndrome of isolated aldosterone deficiency, an autosomal recessive disorder caused by aldosterone synthase deficiency, is also associated with normal plasma cortisol and high plasma renin activity.[15]

Isolated mineralocorticoid deficiency in adults is usually seen as an acquired syndrome referred to as SAD, in which plasma renin activity is usually low and plasma cortisol is normal. There are patients with SAD, however, in whom plasma renin activity is normal or even high (see Table 24–1).

### Combined Mineralocorticoid and Glucocorticoid Deficiency

Patients with combined deficiencies of mineralocorticoid and glucocorticoid hormones usually present with the characteristic features of Addison disease or adrenal insufficiency. These include the development of hypotension, hyponatremia, and hyperkalemia. As a result of aldosterone deficiency, these patients develop volume contraction, which can lead to the development of frank hypotension or at least postural hypotension. Plasma renin activity is increased because of decreased extracellular volume secondary to salt wastage. Prerenal azotemia may also develop as a result of salt wastage, but renal function in these patients is otherwise normal. Hyponatremia is a prominent feature and results from impaired urinary diluting capacity secondary to the absence of glucocorticoid hormones. Impaired distal fluid delivery owing to volume contraction also plays a role in the development of hyponatremia.

The combination of hyponatremia and hyperkalemia in a patient with low blood pressure should prompt the search for Addison disease. Hyperpigmentation, although characteristic of patients with Addison disease, may not be present with moderate adrenal insufficiency and often is difficult to evaluate in African American patients. The diagnosis of adrenal insufficiency is usually established by the finding of a low plasma cortisol level that does not increase normally in response to ACTH administration.

Numerous conditions can result in Addison disease. The most common cause of Addison disease is the primary or idiopathic form of adrenal insufficiency, which is probably an autoimmune disease.[15] Other classic causes of Addison disease, such as tuberculosis and other infectious conditions, should also be considered. Human immunodeficiency virus (HIV) infection has been implicated as a cause of adrenal insufficiency. Patients who have undergone bilateral adrenalectomy for treatment of breast cancer develop a form of acquired adrenal insufficiency.[5] Adrenal insufficiency can also result from hemorrhage into the adrenal gland in patients receiving anticoagulants.

The most common inherited disorder of aldosterone biosynthesis, congenital adrenal hyperplasia, is due to deficiency of 21-hydroxylase (see Fig. 24–1).[29–36] Infants with this disorder usually present with signs of adrenal insufficiency (hyponatremia, dehydration, hyperkalemia) within the first 2 weeks of life; this can progress to shock or even death if untreated.[23, 29] The disorder is more easily recognized in affected females,

**TABLE 24–1.** Causes of Aldosterone Deficiency

| Aldosterone 1 Glucocorticoid Deficiency* | Selective Aldosterone Deficiency† |
|---|---|
| Addison disease | ***Low Plasma Renin Activity*** |
| 21-Hydroxylase deficiency | Hyporeninemic hypoaldosteronism |
| 3 β-Hydroxylase deficiency | Prostaglandin synthase inhibitors |
| 1 β-Hydroxylase deficiency | Atrial natriuretic peptide excess |
| Cholesterol desmolase deficiency | Cyclosporin A |
| Bilateral adrenalectomy | ***Normal Plasma Renin Activity*** |
| Adrenal gland hemorrage | Normoreninemic hypoaldosteronism |
| | ***High Plasma Renin Activity*** |
| | Isolated aldosterone deficiency (Aldosterone synthase deficiency) |
| | Hyperreninemic hypoaldosteronism in the critically ill |
| | Angiotensin-converting enzyme inhibitors and angiotensin II blockers |
| | Heparin therapy |

* Low cortisol, high plasma renin activity.
† Normal cortisol.

who usually have masculinized genitalia at birth due to excess secretion of fetal adrenal androgens. Males with this deficiency appear normal but develop premature puberty.[23, 29] The diagnosis is confirmed by the finding of elevated serum 17-hydroxyprogesterone, the substrate for the absent enzyme (see Fig. 24–1).

Most patients with the salt-wasting form of congenital adrenal hyperplasia have mutations in the 21-hydroxylase gene on both chromosomes, which prevents synthesis of the enzyme.[23, 30] Interestingly, salt wasting often improves with age for unknown reasons, even in patients predicted to have a completely nonfunctional 21-hydroxylase gene. Deficiencies of cholesterol desmolase[31] and 3 β-hydroxysteroid dehydrogenase[32] may also cause salt wasting. These forms of congenital adrenal hyperplasia are very rare compared with 21-hydroxylase deficiency and are distinguished from it by signs of sex steroid deficiency (i.e., ambiguous genitalia in genetic males) rather than androgen excess.

## Isolated Aldosterone Deficiency

In recent years, the molecular basis of the terminal pathway of aldosterone biosynthesis has been elucidated.[37] Aldosterone biosynthesis requires 11 β-hydroxylation of 11-deoxycortosterone to form corticosterone, hydroxylation at position C-18 to form 18-hydroxycorticosterone (18-OHB), and finally oxidation at position C-18 (see Fig. 24–1). One single cytochrome P450 enzyme (aldosterone synthase) catalyzes all three reactions in the zona glomerulosa; therefore, synthesis of cortisol is not affected by deficiency of this enzyme (see Fig. 24–1). The coding gene for aldosterone synthase is termed *CYP11B2*.[37]

Two inborn errors of terminal aldosterone biosynthesis characterized by overproduction of corticosterone and deficient synthesis of aldosterone have been described.[37–47] These include corticosterone methyloxidase I (CMO I) deficiency, in which conversion of β to 18-OHB is defective, and corticosterone methyloxidase II (CMO II) deficiency, in which there is an impairment in the conversion of 18-OHB to aldosterone (see Fig. 24–1).[43, 46, 47] In type I deficiency, 18-OHB concentrations are normal or decreased, whereas in type II deficiency, they are elevated. Plasma renin activity is typically elevated. Both deficiencies are caused by mutations in the gene encoding aldosterone synthase (*CYP IIB2*).[23, 46, 47]

Patients with aldosterone synthase mutations (or CMO deficiency) develop an autosomal recessive disorder; they may have potentially fatal electrolyte abnormalities as neonates or a variable degree of hyponatremia and hyperkalemia combined with poor growth in childhood.[41–45] These patients, however, are usually asymptomatic as adults.[44, 45]

The *DAX1* gene, which encodes an orphan member of the nuclear receptor superfamily, is expressed in the adrenal cortex, gonads, hypothalamus, and anterior pituitary.[48, 49] Mutations in the *DAX1* gene in humans have been reported to cause the X-linked cytomegalic form of adrenal hypoplasia congenita, a rare disorder characterized by impaired development of the adrenal cortex and hypogonadotropic hypogonadism.[48] A case of delayed-onset adrenal insufficiency and incomplete hypogonadotropic hypogonadism was recently associated with a novel missense mutation in the *DAX1* gene.[49]

Treatment of isolated aldosterone deficiency consists of administration of salt or the administration of 9-α-fluorohydrocortisone (0.05 to 0.3 mg daily), or both. The return of plasma renin levels to normal is evidence of a good response. With increasing age, the salt-losing manifestations improve, and it may appear that therapy can be discontinued. However, levels of plasma renin rise and growth decelerates, indicating chronic salt depletion, if treatment is discontinued. The biosynthetic defect persists and can be demonstrated in adults.[43]

## Selective Aldosterone Deficiency

In patients with this syndrome, the deficiency of aldosterone is usually considered secondary, in contrast to the mineralocorticoid deficiency syndromes just described, in which the aldosterone deficiency is a primary event. Glucocorticoid production is normal.[15] Low aldosterone production in patients with SAD is usually associated with low plasma renin activity, but it can also be associated with normal or even high levels of plasma renin activity (see Table 24–1). For instance, heparin causes a decrease in aldosterone synthesis and is thus associated with a reactive increase in plasma renin activity. In critically ill patients, plasma renin levels are very high, yet aldosterone deficiency is present.[50]

The clinical features associated with SAD are typified by the syndrome of hyporeninemic hypoaldosteronism, which accounts for the majority of cases of SAD. This entity, first described by Hudson and colleagues,[51] is now recognized as the most frequent cause of chronic hyperkalemia other than iatrogenic hyperkalemia.[1–4, 6–11, 52–57] Patients present with moderate hyperkalemia (in the range of 5.5 to 6.5 mEq/L), which is usually not associated with electrocardiographic abnormalities. In some cases, hyperkalemia may be intermittent. Most patients are middle-aged or elderly, have cardiovascular disease, and have moderate renal insufficiency (plasma creatinine level 2 to 5 mg/dL). The existence of these comorbid conditions may explain the lack of renal salt wasting, which would otherwise be expected in someone with aldosterone deficiency. Salt wasting may occur if the levels of aldosterone are vanishingly low, and when the glomerular filtration rate (GFR) is normal.

The development of hyperkalemic hyperchloremic metabolic acidosis in these patients is common and is present in about 75% of cases.[4, 10, 11] The term *type IV RTA* is also used to designate this entity.[2, 18] Whereas

**TABLE 24–2.** Potential Causes of Selective Aldosterone Deficiency

| |
|---|
| Decreased renal renin production (see Table 24–3) |
| Deficiency in adrenal renin or other components of the autocrine adrenal renin-angiotensin system |
| Adrenal gland unresponsiveness to angiotensin II |
| Excess natriuretic peptides |
| Acquired angiotensin-converting enzyme deficiency? |
| Acquired biosynthetic defects in aldosterone synthesis |
| Aldosterone synthase deficiency? |

most patients with adrenal insufficiency are hypotensive or exhibit postural hypotension, patients with selective aldosterone deficiency have normal or elevated arterial blood pressure. Postural hypotension, however, can be seen in patients with selective aldosterone deficiency—usually diabetic subjects, who have severe autonomic dysfunction.[15]

The pathogenesis of SAD has not been completely elucidated, and several factors, not mutually exclusive, seem to be involved (Table 24–2). Following is a discussion of various mechanisms that have been implicated as a cause of aldosterone (see Table 24–2) and renin (Table 24–3) deficiency (or both). We discuss them on the basis of whether the presumed defect affects primarily the kidney or the adrenal gland.

## PATHOGENIC MECHANISMS INVOLVING THE KIDNEY

The majority of patients with SAD have low levels of plasma renin activity.[1–11, 56–58] The mechanisms underlying decreased plasma renin activity in patients with hyporeninemic hypoaldosteronism are not fully understood. It is possible that various mechanisms resulting in hyporeninemia may be altered in different patients. Renin release by the juxtaglomerular apparatus normally involves three distinct mechanisms: the renal vascular baroreceptor, the macula densa, and the sympathetic nervous system. The renal vascular baroreceptor senses changes in either renal perfusion pressure or vascular wall tension to alter the release of renin. A decrease in perfusion pressure increases renin release, and vice versa. The macula densa, located at the distal end of the ascending limb of the loop of Henle, recognizes differences in the distal delivery of sodium chloride as a mechanism to modulate renin secretion. The sympathetic nervous system stimulates renin secretion by direct activation of β-adrenergic receptors in the juxtaglomerular apparatus.[59] It is possible that defects in one or more of these pathways lead to hyporeninemia in the syndrome of SAD.

That chronic renin deficiency is the primary factor responsible for decreased aldosterone secretion by the adrenal gland is suggested by several lines of evidence.[5] The type of renal disease seen in patients afflicted with this syndrome often involves chronic tubulointerstitial fibrosis, which may explain low renin production as a result of involvement of the renin secretory cells of the juxtaglomerular apparatus. Vascular lesions such as those seen in diabetic nephropathy may result in hyalinization of the afferent arteriole and arteriolar sclerosis and ultimately damage to the juxtaglomerular cells.[60] The high prevalence of SAD among diabetic patients supports this view.[58, 61] The sluggish rise in plasma renin activity observed in patients with SAD in response to sodium restriction, upright posture, and furosemide administration is also consistent with renin deficiency secondary to damage to the juxtaglomerular apparatus.

In addition to structural damage to the juxtaglomerular apparatus, various other mechanisms for hyporeninemia in patients with SAD have been proposed (see Table 24–3). A defect in the conversion of inactive (big) renin to active renin may be involved; in support of this possibility, some patients with SAD have an increased ratio of inactive to active renin.[62] Another possibility is that plasma renin activity is suppressed as a result of chronic volume expansion associated with chronic renal insufficiency.[63] The levels of plasma renin activity observed in SAD patients after diuretic treatment, however, are lower than those seen in normal subjects on similar diuretic therapy, suggesting that volume expansion alone cannot account for renin supression. Alternatively, renin release may be inhibited by natriuretic peptides. In patients with SAD, volume expansion associated with renal insufficiency and hypertension may provide a stimulus for excess ANP, which, in turn, suppresses both renin and aldosterone secretion. Autonomic insufficiency may play an important role in causing renin deficiency, particularly in diabetic subjects.[61, 64] Hyperkalemia may decrease renal renin production, although this does not seem to play a major role, because correction of hyperkalemia does not increase plasma renin activity in patients with SAD. Another factor to be considered is the normal decrease in plasma renin activity that occurs with advancing age.[65] That the incidence of hyporeninemic hypoaldosteronism is high in elderly individuals supports aging as an additional cause of renin deficiency. Prostaglandins are known to stimulate renin release, and prostaglandin deficiency, tied to the use of nonsteroidal anti-inflammatory drugs (NSAIDs), is associated with a syndrome that resembles hyporeninemic hypoaldosteronism.[66–69] NSAIDs have been used in studies to determine the effects of prostaglandins on renin secretion. For instance, one study in dogs showed that a 50% reduction of renal perfusion increased renal venous renin activity from 3.1 ± 0.6 to 13.1 ± 3.8 ng of angiotensin I/mL per hour within 10 minutes, but this increase in renin activity could be abolished by

**TABLE 24–3.** Possible Causes of Hyporeninemia

| |
|---|
| Atrophy of or damage to juxtaglomerular apparatus |
| Defect in conversion of inactive renin to active renin |
| Volume expansion from decreased glomerular filtration rate |
| Autonomic insufficiency/or decreased sympathetic tone |
| Excess atrial natriuretic peptide |
| Prostaglandin deficiency |
| Hyperkalemia |
| Decreased renin with advancing age |

pretreatment with indomethacin.[68] It seems clear that prostaglandins are important regulators of renin secretion, and their deficiency may lead to impaired renin release and thus inhibition of angiotensin II–dependent aldosterone production.

## PATHOGENIC MECHANISMS INVOLVING THE ADRENAL GLAND

Whereas the preceding considerations emphasize the role of renal renin deficiency in the development of the syndrome of SAD, the following considerations underscore the importance of defects at the level of the adrenal gland in the pathogenesis of this syndrome (see Table 24–2).

If damage to the juxtaglomerular apparatus were solely responsible for renin deficiency and thus the sole cause of aldosterone deficiency in patients with selective aldosterone deficiency, one would expect a normal increase in plasma aldosterone levels in response to angiotensin II infusions. This has not been the case in some patients studied.[55, 70] Schambelan and coworkers suggested that a blunted rise in aldosterone in response to angiotensin II infusion could be explained on the basis of atrophy of the zona glomerulosa of the adrenal gland.[55] In other words, chronic understimulation secondary to chronic renin deficiency would result in functional atrophy of the zona glomerulosa of the adrenals.

Hyperkalemia is an important stimulus for aldosterone release.[71–73] The fact that hyperkalemia fails to correct the aldosterone deficit in patients with SAD suggests a primary role for altered adrenal gland function. The precise mechanism whereby hyperkalemia stimulates aldosterone release has not been completely elucidated. Importantly, increases in plasma potassium increase adrenal renin, although they decrease renal renin.[24, 25] Aldosterone release by isolated adrenal glomerulosa cells increases in response to an increase in potassium only in the presence of adequate levels of angiotensin II. If angiotensin II formation is blocked, increasing the plasma potassium level fails to raise aldosterone secretion normally.[74]

In keeping with this concept, in normal dogs in which angiotensin II formation was blocked by the administration of captopril, an angiotensin-converting enzyme (ACE) inhibitor, an infusion of potassium failed to increase plasma aldosterone levels.[75] The results of this early study in dogs clearly demonstrated that stimulation of aldosterone secretion by potassium is dependent on angiotensin II.[75] Therefore, it is possible that plasma aldosterone levels do not increase toward normal as hyperkalemia develops in patients with SAD because of the associated renin and thus angiotensin II deficiency.

The deficiency in renin formation may be at the level of the kidney, the adrenal gland, or both, causing hyporesponsiveness of the adrenal gland to the potassium stimulus for aldosterone release. That SAD develops in a sizable number of patients in whom plasma renin levels (and presumably angiotensin II levels) are normal or elevated could be better explained if the deficiency were at the level of the adrenal gland, where potassium normally stimulates renin formation.

In addition to renin deficiency, insulin deficiency or resistance could play a role in the development of SAD and would explain, in part, the high prevalance of SAD in diabetic subjects. Insulin not only lowers plasma potassium directly but also may be necessary for appropriate aldosterone release. It is possible that insulin stimulates aldosterone release by translocating potassium into adrenal gland cells. Anephric patients are able to regulate aldosterone in response to changes in serum potassium.[72] This observation suggests that renin deficiency alone cannot completely explain the failure of patients with selective hypoaldosteronism to make aldosterone when they are hyperkalemic, or it suggests that there is another source of renin. It is likely that in anephric subjects, renin is produced by the adrenal gland in considerable amounts, as has been shown in nephrectomized rats.[24, 25]

Natriuretic peptides inhibit both renin and aldosterone secretion.[76] ANP appears to displace the dose-response curve of aldosterone secretion to ACTH infusion to the right. In the rat, specific receptors for ANP in the adrenal capsule have been found.[77] Infusions of ANP suppress aldosterone secretion.[78–80] These studies suggest that ANP both has an indirect effect in inhibiting aldosterone through ACTH and causes a direct inhibition of aldosterone secretion. Thus, increased ANP levels may play a role in the pathogenesis of hypoaldosteronism. Several studies in humans have also demonstrated the effect of ANP on aldosterone secretion, plasma renin activity, and potassium homeostasis.[76, 81–83] In one study, ANP nearly completely prevented the aldosterone increase produced by a potassium chloride infusion in seven patients. Moreover, eight hyperkalemic patients with hypoaldosteronism were found to have markedly elevated levels of ANP (1186 ± 340 pmol/L, compared with 93 ± 10 pmol/L in healthy elderly control patients).[76] In a separate study, six healthy patients were infused with α-human ANP, which not only caused diuresis and natriuresis but also diminished renin and aldosterone secretion.[80] Plasma renin activity and plasma aldosterone were found to decrease in parallel when patients were on high-sodium (200 mmol/day) diets, which also increased ANP levels. Interestingly, while ANP was being infused, there was a significant rise in plasma norepinephrine, but even this sympathetic stimulus did not cause increased production of plasma renin activity and aldosterone.[78]

There is also evidence that aldosterone is under the inhibitory influence of dopamine.[83] It is therefore theoretically possible that dopamine excess could be a cause of aldosterone deficiency in some patients. A defect in one of the steps of aldosterone biosynthesis has been reported occasionally in patients with aldosterone deficiency. Whether such a defect occurs in a substantial number of patients with SAD or is a rarity is not known.

In summary, although several factors can be invoked in the pathogenesis of SAD, it seems clear that renin deficiency plays a key role in this syndrome. As a

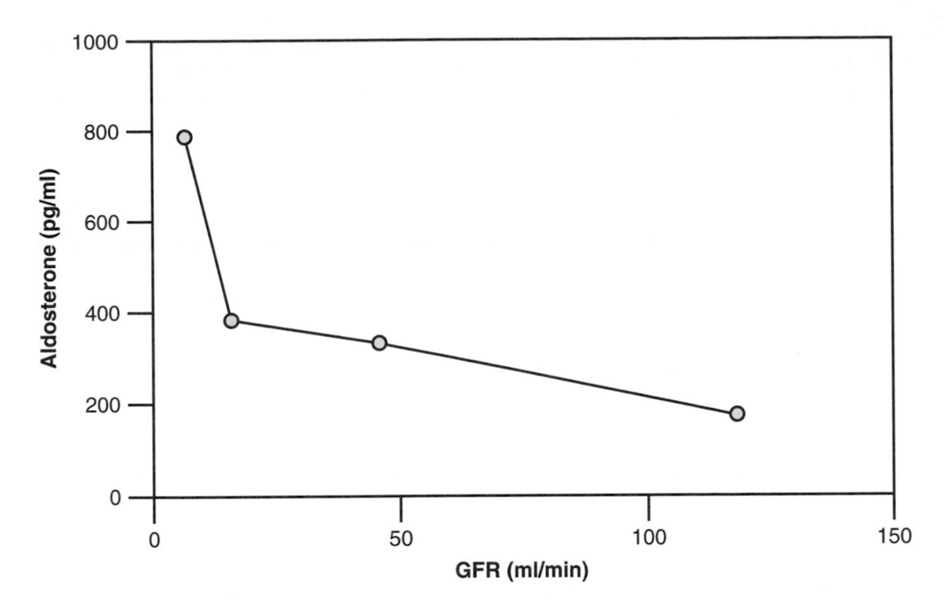


**FIGURE 24–3** ■ Aldosterone levels versus glomerular filtration rate (GFR). (Data adapted from Hene RJ, Boer P, Koomans HA: Plasma aldosterone concentrations in chronic renal disease. Kidney Int 21:98–101, 1982.)

result of renin deficiency, angiotensin II formation is supressed, leading to impaired aldosterone formation. Whether the key determinant is deficiency of renin at the level of the kidney or the adrenal gland is not clear. In either situation, the formation of angiotensin II, the major stimulus for adrenal gland aldosterone formation, would be impaired. The role of renin is further underscored by the finding that angiotensin II is required ("permissive" effect) for hyperkalemia to stimulate aldosterone formation by zona glomerulosa cells in the adrenal gland. Finally, specific defects in the last few steps of adrenal aldosterone synthesis need to be considered, particularly in the minority of patients with SAD in whom plasma renin activity levels are high rather than low. There are no systematic studies, to our knowledge, that have addressed this possibility. An acquired form of hypoaldosteronism caused by heparin, however, provides an example of such a defect.[84–94]

## THE LINK BETWEEN SELECTIVE ALDOSTERONE DEFICIENCY AND CHRONIC RENAL INSUFFICIENCY

The majority of patients with the syndrome of SAD exhibit some degree of chronic renal impairment. There are essentially two possibilities. First, progressive loss of nephrons may unmask a latent defect in the formation of aldosterone. Alternatively, deficiency of aldosterone may develop pari passu with the chronic loss of GFR in some patients. We favor the latter possibility. It seems logical to expect that with chronic reductions in GFR, an increased amount of aldosterone would be required to maintain potassium homeostasis. Indeed, there are data showing that aldosterone increases with progressive loss of GFR (Fig. 24–3).[95] Such an increase in aldosterone would help facilitate the adaptive increase in potassium secretion per remaining nephron, which is characteristic of chronic renal insufficiency. An increase in potassium excretion per nephron can be inferred from the relationship between fractional potassium secretion and GFR (Fig. 24–4), and indeed, patients with uncomplicated chronic renal insufficiency do not develop hyperkalemia until the GFR falls to very low levels (usually <10 mL/min). Hence, the presence of hyperkalemia in patients with moderate chronic renal insufficiency should prompt the search for a specific cause, such as SAD or obstructive nephropathy.[1–15] We think that the syndrome of SAD in most cases is simply the result of lack of a normal adaptive increase in aldosterone production and renal potassium secretion in some patients with chronic renal insufficiency (see Fig. 24–4).

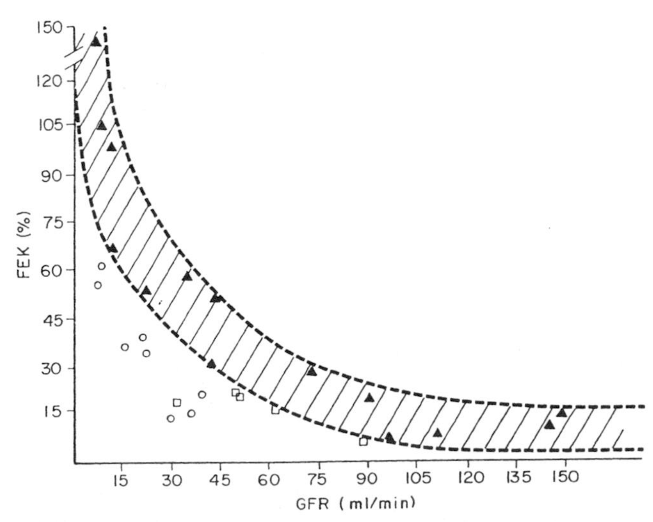


**FIGURE 24–4** ■ Nomogram relating fractional potassium excretion (FEK) to glomerular filtration rate (GFR). Values from patients with an intact hormonal and renal tubular secretory mechanism for potassium (*solid triangles*) are used to delineate the hatched area. The *open squares* and *circles* indicate patients with selective aldosterone deficiency and renal tubular secretory defects, respectively. (From Batlle DC, Arruda JAL, Kurtzman NA: Hyperkalemic distal renal tubular acidosis associated with obstructive uropathy. N Engl J Med 304:373–380, 1981.)

It should be noted that patients with SAD have levels of plasma aldosterone that usually fall within the low range of normal (4 to 40 ng/dL). This "normal" level, however, is inappropriately low, considering the presence of hyperkalemia and impaired GFR. Moreover, a state of relative tubular unresponsiveness to aldosterone could be present as a result of damage to principal cells and their mineralocorticoid receptors, owing to tubulointerstitial fibrosis and progressive nephron loss. Therefore, a low-normal plasma aldosterone level should be considered inappropriately low in the setting of hyperkalemia and chronic renal insufficiency, and thus a state of hypoaldosteronism is present.[6] In many such patients, there is evidence of tubulointerstitial nephropathy, which may affect the juxtaglomerular apparatus, leading to impaired renin release and thereby an impairment in aldosterone production. The adrenal gland may not compensate, despite a rise in plasma potassium, because renal renin is needed for the formation of angiotensin II, which in turn is required for hyperkalemia to stimulate aldosterone release. The ensuing failure to increase aldosterone despite chronic renal insufficiency results in the development of hyperchloremic acidosis and hyperkalemia (the key features of the syndrome of SAD or type IV RTA).

Moreover, some of the causes of renin deficiency listed in Table 24–3 are present in many patients with chronic renal insufficiency (e.g., volume expansion, excess ANP, advancing age). In individuals with chronic renal insufficiency and impaired renal renin production, the adrenal gland may assume a compensatory role by providing a significant amount of renin. In support of this concept, adrenal renin increases after bilateral nephrectomy,[25] and aldosterone levels may be normal in anephric patients.[96, 97] Therefore, it is possible that the adrenal gland assumes a prominent role in renin secretion in patients with chronic renal impairment and that when this adaptation fails, the syndrome of SAD ensues as a result of not only renal renin deficiency but also adrenal renin deficiency.

## Hyperkalemic Distal Renal Tubular Acidosis

Patients with hyperkalemic dRTA present with clinical findings that are often indistinguishable from those of patients with SAD—namely, hyperkalemic hyperchloremic metabolic acidosis, usually in the setting of preexisting chronic renal disease of mild to moderate severity (GFR 20 to 60 mL/min).

Aldosterone levels may be low, normal, or high in patients with hyperkalemic dRTA. The distinguishing feature of this entity is that urine pH cannot be lowered below 5.5 despite acidemia. This is in contrast to patients with SAD, whose urine pH can be lowered below 5.5. Moreover, urine pH in subjects with hyperchloremic dRTA remains inappropriately alkaline in response to stimulation of sodium-dependent distal acidification with either sodium sulfate or loop diuretics.[6–14]

Hyperkalemic dRTA has been well characterized in some patients with obstructive uropathy, sickle-cell disease, and other types of interstitial nephritis of various causes.[6–15, 98–100] Hyperchloremic metabolic acidosis with and without hyperkalemia has been seen in association with chronic "rejection" in renal transplant patients not treated with cyclosporin A or FK506.[13] This may represent the diffuse tubulointerstitial involvement that accompanies the chronic "rejection" process.

Patients with both SAD and hyperkalemic dRTA have low urinary ammonium excretion. The low rate of ammonium excretion observed in patients with SAD has been ascribed, in part, to hyperkalemia.[3] This effect of hyperkalemia has been documented by amelioration of the metabolic acidosis pari passu with an increase in ammonium excretion during correction of hyperkalemia in some patients with SAD.[2, 3] The effect of fludrohydrocortisone, a potent mineralocorticoid, on plasma potassium in a patient with aldosterone deficiency is illustrated in Figure 24–5. The administration of fludrohydrocortisone results in amelioration of the metabolic acidosis and hyperkalemia and is associated with an increase in ammonium excretion. The increase in ammonium excretion may be a direct result of the lowering of plasma potassium or a direct effect on ammonia production, or both. The observation that patients with hyperkalemic dRTA and normal plasma aldosterone levels have a rate of ammonium excretion higher than that of patients with pure SAD supports the concept of an effect of aldosterone independent of potassium, because plasma potassium levels were similar in both groups.[7]

## Diagnostic Work-up and Treatment

A minimal work-up includes determination of urinary pH during acidosis and measurement of urinary potassium, sodium, and chloride excretion in a spot urine sample. The urinary anion gap can be used to calculate urinary ammonium, which is very low in patients with SAD and hyperkalemic dRTA.[101–103] A 24-hour urine collection for measurement of creatinine clearance, titratable acid, sodium, potassium, and ammonia excretion should be obtained while the patient ingests a known diet (e.g., 150 to 200 mEq of sodium, 40 to 60 mEq of potassium).

Measurement of plasma renin activity and plasma or urinary aldosterone level should be obtained as well. If the values are low, measurements should be repeated after either sodium restriction or acute furosemide administration.[11, 12] Patients with SAD have a subnormal rise in plasma aldosterone in response to either of these maneuvers.[11] In an attempt to take into account the effect of plasma potassium on aldosterone secretion, the ratio of plasma aldosterone to plasma potassium or urinary aldosterone to plasma potassium has been used.[4, 6, 10, 11] These ratios are useful, though artificial, because one does not know with certainty the precise relationship between aldosterone and plasma potassium in chronically hyperkalemic subjects. We use a plasma aldosterone–plasma potassium ratio above 3

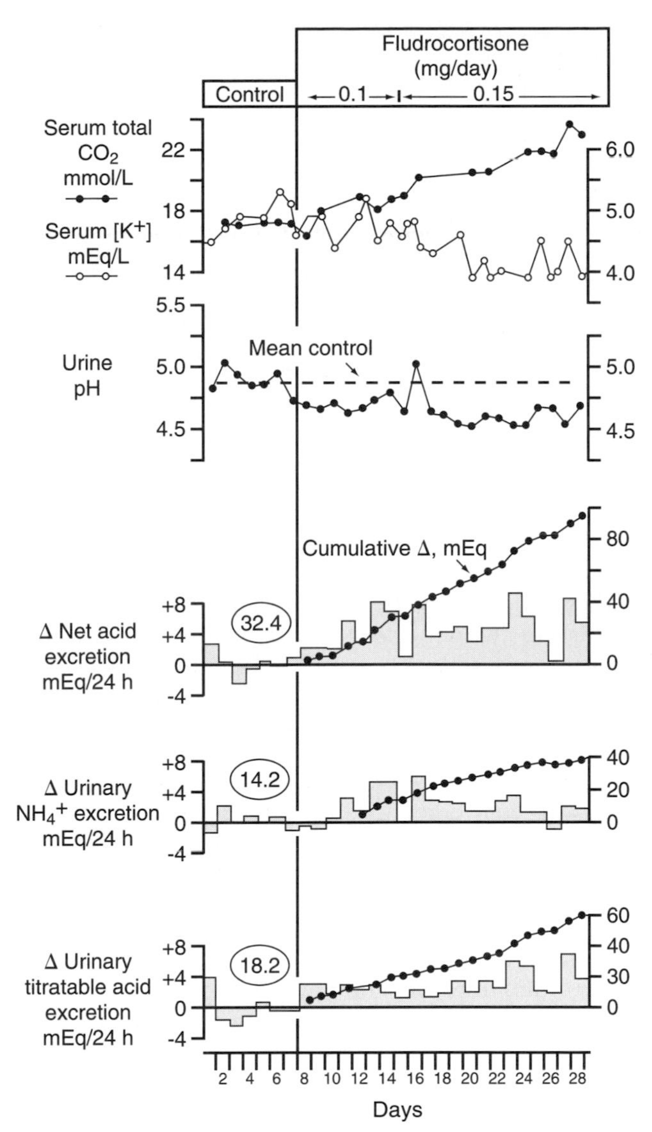


**FIGURE 24–5** ■ Effect of fludrocortisone on serum potassium, serum total carbon dioxide ($CO_2$), urine pH, and acid excretion in one patient with hyporeninemic hypoaldosteronism. (From Sebastian A, Schambelan M, Lindenfeld S, et al: Amelioration of metabolic acidosis with fludrocortisone therapy in hyporeninemic hypoaldosteronism. N Engl J Med 297:576–583, 1977.)

as evidence of a "normal" aldosterone response and thus to rule out aldosterone deficiency.[4, 10, 11, 14]

Both patients with SAD and patients with hyperkalemic dRTA have low fractional potassium excretion (see Fig. 24–4). In patients with hyperkalemic dRTA, potassium excretion fails to increase in response to maneuvers that should stimulate potassium excretion, such as the administration of sodium sulfate or a loop diuretic.[7, 14] The administration of acetazolamide, a diuretic that normally increases potassium excretion by increasing distal sodium and bicarbonate delivery, also fails to increase potassium excretion in such patients.[7, 10] The unresponsiveness to all these maneuvers is in contrast to patients with SAD, in whom mineralocorticoid administration or diuretic administration results in an increase in potassium excretion.[11]

Long-term therapy must be planned carefully, according to the specific pathophysiologic disturbance. For the treatment of SAD, fludrocortisone, at an initial dose of 0.1 mg/day, should be administered. The ameliorative effect of this mineralocorticoid on plasma potassium levels and acid-base balance is well illustrated in one of the patients studied by Sebastian and colleagues (see Fig. 24–5).[2] Because many patients with SAD are elderly and hypertensive, however, mineralocorticoid therapy, by causing salt retention, may exaggerate the hypertension and precipitate congestive heart failure. If mineralocorticoids are given to elderly and hypertensive patients, weekly determinations of weight and weekly physical examinations are mandatory, at least during the first few weeks of therapy. Diuretics such as loop-acting diuretics further enhance the effect of mineralocorticoids, probably by enhancing distal sodium delivery and thus potassium excretion.[11, 18] Asymptomatic patients with moderate hyperkalemia should not be given a mineralocorticoid if hypertension or cardiac insufficiency is present. The development of edema usually indicates the need to discontinue the mineralocorticoid. In younger patients with SAD and normal cardiac reserve, a mineralocorticoid should be given whenever plasma potassium is elevated.

## ALDOSTERONE RESISTANCE

True aldosterone resistance should be manifested by the clinical features of aldosterone deficiency (hyperkalemia, metabolic acidosis) despite elevated levels of aldosterone. Moreover, the administration of physiologic doses of exogenous mineralocorticoids should fail to correct the electrolyte abnormalities. The term *pseudohypoaldosteronism* is usually used to describe the aldosterone resistance that develops as an inherited disorder (Fig. 24–6). Two very different clinical syndromes, now referred to as type I and type II pseudohypoaldosteronism, have been well described. Although both syndromes result in hyperkalemia and metabolic acidosis, the clinical presentation of and genetic basis for these two entities differ greatly, as discussed later (Table 24–4). In addition to these inherited disorders, a state of tubular resistance to aldosterone resulting in hyperkalemic metabolic acidosis occurs in acquired renal diseases such as chronic obstructive uropathy and other tubulointerstitial nephropathies. In such conditions there appears to be diffuse distal tubular damage, resulting in a picture of hyperkalemic dRTA; thus, these conditions are not discussed here.

### Pseudohypoaldosteronism Type I

A syndrome of pseudohypoaldosteronism of infancy, manifested by salt wasting and failure to thrive, was described by Cheek and Perry in 1958.[104] The spectrum of clinical manifestations varies from severely affected patients who die in infancy to asymptomatic carriers.[105] Typically, infants present with weight loss, dehydration, hypotension, failure to thrive, high uri-

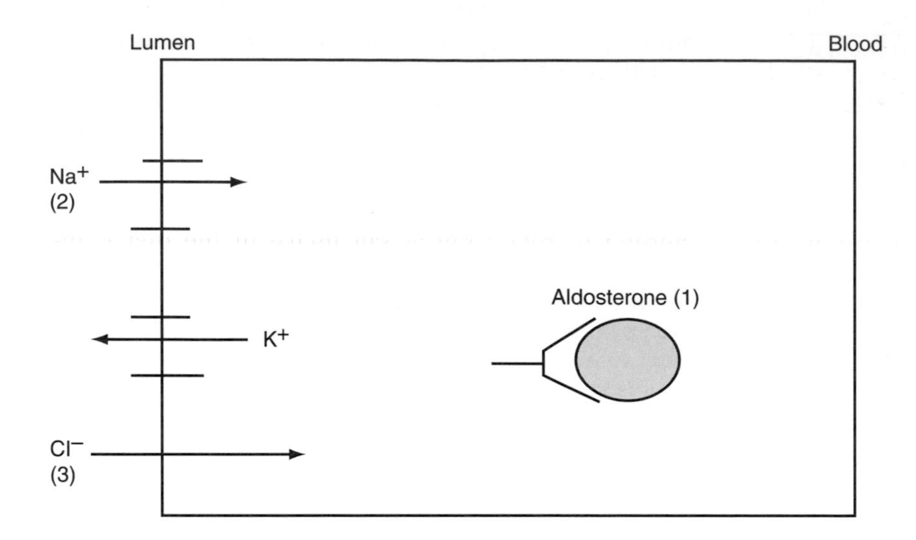


**FIGURE 24–6** ■ Types of aldosterone resistance: (1) receptor level: pseudohypoaldosteronism type Ia, (2) sodium channel defect: pseudohypoaldosteronism type Ib, (3) chloride shunt: pseudohypoaldosteronism type II.

nary sodium despite volume depletion and hypotension, a non–anion gap metabolic acidosis, and hyperkalemia. Plasma and urine aldosterone levels are elevated, and plasma renin activity is increased.[106] More recently, this syndrome has been designated as primary pseudohypoaldosteronism type I (PHA I).[106]

Pseudohypoaldosteronism usually occurs during infancy and is associated with normal renal and adrenal function. This disease can be inherited in either an autosomal dominant or an autosomal recessive mode (see Table 24–4). The autosomal dominant form (type IA) is usually mild, and many of these individuals are asymptomatic carriers. The autosomal recessive form of the disease (type IB), in contrast, is characterized by severe salt wasting, hyperkalemia, and failure to thrive; if left untreated, it can lead to death. Treatment of patients with PHA I requires sodium chloride supplementation in the diet and sometimes potassium-binding resins to correct the hyperkalemia.[107] Clinical improvement is normally seen within 10 to 14 days of salt supplementation.

A syndrome of pure aldosterone resistance implies the presence of a defect at the level of the mineralocorticoid receptor that binds aldosterone or another protein that is the target of aldosterone action. In early studies, aldosterone receptor activity was evaluated in circulating lymphocytes.[108] One study involved nine symptomatic patients from eight families who presented in early infancy with salt-wasting syndrome and markedly elevated levels of plasma renin activity and aldosterone.[108] Type I aldosterone receptors on peripheral mononuclear leukocytes were reduced (0 to 75 receptors/cell) compared with normal subjects (100 to 400 receptors/cell). After screening family members, it was determined that in four of the families the defect was transmitted in an autosomal recessive fashion, while in the other four families the disease was transmitted in an autosomal dominant fashion.[108] More recently, mutations in the mineralocorticoid receptor (MLR) gene encoding the receptor protein have been identified.[109] MLR mutations such as frameshift mutations, premature termination mutations, and splice site mutations were found in four of the six dominant kindreds studied and in some sporadic cases, whereas normal control subjects did not have these mutations. The MLR mutations cosegregated with PHA I, supporting this gene's role in causing PHA I.[109] Affected parents were all heterozygotes for one of these mutations and transmitted the mutant alleles to all nine affected infants. The odds of this occurring by chance alone are 1 in 512.[109] However, MLR mutations in several of the autosomal dominant and sporadic cases have not been identified. This raises the possibility that additional genes or cofactors are involved in the pathogenesis of the disease.[110]

Not all subjects with PHA I appear to have an MLR defect. Defects in the amiloride-sensitive epithelial sodium channel (ENaC) lead to decreased luminal absorption of sodium and hence increased urinary salt wasting. Mutations in ENaC have been identified and associated with PHA I.[111] Electrogenic transepithelial sodium transport is the rate-limiting step in sodium reabsorption in the distal nephron. In the kidney, this electrogenic sodium transport is positively regulated by aldosterone and is mediated by ENaC.[111] Using single-strand conformational polymorphism of all coding exons of α-, β-, and γ-subunits of ENaC, Chang and

**TABLE 24–4.** Causes of Pseudohypoaldosteronism or True Aldosterone Resistance

| | Mode of Inheritance | Genetic Defects | Clinical Features |
|---|---|---|---|
| Pseudohypoaldosteronism type IA | Dominant | Mineralocorticoid receptor | Milder phenotype, may resolve with time |
| Pseudohypoaldosteronism type IB | Recessive | Epithelial sodium channel | Severe phenotype |
| Pseudohypoaldosteronism type II | Dominant | Unknown | Hypertension, short stature, responsive to thiazides |

coworkers identified defects in both the α- and β-subunits in five of seven kindreds with the disease.[111] All the kindreds with the defect in the ENaC showed an autosomal recessive mode of transmission.[111]

Pradervand and colleagues studied mice that showed low levels of the β-subunit of ENaC mRNA expression in the kidney.[112] With normal salt intake, these mice had normal growth rates. However, in vivo, adult ENaC-β homozygous mice exhibited a significantly reduced ENaC activity in the colon and elevated plasma aldosterone levels, suggesting hypovolemia in PHA I.[112] This phenotype was clinically silent, as these mice showed no weight loss, normal plasma sodium and potassium concentrations, normal blood pressure, and a compensated metabolic acidosis. On low-salt diets, ENaC-mutant mice developed clinical symptoms of PHA I (weight loss, hyperkalemia, decreased blood pressure), indicating that the β-subunit of ENaC is required for sodium conservation during salt deprivation.[112]

An autosomal recessive form of PHA I in some individuals is associated with decreased activity of $Na^+,K^+$ ATPase.[105] Decreased $Na^+,K^+$ ATPase activity leads to inhibition of potassium secretion in the distal tubule, which results in hyperkalemia and acidosis.[109] In newborn twins who presented with the syndrome of hyperkalemia and hyponatremia, red blood cell $Na^+,K^+$ ATPase was very low at the time of diagnosis, while serum aldosterone and plasma renin activity were elevated. A control infant with hypoaldosteronism was found to have normal $Na^+,K^+$ ATPase activity, as did the 50 control subjects without any form of this disease.[105] It is not yet known if the low level of $Na^+,K^+$ ATPase activity is due to aldosterone unresponsiveness, which can cause reduction in $Na^+,K^+$ ATPase activity, or to an actual defect in the $Na^+,K^+$ ATPase gene.[105]

Mutations in the actual genes encoding the $Na^+,K^+$ ATPase receptor protein have not yet been identified. It is possible that the reduced number of $Na^+,K^+$ ATPase receptors is secondary to reduced ENaC activity, which, in turn, causes decreased cell $Na^+$ entry and thus a decrease in $Na^+,K^+$ ATPase activity. It is unknown, however, if this is the case, because these patients were not tested for ENaC gene mutations. Mutations within the $Na^+,K^+$ ATPase gene seem to be an unlikely cause of PHA I, because $Na^+,K^+$ ATPase proteins are ubiquitous and would be expected to cause widespread clinical symptoms possibly not compatible with life. For instance, $Na^+,K^+$ ATPase is present in cardiac myocytes and is necessary for appropriate contractile function of the myocardium. If this enzyme were truly deficient, patients with PHA I would be expected to present not only with hypotension, hyperkalemia, and metabolic acidosis but also with congestive heart failure and arrhythmias. Further work is necessary to elucidate whether there are any mutations within the $Na^+,K^+$ ATPase gene in patients with pseudohypoaldosteronism.

The presence of a mild form of PHA I and subsequent improvement in patients with MLR mutations, but not in those with the ENaC mutation, suggests the possibility that there is partial receptor function, receptor-independent ENaC activity, or diminished need for aldosterone with advanced age. Diminished need for aldosterone with increasing age is a likely possibility, because infants typically are on low-salt diets (breast milk or standard formula) and thus need high levels of aldosterone to conserve sodium chloride, whereas adults may not need very high levels of aldosterone to retain salt as salt intake in the diet is increased. Support for a decreased need for aldosterone with increasing age comes from patients with congenital hypoaldosteronism due to aldosterone synthase deficiency, who, like patients with PHA I, improve with age.[46, 47] Patients with the ENaC mutation may not improve as dramatically with increased salt intake because, regardless of sodium intake, the kidney still maintains a diminished capacity to absorb sodium chloride via a nonfunctional ENaC transporter.[109] Interestingly, recovery at the age of 2 or 3 years appears to be part of the evolution of the disease, which may be related to increased salt intake.[106]

## Pseudohypoaldosteronism Type II (Gordon Syndrome)

Pseudohypoaldosteronism type II (PHA II), similarly to PHA I, presents with hyperkalemia and non–anion gap metabolic acidosis. However, unlike PHA I patients, PHA II patients typically present in adolescence or adulthood with hypertension, short stature, and low or normal renin and aldosterone.[113, 114] Neonates with this syndrome have been described more recently.[115] Patients with PHA II are able to conserve sodium (UNa $<10$ mEq/L). Increased levels of urine sodium, by contrast, are typical of PHA I.[116] In diagnosing PHA II, it is important to recognize that there is normal aldosterone secretion in response to renin production. Renal resistance to the effects of mineralocorticoids through the administration of fludrocortisone or deoxycorticosterone should be evident as well. Patients with PHA II remain hyperkalemic even with prolonged administration of mineralocorticoids.

The disease is generally inherited in an autosomal dominant fashion.[113, 114] The defect in these patients appears to be due to increased distal tubular reabsorption of chloride, termed a *chloride shunt*.[117, 118] Because of increased chloride and hence sodium reabsorption in the distal tubule, the body attains a hypervolemic state, resulting in hypertension and suppression of renin and aldosterone. The combination of decreased sodium delivery to the collecting tubule and decreased aldosterone levels contributes to hyperkalemia and metabolic acidosis.[117]

Take and coworkers tested the hypothesis that enhanced distal tubular chloride reabsorption is responsible for the syndrome.[118] Three patients (a middle-aged man and two of his three children) were infused with sodium chloride, sodium sulfate, and sodium bicarbonate. Normal controls displayed kaliuresis with all three infusions, whereas the patients with PHA II excreted significant amounts of urinary potassium when infused with sodium bicarbonate and sodium sulfate but not when they were infused with sodium chloride. In addition, urinary excretion of both sodium and chloride were diminished only when the patients were infused with sodium chloride. These findings confirmed similar findings in the patient studied extensively several years earlier by Schambelan and colleagues.[117]

The features of this disease clearly suggest a transporter defect in proteins involved in chloride transport. Possible proteins responsible for this disease are the $Na^+$-$Cl^-$ cotransporter, the Na-K-2Cl cotransporter, an unknown chloride channel, and the $Cl^-$-$HCO_3^-$ exchanger (*AE1*) protein. Overactivity of the thiazide-sensitive $Na^+$-$Cl^-$ cotransporter could best explain this disease and particularly the exquisite sensitivity to thiazide therapy. Simon and coworkers, however, did not find evidence of mutations in this protein.[119] Oversensitivity of the $Na^+$-$K^+$-$2Cl^-$ cotransporter in the thick ascending limb of the loop of Henle is another mechanism that could cause PHA II, but mutations in this gene have not been found.[115] However, studies in mice demonstrate that increased activity of the $Na^+$-$K^+$-$2Cl^-$ cotransporter in vascular smooth muscle can lead to hypertension, suggesting that increased activity of this exchanger could indeed be responsible for PHA II. Mutations in the $Cl^-$-$HCO_3^-$ exchanger and in unknown chloride channels have not been reported.[120] Linkage analysis in eight PHA II families showing autosomal dominant transmission demonstrated locus heterogeneity of this trait, with a multilocus lod score of 8.1 for linkage of PHA II to chromosomes 1q31-q42 and 17p11-q21. No other chromosomal region showed significant evidence of linkage.[120] In any case, further investigation is needed to determine whether all PHA II families link to one of these two loci and to define the location of genes causing PHA II.

One study established that mutations in two members of the WNK family of serine-threonine kinases cause PHA II, with the evidence strongly supporting a genetic gain-of-function mechanism.[120b] The clustering of WNK4 mutations in a highly conserved domain suggests that they disrupt an interaction at this site required for the normal regulation of WNK4 function. These kinases localize to distal nephron segments presumed to be the site of altered electrolyte transport in PHA II.[120b] The action of these kinases may serve to increase transcellular or paracellular chloride conductance in the collecting duct, thereby increasing salt reabsorption and intravascular volume, while concomitantly dissipating the electrical gradient and diminishing $K^+$ and $H^+$ secretion. Another possibility is that the mutant kinases cause constitutive activity of the electroneutral NaCl cotransporter in the distal tubule.[120b]

Patients with PHA II have responded to treatment with thiazide diuretics, sometimes in combination with a low-sodium diet.[121] In one study, all 10 patients treated with thiazides had a decline in blood pressure and normalization of serum potassium levels.[113] Furosemide treatment also corrects the disorder, although patients appear to be more sensitive to thiazides.[113] Discontinuation of thiazide therapy results in recurrence of hypertension, metabolic acidosis, and hyperkalemia.[113] Diuretics presumably work in these patients by increasing sodium chloride delivery to the distal tubule, thereby allowing for maximal potassium secretion.[116] Salt restriction also normalizes blood pressure and corrects the hyperkalemia in some patients, but not as consistently as thiazide therapy. In one patient with PHA II, all the abnormalities corrected with long-term salt restriction therapy alone.[121] More patients need to be studied to determine whether salt restriction, in the absence of diuretic therapy, is an appropriate treatment for PHA II.

The exquisite response to thiazides can best be explained on the basis of a defect in the thiazide-sensitive $Na^+$-$Cl^-$ cotransporter. Because such a defect has been excluded in the patients studied to date, one has to consider other explanations of how thiazides work in this rare syndrome. Enhanced distal chloride reabsorption, the key transport derangement suspected in this disease, could be overcome when sodium chloride delivery to the collecting tubule is increased by thiazide diuretics. That is, much of the delivered sodium would be reabsorbed through the sodium channel, whereas the chloride would not be reabsorbed at the same rate through the aberrant pathway. In this scenario, loop diuretics should be equally effective, at least on an acute basis, as thiazide diuretics. Fewer patients have been studied using furosemide than thiazide diuretics, and of those studied, some had an adequate response. Perhaps thiazides are better than loop diuretics simply because they are longer acting and better antihypertensive agents. Alternatively, the enhanced chloride transporter may be sensitive to inhibition by thiazides but not by loop diuretics, for which there is no evidence at this time. Moreover, it is not clear how salt restriction improves the hyperkalemia in these patients, although it is easier to see how it ameliorates the hypertension. The iatrogenic causes of hyperkalemia are listed in Table 24–5.

## NONSTEROIDAL ANTI-INFLAMMATORY DRUGS

Chronic use of NSAIDs has been associated with hyporeninemic hypoaldosteronism.[122] Severe and even life-threatening hyperkalemia has occasionally been reported in susceptible people, most notably persons with diabetes and those taking potassium-sparing diuretics or ACE inhibitors in addition to NSAIDs. Unexpected or unrecognized hyperkalemia is of great clinical importance because many patients take over-the-

**TABLE 24–5.** Iatrogenic causes of Renal Hyperkalemia

| Aldosterone Deficiency | Aldosterone "Resistance" |
|---|---|
| Nonsteroidal anti-inflammatory drugs | Cyclosporin A |
| Angiotensin–converting enzyme inhibitors | FK506 (tacrolimus) |
| Angiotensin II blockers | Amiloride |
| Heparin | Triamterene |
| Cyclosporin A | Trimethoprim |
| FK506 (tacrolimus) | Pentamidine |

counter NSAIDs without consulting their physicians. NSAIDs are the most widely used class of drugs, with approximately 50 to 60 million people in the United States alone using them.[122] The introduction of a new class of NSAIDs, the selective COX-2 inhibitors, which have fewer adverse gastrointestinal side effects, will likely result in increased use of these agents.

In an early report of a patient who presented with hyperkalemia associated with hyporeninemic hypoaldosteronism, urinary excretion of both prostaglandin E (PGE) and prostaglandin F (PGF) was substantially depressed when compared with nine control individuals.[122] Because prostaglandins are important regulators of renin secretion, they have an impact on aldosterone production as well. Thus, their inhibition may cause a functional state of aldosterone deficiency. Plasma potassium may increase if there is an associated decline in renal function due to preexisting renal disease oras a result of a fall in GFR due to prostaglandin inhibition.

Prostaglandins are the sole mediators of renin release secondary to the stimulation of the renal baroreceptors and the macula densa. Inhibition of prostaglandin synthesis appears to result in diminished renin secretion via these two mechanisms. Prostaglandin-mediated release of renin via β-adrenergic stimulation appears to occur in rats and cats but, to our knowledge, has not been reported in humans.[59, 69]

By inhibiting both isoforms of COX, all the nonselective inhibitors have relatively similar actions on the kidney. Because COX-1 and COX-2 are located in distinct regions of the kidney, blockade of one or two of these enzymes may have differing effects. Prostaglandins produced by COX-1 ($PGI_2$, $PGE_2$, and $PGD_2$) affect primarily renal homeostatic mechanisms, including dilatation of the renal vascular bed to increase renal perfusion.[123] $PGI_2$ and $PGE_2$ also serve as a counterbalance to the renin-angiotensin-aldosterone system, specifically, angiotensin II–mediated renal vasoconstriction, as well as increased salt and water retention related to increased aldosterone production.

To our knowledge, hyperkalemia has not been reported with use of the newer COX-2 inhibitors. This is somewhat surprising, because their renal effects are apparently similar to the nonselective nonsteroidal agents, including inhibition of renin release. In a study in humans, Stichtenoth and colleagues showed that meloxicam inhibits furosemide-stimulated renin release, suggesting that in humans, COX-2 is responsible for prostaglandin-mediated renin release.[124] Moreover, in COX-2 knockout mice, levels of renin mRNA and renin protein, as well as renin enzyme activities, are significantly reduced when compared with wild-type mice.[125] In rabbits, sodium chloride–dependent stimulation of renin secretion was unaffected by COX-1 inhibition, whereas COX-2 in epithelial cells is a critical component of macula densa control of renin secretion.[126] Interestingly, COX-2–derived metabolites are involved in the regulation of sodium excretion in dogs on a normal or low-sodium diet but are not involved in the maintenance of high renin levels during a long-term decrease in sodium intake.[127] From the latter finding, one could extrapolate that with chronic COX-2 inhibition, renin formation is not inhibited to any major extent and, therefore, hyperkalemia would not be seen.

$PGI_2$ (or prostacyclin) stimulates renin release.[123] When $PGI_2$ is suppressed, a state of hyporeninemic hypoaldosteronism, similar to that seen in type IV RTA, may develop. The renin-stimulating prostaglandins $PGI_2$ and $PGE_2$ are produced primarily by COX-1. Renal $PGE_2$ synthesis has been shown to be reduced by 30% in indomethacin-treated patients but unaffected by meloxicam, a selective COX-2 inhibitor.[124] In rats, indomethacin reduced urinary $PGE_2$ excretion by 70%, while NS398 (a selective COX-2 inhibitor) did not alter $PGE_2$ excretion.[128] Systematic comparative studies examining renin and aldosterone levels as well as urinary potassium excretion in subjects treated with COX-2 inhibitors and NSAIDs are needed to clarify this issue. One recently published randomized, controlled trial studying 75 patients showed that NSAIDs and rofecoxib did not cause clinically significant hyperkalemia, although both caused statistically significant reductions in GFR.[129] Aldosterone and renin levels were not reported in this study. In addition, the patients did not have preexisting renal insufficiency, so they were unlikely to develop hyperkalemia.

At this time, hyperkalemia should be viewed as a potential complication of selective COX-2 inhibitors, as has been widely reported with NSAID use, if they are given to patients at risk, even though it has not been reported. The lack of reported cases of hyperkalemia may simply reflect the relatively recent introduction of COX-2 inhibitors in clinical practice. However, COX-2 inhibitors may have less of an inhibiting effect on the renin-stimulating prostaglandins $PGE_2$ and $PGI_2$ and thus may have less of an effect on aldosterone secretion. Particularly, chronic COX-2 inhibition may not have an effect on renin secretion, which could explain why hyperkalemia has not been reported widely with the chronic use of COX-2 inhibitors.

## ANGIOTENSIN II–CONVERTING ENZYME INHIBITORS AND ANGIOTENSIN II BLOCKERS

In humans, ACE deficiency, most commonly encountered in patients treated with ACE inhibitors, may result in hypoaldosteronism and hyperkalemia. The administration of ACE inhibitors initially is accompanied by a reduction in serum aldosterone, but this is attenuated with continued therapy.[24, 130, 131] In one study, serum aldosterone levels initially decreased by 85% after ACE inhibitor therapy was begun, but after 6 months of treatment, serum aldosterone normalized to baseline levels.[132] Other studies showed that serum aldosterone either increases or normalizes after chronic ACE inhibition.[132–135] Interestingly, we found that fosinopril did not suppress serum aldosterone levels at either 8 or 12 weeks of therapy in patients with proteinuric renal disease in whom renal function was moderately impaired, although serum ACE activity was effectively decreased.[136]

The level of hypoaldosteronism resulting from various ACE inhibitors may depend on their tissue specificity.[24] In other words, because the various ACE inhibitors exhibit different degrees of ACE inhibition at the tissue level, it is reasonable to postulate that angiotensin II–dependent aldosterone production will be inhibited to a lesser degree by agents that have low tissue specificity for the adrenal gland. To our knowledge, no systematic study has been undertaken to determine specific ACE inhibition in the adrenal gland, as has been done in the aorta, heart, kidney, and brain. A few studies have included measurements of adrenal ACE activity after administration of an ACE inhibitor (reviewed in reference 24). For instance, the acute administration of trandolapril and lisinopril resulted in adrenal ACE activity inhibition by more than 90%. By contrast, enalapril inhibited adrenal ACE activity by only 30% to 35%.[137, 138] In addition, after 4 weeks of treatment with enalapril or perindopril, adrenal ACE activity was no different from that in control individuals.[139] If ACE activity is not inhibited in the adrenal glands, aldosterone should be produced, preventing the life-threatening hyperkalemia that patients with chronic renal insufficiency often encounter.[24]

More recently, the effect of the angiotensin receptor blocker (ARB) valsartan on aldosterone and potassium was studied by Bakris and colleagues.[140] In a randomized, double-blind, controlled study, valsartan did not raise serum potassium to the same degree as did lisinopril, an ACE inhibitor. This difference was related to a smaller reduction in plasma aldosterone by valsartan and was not related to changes in GFR.[140] The authors concluded that increases in serum potassium are less likely with ARB than with ACE inhibitor therapy in patients with renal insufficiency.[140] Whether ARBs cause hyperkalemia less often than all ACE inhibitors still needs to be demonstrated for the many agents available. As mentioned earlier, lisinopril inhibits adrenal ACE activity by 90%, whereas enalapril inhibits adrenal activity by only 30% to 35%.[24] Thus, there is a possibility that lisinopril is more likely to cause hyperkalemia than are other ACE inhibitors and ARB agents. Aside from specific differences between ACE inhibitors and ARBs, it seems reasonable to assume that ARBs are less likely to produce hyperkalemia than are ACE inhibitors.

## HEPARIN

Heparin and heparinoid compounds, commonly used for their anticoagulant properties, have been clearly associated with hypoaldosteronism and hyperkalemia.[84–91] Studies using mice adrenal glands have shown that heparin inhibits aldosterone production by the adrenal glomerulosa. In one study, heparin at doses of 0.1 and 0.3 IU/mL blocked aldosterone production stimulated by angiotensin II but not by potassium.[92] At higher doses of 1 and 10 IU/mL, aldosterone production was inhibited even in the presence of angiotensin II, ACTH, and potassium.[92] This study suggests that at lower concentrations, heparin inhibits only the adrenal glomerulosa directly, while at higher concentrations, heparin inhibits all the stimulating actions of angiotensin II, ACTH, and potassium.[92] Animal studies have also shown a visible reduction in the width of the zona glomerulosa after 2 weeks of heparin administration, and more dramatic reduction after 4 weeks of therapy.[85] Further studies in rats have confirmed that plasma aldosterone is significantly decreased after heparin administration.[93]

Studies with human subjects also have shown that heparin inhibits adrenal aldosterone production. For instance, in one study of 20 patients, plasma aldosterone levels were reduced from 74 ± 21 pg/mL before treatment to 37 ± 11 pg/mL after at least 4 days of heparin treatment.[86] Case reports have shown that plasma aldosterone is reduced during heparin therapy despite hyperkalemia and hyperreninism, two powerful stimulants of aldosterone release.[85, 88] Potassium and aldosterone levels usually normalize after discontinuation of heparin. In one human subject treated with heparin for 4 years, the zona glomerulosa was found to be completely atrophied at autopsy, suggesting that heparin directly interferes with aldosterone biosynthesis in the adrenal glands.[94]

Interestingly, not only therapeutic doses of heparin but also low-dose heparin used for prophylaxis of deep vein thrombosis has been associated with decreased aldosterone production. In one study, in five healthy human subjects, 5000 units of subcutaneous heparin administered every 12 hours resulted in a decrease in plasma aldosterone (from 17 to 6.6 ng/dL on day 5 and to 4.3 ng/dL on day 10).[91] Even stimulation with furosemide and 4 hours of ambulation did not result in increased aldosterone levels.[91]

With the recent widespread use of low-molecular-weight heparin (LMWH) as an anticoagulant, studies to observe its effect on aldosterone have been conducted. Although one study initially showed that LMWH did not affect aldosterone levels,[141] since then, there have been numerous studies showing that LMWH, like conventional heparin, reduces serum aldosterone levels.[87, 89, 90] For instance, in a study of 27 patients, LMWH was found to decrease plasma aldosterone concentrations by 43.9% after 4 days of treatment.[89] Moreover, in four of these patients, plasma aldosterone became undetectable during treatment. Serum potassium also increased significantly during treatment and normalized after treatment was discontinued.[89] In this and other studies,[90] plasma renin activity was not reduced, suggesting that LMWH, like conventional heparin, directly inhibits the synthesis of aldosterone by the adrenal glomerulosa.

Most measurements of urinary mineralocorticoid metabolites following administration of heparinoids have shown normal to slightly reduced levels of corticosterone, with subnormal levels of 18-hydroxycorticosterone and aldosterone.[85] This suggests that heparin impairs aldosterone synthesis by inhibiting 18-hydroxylase (see Fig. 24–1). The mechanism whereby heparin and heparinoid compounds cause zona glomerulosa atrophy thus seems to be related to the inhibition of 18-hydroxylase.[87]

## CALCINEURIN INHIBITORS: CYCLOSPORIN A AND TACROLIMUS

Cyclosporin A (CsA) and tacrolimus administration has been shown to cause hyperkalemia.[142–144] Early trials pointed out that patients treated with CsA in doses of 15 mg/kg/day had significantly higher serum potassium levels than did those treated with prednisone or azathioprine.[145] Hamilton and associates showed that lower-dose CsA therapy (5.9 mg/kg/day) can also result in elevation of the mean serum potassium (3.8 mEq/L in azathioprine- and prednisone-treated patients, versus 4.7 mEq/L in CsA-treated patients).[146]

In the rat, urinary potassium excretion is markedly reduced, out of proportion to the reduction in GFR, in rats treated with CsA.[147] Hydrogen ion secretion was found to be reduced, suggesting a hyperkalemic type of dRTA. Kamel and colleagues reported similar findings in humans.[148] Twelve patients treated with CsA with normal renal function were found to have hyperkalemia. Their renal response to hyperkalemia was inappropriate because the transtubular potassium gradient was only 4.3 ± 0.4, compared with 13 ± 1.2 after 50 mmol of potassium chloride was given to control subjects.[147] The newer calcineurin and potent immunosuppressive drug FK506 also has been associated with hyperkalemia. In one study, 65% of liver transplant patients developed hyperkalemia on therapeutic doses of FK506.[149]

The mechanisms by which calcineurin inhibitors affect potassium secretion are not fully understood. CsA and FK506 inhibit renal $Na^+,K^+$ ATPase activity, which may lead to hyperkalemia. CsA-induced inhibition of $Na^+,K^+$ ATPase activity in the cortical collecting duct (CCD) and outer medullary collecting duct could decrease the sodium gradient needed for potassium ion secretion and/or the cellular uptake of potassium and therefore cellular potassium available for secretion, thereby contributing to the hyperkalemia observed in the clinical setting.[150] Lea and colleagues proposed that in rat cells, CsA and FK506 bind to immunophilins in T cells to form receptor complexes that inhibit the phosphatase activity of calcineurin.[151, 152] Because calcineurin activitates $Na^+,K^+$ ATPase through dephosphorylation, these drugs inhibit sodium ion pump activity through the inhibition of calcineurin. In fact, in the CCD, a dose response of FK506 concentrations showed that therapeutic doses of 3 ng/mL significantly inhibited $Na^+,K^+$ ATPase activity by 61%.[151] In addition, Tumlin and coworkers demonstrated that CsA specifically inhibits $Na^+,K^+$ ATPase activity in the CCD, mTAL, and outer medullary collecting duct. In the CCD, inhibition of $Na^+,K^+$ ATPase activity was dose dependent and occurred at concentrations commonly associated with clinical CsA toxicity (600 to 2500 ng/mL).

The striking impairment in potassium secretion that we observed in rats infused with potassium is also suggestive of an impairment in $Na^+,K^+$ ATPase activity.[147] In a series of experiments in rats given CsA intraperitoneally, we found not only a significant reduction in potassium excretion but also an impairment in hydrogen ion secretion.[147] Furthermore, CsA-treated rats displayed a striking defect in their ability to excrete potassium in response to a graded infusion, which increased plasma potassium above 8 mEq/L. The fact that CsA resulted in a defect in both hydrogen and potassium secretion was taken as evidence of decreased sodium transport in the distal nephron (i.e., voltage-dependent defect).[147] Such a defect occurs whenever sodium reabsorption through the sodium channel in principal cells of the collecting tubule is impaired or when sodium delivery to the collecting tubule is decreased. The latter mechanism may be operative in CsA-treated subjects, as shown by Laine and Holmberg.[153] In their study, 11 of 24 renal transplant patients receiving CsA were found to be hyperkalemic. Serum potassium concentration correlated inversely with lithium clearance, suggesting that decreased sodium delivery to the distal tubule results in decreased potassium secretion.[153]

Another mechanism whereby CsA could cause hyperkalemia is a direct inhibition of potassium channels in principal cells of the cortical collecting tubule. In one study done on rabbit cortical collecting tubule principal cells, basolateral exposure to CsA inhibited the activity of the apical membrane channels responsible for physiologic potassium ion secretion.[154] Inhibition of apical secretory potassium ion channels by CsA could contribute to decreased kaliuresis and clinical hyperkalemia observed in patients on CsA therapy.

The role of the renin-angiotensin-aldosterone axis in CsA- and FK506-induced hyperkalemia has also been addressed. In one early study, seven patients who had renal allografts and were treated with CsA had persistent hyperkalemia for several months.[142] Interestingly, all the patients had a hyperkalemic non–anion gap metabolic acidosis. Plasma aldosterone levels were within the normal range in five patients and elevated in two patients. The data demonstrated that aldosterone levels were relatively low for the degree of hyperkalemia in most patients. Plasma renin activity was also low or low-normal in six of the seven patients even in the presence of sodium restriction, indicative of a hyporeninemic state. Of note, five of these six patients were on β-blockers, which are known to inhibit renin release, but one patient who was not receiving a β-blocker also had low renin levels.[142]

Bantle and coworkers studied 10 renal transplant recipients treated with CsA and also noted decreased renin and aldosterone levels in these patients.[143] After stimulation by a low-sodium diet and furosemide, CsA-treated patients had lower plasma renin activity (supine and standing) and lower plasma aldosterone levels. After administration of a potassium chloride load, CsA-treated patients excreted 52% ± 7.1% of the potassium load in 6 hours, compared with excretion of 67% ± 7.0% by the azathioprine-treated patients. There was no difference in plasma aldosterone levels in response to the potassium load in the two groups. These data suggest that CsA causes suppression of plasma renin activity and a tubular insensitivity to aldosterone, both of which may impair potassium excretion.[143]

In a study of 12 hyperkalemic renal transplant patients, Kamel and associates showed that the transtubular potassium gradient remained low even after fludrocortisone therapy (5.6 ± 0.6 in patients, versus 12 ± 1 in control individuals), suggesting a tubular resistance to aldosterone. Bantle and coworkers demonstrated that urinary potassium excretion relative to plasma aldosterone concentration was significantly less in CsA-treated patients, indicative of some degree of renal tubular aldosterone resistance.[143] It seems that a combination of aldosterone deficiency and "resistance" caused by various tubular effects of aldosterone causes the hyperkalemic metabolic acidosis frequently seen in patients treated with CsA.

Interestingly, hyperreninemic hypoaldosteronism has also been reported to cause hyperkalemia in CsA-treated animals but not in humans.[155, 156] In rats, 2 weeks of intragastric administration of low- and high-dose CsA resulted in large increases in plasma renin concentration (23 ± 5, 70 ± 12, and 79 ± 11 ng/mL/hr in control rats and in rats receiving 5 and 20 mg of CsA, respectively), with no concomitant increase in plasma aldosterone. In vitro angiotensin II–stimulated aldosterone secretion by zona glomerulosa cells obtained from CsA-treated rats was also reduced. In contrast, in vitro aldosterone response to graded increments of potassium or ACTH was preserved in CsA-treated rats. When added in vitro to zona glomerulosa cells from untreated rats, CsA also attenuated angiotensin II–stimulated aldosterone secretion but did not affect potassium- or ACTH-mediated aldosterone production (Fig. 24–7). Therefore, CsA-induced hyperreninemic hypoaldosteronism in the rat appears to be due to blockade of angiotensin II–mediated aldosterone production.[155] The increased renin production in CsA-treated animals appears to be due to JGA hyperplasia.[157, 158] In humans, JGA hyperplasia has been observed early after starting CsA therapy following heart transplantation but has not been seen in kidney or bone marrow recipients or diabetic patients.[159]

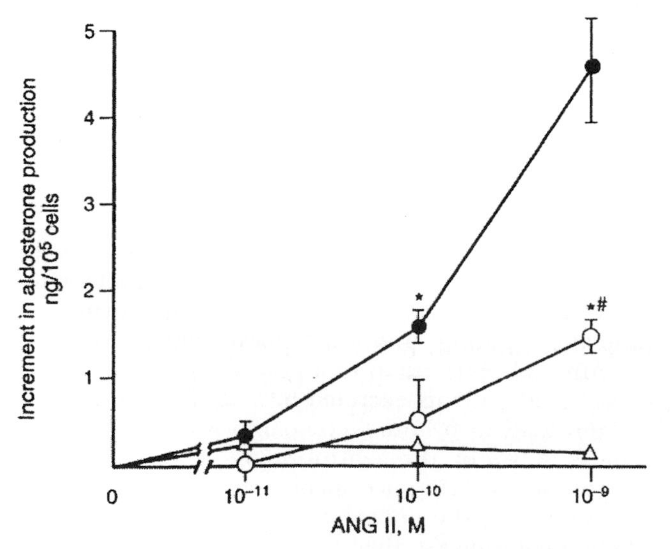


**FIGURE 24–7** ■ In vitro angiotensin II (ANG II)–stimulated aldosterone secretion by zona glomerulosa cells from control and cyclosporin A (CsA)–treated rats. Each data point represents a mean of triplicate incubates derived from a pool of zona glomerulosa cells from seven rats in a single experiment. *Solid circles,* controls; *open circles,* rats given CsA 5mg/kg; *open triangles,* rats given CsA 20 mg/kg. *Asterisks* indicate $P < 0.5$ compared with control group. (From Stern N, Lustig S, Petrasek D, et al: Cyclosporin A–induced hyperreninemic hypoaldosteronism: A model of adrenal resistance to angiotensin II. Hypertension 9 (suppl III): III-31–III-35, 1987.)

## SODIUM CHANNEL INHIBITORS: TRIMETHOPRIM AND PENTAMIDINE

Trimethoprim (TMP) is a recognized cause of hyperkalemia.[160–168] Hyperkalemia has been observed in 20% to 53% of HIV-infected patients receiving high doses of TMP while being treated for *Pneumocystis carinii* pneumonia.[164] In this setting, hyperkalemia was associated with an inappropriate decrease in kaliuresis and was not related to renal failure, adrenal insufficiency, or tubulointerstitial disease. However, patients with preexisting renal dysfunction are much more likely to develop clinically significant hyperkalemia than are patients with normal renal function.[161]

TMP directly interferes with ion transport in the distal nephron.[164, 169] It is now widely recognized that TMP acts like amiloride, a potassium-sparing diuretic, to block apical membrane sodium channels in the distal nephron. As a result, the transepithelial voltage is reduced, and potassium secretion is diminished. Evidence for this came from the studies of Choi[164] and Velazquez[160] and their colleagues. Velazquez demonstrated that rats infused with TMP had decreased urinary potassium excretion and increased urinary sodium excretion.[160] Also, there was a dose-dependent decrease in the transepithelial voltage in rat distal tubules microperfused with TMP. In this study, intravenous TMP decreased potassium excretion by 40%. Choi used the A6 cell line cultured from the toad distal nephron to demonstrate that TMP reversibly inhibited amiloride-sensitive sodium transport.[164] The inhibition of potassium secretion and depolarization of the transepithelial voltage during perfusion with TMP indicate that this medication blocks sodium channels in the luminal membrane of the mammalian distal tubule in a manner similar to amiloride. In addition, TMP has been shown to inhibit renal $Na^+,K^+$ ATPase activity, whereas it has no effect on $H^+$ ATPase activity.[170] Whether this is a primary effect or, more likely, an effect secondary to inhibition of apical sodium transport has not been elucidated.

The concentrations of TMP that inhibit sodium channel transport and decrease potassium excretion in the experimental studies just described are similar to those in the urine of humans treated with high- and standard-dose TMP.[165] In one elderly patient with preexisting renal failure, hyperkalemia developed with a dose of 360 mg/day of TMP.[166] In a retrospective study of 80 patients treated with trimethoprim and sulfamethoxazole (TMP-SMX), it was found that standard-dose TMP-SMX causes an increase in serum potassium.[167] The serum potassium concentration peaked after approximately 5 days of treatment. Moreover, the hyperkalemia that developed reached high levels (>5.5 mEq/L) in 21% of the patients studied.[165, 167]

From the foregoing, it is clear that TMP is one of the best-studied causes of iatrogenic hyperkalemia.

One question that arises is whether this compound causes isolated hyperkalemia or whether it causes the complete picture of hyperkalemic metabolic acidosis. Theoretically, inhibition of the sodium channel should decrease both hydrogen ion and potassium secretion and therefore cause a voltage-dependent type of hyperkalemic dRTA. In reviewing the literature, however, we found that acidosis is not a prominent feature of hyperkalemic patients receiving TMP-SMX; in fact, it is often absent.[160–170] This suggests that inhibition of the sodium channel has a greater impact on potassium secretion than on hydrogen ion secretion, or that hydrogen ion secretion in the outer medullary collecting duct compensates for the inhibition of hydrogen ion secretion caused by inhibition of sodium transport in the cortical collecting tubule. We proposed this explanation in the past to explain the lack of acidosis in lithium-treated patients given amiloride to treat polyuria.[171] In contrast, Lin and associates reported a case of dRTA and hyperkalemia in a patient receiving standard doses of TMP-SMX.[162] This patient's urine pH did not decrease with furosemide, and potassium excretion also remained low, consistent with a voltage-dependent defect. In addition, bicarbonate diuresis did not increase the difference in $P_{CO_2}$ between urine and blood (>20 mm Hg).[162] Plasma aldosterone was not reduced, further excluding aldosterone deficiency. Moreover, this patient had some evidence of salt wastage and hyponatremia, as expected in a true voltage-dependent dRTA. Other cases of metabolic acidosis developing in TMP-treated patients were in the setting of low levels of plasma aldosterone.[168, 172]

TMP, like the potassium-sparing diuretics amiloride and triamterene, is a heterocyclic weak base that exists primarily in its protonated form. Accordingly, it has been proposed that the decrease in kaliuresis caused by TMP could be prevented or attenuated by alkalinizing the luminal fluid in the CCD, thereby converting TMP from its cationic, active form to an electroneutral, inactive form.[173] TMP-induced inhibition of transepithelial sodium ion transport was examined in A6 distal nephron cells by analysis of short-circuit current. The antikaliuretic effect of TMP was examined in vivo in rats pretreated with deoxycorticosterone and with $NH_4Cl$ to lower urine pH, and in rats also receiving azetazolamide to raise urine pH.[173] The concentration of TMP required to inhibit the amiloride-sensitive component of short-circuit current by 50% was 340 μM at pH 8.2 and 50 μM at pH 6.3.[173] In vivo, TMP caused a greater than 50% reduction in potassium excretion, due primarily to a fall in the potassium concentration in the lumen of the terminal CCD. This effect of TMP was markedly attenuated when the urine was made alkaline by acetazolamide.[173] The authors concluded that it is the charged, protonated species of TMP that blocks epithelial sodium channels. Increasing urinary pH decreases the concentration of the charged species of TMP and minimizes its antikaliuretic effect. Therefore, there is a rationale to give alkali to treat or prevent the potassium-retaining effects of protonated TMP, although studies in humans demonstrating the benefit of this interaction are lacking.

Pentamidine, like TMP, is associated with hyperkalemia.[174, 175] Causative mechanisms involve the blockade of apical sodium ion channels in a manner similar to amiloride, as well as hyporeninemic hypoaldosteronism. Kleyman and coworkers studied distal nephron ion transport in an amphibian distal nephron cell line (A6) and primary cultures of rabbit cortical collecting tubules.[174] Various concentrations of pentamidine bathing the luminal surface of the A6 distal nephron cells caused a dose-dependent inhibition of the amiloride-sensitive short-circuit current. The inhibition developed quickly, and 50% blockage of the amiloride-sensitive short-circuit current occurred with 700 μM of pentamidine at a pH of 7.4.[174] Similar results were observed in rabbit luminal membrane channels. By contrast, when pentamidine was exposed to the apical, cell-attached patches on principal cells of primary cultured rabbit cortical collecting tubules, addition of 1 μM of pentamidine to the serosal bath did not significantly affect sodium ion channel activity in the patches. These findings indicate that luminal pentamidine inhibits distal nephron reabsorption of sodium ion by blocking apical sodium ion channels in a manner similar to potassium-sparing diuretics such as amiloride and triamterene. This results in a decrease in the electrochemical gradients that drive secretion of distal nephron potassium ion.[174] Because pentamidine is eliminated through urinary excretion, this renal tubular effect provides a mechanism for pentamidine-induced hyperkalemia. Additionally, an aldosterone-mediated effect has been noted in some hyperkalemic patients. In one study, AIDS patients who were receiving pentamidine clinically resembled patients with type IV RTA.[175] Interestingly, the same metabolic abnormalities recurred in four patients who received more than one course of pentamidine therapy. Plasma renin activity and serum aldosterone were also low in two of the patients in whom these parameters were tested.[175]

Adrenal insufficiency may also contribute to the hyperkalemia seen in AIDS patients.[176] About 50% of patients with advanced AIDS have pathologic evidence of necrotizing adrenalitis, although the degree of adrenal destruction is usually less than 50%. Clinically, adrenal insufficiency occurs in less than 5% of AIDS patients, as 90% of the adrenal cortex must be destroyed in order to develop clinical signs and symptoms. A shift from mineralocorticoid and androgen production to glucocorticoid production occurs, possibly as a response to the stress of severe illness.[176] Subclinical hypoadrenalism combined with pentamidine and/or TMP-SMX administration leads to hyperkalemia and sometimes metabolic acidosis.

## REFERENCES


1. Perez GO, Oster JR, Vaamonde CA: Renal acidosis and renal potassium handling in selective hypoaldosteronism. Am J. Med 57:809–816, 1974.
2. Sebastian A, Schambelan M, Lindenfeld S, et al: Amelioration of metabolic acidosis with fludrocortisone therapy in hyporeninemic hypoaldosteronism. N Engl J Med 297:576–583, 1977.

3. Szylman P, Better OS, Chaimowitz C, et al: Role of hyperkalemia in the metabolic acidosis of isolated hypoaldosteronism. N Engl J Med 294:361–365, 1976.
4. Schambelan M, Sebastian A, Biglieri EG: Prevalence, pathogenesis, and functional significance of aldosterone deficiency in hyperkalemic patients with chronic renal insufficiency. Kidney Int 17:89–101, 1980.
5. Sebastian A, Sutton JM, Hulter HN, et al: Effect of mineralocorticoid replacement therapy on renal acid-base homeostasis in adrenalectomized patients. Kidney Int 18:762–773, 1980.
6. Batlle DC: Hyperkalemic hyperchloremic metabolic acidosis associated with selective aldosterone deficiency and distal renal tubular acidosis. Semin Nephrol 1:260–274, 1981.
7. Batlle DC, Arruda JAL, Kurtzman NA: Hyperkalemic distal renal tubular acidosis associated with obstructive uropathy. N Engl J Med 304:373–380, 1981.
8. Batlle DC, Itsarayoungyuen K, Arruda JAL, et al: Hyperkalemic hyperchloremic metabolic acidosis in sickle cell hemoglobinopathies. Am J Med 72:188–192, 1982.
9. Batlle DC, Sehy JT, Roseman MK, et al: Clinical and pathophysiological spectrum of acquired distal renal tubular acidosis. Kidney Int 20:389–396, 1981.
10. Arruda JAL, Batlle DC, Sehy JT, et al: Hyperkalemia in renal insufficiency: Role of aldosterone and tubular unresponsiveness to aldosterone. Am J Nephrol 1:160–167, 1981.
11. Batlle DC: Sodium-dependent urinary acidification in patients with aldosterone deficiency and adrenalectomized rats. Metabolism 35:852–860, 1986.
12. Batlle DC: Segmental characterization of defects in collecting tubule acidification. Kidney Int 30:545–553, 1986.
13. Batlle DC, Moses MF, Maniligod J, et al: The pathogenesis of hyperchloremic metabolic acidosis associated with renal transplantation. Am J Med 70:786–796, 1981.
14. Schlueter W, Keilani T, Hizon M, et al: On the mechanism of impaired distal acidification in hyperkalemic renal tubular acidosis: Evaluation with amiloride and bumetanide. J Am Soc Nephrol 3:953–964, 1992.
15. Batlle DC, Kurtzman NA: Clinical disorders of aldosterone metabolism. Dis Mon 30:1–55, 1984.
16. Kurtzman NA: Renal tubular acidosis: A constellation of syndromes. Hosp Pract 2:173–188, 1987.
17. Kurtzman NA: Disorders of distal acidification. Kidney Int 38: 720–727, 1990.
18. Sebastian A, Schambelan M, Sutton J: Amelioration of hyperchloremic acidosis with furosemide therapy in patients with chronic renal insufficiency and type IV renal tubular acidosis. Am J Nephrol 4:287–300, 1984.
19. Rastogi S, Bayliss JM, Nascimento L, Arruda JAL: Hyperkalemic renal tubular acidosis: Effect of furosemide in humans and in rats. Kidney Int 28:801–807, 1985.
20. DuBose TD Jr, Catflisch CR: Effect of selective aldosterone deficiency on acidification in nephron segments of the rat inner medulla. J Clin Invest 82:1624–1632, 1988.
21. DuBose TD Jr, Catflisch CR: Validation of the difference in urine and blood $CO_2$ tension during bicarbonate loading as an index of distal nephron acidification in experimental models of distal renal tubular acidosis. J Clin Invest 75:1116–1123, 1985.
22. DuBose TD Jr: Hyperkalemic hyperchloremic metabolic acidosis: Pathophysiologic insights. Kidney Int 51:591–602, 1997.
23. White PC: Mechanisms of disease: Disorders of aldosterone biosynthesis and action. N Engl J Med 331:250–258, 1994.
24. Schlueter W, Keilani T, Batlle DC: Tissue renin angiotensin systems: Theoretical implications for the development of hyperkalemia using angiotension-converting enzyme inhibitors. Am J Med Sci 307(suppl):581–586, 1994.
25. Doi Y, Atarashi K, Franco-Saenz R, Mulrow PJ: Effect of changes in sodium or potassium balance, and nephrectomy, on adrenal renin and aldosterone concentrations. Hypertension 6(suppl 1):124–129, 1984.
26. Mulrow PJ: Adrenal renin: A possible local hormonal regulator of aldosterone production. Yale J Biol Med 62:503–510, 1989.
27. Shier DN, Kusano E, Stone GD, et al: Production of renin, angiotensin II, and aldosterone by adrenal explante cultures: Response to potassium and converting enzyme inhibition. Endocrinology 125:486–491, 1989.
28. Cannon PJ, Ames RP, Laragh JH: Relation between potassium balance and aldosterone secretion in normal subjects and in patients with hypertensive or renal tubular disease. J Clin Invest 45:865–879, 1966.
29. Oelkers W: Adrenal insufficiency. N Engl J Med 335:1206–1212, 1996.
30. White PC, New MI. Genetic basis of endocrine disease 2: Congenital adrenal hyperplasia due to 21-hydroxylase deficiency. J Clin Endocrinol Metab 74:6–11, 1992.
31. Lin D, Gitelman SE, Saenger P, Miller WL: Normal genes for the cholesterol side chain cleavage enzyme, P450scc, in congenital lipoid adrenal hyperplasia. J Clin Invest 88:1955–1962, 1991.
32. Rheaume E, Simard J, Morel Y, et al: Congenital adrenal hyperplasia due to point mutations in the type II 3b-hydroxysteroid dehydrogenase gene. Nat Genet 1:239–245, 1992.
33. Wilson RC, Mercado AB, Cheng KC, New MI: Steroid 21-hydroxylase deficiency: Genotype may not predict phenotype. J Clin Endocrinol Metab 80:2322–2329, 1995.
34. Binder G, Wollmann H, Schwarze CP, et al: X-linked congenital adrenal hypoplasia: New mutations and long-term follow-up in three patients. Clin Endocrinol (Oxf) 53:249–255, 2000.
35. New MI: Steroid 21-hydroxylase deficiency (congenital adrenal hyperplasia). Am J Med 98:2S–8S, 1995.
36. White PC, Speiser PW: Congenital adrenal hyperplasia due to 21-hydroxylase deficiency. Endocr Rev 21:245–291, 2000.
37. Peter M, Sippell WG: Congenital hypoaldosteronism: The Visser-Cost syndrome revisited. Pediatr Res 39:554–560, 1996.
38. Pascoe L, Curnow KM, Slutsker L, et al: Mutations in the human CYP11B2 (aldosterone synthase) gene causing corticosterone methyloxidase II deficiency. Proc Natl Acad Sci U S A 89:4996–5000, 1992.
39. Portrat-Doyen S, Tourniaire J, Richard O, et al: Isolated aldosterone synthase deficiency caused by simultaneous E198D and V386A mutations in the CYP11B2 gene. J Clin Endocrinol Metab 83:4156–4161, 1998.
40. Muller J: Regulation of aldosterone biosynthesis: The end of the road? Clin Exp Pharmacol Physiol Suppl 25:S79–S85, 1998.
41. Peter M, Fawaz L, Drop SLS, et al: Hereditary defect in biosynthesis of aldosterone: Aldosterone synthase deficiency 1964–1997. J Clin Endocrinol Metab 82:3525–3528, 1997.
42. Peter M, Partsch C-J, Sippell WG: Multisteroid analysis in children with terminal aldosterone biosynthesis defects. J Clin Endocrinol Metab 80:1622–1627, 1995.
43. Lee PDK, Patterson BD, Hintz RL, et al: Biochemical diagnosis and management of corticosterone methyloxidase type II deficiency. J Clin Endocrinol Metab 62:225–229, 1986.
44. Ulick S, Wang JZ, Morton DH: The biochemical phenotypes of two inborn errors in the biosynthesis of aldosterone. J Clin Endocrinol Metab 74:1415–1420, 1992.
45. Rosler A: The natural history of salt-wasting disorders of adrenal and renal origin. J Clin Endocrinol Metab 59:689–700, 1984.
46. Mitsuuchi Y, Kawamoto T, Miyahara K, et al: Congenitally defective aldosterone biosynthesis in humans: Inativation of the P-$450^{C18}$ gene (CYP11B2) due to nucleotide deletion in CMO I deficient patients. Biochem Biophys Res Commun 190:864–869, 1993.
47. Pascoe L, Curnow KM, Slutsker L, et al: Mutations in the human CYP11B2 (aldosterone synthase) gene causing corticosterone methyloxidase II deficiency. Proc Natl Acad Sci U S A 89:4996–5000, 1992.
48. Zanaria E, Muscatelli F, Bardoni B, et al: An unusual member of the nuclear hormone receptor superfamily responsible for X-linked adrenal hypoplasia congenita. Nature 372:635–641, 1994.
49. Tabarin A, Achermann JC, Recan D, et al: A novel mutation in DAX1 causes delayed-onset adrenal insufficiency and incomplete hypogonadotropic hypogonadism. J Clin Invest 105:321–328, 2000.
50. Davenport MW, Zipser RD: Association of hypotension with hyper-reninemic hypoaldosteronism in the critically ill patient. Arch Intern Med 143:735–737, 1983.
51. Hudson JB, Chobanian AW, Relman AS: Hypoaldosteronism: A clinical study of a patient with an isolated adrenal mineralocor-

ticoid deficiency, resulting in hyperkalemia and Stokes-Adams attacks. N Engl J Med 257:529, 1957.
52. Posner JB, Jacobs DR: Isolated aldosteronism I. Clinical entity with manifestations of persistent hyperkalemia, periodic paralysis, salt-losing tendency, and acidosis. Metabolism 13:513, 1964.
53. Skanse B, Hokfelt B: Hypoaldosteronism with otherwise intact adrenocortical function, resulting in a characteristic clinical entity. Acta Endocrinol 28:29, 1958.
54. Weidmann P, Reinhart R, Maxwell MH, et al: Syndrome of hyporeninemic hypoaldosteronism and hyperkalemia in renal disease. J Clin Endocrinol Metab 36:965–977, 1973.
55. Schambelan M, Stockigt JR, Biglieri EG: Isolated hypoaldosteronism in adults: A renin-deficiency syndrome. N Engl J Med 287:573–578, 1972.
56. Tan SY, Burton M: Hyporeninemic hypoaldosteronism: An overlooked cause of hyperkalemia. Arch Intern Med 141:30–33, 1981.
57. Vagnucci AH: Selective aldosterone deficiency. J Clin Endocrinol Metab 29:279–289, 1969.
58. Perez GO, Lespier L, Jacobi J, et al: Hyporeninemia and hypoaldosteronism in diabetes mellitus. Arch Intern Med 137:852–855, 1977.
59. Gerber JG, Olson RD, Nies AS: Interrelationship between prostaglandins and renin release. Kidney Int 19:816–821, 1981.
60. Schindler AM, Sommers SC: Diabetic sclerosis of the renal juxtaglomerular apparatus. Lab Invest 15:877–884, 1966.
61. Tuck ML, Sambhi MP, Levin L: Hyporeninemic hypoaldosteronism in diabetes mellitus: Studies of the autonomic nervous system's control of renin release. Diabetes 28:237–241, 1979.
62. DeLeiva A, Christlieb AR, Melby JC, et al: Big renin and biosynthetic defect of aldosterone in diabetes mellitus. N Engl J Med 295:639–643, 1976.
63. Oh MS, Carroll HJ, Clemmons JE, et al: A mechanism for hyporeninemic hypoaldosteronism in chronic renal disease. Metabolism 23:1157–1166, 1974.
64. Christlieb AR, Munichoodappa C, Braaten JT: Decreased response of plasma renin activity to orthostasis in diabetic patients with orthostatic hypotension. Diabetes 23:835–840, 1974.
65. Weidman P, Beretta-Piccoli C, Zhgler WH, et al: Age versus urinary sodium for judging renin, aldosterone, and catecholamine levels: Studies in normal subjects and patients with essential hypertension. Kidney Int 14:619–629, 1978.
66. Oates JA, Whorton AR, Gerkens JF, et al: The participation of prostaglandins in the control of renin release. Fed Proc 38: 72–74, 1978.
67. Lijnen P, Staessen J, Fagard R, Amery A: Effect of prostaglandin inhibition by indomethacin on plasma active and inactive renin concentration in men. Can J Physiol Pharmacol 69:1355–1359, 1991.
68. Data JL, Gerber JG, Crump WJ, et al: The prostaglandin system—a role in canine baroreceptor control of renin release. Circ Res 42:454–458, 1978.
69. Henrich WL: Role of prostaglandins in renin secretion. Kidney Int 19:822–830, 1981.
70. Weidman P, Maxwell MH, Rowe P, et al: Role of the renin-angiotensin-aldosterone system in the regulation of plasma potassium in chronic renal failure. Nephron 15:35, 1975.
71. Bayard F, Cooke CR, Tiller DJ, et al: The regulation of aldosterone secretion in anephric man. J Clin Invest 50:1585–1595, 1971.
72. Cooke CR, Horvath JS, Moore MA, et al: Modulation of plasma aldosterone concentration by plasma potassium in anephric man in the absence of a change in potassium balance. J Clin Invest 52:3028–3032, 1973.
73. Davis JO, Urquhart J, Higgins JT Jr: The effects of alterations of plasma sodium and potassium concentration on aldosterone secretion. J Clin Invest 42:597, 1963.
74. Fredlund P, Saltman S, Kondo T, et al: Aldosterone production by isolated glomerulosa cells: Modulation of sensitivity to angiotensin II and ACTH by extracellular potassium concentration. Endocrinology 100:481–486, 1977.
75. Pratt JH: Role of angiotensin II in potassium-mediated stimulation of aldosterone secretion in the dog. J Clin Invest 70: 667–672, 1982.
76. Clark BA, Brown RS, Epstein FH: Effect of atrial natriuretic peptide on potassium stimulated aldosterone secretion: Potential relevance to hypoaldosteronism in man. J Clin Endocrinol Metab 75:399–403, 1992.
77. Schriffrin EL, Chartier L, Thibault G, et al: Vascular and adrenal receptors for atrial natriuretic factor in the rat. Circ Res 56:801–807, 1985.
78. Tuchelt H, Eschenhagen G, Bahr V, et al: Role of atrial natriuretic factor in changes in the responsiveness of aldosterone to angiotensin II secondary to sodium loading and depletion in man. Clin Sci 79:57–65, 1990.
79. Anderson JV, Struthers AD, Payne NN, et al: Atrial natriuretic peptide inhibits the aldosterone response to angiotensin II in man. Clin Sci 70:507–512, 1986.
80. Cuneo RC, Espiner A, Nicholls MG, et al: Renal, hemodynamic, and hormonal responses to natriuretic peptide infusions in normal man, and effects of sodium intake. J Clin Endocrinol Metab 63:946–953, 1986.
81. Chartier L, Schiffrin EL: Atrial natriuretic peptide inhibits the stimulation of aldosterone secretion by ACTH in vitro and in vivo. Soc Exp Biol Med 182:132–136, 1986.
82. Ferri C, Baldoncini RA, Bellini C, et al: Hormonal and renal responses to atrial natriuretic peptide infusion in low-renin hypertension. Am J Nephrol 15:222–229, 1995.
83. Carey RM, Thorner MO, Ortt EM: Effects of metoclopramide and bromocriptine on the renin-angiotension-aldosterone system in man: Dopaminergic control of aldosterone. J Clin Invest 63:727–735, 1979.
84. Oster JR, Singer I, Fishman LM: Heparin-induced aldosterone suppression and hyperkalemia. Am J Med 98:575–586, 1995.
85. Phelps KR, Oh MS, Carroll HJ: Heparin-induced hyperkalemia: Report of a case. Nephron 24:254–258, 1980.
86. O'Kelly R, Magee F, McKenna TJ: Routine heparin therapy inhibits adrenal aldosterone production. J Clin Endocr Soc 56: 108–112, 1983.
87. Siebels M, Andrassy K, Vecsei P, et al: Dose dependent suppression of mineralocorticoid metabolism by different heparin fractions. Thromb Res 66:467–473, 1992.
88. Leehey D, Gantt C, Lim V: Heparin-induced hypoaldosteronism. JAMA 246:2189–2190, 1981.
89. Levesque H, Verdier S, Caileux N, et al: Low molecular weight heparins and hypoaldosteronism. BMJ 300:1438–1439, 1990.
90. Cailleux N, Moore N, Levesque H, et al: A low molecular weight heparin decreases plasma aldosterone in patients with primary hyperaldosteronism. Br J Clin Pharmacol 43:185–187, 1992.
91. Sherman RA, Ruddy MC: Suppression of aldosterone production by low-dose heparin. Am J Nephrol 6:165–168, 1986.
92. Azukizawa S, Uchida K, Imaizumi N, et al: Direct effects of heparin on basal and stimulated aldosterone production in rat adrenal glomerulosa cells. J Steroid Biochem 25:455–457, 1986.
93. Susic D, Mandal AK, Jovovic D, et al: Antihypertensive action of heparin: Role of the renin-angiotensin-aldosterone system and prostaglandins. J Clin Pharmacol 33:342–347, 1993.
94. Wilson ID, Goetz FC: Selective hypoaldosteronism after prolonged heparin administration. Am J Med 36:635–640, 1964.
95. Hene RJ, Boer P, Koomans HA: Plasma aldosterone concentrations in chronic renal disease. Kidney Int 21:98–101, 1982.
96. Cope CL, Pearson J: Aldosterone secretion in severe renal failure. Clin Sci 25:331, 1963.
97. Schrier RW, Regal E: Influence of aldosterone on sodium, water and potassium metabolism in chronic renal disease. Kidney Int 1:156–168, 1972.
98. Cogan MG, Arieff AI: Sodium wasting, acidosis and hyperkalemia induced by methicillin interstitial nephritis: Evidence for selective distal tubular dysfunction. Am J Med 64:500–507, 1978.
99. Luke RG, Allison ME, Davidson JF, et al: Hyperkalemia and renal tubular acidosis due to renal amyloidosis. Ann Intern Med 70:1211–1217, 1969.
100. Rado JP, Szende L, Szucs L: Hyperkalemia unresponsive to massive doses of aldosterone and renal tubular acidosis in a patient with chronic interstitial nephritis: Clinical and experimental studies. J Med 7:481–510, 1976.
101. Batlle DC, Hizon M, Cohen E, et al: The use of the urinary anion gap in the diagnosis of hyperchloremic acidosis. N Engl J Med 318:594–599, 1988.

102. Batlle DC, Flores G: Underlying defects in distal renal tubular acidosis: New understandigs. Am J Kidney Dis 27:896–915, 1996.
103. Wadi N, et al: Suki and Massry's Therapy of Renal Disorders and Related Disorders, 3rd ed. Kluwer Academic Publishers, Philadelphia, 1997.
104. Cheek DB, Perry JW: A salt wasting syndrome in infancy. Arch Dis Child 33:252–256, 1958.
105. Bistritzer T, Evans S, Cotariu D, et al: Reduced $Na^+$, $K^+$-ATPase activity in patients with pseudohypoaldosteronism. Pediatr Res 35:372–375, 1994.
106. Zennaro MC, Borensztein P, Soubrier F, et al: The enigma of pseudohypoaldosteronism. Steroids 94:96–99, 1994.
107. Kuhnle U, Hinkel GK, Hubl W, Reichelt T: Pseudohypoaldosteronism: Family studies to identify asymptomatic carriers by stimulation of the renin-aldosterone system. Horm Res 46: 124–129, 1996.
108. Kuhnle U, Nielsen D, Tietze H, et al: Pseudohypoaldosteronism in eight families: Different forms of inheritance are evidence for various genetic defects. J Clin Endocrinol Metab 70:638–641, 1992.
109. Geller DS, Rodriguez-Soriano J, Boado AV, et al: Mutations in the mineralocorticoid receptor gene cause autosomal dominant pseudohypoaldosteronism type I. Nat Genet 19:279–281, 1998.
110. Armanini D, Karbowiak I, Zennaro CM, et al: Pseudohypoaldosteronism: Evaluation of type I receptors by radioreceptor assay and by antireceptor antibodies. Steroids 60:161–163, 1995.
111. Chang SS, Grunder S, Hanukoglu A, et al: Mutations in subunits of the epithelial sodium channel cause salt wasting with hyperkalaemic acidosis, pseudohypoaldosteronism type I. Nat Genet 12:248–253, 1996.
112. Pradervand S, Barker PM, Wang Q, et al: Salt restriction induces pseudohypoaldosteronism type I in mice expressing low levels of the B-subunit of the amiloride-sensitive epithelial sodium channel. PNAS Online 96:1732–1737, 1999.
113. Gordon RD: Syndrome of hypertension and hyperkalemia with normal glomerular filtration rate. Hypertension 8:93–102, 1986.
114. Kuhnle U: At the cutting edge—pseudohypoaldosteronism: Mutation found, problem solved? Mol Cell Endocrinol 133: 77–80, 1997.
115. Gereda JE, Bonilla-Felix M, Kalil B, DeWitt SJ: Neonatal presentation of Gordon syndrome. J Pediatr 129:615–617, 1996.
116. Throckmorton DC, Bia Johnson M: Pseudohypoaldosteronism: Case report and discussion of the syndrome. Yale J Biol Med 64:247–254, 1991.
117. Schambelan M, Sebastian A Jr, Rector FC: Mineralocorticoid-resistant renal hyperkalemia without salt wasting (type II pseudohypoaldosteronism): Role of increased renal chloride reabsorption. Kidney Int 19:716–727, 1981.
118. Take C, Ikeda K, Kurasawa T, Kurokawa K: Increased chloride reabsorption as an inherited renal tubular defect in familial type II pseudohypoaldosteronism. N Engl J Med 324:472–476, 1991.
119. Simon DB, Farfel Z, Ellison D, et al: Examination of the thiazide-sensitive $Na^+$-$Cl^-$ contransporter as a candidate gene in Gordon's syndrome [abstract]. J Am Soc Nephrol 6:632, 1995.
120. Mansfield TA, Simon DB, Farfel Z, et al: Multilocus linkage of familial hyperkalemia and hypertension. Nat Genet 16:202–205, 1997.
120b. Wilson FH, Disse-Nicodeme S, Choate KA, et al. Human hypertension caused by mutations in WNK kinases. Science 293: 1107–1112, 2001.
121. Gordon RD, Geddes RA, Pawsey CGK, O'Halloran MW: Hypertension and severe hyperkalaemia associated with suppression of renin and aldosterone and completely reversed by dietary sodium restriction. Aust Ann Med 4:287–294, 1970.
122. Whelton A: Nephrotoxicity of non-steroidal anti-inflammatory drugs: Physiologic foundations and clinical implications. Am J Med 106:12s–24s, 1999.
123. Jacobson EJ: Weighing the renal effects of NSAIDs and COX-2 inhibitors. Clin Dilemmas 1:1–12, 2000.
124. Stichtenoth DO, Wagner B, Frolich JC: Effect of selective inhibition of the inducible cyclooxygenase on renin release in healthy volunteers. J Investig Med 46:290–296, 1998.
125. Yang T, Endo Y, Huang YG, et al: Renin expression in COX-2 knockout mice on normal or low-salt diets. Am J Physiol Renal Physiol 279:F819–F825, 2000.
126. Traynor TR, Smart A, Briggs JP, Schnermann J: Inhibition of macula densa–stimulated renin secretion by pharmacological blockade of cyclooxygenase-2. Am J Physiol Renal Physiol 277: F706–F710, 1999.
127. Rodriguez R, Llinas MT, Gonzalez JD, et al: Renal changes induced by a cyclooxygenase-2 inhibitor during normal and low sodium intake. Hypertension 36:276–281, 2000.
128. Harding P, Carretero OA, Beierwaltes WH: Chronic cyclooxygenase-2 inhibition blunts low sodium–stimulated renin without changing renal haemodynamics. Hypertension 18:1107–1113, 2000.
129. Swan SK, Rudy DW, Lasseter KC, et al: Effect of cyclooxygenase-2 inhibition on renal function in elderly persons receiving a low-salt diet: A randomized controlled trial. Ann Intern Med 133:1–9, 2000.
130. Textor SC, Bravo EL, Fouad FM, Tarazi RC: Hyperkalemia in azotemic patients during angiotensin-converting enzyme inhibition and aldosterone reduction with captopril. Am J Med 73: 719–725, 1982.
131. Atlas SA, Case DB, Sealey JE, et al: Interruption of the renin-angiotensin system in hypertensive patients by captopril induces sustained reduction in aldosterone secretion, potassium retention and natriuresis. Hypertension 1:274–280, 1979.
132. Lijnen P, Staessen J, Fagard R, Amery A: Increase in plasma aldosterone during prolonged captopril treatment. Am J Cardiol 49:1561–1563, 1982.
133. Hodsman GP, Brown JJ, Cumming AMM, et al: Enalapril (MK421) in the treatment of hypertension with renal artery stenosis. J Hypertens 1(suppl 1):109–117, 1983.
134. Biollaz J, Brunner HR, Gavras I, et al: Antihypertensive therapy with MK 421: Angiotensin II–renin relationships to evaluate efficacy of converting enzyme blockade. J Cardiovasc Pharmacol 4:966–972, 1982.
135. Ruilope LM, Miranda B, Morales JM, et al: Converting enzyme inhibition in chronic renal failure. Am J Kidney Dis 13:120–126, 1989.
136. Keilani T, Schlueter W, Molteni A, Batlle DC: Converting enzyme inhibition with fosinopril does not suppress plasma aldosterone and may not cause hyperkalemia despite moderate renal impairment [abstract]. J Am Soc Nephrol 2:281, 1998.
137. Chevillard C, Brown NL, Mathieu M-N, et al: Differential effects of oral trandolapril and enalapril on rat tissue angiotensin-converting enzyme. Eur J Pharmacol 147:23–28, 1988.
138. Sakaguchi K, Chai SY, Jackson B, et al: Inhibition of tissue angiotensin converting enzyme: Quantitation by autoradiography. Hypertension 11:230–238, 1988.
139. Unger T, Ganten D, Lang RE: Tissue converting enzyme and cardiovascular actions of converting enzyme inhibitors. J Cardiovasc Pharmacol 8(suppl 10):S75–S81, 1982.
140. Bakris GL, Siomos M, Richardson D, et al: ACE inhibition or angiotensin receptor blockade: Impact on potassium in renal failure. Kidney Int 58:2084–2092, 2000.
141. Marcelli JM, Lalau JD, Abourachid H, et al: Unlike heparin, low-molecular weight heparin does not suppress aldosterone production. Horm Metab Res 21:402, 1989.
142. Adu D, Michael J, Turney J, McMaster P: Hyperkalemia in cyclosporin-treated renal allograft recipients. Lancet 1:370–372, 1983.
143. Bantle JP, Nath KA, Sutherland DER, et al: Effects of cyclosporine on the renin-angiotensin-aldosterone system and potassium excretion in renal transplant recipients. Arch Intern Med 145: 505–508, 1985.
144. Woo M, Przepiorka D, Ipoliti C, et al: Toxicities of tacrolimus and cyclosporin A after allogeneic blood stem cell transplantation. Bone Marrow Transplant 20:1095–1098, 1997.
145. Sutherland DER, Strand M, Fryd DS: Comparison of cyclosporin versus azathioprine–anti-lymphocyte globulin in renal transplantation. Am J Kidney Dis 3:456–461, 1984.
146. Hamilton DV, Evans DB, Henderson RG: Nephrotoxicity and metabolic acidosis in transplant patients on cyclosporin A. Proc EDTA 18:400–419, 1981.
147. Batlle DC, Gutterman C, Tarka J, Prasad R: Effect of short-

term cyclosporin A administration on urinary acidification. Clin Nephrol 25(suppl 1):S62–S69, 1986.
148. Kamel KS, Ethler JH, Quaggin S, et al: Studies to determine the basis for hyperkalemia in recipients of a renal transplant who are treated with cyclosporine. J Am Soc Nephrol 2:1279–1284, 1992.
149. Allesiani M, Cillo U, Fung J: Adverse effects of FK-506 overdosage after liver transplantation. Transplant Proc 25:628–634, 1993.
150. Tumlin JA, Sands JM: Nephron segment-specific inhibition of $Na^+/K^+$-ATPase activity by cyclosporin A. Kidney Int 43:246–251, 1993.
151. Lea JP, Sands JM, Tumlin JA: Calcineurin: The key to immunosuppressive drug-induced inhibition of Na/K-ATPase activity. JASN Abstracts 4:871, 1993.
152. Mihatsch MJ, Morozumi KM, Yamaguchi Y, et al: The side-effects of ciclosporine-A and tarcrolimus. Clin Nephrol 49: 356–363, 1998.
153. Laine J, Holmberg C: Renal and adrenal mechanisms in cyclosporine-induced hyperkalaemia after renal transplantation. Eur J Clin Invest 25:670–676, 1995.
154. Ling BN, Eaton DC: Cyclosporin A inhibits apical secretory $K^+$ channels in rabbit cortical collecting tubule principal cells. Kidney Int 44:974–984, 1993.
155. Stern N, Lustig S, Petrasek D, et al: Cyclosporin A–induced hyperreninemic hypoaldosteronism: A model of adrenal resistance to angiotensin II. Hypertension 9(suppl III):III-31–III-35, 1987.
156. Lustig S, Stern N, Eggena P, et al: Effect of cyclosporin on blood pressure and renin-aldosterone axis in rats. Am J Physiol 253:H1596–H1600, 1987.
157. Gillum DM, Truong L, Tasby J, et al: Chronic cyclosporine nephrotoxicity: A rodent model. Transplantation 46:285–292, 1988.
158. Nitta K, Friedman AL, Nicastri AD, et al: Granular juxtaglomerular cell hyperplasia caused by cyclosporine. Transplantation 44:417–421, 1987.
159. Mason J, Muller-Schweinitzer E, Dupont M, et al: Cyclosporine and the renin-angiotensin system. Kidney Int 39(suppl 32):S-28–S-32, 1991.
160. Velazquez H, Perazella A, Wright FS, Ellison DH: Renal mechanism of trimethoprim-induced hyperkalemia. Ann Intern Med 119:296–301, 1993.
161. Ellison DH: Hyperkalemia and trimethoprim-sulfamethoxazole. Am J Kidney Dis 29:959–965, 1997.
162. Lin SH, Kuo AA, Yu FC, Lin YF: Reversible voltage-dependent distal renal tubular acidosis in a patient receiving standard doses of trimethoprim-sulphamethoxazole. Nephrol Dial Transplant 12:1031–1033, 1997.
163. Marinella MA: Trimethoprim-induced hyperkalemia: An analysis of reported cases. Gerontology 45:209–212, 1999.
164. Choi MJ, Fernandez PC, Patnaik A, et al: Brief report: Trimethoprim-induced hyperkalemia in a patient with AIDS. N Engl J Med 328:703–706, 1993.
165. Perazella MA, Buller GK: Hyperkalemia and trimethoprim-sulfamethaxozole. Am J Kidney Dis 29:959–965, 1997.
166. Funai N, Shimamoto Y, Matsuzaki M, et al: Hyperkalemia with renal tubular dysfunction by sulfamethoxazole-trimethoprim for *Pneumocystis carinii* pneumonia in patients with lymphoid surgery. Haematologia 25:137–141, 1993.
167. Alappan R, Perazella MA, Buller GK: Hyperkalemia in hospitalized patients treated with trimethoprim-sulfamethoxazole. Ann Intern Med 124:316–320, 1996.
168. Sheehan MT, Wen SF: Hyperkalemic renal tubular acidosis induced by trimethoprim/sulfamethoxazole in an AIDS patient. Clin Nephrol 50:188–193, 1998.
169. Schlanger LE, Kleyman TR, Ling BN: $K^+$-sparing diuretic actions of trimethoprim: Inhibition of $Na^+$ channels in A6 distal nephron cells. Kidney Int 45:1070–1076, 1994.
170. Eiam-Ong S, Kurtzman A, Sabatini S: Studies on the mechanism of trimethoprim-induced hyperkalemia. Kidney Int 49: 1372–1378, 1996.
171. Batlle DC, Von Riotte A, Gaviria M, Grupp M: Amelioration of polyuria in patients on chronic lithium therapy by a specific approach using amiloride. N Engl J Med 312:408–414, 1985.
172. Kalin MF, Poretxky L, Seres DS, Zurnoff B: Hyporeninemic hypoaldosteronism associated with acquired immune deficiency syndrom. Am J Med 82:1035–1038, 1987.
173. Schreiber M, Schlanger LE, Chen CB, et al: Antikaliuretic action of trimethoprim is minimized by raising urine pH. Kidney Int 49:82–87, 1996.
174. Kleyman TR, Roberts C, Ling BN: A mechanism for pentamidine-induced hyperkalemia: Inhibition of distal nephron sodium transport. Ann Intern Med 122:103–106, 1995.
175. Lachaal M, Venuto RC: Nephrotoxicity and hyperkalemia in patients with acquired immunodeficiency syndrome treated with pentamidine. Am J Med 87:260–263, 1989.
176. Carey RM: The changing clinical spectrum of adrenal insufficiency. Ann Intern Med 127:1103–1105, 1997.

Section V
# *Divalent Ions*

## CHAPTER 25

# Renal Regulation of Calcium, Phosphate, and Magnesium

Clara E. Magyar, PhD ▪ Peter A. Friedman, PhD

Calcium, phosphate, and magnesium are multivalent cations that are important for many vital and complex biologic and cellular functions. In humans, the kidneys play a major role in the homeostasis of these ions. Gastrointestinal absorption is balanced by renal excretion. When body stores of these ions decline significantly, gastrointestinal absorption, bone resorption, and renal tubular reabsorption increase to normalize their levels. Renal regulation of these ions occurs through glomerular filtration and tubular reabsorption and/or excretion and is therefore an important determinant of plasma ion concentrations. Under physiologic conditions, the whole-body balance of calcium, phosphate, and magnesium is maintained by fine adjustments of urinary excretion to equal the net intake.

This chapter discusses how calcium, phosphate, and magnesium are handled by the kidney, with emphasis on the cellular and molecular mechanisms governing these processes. In addition, the roles of hormones and other factors regulating the urinary excretion of these ions are examined.

## CALCIUM CHEMISTRY

The calcium ion is ideally suited as a molecular trigger for receptor signaling. Its high coordination number of 6 to 8 facilitates the ability to cross-link proteins.[1] Such cross-linking of osseous structural proteins is enhanced at the relatively high calcium concentrations found in extracellular fluid. Despite these virtues, the proper functioning of a variety of proteins and macromolecules would be impaired if intracellular ionized calcium ($[Ca^{2+}]_i$) were of the same order as the extracellular concentration. Owing to low intracellular levels, changes in calcium activity can function as first or second messengers to activate downstream targets. Intracellular microcrystallization and precipitation of calcium phosphate are avoided by keeping $[Ca^{2+}]_i$ low.

### Serum Calcium

In adults, plasma calcium concentration averages 2.5 mmol/L (5 mEq/L, or 10 mg/dL)* and is found in three forms: protein bound, complexed, and ionized. The relative proportions of the various calcium fractions are shown in Figure 25–1, and the associated calcium concentrations are summarized in Table 25–1. Forty percent of the serum calcium is bound to plasma proteins, mostly to albumin,[2] with smaller percentages bound to globulins.[3] Ten percent of the serum calcium is in the form of complexes with polyvalent anions. The main calcium complexes are formed by ion pairing with bicarbonate ($CaHCO_4^{2-}$), phosphate, and sulfate or with low-molecular-weight organic anions such as citrate.[4] Concentrations of ionized calcium, the complexing anion, and the ambient pH determine the degree of ion pair formation. Only diffusible calcium (i.e., ionized and complexed calcium) is filtered at the glomerulus. Also, only diffusible calcium crosses cell membranes and is the biologically relevant form of the ion.

The ultrafilterable and ionized fractions of calcium are affected by changes in the total serum calcium concentration, blood pH, plasma protein concentration, and concentration of complexing anions. Increases in the total serum calcium concentration are usually accompanied by concomitant elevations in the concentration of ultrafilterable calcium, at least up to a total concentration of about 4 mM.[5,6] Serum protein levels tend to parallel changes in the total serum calcium concentration, so that the ultrafilterable fraction remains constant.[7–9] In severe hypoproteinemia, however, the ultrafilterable fraction increases.[10,11]

The concentration of ionized $Ca^{2+}$ varies inversely with blood pH. Ionized $Ca^{2+}$ is increased in acidosis and decreased in alkalosis. Ionized $Ca^{2+}$ concentrations also change inversely with changes in serum anions. Elevation of phosphate, citrate, sulfate, or bi-

*Concentrations of calcium and phosphate are expressed in SI units (mmol/L). The relations between different units are compared in Table 25–1. Although more traditional units remain in use, they are confusing for multivalent ions and, in the case of Pi, are ambiguous because the concentration of the different forms is dependent on pH.

**TABLE 25–1.** Chemical Forms of Calcium in Plasma

| | Concentration | | |
|---|---|---|---|
| Form | *mmol/L* | *mg/dL* | % of Total |
| Protein bound | 1.15 | 4.6 | 46 |
| Ultrafilterable | 1.35 | 5.4 | 54 |
| Ionized | 1.10 | 4.4 | 44 |
| Complexed | 0.25 | 1.0 | 10 |
| **Total** | **2.50** | **10** | **100** |

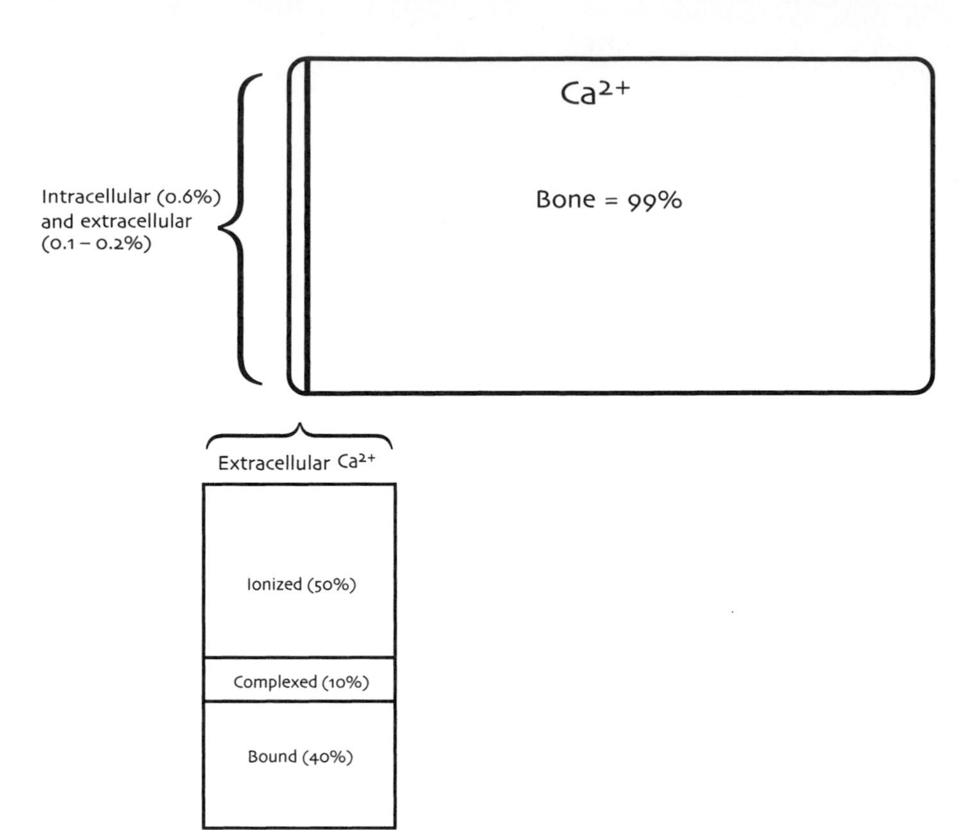


**FIGURE 25–1** ■ Distrubution and chemical forms of calcium in serum. Of total body calcium, 99% is found in bone and hard tissue, with approximately 1% in serum. The extracellular serum calcium concentration, 10 mg/dL or 2.5 mM, can be divided into three pools: ionized calcium (50%), that which is complexed with small anions (10%), and protein bound (40%). The first two moieties (i.e., ionized and complexed) represent the calcium that is filtered at the glomerulus and subject to tubular absorption as it passes through the nephron.

carbonate decreases the serum ionized calcium secondary to augmented formation of calcium complexes.[12]

The concentration of calcium in the extracellular fluid represents a dynamic balance between intestinal absorption, renal reabsorption, and osseous resorption. Symptoms of hypocalcemia vary in relation to the ionized serum calcium concentration. Mild reductions in plasma calcium are associated with paresthesia and muscle cramps; more severe decreases in calcium may induce seizures. Increases in plasma calcium, in contrast, have been implicated in mental status changes, attenuation of the renal effects of parathyroid hormone (PTH), antidiuretic action of vasopressin, and reduced renal concentrating capacity.[13, 14] Assuming a daily dietary calcium intake of 1000 mg, net intestinal absorption averages 200 mg, with the remaining 800 mg excreted in the feces. When in balance, net intestinal absorption is matched by urinary excretion, and calcium accretion and loss from bone are equal. Thus, approximately 200 mg of calcium is excreted daily. In adults, net calcium balance is effectively zero, suggesting that in the absence of a calcium challenge such as lactation, the kidneys represent an important regulatory site of calcium metabolism.[15, 16]

## PHOSPHATE CHEMISTRY

Phosphate is found in both inorganic and organic forms. Organic forms include phospholipids and various organic esters. There are four forms of inorganic orthophosphate that, in principle, can be present in biologic solutions in pH-dependent equilibrium: $H_3PO_4$, $H_2PO_4^-$, $HPO_4^{2-}$, and $PO_4^{3-}$. However, only $HPO_4^{2-}$ and $H_2PO_4^-$ are present in significant concentrations at physiologic pH. The ratio of the two is determined by the Henderson relation:

$$\frac{HPO_4^{2-}}{H_2PO_4^-} = 10^{pH-pKa}$$

The dissociation constant, pKa, for phosphate is 6.8. Thus, at a pH of 7.4, the ratio of $HPO_4^{2-}$ to $H_2PO_4^-$ is essentially 4:1, and the plasma phosphate has an intermediate valence of 1.8.† The abbreviation Pi is used here to refer to aggregate inorganic phosphate.

### Serum Phosphate

As in the case of calcium, not all serum Pi is ultrafilterable. Ninety percent of Pi, whether ionized or complexed with calcium, magnesium, or sodium, is filtered at the glomerulus. Approximately 10% of the remaining plasma Pi is bound to protein and is not filtered. Increases in calcium or Pi decrease ultrafilterable Pi, most likely due to the formation of high-molecular-weight protein complexes. The reduction of ultrafilterable Pi is counterbalanced by the Gibbs-Donnan effect, which raises the Pi concentration in

†The net valence is calculated from the total number of negative charges, (2 × 4) + 1, divided by the number of molecules, 4 + 1, as determined by the Henderson relation, that is, 9/5 = 1.8. Thus, at pH 7.4, 1 mmol of phosphorus = 1.8 mEq.

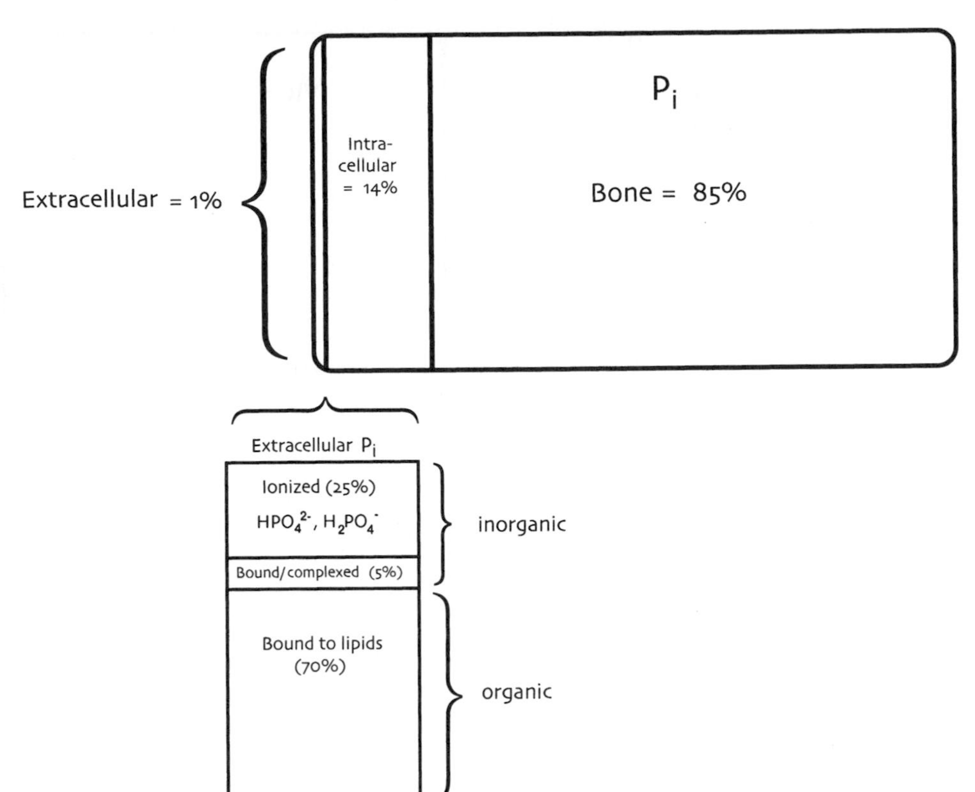


**FIGURE 25–2** ■ Distribution and chemical forms of phosphate in serum. Of total body phosphate, 85% is found in bone and hard tissue; 14% is found inside cells; and approximately 1% is found in serum. Both inorganic (30%) and organic (70%) forms are present in serum. Only the inorganic form is measured. The total serum Pi (3 to 4 mg/dL) can be divided into three pools; ionized (25%); complexed/protein bound (5%); and lipid bound (70%). The complexed and ionized forms are filtered at the glomerulus and subjected to tubular absorption as they traverse the nephron.

the ultrafiltrate. Correcting the volume occupied by plasma proteins (7%) raises the ultrafiltrate Pi concentration by an additional 7.5%, negating the effect of the reduction in protein-bound Pi. Both in vivo and in vitro measurements show that the ratio of ultrafilterable Pi to total plasma Pi is close to 1.[17] The relative proportions of the various phosphate forms are shown in Figure 25–2.

## MAGNESIUM CHEMISTRY

Magnesium is the second most abundant divalent cation in the body. It plays a role in many biochemical interactions, such as activation of enzymes and regulation of protein synthesis. Fifty percent to 67% of total body magnesium is in mineralized bone, and 40% to 50% resides in the intracellular compartment. Only 1% to 2% is found in the extracellular fluid. Most of the intracellular magnesium is bound within membranes of organelles to various metalloenzymes, proteins, and phosphate compounds, including nucleic acids and lipids.

### Serum Magnesium

Plasma magnesium in adults averages 1 mM and is distributed in three forms. Figure 25–3 shows the relative proportions of the various forms of magnesium. Approximately 55% is ionized, 15% is complexed to anions (e.g., bicarbonate, citrate, phosphate, and sulfate), and the remaining 30% is bound to protein, primarily albumin. The ionized fraction is thought to be the most important moiety, although both ionized and complexed magnesium are freely filtered at the glomerulus.

Magnesium distribution is affected mainly by alterations in plasma magnesium, plasma calcium, and blood pH. Because the ultrafilterable fraction of magnesium increases linearly with plasma magnesium concentrations, the percentage of total magnesium ultrafiltrate is unchanged by hypermagnesemia or hypomagnesemia.[18]

## CALCIUM TRANSPORT ALONG THE NEPHRON

Regulation of extracellular calcium homeostasis requires the daily urinary excretion of approximately 200 mg of calcium. The amount of calcium excreted is the difference between the filtered load and the amount reabsorbed. In healthy adults, of the 14,000 mg/day of calcium that is filtered at the glomerulus, less than 1% to 2%, or 140 to 280 mg/day, is excreted in the urine, with the remainder reabsorbed.

Calcium—unlike phosphate and magnesium, which display saturable absorptive kinetics—does not exhibit a tubule maximum, suggesting that the majority of calcium transport is passive.

The major sites of calcium reabsorption are the proximal tubules, thick ascending limbs, and distal tubules, with final adjustments of calcium excretion occurring in the collecting ducts, where transport may

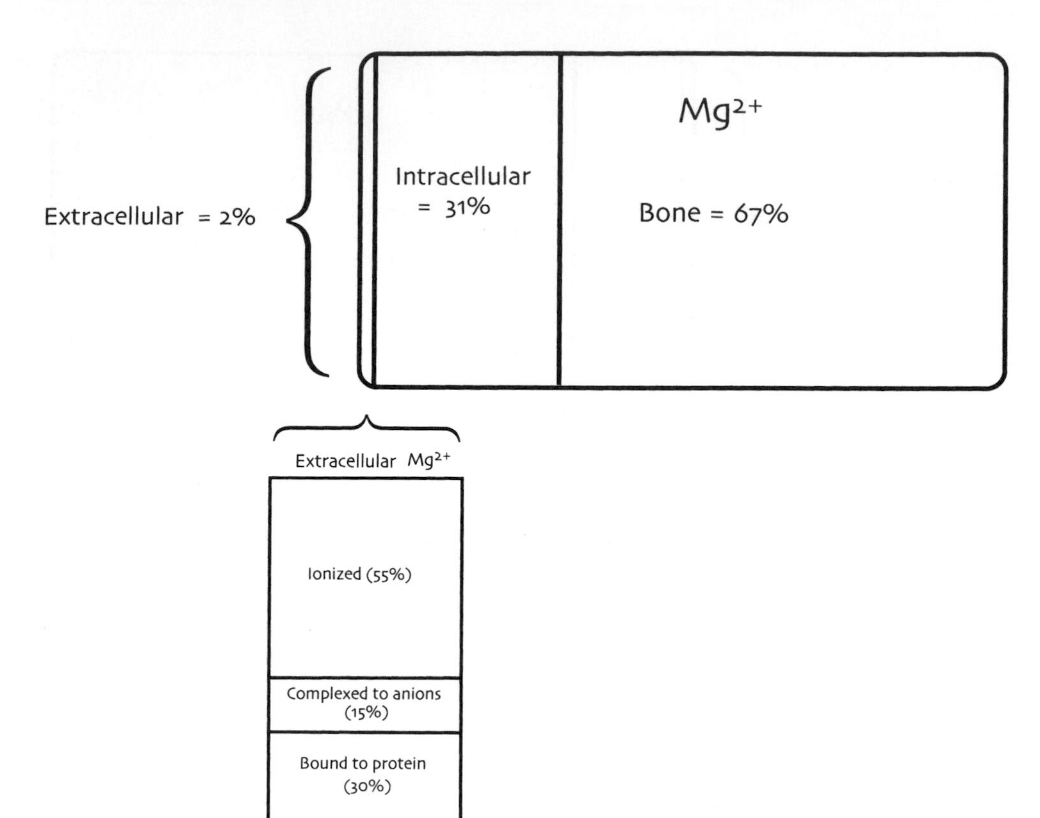


**FIGURE 25–3** ■ Distribution and chemical forms of magnesium in serum. Of total body magnesium, 67% is found in bone and hard tissue; 31% is found inside cells; and approximately 2% is found in serum. Total serum magnesium concentrations (1.5 to 2.5 mg/dL) can be divided into three pools: (1) ionized (55%), (2) complexed (15%), and (3) protein bound (30%). The complexed and ionized forms are filtered at the glomerulus and subjected to tubular absorption.

be absorptive or secretory. Calcium that is not bound to serum proteins, about 60%, is filtered at the glomerulus. Sixty percent to 70% of the ultrafiltrate, composed of ionized and complexed $Ca^{2+}$, is reabsorbed by the proximal tubules, 20% by the thick ascending limbs, and 5% to 10% by the distal tubules. Only 0.5% to 1.5% of the filtered calcium is excreted in the urine. Glomerular ultrafiltration of calcium is depressed by PTH. This leads to reduced single-nephron filtration rates and contributes to the calcium-sparing effects of PTH.[19, 20] The inhibitory action of PTH is mediated by the type 1 and type 2 PTH receptors in the glomerulus.[21–23]

## Proximal Convoluted Tubules

Approximately 60% of the filtered calcium is reabsorbed by the end of the proximal tubule.[24] Proximal tubular calcium reabsorption is thought to occur mainly by passive diffusion and solvent drag, with calcium moving through the paracellular pathway.[25, 26] This conclusion is based on the observation that, under most circumstances, the ratio of calcium in proximal tubule fluid to that in the glomerular filtrate is 1:1.2. A small but significant component of active calcium transport was observed in proximal tubules when measured in the absence of the driving force necessary for passive calcium movement and fluid absorption.[26–28] In contrast, active transport of calcium proceeds in a two-step process, with calcium entry from the tubular lumen across the apical membrane and exit through the basolateral membrane. This active transport component is generally considered to constitute approximately 10% to 15% of total proximal tubule calcium reabsorption. A schematic representation of these processes in the proximal tubules is shown in Figure 25–4.

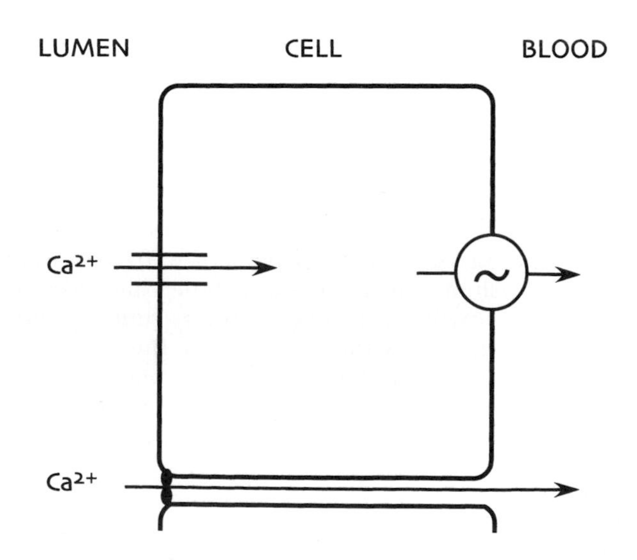


**FIGURE 25–4** ■ Model of proximal tubular calcium absorption. Most calcium is absorbed by passive mechanisms through the paracellular pathway. Some evidence supports the presence of a small component of active, transcellular calcium transport. The plasma membrane $Ca^{2+}$-ATPase (PMCA) is expressed in basolateral plasma membranes.

## Thick Ascending Limbs

Approximately 20% to 25% of the filtered calcium is reabsorbed by the medullary and cortical thick ascending limbs of the loop of Henle. Both passive and active transport mechanisms contribute to calcium absorption (Fig. 25–5). The passive component of calcium transport is driven by changes in the transepithelial voltage, which is established by sodium chloride (NaCl) reabsorption. As NaCl is absorbed along the length of the thick limb, a large diffusion voltage is generated between the lumen and the peritubular fluid; this establishes the characteristic lumen-positive transepithelial voltage and generates the driving force for passive calcium absorption.[29–32] In thick ascending limbs, calcium reabsorption increases in parallel with increases in the lumen-positive transepithelial voltage. Thus, under resting conditions, calcium absorption is thermodynamically passive and proceeds through the paracellular pathway.

Two lines of evidence support the presence of an active, hormone-stimulated component of calcium reabsorption in the thick ascending limbs. First, calcium flux ratios are greater than predicted for simple diffusion by the Ussing flux ratio expression.[33–35] Second, PTH stimulates active calcium absorption in the absence of a transepithelial voltage.[31, 36]

**Bartter Syndrome and Calcium Transport by Thick Ascending Limbs.** Bartter syndrome is characterized by hypokalemic metabolic alkalosis, with accompanying renal sodium wasting and enhanced calcium excretion. Various forms of Bartter syndrome are caused by mutations in genes encoding different proteins. One form occurs from a mutation of the gene encoding the apical membrane, bumetanide-sensitive $Na^+$-$K^+$-$2Cl^-$ cotransporter (NKCC2), *SLC12A1*.[37] Other forms are caused by an inactivating mutation of the ClC-Kb chloride channel gene *CLCNKB*, or the ATP-sensitive ROMK $K^+$ channel gene *KCNJ1*.[38, 39] Irrespective of the mutated genes, all patients with Bartter syndrome present with elevated calcium excretion. Curiously, those with NKCC2 or ROMK mutations tend to exhibit nephrocalcinosis, whereas patients with ClC-Kb mutations do not. The underlying mechanism for these differing phenotypes remains to be elucidated.

## Distal Convoluted Tubules

The distal convoluted tubule absorbs 5% to 10% of the filtered calcium. The tubule fluid-to-ultrafilterable $Ca^{2+}$ (TF/UF)$Ca^{2+}$ ratio is 0.6 to 0.7 at the beginning of the rat distal convoluted tubule and falls to about 0.3 at the point where the distal tubule joins with a cortical collecting duct.[24, 40] Calcium absorption is active, because it proceeds against both chemical and electrical gradients.[40]

Active calcium reabsorption in the distal convoluted tubules occurs through the transcellular pathway. Calcium entry across the apical plasma membrane proceeds through dihydropyridine-sensitive calcium channels, with basolateral exit mediated by the $Na^+$-$Ca^{2+}$ exchanger and the plasma membrane $Ca^{2+}$-ATPase.[41–43] Electrophysiologic patch clamp studies of distal tubule cells from the mouse, rabbit, and pig provide direct evidence that calcium channels mediate calcium entry in this portion of the nephron.[41, 43–45] One such voltage-gated channel, ECaC, was recently implicated

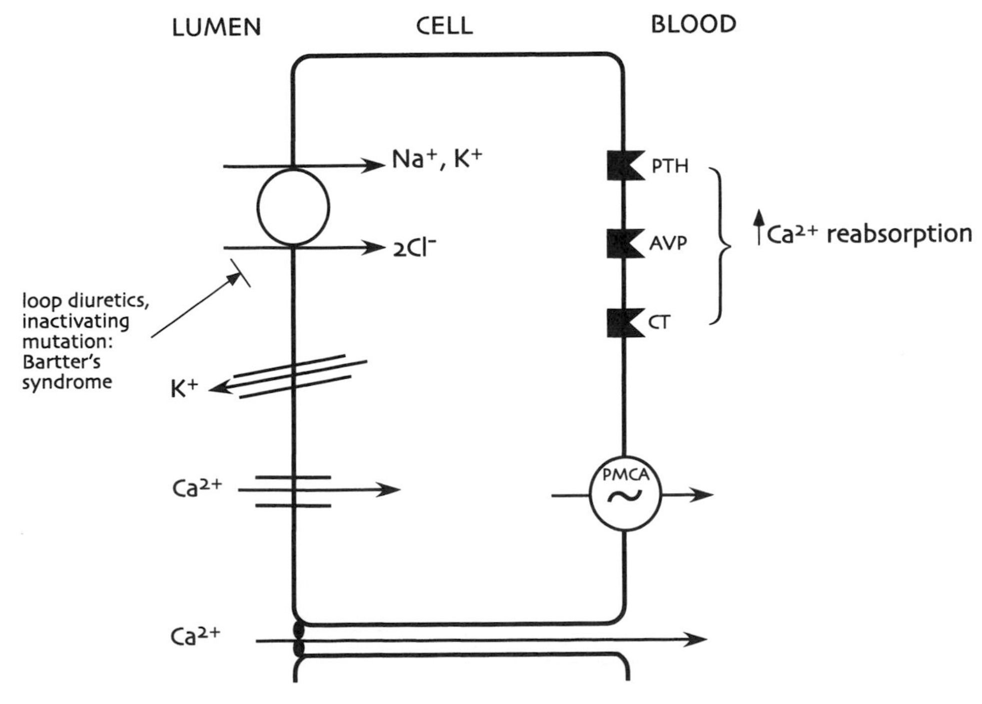


**FIGURE 25–5** ■ Model of calcium absorption by thick ascending limbs. Calcium absorption proceeds through both an active, transcellular pathway and by a passive, paracellular pathway. Only transport pathways relevant to calcium absorption are shown. Resting (i.e., basal) absorption is passive and is driven by the ambient electrochemical gradient for calcium. Calcitropic hormones such as parathyroid hormone (PTH) and calcitonin (CT) stimulate active cellular calcium absorption in cortical and medullary thick ascending limbs, respectively. Passive calcium reabsorption is stimulated indirectly by activation of the Na-K-2Cl cotransporter by other hormones such as arginine vasopressin (AVP). Inhibition of Na-K-2Cl cotransport by loop diuretics or in Bartter syndrome decreases the transepithelial voltage, thus diminishing passive calcium absorption.

as a candidate for the calcium entry channel.[46–48] ECaC has six putative transmembrane-spanning domains and consensus sites for potential phosphorylation by protein kinases A and C. Both amino and carboxy termini are predicted to be intracellular. ECaC bears no resemblance to other epithelial ion channels, although it shares some similarities with capsaicin receptors, which are calcium-permeable, nonselective cation channels.[49] Its role in normal calcium maintenance remains to be determined.

The distal convoluted tubule is the major site of hormone- and diuretic-regulated calcium absorption. Unlike in the proximal tubules or thick ascending limbs, sodium transport and calcium transport are inversely related in the distal convoluted tubules, where increases in sodium absorption are accompanied by decreases in calcium absorption, and, conversely, decreases in sodium are attended by increases in calcium. Examples of the dissociation of calcium and sodium transport include calcium transport stimulation by membrane hyperpolarization in response to PTH, thiazide diuretics, and amiloride.[50–53] A schematic representation of these processes in the distal convoluted tubules is shown in Figure 25–6.

**Gitelman Syndrome and Calcium Transport by Distal Tubules.** Patients with a variant of Bartter syndrome first described by Gitelman and colleagues also present with salt wasting, hypokalemia, and hypermagnesuria but exhibit diminished calcium excretion.[54, 55] An inactivating mutation of the apical membrane Na-Cl cotransporter gene *SLC12A3*, which is located on human chromosome 16, is the cause of Gitelman syndrome.[38] The hypocalciuria of Gitelman syndrome results from diminished NaCl cotransport, which hyperpolarizes the apical cell membrane and stimulates $Ca^{2+}$ entry.

### Connecting and Collecting Tubules

Less than 5% of the filtered calcium is reabsorbed by the cortical collecting tubules. Calcium transport is described as absorptive in some reports and as secretory in others, and it is considered to occur passively.[56, 57] Although PTH receptors are present in this segment,[21] their function is uncertain, as PTH has no effect on the rate of calcium reabsorption.[58]

## REGULATION OF RENAL CALCIUM TRANSPORT

### Parathyroid Hormone

Many physiologic, pharmacologic, and pathologic factors influence renal calcium absorption (Table 25–2). The most important physiologic regulator is PTH, which stimulates calcium absorption. In the absence of PTH or in cases of PTH deficiency, decreased calcium reabsorption is observed. Increased calcium reabsorption due to PTH is seen in the cortical thick limbs, distal convoluted tubules, and, in some species, connecting tubules. Although PTH generally has little to no effect on sodium excretion, acute administration of the hormone may augment sodium excretion.[59, 60] This effect is due to decreased proximal tubule sodium reabsorption.[61, 62]

In distal convoluted tubule cells, PTH-stimulated calcium entry occurs through apical membrane, dihydropyridine-sensitive calcium channels. It has now been established that PTH-stimulated calcium reabsorption is limited to distal nephron segments, where activation of both protein kinase A and protein kinase

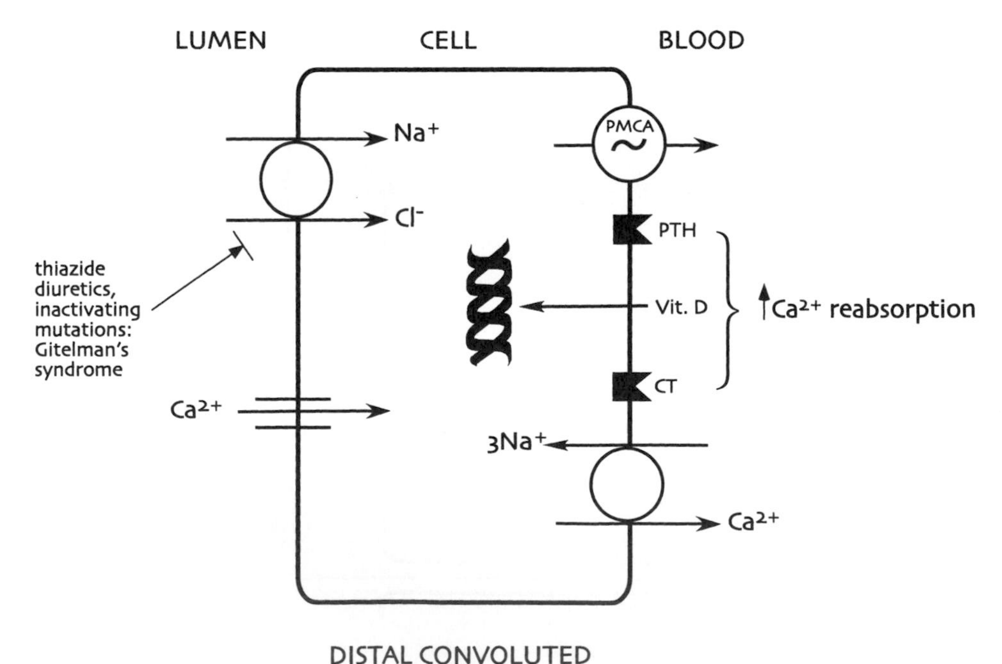


**FIGURE 25–6** ■ Model of calcium absorption by distal convoluted tubules. Apical calcium entry across the plasma membrane proceeds through dihydropyridine-sensitive calcium channels with basolateral exit occurring through a combination of the plasma membrane $Ca^{2+}$-ATPase (PMCA) and $Na^{+}$-$Ca^{2+}$ exchanger. Calcium absorption is entirely transcellular. Calcitropic hormones such as parathyroid hormone (PTH) and calcitonin (CT) stimulate calcium absorption. $1,25(OH)_2D_3$ (vitamin D) stimulates calcium absorption through the activation of nuclear transcription factors. Inhibition of the apical Na-Cl cotransporter by thiazide diuretics or in Gitelman syndrome, which hyperpolarizes the membrane, indirectly stimulates calcium absorption.

**TABLE 25–2.** Factors Regulating Renal Calcium Transport

| Tubule Segment | Normal Fractional Absorption (%) | Increased Calcium Absorption | Decreased Calcium Absorption |
|---|---|---|---|
| Proximal tubule | 61 | Volume contraction, phosphate loading | Volume expansion, phosphate depletion, hypercalcemia, PTH, acetazolamide |
| Descending thin limb | 9 | | Osmotic diuretics |
| Thick ascending limb | 20 | PTH, calcitonin | Furosemide, bumetanide |
| Distal convoluted tubule | 5 | PTH, calcitonin, thiazide diuretics, amiloride, phosphate loading, alkalosis, mineralocorticoid depletion | Acidosis |
| Collecting duct | 3 | | |
| Excreted in urine | <1 | | |

PTH, parathyroid hormone.

C is necessary.[63] Nephrogenous cyclic adenosine monophosphate (cAMP) formation by PTH is observed only in proximal tubules, where the hormone has no effect on calcium absorption but plays a role in other transport and metabolic effects.

PTH action in the kidney is mediated by the type 1 PTH receptor (PTH1R), which also binds PTH-related peptide (PTHrP). PTH1R mRNA transcripts are present in glomeruli, proximal convoluted and straight tubules, thick ascending limbs, distal convoluted tubules, and variably in cortical collecting ducts.[21, 22] A second, type 2, PTH receptor (PTH2R) has also been identified. This receptor responds only to PTH and not to PTHrP and is not expressed in renal tubular cells.[23, 64]

## Parathyroid Hormone–Related Peptide

PTHrP has high homology to PTH within the first 13 amino acids[65] and has comparable effects on kidney.[66, 67] The PTHrP gene in the kidney is expressed in proximal and distal convoluted tubules and in cortical collecting ducts.[68] Its effects on renal calcium reabsorption are similar to those seen in humoral hypercalcemia of malignancy and hyperparathyroidism. PTHrP is thought to contribute to the hypercalcemia observed in some cancer patients. There is still some debate regarding the effects of PTHrP on renal calcium reabsorption. PTHrP(1–36) infusion causes hypercalcemia and decreases calcium excretion,[69–71] as does implantation of PTHrP-secreting human lung tumor cells into mice.[72] In humoral hypercalcemia of malignancy, an increased calcium load is presented to the kidney secondary to calcium mobilization from bone; this further complicates interpretation of the effects of PTHrP on renal calcium absorption. Although reports of higher rates of calcium excretion in humoral hypercalcemia of malignancy than in hyperparathyroidism are not uncommon,[73] when normalized for the change in filtered calcium, PTHrP generally reduces calcium excretion.[74, 75]

## Vitamin D

In addition to exerting actions on intestine and bone, vitamin D enhances renal calcium reabsorption. Its metabolite 1,25-dihydroxycholecalciferol [$1,25(OH)_2D_3$] which is formed by 1α-hydroxylation of 25-hydroxycholecalciferol [$25(OH)D_3$] in proximal tubules, mediates the physiologic actions.[76, 77] 25(OH)D-1α-Hydroxylase is tightly regulated by PTH (in proximal tubules), calcitonin (in proximal straight tubules), hypophosphatemia (stimulating activity), and hypercalcemia (inhibiting activity).[77, 78]

Vitamin D's action on renal calcium reabsorption is thought to occur in distal tubules, although evidence for this is limited.[79] In support of this view, $1,25(OH)_2D_3$-binding studies in rat kidney demonstrated primary localization to distal convoluted tubules and connecting tubules, with decreased labeling in medullary and cortical thick ascending limbs.[80, 81] Calbindin $D_{28K}$, a vitamin D–stimulated calcium-binding protein thought to facilitate cellular calcium diffusion, is also found in distal convoluted and connecting tubules.[82, 83] This provides further support for the localization of vitamin D action.

Although $1,25(OH)_2D_3$ has no effect on proximal tubule calcium transport, it increases proximal phosphate reabsorption.[79, 84, 85] Increases in calcium reabsorption in response to $1,25(OH)_2D_3$ occur in distal convoluted tubules.[86] Bindels and coworkers demonstrated a direct effect of $1,25(OH)_2D_3$ on calcium transport in a rabbit connecting and cortical collecting duct cell culture model.[82] PTH did not enhance the action of $1,25(OH)_2D_3$, suggesting that they share a common mechanism of action.

## Hypercalcemia

Hypercalcemia results in increased renal calcium excretion. This occurs despite a fall in the glomerular capillary ultrafiltration coefficient, $K_f$, leading to a decreased single-nephron and whole-kidney glomerular filtration rate (GFR)—in conditions in which PTH is high.[19, 20, 87] Both PTH1R and PTH2R are expressed in glomerular cells.[22, 88, 89]

The increased calcium and sodium excretion, along with reduced GFR, observed with calcium infusion is partially due to inhibition of proximal tubule solute reabsorption.[5, 6, 19, 90] Elevation of serum calcium suppresses PTH secretion[5] and thereby decreases calcium reabsorption at hormone-sensitive sites in the cortical thick ascending limbs and distal convoluted tubules. Hypercalcemia also directly inhibits calcium reabsorption by the thick ascending limbs of the loop of Henle.[30, 91] This effect may be mediated directly or indirectly by the calcium-sensing receptor (CaSR), a member of the superfamily of G protein–coupled receptors, activating phospholipase C and also inhibiting adenylyl cyclase in target tissues.[92] The physiologic relevance of the CaSR to renal calcium transport has been established by identifying hyper- and hypocalcemic disorders resulting from CaSR mutations: familial hypocalciuric hypercalcemia and neonatal severe hyperparathyroidism result from inactivating CaSR mutations,[93] whereas activating mutations cause autosomal dominant hypocalcemia.[94]

# PHOSPHATE TRANSPORT ALONG THE NEPHRON

Renal Pi homeostasis is regulated primarily by controlling absorption by the proximal tubules. Pi absorption by the proximal nephron is transcellular and involves uptake across the apical brush border membrane (BBM), diffusion through the cell, and efflux across the basolateral membrane (Fig. 25–7). Notably, this pattern is essentially opposite that of calcium absorption, which is virtually all paracellular. Pi uptake across the apical membrane is coupled to $Na^+$, which enters proximal tubule cells down its electrochemical gradient. The $Na^+$ electrochemical gradient is maintained by low intracellular $Na^+$ levels, caused by the continuous basolateral extrusion of $Na^+$ driven by the basolateral membrane $Na^+,K^+$-ATPase. $Na^+$-dependent Pi uptake is the rate-limiting step in Pi absorption and the major site of its regulation. The cellular mechanisms involved in Pi efflux across basolateral membranes have not been elucidated but may be mediated by anion exchange. Under conditions of a normal Pi diet and intact parathyroid glands, approximately 80% of the filtered Pi is absorbed, and the remaining 20% is excreted.

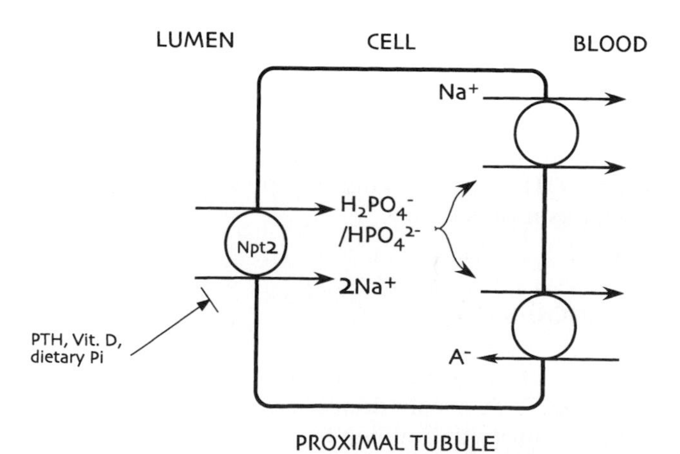


**FIGURE 25–7** ■ Model of proximal tubule Pi absorption. Pi absorption occurs by a transcellular pathway. Apical entry proceeds through the type I (not shown) and, primarily, type II $Na^+$-Pi cotransporters and is inhibited by parathyroid hormone (PTH), increased Pi stores, and $1,25(OH)_2D_3$ (vitamin D). The membrane localization of the type III cotransporters has not yet been established but has been assigned to the basolateral membrane, consistent with their presumed function as "housekeeping" proteins and basolateral Pi efflux, which may also be mediated by an anion exchanger.

## Tubular Pi Transport

Micropuncture studies demonstrated that 60% to 70% of the filtered Pi is absorbed by the late proximal convoluted tubule,[95, 96] with three times as much occurring in proximal straight tubules as in proximal convoluted tubules.[97] Absorption was not affected by replacing bicarbonate with chloride. However, luminal calcium had a profound effect on proximal Pi absorption, increasing unidirectional lumen-to-bath transport by almost twofold.[98] Although calcium has been postulated to modulate the anion affinity of the $Na^+$-Pi cotransporter, the identification of CaSRs at the luminal surface of proximal tubules[21] suggests that the regulatory action may be exerted by the receptor.

Pi absorption by the distal nephron is controversial. Evidence from micropuncture studies suggests that up to 10% of the filtered Pi is absorbed by the distal convoluted tubules.[99] Others have failed to uncover evidence of distal Pi transport.[100] Terminal nephron segments may participate in tubular Pi transport, because a higher fraction of filtered Pi remains in late distal tubules than appears in the final urine.[99–101] In summary, although the proximal tubules are the major sites of Pi absorption, the extent of Pi absorption by distal and terminal nephrons is uncertain.

## Molecular Biology of Renal $Na^+$-Pi Cotransport

Three families of $Na^+$-Pi cotransporters have been identified. Through the use of expression and homology cloning, type I (Npt1)[102, 103] and type II (Npt2)[104] transporters from several mammalian species were isolated.[105, 106] They are expressed primarily in the apical membrane of proximal tubule cells, where the bulk of filtered Pi is absorbed. However, the coupling and regulation of the two transporters are quite distinct (see later). The type III $Na^+$-Pi cotransporters (Pit1 and Pit2) are ubiquitously expressed in mammalian cells, are cell surface retroviral receptors, and are thought to serve a housekeeping role in cellular Pi homeostasis.[107]

### TYPE I $Na^+$-Pi COTRANSPORTER

The Npt1 gene (*SLC17A1*) maps to human chromosome region 6p22.[108] Its cDNA encodes a protein of 465 amino acids with seven to nine putative membrane-spanning segments.[102] Npt1 transcripts have been identified throughout the proximal tubule[109] and constitute approximately 15% of total $Na^+$-Pi cotransporter mRNA in mouse kidney.[110]

Electrophysiologic studies demonstrate that Npt1 mediates electroneutral $Na^+$-Pi cotransport at lower extracellular Pi concentrations (<3 mM).[111] In addition, Npt1 mediates the transport of organic anionic drugs, such as penicillin, and induces a $Cl^-$ conductance.[111] These findings suggest that Npt1 not only functions as a $Na^+$-Pi cotransporter but also serves as a channel for $Cl^-$ transport and for the excretion of anionic xenobiotics.

### TYPE II $Na^+$-Pi COTRANSPORTER

The type II family of $Na^+$-Pi cotransporters consists of type IIa (Npt2), which is expressed exclusively in the renal proximal tubule,[104] and type IIb, which is located in the apical membrane of the intestinal and lung epithelia.[112] The type II cotransporters share only 20% homology with type I transporters and are structurally and genetically distinct. The type IIa and type IIb $Na^+$-Pi cotransporters have an overall homology of approximately 60%, with major differences residing at the COOH terminus. Npt2 proteins, comprising approximately 635 amino acids, are predicted to span the membrane eight times.[104] Both the human and the murine Npt2 genes have been cloned,[113] and the human gene (*SLC34A1*) has been mapped to chromosome region 5q35.[114]

Npt2 accounts for approximately 85% of total Pi transporter mRNA in mouse kidney.[110] Expression of Npt2 cotransporter mRNA is restricted to proximal tubule cells,[115, 116] where Npt2 protein is found in the BBM.[116, 117] The relative abundance of Npt2 protein in $S_1$, $S_2$, and $S_3$ proximal tubule segments and between superficial and juxtamedullary proximal tubules depends on the ambient PTH, pH, and physiologic or pathophysiologic state of the cells or tissue. Npt2 expression in *Xenopus laevis* oocytes demonstrated Npt2-mediated Pi transport with the classic characteristics of renal BBM $Na^+$-Pi cotransport, high Pi affinity (~0.1 mM), a stoichiometry of $3Na^+$:1Pi, pH-dependent Npt2-mediated $Na^+$-Pi cotransport, and Pi-induced inward currents stimulated by increasing pH.[104, 118]

The topology and membrane targeting signals for newly synthesized Npt2 have recently been identified. Both $NH_2$- and COOH-terminal ends of the protein are located in the cytoplasm, whereas transmembrane loops connecting segments 1 and 2, and 3 and 4, are extracellular.[119]

Polarized targeting of Npt2 is a highly specific process that depends on both the amino acid sequence of the transporter (most likely the COOH terminal for apical targeting of Npt2) and the cell line in which it is expressed.

In the rat kidney, three truncated Npt2-related mRNA isoforms are generated by alternative gene splicing. NaPi-2α encodes a 337–amino acid protein, NaPi-2β encodes a 327–amino acid product, and NaPi-2γ encodes a 268–amino acid protein.[120] $Na^+$-Pi cotransport activity was not observed when *Xenopus* oocytes were injected with NaPi-2α, β, or γ cRNA alone. Upon coexpression of Npt2 with NaPi-2α or NaPi-2γ, transport activity was partially or completely inhibited, respectively, whereas coexpression of Npt2 with NaPi-2β resulted in full transporter activity. This suggests that the α and γ subunits function as dominant-negative inhibitors of Npt2.

Targeted mutagenesis was used to knock out the Npt2 gene in mice in order to examine the role of Npt2 in Pi homeostasis.[121] The null mutant mice exhibited increased urinary Pi excretion, an 85% decrease in BBM $Na^+$-Pi cotransport, hypophosphatemia, and an appropriate elevation in serum $1,25(OH)_2D_3$ concentration, with accompanying hypercalcemia, hypercalciuria, and hypoparathyroidism. The heterozygous Npt2+/− mice had normal levels of BBM $Na^+$-Pi cotransporter protein, although the mRNA abundance was half that observed in the wild-type mice. Urinary Pi excretion and serum $1,25(OH)_2D_3$ levels were modestly elevated, yet serum Pi was normal.

### TYPE III $Na^+$-Pi COTRANSPORTERS

Two novel $Na^+$-Pi cotransporters were recently described in the mammalian kidney. Although both are cell surface viral receptors, they mediate high-affinity (Km = 25 μM), electrogenic, Na-dependent Pi transport when expressed in *Xenopus* oocytes.[122] Gibbon ape leukemia virus (Glvr-1, Pit-1) and amphoteric murine retrovirus (Ram-1, Pit-2) are ubiquitously expressed in mammalian tissues, including brain, liver, muscle, heart, thymus, and bone marrow. Pit-1 and Pit-2 do not share any sequence similarity, despite their substrate specificity, and represent less than 1% of the total $Na^+$-Pi cotransporter mRNA in the mouse kidney.[110] However, they account for approximately 80% of total-body $Na^+$-Pi cotransporter mRNA.[123]

## REGULATION OF RENAL Pi TRANSPORT

### Parathyroid Hormone

PTH is the major hormonal regulator of Pi homeostasis and renal Pi transport. Renal Pi absorption by proximal convoluted and straight tubules is inhibited by PTH. Conversely, parathyroidectomy increases renal Pi reabsorption. PTH produces a greater inhibition of Pi transport in proximal straight tubules than in proximal convoluted tubules.[124]

PTH regulates the amount of Npt2 present in the BBM rather than changing the transporter activity. Treatment with PTH, in both animals and cell lines, induces the endocytosis of Npt2 from the BBM.[62,125,126] Microtubules have been implicated in this process, because treatment with paclitaxel (Taxol) blocked the inhibitory effect of PTH.[127, 128]

PTH acts through the PTH1R, stimulating adenylyl cyclase and phospholipase C, with subsequent activation of protein kinase A and protein kinase C.[129–131] Stimulation of either kinase inhibits $Na^+$-Pi cotransport, although protein kinase A activation alone only downregulates transporter number.[132]

Inhibition of both protein kinase A and protein kinase C is required for the complete inhibition of PTH-dependent Pi transport.[133, 134] To examine the role of these kinases in the control of PTH-dependent inhibition of $Na^+$-Pi cotransport, all the Npt2 protein kinase C consensus phosphorylation sites were mutated (Npt2 contains no protein kinase A sites) and expressed in *Xenopus* oocytes.[135] $Na^+$-Pi cotransport was not affected by the alterations of the phosphorylation sites. Additionally, when protein kinase C was directly activated with a phorbol ester, $Na^+$-Pi cotransport activity was inhibited in both the wild-type and the mutant cotransporters, suggesting that protein kinase C does not act directly on the $Na^+$-Pi cotransporter but acts through an indirect mechanism, such as phosphorylation of intermediate regulatory proteins.

Recent work demonstrated that the addition of PTH(1–34) (which signals through both protein kinase A and protein kinase C pathways) to either the apical or the basolateral surface of isolated perfused proximal tubules caused internalization of Npt2.[117] Conversely, PTH(3–34), which signals only through the protein kinase C pathway, had an effect when added apically but not basolaterally. Taken together, these data indicate that Npt2 activity and internalization are regulated by cAMP-dependent and -independent mechanisms, and that functional PTH receptors are located on both the apical and the basolateral membranes of the proximal tubule.

The mitogen-activated protein kinase (MAPK) ERK (extracellular signal-regulated kinase) plays an active role in PTH regulation of renal $Na^+$-Pi cotransport.[136] PTH stimulates ERK activity in a dose-dependent manner, and the MAPK inhibitor PD98059 reduces PTH inhibition of $Na^+$-Pi cotransport in the absence of Npt2 protein downregulation. This suggests that ERK action on Npt2 occurs through a mechanism independent of protein internalization.

## 1,25-Dihydroxyvitamin $D_3$

$1,25(OH)_2D_3$ may exert either phosphaturic or Pi-sparing effects, based on the state of Pi balance. During hypophosphatemia due to vitamin D deficiency or Pi deprivation, or when basal urinary Pi excretion is high (e.g., volume expansion or administration of PTH or calcitonin), $1,25(OH)_2D_3$ is antiphosphaturic. Conversely, $1,25(OH)_2D_3$ is phosphaturic during hyperphosphatemia or Pi-replete states. These opposing responses demonstrate the complexity of renal tubular Pi transport and the indirect effects on Pi homeostasis. Varying the duration of $1,25(OH)_2D_3$ administration also affects Pi transport. Acute $1,25(OH)_2D_3$ administration alters membrane lipid composition and increases renal $Na^+$-Pi cotransport, whereas chronic administration increases intestinal Pi and results in a positive Pi balance.[137, 138]

Npt2 has been implicated as a target of $1,25(OH)_2D_3$ regulation. In vitamin D–deficient, but not parathyroidectomized, rats, $1,25(OH)_2D_3$ increased renal Npt2-mediated cotransport, mRNA, and protein levels.[139]

## Other Hormones

A number of other hormones also target Npt2 in the regulation of renal Pi handling. Thyroid hormone[140] and insulin-like growth factor I[141] increase BBM $Na^+$-Pi cotransport, whereas dexamethasone[142] and epidermal growth factor[143] decrease transport. Generally, thyroid hormone and glucocorticoid effects are mediated by altering gene transcription. For example, administration of $T_3$ to immature hypothyroid rats stimulated renal BBM $Na^+$-Pi cotransport through an increase in Npt2 mRNA, protein, and gene expression.[144] Conversely, dexamethasone did not affect Npt2 gene transcription, nor did insulin-like growth factor I or epidermal growth factor.[145]

Stanniocalcins (STC1, STC2) can also regulate renal Pi transport. First isolated from the corpuscles of Stannius in bony fish, where it was shown to play a role in calcium and phosphate homeostasis,[146] stanniocalcin is found in cortical thick ascending limbs, distal convoluted tubules, and cortical and medullary collecting ducts in humans and rodents.[147, 148] STC1 decreased absolute and fractional Pi excretion and increased BBM $Na^+$-Pi cotransport without affecting the renal excretion of other ions, plasma electrolytes, renal blood flow, GFR, or blood pressure.[149] STC2 has also been shown to inhibit $Na^+$-Pi cotransport in opossum kidney (OK) cells.[150, 151] Although these studies implicate Npt2 as a target for stanniocalcin, the role of stanniocalcin in the maintenance of Pi homeostasis remains to be established.

## pH Regulation of Pi Transport

Proximal tubule Pi absorption is highly dependent on pH. When pH is increased from 6 to 8, BBM vesicular $Na^+$-Pi cotransport is stimulated 10- to 20-fold.[152] This effect is sodium dependent and is greatest at low sodium concentrations and diminished at high sodium concentrations.[152] The affinity for sodium but not for Pi is affected by pH.[153, 154]

## Dietary Pi

Dietary Pi intake is a major regulator of renal Pi homeostasis. During Pi deprivation, apical BBM $Na^+$-Pi cotransport increases, with a concomitant increase in Pi reabsorption. Renal Pi conservation is also driven by rapid growth, pregnancy, and lactation, whereas chronic renal failure, growth cessation, or a high dietary intake reduces Pi absorption.[155, 156]

Alterations of $Na^+$-Pi cotransport due to dietary Pi restriction or supplementation occur within hours; are independent of changes in PTH, $1,25(OH)_2D_3$, or serum calcium levels; and are associated with an increase in the $V_{max}$ of $Na^+$-Pi cotransport, without a change in the Km, indicating an increase in transporter number but not transporter activity.[157] Various studies have demonstrated that Pi intake regulates Npt2 gene expression. In OK cells, an increase in Npt2 protein levels, but not mRNA levels, was observed with both acute and chronic exposure to low extracellular Pi.[158] Low Pi has no effect on Npt2 promoter activity, consistent with the absence of an effect on mRNA abundance.[145] In response to acute exposure to low extracellular Pi, Npt2 is rapidly recruited to the apical BBM through a microtubule-dependent mechanism,[159] whereas in response to elevated Pi levels, Npt2 is internalized through a microtubule-independent mechanism into an endosomal compartment, where it can be targeted for lysosomal degradation.[158]

### Inherited Disorders of Renal Pi Transport

X-linked hypophosphatemia (XLH), autosomal dominant hypophosphatemic rickets (ADHR), and hereditary hypophosphatemic rickets with hypercalciuria (HHRH) are characterized by rachitic bone disease, decreased growth rate and short stature, hypophosphatemia, and renal Pi wasting.[160]

Two mouse models of XLH, *Hyp* and *Gy*, exhibit hypophosphatemia secondary to decreased renal BBM $Na^+$-Pi cotransport from decreased Npt2 mRNA and protein.[161, 162] Mutations of *PHEX* (Pi-regulating gene with homology to endopeptidases on the X chromosome) are responsible for the mouse model of XLH[163,164] and XLH in humans.[165] More than 100 disease-causing mutations have been identified in the *PHEX* gene to date.[166] The fact that *PHEX* is expressed primarily in bone and not kidney[163, 167] implicates the putative endopeptidase in the processing or degrading of a peptide hormone that regulates skeletal mineralization and renal Pi handling.

ADHR was mapped to human chromosome 12q13,[168] and the associated Pi-regulating gene was recently cloned.[169] Unlike XLH and ADHR, HHRH patients present with appropriately elevated serum $1,25(OH)_2D_3$ levels in response to hypophosphatemia and hypercalciuria. HHRH is thought to be primarily a renal Pi-wasting disorder, because everything but the renal abnormality can be corrected with Pi supplementation.[160] Mice homozygous for the disrupted Npt2 gene exhibit a similar phenotype as HHRH patients,[121] suggesting that the Npt2 gene could be a candidate for HHRH.

## MAGNESIUM TRANSPORT ALONG THE NEPHRON

Seventy percent to 80% of total-body magnesium (ionized and complexed fraction) is freely filtered by the glomerulus. At a normal GFR and plasma magnesium concentration, approximately 97% of the filtered magnesium is reabsorbed along the nephron, and only 3% is excreted in the urine. Micropuncture studies have demonstrated that of the filtered magnesium, only 15% to 20% is reabsorbed by the proximal tubule, 65% to 75% by the thick ascending limbs of the loop of Henle, and 5% by the distal nephron.

Whole-kidney clearance studies in humans and dogs suggest the presence of a tubule maximum for magnesium reabsorption.[170, 171] In dogs with intact parathyroid glands, PTH increased the tubule maximum. With high extracellular calcium levels or during volume expansion, the tubule maximum decreased.[170] Although there does not appear to be a tubule maximum in the proximal tubule, magnesium transport in the distal segments is limited by the high plasma (peritubular) magnesium concentration,[172] accounting for the apparent tubule maximum observed in clearance studies.[170, 171]

### Tubular Magnesium Transport

#### PROXIMAL TUBULES

Approximately 20% of filtered magnesium is reabsorbed by the proximal convoluted tubules, compared with 60% to 70% of filtered sodium, calcium, and water.[173] The ratio of magnesium in the tubules to that in plasma increases along the length of the proximal tubule as water is reabsorbed.[174–176] Fractional magnesium reabsorption is invariant, even with volume expansion,[177] administration of diuretics,[178] or increased plasma calcium.[6] This suggests that relative to sodium and water, the permeability to magnesium is low in the proximal tubule, and magnesium transport is most likely a passive process in this portion of the nephron.

#### THICK ASCENDING LIMBS

The major site of magnesium reabsorption is in the thick ascending limbs. In vivo and in vitro microperfusion studies demonstrated that approximately 80% of the magnesium leaving the proximal tubule is reabsorbed in the thick ascending limb.[30, 56, 172] Magnesium transport increases proportionately with increasing luminal concentrations of up to 5 mM, although, regardless of luminal concentration, there is decreased magnesium reabsorption with increased plasma concentrations.[30, 172]

##### *Magnesium Transport and Wasting by Thick Ascending Limbs*

Passive, paracellular diffusion is the principal mechanism of magnesium transport by the thick ascending limbs (Fig. 25–8). Passive magnesium transport is driven by the lumen-positive transepithelial voltage generated by the apical $Na^+$-$K^+$-$2Cl^-$ cotransporter and basolateral sodium efflux via the $Na^+$,$K^+$-ATPase and electrogenic recycling of potassium across the apical cell membrane. Thus, loop diuretics such as furosemide and bumetanide decrease magnesium, calcium,

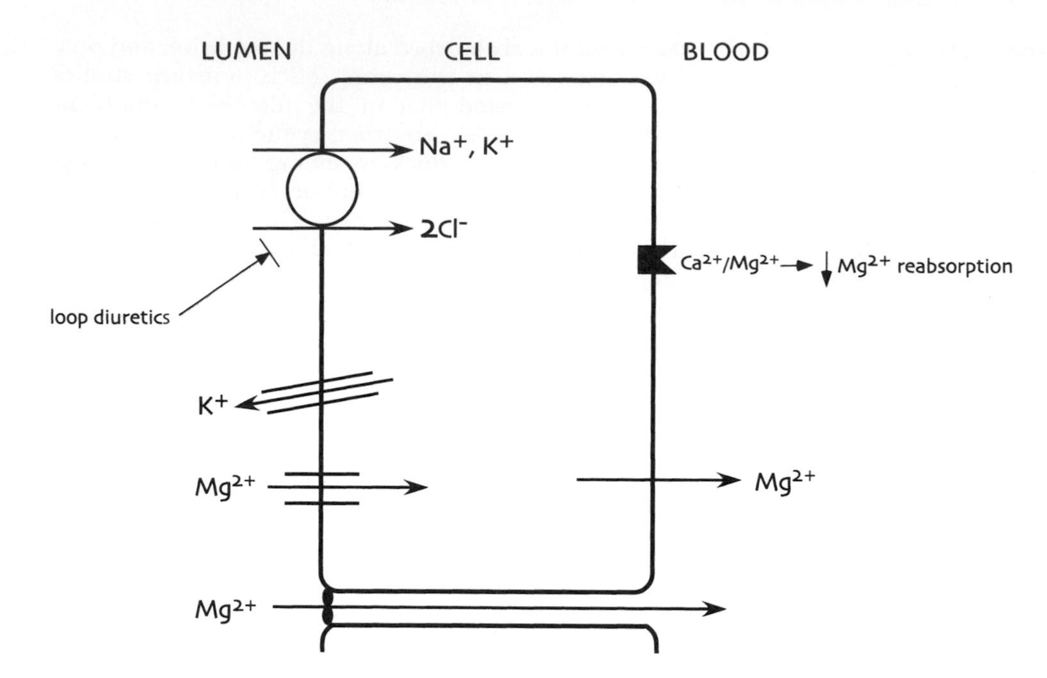


**FIGURE 25–8** ■ Model of magnesium absorption by thick ascending limbs. Magnesium absorption proceeds predominantly through the paracellular pathway although an active component may exist. Inhibition of $Na^+$-$K^+$-$2Cl^-$ cotransport by loop diuretics decreases the transepithelial voltage, thus diminishing passive magnesium absorption. Activation of the calcium-sensing receptor, by increased plasma magnesium or calcium, is also thought to play a role in decreased magnesium absorption.

and sodium reabsorption secondary to inhibiting $Na^+$-$K^+$-$2Cl^-$ cotransport, thereby suppressing the transepithelial voltage that favors magnesium reabsorption.[179]

There may be an active component of magnesium transport in thick limbs as well. This is suggested by work demonstrating increased magnesium reabsorption upon administration of glucagon or antidiuretic hormone, with little or no change in the transepithelial voltage.[180, 181] The cellular mechanisms involved in magnesium efflux across basolateral membranes in thick ascending limbs have not been elucidated.

Patients with Bartter syndrome, one form of which is caused by inactivating mutations in the $Na^+$-$K^+$-$2Cl^-$ cotransporter, are hypercalciuric, with only one third having hypomagnesemia.[37] Although symptoms are identical to those seen with chronic loop diuretic therapy, most patients surprisingly do not exhibit magnesium wasting.

Recent work by Simon and colleagues[182] identified a form of inherited magnesium wasting. Through positional cloning, they determined that mutations in paracellin-1, a protein related to the claudin family of tight junction proteins, is expressed in tight junctions along the thick ascending limb. Their work suggests that paracellin-1 may be a component in a selective paracellular conductive pathway for magnesium. Calcium transport in the thick limbs may also involve paracellin-1, inasmuch as patients with congenital magnesium wasting are generally hypercalciuric.[183] This finding, coupled with the effects of loop diuretics on magnesium transport, could contribute to the magnesium wasting sometimes observed in Bartter syndrome.

Hypercalcemia increases magnesium excretion to a greater extent than it does calcium excretion.[91] Fractional urinary excretion of calcium increased from 0.2% to 8.3%, whereas magnesium increased from 15% to 39%, in thyroparathyroidectomized rats following acute elevation of extracellular calcium concentration. In thick ascending limbs, the fractional reabsorption of magnesium decreased from 78% in control animals to 35% in the hypercalcemic animals.[91] This suggests that both magnesium and calcium may be transported by passive, paracellular means in this segment of the nephron. The reduction of isotonic reabsorption in the proximal tubule by hypercalcemia resulted in a greater delivery of calcium and magnesium to the thick ascending limb.[91] The extracellular CaSR, which is located on the apical membrane of the thick ascending limb, also binds magnesium. In conditions of high plasma magnesium or calcium, it is thought to play a role in the inhibition of passive magnesium transport by inhibiting the $Na^+$-$K^+$-$2Cl^-$ cotransporter, thus decreasing the driving force for magnesium transport.[184]

Familial hypocalciuric hypercalcemia is caused by inactivating mutations in the CaSR, resulting in inappropriate PTH.[93, 185] These patients also exhibit mild hypermagnesemia as a consequence of the impaired response in the thick ascending limbs to the hypercalcemia from the inactive CaSR. Conversely, with activating mutations of the CaSR, as seen with autosomal dominant hypoparathyroidism,[186] most patients present with mild hypomagnesemia,[187] which can be explained by diminished magnesium absorption by the thick ascending limbs.

Hypermagnesuria and hypercalcemia can also be caused by phosphate depletion.[188, 189] Studies by Wong and colleagues[190] demonstrated that the defect in magnesium reabsorption by the thick limbs and distal tubules of phosphate-depleted dogs can be corrected by infusion of PTH or phosphate, which causes parallel increases in calcium and magnesium reabsorption.

### DISTAL CONVOLUTED TUBULES AND COLLECTING TUBULES

Micropuncture studies of the distal tubule demonstrate that less than 10% of the filtered magnesium is reabsorbed by the distal nephron.[172, 175] In immortalized distal convoluted cells, magnesium entry accompanies membrane hyperpolarization induced by amiloride or chlorothiazide.[52, 191] As depicted in Figure 25–9, magnesium entry is inhibited by dihydropyridine channel blockers.[192] PTH, vasopressin, and glucagon also stimulate magnesium entry, presumably through an adenylate cyclase–dependent mechanism.[191, 193, 194] Magnesium transport within distal tubules is thought to be active and transcellular, because of the negative transepithelial voltage and high epithelial resistance.[195]

Little magnesium transport occurs in the collecting duct system. A comparison of urinary magnesium excretion to that remaining in the late distal tubule found that only 1% to 3% of the filtered load of magnesium is reabsorbed in these terminal segments.[18, 101] Other investigators detected little to no magnesium transport by sampling early and late collecting tubule segments or by applying microcatheterization techniques to inner medullary collecting ducts.[196, 197]

Although inhibition of the distal convoluted tubule Na-Cl cotransporter (NCC) by chronic thiazide treatment leads to decreased magnesium reabsorption, the mechanism by which this occurs is unclear. It is thought to result from the accompanying hypokalemia observed with thiazide treatment.[193] Patients with Gitelman syndrome—a variant of Bartter syndrome that mirrors chronic thiazide use—present with hypokalemic metabolic alkalosis, as do those with Bartter syndrome, but they also have hypocalciuria and hypomagnesemia. Mutations in afflicted individuals have been located to the gene encoding the thiazide-sensitive Na-Cl cotransporter.[38, 198, 199] Interestingly, in a mouse knockout model in which the Na-Cl cotransporter gene is deleted, the animals develop hypocalciuria and hypomagnesemia, but not the accompanying hypokalemia observed in patients with Gitelman syndrome.[200] This suggests that a mechanism besides hypokalemia is involved in the magnesium wasting observed with Gitelman syndrome.

## Hormonal Regulation

PTH, which stimulates calcium absorption and inhibits Pi absorption in renal tubules, plays a significant role in the renal handling of magnesium. PTH administration to hypoparathyroid humans, as well as in experimental animal models, increases the reabsorption of both magnesium and calcium.[60, 170, 201, 202] Although micropuncture studies demonstrate only small effects of PTH on magnesium reabsorption by the thick limbs,[172, 178, 203] studies in the hamster show that PTH and cAMP activate magnesium reabsorption.[204] PTH-sensitive magnesium transport has been reported in cortical thick limbs.[56]

Calcitonin, another calcitropic hormone, has been shown to enhance magnesium reabsorption in the loop of Henle.[205] However, this appears to be due to the resultant hypocalcemia, because the effect was not seen if calcium levels were returned to normal.

Although the bulk of filtered magnesium is reabsorbed in thick ascending limbs, the distal tubule also plays an important role in the final adjustments of renal magnesium handling. The number of inherited disorders affecting magnesium transport emphasizes

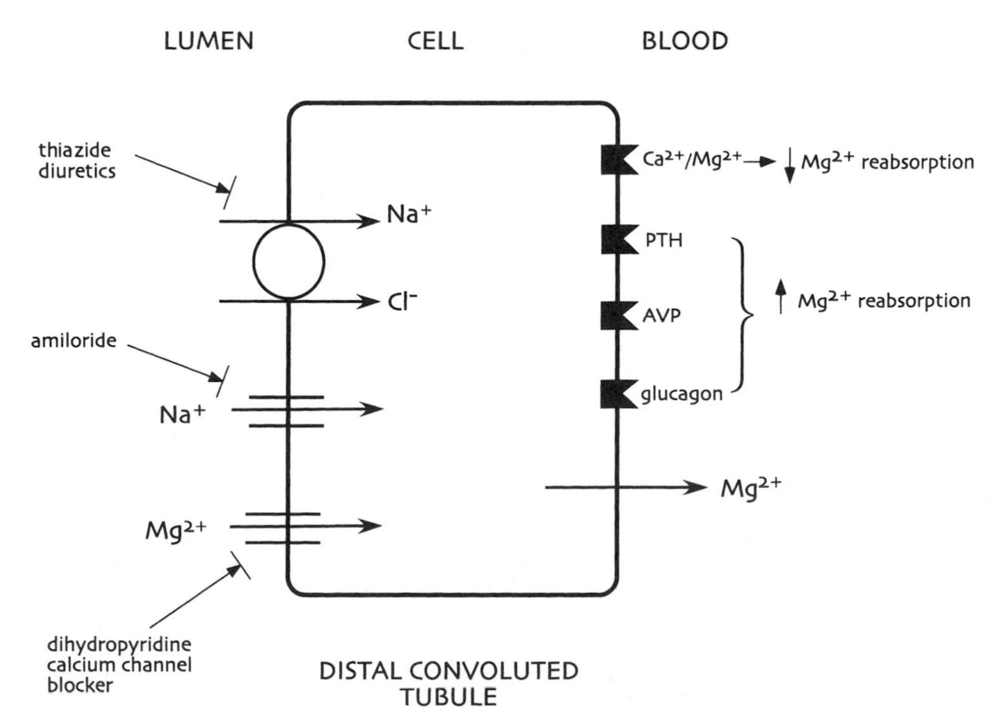


**FIGURE 25–9** ■ Model of magnesium absorption by distal convoluted tubules. Apical magnesium entry is stimulated by hyperpolarizing agents, such as amiloride or thiazide diuretics, and inhibited by dihydropyridine-type calcium channel blockers. Peptide hormone stimulation of magnesium absorption by parathyroid hormone (PTH), arginine vasopressin (AVP), and glucagon is thought to occur through an adenylate cyclase–dependent mechanism. Activation of the calicum-sensing receptor diminishes magnesium absorption.

the importance of magnesium handling in the distal tubule. Greater understanding of these disorders can be achieved once the transport properties are defined.

## REFERENCES


1. Williams RJP: Calcium chemistry and its relation to biological function. Symp Soc Exp Biol 30:1–17, 1976.
2. Moore EW: Ionized calcium in normal serum, ultrafiltrates, and whole blood determined by ion-exchange electrodes. J Clin Invest 49:318–334, 1970.
3. Pfordte K, Ponsold W: Uber die calcium-serumprotein-bindung. Endokrinologie 57:230–236, 1971.
4. Walser M: Ion association. VI. Interactions between calcium, magnesium, inorganic phosphate, citrate and protein in normal human plasma. J Clin Invest 40:723–730, 1961.
5. Edwards BR, Sutton RAL, Dirks JH: Effect of calcium infusion on renal tubular reabsorption in the dog. Am J Physiol 227: 13–18, 1974.
6. Le Grimellec C, Roinel N, Morel F: Simultaneous Mg, Ca, P, K, Na and Cl analysis in rat tubular fluid. III. During acute Ca plasma loading. Pflugers Arch 346:171–188, 1974.
7. Marshall RW: Plasma fractions. In Nordin BEC (ed): Calcium, Phosphate and Magnesium Metabolism. Edinburgh, Churchill Livingstone, 1976, pp 162–185.
8. Loeb RF: The effect of pure protein solutions and of blood serum on the diffusibility of calcium. J Gen Physiol 8:451–461, 1926.
9. Peterson NA, Feigen GA, Crimson JM: Effect of pH on interaction of calcium ions with serum proteins. Am J Physiol 201: 386–392, 1961.
10. Terepka AR, Dewey PA, Toribara TY: The ultrafiltrable calcium of human serum. II. Variations in disease states and under experimental conditions. J Clin Invest 37:87–98, 1957.
11. Hopkins T, Howard JE, Eisenberg H: Ultrafiltration studies on calcium and phosphorous in human serum. Bull Johns Hopkins Hosp 91:1–21, 1952.
12. Walser M: Divalent cations: Physicochemical state in glomerular filtrate and urine and renal excretion. In Orloff J, Berliner RW (eds): Handbook of Physiology, Section 8: Renal Physiology, 1st ed. Washington, DC, American Physiological Society, 1973, pp 555–586.
13. Takaichi K, Kurokawa K: High $Ca^{2+}$ inhibits peptide hormone-dependent cAMP production specifically in thick ascending limbs of Henle. Miner Electrolyte Metab 12:342–346, 1986.
14. Gill JR Jr, Bartter FC: On the impairment of renal concentrating ability in prolonged hypercalcemia and hypercalciuria in man. J Clin Invest 40:716–722, 1961.
15. Peacock M, Robertson WG, Nordin BEC: Relation between serum and urinary calcium with particular reference to parathyroid activity. Lancet 1:384–386, 1969.
16. Stewart AF: Hypercalcemic and hypocalcemic states. In Seldin DW, Giebisch G (eds): The Kidney: Physiology and Pathophysiology, 2nd ed. New York, Raven Press, 1992, pp 2431–2460.
17. Harris CA, Baer PG, Chirito E, Dirks JH: Composition of mammalian glomerular filtrate. Am J Physiol 227:972–976, 1974.
18. Carney SL, Wong NL, Quamme GA, Dirks JH: Effect of magnesium deficiency on renal magnesium and calcium transport in the rat. J Clin Invest 65:180–188, 1980.
19. Humes HD, Ichikawa I, Troy JL, Brenner BM: Evidence for a parathyroid hormone–dependent influence of calcium on the glomerular ultrafiltration coefficient. J Clin Invest 61:32–40, 1978.
20. Ichikawa I, Humes HD, Dousa TP, Brenner BM: Influence of parathyroid hormone on glomerular ultrafiltration in the rat. Am J Physiol 234:F393–F401, 1978.
21. Riccardi D, Lee WS, Lee K, et al: Localization of the extracellular $Ca^{2+}$-sensing receptor and PTH/PTHrP receptor in rat kidney. Am J Physiol 271:F951–F956, 1996.
22. Yang TX, Hassan S, Huang YNG, et al: Expression of PTHrP, PTH/PTHrP receptor, and $Ca^{2+}$-sensing receptor mRNAs along the rat nephron. Am J Physiol 272:F751–F758, 1997.
23. Usdin TB: Evidence for a parathyroid hormone-2 receptor selective ligand in the hypothalamus. Endocrinology 138:831–834, 1997.
24. Lassiter WE, Gottschalk CW, Mylle M: Micropuncture study of renal tubular reabsorption of calcium in normal rodents. Am J Physiol 204:771–775, 1963.
25. Bourdeau JE: Calcium transport across the pars recta of cortical segment 2 proximal tubules. Am J Physiol 251:F718–F724, 1986.
26. Bomsztyk K, George JP, Wright FS: Effects of luminal fluid anions on calcium transport by proximal tubule. Am J Physiol 246:F600–F608, 1984.
27. Rouse D, Ng RCK, Suki WN: Calcium transport in the pars recta and thin descending limb of Henle of rabbit perfused in vitro. J Clin Invest 65:37–42, 1980.
28. Ullrich KJ, Rumrich G, Kloss S: Active $Ca^{2+}$ reabsorption in the proximal tubule of the rat kidney: Dependence on sodium- and buffer transport. Pflugers Arch 364:223–228, 1976.
29. Bourdeau JE, Burg MB: Voltage dependence of calcium transport in the thick ascending limb of Henle's loop. Am J Physiol 236:F357–F364, 1979.
30. Shareghi GR, Agus ZS: Magnesium transport in the cortical thick ascending limb of Henle's loop of the rabbit. J Clin Invest 69:759–769, 1982.
31. Friedman PA: Basal and hormone-activated calcium absorption in mouse renal thick ascending limbs. Am J Physiol 254:F62–F70, 1988.
32. Dietl P, Oberleithner H: $Ca^{2+}$ transport in diluting segment of frog kidney. Pflugers Arch 410:63–68, 1987.
33. Suki WN, Rouse D, Ng RCK, Kokko JP: Calcium transport in the thick ascending limb of Henle: Heterogeneity of function in the medullary and cortical segments. J Clin Invest 66:1004–1009, 1980.
34. Rocha AS, Magaldi JB, Kokko JP: Calcium and phosphate transport in isolated segments of rabbit Henle's loop. J Clin Invest 59:975–983, 1977.
35. Imai M: Calcium transport across the rabbit thick ascending limb of Henle's loop perfused in vitro. Pflugers Arch 374: 255–263, 1978.
36. Bourdeau JE, Burg MB: Effect of PTH on calcium transport across the cortical thick ascending limb of Henle's loop. Am J Physiol 239:F121–F126, 1980.
37. Simon DB, Karet FE, Hamdan JM, et al: Bartter's syndrome, hypokalaemic alkalosis with hypercalciuria, is caused by mutations in the Na-K-2Cl cotransporter NKCC2. Nat Genet 13: 183–188, 1996.
38. Simon DB, Nelson-Williams C, Bia MJ, et al: Gitelman's variant of Bartter's syndrome, inherited hypokalaemic alkalosis, is caused by mutations in the thiazide-sensitive Na-Cl cotransporter. Nat Genet 12:24–30, 1996.
39. Simon DB, Karet FE, Rodriguez-Soriano J, et al: Genetic heterogeneity of Bartter's syndrome revealed by mutations in the $K^+$ channel, ROMK. Nat Genet 14:152–156, 1996.
40. Costanzo LS, Windhager EE: Calcium and sodium transport by the distal convoluted tubule of the rat. Am J Physiol 235: F492–F506, 1978.
41. Matsunaga H, Stanton BA, Gesek FA, Friedman PA: Epithelial $Ca^{2+}$ channels sensitive to dihydropyridines and activated by hyperpolarizing voltages. Am J Physiol 267:C157–C165, 1994.
42. Bacskai BJ, Friedman PA: Activation of latent $Ca^{2+}$ channels in renal epithelial cells by parathyroid hormone. Nature 347: 388–391, 1990.
43. Poncet V, Merot J, Poujeol P: A calcium-permeable channel in the apical membrane of primary cultures of the rabbit distal bright convoluted tubule. Pflugers Arch 422:112–119, 1992.
44. Saunders JCJ, Isaacson LC: Patch clamp study of Ca channels in isolated renal tubule segments. In Pansu D, Bronner F (eds): Calcium Transport and Intracellular Calcium Homeostasis. Berlin, Springer-Verlag, 1990, pp 27–34.
45. Lau K, Quamme G, Tan S: Patch-clamp evidence for a Ca channel in apical membrane of cortical thick ascending limb (cTAL) and distal tubule (DT) cells. J Am Soc Nephrol 2: 775, 1991.
46. Vennekens R, Hoenderop JG, Prenen J, et al: Permeation and gating properties of the novel epithelial $Ca^{2+}$ channel. J Biol Chem 275:3963–3969, 2000.
47. Hoenderop JGJ, van der Kemp AWCM, Hartog A, et al: The

epithelial calcium channel, ECaC, is activated by hyperpolarization and regulated by cytosolic calcium. Biochem Biophys Res Commun 261:488–492, 1999.

48. Hoenderop JGJ, van der Kemp AWCM, Hartog A, et al: Molecular identification of the apical $Ca^{2+}$ channel in 1,25-dihydroxyvitamin $D_3$–responsive epithelia. J Biol Chem 274:8375–8378, 1999.
49. Caterina MJ, Schumacher MA, Tominaga M, et al: The capsaicin receptor: A heat-activated ion channel in the pain pathway. Nature 389:816–824, 1997.
50. Gesek FA, Friedman PA: Mechanism of calcium transport stimulated by chlorothiazide in mouse distal convoluted tubule cells. J Clin Invest 90:429–438, 1992.
51. Gesek FA, Friedman PA: On the mechanism of parathyroid hormone stimulation of calcium uptake by mouse distal convoluted tubule cells. J Clin Invest 90:749–758, 1992.
52. Dai L-J, Friedman PA, Quamme GA: Mechanisms of amiloride stimulation of $Mg^{2+}$ uptake in immortalized mouse distal convoluted tubule cells. Am J Physiol 272:F249–F256, 1997.
53. Friedman PA, Gesek FA: Stimulation of calcium transport by amiloride in mouse distal convoluted tubule cells. Kidney Int 48:1427–1434, 1995.
54. Gitelman HJ, Graham JB, Welt LG: A new familial disorder characterized by hypokalemia and hypomagnesemia. Trans Assoc Am Physicians 79:221–235, 1966.
55. Bettinelli A, Bianchetti MG, Girardin E, et al: Use of calcium excretion values to distinguish two forms of primary renal tubular hypokalemic alkalosis: Bartter and Gitelman syndromes. J Pediatr 120:38–43, 1992.
56. Shareghi GR, Stoner LC: Calcium transport across segments of the rabbit distal nephron in vitro. Am J Physiol 235:F367–F375, 1978.
57. Bourdeau JE, Hellstrom-Stein RJ: Voltage-dependent calcium movement across the cortical collecting duct. Am J Physiol 242: F285–F292, 1982.
58. Shimizu T, Yoshitomi K, Nakamura M, Imai M: Effects of PTH, calcitonin, and cAMP on calcium transport in rabbit distal nephron segments. Am J Physiol 259:F408–F414, 1990.
59. Aurbach GD, Heath DA: Parathyroid hormone and calcitonin regulation of renal function. Kidney Int 6:331–345, 1974.
60. Massry SG, Coburn JW, Friedler RM, et al: Relationship between the kidney and parathyroid hormone. Nephron 15:197–222, 1975.
61. Jespersen B, Randlov A, Abrahamsen J, et al: Effects of PTH(1–34) on blood pressure, renal function, and hormones in essential hypertension—the altered pattern of reactivity may counteract raised blood pressure. Am J Hypertens 10:1356–1367, 1997.
62. Zhang YB, Norian JM, Magyar CE, et al: In vivo PTH provokes apical NHE3 and NaPi2 redistribution and Na-K-ATPase inhibition. Am J Physiol Renal Physiol 276:F711–F719, 1999.
63. Friedman PA, Coutermarsh BA, Kennedy SM, Gesek FA: Parathyroid hormone stimulation of calcium transport is mediated by dual signaling mechanisms involving protein kinase A and protein kinase C. Endocrinology 137:13–20, 1996.
64. Usdin TB, Gruber C, Bonner TI: Identification and functional expression of a receptor selectively recognizing parathyroid hormone, the PTH2 receptor. J Biol Chem 270:15455–15458, 1995.
65. Wysolmerski JJ, Stewart AF: The physiology of parathyroid hormone–related protein: An emerging role as a developmental factor. Annu Rev Physiol 60:431–460, 1998.
66. De Papp AE, Stewart AF: Parathyroid hormone–related protein: A peptide of diverse physiologic functions. Trends Exp Med 4:181–187, 1993.
67. Dunbar ME, Wysolmerski JJ, Broadus AE: Parathyroid hormone–related protein: From hypercalcemia of malignancy to developmental regulatory molecule. Am J Med Sci 312:287–294, 1996.
68. Kramer S, Reynolds FH Jr, Castillo M, et al: Immunological identification and distribution of parathyroid hormone–like protein polypeptides in normal and malignant tissues. Endocrinology 128:1927–1937, 1991.
69. Ebeling PR, Adam WR, Moseley JM, Martin TJ: Actions of synthetic parathyroid hormone–related protein(1–34) on the isolated rat kidney. J Endocrinol 120:45–50, 1989.
70. Rizzoli R, Caverzasio J, Chapuy MC, et al: Role of bone and kidney in parathyroid hormone–related peptide–induced hypercalcemia in rats. J Bone Miner Res 4:759–765, 1989.
71. Stewart AF, Mangin M, Wu T, et al: Synthetic human parathyroid hormone–like protein stimulates bone resorption and causes hypercalcemia in rats. J Clin Invest 81:596–600, 1988.
72. Kukreja SC, Shevrin DH, Wimbiscus SA, et al: Antibodies to parathyroid hormone–related protein lower serum calcium in athymic mouse models of malignancy-associated hypercalcemia due to human tumors. J Clin Invest 82:1798–1802, 1988.
73. Stewart AF, Horst R, Deftos LJ, et al: Biochemical evaluation of patients with cancer-associated hypercalcemia: Evidence for humoral and nonhumoral groups. N Engl J Med 303:1377–1383, 1980.
74. Heller SR, Hosking DJ: Renal handling of calcium and sodium in metastatic and non-metastatic malignancy. BMJ 292:583–586, 1986.
75. Ralston SH, Fogelman I, Gardner MD, et al: Hypercalcaemia of malignancy: Evidence for a nonparathyroid humoral agent with an effect on renal tubular handling of calcium. Clin Sci 66:187–191, 1984.
76. Kawashima H, Torikai S, Kurokawa K: Localization of 25-hydroxyvitamin $D_3$ 1α-hydroxylase and 24-hydroxylase along the rat nephron. Proc Natl Acad Sci U S A 78:1199–1203, 1981.
77. Holick MF: Vitamin D: Photobiology, metabolism, and clinical applications. In DeGroot LJ, Besser M, Burger HG, et al (eds): Endocrinology, 3rd ed. Philadelphia, WB Saunders, 1995, pp 990–1014.
78. Suda T, Shinki T, Kurokawa K: The mechanisms of regulation of vitamin D metabolism in the kidney. Curr Opin Nephrol Hypertens 3:59–64, 1994.
79. Egel J, Pfanstiel J, Puschett JB: Effects of 1,25-dihydroxyvitamin $D_3$ on membrane transport and intermediary metabolism. Miner Electrolyte Metab 11:62–68, 1985.
80. Kawashima H, Kurokawa K: Localization of receptors for 1,25-dihydroxyvitamin $D_3$ along the rat nephron: Direct evidence for presence of the receptors in both proximal and distal nephron. J Biol Chem 257:13428–13432, 1982.
81. Stumpf WE, Sar M, Narbaitz R, et al: Cellular and subcellular localization of 1,25-$(OH)_2$-vitamin $D_3$ in rat kidney: Comparison with localization of parathyroid hormone and estradiol. Proc Natl Acad Sci U S A 77:1149–1153, 1980.
82. Bindels RJM, Hartog A, Timmermans J, van Os CH: Active $Ca^{2+}$ transport in primary cultures of rabbit kidney CCD: Stimulation by 1,25-dihydroxyvitamin $D_3$ and PTH. Am J Physiol 261: F799–F807, 1991.
83. Christakos S, Gabrielides C, Rhoten WB: Vitamin D–dependent calcium binding proteins: Chemistry, distribution, functional considerations, and molecular biology. Endocr Rev 10:3–26, 1989.
84. Bouhtiauy I, Lajeunesse D, Brunette MG: Effect of vitamin D depletion on calcium transport by the luminal and basolateral membranes of the proximal and distal nephrons. Endocrinology 132:115–120, 1993.
85. Kurnik BR, Hruska KA: Effects of 1,25-dihydroxycholecalciferol on phosphate transport in vitamin D–deprived rats. Am J Physiol 247:F177–F184, 1984.
86. Winaver J, Sylk DB, Robertson JS, et al: Micropuncture study of the acute renal tubular transport effects of 25-hydroxyvitamin $D_3$ in the dog. Miner Electrolyte Metab 4:178–188, 1980.
87. Marchand GR: Effect of parathyroid hormone on the determinants of glomerular filtration in dogs. Am J Physiol 248:F482–F486, 1985.
88. Usdin TB, Hilton J, Vertesi T, et al: Distribution of the parathyroid hormone 2 receptor in rat: Immunolocalization reveals expression by several endocrine cells. Endocrinology 140:3363–3371, 1999.
89. Lee KC, Brown D, Ureña P, et al: Localization of parathyroid hormone–related peptide receptor mRNA in kidney. Am J Physiol 270:F186–F191, 1996.
90. Massry SG, Coburn JW, Chapman LW, Kleeman CR: Role of serum Ca, parathyroid hormone, and NaCl infusion on renal Ca and Na clearances. Am J Physiol 214:1403–1409, 1968.
91. Quamme GA: Effect of hypercalcemia on renal tubular han-

dling of calcium and magnesium. Can J Physiol Pharmacol 60: 1275–1280, 1982.
92. Brown EM: Physiology and pathophysiology of the extracellular calcium-sensing receptor. Am J Med 106:238–253, 1999.
93. Pollak MR, Brown EM, Chou Y-HW, et al: Mutations in the human $Ca^{2+}$-sensing receptor gene cause familial hypocalciuric hypercalcemia and neonatal severe hyperparathyroidism. Cell 75:1297–1303, 1993.
94. Pollak MR, Seidman CE, Brown EM: Three inherited disorders of calcium sensing. Medicine 75:115–123, 1996.
95. Staum BB, Hamburger RJ, Goldberg M: Tracer microinjection study of renal tubular phosphate reabsorption in the rat. J Clin Invest 51:2271–2276, 1972.
96. Strickler JC, Thompson DD, Klose RM, Giebisch G: Micropuncture study of inorganic phosphate excretion in the rat. J Clin Invest 43:1596–1607, 1964.
97. Dennis VW, Woodhall PB, Robinson RR: Characteristics of phosphate transport in isolated proximal tubule. Am J Physiol 231:979–985, 1976.
98. Rouse D, Suki WN: Modulation of phosphate absorption by calcium in the rabbit proximal convoluted tubule. J Clin Invest 76:630–636, 1985.
99. Pastoriza-Munoz E, Colindres RE, Lassiter WE, Lechene C: Effect of parathyroid hormone on phosphate reabsorption in rat distal convolution. Am J Physiol 235:F321–F330, 1978.
100. Lang F, Greger R, Marchand GR, Knox FG: Stationary microperfusion study of phosphate reabsorption in proximal and distal nephron segments. Pflugers Arch 368:45–48, 1977.
101. de Rouffignac C, Morel F, Moss N, Roinel N: Micropuncture study of water and electrolyte movements along the loop of Henle in psammomys with special reference to magnesium, calcium and phosphorus. Pflugers Arch 344:309–326, 1973.
102. Werner A, Moore ML, Mantei N, et al: Cloning and expression of cDNA for a Na/Pi cotransport system of kidney cortex. Proc Natl Acad Sci U S A 88:9608–9612, 1991.
103. Chong SS, Kozak CA, Liu L, et al: Cloning, genetic mapping, and expression analysis of a mouse renal sodium-dependent phosphate cotransporter. Am J Physiol 268:F1038–F1045, 1995.
104. Magagnin S, Werner A, Markovich D, et al: Expression cloning of human and rat renal cortex $Na/P_i$ cotransport. Proc Natl Acad Sci U S A 90:5979–5983, 1993.
105. Murer H, Forster I, Hernando N, et al: Posttranscriptional regulation of the proximal tubule NaPi-II transporter in response to PTH and dietary $P_i$. Am J Physiol 277:F676–F684, 1999.
106. Murer H, Biber J: A molecular view of proximal tubular inorganic phosphate ($P_i$) reabsorption and of its regulation. Pflugers Arch 433:379–389, 1997.
107. Kavanaugh MP, Kabat D: Identification and characterization of a widely expressed phosphate transporter/retrovirus receptor family. Kidney Int 49:959–963, 1996.
108. Kos CH, Tihy F, Murer H, et al: Comparative mapping of $Na^+$-phosphate cotransporter genes, NPT1 and NPT2, in human and rabbit. Cytogenet Cell Genet 75:22–24, 1996.
109. Custer M, Meier F, Schlatter E, et al: Localization of NaPi-1, a $Na-P_i$ cotransporter, in rabbit kidney proximal tubules. I. mRNA Localization by reverse transcription/polymerase chain reaction. Pflugers Arch 424:203–209, 1993.
110. Tenenhouse HS, Roy S, Martel J, Gauthier C: Differential expression, abundance, and regulation of $Na^+$-phosphate cotransporter genes in murine kidney. Am J Physiol 275:F527–F534, 1998.
111. Busch AE, Schuster A, Waldegger S, et al: Expression of a renal type I sodium/phosphate transporter (NaPi-1) induces a conductance in *Xenopus* oocytes permeable for organic and inorganic anions. Proc Natl Acad Sci U S A 93:5347–5351, 1996.
112. Hilfiker H, Kvietikova I, Hartmann CM, et al: Characterization of the human type II $Na/P_i$-cotransporter promoter. Pflugers Arch 436:591–598, 1998.
113. Hartmann CM, Hewson AS, Kos CH, et al: Structure of murine and human renal type II $Na^+$-phosphate cotransporter genes (Npt2 and NPT2). Proc Natl Acad Sci U S A 93:7409–7414, 1996.
114. Kos CH, Tihy F, Econs MJ, et al: Localization of a renal sodium-phosphate cotransport gene to human chromosome 5q35. Genomics 19:176–177, 1994.
115. Ritthaler T, Traebert M, Lötscher M, et al: Effects of phosphate intake on distribution of type II $Na/P_i$ cotransporter mRNA in rat kidney. Kidney Int 55:976–983, 1999.
116. Custer M, Lötscher M, Biber J, et al: Expression of $Na-P_i$ cotransport in rat kidney: Localization by RT-PCR and immunohistochemistry. Am J Physiol 266:F767–F774, 1994.
117. Traebert M, Roth J, Biber J, et al: Internalization of proximal tubular type II Na-P(i) cotransporter by PTH: Immunogold electron microscopy. Am J Physiol 278:F148–F154, 2000.
118. Forster I, Hernando N, Biber J, Murer H: The voltage dependence of a cloned mammalian renal type II Na+/Pi cotransporter (NaPi-2). J Gen Physiol 112:1–18, 1998.
119. Lambert G, Traebert M, Hernando N, et al: Studies on the topology of the renal type II NaPi-cotransporter. Pflugers Arch 437:972–978, 1999.
120. Tatsumi S, Miyamoto K, Kouda T, et al: Identification of three isoforms for the $Na^+$-dependent phosphate cotransporter (NaPi-2) in rat kidney. J Biol Chem 273:28568–28575, 1998.
121. Beck L, Karaplis AC, Amizuka N, et al: Targeted inactivation of Npt2 in mice leads to severe renal phosphate wasting, hypercalciuria, and skeletal abnormalities. Proc Natl Acad Sci U S A 95:5372–5377, 1998.
122. Kavanaugh MP, Miller DG, Zhang W, et al: Cell-surface receptors for gibbon ape leukemia virus and amphotropic murine retrovirus are inducible sodium-dependent phosphate symporters. Proc Natl Acad Sci U S A 91:7071–7075, 1994.
123. Tenenhouse HS, Gauthier C, Martel J, et al: $Na^+$-phosphate cotransport in mouse distal convoluted tubule cells: Evidence for Glvr-1 and Ram-1 gene expression. J Bone Miner Res 13: 590–597, 1998.
124. Haas JA, Berndt T, Knox FG: Nephron heterogeneity of phosphate reabsorption. Am J Physiol 234:F287–F290, 1978.
125. Kempson SA, Lötscher M, Kaissling B, et al: Parathyroid hormone action on phosphate transporter mRNA and protein in rat renal proximal tubules. Am J Physiol 268:F784–F791, 1995.
126. Jankowski M, Biber J, Murer H: PTH-induced internalization of a type IIa $Na/P_i$ cotransporter in OK-cells. Pflugers Arch 438:689–693, 1999.
127. Malmström K, Murer H: Parathyroid hormone regulates phosphate transport in OK cells via an irreversible inactivation of a membrane protein. FEBS Lett 216:257–260, 1987.
128. Lötscher M, Scarpetta Y, Levi M, et al: Rapid downregulation of rat renal $Na/P_i$ cotransporter in response to parathyroid hormone involves microtubule rearrangement. J Clin Invest 104:483–494, 1999.
129. Hruska KA, Moskowitz D, Esbrit P, et al: Stimulation of inositol trisphosphate and diacylglycerol production in renal tubular cells by parathyroid hormone. J Clin Invest 79:230–239, 1987.
130. Jüppner H, Abou-Samra AB, Freeman M, et al: A G protein–linked receptor for parathyroid hormone and parathyroid hormone–related peptide. Science 254:1024–1026, 1991.
131. Abou-Samra AB, Jüppner H, Force T, et al: Expression cloning of a common receptor for parathyroid hormone and parathyroid hormone–related peptide from rat osteoblast-like cells: A single receptor stimulates intracellular accumulation of both cAMP and inositol trisphosphates and increases intracellular free calcium. Proc Natl Acad Sci U S A 89:2732–2736, 1992.
132. Lederer ED, Sohi SS, Mathiesen JM, Klein JB: Regulation of expression of type II sodium-phosphate cotransporters by protein kinases A and C. Am J Physiol Renal Physiol 275:F270–F277, 1998.
133. Segal JH, Pollock AS: Transfection-mediated expression of a dominant cAMP-resistant phenotype in the opossum kidney (OK) cell line prevents parathyroid hormone–induced inhibition of Na-phosphate cotransport: A protein kinase-A–mediated event. J Clin Invest 86:1442–1450, 1990.
134. Pfister MF, Forgo J, Ziegler U, et al: cAMP-Dependent and -independent downregulation of type $IINa-P_i$ cotransporters by PTH. Am J Physiol Renal Physiol 276:F720–F725, 1999.
135. Hayes G, Busch AE, Lang F, et al: Protein kinase C consensus sites and the regulation of renal $Na/P_i$-cotransport (NaPi-2) expressed in *Xenopus laevis* oocytes. Pflugers Arch 430:819–824, 1995.
136. Lederer ED, Sohi SS, McLeish KR: Parathyroid hormone stimulates extracellular signal-regulated kinase (ERK) activity

through two independent signal transduction pathways: Role of ERK in sodium-phosphate cotransport. J Am Soc Nephrol 11:222–231, 2000.

137. Kurnik BR, Huskey M, Hruska KA: 1,25-Dihydroxycholecalciferol stimulates renal phosphate transport by directly altering membrane phosphatidylcholine composition. Biochim Biophys Acta 917:81–85, 1987.
138. Elgavish A, Rifkind J, Sacktor B: In vitro effects of vitamin $D_3$ on the phospholipids of isolated renal brush border membranes. J Membr Biol 72:85–91, 1983.
139. Taketani Y, Segawa H, Chikamori M, et al: Regulation of type II renal $Na^+$-dependent inorganic phosphate transporters by 1,25-dihydroxyvitamin $D_3$—identification of a vitamin D–responsive element in the human NAPI-3 gene. J Biol Chem 273:14575–14581, 1998.
140. Sorribas V, Markovich D, Verri T, et al: Thyroid hormone stimulation of Na/Pi-cotransport in opossum kidney cells. Pflugers Arch 431:266–271, 1995.
141. Caverzasio J, Bonjour JP: Insulin-like growth factor I stimulates Na-dependent Pi transport in cultured kidney cells. Am J Physiol 257:F712–F717, 1989.
142. Levi M, Shayman JA, Abe A, et al: Dexamethasone modulates rat renal brush border membrane phosphate transporter mRNA and protein abundance and glycosphingolipid composition. J Clin Invest 96:207–216, 1995.
143. Arar M, Baum M, Biber J, et al: Epidermal growth factor inhibits Na-Pi cotransport and mRNA in OK cells. Am J Physiol 268:F309–F314, 1995.
144. Alcalde AI, Sarasa M, Raldua D, et al: Role of thyroid hormone in regulation of renal phosphate transport in young and aged rats. Endocrinology 140:1544–1551, 1999.
145. Hilfiker H, Hartmann CM, Stange G, Murer H: Characterization of the 5'-flanking region of OK cell type II Na-$P_i$ cotransporter gene. Am J Physiol 274:F197–F204, 1998.
146. Wagner GF, Jaworski EM, Haddad M: Stanniocalcin in the seawater salmon: Structure, function, and regulation. Am J Physiol Regul Integr Comp Physiol 274:R1177–R1185, 1998.
147. Wagner GF, Guiraudon CC, Milliken C, Copp DH: Immunological and biological evidence for a stanniocalcin-like hormone in human kidney. Proc Natl Acad Sci U S A 92:1871–1875, 1995.
148. Chang ACM, Dunham MA, Jeffrey KJ, Reddel RR: Molecular cloning and characterization of mouse stanniocalcin cDNA. Mol Cell Endocrinol 124:185–187, 1996.
149. Wagner GF, Vozzolo BL, Jaworski E, et al: Human stanniocalcin inhibits renal phosphate excretion in the rat. J Bone Miner Res 12:165–171, 1997.
150. Chang ACM, Reddel RR: Identification of a second stanniocalcin cDNA in mouse and human: Stanniocalcin 2. Mol Cell Endocrinol 141:95–99, 1998.
151. Ishibashi K, Miyamoto K, Taketani Y, et al: Molecular cloning of a second human stanniocalcin homologue (STC2). Biochem Biophys Res Commun 250:252–258, 1998.
152. Amstutz M, Mohrmann M, Gmaj P, Murer H: Effect of pH on phosphate transport in rat renal brush border membrane vesicles. Am J Physiol 248:F705–F710, 1985.
153. Busch A, Waldegger S, Herzer T, et al: Electrophysiological analysis of $Na^+$/Pi cotransport mediated by a transporter cloned from rat kidney and expressed in *Xenopus* oocytes. Proc Natl Acad Sci U S A 91:8205–8208, 1994.
154. Hartmann CM, Wagner CA, Busch AE, et al: Transport characteristics of a murine renal Na/$P_i$-cotransporter. Pflugers Arch 430:830–836, 1995.
155. Brazy PC, McKeown JW, Harris RH, Dennis VW: Comparative effects of dietary phosphate, unilateral nephrectomy, and parathyroid hormone on phosphate transport by the rabbit proximal tubule. Kidney Int 17:788–800, 1980.
156. Knox FG, Haas JA, Haramati A: Nephron sites of adaptation to changes in dietary phosphate. Adv Exp Med Biol 151:13–19, 1982.
157. Lötscher M, Wilson P, Nguyen S, et al: New aspects of adaptation of rat renal Na-Pi cotransporter to alterations in dietary phosphate. Kidney Int 49:1012–1018, 1996.
158. Pfister MF, Hilfiker H, Forgo J, et al: Cellular mechanisms involved in the acute adaptation of OK cell Na/$P_i$-cotransport to high- or low-$P_i$ medium. Pflugers Arch 435:713–719, 1998.
159. Lötscher M, Kaissling B, Biber J, et al: Role of microtubules in the rapid regulation of renal phosphate transport in response to acute alterations in dietary phosphate content. J Clin Invest 99:1302–1312, 1997.
160. Rasmussen H, Tenenhouse HS: Mendelian hypophosphatemias. In Scriver CR, Beaudet AL, Sly WS, Valle D (eds): The Metabolic and Molecular Basis of Inherited Disease, 7th ed. New York, McGraw-Hill, 1995, pp 3717–3745.
161. Tenenhouse HS, Werner A, Biber J, et al: Renal $Na^+$-phosphate cotransport in murine X-linked hypophosphatemic rickets: Molecular characterization. J Clin Invest 93:671–676, 1994.
162. Beck L, Meyer RA Jr, Meyer MH, et al: Renal expression of $Na^+$ phosphate cotransporter mRNA and protein: Effect of the Gy mutation and low phosphate diet. Pflugers Arch 431: 936–941, 1996.
163. Beck L, Soumounou Y, Martel J, et al: Pex/PEX tissue distribution and evidence for a deletion in the 3' region of the Pex gene in X-linked hypophosphatemic mice. J Clin Invest 99: 1200–1209, 1997.
164. Strom TM, Francis F, Lorenz B, et al: Pex gene deletions in Gy and Hyp mice provide mouse models for X-linked hypophosphatemia. Hum Mol Genet 6:165–171, 1997.
165. Consortium TH: A gene (PEX) with homologies to endopeptidases is mutated in patients with X-linked hypophosphatemic rickets. Nat Genet 11:130–136, 1995.
166. Sabbagh Y, Jones AO, Tenenhouse HS: PHEXdb, a locus-specific database for mutations causing X-linked hypophosphatemia. Hum Mutat 16:1–6, 2000.
167. Ruchon AF, Marcinkiewicz M, Siegfried G, et al: Pex mRNA is localized in developing mouse osteoblasts and odontoblasts. J Histochem Cytochem 46:459–468, 1998.
168. Econs MJ, McEnery PT, Lennon F, Speer MC: Autosomal dominant hypophosphatemic rickets is linked to chromosome 12p13. J Clin Invest 100:2653–2657, 1997.
169. Consortium TA: Autosomal dominant hypophosphataemic rickets is associated with mutations in FGF23. Nat Genet 26:345–348, 2000.
170. Massry S, Coburn JW, Kleeman CR: Renal handling of magnesium in the dog. Am J Physiol 216:1460–1467, 1969.
171. Rude R, Bethune JE, Singer FR: Renal tubular maximum for magnesium in normal, hyperparathyroid, and hypoparathyroid man. J Clin Endocrinol Metab 51:1425–1431, 1980.
172. Quamme GA, Dirks JH: Intraluminal and contraluminal magnesium on magnesium and calcium transfer in the rat nephron. Am J Physiol 238:F187–F198, 1980.
173. Le Grimellec C, Roinel N, Morel F: Simultaneous Mg, Ca, P, K, Na and Cl analysis in rat tubular fluid. I. During perfusion of either inulin or ferrocyanide. Pflugers Arch 340:181–196, 1973.
174. Quamme GA, Smith CM: Magnesium transport in the proximal straight tubule of the rabbit. Am J Physiol 246:F544–F550, 1984.
175. Brunette M, Vigneault N, Carriere S: Micropuncture study of magnesium transport along the nephron in the young rat. Am J Physiol 227:891–896, 1974.
176. Brunette M, Vigneault N, Carriere S: Micropuncture study of renal magnesium transport in magnesium-loaded rats. Am J Physiol 229:1695–1701, 1975.
177. Poujeol P, Chabardes D, Roinel N, de Rouffignac C: Influence of extracellular fluid volume expansion on magnesium, calcium and phosphate handling along the rat nephron. Pflugers Arch 365:203–211, 1976.
178. Wong NLM, Quamme GA, Sutton RA, Dirks JH: Effects of mannitol on water and electrolyte transport in the dog kidney. J Lab Clin Med 94:683–692, 1979.
179. Quamme G: Effect of furosemide on calcium and magnesium transport in the rat nephron. Am J Physiol 241:F340–F347, 1981.
180. Wittner M, Erickson AE, Wangemann P, et al: Differential effect of ADH on sodium, chloride, potassium, calcium and magnesium transport in cortical and medullary thick ascending limbs of mouse nephron. Pflugers Arch 412:516–523, 1988.
181. Di Stefano A, Wittner M, Nitschke R, et al: Effects of glucagon on $Na^+$, $Cl^-$, $K^+$, $Mg^{2+}$, and $Ca^{2+}$ transports in cortical and medullary thick ascending limbs of mouse kidney. Pflugers Arch 414:640–646, 1989.
182. Simon DB, Lu Y, Choate KA, et al: Paracellin-1, a renal tight

junction protein required for paracellular $Mg^{2+}$ resorption. Science 285:103–106, 1999.
183. Praga M, Vara J, Gonzalez-Parra E, et al: Familial hypomagnesemia with hypercalciuria and nephrocalcinosis. Kidney Int 47: 1419–1425, 1995.
184. Hebert SC, Brown EM, Harris HW: Role of the $Ca^{2+}$-sensing receptor in divalent mineral ion homeostasis. J Exp Biol 200: 295–302, 1997.
185. Chou Y-HW, Pollak MR, Brandi ML, et al: Mutations in the human $Ca^{2+}$-sensing-receptor gene that cause familial hypocalciuric hypercalcemia. Am J Hum Genet 56:1075–1079, 1995.
186. Pollak MR, Brown EM, Estep HL, et al: Autosomal dominant hypocalcaemia caused by a $Ca^{2+}$-sensing receptor gene mutation. Nat Genet 8:303–307, 1994.
187. Pearce S, Williamson C, Kifor O, et al: A familial syndrome of hypocalcemia with hypercalciuria due to mutations in the calcium-sensing receptor. N Engl J Med 335:1115–1122, 1996.
188. Kreusser W, Kurokawa K, Aznar E, et al: Effect of phosphate depletion on magnesium homeostasis in rats. J Clin Invest 61: 573–581, 1978.
189. Sachtjen E, Meyer WA, Massry SG: Evidence of magnesium secretion during phosphate depletion in the rat. Proc Soc Exp Biol Med 162:416–419, 1979.
190. Wong NLM, Quamme GA, O'Callaghan TJ, et al: Renal tubular transport in phosphate depletion: A micropuncture study. Can J Physiol Pharmacol 58:1063–1071, 1980.
191. Dai L-J, Friedman PA, Quamme GA: Cellular mechanisms of chlorothiazide and cellular potassium depletion on $Mg^{2+}$ uptake in mouse distal convoluted tubule cells. Kidney Int 51: 1008–1017, 1997.
192. Quamme GA, Dai L-J, Huysmans D: Presence of a novel influx pathway for $Mg^{2+}$ in MDCK cells. Am J Physiol 259:C521–C525, 1990.
193. Quamme GA: Renal magnesium handling: New insights in understanding old problems. Kidney Int 52:1180–1195, 1997.
194. Dai LJ, Bapty B, Ritchie G, Quamme GA: Glucagon and arginine vasopressin stimulate $Mg^{2+}$ uptake in mouse distal convoluted tubule cells. Am J Physiol 274:F328–F335, 1998.
195. de Rouffignac C, Quamme G: Renal magnesium handling and its hormonal control. Physiol Rev 74:305–322, 1994.
196. Bengele HH, Alexander EA, Lechene CP: Calcium and magnesium transport along the inner medullary collecting duct of the rat. Am J Physiol 239:F24–F29, 1980.
197. Brunette M, Vigneault N, Carriere S: Magnesium handling by the papilla of the young rat. Pflugers Arch 373:229–235, 1978.
198. Mastroianni N, Bettinelli A, Bianchetti M, et al: Novel molecular variants of the Na-Cl cotransporter gene are responsible for Gitelman syndrome. Am J Hum Genet 59:1019–1026, 1996.
199. Takeuchi K, Kure S, Kato T, et al: Association of a mutation in thiazide-sensitive Na-Cl cotransporter with familial Gitelman's syndrome. J Clin Endocrinol Metab 81:4496–4499, 1996.
200. Schultheis PJ, Lorenz JN, Meneton P, et al: Phenotype resembling Gitelman's syndrome in mice lacking the apical $Na^{+}$-$Cl^{-}$ cotransporter of the distal convoluted tubule. J Biol Chem 273: 29150–29155, 1998.
201. Harris CA, Burnatowska MA, Seely JF, et al: Effects of parathyroid hormone on electrolyte transport in the hamster nephron. Am J Physiol 236:F342–F348, 1979.
202. Bethune J, Turpin RA, Inoue H: Effect of parathyroid hormone extract on divalent ion excretion in man. J Clin Endocrinol Metab 28:673–678, 1968.
203. Kuntziger H, Amiel C, Roinel N, Morel F: Effects of parathyroidectomy and cyclic AMP on renal transport of phosphate, calcium and magnesium. Am J Physiol 227:905–911, 1974.
204. Burnatowska MA, Harris CA, Sutton RAL, Dirks JH: Effects of PTH and cAMP on renal handling of calcium, magnesium, and phosphate in the hamster. Am J Physiol 233:F514–F518, 1977.
205. Quamme GA: Effect of calcitonin on calcium and magnesium absorption in rat nephron. Am J Physiol 238:E573–E578, 1980.

CHAPTER 26

# Abnormal Calcium and Magnesium Metabolism

Sanford Reikes, MD ▪ Esther A. González, MD ▪ Kevin J. Martin, MB, BCh

## CALCIUM METABOLISM

Calcium is the most abundant divalent cation in the body and plays a major role not only in the structure of the skeleton but also as a regulator of a variety of cellular functions, by virtue of its role as an extracellular and intracellular messenger.[1, 2] Approximately 99% of the body's calcium is in bone and therefore is not available for the regulation of calcium homeostasis. The remaining 1% of calcium is distributed in soft tissues, teeth, and the extracellular fluid.

In normal humans, calcium balance is maintained in spite of a wide range of intakes, as a result of the interaction of several homeostatic mechanisms that involve the regulation of intestinal, renal, and skeletal function. Plasma calcium ranges from 8.8 to 10.4 mg/dL and consists of three fractions: protein-bound calcium represents approximately 40% of total serum calcium; approximately 10% of total serum calcium circulates as a complex of various anions, including phosphate, bicarbonate, and citrate; and the remaining fraction is ionized calcium, representing approximately 50% of total serum calcium. The last fraction is the physiologically important component available for transport and the regulation of cellular processes. This component, together with the complexed fraction, is ultrafilterable.

Although ionized calcium can easily be measured directly, in some circumstances, one can approximate the measurement by correcting total serum calcium for changes in serum protein concentrations and changes in blood pH.[3–6] For example, for every gram per deciliter that serum albumin differs from 4 g/dL, serum calcium should be adjusted by 0.8 mg/dL. For a pH increment of 0.1, serum calcium should be decreased by 0.12 mg/dL.

### Calcium Homeostasis

Plasma calcium concentration is maintained within a narrow range by an integration of intestinal calcium absorption, renal calcium reabsorption, and the deposition and release of calcium from bone. These three important processes are regulated by the major calciotropic hormones parathyroid hormone (PTH) and vitamin D and, to a lesser extent, by calcitonin. Calcium balance is illustrated in Figure 26–1, which depicts that with a 1000-mg calcium intake, approximately 400 mg will be absorbed in the intestine and 200 mg secreted, for a net absorption of 200 mg. Deposition and mobilization of 200 mg from bone also occur in the normal state, and neutral balance can be achieved by the excretion of 200 mg by the kidney. Obviously, during skeletal growth, there is a need for positive calcium balance, and considerable quantities of calcium can be deposited on a daily basis in the growing skeleton.

In spite of the large influx to and efflux from the extracellular fluid, the serum concentration of ionized calcium remains tightly controlled. This control is exerted primarily by the function of the parathyroid glands, which monitor plasma calcium and alter PTH secretion in response to changes, as illustrated in Figure 26–2. Thus, increases in PTH stimulate bone resorption, resulting in the release of both calcium and phosphorus. PTH acts on the kidney to increase the reabsorption of calcium and stimulates the production of calcitriol, which in turn acts on the intestine to increase the absorption of calcium and phosphorus. The increased influx of phosphorus from mobilization of bone and greater phosphate transport in the intestine is excreted by the actions of PTH on the kidney, thereby achieving homeostasis.

The mechanism of calcium sensing by the parathyroid gland has been elucidated in recent years and depends on a G protein–coupled calcium-sensing receptor.[7] This G protein–coupled receptor plays a key role in the regulation of plasma calcium and is responsible for mediation of the known effects of calcium on parathyroid and renal function. The physiologic relevance of this receptor has been demonstrated by the identification of both inactivating and activating mutations, which result in distinctive clinical syndromes.[8, 9]

### Calcium Metabolism and Bone

The skeleton undergoes a continuous process of remodeling throughout life. There is constant mobilization of calcium from bone and deposition of calcium in newly formed bone matrix. These processes of resorption and mineralization are closely coupled, and disturbances of this coupling are seen in the presence of disease. PTH is the major regulator of bone turnover; it acts primarily on the osteoblast and indirectly affects osteoclast function.[10] The nature of the interaction between osteoblasts and osteoclasts has recently been elucidated with the discovery of the RANK/RANKL/OPG system.[11, 12] It has been demonstrated that osteoclast precursors express a receptor (*r*eceptor *a*ctivator of *NFk*B [RANK]) that must interact with a protein ligand (RANK-ligand, [RANKL]) on the surface of osteoblast-like cells to allow the differentiation of the precursor into mature osteoclasts. Osteoblast-like cells also secrete a soluble receptor (osteoproteg-

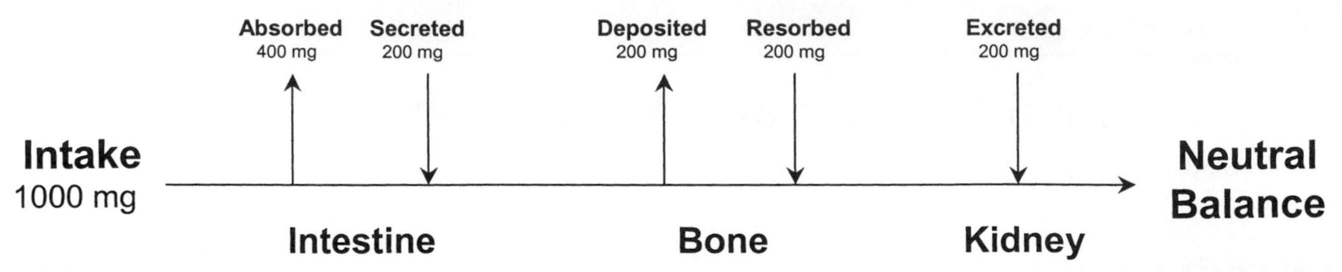


**FIGURE 26–1** ■ Calcium balance. On a usual daily intake of 1000 mg of calcium, there is a net absorption of 200 mg in the intestine. Skeletal balance is neutral. The kidney excretes 200 mg and maintains overall balance.

erin [OPG]) that can interact with RANKL and inhibit osteoclastogenesis by preventing the interaction of osteoclast precursors with RANKL on the osteoblast surface. This system is under the regulation of a variety of hormones, growth factors, and cytokines.[13–15]

Like PTH, the principal target cell for the actions of vitamin D metabolites, such as 1,25-dihydroxyvitamin vitamin $D_3$ (calcitriol), is the osteoblast. Calcitriol has been demonstrated to affect many genes in bone cells, but its major effect on bone mineralization may be the result of its actions to regulate plasma concentrations of calcium and phosphorus, as demonstrated by recent studies in the vitamin D receptor knockout mouse.[16, 17]

Bone remodeling is also regulated by a variety of other hormones, such as insulin, growth hormone, calcitonin, glucocorticoids, insulin-like growth factor I, sex hormones, thyroid hormones, and a host of locally produced cytokines and growth factors. A detailed discussion of this complex physiology is beyond the scope of this chapter, and excellent reviews on this topic are available.[18]

## Intestinal Calcium Absorption

Net intestinal absorption of calcium is approximately 30% of normal intake, but the efficiency of absorption increases as dietary calcium is reduced. This enables calcium balance to be maintained, even at very low dietary calcium intakes.[19] Vitamin D is the major regulator of intestinal calcium absorption. Absorption of calcium across the intestinal mucosa appears to involve an active transcellular transport process, as well as a component of passive paracellular diffusion. Active transport of calcium occurs in the duodenum and upper jejunum, and passive absorption appears to occur throughout the entire small intestine and the colon. Although vitamin D can affect absorp-

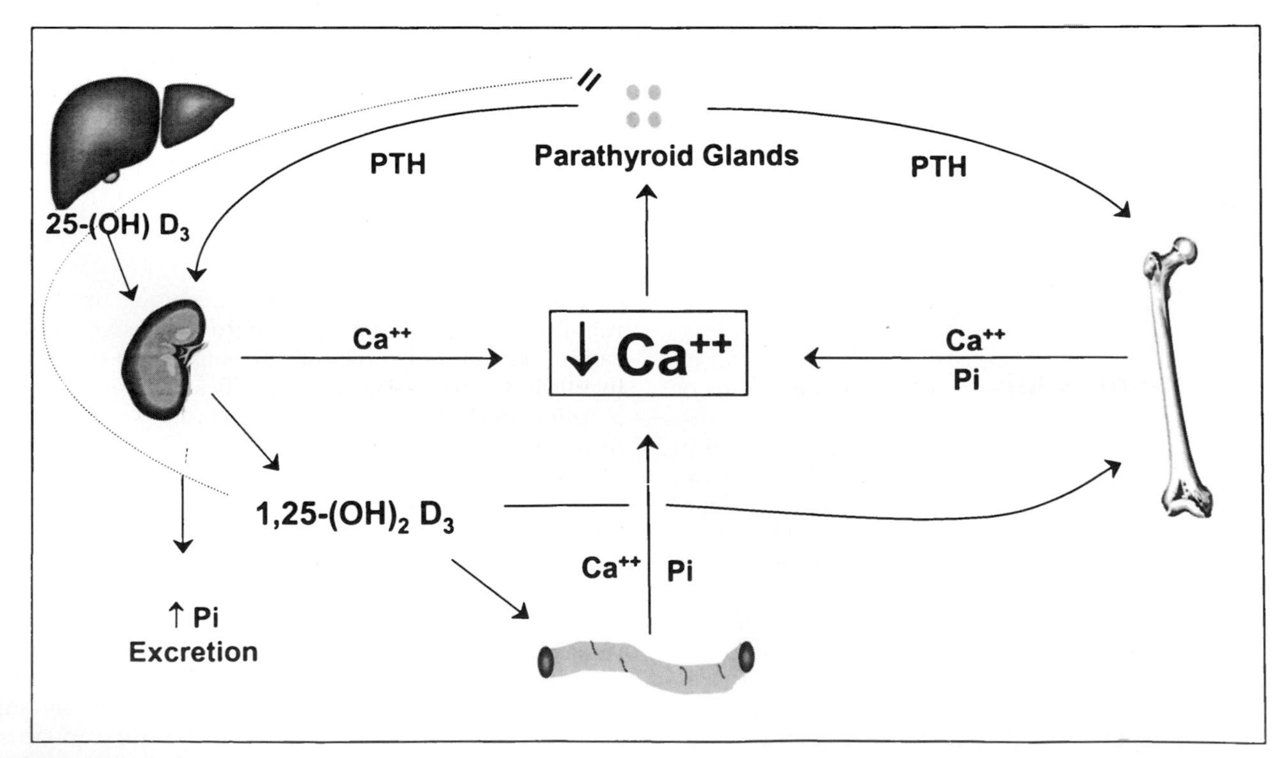


**FIGURE 26–2** ■ Integrated response to a decrease in ionized calcium. Parathyroid hormone acts directly on the kidney and bone and acts indirectly on the intestine by increasing the production of calcitriol in order to restore normocalcemia.

tion in all segments, the duodenum is the most responsive segment. The active absorption of calcium involves movement across the apical membrane, transport across the cytosol of the cell, and extrusion across the basolateral membrane.[20, 21] Following the initial entry step, the calcium is bound to a calcium-binding protein, calbindin-$D_{9K}$, which likely protects against the toxic effects of high calcium concentrations on cellular function, and likely transports the calcium across the cell to the basolateral membrane, where adenosine triphosphate (ATP)–dependent calcium-ATPase (PMCA) and the sodium-calcium exchanger (NCX) transporters facilitate the extrusion of calcium from the cell.[22] The plasma membrane calcium transporter and calbindin appear to be vitamin D dependent.[23] Thus, the major regulator of intestinal calcium absorption is calcitriol. Recent findings have begun to clarify the nature of the initial entry step by identifying a calcium transporter in the intestine, CaT1,[24] which is closely related but not identical to the epithelial calcium channel (ECaC) first described in rabbit kidney and initially thought to be present in intestine as well.[25, 26]

Calcitriol appears to act in the intestine by both genomic and nongenomic mechanisms. The latter, known as transcaltachia, occurs very rapidly (within seconds to minutes) and is thought to be too rapid to be the result of gene transcription.[27, 28] Although vitamin D is undoubtedly the most important regulator, many other factors can influence the absorption of calcium by the intestine, either directly or indirectly. The components of the diet, such as phosphate, oxalate, long-chain fatty acids, lysine, arginine, and lactose, can all influence calcium absorption in the intestine.

## Renal Handling of Calcium

The kidney plays a key role in the maintenance of overall calcium homeostasis, both by excreting calcium from the body and by converting vitamin D to its active metabolite, calcitriol.[29] Thus, the kidney needs to excrete an amount of calcium that is equal to the daily net intestinal calcium absorption. The excretion of calcium by the kidney begins with the filtration of the ultrafilterable fraction of plasma calcium at the level of the glomerulus. Because the filtered load of calcium is more than 10,000 mg/day, approximately 98% of this needs to be reabsorbed along the nephron to allow the excretion of the 200 mg/day required to maintain balance. Approximately 60% to 70% of filtered calcium is reabsorbed in the proximal convoluted tubule, 20% in the thick ascending limb of the loop of Henle, 5% to 10% in the distal tubule and connecting tubule, and 4% in the collecting duct.[30]

Calcium absorption in the proximal tubule and the thick ascending limb is predominantly through a paracellular and therefore passive pathway. There is some suggestion that an active component may also exist in the early proximal tubule as well as in the $S_3$ segment, but this has not been characterized. The calcium-sensing receptor has been localized to the proximal tubule brush border, but its role in calcium absorption in this segment has not been defined.[31]

Calcium absorption in the distal nephron occurs against an electrochemical gradient, and because the tight junctions are relatively impermeable to calcium, an active transcellular pathway is required. In this segment, similar to the intestine, transcellular calcium transport is believed to have three components: entry of calcium across the apical membrane; diffusion of calcium across the cell, bound to a calcium-binding protein, calbindin-$D_{28K}$; and finally, extrusion of calcium at the basolateral membrane. Progress on elucidating the molecular nature of the influx pathway has clarified our understanding of calcium absorption in the distal nephron. Recently, an expression cloning strategy in *Xenopus* oocytes yielded an ECaC that appears to fulfill the characteristics required for this transport mechanism.[25, 26] Other studies confirmed these findings in the rat and demonstrated that the initial localization of ECaC to the intestine may have been the result of detection of the closely related CaT1, which has significant homology but is not identical to the renal ECaC or CaT2.[32] The integrated transport scheme is illustrated in Figure 26–3. ECaC is localized at the apical domain of the distal tubular segments of the mammalian kidney. ECaC colocalizes with calbindin-$D_{28K}$–positive segments of the renal tubule. ECaC contains potential regulatory sites for protein kinase C and protein kinase A, as well as cyclic guanosine monophosphate–dependent protein kinase, and the functional and pharmacologic properties of ECaC appear to be consistent with the characteristics described for transcellular calcium transport in cells from the distal nephron. Thus, there is substantial evidence that ECaC is the mechanism of apical calcium entry.

Calcium extrusion mechanisms of the basolateral membrane of the cells involve two transporters: NCX and PMCA.[33, 34] NCX-1 is the isoform expressed in the kidney, and it, too, is restricted to the distal nephron, where it localizes in the basolateral membrane. PMCAs also exist in a number of isoforms, some of which are ubiquitously expressed.[33] It is likely that PMCA-1 is the isoform that participates in the process of transcellular calcium transport, because it is expressed in the small intestine as well as in the distal nephron segments involved in active calcium transport.[35] Studies in cells from the distal nephron have confirmed that the major calciotropic hormones PTH, calcitriol, and calcitonin regulate calcium transport processes, but such studies also suggest that other hormones may play a role in the regulation of calcium transport, including vasopressin, prostaglandin $E_2$, adenosine, ATP, nitric oxide, and atrial natriuretic peptide.[35] The role of ECaC abnormalities in human disease, such as hypercalciuria, remains to be demonstrated, but it is attractive to consider this as a target gene because of the association of both intestinal and renal transport abnormalities in hypercalciuria. Similarly, studies in vitro suggest that ECaC could account for the observation of acidosis-induced hypercalciuria, in that at low pH, calcium

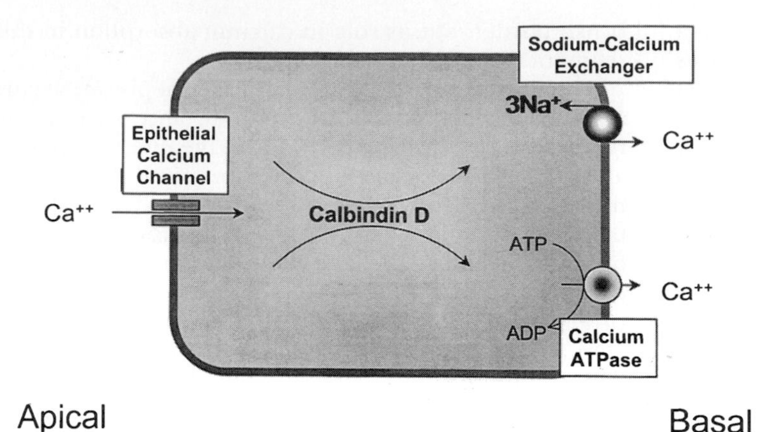


Epithelial calcium channels: ECaC1, ECaC2, CaT1, CaT2
Sodium-calcium exchanger: NCX1
Calcium ATPase : PMCA

**FIGURE 26–3** ■ Calcium absorption in the distal nephron. Calcium entry at the apical membrane is through the epithelial calcium channel (ECaC). Intracellular calcium transport involves calbindin $D_{28K}$. Calcium extrusion at the basolateral membrane is by the sodium-calcium exchanger (NCX1) and calcium ATPase (PMCA1).

entry through ECaC is limited.[25] Further studies are necessary to clarify these issues.

### FACTORS INFLUENCING THE RENAL HANDLING OF CALCIUM

Renal calcium excretion is influenced by many factors, including ambient serum calcium, state of the extracellular volume, changes in acid-base balance, vitamin D and PTH levels, and use of diuretics.[30] Hypercalcemia is generally associated with an increase in calcium excretion because of an increase in the filtered load and a decrease in the tubular reabsorption of calcium. Although hypercalcemia can decrease the glomerular filtration rate (GFR) and therefore tends to offset the increase in filtered load, hypercalcemia also causes a decline in tubular reabsorption of calcium by both PTH-dependent and PTH-independent effects. Hypercalcemia is associated with a decrease in calcium reabsorption in the proximal tubule, although the mechanism is not well understood. In the thick ascending limb, hypercalcemia activates the calcium-sensing receptor located on the basolateral membrane, which results in a decrease in calcium absorption by altering the activity of the $Na^+$-$K^+$-$2Cl^-$ transporter.[36] Reduced activity of this transporter results in a decrease in the lumen-positive potential difference and, consequently, decreases calcium reabsorption. The effects of hypercalcemia on calcium reabsorption in the distal nephron are likely due to a decrease in PTH resulting in decreased calcium reabsorption in the distal nephron segments. Hypocalcemia decreases renal calcium excretion by decreasing the filtered load and enhancing the tubular reabsorption of calcium. Some of the enhancement in renal calcium reabsorption occurs as a consequence of increased levels of PTH, which increase calcium reabsorption in the distal nephron.

Expansion of the extracellular fluid is associated with an increase in the excretion of sodium, chloride, and calcium, whereas the reciprocal effects are seen with volume contraction. The precise mechanisms of this effect are closely interrelated with the effects of sodium reabsorption and the compensatory changes that occur as a result of volume expansion. Acute and chronic metabolic acidosis is often associated with an increase in calcium excretion, independent of changes in PTH.[37] Part of the calciuria may be due to mobilization of calcium from bone, as hydrogen ion is buffered in the skeleton; however, direct effects of acidosis on tubular calcium resorption also play a role.[37] The recent studies on ECaC are also consistent with acidosis directly decreasing the apical entry of calcium in the distal nephron.[25] Although the effects of PTH and calcium on calcium absorption in the kidney have been well described, the effects of vitamin D metabolites on calcium transport are controversial and are likely to be deeply entwined with the effects on calbindin. The direct effects of vitamin D metabolites on overall calcium handling in the kidney are not well defined.[30]

Loop diuretics decrease calcium absorption as a result of inhibition of the transport of sodium chloride at the $Na^+$-$K^+$-$2Cl^-$ transporter in the ascending loop of Henle. Thiazide diuretics, which act in the distal tubule, are associated with hypocalciuria.[38, 39]

## HYPERCALCEMIA

In general, the term *hypercalcemia* implies that the concentration of serum ionized calcium is greater than 1.27 mmol/L or that total serum calcium is greater than 10.4 mg/dL. Hypercalcemia has been reported to be present in 0.1% of the general population, and a much higher prevalence is expected in hospitalized patients. Malignancy and hyperparathyroidism are the most common causes of hypercalcemia, accounting for up to 80% to 90% of cases, and their prevalence differs among patient populations.[40] Hypercalcemia due to primary hyperparathyroidism is most commonly found in nonhospitalized patients, whereas hypercalcemia related to malignancy is more prevalent among hospitalized patients.

## Clinical Features of Hypercalcemia

The clinical manifestations of hypercalcemia are nonspecific, vary greatly in severity, and affect a variety of organ systems (Table 26–1). The expression of hypercalcemic features in a particular patient depends on the magnitude of the elevation in serum calcium, as well as on the evolution and nature of the underlying disorder. Thus, patients in whom hypercalcemia develops rapidly are more likely to be symptomatic, and patients with certain hypercalcemic disorders may manifest characteristic clinical features of hypercalcemia. The most frequent manifestations of hypercalcemia include neurologic, renal, cardiovascular, and gastrointestinal complications.

Polyuria is the most common renal manifestation of hypercalcemia. The impaired urinary concentrating ability is thought to involve the actions of the calcium receptor.[41, 42] Thus, activation of this receptor by an elevated serum calcium level may result in decreased transport of sodium chloride in the thick ascending limb of the loop of Henle, resulting in decreased countercurrent multiplication and ultimately affecting urinary concentrating ability. In addition, activation of the calcium receptor in the collecting duct may blunt the response of this nephron segment to antidiuretic hormone. Hypercalcemia can cause both acute and chronic renal insufficiency. The acute decrease in GFR may be related to the natriuretic effect of hypercalcemia, which leads to diuresis and volume contraction. In addition, a direct effect of serum calcium on smooth muscle cells may lead to renal vasoconstriction.[43] Correction of hypercalcemia in these circumstances results in normalization of the GFR. Chronic renal insufficiency is characterized by calcium deposition and interstitial fibrosis. Hypercalciuria may in some cases precede hypercalcemia, because extracellular calcium may have a calciuric effect by acting on the calcium receptor on the thick ascending limb of the loop of Henle.[44] Both nephrolithiasis and nephrocalcinosis may occur as a result of hypercalciuria.

**TABLE 26–1.** Clinical Manifestations of Hypercalcemia

| Renal | Cardiovascular |
|---|---|
| Impaired urinary concentration | Hypertension |
| Renal insufficiency | Bradycardia |
| Acute | Shortened QT interval |
| Chronic | **Gastrointestinal** |
| Nephrocalcinosis | Anorexia |
| Nephrolithiasis | Nausea |
| **Neurologic** | Vomiting |
| Lethargy | Constipation |
| Drowsiness | Peptic ulcer disease |
| Confusion | Pancreatitis |
| Irritability | |
| Stupor | |
| Coma | |
| Convulsions | |
| Paresthesias | |
| Muscle weakness | |
| Tetany | |

**TABLE 26–2.** Disorders Associated with Hypercalcemia

| PTH Related | Renal Failure and Transplant Related |
|---|---|
| Primary hyperparathyroidism | Recovery from acute renal failure |
| Adenoma | Chronic renal failure |
| Hyperplasia | Post-transplant |
| Carcinoma | **Non–PTH-Related Endocrine** |
| MEN syndromes (1, 2A) | Hyperthyroidism |
| FHH | Pheochromocytoma |
| **Malignancy Related** | Adrenal insufficiency |
| Humoral hypercalcemia of malignancy | **Miscellaneous** |
| PTHrP mediated | Granulomatous disorders |
| Calcitriol mediated | Milk-alkali syndrome |
| Osteolytic metastases | Immobilization |
| **Drug Related** | Paget disease |
| Vitamin D compounds | Jansen disease |
| Thiazide diuretics | |
| Lithium | |
| Vitamin A | |

FHH, familial hypocalciuric hypercalcemia; MEN, multiple endocrine neoplasia; PTH, parathyroid hormone; PTHrP, parathyroid hormone–related peptide.

Neurologic complications are commonly present. Patients often present with lethargy, drowsiness, confusion, and, in more severe cases, convulsions, stupor, and coma. Signs of neuromuscular irritability include paresthesias and tetany. The cardiovascular complications of hypercalcemia include hypertension, bradycardia, and shortened QT interval. Hypercalcemia is also associated with a variety of gastrointestinal manifestations, including anorexia, nausea, vomiting, constipation, peptic ulcer disease, and pancreatitis.

## Disorders Associated with Hypercalcemia

As mentioned earlier, the most common disorders leading to hypercalcemia fall into two groups: parathyroid related and malignancy related (Table 26–2). Less common causes of hypercalcemia include drugs, milk-alkali syndrome, granulomatous disorders, and Paget disease. Patients with renal disease may have hypercalcemia due to multiple factors related to medical therapy, dialysis, and transplantation.

### PARATHYROID-RELATED HYPERCALCEMIA

#### *Primary Hyperparathyroidism*

Primary hyperparathyroidism is characterized by hypercalcemia and hypophosphatemia as a result of increased secretion of PTH.[45] It affects approximately 1 in 500 individuals and is the leading cause of hypercalcemia. The diagnosis is often made before the development of symptoms related to excess PTH, owing to the availability of routine measurements of serum calcium. Primary hyperparathyroidism is caused by a single adenoma in approximately 85% of cases; diffuse hyperplasia of all four glands and parathyroid carcinoma account for the remaining 10% and 5%, respectively. A subset of patients with primary hyperparathyroidism have other endocrine abnormalities related to the multiple endocrine neoplasia (MEN) syndromes. MEN 1 (Wermer syndrome) consists of primary hyperparathyroidism most often due to diffuse parathyroid gland hyperplasia, benign pituitary tumors, and tumors of the endocrine pancreas, especially gastrinomas, which are often associated with peptic ulcer disease (Zollinger-Ellison syndrome).[46] MEN 2A refers to the presence of primary hyperparathyroidism, pheochromocytoma, and medullary carcinoma of the thyroid. Both conditions are inherited as autosomal dominant traits.[47] Hypercalcemia in patients with hyperparathyroidism results from the effects of PTH in its target organs. Thus, PTH increases bone resorption, increases renal calcium reabsorption, and increases intestinal calcium absorption. The last effect of PTH is indirect and is due to increased renal 1 α-hydroxylase activity, which in turn increases the level of calcitriol in the serum, thus enhancing intestinal calcium absorption.

**Pathogenesis of Primary Hyperparathyroidism.** The pathogenesis of primary hyperparathyroidism remains largely unknown. Linkage analysis and molecular genetic studies in the MEN syndromes have provided some insight into the molecular defects involved in the genesis of these disorders and have suggested potential mechanisms for the pathogenesis of sporadic hyperparathyroidism.[48] At least two molecular defects are thought to be involved in the development of hyperparathyroidism: loss of function of a tumor suppressor gene, and overactivity of a growth-promoting gene.

MEN 1 is caused by germline mutations of the MEN 1 gene (*menin*), a tumor suppressor gene, located on chromosome 11. Affected individuals inherit one allele as an autosomal dominant trait. Loss of the second allele by a somatic event renders the cell unable to regulate growth, resulting in monoclonal expansion and tumor development. Somatic mutations in the MEN 1 gene are present in approximately 25% of spontaneous parathyroid adenomas, implying similar defects in these two forms of hyperparathyroidism.[49, 50] A second mechanism of unregulated growth—activation of a growth-promoting gene—may also play a role in the pathogenesis of primary hyperparathyroidism. In these patients, the PTH gene is rearranged as a result of pericentric inversion of chromosome 11.[51, 52] The translocation results in the formation of a gene, *PRAD 1* (*p*arathyroid gene *r*earrangement in *ad*enoma), which is driven by the regulatory region of the PTH gene. PRAD 1 was subsequently found to be cyclin D1, a regulator of the cell cycle. Thus, excessive expression of PRAD 1 driven by the PTH promoter leads to unregulated cellular proliferation. This defect has been observed in approximately 20% of patients with parathyroid adenomas.[53] The defect in MEN 2A has also been identified. It involves activating mutations of a proto-oncogene, RET, which encodes a tyrosine kinase.[54, 55] Genetic screening for germline mutations of the RET gene in affected families makes it possible to identify affected patients and refer them to surgery early, in order to prevent the development of medullary carcinoma of the thyroid.[56, 57] Other genetic abnormalities are likely to be involved in hyperparathyroidism.[58–62] The mechanisms involved in the development of parathyroid carcinoma appear to be different from those responsible for adenoma formation. Thus, loss of the retinoblastoma tumor supressor gene has been implicated in the development of parathyroid carcinoma.[63–65]

Studies using parathyroid cells from patients with primary hyperparathyroidism have demonstrated a shift in the set-point for PTH release. That is, a higher extracellular calcium concentration is required to achieve a 50% decrease in PTH secretion. This finding suggests an abnormality in the parathyroid calcium-sensing receptor, and although a search for mutations in this receptor in patients with primary hyperparathyroidism has yielded negative results,[66, 67] studies have demonstrated decreased expression of the calcium receptor in parathyroid adenoma.[68, 69] It remains unclear whether decreased expression of the calcium-sensing receptor precedes adenoma formation or occurs as a consequence of cellular dedifferentiation.

**Signs and Symptoms Associated with Primary Hyperparathyroidism.** Approximately half the patients with primary hyperparathyroidism are asymptomatic. This is largely due to early diagnosis of the disorder with routine measurements of serum calcium. The most frequent manifestations of hyperparathyroidism relate to the kidneys and bones. Urinary tract obstruction, infections, and chronic renal insufficiency may occur as a result of nephrolithiasis. The usual composition of kidney stones in hyperparathyroidism is either calcium oxalate or calcium phosphate. Deposition of calcium in the renal parenchyma leads to nephrocalcinosis, which may cause chronic renal insufficiency. The characteristic bone lesion of hyperparathyroidism is osteitis fibrosa cystica, which exhibits an increased number of osteoclasts, decreased number of trabeculae, and marrow fibrosis. Symptomatic patients may also have neurologic, muscular, and gastrointestinal manifestations.

**Diagnosis and Management of Primary Hyperparathyroidism.** The diagnostic evaluation of primary hyperparathyroidism often follows the incidental finding of hypercalcemia or the evaluation of hypercalciuria. Hypophosphatemia is usually present unless the patient has developed advanced renal insufficiency. The diagnosis of hyperparathyroidism relies on the measurement of serum calcium and circulating PTH levels. The introduction of an intact PTH assay allows a high level of diagnostic accuracy,[70] and further refinements may become available in the near future.[71, 72] The diagnosis of parathyroid carcinoma is difficult to make before histologic examination of the tissue; however, severe hypercalcemia with total serum calcium concentrations in the range of 14 to 15 mg/dL is often encountered with carcinoma.

Primary hyperparathyroidism may be managed medically or surgically. Recent studies comparing the outcome of surgery versus medical management strongly point toward surgery as the treatment of choice, because a good proportion of asymptomatic patients will have disease progression.[73, 74] In general, asymptomatic patients older than 50 years of age with only minimal hypercalcemia and well-preserved renal function and bone mass may be offered the option of close medical follow-up; however, at least 25% of patients will progress, and it should be emphasized that surgical correction of primary hyperparathyroidism is always an acceptable approach, because the procedure carries a high success rate with low morbidity and mortality.

The specific procedure to be performed depends on the findings at the time of surgical exploration. There is controversy whether all four glands should be biopsied at the time of surgery.[75, 76] The conservative approach is based on the fact that typically only one gland is abnormal. Thus, if the enlarged gland is identified and a second gland is normal, no further intervention is required. The risk of this approach is that hyperparathyroidism is likely to recur if additional abnormal parathyroid tissue is missed and therefore not removed. The more aggressive approach involves the identification of all four glands and removal of most of the parathyroid tissue. Most of the surgical literature favors an intermediate approach whereby all four glands are explored and only abnormal parathyroid tissue is removed. When only one gland is found to be abnormal, removal of the adenoma is usually curative, and recurrence of hyperparathyroidism is rare. In cases of diffuse hyperplasia and multiple gland involvement, all the glands must be identified, and either three and a half or all four glands are removed, with immediate autotransplantation of a portion of a parathyroid gland in the muscle or subcutaneous tissue of the forearm.[77, 78] On the rare occasion when carcinoma is encountered, wide excision should be performed, avoiding rupture of the capsule. If no abnormal glands are identified in the neck at the time of exploration, it implies that there are additional glands in unusual locations, and a variety of imaging techniques are available to aid in the identification of these ectopic parathyroid glands, including ultrasonography, computed tomography, magnetic resonance imaging, and nuclear medicine studies.[79–83] These studies are not performed routinely before parathyroidectomy except when surgical exploration fails to identify the abnormal gland or in the setting of recurrent hyperparathyroidism.

A decrease in serum calcium is expected to occur within the first 24 hours following successful parathyroidectomy. The degree of postoperative hypocalcemia varies, depending on both the extent of the surgical procedure and the severity of the bone disease. Patients with well-preserved bone mineral and normal renal function may have only mild decreases in serum calcium, whereas those with severe osteitis fibrosa and extensive surgery may have profound hypocalcemia. Symptomatic hypocalcemia following parathyroidectomy requires intravenous (IV) calcium administration with or without the use of calcitriol.

***Familial Hypocalciuric Hypercalcemia and Neonatal Severe Hyperparathyroidism***

Familial hypocalciuric hypercalcemia (FHH) is an autosomal dominant disorder characterized by moderate chronic hypercalcemia and low urinary calcium excretion (urinary calcium-to-creatinine ratio $<0.01$).[84] The serum calcium is usually between 10.5 and 12.5 mg/dL, and the typical features of hypercalcemia are rarely present. Low urinary calcium excretion is an important finding, as it distinguishes this disorder from primary hyperparathyroidism. The levels of PTH are within the normal range in most patients; however, they are inappropriately high relative to the level of serum calcium. Approximately one fifth of patients have elevated PTH levels.

The pathophysiology of FHH involves abnormal sensing of calcium concentration by the parathyroid glands and the kidneys as a result of inactivating mutations in the calcium-sensing receptor.[8] The defective receptors are unable to sense calcium concentrations, and they function as if hypocalcemia were present. This abnormality leads to increased PTH secretion and increased renal tubular calcium reabsorption. Patients with FHH are usually asymptomatic and are detected as a result of genetic screening after a family member is diagnosed with hyperparathyroidism. Because the hypercalcemia of FHH is benign and does not respond to parathyroidectomy, it is important to differentiate this disorder from primary hyperparathyroidism.

Neonatal severe hyperparathyroidism is a rare disorder often found in the offspring of kindreds with FHH, and it represents defects in both alleles of the calcium receptor.[85] It is characterized by severe hyperparathyroidism and life-threatening hypercalcemia. Treatment requires parathyroidectomy; the disorder is lethal without surgical intervention.

## MALIGNANCY-RELATED HYPERCALCEMIA

Malignancy is the second most common cause of hypercalcemia. The mechanism underlying malignancy-related hypercalcemia involves either a direct invasion of bone by tumor or an indirect effect of the tumor on bone via the production of circulating factors that promote bone resorption.[86, 87] The latter is commonly referred to as humoral hypercalcemia of malignancy (HHM). By the time hypercalcemia becomes evident, the malignancy is usually advanced, and the presence of hypercalcemia is a poor prognostic factor. A variety of malignancies are associated with HHM by the production of PTH-related peptide (PTHrP), including renal cell, squamous cell, breast, and ovarian carcinoma. PTHrP shares similarity with PTH in the first 13 amino acids, and it interacts with the PTH receptor in bone and kidney.[88] If PTHrP-mediated HHM is suspected, the diagnosis is confirmed by measuring circulating PTHrP levels.[89, 90]

Malignant lymphomas may also cause HHM, but in this case, the humoral factor produced is calcitriol, which promotes intestinal calcium absorption and increases osteoclastic bone resorption.[91] Direct involvement of the bone by metastatic disease is responsible for hypercalcemia in most cases of advanced carcinoma of the breast and prostate. Multiple myeloma may be associated with extensive bone destruction; however, hypercalcemia is rarely present in the absence of renal insufficiency. The mediators of osteoclastic bone resorption in multiple myeloma include interleukin-1β, interleukin-6, and tumor necrosis factor-α.[92–94] Hypercalcemia of malignancy usually improves with reduction of tumor mass.

## DRUG-RELATED HYPERCALCEMIA

Commonly used drugs that may cause hypercalcemia include vitamin D compounds, thiazide diuretics, vitamin A, lithium, and calcium supplements.[95–99] The last are more likely to cause hypercalcemia in the setting of chronic renal failure. Large doses of vitamin D or any of its metabolites may cause hypercalcemia as a result of increased intestinal calcium absorption and bone resorption. Patients requiring large doses of vitamin D for treatment of hypoparathyroidism are at especially high risk for the development of hypercalcemia. Interestingly, in these circumstances, the levels of 25-hydroxyvitamin $D_3$ are markedly elevated, but the levels of calcitriol, the most active form of vitamin D, may be only mildly elevated, suggesting the involvement of vitamin D metabolites other than calcitriol in the development of hypercalcemia. Hypercalcemia in this setting responds to glucocorticoids and dietary calcium restriction.

It is well recognized that thiazide diuretics can cause hypercalcemia. This usually occurs in patients with underlying disorders that promote bone resorption or during vitamin D therapy.[96] The exact mechanisms involved in the development of thiazide-induced hypercalcemia are not clear, but it appears that increased renal tubular calcium reabsorption occurs as a result of volume contraction. Lithium therapy is another well-known cause of hypercalcemia and is associated with high levels of PTH. The mechanism of lithium-induced hypercalcemia appears to involve alterations in the set-point for PTH secretion.[100]

Excessive consumption of vitamin A may promote the development of hypercalcemia, likely due to increased osteoclastic bone resorption. Most cases of vitamin A intoxication are due to excessive consumption of vitamin supplements.[95] As is the case with vitamin D intoxication, this form of hypercalcemia responds to therapy with glucocorticoids.

Calcium salts are used in high doses as phosphate binders in patients with chronic renal failure and are a common cause of hypercalcemia in this patient population, especially when combined with the use of calcitriol. The latter is also an important cause of hypercalcemia in patients with chronic renal failure.

## NON–PARATHYROID HORMONE–RELATED ENDOCRINE HYPERCALCEMIA

Several endocrine disorders such as hyperthyroidism, pheochromocytoma, and adrenal insufficiency are known to be associated with hypercalcemia. Hypercalcemia may occur in up to 20% of patients affected with hyperthyroidism.[101] Excess thyroid hormone may cause increased bone turnover, with the rate of bone resorption exceeding the rate of bone formation.[102] The hypercalcemia is usually mild and responds to successful treatment of the hyperthyroid state.

Pheochromocytoma may also be associated with hypercalcemia in the absence of MEN syndromes.[103] The fact that the hypercalcemia is usually corrected by removing the tumor and not by pharmacologic blockade of catecholamine synthesis suggests that the production of a humoral factor by the tumor cells is the cause of hypercalcemia in these patients. This humoral factor appears to be PTHrP, because both the protein and mRNA have been demonstrated in tumor tissue.[104–106]

Adrenal insufficiency is an unusual cause of hypercalcemia.[107] Although several mechanisms have been proposed, there is no clear explanation for this abnormality; however, it responds to therapy with glucocorticoids. Other endocrine disorders that have been associated with hypercalcemia include acromegaly and pancreatic islet cell tumors.

## OTHER CAUSES OF HYPERCALCEMIA

### *Granulomatous Disorders*

Sarcoidosis is a systemic disorder of unclear cause characterized by the presence of noncaseating granulomas in a variety of organs. It may be complicated by hypercalcemia in up to 25% of cases.[108] Hypercalciuria is a more common finding in these patients, and in some instances, it may precede the development of hypercalcemia. Renal complications of hypercalciuria such as nephrocalcinosis and nephrolithiasis are common. In addition, sarcoidosis may affect the kidney directly and lead to renal insufficiency as a result of granulomatous interstitial nephritis.[109] The development of hypercalcemia in sarcoidosis involves increased production of calcitriol of extrarenal origin. The macrophages from sarcoid granulomas have 1 α-hydroxylase activity and can therefore 1 α-hydroxylate 25-hydroxyvitamin $D_3$, resulting in increased synthesis of calcitriol.[110–112] The generation of calcitriol by macrophages in sarcoidosis appears to be less tightly regulated than renal synthesis, owing to defects in a number of steps involved in vitamin D metabolism. Glucocorticoids are effective in decreasing abnormal calcitriol production and are used as first-line therapy for hypercalcemia in this patient population.[113] Other agents used to treat hypercalcemia in sarcoidosis include chloroquine and ketoconazole.[114, 115] In addition to drug therapy, avoidance of excessive sun exposure and restriction of dietary calcium intake and vitamin D may help control the hypercalcemia.

Hypercalcemia has also been described in a variety of infectious granulomatous disorders such as disseminated candidiasis, disseminated coccidioidomycosis, histoplasmosis, leprosy, tuberculosis, and berylliosis. As is the case with sarcoidosis, the pathogenesis of hypercalcemia in these diseases is related to the unregulated production of calcitriol by the activated macrophages in the granulomatous lesions.

### *Milk-Alkali Syndrome*

The milk-alkali syndrome is characterized by hypercalcemia, alkalemia, nephrocalcinosis, and renal insufficiency.[116, 117] It is caused by excessive consumption of calcium and absorbable antacids, and it was formerly encountered among patients with peptic ulcer disease who consumed large amounts of milk and calcium carbonate to relieve their symptoms. As expected, the milk-alkali syndrome has decreased in frequency since the introduction of other therapies for peptic ulcer disease. The reason for the development of this syndrome in the setting of calcium and alkali intake remains unclear; however, there is evidence that alkalemia impairs urinary calcium excretion. The resultant hypercalcemia may provoke natriuresis and result in volume contraction, which in turn increases bicarbonate reabsorption, exacerbating the alkalemia. Coexisting renal insufficiency is an important contributor, because urinary calcium excretion may be impaired in this setting. Hyperphosphatemia is also a complication of the milk-alkali syndrome and is due to impaired renal phosphate excretion in the presence of renal insufficiency in combination with the oral consumption of phosphate present in milk. Metastatic calcification may occur as a result of hypercalcemia and hyperphosphatemia in the setting of metabolic alkalosis.

### *Immobilization*

Long-term immobilization may cause hypercalcemia, especially in patients with high bone turnover, such as children or adults with Paget disease. Concurrent biochemical findings include hypercalciuria, which can be severe at times; hyperphosphatemia; and low levels of calcitriol and PTH. The mechanisms underlying the development of hypercalcemia in immobilized patients has not been clearly elucidated, but it appears to involve uncoupling of the processes of bone formation and bone resorption such that there is increased mobilization of skeletal calcium. The hypercalcemia usually resolves with resumption of ambulation, and it may also be controlled with the use of glucocorticoids, calcitonin, and bisphosphonates.[118–120]

### *Paget Disease*

Paget disease affects approximately 1% of the population older than 45 years of age. It is a chronic, focal skeletal disorder characterized by increased bone remodeling at multiple sites, leading to abnormally high bone formation and bone resorption rates, which result in skeletal deformities and pathologic fractures.[121] The underlying abnormality in Paget disease arises in the osteoclasts, which are large and hypernucleated and have been found to contain inclusion bodies similar to those present in virus-infected cells. This finding suggests a viral cause in the pathogenesis of Paget disease, which is supported by recent studies demonstrating that a pagetic phenotype can be induced in osteoclasts expressing the measles virus nucleocapsid.[122]

### *Jansen Disease*

Jansen-type metaphyseal chondrodysplasia is a rare disorder characterized by a variety of developmental defects involving the skeleton, such as bowed legs, short stature, and cystic bone lesions. Hypercalcemia and hypophosphatemia are also features of this disorder. Children with this disorder rarely survive to adulthood. The molecular basis for Jansen disease has recently been elucidated, and it is caused by mutations in the gene coding for the PTH receptor, which result in overactivity of the receptor without requiring PTH for stimulation.[123, 124]

## HYPERCALCEMIA RELATED TO RENAL FAILURE

The diuretic phase of acute renal failure may be accompanied by hypercalcemia. The proposed mechanisms responsible for hypercalcemia during recovery from renal failure due to rhabdomyolysis are as follows: Early in the course of rhabdomyolysis, the hyperphosphatemia resulting from tissue injury and from renal phosphate retention causes hypocalcemia due to calcium deposition in soft tissues. The hypocalcemia stimulates PTH release, and the high levels of PTH in turn increase the activity of 1 $\alpha$-hydroxylase, resulting in increased synthesis of calcitriol.[125] During the polyuric phase of renal failure, the hyperphosphatemia resolves, and the soft tissue calcium deposits are mobilized. Although the hyperparathyroidism and the high levels of calcitriol may contribute to hypercalcemia, it appears that the mobilization of calcium from ectopic sites plays the major role in the development of hypercalcemia in this setting.[125–129]

Hypercalcemia in the setting of chronic renal failure largely results from efforts to control secondary hyperparathyroidism. With progressive renal failure, there is a tendency to develop hyperparathyroidism due to several factors, including hyperphosphatemia, decreased levels of calcitriol, hypocalcemia, intrinsic abnormalities of the parathyroid glands, and skeletal resistance to the actions of PTH.[130] The management of hyperparathyroidism in chronic renal failure involves the use of phosphate binders to control the hyperphosphatemia.[131, 132] Aluminum hydroxide was widely used for this purpose in the past, and it can cause hypercalcemia associated with decreased bone turnover. The use of aluminum has decreased dramatically in recent years in view of its toxicity (to the central nervous system and bone),[133] and calcium-containing salts, often used in large doses, are now administered as phosphate binders and contribute to the hypercalcemia of chronic renal failure.

Another important aspect in the management of secondary hyperparathyroidism in chronic renal failure is the administration of calcitriol or its newer analogues.[134–136] Thus, the simultaneous administration of calcium-containing phosphate binders and potent vitamin D compounds may lead to hypercalcemia in this patient population. In advanced stages of secondary hyperparathyroidism, marked parathyroid gland hyperplasia may occur, which may be associated with hypercalcemia. At this stage, the decreased expression of parathyroid calcium receptors as well as vitamin D receptors renders the excessive PTH secretion extremely resistant to medical therapy, and surgical intervention must be considered.

### HYPERCALCEMIA FOLLOWING RENAL TRANSPLANTATION

Patients with uremic hyperparathyroidism and advanced parathyroid hyperplasia are at high risk for developing hypercalcemia following successful renal transplantation.[137, 138] Most commonly, the hypercalcemia is mild, and it resolves within 12 to 24 months. The hypercalcemia following kidney transplantation is thought to occur as a result of the marked increase in parathyroid gland mass rather than true glandular autonomy. In cases of severe hypercalcemia, renal function may be compromised, and surgical parathyroidectomy is the treatment of choice. Patients with chronic renal failure and refractory, severe secondary hyperparathyroidism who are candidates for living, related-donor kidney transplants may benefit from parathyroidectomy before surgery to protect the graft from the adverse effects of hypercalcemia following surgery.

## Approach to the Patient with Hypercalcemia

All patients with hypercalcemia should undergo an investigation in search of the underlying cause (Fig. 26–4). A complete history and physical examination accompanied by routine biochemical studies, urinalysis, and chest radiograph are particularly helpful in the initial evaluation, because hypercalcemia of malignancy is often associated with an advanced process that rarely escapes detection after a basic clinical evaluation. In the presence of malignancy, measurement of PTHrP and calcitriol levels and skeletal imaging studies are useful in differentiating the specific mechanisms involved in the hypercalcemia. If no evidence of malignancy is found, the level of intact PTH should be obtained. Elevated PTH in the setting of hypercalcemia is diagnostic of hyperparathyroidism. A urine calcium-to-creatinine ratio is useful in differentiating primary hyperparathyroidism from FHH. In the absence of hyperparathyroidism or malignancy, less common causes of hypercalcemia should be considered, such as vitamin D toxicity and sarcoidosis, which can be evaluated by checking the levels of vitamin D and angiotensin-converting enzyme, respectively.

## General Principles of Management

Acutely, hypercalcemia responds well to medical therapy; however, on a chronic basis, successful management is less likely unless the underlying cause of hypercalcemia is corrected. The pharmacologic options for the treatment of hypercalcemia are best guided by an understanding of the basic pathogenetic process. Because hypercalcemia may be the result of increased intestinal calcium absorption, increased bone resorption, or impaired urinary calcium excretion, the choice of therapy should be directed toward counteracting the particular mechanism involved. Thus, hypercalcemia in patients with osteolytic metas-

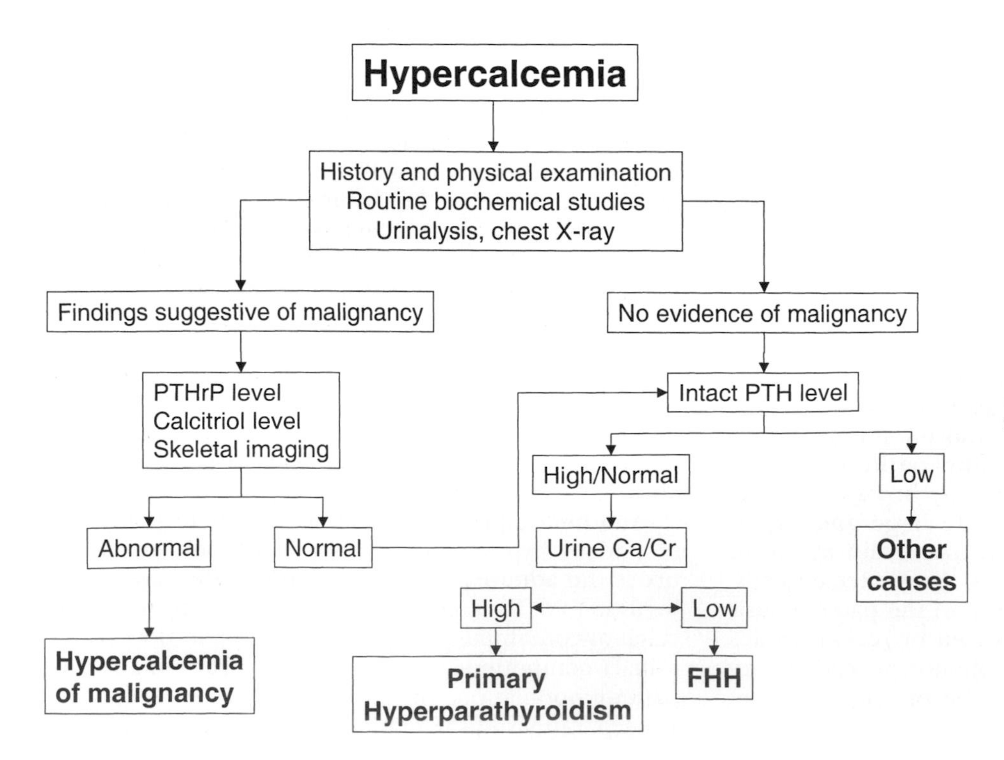


**FIGURE 26–4** ■ Scheme for the evaluation of hypercalcemia. (For a full description, see the text.)

tasis is better handled by adding an antiresorptive agent than by restricting dietary calcium. Conversely, in patients with sarcoidosis, restriction of dietary calcium is beneficial.

In general, a patient with severe and symptomatic hypercalcemia requires the prompt institution of effective therapy. Because dehydration frequently accompanies hypercalcemia, and the resultant decrease in GFR leads to impaired calcium clearance, restoration of extracellular fluid volume is an effective means of increasing urinary calcium excretion. Thus, the IV administration of isotonic saline is often accompanied by the use of loop diuretics to enhance urinary calcium excretion, and the latter can be further enhanced by increasing urinary sodium excretion.

Inhibition of bone resorption can be achieved with a variety of agents, including bisphosphonates, calcitonin, gallium nitrate, and plicamycin. The bisphosphonates are concentrated in areas of high bone turnover and inhibit osteoclastic bone resorption by interfering with both the development and the activity of osteoclasts. These agents have become the treatment of choice in hypercalcemia of malignancy.[139–142] Bisphosphonates may cause renal insufficiency and should be used carefully in patients with impaired renal function. Calcitonin is another effective inhibitor of osteoclastic bone resorption, and it has a rapid onset of action, although the effect is only transient. Gallium nitrate is a potent inhibitor of bone resorption, but its use is contraindicated in the presence of renal insufficiency.[143] Plicamycin impairs osteoclast function, but it is rarely used owing to its multiple side effects, including liver, kidney, and bone marrow toxicity.[144]

Glucocorticoids are particularly useful in the management of hypercalcemia associated with increased intestinal calcium absorption, such as in sarcoidosis, and the complications that arise from the long-term use of these agents in chronic disorders are well known. Limited sun exposure and dietary calcium restriction are also important measures in the management of hypercalcemia related to increased intestinal calcium absorption.

As discussed earlier, for hypercalcemia secondary to primary hyperparathyroidism, surgical intervention is the preferred approach because it has been shown to prevent further complications of the hyperparathyroid state. The use of calcimimetic agents, compounds that activate the calcium receptor and therefore suppress PTH secretion, may provide an option in the future for selected patients with hyperparathyroidism.[145]

Hypercalcemia in patients with renal failure may require a different approach, owing to their inability to adequately excrete a sodium load. In this case, acute hemodialysis using a dialysate containing a low calcium concentration may be necessary.[146] The commonly used bone antiresorptive agents such as bisphosphonates and gallium nitrate are not recommended in patients with renal insufficiency, thus adding to the difficulty in managing these patients. Fortunately, hemodialysis is an effective and safe alternative for patients with symptomatic hypercalcemia in the setting of renal impairment.

# HYPOCALCEMIA

Chronic hypocalcemia is encountered less often than hypercalcemia. A total serum calcium concentration below the normal range may be indicative of true hypocalcemia—that is, a low ionized calcium concentration—or it may be secondary to hypoalbuminemia, in which case, true hypocalcemia is not present. In the latter situation, hypocalcemia is excluded by the finding of a normal ionized calcium concentration. A variety of clinical conditions are associated with transient hypocalcemia in hospitalized patients, including sepsis, pancreatitis, transfusions with citrated blood, and respiratory alkalosis related to hyperventilation. The last may be encountered in the setting of lung disease, cardiovascular disease, central nervous system disorders, or any condition associated with stress or pain. Chronic hypocalcemia is most commonly related to abnormalities of the major hormones involved in calcium homeostasis, namely, PTH and vitamin D. Patients with clinical disorders associated with chronic hypocalcemia are usually symptomatic and require long-term therapy.

## Clinical Features of Hypocalcemia

As is the case with hypercalcemia, the manifestations of hypocalcemia vary greatly at a given level of serum calcium. The most common signs and symptoms are neuromuscular. Patients may experience muscle cramps, acral and circumoral paresthesias, and, in more severe cases, laryngeal spasm, seizures, mental changes, and even coma. The Chvostek and Trousseau signs may be present in patients with latent tetany. Psychiatric manifestations of hypocalcemia include mental status changes, anxiety, irritability, depression, and hallucinations. Increased intracranial pressure may develop in patients with long-standing hypocalcemia, which can be associated with papilledema. Cardiovascular manifestations may be present in the form of hypotension and congestive heart failure. Electrocardiogram abnormalities related to hypocalcemia include prolonged QT interval, arrhythmias, and heart block. Other manifestations of chronic hypocalcemia involve the skin, hair, nails, and teeth; thus, patients may have dry skin, dermatitis, coarse hair, alopecia, brittle nails, dental caries, and hypoplastic teeth. In general, the clinical manifestations of hypocalcemia are easily reversible by adequate therapy.

## Disorders Associated with Hypocalcemia

Most of the causes of hypocalcemia are related to abnormalities of PTH and vitamin D systems (Table 26–3). Patients may have low circulating levels of PTH, or they may be resistant to the actions of the hormone. Vitamin D deficiency, abnormal vitamin D metabolism, and vitamin D resistance may also cause hypocalcemia.

**TABLE 26–3.** Disorders Associated with Hypocalcemia

| Parathyroid Hormone Related | Renal Disease Related |
|---|---|
| Hypoparathyroidism | Acute renal failure |
| Genetic | Chronic renal failure |
| Calcium receptor gene defects | Nephrotic syndrome |
| PTH gene defects | **Miscellaneous** |
| DiGeorge syndrome | Sepsis |
| Acquired | Pancreatitis |
| Neck surgery/irradiation | Osteoblastic metastases |
| Infiltrative | Hungry bone syndrome |
| Magnesium disorders | Transfusion with citrated blood |
| Target organ resistance to PTH | Acute respiratory alkalosis |
| Pseudohypoparathyroidism types Ia, Ib, Ic, II | Medications |
| Magnesium depletion | |
| **Vitamin D Related** | |
| Vitamin D deficiency | |
| Nutritional | |
| Malabsorption | |
| Lack of sun exposure | |
| Altered vitamin D metabolism | |
| Liver disease | |
| Chronic renal failure | |
| Hyperphosphatemia | |
| VDDR I | |
| Vitamin D resistance | |
| VDDR II | |

PTH, parathyroid hormone; VDDR, vitamin D–dependent rickets.

In critically ill patients, sepsis, pancreatitis, blood transfusions, and respiratory alkalosis due to hyperventilation are associated with hypocalcemia. Patients with renal insufficiency are also prone to developing hypocalcemia from a variety of causes, including hyperphosphatemia and calcitriol deficiency.

## PARATHYROID HORMONE–RELATED HYPOCALCEMIA

### *Hypoparathyroidism*

In a small proportion of patients with hypoparathyroidism, there is a hereditary basis for their disorder, and in only a few kindreds has the molecular defect been characterized. Among the genetic causes of hypoparathyroidism, gain-of-function mutations of the extracellular calcium-sensing receptor are the most common. Unlike the mutations responsible for FHH, the mutations found in these patients result in inappropriate activation of the calcium receptor with respect to serum calcium. As a result, PTH secretion may be suppressed by serum calcium concentrations below the normal range. This condition is referred to as autosomal dominant hypoparathyroidism or autosomal dominant hypocalcemia[147] and is characterized by hypocalcemia and PTH levels in the normal range but inappropriately low for the degree of hypocalcemia. Treatment with calcium supplements and vitamin D is advisable only for those patients with severe symptoms related to hypocalcemia, as these agents may exacerbate hypercalciuria.[9] The hypercalciuria is due to the effects of overactivity of the calcium receptor in the renal tubule, which would favor urinary calcium excretion. Defects in the pre-pro-PTH gene as well as in the PTH gene have been described in kindreds with hereditary hypoparathyroidism.[148, 149] Hereditary hypoparathyroidism may also occur in association with other genetic abnormalities, such as those present in DiGeorge syndrome, which is due to defective development of the thymus and the parathyroid glands and is characterized by neonatal hypoparathyroidism, cardiovascular defects, thymic aplasia, and abnormal facies.[150]

Most commonly, chronic acquired hypoparathyroidism results from surgical excision of the parathyroid glands or from injury to the glands during neck surgery or irradiation.[151–153] Frequently, transient hypoparathyroidism occurs after partial parathyroidectomy, as discussed earlier. Magnesium deficiency may result in hypocalcemia by two mechanisms: impaired PTH release, and resistance to PTH in target organs. In these patients, hypocalcemia may be reversed by correcting the hypomagnesemia.[154, 155] Hypocalcemia has also been reported to occur in cases of magnesium excess, such as during the administration of magnesium sulfate for the treatment of preeclampsia.[156] Infiltrative disorders affecting the parathyroid glands, such as neoplasia, granulomatous disorders, and hemochromatosis, are relatively rare causes of acquired hypoparathyroidism.

### *Target Organ Resistance to Parathyroid Hormone*

*Pseudohypoparathyroidism* is the term used to describe conditions characterized by biochemical features of PTH deficiency, such as hypocalcemia and hyperphosphatemia, in the presence of high circulating levels of PTH. Two types of pseudohypoparathyroidism have been described (Table 26–4). Type I is characterized by decreased urinary cyclic adenosine monophosphate (cAMP) production and decreased urinary phosphate excretion in response to PTH. It has been classified into three subtypes. Type Ia refers to patients with the biochemical findings of pseudohypoparathyroidism and the somatic characteristics of Albright hereditary

**TABLE 26–4.** Classification of Pseudohypoparathyroidism

| Type | AHO Features | Urinary Phosphorus | Urinary cAMP | Molecular Defect | Hormone Resistance | Inheritance |
|---|---|---|---|---|---|---|
| Ia | Yes | Decreased | Decreased | Gsα gene mutations | Generalized | Autosomal dominant |
| Ib | No | Decreased | Decreased | ? | PTH | Autosomal dominant |
| Ic | Yes | Decreased | Decreased | ? | Generalized | Autosomal dominant |
| II | No | Decreased | Normal | ? | PTH | Sporadic |

AHO, Albright hereditary osteodystrophy; cAMP, cyclic adenosine monophosphate; PTH, parathyroid hormone.

osteodystrophy, that is, short stature, mental retardation, round face, and shortening of the metacarpals and metatarsals. The cellular abnormality in this disorder has been characterized, and it is due to mutations in the gene coding for the α subunit of the stimulatory G protein (Gsα); as expected, resistance to multiple peptide hormones is also a feature of this disorder.[157, 158] Type Ib is characterized by resistance to PTH but no features of Albright hereditary osteodystrophy or multihormone resistance, which initially suggested that it resulted from mutations of the PTH receptor; however, recent studies have excluded this possibility, and the basis for PTH resistance in these patients remains an enigma.[159, 160] Patients with type Ic pseudohypoparathyroidism have all the biochemical and somatic features found in type Ia, with normal activity of Gsα; however, there appears to be a defect in receptor-cyclase coupling activity or in the catalytic unit of adenylate cyclase.[161, 162]

Type II pseudohypoparathyroidism refers to the presence of PTH resistance in target tissues in the presence of a normal cAMP response to PTH.[163] Thus, the defect in these patients occurs distal to the generation of cAMP. Unlike type I pseudohypoparathyroidism, which is inherited in an autosomal dominant fashion, type II occurs sporadically, without a clear familial inheritance pattern. The term *pseudohypohyperparathyroidism* is used to describe a subset of individuals with features of pseudohypoparathyroidism but lacking PTH resistance at the level of the bone. Affected individuals develop osteitis fibrosa cystica. Successful treatment of the hyperparathyroidism in patients with this disorder results in normalization of bone turnover.[164]

## VITAMIN D–RELATED HYPOCALCEMIA

Vitamin D deficiency due to malnutrition is thought to be a relatively rare problem in the United States because of the addition of this vitamin to dairy products; however, recent studies suggest that hypovitaminosis D may be more prevalent than previously reported.[165] There also appears to be a high incidence of vitamin D deficiency among elderly patients, especially in areas with limited sun exposure, because the presence of sunlight is required for the production of vitamin $D_3$ from 7-dehydrocholesterol in the skin. In addition to dietary deficiency and lack of exposure to the sun, intestinal malabsorption due to a variety of gastrointestinal disorders is a well-recognized cause of vitamin D deficiency. In the United States, gastric surgery is the most common gastrointestinal abnormality leading to vitamin D deficiency. Hypocalcemia and osteomalacia occur in approximately one tenth of patients following subtotal gastrectomy and gastrojejunostomy.[166] A much higher incidence of hypocalcemia is encountered in the subset of patients with bone pain and overt osteomalacia.

Altered vitamin D metabolism can result from a variety of reasons and may be associated with hypocalcemia. Although rare, hypocalcemia may occur in patients with hepatic disease due to impaired 25-hydroxylation of vitamin D. Hypocalcemia is also a feature in patients with renal insufficiency owing to decreased renal 1-α-hydroxylase activity and impaired production of 1,25-dihydroxyvitamin $D_3$. Hyperphosphatemia may induce hypocalcemia by inhibiting 1-α-hydroxylase and by causing the precipitation of calcium from serum. Vitamin D–dependent rickets type I (VDDR I) is a rare genetic disorder inherited as an autosomal recessive trait and characterized by hypocalcemia, skeletal deformities, secondary hyperparathyroidism, and low levels of 1,25-dihydroxyvitamin $D_3$. Patients responded to physiologic doses of 1,25-dihydroxyvitamin $D_3$, which suggested that the defect in this form of rickets was a deficiency in 1-α-hydroxylase, and indeed, the gene for this enzyme has been found to be defective in these patients.[167]

In addition to deficiency and abnormal metabolism of vitamin D, resistance to the hormone may result in hypocalcemia. Vitamin D–dependent rickets type II (VDDR II) is an autosomal recessive disorder with features similar to those found in VDDR I, except that in these patients, levels of 1,25-dihydroxyvitamin $D_3$ are elevated.[168] Thus, in this condition, there is end-organ resistance to the effects of the hormone, and the patients have low calcium levels and high levels of phosphorus and PTH. Mutations in the gene for the vitamin D receptor have been identified in patients with VDDR II.[169–171]

## HYPOCALCEMIA RELATED TO RENAL DISEASE

Patients with renal disease are at high risk for the development of hypocalcemia due to a variety of factors. In the setting of acute renal failure associated with rhabdomyolysis, patients may develop severe hyperphosphatemia from both excessive release of phosphorus from the damaged tissue and impaired excretion of phosphorus by the malfunctioning kidney. The released phosphorus complexes with serum calcium and may cause hypocalcemia.

Advanced chronic renal insufficiency may be associated with hypocalcemia due to the accompanying hyperphosphatemia and low levels of calcitriol. Calcitriol deficiency can be explained by several mechanisms. First, with decreasing renal mass, there is decreased activity of 1-α-hydroxylase. Second, as GFR decreases, there is decreased delivery of 25-hydroxyvitamin $D_3$ to the proximal tubular cell; thus, less substrate is available for conversion to calcitriol.[172] Finally, hyperphosphatemia, a common finding in patients with chronic renal failure, decreases the synthesis of calcitriol by inhibiting 1-α-hydroxylase activity. The resultant low levels of 1,25-dihydroxyvitamin $D_3$ lead to decreased intestinal calcium absorption and hypocalcemia. Decreased GFR leads to retention of phosphorus by the renal tubules, and, in addition to decreasing 1-α-hydroxylase activity, hyperphosphatemia per se may cause hypocalcemia due to the formation of complexes with calcium.

Patients with renal disease associated with the nephrotic syndrome may also have hypocalcemia, even if the GFR is well preserved and thus low levels of calcitriol and hyperphosphatemia are not contributing factors. Hypocalcemia in these patients is thought to be secondary to low levels of 25-hydroxyvitamin $D_3$ as a result of losses of the vitamin and its binding protein in the urine.

### OTHER CAUSES OF HYPOCALCEMIA

Hypocalcemia is particularly prevalent in critically ill patients. There is a high incidence of hypocalcemia in patients with acute pancreatitis; this is thought to be partially due to saponification of the degraded fatty tissue in the pancreatic bed. The mechanisms involved in the development of hypocalcemia in sepsis are not well understood. Transfusions with citrated blood and citrate administration during plasmapheresis are relatively rare causes of hypocalcemia. The "hungry bone syndrome" may be associated with profound hypocalcemia following parathyroidectomy, especially in the setting of severe osteitis fibrosa cystica. Hypocalcemia may also be associated with certain malignancies, including breast and prostate cancer, which may metastasize to the bone and cause increased osteoblastic activity with increased bone formation and hypocalcemia.[173, 174] Drug-related hypocalcemia is not commonly encountered but may result from agents used in the treatment of hypercalcemia, such as bisphosphonates, calcitonin, and plicamycin. A variety of anticonvulsant agents may cause hypocalcemia by interfering with vitamin D metabolism.[175, 176] The use of anti-infectious and chemotherapeutic compounds such as ketoconazole and cisplatin has also been associated with hypocalcemia.

## Approach to the Patient with Hypocalcemia

The diagnosis of hypocalcemia is established by the presence of low ionized serum calcium, which is usually measured to confirm the diagnosis after finding a low total serum calcium concentration. Total serum calcium can be corrected for hypoalbuminemia by increasing the measured calcium by 0.8 mg/dL for each gram per deciliter reduction of albumin. Once the presence of hypocalcemia has been confirmed, the duration of hypocalcemia and the setting in which it occurs may offer clues to the underlying cause. For example, in critically ill patients, hypocalcemia may be related to sepsis, pancreatitis, or transfusions with citrated blood. Long-standing hypocalcemia is often related to PTH or vitamin D abnormalities. Because some of these disorders are hereditary, a family history is important, as is the presence of other associated features, such as those found in Albright hereditary osteodystrophy. An adult with hypocalcemia of recent onset is unlikely to have a hereditary disorder, in which case a careful nutritional, surgical, and medication history may be helpful. In the presence of renal disease, hypocalcemia is usually due to the functional renal abnormality, such as phosphate retention and decreased synthesis of calcitriol.

Determination of serum phosphorus and magnesium may also offer helpful clues. If hypomagnesemia is encountered, a 24-hour urine collection for magnesium helps differentiate between renal magnesium wasting and other causes of hypomagnesemia. The presence of hyperphosphatemia suggests hypoparathyroidism. The diagnosis of the underlying disorder causing hypocalcemia is usually made by measuring the levels of PTH and vitamin D metabolites. Low or inappropriately normal PTH levels are indicative of hypoparathyroidism. Elevated PTH levels suggest resistance to the hormone due to pseudohypoparathyroidism or vitamin D–related disorders, for example. Measurement of 25-hydroxyvitamin $D_3$ and 1,25-dihydroxyvitamin $D_3$ is very helpful. Low 25-hydroxyvitamin $D_3$ suggests nutritional vitamin D deficiency, lack of exposure to sunlight, intestinal malabsorption, or the nephrotic syndrome. In conditions associated with PTH resistance, decreased intake or metabolism of vitamin D, and renal insufficiency, the level of 1,25-dihydroxyvitamin $D_3$ is expected to be decreased. Measuring urinary cAMP and phosphorus in response to PTH confirms the diagnosis in patients with suspected pseudohypoparathyroidism.

## General Principles of Management

As is the case with hypercalcemia, successful treatment of hypocalcemia relies on management of the underlying cause. Acute symptomatic hypocalcemia represents a medical emergency, and immediate therapy with IV calcium preparations is justified. Calcium gluconate is preferred over calcium chloride because of the risk of thrombophlebitis and tissue necrosis associated with the latter. If hypomagnesemia is present, magnesium can be supplemented either orally or intravenously, depending on its severity. The treatment of chronic hypocalcemia, which is usually due to postsurgical hypoparathyroidism or vitamin D deficiency, focuses on the administration of oral calcium and vitamin D compounds, with the goal of increasing intestinal calcium absorption. Patients may require a daily dose of 2 to 4 g of elemental calcium. For the management of hypoparathyroidism, oral calcitriol is usually effective, but close monitoring of calcium is required. It is important to add calcium to vitamin D therapy because of the potential for osteopenia due to excessive bone resorption. In the absence of PTH, the use of vitamin D compounds is often associated with hypercalciuria; thus, frequent monitoring is necessary to assess the effectiveness of therapy as well as urinary calcium excretion. Thiazide diuretics may be useful in this regard because of their hypocalciuric properties.[39]

# MAGNESIUM METABOLISM

Disorders of magnesium homeostasis are commonly encountered in clinical practice. Magnesium is critical to a diverse group of cellular processes, including ATP use, cell membrane function, protein synthesis, mitochondrial function, and hormone secretion; it is second only to potassium in concentration as an intracellular cation. Diverse organ systems are affected by deficient or excess serum magnesium, but the most clinically significant hazards of hypo- or hypermagnesemia are due to alterations in the function of excitable membranes in nerve, muscle, and the cardiac conducting system. Furthermore, abnormal serum magnesium levels can secondarily affect calcium and potassium metabolism, potentially causing further derangements in neuromuscular and cardiovascular physiology.

The magnesium content of the adult human body varies from 11.4 to 17.5 mmol/kg (277 to 425 mg/kg).[177] Only 1% to 2% of this magnesium is extracellular, and approximately one third of the extracellular magnesium is bound to plasma proteins.[178] The normal total serum magnesium level ranges from 1.4 to 2 mEq/L (0.7 to 1 mmol/L). The majority of the body's magnesium is contained within bone, muscle, and erythrocytes, and it exchanges very slowly with extracellular magnesium.[179] Therefore, skeletal and intracellular magnesium is an ineffective buffer in the setting of acute extracellular magnesium losses. The average dietary intake of magnesium is about 20 to 40 mEq/day, of which approximately one third is absorbed by the gastrointestinal tract, primarily in the small bowel.[180] Magnesium present in fluids secreted into the gastrointestinal tract (~3.4 mEq/day) is also reabsorbed. Approximately 80% of total serum magnesium is filtered by the glomerulus, and subsequently all but 3% of filtered magnesium is reabsorbed by the renal tubules, most avidly by the cortical thick ascending limb of the loop of Henle and the distal tubule. The nephron is the primary site of magnesium regulation, responding to changes in serum ionized magnesium ($Mg^{2+}$) levels and various other influences, such as hormones, serum pH, and calcium levels. Magnesium has been labeled an "orphan" ion, because there are no hormones specifically dedicated to its regulation. However, the nephron appears to be capable of responding directly to changes in $Mg^{2+}$ concentration. In general, changes in magnesium intake are matched by changes in renal tubular reabsorption, so that overall balance is achieved. Recently, molecular biology techniques have been applied to genetic disorders of magnesium metabolism, leading to the discovery of novel magnesium transport molecules and regulatory pathways. It is reasonable to expect that past and future studies of disorders of magnesium homeostasis will provide new opportunities for therapeutic interventions for diverse diseases of fluid and electrolyte metabolism.

# HYPOMAGNESEMIA

## Epidemiology

Hypomagnesemia is a common electrolyte abnormality in hospitalized patients. Wong and colleagues found hypomagnesemia in 11% of hospital inpatients.[181] The frequency of hypomagnesemia appears to be even higher in critically ill patients and may reach 60% in patients admitted to medical or surgical intensive care units.[182, 183] Hospitalized patients with low serum magnesium have a higher mortality rate inside or outside the intensive care unit.[184] The chronically ill population is also at increased risk for hypomagnesemia. Hypomagnesemia was present in 9.7% of mostly elderly residents of long-term medical care facilities.[185] As described in detail later, many conditions that are present in acute or chronic illness are associated with hypomagnesemia (Table 26–5), explaining its high prevalence in these populations.

**TABLE 26–5.** Causes of Hypomagnesemia

| Nutritional Deficiency | Miscellaneous |
|---|---|
| Magnesium-deficient diet | Acute pancreatitis |
| Protein-caloric malnutrition | Diabetes mellitus |
| **Gastrointestinal Magnesium Loss** | Hyperthyroidism |
| Crohn disease | Hyperaldosteronism |
| Whipple disease | Hyperparathyroidism |
| Ulcerative colitis | Postparathyroidectomy |
| Celiac disease | Cardiopulmonary bypass |
| Short bowel syndrome | Transfusions |
| Intestinal fistulas, drains, or bypass surgery | Extensive burns |
| Familial magnesium malabsorption | Pregnancy |
| **Renal Magnesium Loss** | Lactation |
| Hereditary magnesium wasting | |
| Autosomal recessive hypomagnesemia with hypercalciuria and nephrocalcinosis | |
| Activating mutation of calcium-sensing receptor | |
| Autosomal dominant hypomagnesemia without hypercalciuria | |
| Gitelman syndrome | |
| Magnesium wasting secondary to exposure to exogenous agents | |
| Ethanol | |
| Loop and thiazide diuretics | |
| Aminoglycosides | |
| Amphotericin B | |
| Cisplatin | |
| Cyclosporine | |
| Foscarnet | |

## Defense against Hypomagnesemia

As noted earlier, skeletal and intracellular stores of magnesium exchange very slowly with serum magnesium and are therefore an inefficient defense against hypomagnesemia. The kidney is the primary regulator of serum magnesium, capable of decreasing urinary magnesium concentrations to very low levels in the presence of decreased serum magnesium. Shils fed normal adults magnesium-deficient diets and found that urinary magnesium content fell dramatically within 1 day.[186] By day 7, urinary magnesium had fallen from a baseline of 8 to 16 mEq/day to less than 1 mEq/day. Studies in humans fail to show increased magnesium uptake by the gut after 5 days of magnesium depletion. Although numerous hormones can alter renal magnesium handling, none has been found to serve as a physiologic defense against hypomagnesemia (see references 187 and 188 for a review). The remainder of this section focuses primarily on the mechanism for increased renal reabsorption of magnesium induced through the *direct* actions of decreased serum magnesium on the kidney.

The majority of filtered $Mg^{2+}$ is reabsorbed in the cortical thick ascending limb of the loop of Henle (cTAL) by a paracellular mode of transport driven by lumen-positive transepithelial voltage.[189–191] This lumen-positive voltage is established by the $Na^+$-$2Cl^-$-$K^+$ cotransporter coupled to potassium reentry into the lumen. Evidence supports regulation of $Mg^{2+}$ reabsorption in the cTAL through changes in transepithelial voltage, as well as alterations in paracellular permeability to $Mg^{2+}$.[192–194] Serum $Mg^{2+}$ levels may directly influence cTAL $Mg^{2+}$ reabsorption through interaction with the extracellular $Ca^{2+}$-sensing receptor. This protein has been localized to the cTAL[31] and has been shown to bind $Mg^{2+}$, though with much less affinity than $Ca^{2+}$.[7] Naturally occurring inactivating mutations of this receptor are found in FHH and neonatal severe hyperparathyroidism,[8] and these patients frequently manifest hypermagnesemia.[195, 196] Furthermore, activating mutations of the $Ca^{2+}$-sensing receptor have been found in patients with autosomal dominant hypercalciuric hypocalcemia, and a subset of these patients demonstrates hypomagnesemia.[9]

Binding of $Mg^{2+}$ to the $Ca^{2+}$-sensing receptor has been proposed to reduce the backleak of potassium into the tubular lumen of the cTAL, resulting in decreased lumen-positive potential and therefore decreasing the driving force for $Ca^{2+}$ and $Mg^{2+}$ reabsorption.[44, 197] However, Attie and coworkers demonstrated that patients with FHH had normal magnesium handling following parathyroidectomy, suggesting that the hypermagnesemia and decreased urinary magnesium clearance seen in FHH patients may be mediated by high levels of circulating PTH, rather than by direct actions of $Mg^{2+}$ on the nephron.[198] Evidence supports the existence of a separate regulatory pathway in the cTAL, directly responsive to serum magnesium levels and distinct from the $Ca^{2+}$-sensing receptor–mediated system. In contrast to $Ca^{2+}$-sensing receptor–mediated changes in $Mg^{2+}$ transport, this pathway allows changes in $Mg^{2+}$ reabsorption independent of $Ca^{2+}$ or $Na^+$ transport or circulating PTH levels,[190, 199] and it is likely to be the primary mechanism by which the kidney responds to decreasing serum $Mg^{2+}$.

The distal tubule reabsorbs about 10% of filtered $Mg^{2+}$.[188] Although the absolute quantity of magnesium reabsorption is low, this nephron segment is responsible for adjusting the final concentration of magnesium in the urine. Regulation of magnesium handling in the distal tubule is not as well characterized as that in the cTAL. Evidence from experiments on isolated distal tubule cells supports the existence of transcellular reabsorption of $Mg^{2+}$ in the distal tubule regulated by the extracellular $Mg^{2+}$ concentration.[200, 201] As in the cTAL, the $Ca^{2+}$-sensing receptor has been postulated to play a role in magnesium regulation in the distal tubule.

## Causes of Hypomagnesemia

### NUTRITIONAL DEFICIENCY

Magnesium is an essential mineral with an obligate loss from the body in stool, perspiration, and urine. As a result, diets with a magnesium content less than the amount lost will eventually result in clinically significant magnesium depletion. Humans develop a negative magnesium balance with diets containing less than 0.5 mEq (6 mg) of magnesium per kilogram of body weight.[202] Growing children require proportionally more magnesium in their diets. As outlined earlier, decreased dietary magnesium intake is initially countered by decreased urinary excretion and increased fractional absorption of intestinal magnesium. Data from animal studies indicate that in conditions of magnesium depletion, slow mobilization of $Mg^{2+}$ from the skeleton does occur, buffering against hypomagnesemia.[203]

Magnesium is nearly ubiquitous in food, being present in grains, vegetables, and meats, as well as in "hard" water. However, there is concern that refinement of sugar and cereal grains reduces the $Mg^{2+}$ content of these foods. Similarly, softening of hard water reduces the $Mg^{2+}$ content and may be a factor predisposing individuals to hypomagnesemia.[204] Alcoholics often eat diets deficient in magnesium, and ethanol has been shown to increase magnesium loss in the urine,[205–209] contributing to hypomagnesemia. Protein-calorie malnutrition can lead to hypomagnesemia,[210, 211] especially when associated with metabolic acidosis. Parenteral nutrition with solutions deficient in magnesium can also precipitate hypomagnesemia. At particular risk are patients with excessive magnesium losses, such as those on diuretics, having extensive burns, or undergoing prolonged suctioning of gastrointestinal fluids.

### GASTROINTESTINAL LOSSES

The gastrointestinal tract is the only physiologic route for magnesium entry into the body. Therefore, diseases of the bowel or alterations of the normal course of transit through the intestine can produce hypomagnesemia. Hypomagnesemia can complicate illnesses characterized by severe malabsorption, diarrhea, or steatorrhea, such as Crohn disease, Whipple disease, ulcerative colitis, short bowel syndrome, and celiac disease.[212–218] The magnesium content of stool correlates with fecal fat content, suggesting that insoluble soaps form from $Mg^{2+}$ and fatty acids, thereby preventing magnesium absorption. Lower gastrointestinal tract fluids contain up to 15 mEq/L of magnesium, so chronic diarrhea can produce substantial magnesium losses. Intestinal fistulas, drains, or bypass surgery can also result in magnesium losses.[215, 219] Because a portion of magnesium from the diet and gastrointestinal secretions is absorbed in the colon, ileostomies may result in hypomagnesemia.[215] Acute pancreatitis has also been associated with hypomagnesemia. The mechanism is thought to be similar to that of pancreatitis-induced hypocalcemia: saponification of necrotic fat from the inflamed pancreas.[220, 221] The frequency of pancreatitis-induced hypomagnesemia is difficult to determine precisely, because many cases of acute pancreatitis are induced by alcohol ingestion, which is itself associated with hypomagnesemia.[207–209]

## FAMILIAL MAGNESIUM MALABSORPTION

Familial hypomagnesemia due to specific intestinal malabsorption of magnesium was originally described in 1965 in an infant who presented with seizures and hypocalcemia and depressed serum magnesium.[222] Since then, there have been at least 30 cases reported, frequently in consanguineous families.[223] These patients typically present in infancy, though cases have been diagnosed in older children[224] and adults.[225] Balance studies universally reveal appropriate renal magnesium conservation in the setting of hypomagnesemia, but increased fecal magnesium.[222–229] Hypocalcemia is a frequent finding at initial presentation, but this resolves after serum magnesium levels are restored to normal. Hypomagnesemia of diverse causes is frequently associated with secondary hypocalcemia.

The molecular basis for isolated magnesium malabsorption remains unknown. Oral or enteral supplementation of magnesium is effective for raising serum magnesium concentrations to the normal range, but quantities of magnesium several times higher than that contained in the typical diet must be used to maintain adequate levels.[222–229] It has been suggested, therefore, that carrier-mediated magnesium transport is defective, but passive, concentration-dependent magnesium transport remains intact.[230] The initial preponderance of boys in the case reports of isolated magnesium malabsorption, and the report of a girl with hypomagnesemia and a balanced 9/X translocation,[231] led to speculation about an X-linked mode of inheritance. However, many reports since that time support an autosomal dominant pattern.[223, 227, 232]

As noted earlier, treatment is oral or enteral supplementation of magnesium, often requiring 30 to 35 mg/kg/day of elemental magnesium. Parenteral magnesium may be given in the setting of severe hypocalcemia accompanied by seizures. With chronic magnesium supplementation, the prognosis is generally quite favorable, with normal development described over several years of observation.[233]

## RENAL MAGNESIUM LOSS

Because the kidney is the primary site for magnesium regulation and filters approximately 300 to 350 mEq/day, disruption in renal magnesium reabsorption may result in clinically significant hypomagnesemia. Excessive renal magnesium loss may occur through the actions of various therapeutic agents, metabolic perturbations, renal injuries, or toxic exposures. Genetic abnormalities in magnesium transport are rarer causes of renal magnesium wasting.

### *Primary Renal Magnesium Wasting*

Defects in renal magnesium transport resulting in hypomagnesemia are rarely encountered disorders, often familial, and frequently associated with defects in tubular transport of calcium and potassium as well as disorders of acid-base regulation. These disorders may be divided into three categories: magnesium wasting accompanied by hypercalciuria and a propensity to develop nephrocalcinosis and ocular defects; magnesium wasting with metabolic alkalosis, hypokalemia, and hypocalciuria (Gitelman syndrome); and isolated renal magnesium wasting.

Primary renal magnesium wasting accompanied by hypercalciuria has been described in several kindreds.[234–238] Frequently, relatives of affected individuals demonstrate hypercalciuria,[235, 239] and sporadic cases have been reported.[240, 241] Presentation is typically in childhood or adolescence with tetany or seizure, attributed to hypocalcemia. Nephrocalcinosis and nephrolithiasis are practically universal in this disorder, and renal failure is common. Acidification defects are also frequently encountered, usually distal-type renal tubular acidosis. Distal renal tubular acidosis has been attributed to impaired tubular function as a result of nephrocalcinosis and medullary interstitial nephropathy. Elevated serum PTH levels have also been observed in these patients, presumably secondary to the constant leak of calcium from the kidney. Some patients present with hypokalemia, possibly due to direct effects of hypomagnesemia on potassium transport or secondary hyperaldosteronism.[242] Transmission appears to be autosomal recessive, and consanguineous unions are frequently found in kindreds with this disorder. Recently, a human gene, *PCLN-1,* was identified that codes for paracellin-1, a component of tight junctions in the thick ascending limb of the loop of Henle. Mutations in *PCLN-1* were found in patients with familial hypercalciuric hypomagnesemia from multiple families.[243] It has been suggested that paracellin-1 is, or is part of, a pore conducting the paracellular flow of $Mg^{2+}$ and $Ca^{2+}$ in the thick ascending limb of the loop of Henle. Hypomagnesemia with hypercalciuria and nephrocalcinosis can occur in patients with activating mutations of the $Ca^{2+}$-sensing receptor.[9] In these cases, PTH is suppressed, and hypomagnesemia is mild and not a universal finding.

Gitelman syndrome was first described in 1966 in three individuals (two were sisters) with hypokalemia and metabolic alkalosis associated with renal magnesium wasting and hypocalciuria.[244] These patients can be distinguished from patients with Bartter syndrome, because the latter typically have normal serum magnesium and do not have hypocalciuria.[245, 246] Like Bartter syndrome, Gitelman syndrome demonstrates an autosomal recessive transmission and is characterized by hypokalemic metabolic alkalosis. Gitelman syndrome typically has a milder course than Bartter syndrome and is less likely to present with symptoms in the neonatal period.[246] Patients with Gitelman syndrome may have muscle weakness or carpopedal spasm.[244, 247, 248] As noted earlier, Gitelman syndrome is characterized by hypocalciuria and hypomagnesemia with a high fractional excretion of magnesium, features not observed in Bartter syndrome.

The molecular basis for Gitelman syndrome has been shown to be localized to the thiazide-sensitive NaCl cotransporter (NCCT) in the distal convoluted tubule.[249] Linkage analysis confirms that the disorder maps to the NCCT gene locus on chromosome 16q13.[248] Subsequent researchers have confirmed that numerous different mutations in the gene coding for this transporter result in Gitelman syndrome.[250–254] It has been suggested that impaired sodium reabsorption in the distal tubule results in volume contraction and subsequent hyperaldosteronism, promoting hypokalemia and metabolic alkalosis.[249] The mechanism for magnesium wasting and hypocalciuria in Gitelman syndrome is unknown. Thiazide diuretics impair function of the NCCT and can cause hypocalciuria, but not hypomagnesemia. It has been speculated that decreased sodium transport in the early distal convoluted tubule in Gitelman syndrome results in increased uptake in more distal segments, resulting in decreased function of a putative basolateral $Na^+$-$Mg^{2+}$ exchanger.

Treatment of Gitelman syndrome with magnesium supplements results in improvement in intra- and extracellular magnesium but fails to raise serum magnesium to normal levels. Of note, magnesium supplementation has no effect on hypokalemia, confirming that hypokalemia in Gitelman syndrome is not secondary to hypomagnesemia.

Finally, primary renal magnesium wasting is seen rarely in patients without Gitelman syndrome or nephrocalcinosis.[255–257] An autosomal dominant form has been mapped to chromosome 11q23.[258] Urinary calcium is typically normal in these patients, but it may be elevated in the autosomal dominant form.[256]

## ALCOHOL

Hypomagnesemia is relatively common in alcoholics and is the most common electrolyte disturbance among alcoholics admitted to the hospital.[259] Numerous studies have confirmed the link between hypomagnesemia and ethanol.[205–209] Increased urinary excretion of $Mg^{2+}$ has been demonstrated following acute alcohol ingestion in alcoholic as well as nonalcoholic subjects.[205, 209] Renal magnesium handling was studied in 61 alcoholics after significant hepatic disease had been excluded by biopsy and pancreatitis had been excluded by serum chemistry.[208] Hypomagnesemia was present in 30% of these subjects, and many had hypocalcemia, hypophosphatemia, or acid-base abnormalities. Increased tubular excretion of magnesium was found in 50% of the hypomagnesemic subjects, and abnormalities in the renal handling of calcium, phosphorus, uric acid, and $\beta_2$-microglobulin, as well as acidification of the urine, were observed in many alcoholic subjects. These findings led the authors to speculate that the toxic effects of ethanol may produce generalized tubular dysfunction, rather than specific impairment of $Mg^{2+}$ transport. Of particular note, the abnormal serum and urinary chemistries normalized after 4 weeks of abstinence from ethanol.

## DRUGS

### *Diuretics*

Both loop diuretics and thiazide diuretics have been shown to increase magnesium excretion.[260, 261] By blocking the function of the $Na^+$-$2Cl^-$-$K^+$ cotransporter, loop diuretics diminish the lumen-positive potential that drives paracellular $Mg^{2+}$ transport in the thick ascending limb of the loop of Henle.[194] The mechanism of thiazide diuretic–induced magnesium wasting is not clear. Chlorothiazide actually *increases* $Mg^{2+}$ transport in cultured distal tubule cells.[262] Hypomagnesemia has been reported after loop or thiazide diuretic treatment of hypertension, congestive heart failure, and nephrolithiasis.[263] The degree of decreased serum magnesium is typically very mild, rarely falling below the lower limit of normal, and studies have been hampered by the lack of adequate and comparable controls.[263, 264] There is some evidence that the elderly are especially vulnerable to thiazide-induced hypomagnesemia.[265] Data suggesting that loop or thiazide diuretics cause tissue magnesium depletion have been criticized for faulty methodology and inadequate controls.[264] Of note, potassium-sparing diuretics have been shown to decrease magnesium excretion and are not associated with hypomagnesemia.[255]

### *Antibiotics*

Several commonly used aminoglycosides have been associated with magnesium deficiency, including tobramycin, gentamicin, amikacin, and sisomicin.[266–268] The onset of hypomagnesemia with respect to aminoglycoside dose is highly variable, occurring during the course of drug therapy or several weeks after therapy has been completed, and hypomagnesemia may persist for months after the aminoglycoside has been withdrawn.[269] Hypomagnesemia has been noted in 4.5% of cancer patients receiving aminoglycoside therapy.[267] However, that figure includes only patients with both hypocalcemia and hypomagnesemia and therefore likely underestimates the true incidence of hypomagnesemia. Aminoglycosides have long been known to be nephrotoxic, typically causing injury to the proximal tubule and acute renal failure. However, hypomagnesemia secondary to aminoglycosides appears to be independent of tubular necrosis and renal failure. For example, administration of gentamicin to rats results in vigorous and sustained magnesiuresis and calciuresis within 60 minutes, before any tubular injury occurs.[270] It has been postulated that aminoglycosides exert their magnesium-wasting effect at the level of the thick ascending limb of the loop of Henle.[269]

Although the association of hypomagnesemia with

amphotericin B has been well demonstrated,[271–273] the effect of this agent on urinary excretion of magnesium has not been clearly established. Amphotericin B has been shown to both increase[271] and decrease[274] renal magnesium excretion. In recent years, lipid-associated amphotericin B formulations have been introduced in an effort to limit the nephrotoxic effects of this agent, but they appear to have had little effect in altering the incidence of hypomagnesemia.[273]

Several cases of severe and symptomatic hypomagnesemia have been reported after IV pentamidine therapy.[275–278] Foscarnet used to treat cytomegalovirus retinitis has been associated with hypomagnesemia: 9 of 13 patients treated with foscarnet had decrements in serum $Mg^{2+}$ to levels below 0.49 mmol/L.[279]

***Antineoplastics***

Cisplatin therapy for malignancies is a well-known cause of hypomagnesemia, occurring as early as 2 days after administration of this agent.[280–282] The hypomagnesemia induced by cisplatin is often severe and persistent. Lam and Adelstein found hypomagnesemia in all 28 subjects evaluated, with serum magnesium nadirs as low as 0.12 mmol/L and serum $Mg^{2+}$ levels less than 0.41 mmol/L in almost half the patients.[282] Hypomagnesemia persisted up to 5 months after the end of cisplatin therapy. Chronic hypomagnesemia (mean follow-up of 2.3 years) has been reported in more than 25% of children receiving cisplatin.[283] Administration of cisplatin to rats induces prompt magnesiuresis, an effect that can be prevented by systemic treatment with the flavonoid silibinin.[284, 285] Silibinin treatment in human subjects receiving cisplatin therapy has not been reported. Carboplatin has been used to treat malignancies in place of the more nephrotoxic cisplatin and is less likely to induce severe hypomagnesemia than is cisplatin.[286, 287]

***Cyclosporine***

The immunosuppressant agent cyclosporine has been associated with hypomagnesemia.[288–291] Although magnesium depletion is very common, the effect is usually relatively mild, only lowering serum magnesium to an average of 0.70 mmol/L in one study.[291] Both urinary magnesium wasting and a shift of $Mg^{2+}$ into cells have been shown to cause cyclosporine-associated hypomagnesemia.[291, 292]

### OTHER CAUSES OF HYPOMAGNESEMIA

Diabetes mellitus is associated with hypomagnesemia.[293] Serum magnesium has been correlated to level of glycemic control in type I diabetics.[294, 295] However, Ponder and colleagues[296] found that although diabetic children had increased urinary excretion of magnesium, urinary magnesium did not correlate with serum glucose levels. Hypomagnesemia has not been consistently observed in patients with type II diabetes. In an evaluation of 32 patients with type II diabetes, Mikhail and Ehsanipoor[297] found no difference in total serum magnesium compared with nondiabetics, while Resnick and coworkers[298] found a reduction in serum ionized $Mg^{2+}$ but not total serum magnesium. The physiologic basis for hypomagnesemia in diabetes is far from clear, but insulin has been shown to stimulate absorption of $Mg^{2+}$ by the mouse cortical thick ascending limb[192] and cultured mouse distal convoluted tubule cells.[299] It seems reasonable to speculate that insulin deficiency can result in magnesium wasting in those segments in type I diabetics. Glycosuria, ketoaciduria, hypophosphatemia, and insulin-mediated intracellular $Mg^{2+}$ shifts have also been postulated as mechanisms for diabetes-associated hypomagnesemia.[295, 300]

Other endocrine disorders have been linked to hypomagnesemia, including hyperthyroidism,[301] hyperaldosteronism,[302] and hyperparathyroidism.[303] Hypomagnesemia has been observed following rapid correction of metabolic acidosis[304] or hyperparathyroidism,[305] possibly due to the "hungry bone syndrome" of rapid skeletal mineralization. Hypophosphatemia[306, 307] and hypercalcemia[308] have each been linked to hypomagnesemia. Cardiac surgery requiring cardiopulmonary bypass can result in hypomagnesemia,[309–311] as can massive transfusions of citrate-containing blood products.[312] Severe burns,[313] excessive lactation,[314] and the last trimester of pregnancy[315] have all been associated with magnesium deficiency.

## Evaluation of Magnesium Status

In clinical practice, magnesium status is assessed most commonly by measurement of total serum magnesium. Total serum magnesium has been shown to correlate with skeletal magnesium content,[316] and in most cases, hypomagnesemia indicates significant magnesium depletion. Though convenient, total serum magnesium is not an ideal index of overall magnesium status in any given patient, because less than 1% of total body magnesium is in the serum. Furthermore, approximately one third of serum magnesium is bound to albumin[178] and is therefore unavailable to participate in biochemical processes. It has been suggested that measurement of ionized serum magnesium or intracellular magnesium may provide more clinically relevant information.

The total magnesium content of erythrocytes, skeletal muscle, bone, and mononuclear blood cells has been measured as an indicator of magnesium status. In general, correlation between intracellular magnesium and total serum magnesium concentration is poor.[316–320] The clinical utility of total erythrocyte magnesium concentration is uncertain.[321, 322] Mononuclear blood cell magnesium content correlates poorly with skeletal and cardiac muscle magnesium content.[323] Nevertheless, in some settings, intracellular magnesium concentration may be a more useful index of magnesium status than total serum magnesium. For example, Cohen and Kitzes[318] demonstrated reduced lymphocyte magnesium in patients with magnesium-responsive, digoxin-related tachyarrhythmias, although total serum magnesium was normal. Ryan and colleagues[324] found that diuretic administration in rats resulted in a reduction in lymphocyte magnesium of a similar magnitude to the reduction in magnesium from skeletal and cardiac muscle. At present, the measurement of intracellular magnesium is an investigational technique and is seldom used in clinical practice.

Total serum magnesium consists of three fractions: ionized (free), anion complexed, and protein bound. Because only the ionized form is physiologically active, measurement of this fraction may be a more clinically useful index of magnesium status than total serum magnesium. The range of ionized $Mg^{2+}$ in healthy volunteers is 0.44 to 0.59 mmol/L and correlates loosely with total serum magnesium, although this correlation is stronger in critically ill patients than in normal volunteers.[325] Alterations in protein binding of magnesium may lead to alterations in ionized $Mg^{2+}$ concentrations without changing total serum magnesium levels. Furthermore, in an analogous manner to serum calcium, changes in the concentration of serum albumin may affect total magnesium concentration without disrupting the ionized $Mg^{2+}$ concentration. In fact, ionized $Mg^{2+}$ does decrease as pH rises,[326, 327] and hypoproteinemia is associated with decreased total serum magnesium with normal or elevated ionized $Mg^{2+}$.[327–330] An equation to correct the total magnesium concentration for hypoalbuminemia has been proposed: $Mg_c = Mg_T + 0.05\ (4 - Alb)$, where $Mg_c$ is the corrected magnesium concentration (mmol/L), $Mg_T$ is the measured total magnesium, and Alb is the albumin concentration (g/dL).[328] The increasing availability of magnesium ion–specific electrodes will enable the routine measurement of ionized magnesium, but the role of this test in the clinical arena is uncertain.[331]

The magnesium loading test has been proposed as a means of measuring the magnesium status of patients (Fig. 26–5). This test is based on the ability of the normally functioning kidney to retain magnesium in the setting of magnesium depletion. Retention of an infused magnesium load would imply physiologically relevant magnesium depletion, regardless of the serum magnesium level. This test is particularly useful when magnesium depletion is suspected despite normal serum magnesium levels. In one protocol,[332] 2.4 mg/kg of elemental magnesium is infused over 4 hours. A 24-hour urine collection is initiated simultaneously with the infusion. Excretion of less than 70% of the infused magnesium is considered indicative of functional magnesium deficiency,[332–334] even though total or ionized serum magnesium concentrations may be normal (normomagnesemic magnesium depletion). The magnesium loading test is unreliable in patients with abnormal renal function or those who are receiving medications that alter the renal excretion of magnesium.

In patients with hypomagnesemia, a thorough history and physical examination usually reveal the cause, but in some cases, the origin of the $Mg^{2+}$ deficit remains elusive. In such patients, differentiation between renal losses and gastrointestinal losses can be made by measuring the fractional excretion of $Mg^{2+}$ (FEMg) from a random urine sample. This value can be calculated as follows: $FEMg = (U_{Mg} \times P_{Cr} \times 100)/(0.7 \times P_{Mg} \times U_{cr})$, where U and P refer to the urine and plasma concentrations of magnesium (Mg) and creatinine (Cr). In a study of 74 hypomagnesemic patients,[335] the mean FEMg in subjects with renal magnesium losses was 15% (range, 4% to 48%), whereas the mean FEMg in patients with extrarenal magnesium losses was 1.4% (range, 0.5% to 2.7%). Therefore, in hypomagnesemic patients with normal renal function, FEMg of 4% or greater suggests renal magnesium wasting rather than extrarenal magnesium loss.

## Clinical Features of Hypomagnesemia

### HYPOKALEMIA

Potassium depletion and magnesium depletion often occur together as the result of processes that simultaneously induce negative balances in these two cations. For example, diuretic use is a well-described cause of hypokalemia and hypomagnesemia.[336, 337]

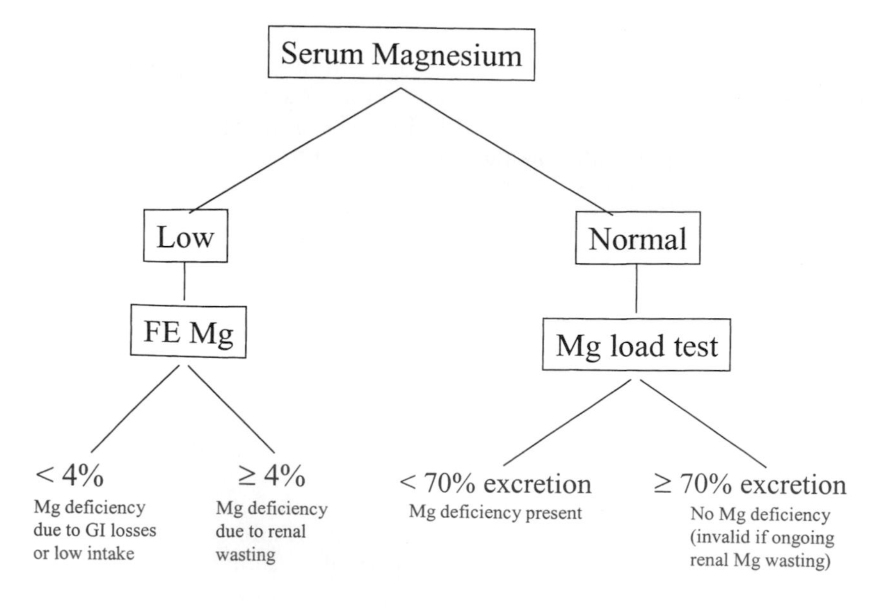


**FIGURE 26–5** ■ Scheme for the evaluation of a suspected magnesium deficiency. (For a full description, see the text.)

Gitelman syndrome promotes renal wasting of both magnesium and potassium.[338] Primary hyperaldosteronism and severe diarrhea can also cause parallel magnesium and potassium deficits. It is clear that magnesium depletion itself can induce hypokalemia. Shils[339] reported increased kaliuresis and hypokalemia after human subjects were maintained on a magnesium-deficient diet. Positive potassium balance was achieved only after the subjects were treated with magnesium. Correlation between serum potassium and magnesium levels has been found in surgical patients[321] and cardiac intensive care unit patients, regardless of whether they were undergoing diuretic therapy.[340] Hypomagnesemia is present in 42% to 61% of hypokalemic hospitalized patients.[306, 341]

The cause of hypomagnesemia-related hypokalemia is not clear. Hypomagnesemia is associated with intracellular potassium depletion.[342, 343] It has been hypothesized that hypomagnesemia might result in decreased cytosolic $Mg^{2+}$ in renal tubular cells and subsequent increased loss of potassium through a magnesium-inhibited potassium channel, perhaps via a magnesium-dependent decrease in ATP activity.[344] Channels exhibiting such characteristics have been found in experimental systems.[345, 346] Hypokalemia in the setting of magnesium depletion can be refractory to potassium repletion unless magnesium is also administered.[339, 347] It is therefore prudent to measure serum magnesium levels in hypokalemic patients, especially if the hypokalemia has proved resistant to potassium supplementation.

## HYPOCALCEMIA

Hypocalcemia is frequently encountered in patients with hypomagnesemia.[222–224, 226–230, 234] Hypomagnesemia is found in about 23% of hypocalcemic patients.[181, 306] In a medical intensive care unit setting, 27% of hypomagnesemic patients with normal renal function had hypocalcemia.[183] In normal human subjects, moderate hypomagnesemia (0.61 mmol/L) results in a decline in serum ionized $Ca^{2+}$ of about 0.05 to 0.07 mmol/L,[348] whereas severe, symptomatic hypocalcemia generally occurs when serum magnesium levels fall below 0.5 mmol/L.[186, 234]

The origin of the hypocalcemia observed in hypomagnesemia is multifactorial. Plasma PTH is often normal or decreased in patients with hypomagnesemia and hypocalcemia,[349, 350] indicating an inappropriate response of the parathyroid glands to low serum calcium. The secretion of PTH is decreased in the presence of hypomagnesemia, whereas synthesis of PTH is unimpaired in this setting.[351] Another factor leading to low serum calcium in hypomagnesemic individuals is skeletal resistance to the actions of PTH,[352, 353] providing an explanation for the observations of Fatemi and coworkers,[348] who found that PTH was *increased* in about one fourth of human subjects fed a low-magnesium diet. Interestingly, these subjects had no change in serum calcium levels, despite an average 68% increase in PTH. Finally, levels of 1,25-dihydroxyvitamin $D_3$ have been shown to be reduced in patients with hypocalcemia and hypomagnesemia.[354] Resistance to the positive effects of PTH on calcitriol synthesis by the kidney has been demonstrated in hypomagnesemic subjects.[348] The importance of low serum calcitriol levels as a cause of hypocalcemia in hypomagnesemic individuals is questionable, because serum calcium is normalized by magnesium therapy before any significant rise in serum calcitriol concentration.[354]

Therapy with IV or oral calcium is generally not effective in raising serum calcium levels unless magnesium is also replaced.[222, 225–227, 229] Magnesium alone has been shown to be beneficial in raising serum calcium levels in conditions of magnesium deficiency.[183, 226, 228] However, gentamicin-induced hypomagnesemia is associated with a hypocalcemia that may not improve with magnesium therapy alone.[267]

## NEUROMUSCULAR MANIFESTATIONS

Hypomagnesemia is most often asymptomatic.[182, 355] Symptoms of neuromuscular irritability such as tetany, seizures, and positive Chvostek and Trousseau signs have been attributed to magnesium depletion. However, hypomagnesemia is often observed in the setting of simultaneous hypocalcemia, hypokalemia, and disorders of acid-base balance. These concomitant metabolic derangements make it difficult to assign specific symptoms to hypomagnesemia alone. For example, in experimental magnesium depletion, a positive Chvostek sign and tetany were commonly observed, but these subjects were universally hypocalcemic.[339] Nevertheless, these neuromuscular manifestations resolved with magnesium supplementation. Patients with familial magnesium malabsorption typically present with seizures in the setting of hypocalcemia and hypomagnesemia.[223, 226]

Neuromuscular symptoms have been reported in individuals with normal serum calcium, including tetany, carpopedal spasm, positive Chvostek and Trousseau signs, hyperreflexia, and seizures,[247, 356–358] as well as athetoid movements,[357] psychiatric changes,[358, 359] vertigo, ataxia, and tremor.[358] A case of focal neurologic deficits (aphasia and hemiparesis) due to severe hypomagnesemia has been reported.[360] Muscle weakness, manifested by decreased isometric muscle strength[361] and diminished respiratory power,[362] has been observed in hypomagnesemia.

The origin of neuromuscular manifestations of magnesium depletion is likely multifactorial, as magnesium plays such a ubiquitous role in intracellular metabolism and membrane physiology. Changes in extracellular magnesium levels alter the excitability of neurons.[363] Depletion of magnesium favors calcium release from the sarcoplasmic reticulum of muscle tissue,[364, 365] favoring contraction. Augmented contraction of vascular smooth muscle via this mechanism may explain the effects of magnesium concentration on blood pressure (see later).

## CARDIOVASCULAR MANIFESTATIONS

### *Electrocardiographic Changes and Arrhythmias*

Several electrocardiographic changes have been attributed to magnesium depletion. Prolongation of the

QRS complex, increased QT interval, and peaked T waves have been reported in hypomagnesemia.[366–368] Flattened or inverted T waves and prominent U waves may accompany more severe magnesium depletion.[366] Because reduced serum potassium and calcium concentrations often accompany hypomagnesemia, it is often difficult to attribute specific electrocardiographic abnormalities to a specific electrolyte abnormality. Arrhythmias in patients without known cardiac disease have been described in those with hypomagnesemia. Data from the Framingham Study indicate an increased risk of complex and frequent (>30/hr) premature ventricular contractions as serum magnesium decreases.[369] Torsades de pointes has been associated with magnesium deficiency and frequently responds to magnesium supplementation.[370–372] It has been speculated that magnesium depletion–induced prolongation of the QT interval confers increased risk of torsades de pointes.

Hypomagnesemia appears to increase the toxic effects of digoxin.[373] Cohen and Kitzes[318] reported an increased frequency of tachyarrhythmias in patients on digoxin who had depressed lymphocyte magnesium. The threshold for cardiac glycoside–induced arrhythmias is reduced in magnesium-deprived monkeys.[374] Not only do patients with magnesium depletion appear to have an increased sensitivity to digoxin, but patients taking digoxin have an increased frequency of hypomagnesemia,[309, 375] perhaps due to frequent diuretic use in this group of patients.

Numerous studies have demonstrated increased arrhythmias in patients with congestive heart failure and magnesium depletion.[376–378] In general, these studies are difficult to interpret, owing to the variable frequency of digoxin use or coexisting hypokalemia due to diuretics. After carefully controlling for serum potassium concentration, Boyd and coworkers[340] found no difference in serum magnesium between cardiac intensive care unit patients who had arrhythmias and those without arrhythmias. However, Gottlieb and colleagues[376] found an increased frequency of premature ventricular contractions and ventricular tachycardia in patients with symptomatic congestive heart failure and magnesium levels below 1.6 mEq/L, with no difference in serum potassium concentrations in patients with or without hypomagnesemia. Furthermore, 1-year survival was 45% in the hypomagnesemic patients, compared with 71% in the normomagnesemic group. Randomized, double-blind, placebo-controlled trials have demonstrated that magnesium supplementation can decrease the frequency of premature ventricular contractions and ventricular tachycardia in patients with symptomatic congestive heart failure, with or without demonstrable hypomagnesemia.[378–380] Magnesium supplementation has also been beneficial in the treatment of multifocal atrial tachycardia due to congestive heart failure or chronic obstructive pulmonary disease.[381]

Patients with acute myocardial infarction (AMI) and magnesium depletion are at increased risk of ventricular arrhythmias, including ventricular fibrillation.[382] Furthermore, AMI itself is associated with reduced serum and tissue magnesium.[382, 383] Administration of magnesium to rats 5 minutes after coronary artery ligation results in a decrease in ventricular tachyarrhythmias.[384] Magnesium therapy was also successful in ameliorating ventricular arrhythmias after reversal of coronary ligation in rats, a model of reperfusion injury.[384] Several randomized, placebo-controlled trials have been published to assess the benefits of IV magnesium supplementation at the time of AMI.[385–390] Several investigators have shown a decrease in ventricular arrhythmias following AMI in patients who received IV magnesium rather than placebo.[386, 387, 390] A meta-analysis of IV magnesium in the setting of AMI reported a 49% reduction in ventricular tachycardia and ventricular fibrillation.[391] Reduction in the incidence of supraventricular tachyarrhythmias has also been demonstrated following magnesium supplementation in the setting of AMI.[389] However, in the 2316-patient LIMIT-2 study,[388] IV magnesium or placebo was initiated upon presentation with AMI. No decrease in tachyarrhythmias was observed with magnesium therapy, although treatment with magnesium was associated with a 24% reduction in mortality at 28 days, compared with placebo. The ongoing Magnesium in Coronaries (MAGIC) trial will attempt to clarify the role of magnesium in the setting of AMI.[392]

Cardiopulmonary bypass during cardiac surgery can significantly reduce serum magnesium (see earlier). In a randomized, placebo-controlled trial, England and colleagues demonstrated that an IV magnesium infusion 30 minutes after finishing cardiopulmonary bypass resulted in significant reduction in postoperative ventricular arrhythmias.[309] In a recent study of children undergoing surgical repair of congenital cardiac defects, IV magnesium reduced the incidence of hemodynamically significant junctional tachycardia, compared with placebo.[393] Magnesium infusion after coronary artery bypass surgery was no better than placebo in reducing the frequency of postoperative atrial fibrillation.[394]

It has been suggested that the salutary effects of magnesium supplementation in preventing arrhythmias may not be entirely related to the replenishment of depleted serum or tissue magnesium stores, but instead may be the result of specific pharmacologic arrhythmia-suppressing properties of magnesium. Kulick and coworkers[395] demonstrated delayed conduction through the atrioventricular node and prolonged PR intervals after magnesium administration to normomagnesemic subjects without known cardiac disease. It is tempting to speculate that magnesium may have antiarrhythmic properties independent of its physiologic role, therefore serving as a drug as well as a nutrient. Because of the apparent increased prevalence of hypomagnesemia in patients with cardiac disease and the associated arrhythmias observed in the setting of magnesium depletion, regular evaluation of magnesium status in these patients, and correction of deficits, is advisable, particularly in patients taking diuretics or digoxin.

***Myocardial Ischemia and Infarction***

There is evidence that magnesium deficiency may result in increased risk for ischemic heart disease. Magnesium retention testing has demonstrated a higher frequency of magnesium depletion in patients with ischemic heart disease compared with controls, whether or not the patients presented with AMI.[383] Increased dietary magnesium has been linked with reductions in atherosclerotic disease and cardiovascular mortality,[396–398] but more recent epidemiologic studies failed to confirm this correlation.[399, 400] A large prospective trial found that the risk of coronary artery disease increased in inverse proportion to serum magnesium.[401] These studies demonstrate an association between magnesium deficiency and coronary artery disease but do not prove that magnesium status plays a role in the pathogenesis of coronary atherosclerosis. Evidence from animal models suggests possible mechanisms for magnesium status to influence the development of coronary atherosclerosis. Magnesium-deficient dogs were found to develop fibrous plaques and calcifications in the media and elastica of the coronary arteries.[402] Rats fed a magnesium-deficient diet developed hypertriglyceridemia and hypercholesterolemia, with reduced high-density lipoprotein and elevated low-density lipoprotein.[403–406] Furthermore, lipoproteins from magnesium-deficient rats were more susceptible to peroxidation and induced more cultured vascular smooth muscle cell proliferation than did those from control rats.[406] Oxidation of apoproteins and proliferation of vascular smooth muscle are thought to be important steps in the development of atherosclerotic plaques.

Magnesium depletion has been associated with vasospasm and platelet aggregation, both of which appear to participate in the pathogenesis of myocardial infarction. Spasm can be induced in isolated dog coronary artery tissue exposed to hypomagnesemic media.[407] Variant (Prinzmetal) angina is the result of coronary vasospasm. Two studies have reported increased magnesium retention in patients with variant angina.[408, 409] Furthermore, magnesium therapy has been demonstrated to terminate attacks of variant angina and prevent induced vasospastic angina.[410–412] Platelets from subjects maintained on a magnesium-deficient diet demonstrated increased reactivity to a thromboxane $A_2$ analogue that corrected after magnesium repletion.[413] Magnesium has been shown to inhibit the synthesis and release of proaggregatory compounds from platelets in vitro.[414]

Magnesium status has important implications for outcome of AMI. Magnesium deficiency has been demonstrated to increase the area of infarction in dogs with ligated coronary arteries.[415] Rats given magnesium supplementation immediately following coronary artery ligation had improved survival compared with rats that received placebo in the setting of AMI.[384] Randomized, controlled trials, including LIMIT-2, have demonstrated a 25% to 80% reduction in mortality when IV magnesium is administered upon presentation with AMI.[386–388, 390] This improved survival was sustained through 2 years of follow-up.[416] However, ISIS-4, a multicenter trial of more than 58,000 subjects, failed to demonstrate a survival benefit in patients receiving magnesium after AMI.[385] This discrepancy has been explained by noting that the magnesium infusion in ISIS-4 may have been given too late to prevent reperfusion injury.[417] Furthermore, 70% of the patients in the ISIS-4 trial received thrombolytic therapy, compared with only 30% of the patients in the LIMIT-2 study. The mortality rate in the control group in the ISIS-4 trial (7.2%) was actually lower than the mortality in the magnesium-treated group in the 2316-patient LIMIT-2 trial (7.8%), which showed a 24% reduction in 30-day mortality.[388] Thus, there may have been a survival benefit to thrombolysis that eclipsed any benefit of magnesium therapy in the ISIS-4 patients. The MAGIC trial in progress now is a multicenter study to evaluate the effect of early magnesium infusion on mortality in suspected AMI.[392] For now, the role of IV magnesium in the setting of AMI is uncertain, but it would certainly be prudent to screen patients with ischemic cardiac disease for hypomagnesemia and replete those with evidence of magnesium deficiency, especially those patients taking digoxin or diuretics.

#### *Hypertension*

Hypomagnesemia may have a role in essential hypertension. Decreased erythrocyte magnesium content has been reported in patients with essential hypertension,[418] although a recent study showed *increased* erythrocyte magnesium in patients with essential hypertension.[419] An inverse relation between blood pressure and serum magnesium was reported in a study of normotensive elderly subjects.[420] An improvement in blood pressure after initiating oral magnesium therapy in hypertensive patients on chronic diuretic therapy has been reported by some[421] but not by others.[422, 423]

## Treatment of Magnesium Deficiency

Administration of magnesium remains the cornerstone of therapy for magnesium deficiency. The dosage and route of administration should be determined by the specific clinical presentation. When renal function is intact, there is a wide margin of safety in administration of magnesium, because any excess will be excreted in the urine, and clinically significant hypermagnesemia in patients with normal renal function is unusual. However, caution must be exercised in administering magnesium to patients with decreased GFR. In magnesium-replete patients who require parenteral nutrition, magnesium balance can be maintained through the addition of 100 to 200 mg of elemental magnesium to the nutrition solution each day, provided that the patient does not have excessive magnesium losses from the kidney or gastrointestinal tract.[424] In patients at risk of magnesium depletion through renal magnesium wasting from diuretic, amphotericin, or aminoglycoside use, addition of amiloride or triamterene can prevent hypomagnesemia.[336, 425, 426]

Patients presenting with symptomatic hypomagnesemia should be treated with parenteral magnesium. It must be appreciated that cellular uptake of magnesium is relatively slow, even in cases of significant magnesium depletion. As a result, parenteral administration of magnesium typically raises the serum magnesium concentration acutely, before total body magnesium repletion has been accomplished. Because serum magnesium concentration is the primary stimulus for magnesium resorption in the thick ascending limb of the loop of Henle, increased magnesium excretion follows an IV or intramuscular (IM) dose. Approximately 50% of administered IV magnesium is lost in the urine.[332–334, 427] Assessment of the total magnesium deficit is difficult, so empirical therapy is usually undertaken, with close attention to the clinical response. It has been suggested that symptomatic magnesium depletion reflects a total magnesium deficit of 1 to 2 mEq/kg of body weight.[427] In symptomatic patients, magnesium sulfate ($MgSO_4$) can be given IV or IM at a dose of 8 to 12 g (0.8 to 1.2 g of elemental magnesium) over the first 24 hours, then 4 to 6 g over 24 hours for each of the next 3 to 5 days.[428] One gram of 50% $MgSO_4$ provides 8.13 mEq or 98 mg of elemental magnesium. Patients presenting with seizures or ventricular arrhythmias can be given 8 to 16 mEq of magnesium over 5 to 10 minutes, followed by a continuous daily infusion of 48 to 64 mEq for 3 to 5 days.[429] In general, if parenteral magnesium is to be given, the IV route is preferable, because IM injections of magnesium are often painful, and absorption may be unpredictable. Intraperitoneal administration has been used in a patient with severe renal magnesium wasting. Infusion of 1 g of $MgSO_4$ in 500 mL of 5% dextrose in water twice a day resulted in increased serum magnesium. Higher doses were associated with severe abdominal pain (B. Bastani, personal communication).

In patients with normal serum magnesium concentrations but demonstrating unexplained hypocalcemia, hypokalemia, tetany, seizures, or arrhythmias, a magnesium tolerance test as described earlier can be diagnostic as well as therapeutic. Patients with greater than 20% retention of the infused dose over 24 hours have probable magnesium deficiency and can be given magnesium replacement therapy, as described earlier. However, results of a magnesium tolerance test may not be available quickly, and the test itself is unreliable in conditions of renal magnesium wasting. Therefore, empirical parenteral magnesium replacement is reasonable in patients with risk factors for magnesium deficiency presenting with typical symptoms or signs, provided that renal function is normal. Three to 5 days of IV magnesium therapy with 32 to 64 mEq/day has been shown to be sufficient to restore normocalcemia in hypocalcemic patients with normal serum magnesium and risk factors for magnesium depletion.[430] Careful observation of serum magnesium level and renal function must accompany parenteral therapy. Development of hypermagnesemia or deterioration of renal function should prompt reduction or cessation of magnesium administration.

Asymptomatic patients with magnesium deficiency and patients who are magnesium replete but have poor dietary intake or ongoing losses can be treated with oral magnesium salts. Numerous oral magnesium preparations are available, and there has been little comparative analysis of individual formulations. In a study of healthy volunteers, administration of 32 mEq/day in one of three oral preparations (magnesium chloride solution, magnesium gluconate tablets, or Slow-Mag magnesium chloride) resulted in increased serum and lymphocyte magnesium, but no difference was observed among the different supplements.[431] Because oral magnesium can cause diarrhea, it is typically given in three to four divided doses. Sustained-release preparations may allow more steady absorption and thus limit urinary loss of administered magnesium.[242] There is some evidence that enteric-coated forms of magnesium may have decreased bioavailability.[432] Patients manifesting only mild symptoms of magnesium depletion can be treated with oral supplementation at an initial total daily dose of 30 to 60 mEq in divided doses. Initial therapy for mild, asymptomatic magnesium deficiency is 10 to 30 mEq/day in divided doses. Therapy can be adjusted based on the patient's symptoms and serum magnesium level or magnesium retention test. Continuous supplementation may be necessary in conditions of persistent magnesium loss.

Conditions associated with renal magnesium wasting are often refractory to supplemental magnesium, because additional magnesium is rapidly excreted in the urine. In patients with renal magnesium wasting from diuretics, aminoglycosides, amphotericin, or cisplatin, addition of amiloride or triamterene may reduce renal tubular loss and restore magnesium balance. These agents may also be useful in treating syndromes of renal magnesium wasting, including Gitelman syndrome.[255, 433]

## HYPERMAGNESEMIA

Under normal conditions, hypermagnesemia is prevented through excretion of excess serum magnesium into the urine. Magnesium loading results in decreased reabsorption from the cTAL, thereby increasing FEMg and maintaining normomagnesemia.[187] Clinically significant magnesium intoxication is therefore encountered primarily in the setting of impaired renal function. Less commonly, very large magnesium loads can overwhelm the renal tubular capacity to maintain magnesium balance, resulting in hypermagnesemia. Hypermagnesemia has been reported to be present in over 9% of hospitalized patients but is relatively underdiagnosed, because magnesium status is not routinely evaluated.[181]

### Causes of Hypermagnesemia

#### RENAL FAILURE

Patients with moderate to severe renal disease have a diminished capacity to excrete magnesium that is roughly proportional to the decline in GFR, making them susceptible to hypermagnesemia. The FEMg rises as renal failure progresses, until renal function declines to a creatinine clearance of approximately 30 mL/min, at which point this adaptive mechanism is overwhelmed, and serum magnesium rises in proportion to the decline in GFR.[434, 435] Patients with end-stage renal disease generally have mild, asymptomatic hypermagnesemia or serum magnesium levels at the upper limit of normal, unless magnesium-containing antacids or laxatives are administered.[434] Use of such agents by patients with decreased creatinine clearance has been associated with severe and symptomatic, or even fatal, hypermagnesemia.[434, 436] It is therefore critical to limit or avoid all magnesium-containing antacids, cathartics, enemas, or infusions in patients with significant renal impairment. If magnesium-based phosphate binders are used in patients on dialysis, dialysate magnesium must be decreased. Excessive dialysate magnesium can precipitate hypermagnesemia, and dialysis-unit water-treatment facilities must be designed and monitored to prevent elevated magnesium concentrations in municipal water sources from contaminating the dialysate.

#### MAGNESIUM INGESTION

Occasionally, ingestion of magnesium as a cathartic or antacid can induce hypermagnesemia in patients with normal renal function. It has been proposed that active gastrointestinal disease predisposes patients to hypermagnesemia from ingestion of magnesium-containing agents,[437] but this assertion is difficult to prove epidemiologically, because these compounds are usually administered specifically for gastrointestinal complaints and bowel preparation preceding endoscopy. Repetitive use of magnesium-containing cathartics to treat suspected drug overdose can result in elevations of serum magnesium in patients with normal renal function.[438] Bowel obstruction or perforated gastric ulcer may be a risk factor for hypermagnesemia from oral magnesium ingestion.[439, 440] Magnesium-containing enemas can substantially elevate the serum magnesium concentration.[441]

#### MAGNESIUM INFUSION

The neuromuscular relaxation produced by hypermagnesemia (see later) has been used for decades to treat preeclampsia and eclampsia, as well as premature labor. Infusions of $MgSO_4$ are administered with the goal of achieving serum magnesium concentrations two to three times the normal level. Few complications have been reported other than hyporeflexia and transient hypocalcemia that may be symptomatic.[442–444]

#### TUBULAR DEFECTS OF MAGNESIUM HANDLING

Mild hypermagnesemia has been described in patients with FHH, a defect in the function of the calcium-sensing receptor.[195, 196] Magnesium can also serve as a ligand for these receptors,[7] and it has been suggested that increases in serum magnesium stimulate calcium-sensing receptors on the basolateral surface of the renal tubule, thereby decreasing resorption of magnesium from the lumen. Therefore, a defect in these receptors would produce elevations in serum magnesium. Another tubular defect in magnesium excretion has been described by Mehrotra and coworkers,[445] characterized by hypokalemic metabolic alkalosis and hypomagnesuria. The molecular basis for this defect has yet to be demonstrated.

#### OTHER CAUSES

Other uncommon causes of hypermagnesemia include lithium ingestion,[446] milk-alkali syndrome, neoplasms with skeletal involvement,[441] theophylline intoxication,[447] and hypothyroidism.[301]

## Clinical Features of Hypermagnesemia

As with hypomagnesemia, the clinical picture of hypermagnesemia is dominated by cardiovascular and neuromuscular symptoms. The sequelae of magnesium excess vary in type and severity as the serum magnesium concentration increases. Hypermagnesemia may have a variety of effects on the cardiovascular system. Magnesium is capable of blocking the entry of calcium into vascular smooth muscle cells.[448] Hypermagnesemia is associated with relaxation of vascular smooth muscle and hypotension.[421, 448] Besides calcium channel blockade, magnesium may induce vascular relaxation through induction of prostacyclin.[449] Mild hypermagnesemia (3–5 mEq/L) may be associated with cutaneous flushing and mild hypotension.[434] Hypotension is more consistently observed at serum magnesium concentrations above 5 mEq/L.[441] Severe, refractory hypotension occurs above 10 mEq/L of serum magnesium.[440, 450, 451] Electrocardiographic changes and bradycardia may accompany hypermagnesemia. Prolonged PR intervals, increased QRS duration, and increased QT intervals occur with variable frequency at magnesium concentrations between 5 and 10 mEq/L.[441, 452] Bradycardia has been reported to occur at levels as low as 4.5 mEq/L.[453] Complete heart block or cardiac arrest may be seen at levels over 15 mEq/L.[436, 441, 450]

The neuromuscular relaxation induced by hypermagnesemia is used in the treatment of premature labor by magnesium infusions. Hypermagnesemia can inhibit acetylcholine release from the presynaptic nerve terminal and can diminish the response to acetylcholine at the motor end plate.[454, 455] The neuromuscular sequelae of hypermagnesemia are hyporeflexia at magnesium levels of 4 to 7 mEq/L, weakness of skeletal musculature at levels above 10 mEq/L,[441] and paralysis of the respiratory musculature at around 14 mEq/L.[456] Complete muscle paralysis without loss of consciousness can occur at magnesium levels of 14.6 to 19.7 mEq/L.[441, 457]

Hypermagnesemia can induce hypocalcemia that may be symptomatic.[442, 458] The hypocalcemia is due in part to inhibition of PTH secretion by acutely increased serum magnesium concentrations.[459, 460] In addition to the more common manifestations described earlier, excess magnesium can result in paralytic ileus,[461] nausea, vomiting, and impaired platelet function.[441]

## Treatment of Hypermagnesemia

In patients with normal renal function, cessation of magnesium ingestion or infusion is usually sufficient to allow serum magnesium levels to return quickly to normal. In severe, symptomatic cases of magnesium intoxication, administration of parenteral calcium (100–200 mg of elemental calcium infused over 5–10 minutes) can transiently antagonize the effects of hypermagnesemia.[441, 451] If elevated magnesium concentrations persist, or the patient has renal failure, hemodialysis or peritoneal dialysis using a dialysate with a low magnesium concentration can rapidly correct the hypermagnesemia.[441]

## REFERENCES


1. Pietrobon D, Di Virgilio F, Pozzan T: Structural and functional aspects of calcium homeostasis in eukaryotic cells. Eur J Biochem 193:599–622, 1990.
2. Brown EM: Extracellular $Ca^{2+}$ sensing, regulation of parathyroid cell function, and role of $Ca^{2+}$ and other ions as extracellular (first) messengers. Physiol Rev 71:371–411, 1991.
3. Thode J, Juul-Jorgensen B, Bhatia HM, et al: Comparison of serum total calcium, albumin-corrected total calcium, and ionized calcium in 1213 patients with suspected calcium disorders. Scand J Clin Lab Invest 49:217–223, 1989; erratum in Scand J Clin Lab Invest 50:113, 1990.
4. Kragh-Hansen U, Vorum H: Quantitative analyses of the interaction between calcium ions and human serum albumin. Clin Chem 39:202–208, 1993.
5. Butler SJ, Payne RB, Gunn IR, et al: Correlation between serum ionised calcium and serum albumin concentrations in two hospital populations. BMJ 289:948–950, 1984.
6. Moore EW: Ionized calcium in normal serum, ultrafiltrates, and whole blood determined by ion-exchange electrodes. J Clin Invest 49:318–334, 1970.
7. Brown EM, Gamba G, Riccardi D, et al: Cloning and characterization of an extracellular Ca(2+)-sensing receptor from bovine parathyroid. Nature 366:575–580, 1993.
8. Pollak MR, Brown EM, Chou YH, et al: Mutations in the human Ca(2+)-sensing receptor gene cause familial hypocalciuric hypercalcemia and neonatal severe hyperparathyroidism. Cell 75: 1297–1303, 1993; see comments.
9. Pearce SH, Williamson C, Kifor O, et al: A familial syndrome of hypocalcemia with hypercalciuria due to mutations in the calcium-sensing receptor. N Engl J Med 335:1115–1122, 1996; see comments.
10. McSheehy PM, Chambers TJ: Osteoblastic cells mediate osteoclastic responsiveness to parathyroid hormone. Endocrinology 118:824–828, 1986.
11. Lacey DL, Timms E, Tan HL, et al: Osteoprotegerin ligand is a cytokine that regulates osteoclast differentiation and activation. Cell 93:165–176, 1998.
12. Suda T, Takahashi N, Udagawa N, et al: Modulation of osteoclast differentiation and function by the new members of the tumor necrosis factor receptor and ligand families. Endocr Rev 20:345–357, 1999.
13. Hofbauer LC, Khosla S, Dunstan CR, et al: Estrogen stimulates gene expression and protein production of osteoprotegerin in human osteoblastic cells. Endocrinology 140:4367–4370, 1999.
14. Hofbauer LC, Gori F, Riggs BL, et al: Stimulation of osteoprotegerin ligand and inhibition of osteoprotegerin production by glucocorticoids in human osteoblastic lineage cells: Potential paracrine mechanisms of glucocorticoid-induced osteoporosis. Endocrinology 140:4382–4389, 1999; see comments.
15. Hofbauer LC, Khosla S, Dunstan CR, et al: The roles of osteoprotegerin and osteoprotegerin ligand in the paracrine regulation of bone resorption. J Bone Miner Res 15:2–12, 2000.
16. Li YC, Amling M, Pirro AE, et al: Normalization of mineral ion homeostasis by dietary means prevents hyperparathyroidism, rickets, and osteomalacia, but not alopecia in vitamin D receptor–ablated mice. Endocrinology 139:4391–4396, 1998.
17. Amling M, Priemel M, Holzmann T, et al: Rescue of the skeletal phenotype of vitamin D receptor–ablated mice in the setting of normal mineral ion homeostasis: Formal histomorphometric and biomechanical analyses. Endocrinology 140:4982–4987, 1999.
18. Bilezikian JP, Raisz LG, Rodan AR: Principles of Bone Biology. San Diego, Calif, Academic Press, 1996.
19. Kumar R: Vitamin D and calcium transport [clinical conference]. Kidney Int 40:1177–1189, 1991.
20. Wasserman RH, Fullmer CS: Vitamin D and intestinal calcium transport: Facts, speculations and hypotheses. J Nutr 125: 1971S–1979S, 1995.
21. Kumar R: Calcium transport in epithelial cells of the intestine and kidney. J Cell Biochem 57:392–398, 1995.
22. Wasserman RH, Chandler JS, Meyer SA, et al: Intestinal calcium transport and calcium extrusion processes at the basolateral membrane. J Nutr 122:662–671, 1992.
23. Wasserman RH, Taylor AN: Vitamin D–dependent calcium-binding protein: Response to some physiological and nutritional variables. J Biol Chem 243:3987–3993, 1968.
24. Peng JB, Chen XZ, Berger UV, et al: Molecular cloning and characterization of a channel-like transporter mediating intestinal calcium absorption. J Biol Chem 274:22739–22746, 1999.
25. Hoenderop JG, van der Kemp AW, Hartog A, et al: Molecular identification of the apical $Ca^{2+}$ channel in 1,25-dihydroxyvitamin D3–responsive epithelia. J Biol Chem 274:8375–8378, 1999.
26. Hoenderop JG, Hartog A, Stuiver M, et al: Localization of the epithelial Ca(2+) channel in rabbit kidney and intestine. J Am Soc Nephrol 11:1171–1178, 2000.
27. Norman AW, Song X, Zanello L, et al: Rapid and genomic biological responses are mediated by different shapes of the agonist steroid hormone, 1-alpha,25$(OH)_2$ vitamin $D_3$. Steroids 64:120–128, 1999.
28. Dormanen MC, Bishop JE, Hammond MW, et al: Nonnuclear effects of the steroid hormone 1 alpha,25$(OH)_2$-vitamin $D_3$: Analogs are able to functionally differentiate between nuclear and membrane receptors. Biochem Biophys Res Commun 201: 394–401, 1994.
29. Kurokawa K: The kidney and calcium homeostasis. Kidney Int Suppl 44:S97–S105, 1994.
30. Suki WN, Lederer ED, Rouse D: Renal transport of calcium, magnesium, and phosphate. In Brenner BM (ed): The Kidney, 6th ed. Philadelphia, WB Saunders, 2000, pp 520–574.
31. Riccardi D, Lee WS, Lee K, et al: Localization of the extracellular Ca(2+)-sensing receptor and PTH/PTHrP receptor in rat kidney. Am J Physiol 271:F951–F956, 1996.
32. Peng JB, Chen XZ, Berger UV, et al: A rat kidney-specific calcium transporter in the distal nephron. J Biol Chem 275: 28186–28194, 2000.
33. Carafoli E, Garcia-Martin E, Guerini D: The plasma membrane calcium pump: Recent developments and future perspectives. Experientia 52:1091–1100, 1996.
34. Friedman PA, Gesek FA: Cellular calcium transport in renal epithelia: Measurement, mechanisms, and regulation. Physiol Rev 75:429–471, 1995.
35. Hoenderop JG, Willems PH, Bindels RJ: Toward a comprehensive molecular model of active calcium reabsorption. Am J Physiol Renal Physiol 278:F352–F360, 2000.
36. Hebert SC, Brown EM, Harris HW: Role of the Ca(2+)-sensing receptor in divalent mineral ion homeostasis. J Exp Biol 200: 295–302, 1997.
37. Stacy BD, Wilson BW: Acidosis and hypercalciuria: Renal mechanisms affecting calcium, magnesium and sodium excretion in the sheep. J Physiol (Lond) 210:549–564, 1970.

38. Brickman AS, Massry SG, Coburn JW: Changes in serum and urinary calcium during treatment with hydrochlorothiazide: Studies on mechanisms. J Clin Invest 51:945–954, 1972.
39. Brickman AS, Coburn JW, Koppel MH, et al: The effect of hydrochlorothiazide administration on serum and urinary calcium in normal, hypoparathyroid and hyperparathyroid subjects: Studies on mechanisms. Isr J Med Sci 7:518–519, 1971.
40. Shoback D: Disorders of calcium and bone and mineral metabolism. In Arieff AI, DeFronzo RA (eds): Fluid, Electrolyte, and Acid-Base Disorders, 2nd ed. New York, Churchill Livingstone, 1995, pp 427–473.
41. Sands JM, Naruse M, Baum M, et al: Apical extracellular calcium/polyvalent cation–sensing receptor regulates vasopressin-elicited water permeability in rat kidney inner medullary collecting duct. J Clin Invest 99:1399–1405, 1997.
42. Hebert SC, Brown EM: The scent of an ion: Calcium-sensing and its roles in health and disease. Curr Opin Nephrol Hypertens 5:45–53, 1996.
43. Erne P, Bolli P, Burgisser E, et al: Correlation of platelet calcium with blood pressure: Effect of antihypertensive therapy. N Engl J Med 310:1084–1088, 1984.
44. Hebert SC: Extracellular calcium-sensing receptor: Implications for calcium and magnesium handling in the kidney. Kidney Int 50:2129–2139, 1996.
45. Silverberg SJ, Bilezikian JP: Evaluation and management of primary hyperparathyroidism. J Clin Endocrinol Metab 81: 2036–2040, 1996; see comments.
46. Metz DC, Jensen RT, Bale AE, et al: Multiple endocrine neoplasia type I: Clinical features and management. In Bilezikian JP, Marcus R, Levine MA (eds): The Parathyroids: Basic and Clinical Concepts. New York, Raven Press, 1994, pp 591–646.
47. Gagel RF: Multiple endocrine neoplasia type II. In Bilezikian JP, Marcus R, Levine MA (eds): The Parathyroids: Basic and Clinical Concepts. New York, Raven Press, 1994, pp 681–698.
48. Phay JE, Moley JF, Lairmore TC: Multiple endocrine neoplasias. Semin Surg Oncol 18:324–332, 2000.
49. Miedlich S, Krohn K, Lamesch P, et al: Frequency of somatic MEN1 gene mutations in monoclonal parathyroid tumours of patients with primary hyperparathyroidism. Eur J Endocrinol 143:47–54, 2000.
50. Heppner C, Kester MB, Agarwal SK, et al: Somatic mutation of the MEN1 gene in parathyroid tumours. Nat Genet 16: 375–378, 1997.
51. Motokura T, Bloom T, Kim HG, et al: A novel cyclin encoded by a bcl1-linked candidate oncogene. Nature 350:512–515, 1991; see comments.
52. Arnold A, Motokura T, Bloom T, et al: The putative oncogene PRAD1 encodes a novel cyclin. Cold Spring Harb Symp Quant Biol 56:93–97, 1991.
53. Hsi ED, Zukerberg LR, Yang WI, et al: Cyclin D1/PRAD1 expression in parathyroid adenomas: An immunohistochemical study. J Clin Endocrinol Metab 81:1736–1739, 1996.
54. Mulligan LM, Kwok JB, Healey CS, et al: Germ-line mutations of the RET proto-oncogene in multiple endocrine neoplasia type 2A. Nature 363:458–460, 1993.
55. Asai N, Iwashita T, Matsuyama M, et al: Mechanism of activation of the RET proto-oncogene by multiple endocrine neoplasia 2A mutations. Mol Cell Biol 15:1613–1619, 1995.
56. Noll WW: Utility of RET mutation analysis in multiple endocrine neoplasia type 2. Arch Pathol Lab Med 123:1047–1049, 1999.
57. Learoyd DL, Messina M, Zedenius J, et al: Molecular genetics of thyroid tumors and surgical decision-making. World J Surg 24:923–933, 2000.
58. Cryns VL, Yi SM, Tahara H, et al: Frequent loss of chromosome arm 1p DNA in parathyroid adenomas. Genes Chromosomes Cancer 13:9–17, 1995.
59. Palanisamy N, Imanishi Y, Rao PH, et al: Novel chromosomal abnormalities identified by comparative genomic hybridization in parathyroid adenomas. J Clin Endocrinol Metab 83:1766–1770, 1998.
60. Tahara H, Smith AP, Gaz RD, et al: Parathyroid tumor suppressor on 1p: Analysis of the p18 cyclin-dependent kinase inhibitor gene as a candidate. J Bone Miner Res 12:1330–1334, 1997.
61. Tahara H, Smith AP, Gaz RD, et al: Loss of chromosome arm 9p DNA and analysis of the p16 and p15 cyclin-dependent kinase inhibitor genes in human parathyroid adenomas. J Clin Endocrinol Metab 81:3663–3667, 1996.
62. Tahara H, Smith AP, Gaz RD, et al: Genomic localization of novel candidate tumor suppressor gene loci in human parathyroid adenomas. Cancer Res 56:599–605, 1996.
63. Szijan I, Orlow I, Dalamon V, et al: Alterations in the retinoblastoma pathway of cell cycle control in parathyroid tumors. Oncol Rep 7:421–425, 2000.
64. Subramaniam P, Wilkinson S, Shepherd JJ: Inactivation of retinoblastoma gene in malignant parathyroid growths: A candidate genetic trigger? Aust N Z J Surg 65:714–716, 1995.
65. Cryns VL, Thor A, Xu HJ, et al: Loss of the retinoblastoma tumor-suppressor gene in parathyroid carcinoma. N Engl J Med 330:757–761, 1994; see comments.
66. Degenhardt S, Toell A, Weidemann W, et al: Point mutations of the human parathyroid calcium receptor gene are not responsible for non-suppressible renal hyperparathyroidism. Kidney Int 53:556–561, 1998.
67. Cetani F, Pinchera A, Pardi E, et al: No evidence for mutations in the calcium-sensing receptor gene in sporadic parathyroid adenomas. J Bone Miner Res 14:878–882, 1999.
68. Kifor O, Moore FD Jr, Wang P, et al: Reduced immunostaining for the extracellular $Ca^{2+}$-sensing receptor in primary and uremic secondary hyperparathyroidism. J Clin Endocrinol Metab 81:1598–1606, 1996; see comments.
69. Gogusev J, Duchambon P, Hory B, et al: Depressed expression of calcium receptor in parathyroid gland tissue of patients with hyperparathyroidism. Kidney Int 51:328–336, 1997.
70. Nussbaum SR, Zahradnik RJ, Lavigne JR, et al: Highly sensitive two-site immunoradiometric assay of parathyrin, and its clinical utility in evaluating patients with hypercalcemia. Clin Chem 33:1364–1367, 1987.
71. Gao P, Scheibel SJ, D'amour P, et al: Measuring the biologically active or authentic whole-parathyroid hormone (PTH) with a novel immunoradiometric assay without cross reaction to the PTH (7–84) fragment. J Bone Miner Res 14:S446, 1999.
72. Brossard JH, Lepage R, Gao P, et al: A new commercial whole-PTH assay free of interference by non-(1–84) parathyroid hormone fragments in uremic samples. J Bone Miner Res 14: S444, 1999.
73. Silverberg SJ, Shane E, Jacobs TP, et al: A 10-year prospective study of primary hyperparathyroidism with or without parathyroid surgery. N Engl J Med 341:1249–1255, 1999; see comments; erratum in N Engl J Med 342:144, 2000.
74. Silverberg SJ, Bilezikian JP, Bone HG, et al: Therapeutic controversies in primary hyperparathyroidism. J Clin Endocrinol Metab 84:2275–2285, 1999.
75. Norton JA, Brennan MF, Wells SA: Surgical management of hyperparathyroidism. In Bilezikian JP, Marcus R, Levine MA (eds): The Parathyroids: Basic and Clinical Concepts. New York, Raven Press, 1994, pp 531–551.
76. Oertli D, Richter M, Kraenzlin M, et al: Parathyroidectomy in primary hyperparathyroidism: Preoperative localization and routine biopsy of unaltered glands are not necessary. Surgery 117:392–396, 1995.
77. Wells SA Jr, Farndon JR, Dale JK, et al: Long-term evaluation of patients with primary parathyroid hyperplasia managed by total parathyroidectomy and heterotopic autotransplantation. Ann Surg 192:451–458, 1980.
78. Chou FF, Chan HM, Huang TJ, et al: Autotransplantation of parathyroid glands into subcutaneous forearm tissue for renal hyperparathyroidism. Surgery 124:1–5, 1998; see comments.
79. Yamashita H, Noguchi S, Futata T, et al: Usefulness of quick intraoperative measurements of intact parathyroid hormone in the surgical management of hyperparathyroidism. Biomed Pharmacother 54(suppl 1):108s–111s, 2000.
80. Dackiw AP, Sussman JJ, Fritsche HA Jr, et al: Relative contributions of technetium Tc 99m sestamibi scintigraphy, intraoperative gamma probe detection, and the rapid parathyroid hormone assay to the surgical management of hyperparathyroidism. Arch Surg 135:550–555; discussion 555–557, 2000.
81. Wilkinson RH Jr, Leight GS Jr, Garner SC, et al: Complementary nature of radiotracer parathyroid imaging and intraopera-

tive parathyroid hormone assays in the surgical management of primary hyperparathyroid disease: Case report and review. Clin Nucl Med 25:173–178, 2000.
82. Ishibashi M, Uchida M, Nishida H, et al: Pre-surgical localization of ectopic parathyroid glands using three-dimensional CT imaging, 99Tcm sestamibi, and 99Tcm tetrofosmin imaging. Br J Radiol 72:296–300, 1999.
83. Miller FR, Netterville JL: Surgical management of thyroid and parathyroid disorders. Med Clin North Am 83:247–259, 1999.
84. Heath DA: Familial hypocalciuric hypercalciuria. In Bilezikian JP, Marcus R, Levine MA (eds): The Parathyroids: Basic and Clinical Concepts. New York, Raven Press, 1994, pp 699–710.
85. Pollak MR, Chou YH, Marx SJ, et al: Familial hypocalciuric hypercalcemia and neonatal severe hyperparathyroidism: Effects of mutant gene dosage on phenotype. J Clin Invest 93: 1108–1112, 1994.
86. Mundy GR, Guise TA: Hypercalcemia of malignancy. Am J Med 103:134–145, 1997; see comments.
87. Goltzman D, Henderson JE: Parathyroid hormone–related peptide and hypercalcemia of malignancy. Cancer Treat Res 89: 193–215, 1997.
88. Segre G: Receptors for parathyroid hormone and parathyroid hormone–related protein multiple endocrine neoplasia type I: Clinical features and management. In Bilezikian JP, Marcus R, Levine MA (eds): The Parathyroids: Basic and Clinical Concepts. New York, Raven Press, 1994, pp 213–238.
89. Wu TJ, Taylor RL, Kao PC: Parathyroid-hormone-related peptide immunochemiluminometric assay: Developed with polyclonal antisera produced from a single animal. Ann Clin Lab Sci 27:384–390, 1997.
90. Ikeda K, Ohno H, Hane M, et al: Development of a sensitive two-site immunoradiometric assay for parathyroid hormone–related peptide: Evidence for elevated levels in plasma from patients with adult T-cell leukemia/lymphoma and B-cell lymphoma. J Clin Endocrinol Metab 79:1322–1327, 1994.
91. Lands RH: Non-Hodgkin's lymphoma, hypercalcemia, and elevated calcitriol levels: A report and review. J Tenn Med Assoc 88:310–311, 1995.
92. Gado K, Domjan G, Hegyesi H, et al: Role of interleukin-6 in the pathogenesis of multiple myeloma. Cell Biol Int 24: 195–209, 2000.
93. Lust JA, Donovan KA: The role of interleukin-1 beta in the pathogenesis of multiple myeloma. Hematol Oncol Clin North Am 13:1117–1125, 1999.
94. Sati HI, Greaves M, Apperley JF, et al: Expression of interleukin-1 beta and tumour necrosis factor-alpha in plasma cells from patients with multiple myeloma. Br J Haematol 104:350–357, 1999.
95. Ragavan VV, Smith JE, Bilezikian JP: Vitamin A toxicity and hypercalcemia. Am J Med Sci 283:161–164, 1982.
96. Strong P, Jewell S, Rinker J, et al: Thiazide therapy and severe hypercalcemia in a patient with hyperparathyroidism. West J Med 154:338–340, 1991.
97. Schwartzman MS, Franck WA: Vitamin D toxicity complicating the treatment of senile, postmenopausal, and glucocorticoid-induced osteoporosis: Four case reports and a critical commentary on the use of vitamin D in these disorders. Am J Med 82: 224–230, 1987.
98. McHenry CR, Rosen IB, Rotstein LE, et al: Lithiumogenic disorders of the thyroid and parathyroid glands as surgical disease. Surgery 108:1001–1005, 1990.
99. Blau EB, Hoyman S: Severe hypercalcemia, renal failure, and medullary nephrocalcinosis secondary to calcium carbonate ingestion [letter]. Pediatr Nephrol 11:391, 1997.
100. Racke F, McHenry CR, Wentworth D: Lithium-induced alterations in parathyroid cell function: Insight into the pathogenesis of lithium-associated hyperparathyroidism. Am J Surg 168: 462–465, 1994.
101. Gordon DL, Suvanich S, Erviti V, et al: The serum calcium level and its significance in hyperthyroidism: A prospective study. Am J Med Sci 268:31–36, 1974.
102. Garnero P, Vassy V, Bertholin A, et al: Markers of bone turnover in hyperthyroidism and the effects of treatment. J Clin Endocrinol Metab 78:955–959, 1994.
103. Hajjar ET, Jaber R: Hypercalcemia in pheochromocytoma. J Med Liban 26:269–272, 1973.
104. Kimura S, Nishimura Y, Yamaguchi K, et al: A case of pheochromocytoma producing parathyroid hormone–related protein and presenting with hypercalcemia. J Clin Endocrinol Metab 70:1559–1563, 1990.
105. Stewart AF, Hoecker JL, Mallette LE, et al: Hypercalcemia in pheochromocytoma: Evidence for a novel mechanism. Ann Intern Med 102:776–779, 1985.
106. Garbini A, Mainardi M, Grimi M, et al: Pheochromocytoma and hypercalcemia due to ectopic production of parathyroid hormone. N Y State J Med 86:25–27, 1986.
107. Montoli A, Colussi G, Minetti L: Hypercalcaemia in Addison's disease: Calciotropic hormone profile and bone histology. J Intern Med 232:535–540, 1992.
108. Bell NH: Endocrine complications of sarcoidosis. Endocrinol Metab Clin North Am 20:645–654, 1991.
109. Casella FJ, Allon M: The kidney in sarcoidosis. J Am Soc Nephrol 3:1555–1562, 1993.
110. Adams JS, Gacad MA: Characterization of 1 alpha-hydroxylation of vitamin $D_3$ sterols by cultured alveolar macrophages from patients with sarcoidosis. J Exp Med 161:755–765, 1985.
111. Adams JS, Singer FR, Gacad MA, et al: Isolation and structural identification of 1,25-dihydroxyvitamin $D_3$ produced by cultured alveolar macrophages in sarcoidosis. J Clin Endocrinol Metab 60:960–966, 1985.
112. Insogna KL, Dreyer BE, Mitnick M, et al: Enhanced production rate of 1,25-dihydroxyvitamin D in sarcoidosis. J Clin Endocrinol Metab 66:72–75, 1988.
113. Chesney RW, Hamstra AJ, DeLuca HF, et al: Elevated serum 1,25-dihydroxyvitamin D concentrations in the hypercalcemia of sarcoidosis: Correction by glucocorticoid therapy. J Pediatr 98:919–922, 1981.
114. Adams JS, Diz MM, Sharma OP: Effective reduction in the serum 1,25-dihydroxyvitamin D and calcium concentration in sarcoidosis-associated hypercalcemia with short-course chloroquine therapy. Ann Intern Med 111:437–438, 1989.
115. Bia MJ, Insogna K: Treatment of sarcoidosis-associated hypercalcemia with ketoconazole. Am J Kidney Dis 18:702–705, 1991.
116. Schuman CA, Jones HWD: The "milk-alkali" syndrome: Two case reports with discussion of pathogenesis. Q J Med 55: 119–126, 1985.
117. Fiorino AS: Hypercalcemia and alkalosis due to the milk-alkali syndrome: A case report and review. Yale J Biol Med 69:517–523, 1996.
118. Gopal H, Sklar AH, Sherrard DJ: Symptomatic hypercalcemia of immobilization in a patient with end-stage renal disease. Am J Kidney Dis 35:969–972, 2000.
119. Massagli TL, Cardenas DD: Immobilization hypercalcemia treatment with pamidronate disodium after spinal cord injury. Arch Phys Med Rehabil 80:998–1000, 1999.
120. Kaul S, Sockalosky JJ: Human synthetic calcitonin therapy for hypercalcemia of immobilization. J Pediatr 126:825–827, 1995.
121. Case records of the Massachusetts General Hospital. Weekly clinicopathological exercises. Case 44-1986. An 80-year-old woman with Paget's disease and severe hypercalcemia after a recent fracture. N Engl J Med 315:1209–1219, 1986.
122. Kurihara N, Reddy SV, Menaa C, et al: Osteoclasts expressing the measles virus nucleocapsid gene display a pagetic phenotype. J Clin Invest 105:607–614, 2000; see comments.
123. Schipani E, Langman C, Hunzelman J, et al: A novel parathyroid hormone (PTH)/PTH-related peptide receptor mutation in Jansen's metaphyseal chondrodysplasia. J Clin Endocrinol Metab 84:3052–3057, 1999.
124. Schipani E, Kruse K, Juppner H: A constitutively active mutant PTH-PTHrP receptor in Jansen-type metaphyseal chondrodysplasia. Science 268:98–100, 1995.
125. Hadjis T, Grieff M, Lockhat D, et al: Calcium metabolism in acute renal failure due to rhabdomyolysis. Clin Nephrol 39: 22–27, 1993.
126. Akmal M, Bishop JE, Telfer N, et al: Hypocalcemia and hypercalcemia in patients with rhabdomyolysis with and without acute renal failure. J Clin Endocrinol Metab 63:137–142, 1986.
127. Akmal M, Goldstein DA, Telfer N, et al: Resolution of muscle calcification in rhabdomyolysis and acute renal failure. Ann Intern Med 89:928–930, 1978.
128. Lane JT, Boudreau RJ, Kinlaw WB: Disappearance of muscular

calcium deposits during resolution of prolonged rhabdomyolysis-induced hypercalcemia. Am J Med 89:523–525, 1990; see comments.
129. Llach F, Felsenfeld AJ, Haussler MR: The pathophysiology of altered calcium metabolism in rhabdomyolysis-induced acute renal failure: Interactions of parathyroid hormone, 25-hydroxycholecalciferol, and 1,25-dihydroxycholecalciferol. N Engl J Med 305:117–123, 1981.
130. González EA, Martin KJ: Renal osteodystrophy: Pathogenesis and management. Nephrol Dial Transplant 10(suppl 3):13–21, 1995.
131. Chertow GM, Burke SK, Dillon MA, et al: Long-term effects of sevelamer hydrochloride on the calcium × phosphate product and lipid profile of haemodialysis patients. Nephrol Dial Transplant 15:559, 2000.
132. Slatopolsky E, Weerts C, Lopez-Hilker S, et al: Calcium carbonate as a phosphate binder in patients with chronic renal failure undergoing dialysis. N Engl J Med 315:157–161, 1986.
133. González E, Martin K: Aluminum and renal osteodystrophy: A diminishing clinical problem. Trends Endocrinol Metab 3: 371–375, 1992.
134. Slatopolsky E, Weerts C, Thielan J, et al: Marked suppression of secondary hyperparathyroidism by intravenous administration of 1,25-dihydroxy-cholecalciferol in uremic patients. J Clin Invest 74:2136–2143, 1984.
135. Martin KJ, González EA, Gellens M, et al: 19-Nor-1-α-25-Dihydroxyvitamin $D_2$ (paricalcitol) safely and effectively reduces the levels of intact PTH in patients on hemodialysis. J Am Soc Nephrol 10:1427–1432, 1998.
136. Tan AU Jr, Levine BS, Mazess RB, et al: Effective suppression of parathyroid hormone by 1 alpha-hydroxy-vitamin $D_2$ in hemodialysis patients with moderate to severe secondary hyperparathyroidism. Kidney Int 51:317–323, 1997.
137. Golconda MS, Larson TS, Kolb LG, et al: 1,25-Dihydroxyvitamin D–mediated hypercalcemia in a renal transplant recipient. Mayo Clin Proc 71:32–36, 1996.
138. Parfitt AM: Hypercalcemic hyperparathyroidism following renal transplantation: Differential diagnosis, management, and implications for cell population control in the parathyroid gland. Miner Electrolyte Metab 8:92–112, 1982.
139. Kutluk T, Akyuz C, Yalcin B, et al: Use of pamidronate in the management of acute cancer-related hypercalcemia in children [letter; comment]. Med Pediatr Oncol 31:39, 1998.
140. Young G, Shende A: Use of pamidronate in the management of acute cancer-related hypercalcemia in children. Med Pediatr Oncol 30:117–121, 1998; see comments.
141. Oiso Y, Tomita A, Hasegawa H, et al: Pamidronate treatment in patients with tumor-associated hypercalcemia: Pharmacological effects and pharmacokinetics. Endocr J 41:655–661, 1994.
142. Gucalp R, Theriault R, Gill I, et al: Treatment of cancer-associated hypercalcemia: Double-blind comparison of rapid and slow intravenous infusion regimens of pamidronate disodium and saline alone. Arch Intern Med 154:1935–1944, 1994; see comments.
143. Warrell RP Jr: Clinical trials of gallium nitrate in patients with cancer-related hypercalcemia. Semin Oncol 18:26–31, 1991.
144. Ahr DJ, Scialla SJ, Kimbali DB Jr: Acquired platelet dysfunction following mithramycin therapy. Cancer 41:448–454, 1978.
145. Silverberg SJ, Bone HG 3rd, Marriott TB, et al: Short-term inhibition of parathyroid hormone secretion by a calcium-receptor agonist in patients with primary hyperparathyroidism. N Engl J Med 337:1506–1510, 1997.
146. Camus C, Charasse C, Jouannic-Montier I, et al: Calcium-free hemodialysis: Experience in the treatment of 33 patients with severe hypercalcemia. Intensive Care Med 22:116–121, 1996.
147. Okazaki R, Chikatsu N, Nakatsu M, et al: A novel activating mutation in calcium-sensing receptor gene associated with a family of autosomal dominant hypocalcemia. J Clin Endocrinol Metab 84:363–366, 1999.
148. Arnold A, Horst SA, Gardella TJ, et al: Mutation of the signal peptide-encoding region of the preproparathyroid hormone gene in familial isolated hypoparathyroidism. J Clin Invest 86: 1084–1087, 1990.
149. Parkinson DB, Thakker RV: A donor splice site mutation in the parathyroid hormone gene is associated with autosomal recessive hypoparathyroidism. Nat Genet 1:149–152, 1992.
150. Raatikka M, Rapola J, Tuuteri L, et al: Familial third and fourth pharyngeal pouch syndrome with truncus arteriosus: DiGeorge syndrome. Pediatrics 67:173–175, 1981.
151. Pattou F, Combemale F, Fabre S, et al: Hypocalcemia following thyroid surgery: Incidence and prediction of outcome. World J Surg 22:718–724, 1998.
152. Wittle LW, Augostini RS, Chizmar WS: The occurrence of chronic hypocalcemia following parathyroidectomy in the green frog, *Rana clamitans.* Gen Comp Endocrinol 80:419–426, 1990.
153. Price JC, Ridley MB: Hypocalcemia following pharyngoesophageal ablation and gastric pull-up reconstruction: Pathophysiology and management. Ann Otol Rhinol Laryngol 97:521–526, 1988.
154. Rude RK, Oldham SB, Singer FR: Functional hypoparathyroidism and parathyroid hormone end-organ resistance in human magnesium deficiency. Clin Endocrinol (Oxf) 5:209–224, 1976.
155. Rude RK, Oldham SB, Sharp CF Jr, et al: Parathyroid hormone secretion in magnesium deficiency. J Clin Endocrinol Metab 47:800–806, 1978.
156. Cruikshank DP, Chan GM, Doerrfeld D: Alterations in vitamin D and calcium metabolism with magnesium sulfate treatment of preeclampsia. Am J Obstet Gynecol 168:1170–1176; discussion 1176–1177, 1993.
157. Miric A, Vechio JD, Levine MA: Heterogeneous mutations in the gene encoding the alpha-subunit of the stimulatory G protein of adenylyl cyclase in Albright hereditary osteodystrophy. J Clin Endocrinol Metab 76:1560–1568, 1993.
158. Levine MA, Ahn TG, Klupt SF, et al: Genetic deficiency of the alpha subunit of the guanine nucleotide-binding protein Gs as the molecular basis for Albright hereditary osteodystrophy. Proc Natl Acad Sci U S A 85:617–621, 1988.
159. Jan de Beur SM, Ding CL, LaBuda MC, et al: Pseudohypoparathyroidism 1b: Exclusion of parathyroid hormone and its receptors as candidate disease genes. J Clin Endocrinol Metab 85: 2239–2246, 2000.
160. Schipani E, Weinstein LS, Bergwitz C, et al: Pseudohypoparathyroidism type Ib is not caused by mutations in the coding exons of the human parathyroid hormone (PTH)/PTH-related peptide receptor gene. J Clin Endocrinol Metab 80:1611–1621, 1995.
161. Farfel Z, Brothers VM, Brickman AS, et al: Pseudohypoparathyroidism: Inheritance of deficient receptor-cyclase coupling activity. Proc Natl Acad Sci U S A 78:3098–3102, 1981.
162. Barrett D, Breslau NA, Wax MB, et al: New form of pseudohypoparathyroidism with abnormal catalytic adenylate cyclase. Am J Physiol 257:E277–E283, 1989.
163. Drezner M, Neelon FA, Lebovitz HE: Pseudohypoparathyroidism type II: A possible defect in the reception of the cyclic AMP signal. N Engl J Med 289:1056–1060, 1973.
164. Tollin SR, Perlmutter S, Aloia JF: Serial changes in bone mineral density and bone turnover after correction of secondary hyperparathyroidism in a patient with pseudohypoparathyroidism type Ib. J Bone Miner Res 15:1412–1416, 2000.
165. Thomas MK, Lloyd-Jones DM, Thadhani RI, et al: Hypovitaminosis D in medical inpatients. N Engl J Med 338:777–783, 1998.
166. Zittel TT, Zeeb B, Maier GW, et al: High prevalence of bone disorders after gastrectomy. Am J Surg 174:431–438, 1997.
167. Fu GK, Lin D, Zhang MY, et al: Cloning of human 25-hydroxyvitamin D-1 alpha-hydroxylase and mutations causing vitamin D–dependent rickets type 1. Mol Endocrinol 11:1961–1970, 1997.
168. Brooks MH, Bell NH, Love L, et al: Vitamin-D-dependent rickets type II: Resistance of target organs to 1,25-dihydroxyvitamin D. N Engl J Med 298:996–999, 1978.
169. Hughes M, Malloy P, Kieback D, et al: Human vitamin D receptor mutations: Identification of molecular defects in hypocalcemic vitamin D resistant rickets. Adv Exp Med Biol 255: 491–503, 1989.
170. Kristjansson K, Rut AR, Hewison M, et al: Two mutations in the hormone binding domain of the vitamin D receptor cause tissue resistance to 1,25 dihydroxyvitamin $D_3$. J Clin Invest 92: 12–16, 1993.
171. Wiese RJ, Goto H, Prahl JM, et al: Vitamin D–dependency

rickets type II: Truncated vitamin D receptor in three kindreds. Mol Cell Endocrinol 90:197–201, 1993.
172. Nykjaer A, Dragun D, Walther D, et al: An endocytic pathway essential for renal uptake and activation of the steroid 25-(OH) vitamin $D_3$. Cell 96:507–515, 1999.
173. Szentirmai M, Constantinou C, Rainey JM, et al: Hypocalcemia due to avid calcium uptake by osteoblastic metastases of prostate cancer. West J Med 163:577–578, 1995.
174. Kukreja SC, Shanmugam A, Lad TE: Hypocalcemia in patients with prostate cancer. Calcif Tissue Int 43:340–345, 1988.
175. Schmitt BP, Nordlund DJ, Rodgers LA: Prevalence of hypocalcemia and elevated serum alkaline phosphatase in patients receiving chronic anticonvulsant therapy. J Fam Pract 18:873–877, 1984.
176. Frame B: Hypocalcemia and osteomalacia associated with anticonvulsant therapy. Ann Intern Med 74:294–295, 1971.
177. Widdowson EM, McCance RA, Spray CM: The chemical composition of the human body. Clin Sci 10:113–125, 1951.
178. Soman SD, Joseph KT, Raut SJ, et al: Studies on major and trace element content in human tissues. Health Phys 19:641–656, 1970.
179. Aikawa JK, Gordon GS, Rhoades EL: Magnesium metabolism in human beings: Studies with $Mg^{28}$. J Appl Physiol 15:503–507, 1960.
180. Wacker WEC, Parisi AF: Magnesium metabolism. N Engl J Med 278:658–663, 1968.
181. Wong ET, Rude RK, Singer FR, et al: A high prevalence of hypomagnesemia and hypermagnesemia in hospitalized patients. Am J Clin Pathol 79:348–352, 1983.
182. Chernow B, Bamberger S, Stoiko M, et al: Hypomagnesemia in patients in postoperative intensive care. Chest 95:391–397, 1989; erratum in Chest 95:1362, 1989.
183. Ryzen E, Wagers PW, Singer FR, et al: Magnesium deficiency in a medical ICU population. Crit Care Med 13:19–21, 1985.
184. Rubeiz GJ, Thill-Baharozian M, Hardie D, et al: Association of hypomagnesemia and mortality in acutely ill medical patients. Crit Care Med 21:203–209, 1993; see comments.
185. Touitou Y, Godard JP, Ferment O, et al: Prevalence of magnesium and potassium deficiencies in the elderly. Clin Chem 33: 518–523, 1987.
186. Shils ME: Experimental production of magnesium deficiency in man. Ann N Y Acad Sci 162:847–855, 1969.
187. Quamme GA: Renal magnesium handling: New insights in understanding old problems. Kidney Int 52:1180–1195, 1997.
188. de Rouffignac C, Quamme G: Renal magnesium handling and its hormonal control. Physiol Rev 74:305–322, 1994.
189. Quamme GA, Dirks JH: Intraluminal and contraluminal magnesium on magnesium and calcium transfer in the rat nephron. Am J Physiol 238:F187–F198, 1980.
190. Shafik IM, Quamme GA: Early adaptation of renal magnesium reabsorption in response to magnesium restriction. Am J Physiol 257:F974–F977, 1989.
191. Brunette MG, Vigneault N, Carriere S: Micropuncture study of renal magnesium transport in magnesium-loaded rats. Am J Physiol 229:1695–1701, 1975.
192. Mandon B, Siga E, Chabardes D, et al: Insulin stimulates $Na^+$, $Cl^-$, $Ca^{2+}$, and $Mg^{2+}$ transports in TAL of mouse nephron: Cross-potentiation with AVP. Am J Physiol 265:F361–F369, 1993.
193. Wittner M, Mandon B, Roinel N, et al: Hormonal stimulation of $Ca^{2+}$ and $Mg^{2+}$ transport in the cortical thick ascending limb of Henle's loop of the mouse: Evidence for a change in the paracellular pathway permeability. Pflugers Arch 423: 387–396, 1993.
194. Di Stefano A, Roinel N, de Rouffignac C, et al: Transepithelial $Ca^{2+}$ and $Mg^{2+}$ transport in the cortical thick ascending limb of Henle's loop of the mouse is a voltage-dependent process. Renal Physiol Biochem 16:157–166, 1993.
195. Marx SJ, Attie MF, Levine MA, et al: The hypocalciuric or benign variant of familial hypercalcemia: Clinical and biochemical features in fifteen kindreds. Medicine 60:397–412, 1981.
196. Law WMJ, Heath HD: Familial benign hypercalcemia (hypocalciuric hypercalcemia): Clinical and pathogenetic studies in 21 families. Ann Intern Med 102:511–5519, 1985.
197. Wang WH, Lu M, Hebert SC: Cytochrome P-450 metabolites mediate extracellular Ca(2+)-induced inhibition of apical K+ channels in the TAL. Am J Physiol 271:C103–C111, 1996.
198. Attie MF, Gill JRJ, Stock JL, et al: Urinary calcium excretion in familial hypocalciuric hypercalcemia: Persistence of relative hypocalciuria after induction of hypoparathyroidism. J Clin Invest 72:667–676, 1983.
199. Dunn MJ, Walser M: Magnesium depletion in normal man. Metabolism 15:884–895, 1966.
200. Dai LJ, Raymond L, Friedman PA, et al: Mechanisms of amiloride stimulation of $Mg^{2+}$ uptake in immortalized mouse distal convoluted tubule cells. Am J Physiol 272:F249–F256, 1997.
201. Quamme GA, Dai LJ: Presence of a novel influx pathway for $Mg^{2+}$ in MDCK cells. Am J Physiol 259:C521–C525, 1990.
202. Seelig MS: The requirements of magnesium by the normal adult—summary and analysis of published data. Am J Clin Nutr 14:342–390, 1964.
203. Alfrey AC, Miller NL, Trow R: Effect of age and magnesium depletion on bone magnesium pools in rats. J Clin Invest 54: 1074–1081, 1974.
204. Marier JR: Magnesium content of the food supply in the modern-day world. Magnesium 5:1–8, 1986.
205. Kalbfleisch JM, Lindeman RD, Ginn HE, et al: Effects of ethanol administration on urinary excretion of magnesium and other electrolytes in alcoholic and normal subjects. J Clin Invest 42:1471–1475, 1963.
206. Heaton FW, Pyrah LN, Beresford CC, et al: Hypomagnesemia in chronic alcoholism. Lancet 2:802–805, 1962.
207. Jones JE, Shane SR, Jacobs WH, et al: Magnesium balance studies in chronic alcoholism. Ann N Y Acad Sci 162:934–946, 1969.
208. De Marchi S, Cecchin E, Basile A, et al: Renal tubular dysfunction in chronic alcohol abuse—effects of abstinence. N Engl J Med 329:1927–1934, 1993.
209. McCollister RJ, Flink EB, Lewis MD: Urinary excretion of magnesium in man following the ingestion of ethanol. Am J Clin Nutr 12:415–420, 1963.
210. Caddell JL, Goddard DR: Studies in protein-calorie malnutrition. I. Chemical evidence for magnesium deficiency. N Engl J Med 276:533–535, 1967.
211. Caddell JL: Magnesium deficiency in protein-calorie malnutrition: A follow-up study. Ann N Y Acad Sci 162:874–890, 1969.
212. Cosnes J, Gendre JP, Evard D, et al: Compensatory enteral hyperalimentation for management of patients with severe short bowel syndrome. Am J Clin Nutr 41:1002–1009, 1985.
213. Fukumoto S, Matsumoto T, Tanaka Y, et al: Renal magnesium wasting in a patient with short bowel syndrome with magnesium deficiency: Effect of 1 alpha-hydroxyvitamin $D_3$ treatment. J Clin Endocrinol Metab 65:1301–1304, 1987.
214. Gerlach K, Morowitz DA, Kirsner JB: Symptomatic hypomagnesemia complicating regional enteritis. Gastroenterology 59: 567–574, 1970.
215. Heaton FW, Clark CG, Goligher JC: Magnesium deficiency complicating intestinal surgery. Br J Surg 54:41–45, 1967.
216. Ament ME: Malabsorption syndromes in infancy and childhood. II. J Pediatr 81:867–884, 1972.
217. Nyhlin H, Dyckner T, Ek B, et al: Magnesium in Crohn's disease. Acta Med Scand Suppl 661:21–25, 1982.
218. Rudman D, Dedonis JL, Fountain MT, et al: Hypocitraturia in patients with gastrointestinal malabsorption. N Engl J Med 303: 657–661, 1980.
219. Hessov I, Hasselblad C, Fasth S, et al: Magnesium deficiency after ileal resections for Crohn's disease. Scand J Gastroenterol 18:643–649, 1983.
220. Ryzen E, Rude RK: Low intracellular magnesium in patients with acute pancreatitis and hypocalcemia. West J Med 152: 145–148, 1990.
221. Hersh T, Siddiqui DA: Magnesium and the pancreas. Am J Clin Nutr 26:362–366, 1973.
222. Paunier L, Radde IC, Kooh SW, et al: Primary hypomagnesemia with secondary hypocalcemia in an infant. Pediatrics 41:385–402, 1968.
223. Shalev H, Phillip M, Galil A, et al: Clinical presentation and outcome in primary familial hypomagnesaemia. Arch Dis Child 78:127–130, 1998.
224. Romero R, Meacham LR, Winn KT: Isolated magnesium malabsorption in a 10-year-old boy. Am J Gastroenterol 91:611–613, 1996.

225. Coenegracht JM, Houben HGJ: Idiopathic hypomagnesemia with hypocalcemia in an adult. Clin Chim Acta 50:349–357, 1974.
226. Abdulrazzaq YM, Smigura FC, Wettrell G: Primary infantile hypomagnesaemia: Report of two cases and review of literature. Eur J Pediatr 148:459–461, 1989.
227. Pronicka E, Gruszczynska B: Familial hypomagnesaemia with secondary hypocalcaemia—autosomal or X-linked inheritance? J Inherit Metab Dis 14:397–399, 1991.
228. Stromme JH, Nesbakken R, Normann T, et al: Familial hypomagnesemia: Biochemical, histological and hereditary aspects studied in two brothers. Acta Paediatr Scand 58:433–444, 1969.
229. Nordio S, Donath A, Macagno F, et al: Chronic hypomagnesemia with magnesium-dependent hypocalcemia. I. A new syndrome with intestinal magnesium malabsorption. Acta Paediatr Scand 60:441–448, 1971.
230. Milla PJ, Aggett PJ, Wolff OH, et al: Studies in primary hypomagnesaemia: Evidence for defective carrier-mediated small intestinal transport of magnesium. Gut 20:1028–1033, 1979.
231. Chery M, Biancalana V, Philippe C, et al: Hypomagnesemia with secondary hypocalcemia in a female with balanced X;9 translocation: Mapping of the Xp22 chromosome breakpoint. Hum Genet 93:587–591, 1994.
232. Walder RY, Shalev H, Brennan TM, et al: Familial hypomagnesemia maps to chromosome 9q, not to the X chromosome: Genetic linkage mapping and analysis of a balanced translocation breakpoint. Hum Mol Genet 6:1491–1497, 1997.
233. Strømme JH, Steen-Johnsen J, Harnaes K, et al: Familial hypomagnesemia—a follow-up examination of three patients after 9 to 12 years of treatment. Pediatr Res 15:1134–1139, 1981.
234. Evans RA, Carter JN, George CR, et al: The congenital magnesium-losing kidney: Report of two patients. Q J Med 50:39–52, 1981.
235. Praga M, Vara J, González-Parra E, et al: Familial hypomagnesemia with hypercalciuria and nephrocalcinosis. Kidney Int 47: 1419–1425, 1995.
236. Michelis MF, Drash AL, Linarelli LG, et al: Decreased bicarbonate threshold and renal magnesium wasting in a sibship with distal renal tubular acidosis (evaluation of the pathophysiological role of parathyroid hormone). Metabolism 21:905–920, 1972.
237. Manz F, Schärer K, Janka P, et al: Renal magnesium wasting, incomplete tubular acidosis, hypercalciuria and nephrocalcinosis in siblings. Eur J Pediatr 128:67–79, 1978.
238. Nicholson JC, Jones CL, Powell HR, et al: Familial hypomagnesaemia—hypercalciuria leading to end-stage renal failure. Pediatr Nephrol 9:74–76, 1995; see comments.
239. Torralbo A, Pina E, Portolés J, et al: Renal magnesium wasting with hypercalciuria, nephrocalcinosis and ocular disorders. Nephron 69:472–475, 1995.
240. Runeberg L, Collan Y, Jokinen EJ, et al: Hypomagnesemia due to renal disease of unknown etiology. Am J Med 59:873–881, 1975.
241. Ulmann A, Hadj S, Lacour B, et al: Renal magnesium and phosphate wastage in a patient with hypercalciuria and nephrocalcinosis: Effect of oral phosphorus and magnesium supplements. Nephron 40:83–87, 1985.
242. Agus ZS: Hypomagnesemia. J Am Soc Nephrol 10:1616–1622, 1999.
243. Simon DB, Lu Y, Choate KA, et al: Paracellin-1, a renal tight junction protein required for paracellular $Mg^{2+}$ resorption. Science 285:103–106, 1999; see comments.
244. Gitelman HJ, Graham JB, Welt LG: A new familial disorder characterized by hypokalemia and hypomagnesemia. Trans Assoc Am Physicians 79:221–235, 1966.
245. Bettinelli A, Bianchetti MG, Girardin E, et al: Use of calcium excretion values to distinguish two forms of primary renal tubular hypokalemic alkalosis: Bartter and Gitelman syndromes. J Pediatr 120:38–43, 1992; see comments.
246. Kurtz I: Molecular pathogenesis of Bartter's and Gitelman's syndromes [clinical conference]. Kidney Int 54:1396–1410, 1998.
247. Bettinelli A, Basilico E, Metta MG, et al: Magnesium supplementation in Gitelman syndrome. Pediatr Nephrol 13:311–314, 1999.
248. Pollak MR, Delaney VB, Graham RM, et al: Gitelman's syndrome (Bartter's variant) maps to the thiazide-sensitive cotransporter gene locus on chromosome 16q13 in a large kindred. J Am Soc Nephrol 7:2244–2248, 1996.
249. Simon DB, Lifton RP: The molecular basis of inherited hypokalemic alkalosis: Bartter's and Gitelman's syndromes. Am J Physiol 271:F961–F966, 1996.
250. Takeuchi K, Kure S, Kato T, et al: Association of a mutation in thiazide-sensitive Na-Cl cotransporter with familial Gitelman's syndrome. J Clin Endocrinol Metab 81:4496–4499, 1996.
251. Mastroianni N, Bettinelli A, Bianchetti M, et al: Novel molecular variants of the Na-Cl cotransporter gene are responsible for Gitelman syndrome. Am J Hum Genet 59:1019–1026, 1996.
252. Lemmink HH, Knoers NV, Károlyi L, et al: Novel mutations in the thiazide-sensitive NaCl cotransporter gene in patients with Gitelman syndrome with predominant localization to the C-terminal domain. Kidney Int 54:720–730, 1998.
253. Kunchaparty S, Palcso M, Berkman J, et al: Defective processing and expression of thiazide-sensitive Na-Cl cotransporter as a cause of Gitelman's syndrome. Am J Physiol 277:F643–F649, 1999.
254. Károlyi L, Ziegler A, Pollak M, et al: Gitelman's syndrome is genetically distinct from other forms of Bartter's syndrome. Pediatr Nephrol 10:551–554, 1996.
255. Bundy JT, Connito D, Mahoney MD, et al: Treatment of idiopathic renal magnesium wasting with amiloride. Am J Nephrol 15:75–77, 1995.
256. Geven WB, Monnens LA, Willems HL, et al: Renal magnesium wasting in two families with autosomal dominant inheritance. Kidney Int 31:1140–1144, 1987.
257. Freeman RM, Pearson E: Hypomagnesemia of unknown etiology. Am J Med 41:645–656, 1966.
258. Meij IC, Saar K, van den Heuvel LP, et al: Hereditary isolated renal magnesium loss maps to chromosome 11q23. Am J Hum Genet 64:180–188, 1999.
259. Elisaf M, Merkouropoulos M, Tsianos EV, et al: Pathogenetic mechanisms of hypomagnesemia in alcoholic patients. J Trace Elem Med Biol 9:210–214, 1995.
260. Leary WP, Reyes AJ, Wynne RD, et al: Renal excretory actions of furosemide, of hydrochlorothiazide and of the vasodilator flosequinan in healthy subjects. J Int Med Res 18:120–141, 1990.
261. Quamme GA: Effect of furosemide on calcium and magnesium transport in the rat nephron. Am J Physiol 241:F340–F347, 1981.
262. Dai LJ, Friedman PA, Quamme GA: Cellular mechanisms of chlorothiazide and cellular potassium depletion on $Mg^{2+}$ uptake in mouse distal convoluted tubule cells. Kidney Int 51: 1008–1017, 1997.
263. Davies DL, Fraser R: Do diuretics cause magnesium deficiency? Br J Clin Pharmacol 36:1–10, 1993.
264. McInnes GT, Yeo WW, Ramsay LE, et al: Cardiotoxicity and diuretics: Much speculation—little substance [editorial]. J Hypertens 10:317–325, 1992; erratum in J Hypertens 10:following H24, 1992.
265. Martin BJ, Milligan K: Diuretic-associated hypomagnesemia in the elderly. Arch Intern Med 147:1768–1771, 1987.
266. Wilkinson R, Lucas GL, Heath DA, et al: Hypomagnesaemic tetany associated with prolonged treatment with aminoglycosides. BMJ 292:818–819, 1986.
267. Keating MJ, Sethi MR, Bodey GP, et al: Hypocalcemia with hypoparathyroidism and renal tubular dysfunction associated with aminoglycoside therapy. Cancer 39:1410–1414, 1977.
268. Bar RS, Wilson HE, Mazzaferri EL: Hypomagnesemic hypocalcemia secondary to renal magnesium wasting. Ann Intern Med 82:646–649, 1975.
269. Shah GM, Kirschenbaum MA: Renal magnesium wasting associated with therapeutic agents. Miner Electrolyte Metab 17:58–64, 1991.
270. Foster JE, Harpur ES, Garland HO: An investigation of the acute effect of gentamicin on the renal handling of electrolytes in the rat. J Pharmacol Exp Ther 261:38–43, 1992.
271. Barton CH, Pahl M, Vaziri ND, et al: Renal magnesium wasting associated with amphotericin B therapy. Am J Med 77:471–474, 1984.

272. Clark AD, McKendrick S, Tansey PJ, et al: A comparative analysis of lipid-complexed and liposomal amphotericin B preparations in haematological oncology. Br J Haematol 103:198–204, 1998; erratum in Br J Haematol 103:1215, 1998.
273. Walsh TJ, Finberg RW, Arndt C, et al: Liposomal amphotericin B for empirical therapy in patients with persistent fever and neutropenia. National Institute of Allergy and Infectious Diseases Mycoses Study Group. N Engl J Med 340:764–771, 1999.
274. Llanos A, Cieza J, Bernardo J, et al: Effect of salt supplementation on amphotericin B nephrotoxicity. Kidney Int 40:302–308, 1991.
275. Shah GM, Alvarado P, Kirschenbaum MA: Symptomatic hypocalcemia and hypomagnesemia with renal magnesium wasting associated with pentamidine therapy in a patient with AIDS. Am J Med 89:380–382, 1990.
276. Wharton JM, Demopulos PA, Goldschlager N: Torsade de pointes during administration of pentamidine isethionate. Am J Med 83:571–576, 1987.
277. Burnett RJ, Reents SB: Severe hypomagnesemia induced by pentamidine. DICP 24:239–240, 1990.
278. Gradon JD, Fricchione L, Sepkowitz D: Severe hypomagnesemia associated with pentamidine therapy. Rev Infect Dis 13: 511–512, 1991.
279. Palestine AG, Polis MA, De Smet MD, et al: A randomized, controlled trial of foscarnet in the treatment of cytomegalovirus retinitis in patients with AIDS. Ann Intern Med 115: 665–673, 1991; see comments.
280. Schilsky RL, Anderson T: Hypomagnesemia and renal magnesium wasting in patients receiving cisplatin. Ann Intern Med 90:929–931, 1979.
281. Daugaard G, Abildgaard U, Holstein-Rathlou NH, et al: Renal tubular function in patients treated with high-dose cisplatin. Clin Pharmacol Ther 44:164–172, 1988.
282. Lam M, Adelstein DJ: Hypomagnesemia and renal magnesium wasting in patients treated with cisplatin. Am J Kidney Dis 8: 164–169, 1986.
283. Ariceta G, Rodriguez-Soriano J, Vallo A, et al: Acute and chronic effects of cisplatin therapy on renal magnesium homeostasis. Med Pediatr Oncol 28:35–40, 1997.
284. Bokemeyer C, Fels LM, Dunn T, et al: Silibinin protects against cisplatin-induced nephrotoxicity without compromising cisplatin or ifosfamide anti-tumour activity. Br J Cancer 74:2036–2041, 1996.
285. Gaedeke J, Fels LM, Bokemeyer C, et al: Cisplatin nephrotoxicity and protection by silibinin. Nephrol Dial Transplant 11: 55–62, 1996.
286. English MW, Skinner R, Pearson AD, et al: Dose-related nephrotoxicity of carboplatin in children. Br J Cancer 81:336–341, 1999.
287. Ettinger LJ, Gaynon PS, Krailo MD, et al: A phase II study of carboplatin in children with recurrent or progressive solid tumors: A report from the Children's Cancer Group. Cancer 73:1297–1301, 1994.
288. Barton CH, Vaziri ND, Martin DC, et al: Hypomagnesemia and renal magnesium wasting in renal transplant recipients receiving cyclosporine. Am J Med 83:693–699, 1987.
289. Vannini SD, Mazzola BL, Rodoni L, et al: Permanently reduced plasma ionized magnesium among renal transplant recipients on cyclosporine. Transpl Int 12:244–249, 1999.
290. June CH, Thompson CB, Kennedy MS, et al: Profound hypomagnesemia and renal magnesium wasting associated with the use of cyclosporine for marrow transplantation. Transplantation 39:620–624, 1985.
291. Nozue T, Kobayashi A, Kodama T, et al: Pathogenesis of cyclosporine-induced hypomagnesemia. J Pediatr 120:638–640, 1992.
292. Barton CH, Vaziri ND, Mina-Araghi S, et al: Effects of cyclosporine on magnesium metabolism in rats. J Lab Clin Med 114: 232–236, 1989; see comments.
293. Mather HM, Nisbet JA, Burton GH, et al: Hypomagnesaemia in diabetes. Clin Chim Acta 95:235–242, 1979.
294. Sjogren A, Floren CH, Nilsson A: Magnesium deficiency in IDDM related to level of glycosylated hemoglobin. Diabetes 35: 459–463, 1986.
295. McNair P, Christensen MS, Christiansen C, et al: Renal hypomagnesaemia in human diabetes mellitus: Its relation to glucose homeostasis. Eur J Clin Invest 12:81–85, 1982.
296. Ponder SW, Brouhard BH, Travis LB: Hyperphosphaturia and hypermagnesuria in children with IDDM. Diabetes Care 13: 437–441, 1990.
297. Mikhail N, Ehsanipoor K: Ionized serum magnesium in type 2 diabetes mellitus: Its correlation with total serum magnesium and hemoglobin A1c levels. South Med J 92:1162–1166, 1999.
298. Resnick LM, Altura BT, Gupta RK, et al: Intracellular and extracellular magnesium depletion in type 2 (non-insulin-dependent) diabetes mellitus. Diabetologia 36:767–770, 1993.
299. Dai LJ, Ritchie G, Bapty BW, et al: Insulin stimulates $Mg^{2+}$ uptake in mouse distal convoluted tubule cells. Am J Physiol 277:F907–F913, 1999.
300. Martin HE, Smith K, Wilson ML: The fluid and electrolyte therapy of severe diabetic acidosis and ketosis. Am J Med 24: 376–389, 1958.
301. Jones JE, Desper PC, Shane SR, et al: Magnesium metabolism in hyperthyroidism and hypothyroidism. J Clin Invest 45:891–900, 1966.
302. Mader IJ, Iseri LT: Spontaneous hypomagnesemia, alkalosis and tetany due to secretion of corticosterone-like mineralocorticoids. Am J Med 19:976–988, 1955.
303. Sutton RA: Plasma magnesium concentration in primary hyperparathyroidism. BMJ 1:529–533, 1970.
304. Frisch LS, Mimouni F: Hypomagnesemia following correction of metabolic acidosis: A case of hungry bones. J Am Coll Nutr 12:710–713, 1993.
305. Heaton FW, Pyrah LN: Magnesium metabolism in patients with parathyroid disorders. Clin Sci 25:475–485, 1963.
306. Whang R, Oei TO, Aikawa JK, et al: Predictors of clinical hypomagnesemia: Hypokalemia, hypophosphatemia, hyponatremia, and hypocalcemia. Arch Intern Med 144:1794–1796, 1984.
307. Kreusser WJ, Kurokawa K, Aznar E, et al: Effect of phosphate depletion on magnesium homeostasis in rats. J Clin Invest 61: 573–581, 1978.
308. Kelepouris E, Agus ZS: Hypomagnesemia: Renal magnesium handling. Semin Nephrol 18:58–73, 1998.
309. England MR, Gordon G, Salem M, et al: Magnesium administration and dysrhythmias after cardiac surgery: A placebo-controlled, double-blind, randomized trial. JAMA 268:2395–2402, 1992; see comments.
310. Speziale G, Ruvolo G, Fattouch K, et al: Arrhythmia prophylaxis after coronary artery bypass grafting: Regimens of magnesium sulfate administration. Thorac Cardiovasc Surg 48:22–26, 2000.
311. Yurvati AH, Sanders SP, Dullye LJ, et al: Antiarrhythmic response to intravenously administered magnesium after cardiac surgery. South Med J 85:714–717, 1992.
312. McLellan BA, Reid SR, Lane PL: Massive blood transfusion causing hypomagnesemia. Crit Care Med 12:146–147, 1984.
313. Broughton A, Anderson IR, Bowden CH: Magnesium-deficiency syndrome in burns. Lancet 2:1156–1158, 1968.
314. Greenwald JH, Dubin A, Cardon L: Hypomagnesemic tetany due to excessive lactation. Am J Med 35:845–860, 1963.
315. Varon ME, Sherer DM, Abramowicz JS, et al: Maternal ventricular tachycardia associated with hypomagnesemia. Am J Obstet Gynecol 167:1352–1355, 1992.
316. Alfrey AC, Miller NL, Butkus D: Evaluation of body magnesium stores. J Lab Clin Med 84:153–162, 1974.
317. Dyckner T, Wester PO: The relation between extra- and intracellular electrolytes in patients with hypokalemia and/or diuretic treatment. Acta Med Scand 204:269–282, 1978.
318. Cohen L, Kitzes R: Magnesium sulfate and digitalis-toxic arrhythmias. JAMA 249:2808–2810, 1983.
319. Ryzen E, Elkayam U, Rude RK: Low blood mononuclear cell magnesium in intensive cardiac care unit patients. Am Heart J 111:475–480, 1986.
320. Elin RJ, Hosseini JM: Magnesium content of mononuclear blood cells. Clin Chem 31:377–380, 1985.
321. Ladefoged K, Hagen K: Correlation between concentrations of magnesium, zinc, and potassium in plasma, erythrocytes and muscles. Clin Chim Acta 177:157–166, 1988.
322. Elin RJ: Assessment of magnesium status. Clin Chem 33:1965–1970, 1987.

323. Wong NL, Sutton RA, Dirks JH: Is lymphocyte magnesium concentration a reflection of intracellular magnesium concentration? J Lab Clin Med 112:721–726, 1988.
324. Ryan MP, Ryan MF, Counihan TB: The effect of diuretics on lymphocyte magnesium and potassium. Acta Med Scand Suppl 647:153–161, 1981.
325. Greenway DC, Hindmarsh JT, Wang J, et al: Reference interval for whole blood ionized magnesium in a healthy population and the stability of ionized magnesium under varied laboratory conditions. Clin Biochem 29:515–520, 1996.
326. Elin RJ, Hristova EN, Cecco SA, et al: Comparison of precision and effect of pH and calcium on the AVL and NOVA magnesium ion-selective electrodes. Scand J Clin Lab Invest Suppl 224:203–210, 1996.
327. Kulpmann WR, Gerlach M: Relationship between ionized and total magnesium in serum. Scand J Clin Lab Invest Suppl 224: 251–258, 1996.
328. Kroll MH, Elin RJ: Relationships between magnesium and protein concentrations in serum. Clin Chem 31:244–246, 1985.
329. Kulpmann WR, Rossler J, Brunkhorst R, et al: Ionised and total magnesium serum concentrations in renal and hepatic diseases. Eur J Clin Chem Clin Biochem 34:257–264, 1996.
330. Saha H, Harmoinen A, Karvonen AL, et al: Serum ionized versus total magnesium in patients with intestinal or liver disease. Clin Chem Lab Med 36:715–718, 1998.
331. Sanders GT, Huijgen HJ, Sanders R: Magnesium in disease: A review with special emphasis on the serum ionized magnesium. Clin Chem Lab Med 37:1011–1033, 1999.
332. Ryzen E, Elbaum N, Singer FR, et al: Parenteral magnesium tolerance testing in the evaluation of magnesium deficiency. Magnesium 4:137–147, 1985; erratum in Magnesium 6:168, 1987.
333. Hebert P, Mehta N, Wang J, et al: Functional magnesium deficiency in critically ill patients identified using a magnesium-loading test. Crit Care Med 25:749–755, 1997.
334. Gullestad L, Midtvedt K, Dolva LO, et al: The magnesium loading test: Reference values in healthy subjects. Scand J Clin Lab Invest 54:23–31, 1994.
335. Elisaf M, Panteli K, Theodorou J, et al: Fractional excretion of magnesium in normal subjects and in patients with hypomagnesemia. Magnes Res 10:315–320, 1997.
336. Ryan MP: Diuretics and potassium/magnesium depletion: Directions for treatment. Am J Med 82:38–47, 1987.
337. Franse LV, Pahor M, Di Bari M, et al: Hypokalemia associated with diuretic use and cardiovascular events in the Systolic Hypertension in the Elderly Program. Hypertension 35:1025–1030, 2000; see comments.
338. Gitelman HJ, Graham JB, Welt LG: A familial disorder characterized by hypokalemia and hypomagnesemia. Ann N Y Acad Sci 162:856–864, 1969.
339. Shils ME: Experimental human magnesium depletion. Medicine 48:61–85, 1969.
340. Boyd JC, Bruns DE, DiMarco JP, et al: Relationship of potassium and magnesium concentrations in serum to cardiac arrhythmias. Clin Chem 30:754–757, 1984.
341. Whang R, Ryder KW: Frequency of hypomagnesemia and hypermagnesemia: Requested vs routine. JAMA 263:3063–3064, 1990; see comments.
342. Whang R, Morosi HJ, Rodgers D, et al: The influence of sustained magnesium deficiency on muscle potassium repletion. J Lab Clin Med 70:895–902, 1967.
343. Dorup I, Clausen T: Correlation between magnesium and potassium contents in muscle: Role of Na(+)-K+ pump. Am J Physiol 264:C457–C463, 1993.
344. Kelepouris E, Kasama R, Agus ZS: Effects of intracellular magnesium on calcium, potassium and chloride channels. Miner Electrolyte Metab 19:277–281, 1993.
345. Matsuda H: Open-state substructure of inwardly rectifying potassium channels revealed by magnesium block in guinea-pig heart cells. J Physiol 397:237–258, 1988.
346. Nichols CG, Ho K, Hebert S: Mg(2+)-dependent inward rectification of ROMK1 potassium channels expressed in *Xenopus* oocytes. J Physiol 476:399–409, 1994.
347. Whang R, Whang DD, Ryan MP: Refractory potassium repletion: A consequence of magnesium deficiency. Arch Intern Med 152:40–45, 1992; see comments.
348. Fatemi S, Ryzen E, Flores J, et al: Effect of experimental human magnesium depletion on parathyroid hormone secretion and 1,25-dihydroxyvitamin D metabolism. J Clin Endocrinol Metab 73:1067–1072, 1991.
349. Rude RK, Oldham SB, Singer FR: Functional hypoparathyroidism and parathyroid hormone end-organ resistance in human magnesium deficiency. Clin Endocrinol 5:209–224, 1976.
350. Chase LR, Slatopolsky E: Secretion and metabolic efficacy of parathyroid hormone in patients with severe hypomagnesemia. J Clin Endocrinol Metab 38:363–371, 1974.
351. Anast CS, Winnacker JL, Forte LR, et al: Impaired release of parathyroid hormone in magnesium deficiency. J Clin Endocrinol Metab 42:707–717, 1976.
352. Estep H, Shaw WA, Watlington C, et al: Hypocalcemia due to hypomagnesemia and reversible parathyroid hormone unresponsiveness. J Clin Endocrinol Metab 29:842–848, 1969.
353. Freitag JJ, Martin KJ, Conrades MB, et al: Evidence for skeletal resistance to parathyroid hormone in magnesium deficiency: Studies in isolated perfused bone. J Clin Invest 64:1238–1244, 1979.
354. Rude RK, Adams JS, Ryzen E, et al: Low serum concentrations of 1,25-dihydroxyvitamin D in human magnesium deficiency. J Clin Endocrinol Metab 61:933–940, 1985.
355. Kingston ME, Al-Siba'i MB, Skooge WC: Clinical manifestations of hypomagnesemia. Crit Care Med 14:950–954, 1986.
356. Wacker WEC, Moore FD, Ulmer DD, et al: Normocalcemic magnesium deficiency tetany. JAMA 180:161–163, 1962.
357. Vallee BL, Warren EC, Wacker WEC, et al: The magnesium-deficiency tetany syndrome in man. N Engl J Med 262:155–161, 1960.
358. Hanna S, Harrison M, MacIntyre I, et al: The syndrome of magnesium deficiency in man. Lancet 2:172–175, 1960.
359. Hall RC, Joffe JR: Hypomagnesemia: Physical and psychiatric symptoms. JAMA 224:1749–1751, 1973.
360. Leicher CR, Mezoff AG, Hyams JS: Focal cerebral deficits in severe hypomagnesemia. Pediatr Neurol 7:380–381, 1991.
361. Stendig-Lindberg G, Bergstrom J, Hultman E: Hypomagnesaemia and muscle electrolytes and metabolites. Acta Med Scand 201:273–280, 1977.
362. Dhingra S, Solven F, Wilson A, et al: Hypomagnesemia and respiratory muscle power. Am Rev Respir Dis 129:497–498, 1984.
363. Frankenhauser B, Meves H: Effect of magnesium and calcium on frog myelinated nerve fiber. J Physiol 142:360–365, 1958.
364. Meissner G, Darling E, Eveleth J: Kinetics of rapid $Ca^{2+}$ release by sarcoplasmic reticulum: Effects of $Ca^{2+}$, $Mg^{2+}$, and adenine nucleotides. Biochemistry 25:236–244, 1986.
365. Stephenson EW: Magnesium effects on activation of skinned fibers from striated muscle. Fed Proc 40:2662–2666, 1981.
366. Arsenian MA: Magnesium and cardiovascular disease. Prog Cardiovasc Dis 35:271–310, 1993.
367. Loeb HS, Pietras RJ, Gunnar RM, et al: Paroxysmal ventricular fibrillation in two patients with hypomagnesemia. Circulation 37:210–215, 1968.
368. Seta K, Kleiger R, Hellerstein EE, et al: Effect of potassium and magnesium deficiency on the electrocardiogram and plasma electrolytes of pure-bred beagles. Am J Cardiol 17:516–519, 1966.
369. Tsuji H, Venditti FJJ, Evans JC, et al: The associations of levels of serum potassium and magnesium with ventricular premature complexes (the Framingham Heart Study). Am J Cardiol 74: 232–235, 1994.
370. Ramee SR, White CJ, Svinarich JT, et al: Torsade de pointes and magnesium deficiency. Am Heart J 109:164–167, 1985.
371. Levine SR, Crowley TJ, Hai HA: Hypomagnesemia and ventricular tachycardia: A complication of ulcerative colitis and parenteral hyperalimentation in a nondigitalized noncardiac patient. Chest 81:244–247, 1982.
372. Topol EJ, Lerman BB: Hypomagnesemic torsades de pointes. Am J Cardiol 52:1367–1368, 1983.
373. Seller RH: The role of magnesium in digitalis toxicity. Am Heart J 82:551–556, 1971.
374. Vitale JJ, Velez H, Guzman C, et al: Magnesium deficiency in the cebus monkey. Circ Res 12:642–650, 1963.
375. Whang R, Oei TO, Watanabe A: Frequency of hypomagnesemia

in hospitalized patients receiving digitalis. Arch Intern Med 145:655–656, 1985.
376. Gottlieb SS, Baruch L, Kukin ML, et al: Prognostic importance of the serum magnesium concentration in patients with congestive heart failure. J Am Coll Cardiol 16:827–831, 1990.
377. Sueta CA, Patterson JH, Adams KFJ: Antiarrhythmic action of pharmacological administration of magnesium in heart failure: A critical review of new data. Magnes Res 8:389–401, 1995.
378. Ceremuzynski L, Gebalska J, Wolk R, et al: Hypomagnesemia in heart failure with ventricular arrhythmias: Beneficial effects of magnesium supplementation. J Intern Med 247:78–86, 2000.
379. Gottlieb SS, Fisher ML, Pressel MD, et al: Effects of intravenous magnesium sulfate on arrhythmias in patients with congestive heart failure. Am Heart J 125:1645–1650, 1993.
380. Sueta CA, Clarke SW, Dunlap SH, et al: Effect of acute magnesium administration on the frequency of ventricular arrhythmia in patients with heart failure. Circulation 89:660–666, 1994; see comments.
381. Cohen L, Kitzes R, Shnaider H: Multifocal atrial tachycardia responsive to parenteral magnesium. Magnes Res 1:239–242, 1988.
382. Dyckner T: Serum magnesium in acute myocardial infarction: Relation to arrhythmias. Acta Med Scand 207:59–66, 1980.
383. Rasmussen HS, McNair P, Goransson L, et al: Magnesium deficiency in patients with ischemic heart disease with and without acute myocardial infarction uncovered by an intravenous loading test. Arch Intern Med 148:329–332, 1988.
384. Komori S, Li B, Matsumura K, et al: Antiarrhythmic effect of magnesium sulfate against occlusion-induced arrhythmias and reperfusion-induced arrhythmias in anesthetized rats. Mol Cell Biochem 199:201–208, 1999.
385. Anonymous: ISIS-4: A randomised factorial trial assessing early oral captopril, oral mononitrate, and intravenous magnesium sulphate in 58,050 patients with suspected acute myocardial infarction. ISIS-4 (Fourth International Study of Infarct Survival) Collaborative Group. Lancet 345:669–685, 1995; see comments.
386. Gyamlani G, Parikh C, Kulkarni AG: Benefits of magnesium in acute myocardial infarction: Timing is crucial. Am Heart J 139: 703, 2000.
387. Raghu C, Peddeswara Rao P, Seshagiri Rao D: Protective effect of intravenous magnesium in acute myocardial infarction following thrombolytic therapy. Int J Cardiol 71:209–215, 1999; see comments.
388. Woods KL, Fletcher S, Roffe C, et al: Intravenous magnesium sulphate in suspected acute myocardial infarction: Results of the second Leicester Intravenous Magnesium Intervention Trial (LIMIT-2). Lancet 339:1553–1558, 1992; see comments.
389. Rasmussen HS, Suenson M, McNair P, et al: Magnesium infusion reduces the incidence of arrhythmias in acute myocardial infarction: A double-blind placebo-controlled study. Clin Cardiol 10:351–356, 1987.
390. Smith LF, Heagerty AM, Bing RF, et al: Intravenous infusion of magnesium sulphate after acute myocardial infarction: Effects on arrhythmias and mortality. Int J Cardiol 12:175–183, 1986.
391. Horner SM: Efficacy of intravenous magnesium in acute myocardial infarction in reducing arrhythmias and mortality: Meta-analysis of magnesium in acute myocardial infarction. Circulation 86:774–779, 1992.
392. Anonymous: Rationale and design of the magnesium in coronaries (MAGIC) study: A clinical trial to reevaluate the efficacy of early administration of magnesium in acute myocardial infarction. The MAGIC Steering Committee. Am Heart J 139: 10–14, 2000.
393. Dorman BH, Sade RM, Burnette JS, et al: Magnesium supplementation in the prevention of arrhythmias in pediatric patients undergoing surgery for congenital heart defects. Am Heart J 139:522–528, 2000.
394. Solomon AJ, Berger AK, Trivedi KK, et al: The combination of propranolol and magnesium does not prevent postoperative atrial fibrillation. Ann Thorac Surg 69:126–129, 2000.
395. Kulick DL, Hong R, Ryzen E, et al: Electrophysiologic effects of intravenous magnesium in patients with normal conduction systems and no clinical evidence of significant cardiac disease. Am Heart J 115:367–373, 1988.
396. Singh RB, Niaz MA, Moshiri M, et al: Magnesium status and risk of coronary artery disease in rural and urban populations with variable magnesium consumption. Magnes Res 10:205–213, 1997.
397. Neri LC, Johansen HL: Water hardness and cardiovascular mortality. Ann N Y Acad Sci 304:203–221, 1978.
398. Altura BT, Brust M, Bloom S, et al: Magnesium dietary intake modulates blood lipid levels and atherogenesis. Proc Natl Acad Sci U S A 87:1840–1844, 1990.
399. Maheswaran R, Morris S, Falconer S, et al: Magnesium in drinking water supplies and mortality from acute myocardial infarction in north west England. Heart 82:455–460, 1999.
400. Elwood PC, Fehily AM, Ising H, et al: Dietary magnesium does not predict ischaemic heart disease in the Caerphilly cohort. Eur J Clin Nutr 50:694–697, 1996.
401. Liao F, Folsom AR, Brancati FL: Is low magnesium concentration a risk factor for coronary heart disease? The Atherosclerosis Risk in Communities (ARIC) Study. Am Heart J 136:480–490, 1998.
402. Vitale JJ, Hellerstein EE, Nakamura M, et al: Effects of magnesium-deficient diet upon puppies. Circ Res 9:387–394, 1961.
403. Rayssiguier Y, Gueux E, Bussiere L, et al: Dietary magnesium affects susceptibility of lipoproteins and tissues to peroxidation in rats. J Am Coll Nutr 12:133–137, 1993.
404. Rayssiguier Y, Gueux E: Magnesium and lipids in cardiovascular disease. J Am Coll Nutr 5:507–519, 1986.
405. Nassir F, Mazur A, Giannoni F, et al: Magnesium deficiency modulates hepatic lipogenesis and apolipoprotein gene expression in the rat. Biochim Biophys Acta 1257:125–132, 1995.
406. Bussiere L, Mazur A, Gueux E, et al: Triglyceride-rich lipoproteins from magnesium-deficient rats are more susceptible to oxidation by cells and promote proliferation of cultured vascular smooth muscle cells. Magnes Res 8:151–157, 1995.
407. Turlapaty PD, Altura BM: Magnesium deficiency produces spasms of coronary arteries: Relationship to etiology of sudden death ischemic heart disease. Science 208:198–200, 1980.
408. Goto K, Yasue H, Okumura K, et al: Magnesium deficiency detected by intravenous loading test in variant angina pectoris. Am J Cardiol 65:709–712, 1990.
409. Igawa A, Miwa K, Miyagi Y, et al: Comparison of frequency of magnesium deficiency in patients with vasospastic angina and fixed coronary artery disease. Am J Cardiol 75:728–731, 1995.
410. Kugiyama K, Yasue H, Okumura K, et al: Suppression of exercise-induced angina by magnesium sulfate in patients with variant angina. J Am Coll Cardiol 12:1177–1183, 1988.
411. Cohen L, Kitzes R: Magnesium sulfate in the treatment of variant angina. Magnesium 3:46–49, 1984.
412. Cohen L, Kitzes R: Prompt termination and/or prevention of cold-pressor-stimulus-induced vasoconstriction of different vascular beds by magnesium sulfate in patients with Prinzmetal's angina. Magnesium 5:144–149, 1986.
413. Nadler JL, Malayan S, Luong H, et al: Intracellular free magnesium deficiency plays a key role in increased platelet reactivity in type II diabetes mellitus. Diabetes Care 15:835–841, 1992; see comments.
414. Hwang DL, Yen CF, Nadler JL: Effect of extracellular magnesium on platelet activation and intracellular calcium mobilization. Am J Hypertens 5:700–706, 1992.
415. Chang C, Varghese PJ, Downey J, et al: Magnesium deficiency and myocardial infarct size in the dog. J Am Coll Cardiol 5: 280–289, 1985.
416. Woods KL, Fletcher S: Long-term outcome after intravenous magnesium sulphate in suspected acute myocardial infarction: The second Leicester Intravenous Magnesium Intervention Trial (LIMIT-2). Lancet 343:816–819, 1994; see comments.
417. Seelig MS, Elin RJ, Antman EM: Magnesium in acute myocardial infarction: Still an open question. Can J Cardiol 14:745–749, 1998.
418. Resnick LM, Gupta RK, Laragh JH: Intracellular free magnesium in erythrocytes of essential hypertension: Relation to blood pressure and serum divalent cations. Proc Natl Acad Sci U S A 81:6511–6515, 1984.
419. Sasaki S, Oshima T, Matsuura H, et al: Abnormal magnesium status in patients with cardiovascular diseases. Clin Sci (Colch) 98:175–181, 2000.

420. Petersen B, Schroll M, Christiansen C, et al: Serum and erythrocyte magnesium in normal elderly Danish people: Relationship to blood pressure and serum lipids. Acta Med Scand 201: 31–34, 1977.
421. Dyckner T, Wester PO: Effect of magnesium on blood pressure. BMJ 286:1847–1849, 1983.
422. Henderson DG, Schierup J, Schodt T: Effect of magnesium supplementation on blood pressure and electrolyte concentrations in hypertensive patients receiving long term diuretic treatment. BMJ 293:664–665, 1986.
423. Cappuccio FP, Markandu ND, Beynon GW, et al: Lack of effect of oral magnesium on high blood pressure: A double blind study. BMJ 291:235–238, 1985.
424. Freeman JB, Wittine MF, Stegink LD, et al: Effects of magnesium infusions on magnesium and nitrogen balance during parenteral nutrition. Can J Surg 25:570–572, 574, 1982.
425. Wazny LD, Brophy DF: Amiloride for the prevention of amphotericin B–induced hypokalemia and hypomagnesemia. Ann Pharmacother 34:94–97, 2000.
426. Purnell J, Houghton DC, Porter GA, et al: Effect of amiloride on experimental gentamicin nephrotoxicity. Nephron 40:166–170, 1985.
427. Flink EB: Therapy of magnesium deficiency. Ann N Y Acad Sci 162:901–905, 1969.
428. al-Ghamdi SM, Cameron EC, Sutton RA: Magnesium deficiency: Pathophysiologic and clinical overview. Am J Kidney Dis 24:737–752, 1994; see comments.
429. Ryzen E: Magnesium homeostasis in critically ill patients. Magnesium 8:201–212, 1989.
430. Ryzen E, Nelson TA, Rude RK: Low blood mononuclear cell magnesium content and hypocalcemia in normomagnesemic patients. West J Med 147:549–553, 1987.
431. White J, Massey L, Gales SK, et al: Blood and urinary magnesium kinetics after oral magnesium supplements. Clin Ther 14: 678–687, 1992.
432. Fine KD, Santa Ana CA, Porter JL, et al: Intestinal absorption of magnesium from food and supplements. J Clin Invest 88: 396–402, 1991.
433. Colussi G, Rombola G, De Ferrari ME, et al: Correction of hypokalemia with antialdosterone therapy in Gitelman's syndrome. Am J Nephrol 14:127–135, 1994.
434. Randall REJ, Cohen MD, Spray CSJ, et al: Hypermagnesemia in renal failure: Etiology and toxic manifestations. Ann Intern Med 61:73–88, 1964.
435. Popovtzer MM, Schainuck LI, Massry SG, et al: Divalent ion excretion in chronic kidney disease: Relation to degree of renal insufficiency. Clin Sci 38:297–307, 1970.
436. Schelling JR: Fatal hypermagnesemia. Clin Nephrol 53:61–65, 2000.
437. Clark BA, Brown RS: Unsuspected morbid hypermagnesemia in elderly patients. Am J Nephrol 12:336–343, 1992.
438. Smilkstein MJ, Steedle D, Kulig KW, et al: Magnesium levels after magnesium-containing cathartics. J Toxicol Clin Toxicol 26:51–65, 1988.
439. McLaughlin SA, McKinney PE: Antacid-induced hypermagnesemia in a patient with normal renal function and bowel obstruction. Ann Pharmacother 32:312–315, 1998.
440. Mordes JP, Swartz R, Arky RA: Extreme hypermagnesemia as a cause of refractory hypotension. Ann Intern Med 83:657–658, 1975.
441. Mordes JP, Wacker WE: Excess magnesium. Pharmacol Rev 29: 273–300, 1977.
442. Mayan H, Hourvitz A, Schiff E, et al: Symptomatic hypocalcaemia in hypermagnesaemia-induced hypoparathyroidism, during magnesium tocolytic therapy—possible involvement of the calcium-sensing receptor. Nephrol Dial Transplant 14:1764–1766, 1999.
443. Eisenbud E, LoBue CC: Hypocalcemia after therapeutic use of magnesium sulfate. Arch Intern Med 136:688–691, 1976.
444. Monif GR, Savory J: Iatrogenic maternal hypocalcemia following magnesium sulfate therapy. JAMA 219:1469–1470, 1972.
445. Mehrotra R, Nolph KD, Kathuria P, et al: Hypokalemic metabolic alkalosis with hypomagnesuric hypermagnesemia and severe hypocalciuria: A new syndrome? Am J Kidney Dis 29: 106–114, 1997.
446. Mellerup ET, Plenge P: Lithium effects on magnesium, calcium, and phosphate metabolism in rats. Int Pharmacopsychiatry 11:190–195, 1976.
447. Eshleman SH, Shaw LM: Massive theophylline overdose with atypical metabolic abnormalities. Clin Chem 36:398–399, 1990.
448. Altura BM, Altura BT, Carella A, et al: $Mg^{2+}$-$Ca^{2+}$ interaction in contractility of vascular smooth muscle: $Mg^{2+}$ versus organic calcium channel blockers on myogenic tone and agonist-induced responsiveness of blood vessels. Can J Physiol Pharmacol 65:729–745, 1987.
449. Nadler JL, Goodson S, Rude RK: Evidence that prostacyclin mediates the vascular action of magnesium in humans. Hypertension 9:379–383, 1987.
450. Qureshi T, Melonakos TK: Acute hypermagnesemia after laxative use. Ann Emerg Med 28:552–555, 1996.
451. Fassler CA, Rodriguez RM, Badesch DB, et al: Magnesium toxicity as a cause of hypotension and hypoventilation: Occurrence in patients with normal renal function. Arch Intern Med 145:1604–1606, 1985.
452. DiCarlo LAJ, Morady F, de Buitleir M, et al: Effects of magnesium sulfate on cardiac conduction and refractoriness in humans. J Am Coll Cardiol 7:1356–1362, 1986.
453. Berns AS, Kollmeyer KR: Magnesium-induced bradycardia [letter]. Ann Intern Med 85:760–761, 1976.
454. Swift TR: Weakness from magnesium-containing cathartics: Electrophysiologic studies. Muscle Nerve 2:295–298, 1979.
455. Castelbaum AR, Donofrio PD, Walker FO, et al: Laxative abuse causing hypermagnesemia, quadriparesis, and neuromuscular junction defect. Neurology 39:746–747, 1989.
456. Cao Z, Bideau R, Valdes RJ, et al: Acute hypermagnesemia and respiratory arrest following infusion of $MgSO_4$ for tocolysis. Clin Chim Acta 285:191–193, 1999.
457. Rizzo MA, Fisher M, Lock JP: Hypermagnesemic pseudocoma. Arch Intern Med 153:1130–1132, 1993; see comments.
458. Cholst IN, Steinberg SF, Tropper PJ, et al: The influence of hypermagnesemia on serum calcium and parathyroid hormone levels in human subjects. N Engl J Med 310:1221–1225, 1984.
459. Navarro JF, Mora C, Jimenez A, et al: Relationship between serum magnesium and parathyroid hormone levels in hemodialysis patients. Am J Kidney Dis 34:43–48, 1999.
460. Zofkova I, Lamberg-Allardt C, Kancheva RL, et al: Effect of hypermagnesemia on the adrenohypophyseal-gonadal function, parathyroid hormone secretion and some other hormonal indicators. Horm Metab Res 25:29–33, 1993.
461. Golzarian J, Scott HWJ, Richards WO: Hypermagnesemia-induced paralytic ileus. Dig Dis Sci 39:1138–1142, 1994.

CHAPTER 27

# Hypophosphatemia and Hyperphosphatemia

Keith A. Hruska, MD

## PHOSPHORUS HOMEOSTASIS

The phosphate anion is ubiquitously distributed throughout the body. It is widely distributed in the form of organic phosphate compounds in cells that play fundamental roles in several aspects of metabolism. The energy required for many cellular reactions, including biosynthesis, derives from hydrolysis of adenosine triphosphate (ATP). Organic phosphates are important components of cell membrane phospholipids. Eighty percent to 85% of body phosphorus is in the skeleton, where it is a component of a rapidly exchangeable ionic pool and a component of the bone mineral hydroxyapatite. Phosphorylation of proteins is a critical mechanism of post-translational modification affecting their function.

Changes in serum phosphorus influence the dissociation of oxygen from hemoglobin through regulation of 2,3-diphosphoglycerate concentrations. The concentration of phosphorus influences the activity of several metabolic pathways such as ammoniagenesis, glycolysis, gluconeogenesis, parathyroid hormone (PTH) secretion, phosphate reabsorption, and the formation of 1,25-dihydroxyvitamin $D_3$ [$1,25(OH)_2D_3$] from 25-hydroxyvitamin $D_3$ [$25(OH)D_3$]. In the extracellular fluid, phosphorus is present predominantly in the inorganic form. The physiologic concentration of serum phosphorus ranges from 2.5 to 4.5 mg/dL (0.9 to 1.45 mM) in adults.[1] In serum, phosphorus exists mainly as the free ion, and only a small fraction (<15%) is protein bound.[2,3] There is a diurnal variation in serum phosphorus of 0.6 to 1 mg/dL, with the nadir occurring between 8 AM and 11 AM. Ingestion of meals rich in carbohydrate decreases serum phosphorus concentrations as a result of movement of phosphorus from the extracellular to the intracellular space.

## Gastrointestinal Absorption of Phosphorus

Approximately 1 g of phosphorus is ingested daily in an average diet in the United States. About 300 mg is excreted in the stool, and 700 mg is absorbed (Fig. 27–1). Most of the phosphorus is absorbed in the duodenum and jejunum, with minimal absorption occurring in the ileum.[4] Phosphorus transport in proximal segments of the small intestine appears to involve both passive and active components and to be under the influence of vitamin D.

The movement of phosphorus from the intestinal lumen to the blood requires (1) transport across the luminal brush border membrane (BBM) of the intestine, (2) transport through the cytoplasm, and (3) transport across the basolateral plasma membrane of the epithelium. The rate-limiting step and the main driving force of absorption is the luminal membrane step.[1]

### ENTEROCYTE MECHANISM OF PHOSPHORUS ABSORPTION

***Luminal Membrane Transport***

The mechanism of transport across the intestinal brush border epithelial membrane involves a sodium-phosphate cotransport system, as suggested by Berner and colleagues[5] and confirmed by the identification of the responsible molecular mechanism, a type IIb sodium-phosphate (Na-Pi) cotransporter, Npt2.[6] The Na-Pi cotransporters represent secondary active forms of ion transport using the energy of the sodium gradient from outside to inside the cell to move the phosphate ion uphill against an electrochemical gradient (Fig. 27–2). The role of $1,25(OH)_2D_3$ and $25(OH)D_3$ in this transport system has been studied by several investigators.[7–10]

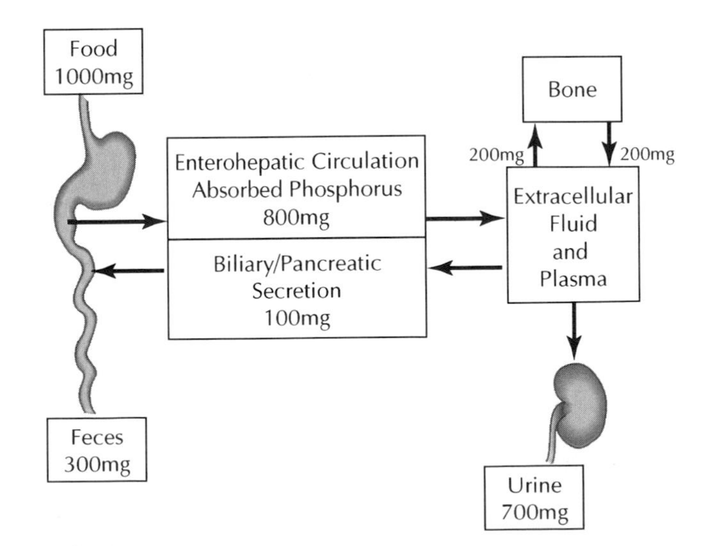


**FIGURE 27–1** ■ Phosphate balance diagram. Approximately 1000 mg of phosphorus is ingested daily in our food and 800 mg is absorbed from the intestine into the enterohepatic circulation. Biliary/pancreatic secretions return approximately 100 mg into the intestinal fluid. Phosphorus leaves the extracellular fluid and plasma compartment by deposition into bone. Bone reabsorption also returns phosphorus into the extracellular fluid. Urinary excretion accounts for the bulk of phosphorus exit, which is equal to intake; in the steady state, human adults are in phosphate balance.

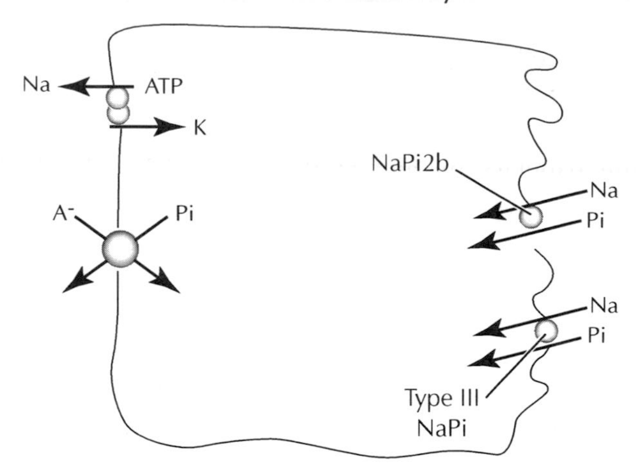


**FIGURE 27–2** ■ Mechanisms of intestinal phosphate absorption. Enterocytic phosphate transport is accomplished by the presence of two classes of phosphate transporters in the luminal membrane of the duodenum and jujunum. The most important class is the NaPi2b isoform of the class II sodium-dependent phosphate transporters. This is responsible for vitamin D–regulated phosphate transport. Following absorption, unknown mechanisms account for transcellular movement of phosphorus, and phosphate exits the basolateral membrane using an organic anion cotransport system to move phosphorus down its electrochemical gradient and organic anions into the cell. The energy for sodium-dependent phosphate transport is established by the sodium-potassium-ATPase, which maintains high intracellular potassium and low intracellular sodium concentrations. The sodium gradient is the energy for the uphill movement of sodium and phosphate transport into the cell.

Murer and Hildmann showed that in vivo administration of 1,25-dihydroxyvitamin D to rabbits affects in vitro uptake of phosphorus by intestinal BBM vesicles.[8] Reduction of endogenous $1,25(OH)_2D_3$ decreased the uptake of phosphorus by approximately 65% in BBM vesicles. This uptake increased threefold after injection of high doses of $1,25(OH)_2D_3$. These studies agree with those of Fuchs and Peterlik, who obtained similar results using chick intestinal epithelial BBM vesicles.[4] Vitamin D stimulates phosphorus absorption by increasing Npt2b gene transcription and by a calcium-dependent duodenal process. Decreased phosphate transport in the intestine of the vitamin D receptor null mouse confirms these results.

Studies of phosphorus accumulation by rat intestinal brush border vesicles demonstrated that at physiologic pH, phosphorus uptake is dependent on luminal sodium and is affected by the transmembrane potential, indicating that, like the renal type II cotransporter NaPi-2, the intestinal type IIb cotransporter, NaPi-2b, is electrogenic.[6] The $K_m$(Pi) of NaPi-2b is approximately 50 μm, a finding that is consistent with the renal transport protein. In contrast to the renal NaPi-2a isoform, the intestinal NaPi-2b cotransporter is less dependent on pH and is slightly more active at acidic pH values. PTH may influence phosphorus absorption in the gut, but it does so indirectly by stimulating the renal synthesis of $1,25(OH)_2D_3$. PTH does not directly affect the activity of NaPi-2b. Low-phosphorus diets increase the absorption of phosphorus from the intestine but may also do so by stimulating the formation of $1,25(OH)_2D_3$. In animals fed a high-phosphorus diet, suppression of $1,25(OH)_2D_3$ may result in decreased intestinal absorption of phosphorus.

#### *Transcellular Movement of Phosphorus*

The second component of transcellular intestinal phosphorus transport involves the movement of phosphorus from the luminal to the basolateral membrane. The cellular events that mediate this transcellular process involve transfer of phosphorus from the membrane to a vesicular compartment and participation of the microtubular network of intestinal cells.[4] Microtubules may be important in conveying phosphorus from the BBM to the basolateral membrane and may be involved in the extrusion of phosphorus at the basolateral membrane from the epithelial cell.

#### *Phosphate Exit at Basolateral Membrane*

Little is known about the mechanisms of phosphorus extrusion at the basolateral membrane of intestinal epithelial cells. The electrochemical gradient for phosphorus favors movement from the intracellular to the extracellular compartment, because the interior of the cell is electrically negative compared with the basolateral external surface.[8] Thus, it has been presumed that the exit of phosphorus across the basolateral membrane represents a mode of passive transport.[11]

## Renal Reabsorption of Phosphorus

Most of the inorganic phosphorus in serum (90% to 95%) is ultrafilterable at the level of the glomerulus. At physiologic levels of serum phosphorus, approximately 7 g of phosphorus is filtered daily by the kidney, of which 80% to 90% is reabsorbed by the renal tubules, and the remainder is excreted in the urine, ≈700 mg on a 1-g phosphorus diet, equal to net absorption (see Fig. 27–1).[12] Thus, in adults at steady state, intake and excretion of phosphorus is in balance.

Micropuncture studies have demonstrated that 60% to 70% of the filtered phosphorus is reabsorbed in the proximal tubule (Fig. 27–3). However, there is also evidence that a significant amount of filtered phosphorus is reabsorbed in distal segments of the nephron.[13] When serum phosphorus levels increase and the filtered load of phosphorus increases, the capacity to reabsorb phosphorus also increases. However, a maximum rate of transport (Tm) for phosphorus reabsorption is obtained, usually at serum phosphorus concentrations of 6 mg/dL. There is a direct correlation between Tm phosphorus values and glomerular filtration rate (GFR), even when the latter covers a broad range.

Micropuncture studies suggest that two different mechanisms are responsible for phosphorus reabsorption in the proximal tubule. In the first third of the proximal tubule, in which only 10% to 15% of the filtered sodium and fluid is reabsorbed, the ratio of tubular fluid (TF) phosphorus to plasma ultrafilterable (UF) phosphorus falls to approximately 0.6. This indi-

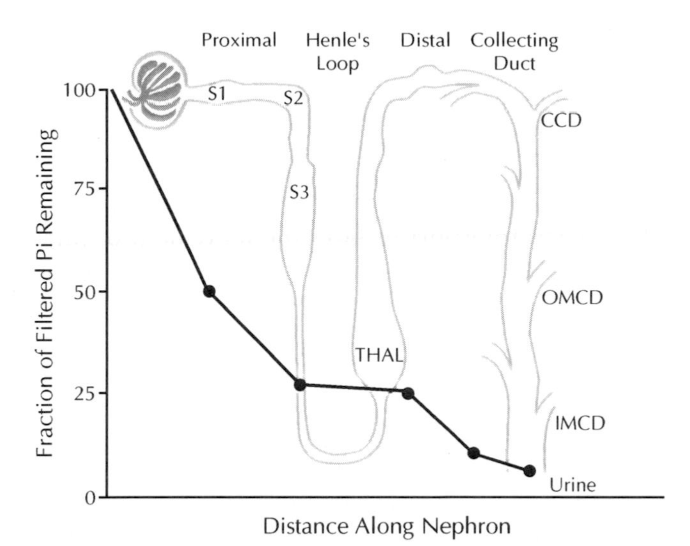


**FIGURE 27–3** ■ Phosphate reabsorption along the nephron. Very early in the proximal tubule, approximately 50% of the filtered phosphate is reabsorbed. Phosphate transport continues in the S2 and S3 portions of the proximal nephron, where an additional 25% is reabsorbed. The loop of Henle does not contribute to phosphate transport. Approximately 15% of the filtered load is reabsorbed in the distal tubule and cortical collecting duct. A small amount of phosphate transport is present in the medullary collecting duct.

cates that the first third of the proximal tubule accounts for approximately 50% of the total amount of phosphorus reabsorbed in this segment of the nephron (see Fig. 27–3). In the last two thirds of the proximal tubule, the reabsorption of phosphorus parallels the movement of salt and water. In the remaining 70% of the pars convoluta, the TF:UF phosphorus ratio remains at 0.6 to 0.7, whereas fluid reabsorption increases to approximately 60% to 70% of the filtered load. Thus, in the last two thirds of the proximal tubule, the TF:UF phosphorus reabsorption is directly proportional to sodium and fluid reabsorption. A significant amount of phosphorus, perhaps on the order of 20% to 30%, is reabsorbed beyond the portion of the proximal tubule that is accessible to micropuncture. There is little phosphorus transport within the loop of Henle,[14] with most transport distal to micropuncture accessibility occurring in the distal convoluted tubule. In this location, Pastoriza-Munoz and coworkers found that approximately 15% of filtered phosphorus is reabsorbed under baseline conditions in animals subjected to parathyroidectomy, but the value falls to about 6% after administration of large doses of PTH.[13]

The collecting duct is a potential site for distal nephron reabsorption of phosphorus.[15–17] Transport in this nephron segment may explain the discrepancy between the amount of phosphorus delivered to the late distal tubule in micropuncture studies and the considerably smaller amount of phosphorus that appears in the final urine of the same kidney. Phosphorus transport in the cortical collecting tubule is independent of regulation by PTH. This is in agreement with the absence of PTH-dependent adenylate cyclase in the cortical collecting tubule.[17]

## COMPARISON OF SUPERFICIAL AND DEEP NEPHRON TRANSPORT

The contribution of superficial and deep nephrons of the kidney to phosphorus homeostasis differs. Nephron heterogeneity in phosphorus handling has been evaluated in a number of conditions by puncture of the papillary tip and of the superficial early distal tubule; the recorded fractional delivery represents deep and superficial nephron function, respectively.

Using this technique, Haramati and colleagues demonstrated that in thyroparathyroidectomized (TPTX) rats fed a normal-phosphorus diet, phosphorus reabsorption is greater in deep than in superficial nephrons, and this heterogeneous handling of phosphorus can be mitigated by both PTH infusion and a low-phosphorus diet.[18, 19] Studies in TPTX rats fed a normalphosphorus diet presented in vivo measurements of maximal tubular reabsorptive capacities of deep and superficial nephrons. Deep nephron values (5.05 pmol/mL/min) were significantly greater than those obtained in superficial nephrons (3.38 pmol/mL/min). These results suggest that the juxtamedullary nephrons are more responsive to body phosphorus requirements than are the superficial nephrons. Also, microinjection of phosphorus tracer into thin ascending and descending limbs of the loop of Henle revealed that only 80% of phosphorus was recovered in the urine, whereas 88% to 100% of phosphorus was recovered when the tracer was injected into the late superficial distal tubule.

They concluded that a significant amount of phosphorus must be reabsorbed by the juxtamedullary distal tubules, or by segments connecting the juxtamedullary distal tubules to the collecting ducts, to account for the discrepant results of superficial nephron injection and injection into the juxtamedullary ascending limb of the loop of Henle. These data seem to support an increased capacity to reabsorb phosphorus in deep as opposed to superficial nephrons.

In summary, phosphorus transport occurs in the distal nephron, particularly in the distal convoluted tubule and cortical collecting tubular system. This transport may be considerable under certain experimental conditions, but the importance of the terminal nephron system in day-to-day phosphorus homeostasis remains to be defined. It is also evident from various micropuncture and microinjection studies that juxtamedullary and superficial nephrons have different capacities for phosphorus transport. The increased responsiveness of the deep nephrons to phosphorus intake suggests that they play a key regulatory role in phosphorus homeostasis.

## CELLULAR MECHANISMS OF PHOSPHATE REABSORPTION IN THE KIDNEY

The apical membrane of renal tubular cells is the initial barrier across which phosphorus and other solutes in the tubular fluid must pass to be transported into the peritubular capillary network. Because the electrical charge of the cell interior is negative to the exterior, and phosphorus concentrations are higher in the cytosol, phosphorus must move against an electrochemical gradient into the cell interior; in contrast, at the antiluminal membrane, the transport of phosphorus into the peritubular capillary is favored by the high intracellular phosphorus concentration and the electronegativity of the cell interior (Fig. 27–4). Studies of apical membrane vesicles have demonstrated cotransport of sodium with phosphate across the BBM, whereas the transport of phosphorus across the basolateral membrane is independent of that of sodium.[20] The apical membrane sodium-phosphate cotransport protein (NaPi-2a) energizes the uphill transport of phosphate across the BBM by the movement of sodium down its electrochemical gradient. The latter gradient is established and maintained by active extrusion of sodium across the basolateral cell membrane into the peritubular capillary through the action of $Na^+$, $K^+$ ATPase (see Fig. 27–2).[21]

Three families of Na-Pi cotransport proteins of the proximal tubule (types I, II, and III) have been cloned using *Xenopus* RNA expression strategies for types I and II[22, 23] and retroviral receptor identification for type III.[24] The NaPi-2 DNA clones encode 80- to 95-kDa proteins that reconstitute sodium-dependent concentrative, or "uphill," transport of phosphate upon chromosomal RNA injection in oocytes[23] or transfection of sf9 cells.[25] The type I cotransporter, NaPi-1, is expressed predominantly in the renal proximal tubule, and it accounts for about 13% of the known Na-Pi cotransporter mRNA in mouse kidney[26] (see Fig. 27–4). NaPi-1 is not regulated by dietary phosphate, and

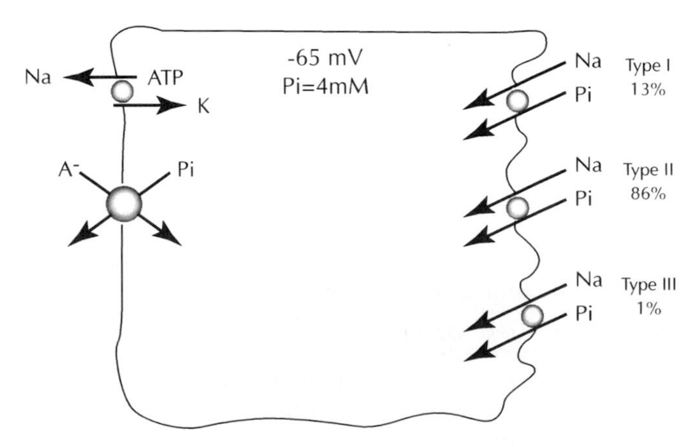


**FIGURE 27–4** ■ Mechanisms of proximal renal tubular cell phosphate transport. The apical membrane of the proximal tubule possesses three types of sodium-dependent phosphate transport proteins. By RNA message, 86% is the type II transporter, which is responsible for physiologic regulation of phosphate reabsorption. The isoform in the proximal tubule is the NaPi2a isoform. Sodium-dependent phosphate transport is a secondary active form of transport that is energized by the sodium gradient, which is established by a basolateral membrane sodium-potassium-ATPase. The mechanism of transcellular phosphate transport is unkown but appears to be related to the microtubular filament system. Exit at the basolateral membrane is accomplished by an inorganic anion cotransport system, thus allowing phosphate to exit down its electrochemical gradient.

studies of NaPi-1 cRNA–injected oocytes revealed that it may function not only as an Na-Pi cotransporter but also as a chloride and organic anion channel.[27]

The NaPi-2 proteins are similar among several species, including human,[22] and several isoforms have been described.[28] Nephron localization of NaPi-2 proteins revealed expression limited to the proximal tubule of superficial and deep nephrons (greater in the latter, concordant with physiologic studies)[22] (see Fig. 27–4).[29] Immunolocalization studies in renal epithelial cells demonstrated apical membrane and subapical membrane vesicle staining,[22] suggesting that a functional pool of transporters is available for insertion or retrieval from the BBM itself. This has been shown to be a major mechanism of inorganic phosphate ($P_i$) transport regulation in response to acute changes in phosphorus and PTH.[22, 30, 31] The NaPi-2 family is upregulated at message and protein levels by chronic feeding of low-$P_i$ diets[28, 32, 33] and is regulated at message and protein levels by PTH.[32–34]

The type III Na-Pi cotransporters were originally identified as retroviral receptors for gibbon ape leukemia virus (Glvr-1) and murine amphotropic virus (Ram-1).[24] They are ubiquitously expressed, and they constitute about 1% of the known Na-Pi cotransporter mRNA in mouse kidney[26] (see Fig. 27–4). Their levels and activity adapt to dietary phosphate changes, and although they are thought to represent "housekeeping" Na-Pi cotransporters, they appear to have critical roles in phosphate transport related to mineralization. They appear to be the major phosphate transporter of osteoblasts, and they are involved in matrix vesicle-related mineralization.[35–37] They are also involved in phosphate regulation of vascular smooth muscle calcification associated with atherosclerosis, diabetes, and chronic renal failure.[38]

Studies of phosphorus exit across the basolateral membrane suggest that it is accompanied by the net transfer of a negative charge and occurs down a favorable electrochemical gradient via sodium-independent mechanisms.[39]

## FACTORS AFFECTING URINARY EXCRETION OF PHOSPHORUS

Several factors are known to affect the urinary excretion of phosphorus. Of the many factors that regulate phosphate transport in the kidney, the most important are phosphate delivery and PTH.

### *Effects of Parathyroid Hormone on Phosphorus Reabsorption in the Kidney*

Parathyroidectomy decreases urinary phosphorus excretion, whereas administration of PTH rapidly increases phosphorus excretion.[39–41] Micropuncture studies indicate that PTH inhibits phosphorus transport in the proximal tubule[42, 43] and probably in segments of the nephron located beyond the proximal tubule.[13] TF:UF phosphorus reaches a value of 0.6 by the $S_2$ segment of the proximal tubule; once achieved, this equilibrium ratio is maintained along the accessible portion of the proximal tubule. Within 6 to 24 hours of parathyroidectomy, the proximal TF:UF phosphorus value falls to 0.2 to 0.4, indicating an increase in phosphorus reabsorption.[43–45] Tubular fluid phosphorus falls progressively with continuous fluid absorption along the length of the tubule, so that by the end of the proximal tubule, the reabsorption of phosphorus is 70% to 85% of the filtered load, resulting in decreased phosphorus delivery to distal segments of the nephron. Because decreased delivery of phosphorus out of the proximal tubule complicates the evaluation of any distal effects of PTH on phosphorus excretion, maneuvers have been designed to increase phosphorus delivery to the distal nephron to study distal effects of parathyroidectomy on phosphorus reabsorption (e.g., phosphorus loading by intravenous infusion).[46, 47]

In a nonphosphorus-loaded, acutely parathyroidectomized animal, virtually all the distal load of phosphorus is reabsorbed by the distal nephron, reducing urinary phosphorus excretion to very low levels.[48, 49] In a phosphorus-loaded animal, the distal reabsorption of phosphorus increases until saturation is approached and urinary phosphorus excretion begins to rise. Acute administration of PTH to phosphorus-loaded, parathyroidectomized dogs sharply lowers distal reabsorption. These experiments indicate that PTH inhibits reabsorption of phosphorus in the distal as well as the proximal nephron.

Administration of PTH in vivo results in decreased rates of sodium-dependent phosphorus transport in BBM vesicles isolated from the kidneys of treated rats.[50, 51] The uptake of D-glucose and sodium was not affected by administration of PTH. Intravenous infusion of dibutyryl cyclic adenosine monophosphate (cAMP) also decreased sodium-dependent phosphorus uptake in isolated brush border vesicles, but neither PTH nor dibutyryl cAMP decreased phosphate transport when added directly to membrane vesicles.[50] These observations suggest that the effects of PTH on renal phosphate transport are mediated through altered functional characteristics (decreased $V_{max}$) of the renal BBM sodium-dependent phosphate transporter.[51]

Cloning of the NaPi-2 cotransport proteins has not completely elucidated the mechanisms of PTH action on phosphate transport as yet. Because the phosphaturic effect of PTH can be reproduced by analogues of cAMP, the intracellular mechanism of phosphate transport regulation is thought to involve the cAMP–protein kinase A signal pathway. However, the Na-Pi transport proteins are not characterized by protein kinase A–mediated phosphorylation sites.[52] Phosphorylation of BBM proteins in vitro occurs in parallel with inhibition of Npt2 cotransport.[51] Parathyroidectomy of rats causes a two- to threefold increase in the Npt2 protein content of BBM vesicles.[34] Immunocytochemistry reveals the increase in protein exclusively in apical BBMs of proximal tubules.[53] PTH treatment for 15 minutes decreases protein levels and decreases the abundance of Npt2-specific messenger RNA (mRNA) by 31%.[54] The rapid actions of PTH are related to endocytic retrieval of transport protein from the BBM. The endocytic vesicular pool of NaPi-2 is associated with microtubules during their traffic to lysosomal degradation.[34, 53]

### *Effects of Changes in Acid-Base Balance on Phosphate Excretion*

The effect of acid-base status on the renal excretion and transport of phosphate is complex. Acute respiratory acidosis increases phosphate excretion, and acute respiratory alkalosis decreases it.[54] These effects occur independently of PTH and plasma or luminal bicarbonate levels.[54] However, other studies suggest that the effects of respiratory acid-base changes may be mediated by changes in plasma phosphate.[54]

Acute metabolic acidosis has minimal effects on phosphate excretion; however, the phosphaturic effect of PTH is blunted.[44] Acute metabolic alkalosis causes an increase in phosphate excretion independent of PTH.[55–59] This effect is due, in part, to volume expansion produced by the infusion of bicarbonate.[56, 57]

Chronic acidosis increases phosphate excretion, again independent of PTH or changes in ionized $Ca^{2+}$.[59–62] The effect appears to be directly on the sodium-dependent phosphate transport mechanism.[63] Chronic alkalosis decreases phosphate excretion, probably by the same mechanism as acidosis, operating in the opposite direction.[55, 64] It has been shown that acute and chronic acidosis in rats decreases the proximal tubule cell luminal membrane expression of the Npt2 cotransporter.[65] It seems that in acute acidosis the transporter is internalized, because the total cortical homogenate cotransporter expression is unchanged. The effects of acid-base perturbations are complex and depend on antecedent dietary intake, the chronicity of the change, and whether the change affects luminal or intracellular pH, or both.

### *Adrenal Hormones*

Administration of pharmacologic amounts of cortisol leads to phosphaturia. Acute adrenalectomy diminishes GFR and increases the reabsorption of phosphorus in the proximal tubule. Frick and Durasin concluded that glucocorticoid hormones could play an important role in the regulation of fractional reabsorption of phosphorus.[66] The current notion that cellular metabolism plays an important role in regulating the proximal tubular reabsorption of phosphorus is relevant to these observations. An effect of glucocorticoid hormones in altering carbohydrate metabolism within the proximal tubular cells could underlie the effects described.

### *Vitamin D*

Controversy still surrounds the regulatory role of vitamin D in renal phosphorus handling. Several past studies demonstrated that the chronic administration of vitamin D to parathyroidectomized animals causes phosphaturia.[67–69] Conversely, other investigators reported that vitamin D acutely stimulates proximal tubular phosphorus transport in both parathyroidectomized and vitamin D–depleted rats.[70] A unifying interpretation of these studies was hampered by the fact that the dosages of vitamin D administered and the status of the serum calcium, phosphorus, and PTH varied considerably from study to study.

Liang and coworkers administered $1,25(OH)_2D_3$ to vitamin D–deficient chicks and subsequently examined the transport characteristics of isolated renal tubule cells.[71] Three hours after the in vivo administration of vitamin D, phosphorus uptake by the cells was significantly increased, whereas 17 hours after the administration of vitamin D, phosphorus uptake was reduced. The serum phosphorus concentration, however, was significantly increased at the 17-hour point, and administration of phosphorus to vitamin D–depleted animals so that their serum phosphorus reached a level comparable to that of the 17-hour vitamin D–replete group resulted in a similar decrease in phosphorus uptake.[71] In response to in vitro preincubation with as little as 0.01 pM of $1,25(OH)_2D_3$, renal cells isolated from vitamin D–deficient chicks demonstrated a specific increase in sodium-dependent phosphorus uptake, which was blocked by pretreatment with actinomycin D. The stimulatory effect was relatively specific for $1,25(OH)_2D_3$, and kinetic analysis indicated that the $V_{max}$ of the phosphorus transport system was increased, whereas the affinity of the system for phosphorus was unaffected.[71]

Kurnik and Hruska also examined the relationship between vitamin D and renal phosphorus excretion in a normocalcemic, normophosphatemic weanling rat model fed a vitamin D–deficient diet.[72] The animals were mildly vitamin D deficient [92 pg/mL of $1,25(OH)_2D_3$ versus 169 pg/mL in controls] but had no evidence of secondary hyperparathyroidism. Clearance studies performed in the basal, partially vitamin D–deficient state showed an increase in both absolute and fractional phosphorus excretion compared with controls. Animals replete with $1,25(OH)_2D_3$ and maintained on diets designed to protect against the development of hyperphosphatemia demonstrated a significant decrease in urinary phosphorus excretion. In other animals that were similarly replete with vitamin D but did not receive dietary adjustment, both the serum phosphorus and the urinary phosphorus excretion levels increased significantly. A third group was fed a normal diet and received smaller doses of $1,25(OH)_2D_3$ (15 pmol/g body weight) for shorter periods of time, and although this dose had no effect on the serum phosphorus concentration, the phosphaturia was completely resolved.

Studies of BBM vesicles prepared from these animals revealed that in the partially vitamin D–deficient state, sodium-dependent phosphorus uptake was significantly reduced, compared with control animals. Animals replete with vitamin D and fed a controlled diet had a greater sodium-dependent phosphorus uptake than did both vitamin D–depleted animals and vitamin D–replete animals not maintained on controlled diets.

The results of this series of studies suggest that the direct action of $1,25(OH)_2D_3$ is to increase renal tubular phosphorus reabsorption. Long-term administration of vitamin D, however, represents a more complex situation. Here, phosphaturia usually occurs due to changes in the filtered load of phosphorus, in the body distribution of phosphorus, or in intracellular phosphorus activity produced by the actions of vitamin D to increase phosphate absorption and plasma phosphate.

#### *Growth Hormone*

An increase in serum phosphorus and a rise in renal phosphorus transport are characteristics of growth hormone excess during the period of rapid growth in children, in cases of acromegaly, or during exogenous growth hormone administration in experimental animals. Hammerman and Hruska reexamined this phenomenon in the BBM vesicle preparation in the dog and demonstrated that growth hormone treatment resulted in an increased sodium-dependent phosphorus transport.[51] These data reassert the importance of BBM phosphorus uptake in regulating overall renal phosphorus reabsorptive capacity. The action of growth hormone is likely mediated by insulin-like growth factor-1.[73]

#### *Alterations in Dietary Phosphorus Intake*

The mechanism by which the kidney conserves phosphorus when dietary phosphorus is reduced or increased is intriguing. Earlier micropuncture studies suggested that the most striking adaptive increase in phosphorus transport occurs in the proximal tubule. Later studies suggested that the entire nephron participates in the reduction of phosphorus excretion during dietary phosphorus deprivation.[43] It has been shown that isolated perfused tubules obtained from rabbits fed a normal- or low-phosphorus diet differ in their capacity to reabsorb phosphate. In normal animals, the proximal convoluted tubule is capable of reabsorbing 7.2 ± 0.8 pmol/mL/min, whereas tubules obtained from phosphorus-deprived animals reabsorb 11.1 ± 1.3 pmol/mL/min. Conversely, animals with a high dietary phosphorus intake show reduced phosphorus reabsorption when the proximal tubules are perfused in vitro (2.7 ± 2.6 pmol/mL/min).

Based on renal BBM preparations, it has been suggested that the effect of reduced dietary phosphorus to stimulate renal phosphorus transport is intrinsic to the renal tubular epithelium and occurs specifically at the BBM Na-Pi cotransporter. Considerable evidence has accrued from studies performed in cell lines isolated from mammalian kidneys, indicating that the adaptation to phosphate supply by the Na-Pi cotransporter is biphasic.[74–76] These studies demonstrated that incubation of cells in a low-phosphate medium results in a twofold increase in sodium-independent phosphate cotransport.

The first phase of adaptation is observed rapidly (within 10 minutes) and is characterized by an increase in the $V_{max}$ of the transporter. This initial phase is independent of new protein synthesis. A slower phase resulting in a doubling of the phosphate transport rate, again through an increase in $V_{max}$, occurs over several hours (maximum ≈ 15 hours) and is inhibited by blocking new protein synthesis. These studies have been interpreted to indicate that the immediate response to reduced phosphate availability is the insertion of new transport units into the BBM from an intracellular store, probably the vesicular pool involved in endocytic traffic of the transporter.[30, 77] Then, through gene transcription and increased Na-Pi protein synthesis, additional units are produced and inserted into the brush border.[29]

Chronic feeding of low-$P_i$ diet increases steady-state mRNA levels of Npt6 in rabbits and Npt2 in rats.[28, 78] Acute $P_i$ deprivation does not affect Npt2 family mRNA levels, compatible with a protein synthesis–independent action related to insertion of new transport proteins from subapical vesicles into the BBM.[30, 77]

***Stanniocalcin***

Stanniocalcin is a new calcium-regulating hormone found in serum and the kidney.[79] Its name derives from its synthesis by the corpuscles of Stannius, endocrine glands found in the kidneys of bony fishes. In mammals, stanniocalcin lowers calcium transport and increases phosphate reabsorption. The bony fishes use this action to increase phosphate deposition into bone and scales. The role of stanniocalcin in human physiology requires elucidation, as does the regulation of its secretion.

***Diuretics***

Acetazolamide inhibits phosphate reabsorption by its effect of decreasing sodium-dependent bicarbonate transport in the proximal tubule, essential for maintenance of the sodium gradient. Furosemide inhibits carbonic anhydrase activity and thus decreases phosphate transport. Similar effects have been demonstrated with the administration of large doses of thiazide diuretics.[80]

# HYPOPHOSPHATEMIA

Hypophosphatemia refers to serum phosphorus concentrations of less than 2.5 mg/dL. Hypophosphatemia usually results from one or a combination of the following factors[81, 82]: (1) increased excretion of phosphorus in the urine, (2) decreased gastrointestinal absorption of phosphorus, or (3) translocation of phosphorus from the extracellular to the intracellular space. The major causes of hypophosphatemia are listed in Table 27–1.

**TABLE 27–1.** Causes of Hypophosphatemia

I. Increased excretion of phosphorus in the urine
   A. Primary hyperparathyroidism
   B. Secondary hyperparathyroidism
   C. Renal tubular defects
   D. Diuretic phase of acute tubular necrosis
   E. Postobstructive diuresis
   F. After renal transplantation
   G. Extracellular fluid volume expansion
   H. Familial
      1. X-linked hypophosphatemia
      2. McCune-Albright syndrome
II. Decrease in gastrointestinal absorption of phosphorus
   A. Malabsorption
   B. Malnutrition—starvation
   C. Administration of phosphate binders
   D. Abnormalities of vitamin D metabolism
      1. Vitamin D deficiency—rickets
      2. Familial
         a. Vitamin D–dependent rickets
         b. X-linked hypophosphatemia
III. Miscellaneous causes; translocation of phosphorus
   A. Diabetes mellitus (during treatment for ketoacidosis)
   B. Severe respiratory alkalosis
   C. Recovery phase of malnutrition
   D. Alcohol withdrawal
   E. Toxic shock syndrome
   F. Leukemia, lymphoma
   G. Severe burns

## Increased Urinary Excretion of Phosphorus

Several pathophysiologic conditions may increase the excretion of phosphorus in the urine. Some of these conditions are characterized by elevated levels of circulating PTH. Because PTH decreases phosphorus reabsorption by the kidney, modest to marked elevations of this hormone may increase urinary excretion of this anion. Decreased tubular reabsorption of phosphorus may also occur without increased levels of PTH and may be due to changes in the reabsorption of salt and water or to renal tubular defects specific for the reabsorption of certain solutes or phosphorus. Hypophosphatemia may also occur in the diuretic phase of acute tubular necrosis or in postobstructive diuresis, presumably owing to a combination of high levels of PTH and decreased tubular reabsorption of salt and water.

### PRIMARY HYPERPARATHYROIDISM

Primary hyperparathyroidism is a common entity in clinical medicine.[83] PTH is secreted in excess of the physiologic needs for mineral homeostasis, owing to either adenomas or hyperplasia of the parathyroid glands.[84] This results in decreased phosphorus reabsorption by the kidney. The losses of phosphorus in the urine result in hypophosphatemia. The degree of hypophosphatemia may vary considerably among patients, because mobilization of phosphorus from bone partially mitigates the hypophosphatemia. Moreover, if the patient ingests large amounts of dietary phosphorus, the degree of hypophosphatemia observed may be mild. Because these patients also have elevated levels of serum calcium, the diagnosis is relatively easy in the majority of cases, based on the finding of elevated levels of immunoreactive PTH.

### SECONDARY HYPERPARATHYROIDISM

Although secondary hyperparathyroidism is present in most patients with chronic renal disease, hyperphosphatemia rather than hypophosphatemia occurs in such patients, owing to decreased phosphorus excretion in the urine as a consequence of the fall in GFR. However, certain conditions characterized by malabsorption of calcium from the gastrointestinal tract may produce hypocalcemia, leading to the development of secondary hyperparathyroidism.[85] The elevated levels of PTH decrease phosphorus reabsorption by the kidney, resulting in hypophosphatemia.

Thus, patients with gastrointestinal abnormalities resulting in calcium malabsorption and secondary hyperparathyroidism have low levels of both serum calcium and phosphorus. In these patients, the hypocalcemia is responsible for the increased release of PTH. In addition, decreased intestinal absorption of phosphorus as a result of the primary gastrointestinal disease may contribute to the decrement in the serum phosphorus level. In general, these patients have urinary losses of phosphorus that are out of proportion to the hypophosphatemia; this is in contrast to patients with predominant phosphorus malabsorption and no secondary hyperparathyroidism, in whom urinary excretion of phosphorus is low.

## RENAL TUBULAR DEFECTS

Several conditions characterized by either single or multiple tubular defects have been described in which phosphorus reabsorption is decreased.[86] In Fanconi syndrome,[86] patients excrete not only increased amounts of phosphorus in the urine but also increased quantities of amino acids, uric acid, and glucose, resulting in hypouricemia and hypophosphatemia. Rare familial forms of hypercalciuria are often associated with one or more of the components of Fanconi syndrome, including hypophosphatemia and hyperphosphaturia.[87–89] Interestingly, these familial syndromes—Dent disease and its variants—are caused by a mutation in the ClCN5 chloride channel,[87, 90] which is an intracellular vesicular channel, perhaps related to the vesicles that harbor the Na-Pi cotransport proteins.[91, 92] There are other conditions in which an isolated defect in the renal tubular transport of phosphorus has been found—for example, in fructose intolerance, an autosomal recessive disorder.[93]

Following renal transplantation, an acquired renal tubular defect may be responsible for the persistence of hypophosphatemia in some patients,[94] although current evidence suggests that an abnormality in *PHEX* gene activity or increased production of phosphatonin is the likely cause of persistent post-transplant hypophosphatemia, rather than an intrinsic renal tubular transport defect (see "X-Linked Hypophosphatemic Rickets").

## DIURETIC PHASE OF ACUTE TUBULAR NECROSIS

Most patients with acute renal failure develop secondary hyperparathyroidism and hyperphosphatemia during the oliguric phase. During the recovery phase of acute renal failure, the combined occurrence of profound diuresis, secondary hyperparathyroidism, and continued use of phosphate binders may lead to the development of severe hypophosphatemia. This hypophosphatemia is usually short-lived, and serum phosphorus levels return to normal as the diuretic phase of acute tubular necrosis subsides.

## POSTOBSTRUCTIVE DIURESIS

A marked phosphaturia may develop in some patients after relief of urinary tract obstruction. This phosphaturia may be severe enough in a few patients to lead to the development of hypophosphatemia.[95]

## POST–RENAL TRANSPLANTATION

Hypophosphatemia, sometimes severe, is common in patients after renal transplantation.[94, 96] Patients undergoing renal transplantation usually have secondary hyperparathyroidism.[94, 96] As the GFR is restored after placement of the graft, the high levels of PTH acting on the transplanted kidney increase phosphorus excretion in the urine.

However, in some patients, a persistent phosphaturia that is out of proportion to the levels of serum phosphorus is observed, even after PTH levels have returned to normal. In these patients, it appears that either a defect in *PHEX* activity or excessive phosphatonin is present (see "X-Linked Hypophosphatemic Rickets"). Thus, hypophosphatemia in the first few days after renal transplantation may result from a combination of factors: (1) continued administration of phosphate binders after the transplant has adequate function, (2) secondary hyperparathyroidism in the presence of near normal GFR, and (3) an abnormality in *PHEX* activity or phosphatonin production.

When phosphate binders are decreased or discontinued and hyperparathyroidism subsides, phosphorus levels usually return to normal in most patients with renal grafts. When this fails to occur, either *PHEX* or phosphatonin appears to be implicated.[94] Prolonged periods of severe hypophosphatemia may cause bone disease characterized by severe osteomalacia in some of these patients.

## EXTRACELLULAR FLUID VOLUME EXPANSION

Expansion of the extracellular fluid volume by the administration of solutions containing sodium increases the urinary excretion of phosphorus. An important mechanism by which extracellular fluid volume expansion produces phosphaturia consists of a fall in ionized calcium and subsequent release of PTH.[97] This condition is probably of minor importance in clinical medicine, and restoration of extracellular fluid volume to normal returns phosphorus reabsorption to physiologic levels.

## X-LINKED HYPOPHOSPHATEMIC RICKETS

This X-linked dominant disorder is characterized by hypophosphatemia, decreased reabsorption of phosphorus by the renal tubule, decreased absorption of calcium and phosphorus from the gastrointestinal tract, and varying degrees of rickets or osteomalacia. Patients with this disorder exhibit normal levels of $1,25(OH)_2D_3$ and reduced Na-Pi transport in the proximal tubule in the face of severe hypophosphatemia. The gene for X-linked hypophosphatemia is not the phosphate transport protein itself, which maps to chromosome 5 in humans[98] and exhibits normal function in isolated BBM preparations from animal models of X-linked hypophosphatemic rickets. The genetic defect for this disorder is in a gene termed *PHEX*, which encodes for a neutral endopeptidase presumed to be responsible for degradation of an as yet unidentified systemic phosphaturic hormone, "phosphatonin."[99] The defective *PHEX* gene product in X-linked hypophosphatemic rickets permits phosphatonin to inhibit renal phosphate absorption, despite persistent hypophosphatemia. Phosphatonin remains to be discovered, but candidate proteins have been suggested.[100]

The role of alterations in vitamin D sensitivity or synthesis in the defective transport of phosphorus observed in both the gut and the kidney has been investigated in the murine homologue of X-linked hypophosphatemia (Hyp).[101] Tenenhouse and Scriver found that administration of small doses of $1,25(OH)_2D_3$ to normal animals significantly increased plasma calcium, plasma phosphorus, and fractional calcium excretion without a change in fractional phosphorus excretion or phosphorus transport, as measured in proximal tubular BBM vesicles.[102] However, there was no response to this dose of $1,25(OH)_2D_3$ in the Hyp mice. At a fivefold higher dose of vitamin D, the familial hypophosphatemic mice did show increased plasma calcium and fractional calcium excretion, as well as increased plasma phosphorus levels, but again there was no change in fractional phosphorus excretion or in sodium-dependent phosphorus transport in BBM vesicles. Although $1,25(OH)_2D_3$ increased phosphorus transport in the intestine, there was no defect of phosphorus transport in the intestine of untreated hypophosphatemic mice. The conclusion from these studies is that vitamin D influences phosphorus homeostasis in Hyp mice by stimulation of phosphorus absorption from the gastrointestinal tract. The defect in renal phosphorus reabsorption was unchanged, despite high levels of vitamin D. These observations are consistent with studies performed in humans with familial hypophosphatemia, in whom the renal reabsorptive defect persists despite correction of growth by administration of vitamin D and oral phosphate supplements.[103]

There is, however, evidence of defective or altered metabolism of vitamin $D_3$ in Hyp mice. Meyer and coworkers found that on a normal diet, plasma $1,25(OH)_2D_3$ levels were the same in Hyp and normal mice,[104] although $25(OH)D_3$ levels were reduced in Hyp mice. Because hypophosphatemia increases plasma $1,25(OH)_2D_3$ levels, the hypophosphatemic mice were resistant to the stimulatory effect of hypophosphatemia. To test this possibility, these authors fed the animals a low-phosphorus diet and found a paradoxical reduction in $1,25(OH)_2D_3$ levels in hypophosphatemic mice. They concluded that Hyp mice have a defective control system for plasma $1,25(OH)_2D_3$ that is unresponsive to a low-phosphate diet stimulus. The issue is further complicated by Beamer and colleagues, who studied the effect of various preparations of vitamin $D_3$ on intestinal transport of phosphorus.[105] The Hyp mice responded to 1α-dihydroxyvitamin $D_3$ but not to $1,25(OH)_2D_3$, suggesting that intestinal phosphorus transport responsiveness is not genetically absent in this model but rather does not respond to normal endogenous levels of $1,25(OH)_2D_3$. Thus, mice with familial hypophosphatemia appear to have impaired metabolism of vitamin D, but this impairment does not cause the renal phosphate transport defect. There is also evidence that the decreased tubular reabsorption of phosphorus is not due to increased PTH levels.[105] The component of renal phosphorus transport that is PTH independent is abnormal and is responsible for the increased phosphaturia. Tenenhouse and associates showed that tissue phosphate levels were normal in Hyp mice, whereas these levels tended to be low in animals with hypophosphatemia secondary to a reduction in dietary phosphorus.[106] It therefore seems that X-linked hypophosphatemia is a selective disorder of the transepithelial transport of phosphate. However, there is no correlation between the degree of hypophosphatemia and the severity of bone disease. Moreover, alterations in vitamin D metabolism cannot be explained solely by the presence of hypophosphatemia. Therefore, an undefined pathologic mechanism related to *PHEX* function involves both abnormal phosphate transport and renal 1-hydroxylase function.

Tenenhouse and associates extended their studies in Hyp mice to demonstrate that the message levels for the Npt2 cotransport protein are reduced by 50% in the renal cortex, similar to the reduction in apical membrane vesicle Npt2 protein levels.[107] However, the mapping of Npt2 and Npt1 to chromosomes 5 and 6, respectively,[98, 108] indicates that these genes are not candidates for the genetic defects leading to X-linked hypophosphatemia or Hyp. X-linked hypophosphatemia and Hyp are caused by abnormal levels of a circulating hormonal factor. Results of the cross-perfusion studies of Meyer and coworkers[109] and the cross-transplantation studies of Nesbitt and colleagues[110] were interpreted to indicate the presence of a circulating factor. Furthermore, Nesbitt's group was unable to demonstrate transmission of the Hyp renal defect by transplanting a Hyp kidney into a normal recipient.[110] Likewise, transplantation of a normal kidney into a Hyp recipient failed to correct the Hyp phenotypic abnormalities. These studies, in addition to studies in oncogenic osteomalacia, suggest that a circulating humoral factor could be capable of producing the Hyp and X-linked hypophosphatemia phenotype. Although it has yet to be discovered, the substance has been named phosphatonin.[111]

The circulating humoral factor hypothesis for the cause of X-linked hypophosphatemia was supported by the discovery of the defective gene, *PHEX*, through positional cloning.[99] The *PHEX* gene product encodes a neutral endopeptidase of the same family as endothelin-converting enzyme, and it is characterized by zinc regulation and a single transmembrane spanning domain. The model proposed by this result suggests that a circulating phosphaturic factor is normally catabolized by the *PHEX* gene product. When *PHEX* is mutated, the phosphaturic factor levels are increased, and hypophosphatemia results.

An interesting aspect of the Hyp phenotype is the presence of a normal sodium-dependent phosphate cotransport in osteoblasts.[112] However, the osteoblasts of Hyp have been shown to be defective in models of endochondral bone formation.[113, 114] Defective mineralization is an important aspect of osteomalacia, and mineralization is controlled by calcium, phosphate, and bone matrix proteins. We have demonstrated defective phosphorylation of a key bone matrix protein, osteopontin, in Hyp mice and abnormally low activity of a protein kinase (casein kinase-II–like activity) responsible for osteopontin phosphorylation.[115, 116] Thus, multiple proteins appear to be defective in the Hyp phenotype. This is compatible with multiple targets of the *PHEX* gene, such as phosphatonin and an inhibitor of casein kinase-II, which achieve greater activity when *PHEX* is defective.[109, 110, 115, 117]

From a therapeutic point of view, the combination of neutral phosphate and $1,25(OH)_2D_3$ has led to improvement of the bone disease in some patients with X-linked hypophosphatemia and in Hyp mice.[118, 119] In patients with X-linked hypophosphatemia, phosphorus is usually administered in four doses, with the total amount ranging between 1 and 4 g/day. Pharmacologic doses of calcitriol on the order of 1 to 3 μg/day may be necessary to correct the skeletal alterations. $1,25(OH)_2D_3$ does not correct the increased fractional excretion of phosphate. The enthusiasm for this regimen is tempered by a high incidence of nephrocalcinosis and occasional renal failure.[118–120]

### AUTOSOMAL DOMINANT HYPOPHOSPHATEMIC RICKETS

Autosomal dominant hypophosphatemic rickets is a rare condition that resembles X-linked hypophosphatemia, except in its inheritance. It has recently become critically important because of positional cloning of the gene responsible for the disorder, fibroblast growth factor 23 (*FGF23*),[100] on chromosome 12p13. *FGF23* is not known to regulate phosphate transport, but it is an attractive candidate for the *PHEX* substrate phosphatonin, which is normally inactivated. It is possible that because of mutations, *FGF23* is resistant to the *PHEX* endopeptidase and circulates in an active form. This is totally speculative at this writing, and discovery of the gene provides the opportunity to investigate how this new factor regulates phosphate transport.

### McCUNE-ALBRIGHT SYNDROME

McCune-Albright syndrome is characterized by the clinical triad of polyostotic fibrous dysplasia, café au lait skin pigmentation, and endocrine or metabolic disorders. The endocrine disorders include autonomous secretion of various hormones such as growth hormone, thyroid hormone, cortisol, estradiol, and testosterone. Rickets and osteomalacia due to hyperphosphaturic hypophosphatemia are prominent components of the syndrome. The disorders of the syndrome share in common an excessive function of cells whose actions are normally regulated by hormones that induce cAMP generation. The molecular basis for the phenotype is an activating mutation of the $G_s\alpha$ protein (the α component of the stimulatory heterotrimeric guanosine triphosphate binding protein) in the cells of affected tissues in patients with the syndrome.[121] Kidney tissue, presumably proximal tubule, from patients has been reported to contain cells with the mutation.[121]

## Decreased Gastrointestinal Absorption

### ABNORMALITIES OF VITAMIN D METABOLISM

Vitamin D and its metabolites play an important role in phosphorus homeostasis.[122] Vitamin D promotes the intestinal absorption of calcium and phosphorus and is necessary to maintain the normal mineralization of bone. Dietary deficiencies of vitamin D increase the amount of osteoid tissue in the skeleton and decrease normal mineralization. Bone mineralization is a complex process that is not completely understood. Normally, the osteoblast is responsible for laying down normal collagen that is well organized and distributed in a lamellar fashion. Between the recently deposited collagen and the old bone is an area called the mineralization front. Initially, amorphous calcium phosphate is deposited in the mineralization front and eventually matures into hydroxyapatite $[Ca_{10}(PO_4)_6(OH)_2]$. Thus, the osteoid tissue changes into bone. Optimal mineralization requires the following: (1) normal bone cell activity, (2) normal supply of minerals, (3) appropriate pH (7.4 to 7.6), (4) normal synthesis and composition of the matrix, and (5) control of inhibitors of calcification.

The appositional growth rate in normal bone is about 1 μm/day, and complete mineralization of the osteoid requires 13 to 21 days. Thus, the thickness of the osteoid usually does not exceed 20 μm. Less than 20% of bone surface is normally covered by osteoid. When a biopsy is performed in a normal subject who previously ingested two doses of tetracycline separately and 3 weeks apart, one normally detects two fluorescent rings or bands, indicating the locations of the mineralization front. In a patient with osteomalacia, usually a single band, no band, or an irregular and spotty uptake of tetracycline is seen. In patients with rickets or osteomalacia, there is a quantitative and qualitative defect in bone mineralization.

### VITAMIN D–DEFICIENT RICKETS

Diets deficient in vitamin D lead to the metabolic disorder known as rickets when it occurs in children and osteomalacia when it appears in adults.[123] Deficiency of vitamin D in childhood results in severe deformities of bone because of rapid growth. These deformities are characterized by soft, loose areas in the skull, known as *craniotabes,* and by costochondral swelling or bending, known as *rachitic rosary.* The chest usually becomes flattened, and the sternum may be pushed forward to form the so-called pigeon chest. Thoracic expansion may be greatly reduced, with impairment of respiratory function. Kyphosis is a common finding. There is remarkable swelling of the joints, particularly the wrists and ankles, with characteristic anterior bowing of the legs; fractures of the greenstick variety may also be seen. In adults, the symptoms are not as striking and are usually characterized by bone pain, weakness, radiolucent areas, and pseudofractures. Pseudofractures represent stretch fractures in which the normal process of healing is impaired, owing to a mineralization defect. Mild hypocalcemia may be present; however, hypophosphatemia is the most frequent biochemical alteration. This metabolic abnormality responds well to administration of small amounts of vitamin D.

## VITAMIN D–DEPENDENT RICKETS

There are recessively inherited forms of vitamin D–refractory rickets. These conditions are characterized by hypophosphatemia, hypocalcemia, elevated levels of serum alkaline phosphatase and, sometimes, generalized aminoaciduria and severe bone lesions. Two main forms of vitamin D–dependent rickets (VDDR) have been characterized. The serum concentrations of $1,25(OH)_2D_3$ differentiate the two types of VDDR. Type I VDDR is due to a mutation in the gene converting $25(OH)D_3$ to $1,25(OH)_2D_3$, the renal 1-hydroxylase enzyme.[124, 125] This condition responds to very large doses of vitamins $D_2$ and $D_3$ (100 to 300 times the normal physiologic doses), or 0.5 to 1 μg/day of $1,25(OH)_2D_3$. Type II VDDR is characterized by an end-organ resistance to $1,25(OH)_2D_3$. Plasma levels of $1,25(OH)_2D_3$ are elevated. This finding, in association with radiographic and biochemical signs of rickets, implies resistance of the target tissue to calcitriol. Cellular defects found in patients with type II VDDR are heterogeneous, providing a partial explanation for the different clinical manifestations of this disorder. Among the cellular defects are (1) decreased number of cytosolic receptors, (2) deficient maximal hormonal binding, (3) deficient hormone-binding affinity, (4) normal hormonal binding but undetectable nuclear localization, and (5) abnormal DNA binding domain for the $1,25(OH)_2D_3$ receptor.[126]

Numerous studies have demonstrated that hereditary type II VDDR is a genetic disease affecting the vitamin D receptor.[127–134] Defects in the hormone-binding domain[127, 128] and the DNA-binding domain[129, 130] have been defined. In addition, several cases of human VDDR have been studied, and no abnormality in the coding region of the vitamin D receptor has been found,[131] suggesting a defect elsewhere in the hormone action pathway. An unexplained feature of this disease in adolescents is the tendency for calcium levels to normalize and for the radiographic abnormalities of rickets to improve; it thus appears that they outgrow the disease. Human VDDR as a genetic defect in the vitamin D receptor varies significantly from other genetic diseases of steroid hormone receptors caused by resistance to thyroid hormone, androgens, and estrogens.[132–134] For instance, individuals heterozygous for vitamin D receptor mutations are apparently completely normal. Second, no dominant negative mutations, which are prominent in thyroid hormone resistance, have been identified as a cause of human VDDR. Thus, much remains to be learned from the genetic analysis of this disease. Treatment of this condition requires large pharmacologic doses of calcium, which overcome the receptor defects and maintain bone remodeling.[130] Studies in mice with targeted disruption of the vitamin D receptor gene, an animal model of type II VDDR, confirm that many aspects of the clinical phenotype are due to decreased intestinal ion transport and can be overcome by adjustments in dietary intake.[135]

## ONCOGENIC OSTEOMALACIA

Oncogenic osteomalacia is a rare syndrome characterized by hypophosphatemia associated with tumors. It was described initially in association with benign mesenchymal tumors; however, more recent reports emphasize its association with malignant tumors.[136–138] The other characteristics of this syndrome are increased phosphate excretion, low plasma $1,25(OH)_2D_3$ concentrations, and osteomalacia. All the biochemical and pathologic abnormalities disappear when the tumor is resected. The tumors associated with this syndrome are thought to secrete a substance that inhibits the renal tubular reabsorption of phosphate and suppresses $25(OH)D_3$ 1α-hydroxylase activity. Whether this factor interacts directly with renal tubular cells is unknown. Cai and coworkers investigated whether the medium in which sclerosing hemangioma cells from a patient with osteogenic osteomalacia were cultured could affect sodium-dependent phosphate transport.[117] They found that the medium inhibited sodium-dependent phosphate transport without increasing cellular concentrations of cAMP. The medium had PTH-like immunoreactivity but no PTH-related protein immunoreactivity, and the action of the tumor medium was not blocked by a PTH antagonist. Plasma $1,25(OH)_2D_3$ concentrations are low in patients with oncogenic osteomalacia, despite the presence of hypophosphatemia,[139–141] which usually increases plasma concentrations of $1,25(OH)_2D_3$ by stimulating renal $25(OH)D_3$ 1α-hydroxylase in a PTH-independent manner.[142] In addition to the hypophosphatemia, deficient production of $1,25(OH)_2D_3$ contributes to the pathogenesis of osteomalacia in these patients. Miyauchi and colleagues reported that $25(OH)D_3$ 1α-hydroxylase activity of cultured renal tubular cells was decreased by incubating the cells with tumor extracts.[143] This supports the concept that the tumor extracts contain a substance that inhibits the formation of $1,25(OH)_2D_3$ in the proximal tubule.

The various studies of oncogenic osteomalacia and some studies associated with X-linked hypophosphatemic rickets support the possibility that a hormone primarily responsible for the regulation of renal phosphate reabsorption is abnormally produced in these conditions. Econs and Drezner called the substance phosphatonin.[111] The similarity between oncogenic osteomalacia and X-linked hypophosphatemia raises the possibility that phosphatonin is the factor normally degraded by the *PHEX* gene product that causes abnormal phosphate transport in X-linked hypophosphatemia and the Hyp mouse.

### MALABSORPTION

Because most of the absorption of phosphorus from the gastrointestinal tract occurs in the duodenum and jejunum, gastrointestinal disorders such as celiac disease, tropical and nontropical sprue, and regional enteritis may decrease the absorption of phosphorus.[85] Phosphorus malabsorption has also been described in patients who have undergone surgical bypass procedures for morbid obesity. The degree of hypophosphatemia varies among patients with intestinal malabsorption, being extremely mild in some cases and severe in others.

### MALNUTRITION

Most of the phosphorus ingested in the diet is present in protein, particularly meat, cheese, milk, and eggs. In many parts of the world where protein consumption is extremely low, hypophosphatemia occurs predominantly in children. Overall growth is retarded, and a number of metabolic abnormalities are present.[144]

### ADMINISTRATION OF PHOSPHATE BINDERS

Certain compounds, mainly aluminum salts (aluminum hydroxide, aluminum carbonate gel) and calcium carbonate, are used in the treatment of hyperphosphatemia.[145] However, when these compounds are given in excess, they may produce profound hypophosphatemia. These gels trap phosphorus in the small intestine and increase the amount of phosphorus in the stool. Patients ingesting large amounts of phosphate binders who are not followed closely may develop phosphate depletion. Over a period of time, such individuals may develop severe weakness, bone pain, and osteomalacia.

## Other Causes of Hypophosphatemia

Reviews of the causes of hypophosphatemia in hospitalized patients attributed the majority of cases to intravenous administration of carbohydrate.[146, 147] However, a wide variety of other causes were found, including diuretic usage, hyperalimentation, alcoholism, respiratory alkalosis, and use of phosphate binders.[148] A 31% incidence of hypophosphatemia was seen in patients admitted to a general medical ward, and a further decrease in serum concentrations occurred in all patients with acute alcoholism 2 to 5 days after admission to a medical ward.[149] Hypophosphatemia is also seen frequently during treatment for diabetic ketoacidosis.[150] When diabetic patients develop ketoacidosis, they usually have increased phosphate excretion in the urine; however, serum phosphate may be slightly elevated owing to acidosis. During the administration of insulin, there is a rapid decrease in glucose levels, with translocation of phosphate from the extracellular to the intracellular space, resulting in hypophosphatemia.

Acute respiratory alkalosis decreases urinary phosphate excretion but produces marked hypophosphatemia.[151] In contrast, patients who receive sodium bicarbonate excrete large amounts of phosphate in the urine; however, the hypophosphatemia that may develop is only moderate in nature. It has been postulated that in respiratory alkalosis there is an increase in intracellular pH with activation of glycolysis and increased formation of phosphate-containing sugars, leading to a precipitous fall in the concentration of serum phosphorus. The mild hypophosphatemia that may be seen during administration of sodium bicarbonate is probably secondary to increased renal phosphate excretion due to a decrease in ionized calcium and release of PTH, as well as to the consequences of extracellular fluid volume expansion.[57]

In addition, new clinical disorders have been identified in which hypophosphatemia is an important aspect of the pathologic condition. Marked hypophosphatemia has been associated with acute leukemia or with lymphomas in the leukemic phase.[152–154] These individuals typically present with hypophosphatemia, normocalcemia, and no evidence of excess PTH activity. Urinary phosphate is typically extremely low. Although kinetic studies have not been performed in this setting, the fact that serum phosphate concentration correlated with a growth phase of the tumors and that hyperphosphatemia was seen when cells were destroyed by chemotherapy or radiotherapy strongly suggests that serum phosphorus was initially used in the rapid growth of new cells. Because these patients are often severely ill and under treatment with glucose infusions as well as antacids and other drugs known to induce hypophosphatemia, they may be at great risk of developing severe acute phosphorus depletion.

Another clinical condition in which hypophosphatemia has been a prominent feature is toxic shock syndrome. Chesney and colleagues described 22 women with this disorder who showed hypocalcemia and hypophosphatemia as prominent manifestations.[155] Whether respiratory alkalosis or staphylococcal sepsis induced the release of substances that were responsible for acute phosphorus shifts into cells is unknown.

Linnquist and coworkers studied in a prospective fashion the importance of hypophosphatemia in patients with severe burns.[156] In 33 patients studied for 2 weeks after injury, transient hypophosphatemia was seen in the second to tenth days in all these individuals. Five of seven patients who died from complications of the terminal injury had severe hypophosphatemia. Because urinary phosphorus excretion was not increased, tissue uptake seems to be the predominant mechanism responsible for the hypophosphatemia.

Levy reported the occurrence of severe hypophosphatemia during the rewarming phase in a profoundly hypothermic patient.[157] In this individual, urinary excretion of phosphorus was minimal, suggesting that a shift of phosphate into the cells occurred as a consequence of rewarming.

Finally, the development of hypophosphatemia as a consequence of refeeding clinically starved patients has been reported. Silvis and coworkers showed that the classic phosphorus depletion syndrome, consisting of paresthesias, weakness, seizures, and hypophosphatemia, can occur in individuals who receive oral caloric supplements following a prolonged period of starvation.[158] To further evaluate this issue, they performed studies in normal dogs who had been starved or had received normal diets and found that the infusion of calories through an intragastric catheter to previously starved animals resulted in a fall in serum phosphorus from an average of 4.8 to 1.6 mg/dL. Nearly 50% of starved animals developed clinical signs of phosphate depletion following oral refeeding. Weinsier and Krumdiek reported two patients who developed phosphorus depletion syndrome in association with cardiopulmonary decompensation following overzealous hyperalimentation after prolonged caloric deprivation.[159]

## Clinical and Biochemical Manifestations of Hypophosphatemia

The manifestations of hypophosphatemia are presented in Table 27–2. It has been suggested that the clinical manifestations of hypophosphatemia and severe phosphorus depletion are related to disturbances in cellular energy and metabolism. Studies have examined the effects of phosphate depletion on cellular energetics and other components of cell function. A study of glycolytic intermediates and adenine nucleotides during insulin treatment of patients with diabetic ketoacidosis emphasized the important effects of insulin-induced cellular phosphate depletion on cell metabolism.[160] These results demonstrated that the reduced level of 2,3-diphosphoglycerate (2,3-DPG) seen during insulin treatment of diabetes is due to intracellular phosphorus depletion producing a decrease in glyceraldehyde-3-phosphate dehydrogenase activity rather than inhibition of the phosphofructokinase enzyme system. Ditzel suggested that repeated transient decreases in red cell oxygen delivery due to reduced 2,3-DPG with insulin-induced hypophosphatemia could contribute, over many years, to the microvascular disease seen in diabetic patients.[161] It should be pointed out that patients with mild degrees of hypophosphatemia are usually asymptomatic. However, if hypophosphatemia is severe—that is, if serum phosphorus levels are below 1.5 mg/dL—a series of hematologic, neurologic, and metabolic disorders may develop. In general, such patients become anorectic and weak, and mild bone pain may be present if the hypophosphatemia persists for several months (see Table 27–2).

**TABLE 27–2.** Clinical and Biochemical Manifestations of Marked Hypophosphatemia

I. Cardiovascular and skeletal muscle
    A. Decreased cardiac output
    B. Muscle weakness
    C. Decreased transmembrane resting potential
    D. Rhabdomyolysis
II. Carbohydrate metabolism
    A. Hyperinsulinemia
    B. Decreased glucose metabolism
III. Hematologic alterations
    A. Red blood cells
        1. Decreased adenosine triphosphate (ATP) content
        2. Decreased 2,3-diphosphoglycerate
        3. Decreased $P_{50}$
        4. Increased oxygen affinity
        5. Decreased life span
        6. Hemolysis
        7. Spherocytosis
    B. Leukocytes
        1. Decreased phagocytosis
        2. Decreased chemotaxis
        3. Decreased bactericidal activity
    C. Platelets
        1. Impaired clot retraction
        2. Thrombocytopenia
        3. Decreased ATP content
        4. Megakaryocytosis
        5. Decreased life span
IV. Neurologic manifestations
    A. Anorexia
    B. Irritability
    C. Confusion
    D. Paresthesias
    E. Dysarthria
    F. Ataxia
    G. Seizures
    H. Coma
V. Skeletal abnormalities
    A. Bone pain
    B. Radiolucent areas (on x-ray)
    C. Pseudofractures
    D. Rickets or osteomalacia
VI. Biochemical and renal manifestations
    A. Low parathyroid hormone levels
    B. Increased 1,25-dihydroxyvitamin $D_3$
    C. Hypercalciuria
    D. Hypomagnesemia
    E. Hypermagnesuria
    F. Hypophosphaturia
    G. Decreased glomerular filtration rate
    H. Decreased maximum rate of transport for bicarbonate
    I. Decreased renal gluconeogenesis
    J. Decreased titratable acid excretion
    K. Increased creatinine phosphokinase
    L. Increased aldolase

Adapted from Slatopolsky E: Pathophysiology of calcium, magnesium, and phosphorus. In Klahr S (ed): The Kidney and Body Fluids in Health and Disease. New York, Plenum, 1983, p 269.

## CARDIOVASCULAR AND SKELETAL MUSCLE MANIFESTATIONS

Severe cardiomyopathy with decreased cardiac output has been described in patients and animals with severe hypophosphatemia.[162, 163] Studies revealed that the resting muscle membrane potential fell, sodium chloride and water content of the tissue increased, and potassium content decreased in severe hypophosphatemia.[164] These values returned to normal after phosphate was administered. Skeletal muscle weakness and electromyographic abnormalities are associated with chronic hypophosphatemia and phosphate depletion. Dogs fed low-phosphate diets for several months developed changes in muscle, rhabdomyolysis, and characteristic increases in their levels of creatinine phosphokinase and aldolase in blood.[165] The syndrome of rhabdomyolysis has been observed in alcoholic patients with hypophosphatemia.[166] Knochel and colleagues showed that myopathy associated with phosphate depletion in dogs led to changes in cell water content, sodium concentration, and transmembrane potential difference.[165] Kretz and associates examined the possibility that changes in calcium transport in the sarcoplasmic reticulum of muscle were responsible for the clinical myopathy seen in acute phosphate depletion.[167] Despite significant hypophosphatemia and a reduction in muscle phosphorus concentration, they found no significant changes in the rate of calcium uptake or calcium-concentrating ability in vesicles prepared from muscle sarcoplasmic reticulum of phosphate-depleted rats. Thus, the role of altered transcellular calcium movements in phosphate-depleted tissues has not been completely understood.

## EFFECTS ON CARBOHYDRATE METABOLISM

Hyperinsulinemia and abnormal glucose metabolism suggesting insulin resistance have been described in phosphate depletion. DeFronzo and Lang used the glucose and insulin clamp technique to study the kinetics of glucose metabolism in patients with a variety of chronic hypophosphatemic conditions, including vitamin D–resistant rickets.[168] When glucose was infused to maintain constant glycemia at 125 mg/dL, hypophosphatemic individuals required 36% less glucose to maintain these glycemic levels than did controls. Also, when euglycemia was achieved by combined insulin and glucose infusion, the hypophosphatemic individuals required 40% less glucose to maintain euglycemia than did controls. Insulin catabolism was apparently unaffected in these hypophosphatemic individuals. These data indicate that hypophosphatemia is associated with impaired glucose metabolism in both hyperglycemic and euglycemic patients.

## HEMATOLOGIC MANIFESTATIONS

Hematologic abnormalities of hypophosphatemia are a major manifestation of this syndrome.[169–171] In addition to defects in the affinity of oxyhemoglobin, leading to generalized tissue hypoxia, there may be increased hemolysis.[172, 173] Quantitative and functional defects have also been described in platelets and leukocytes.[174] These defects lead to diminished platelet aggregation, as well as abnormalities in chemotaxis and phagocytosis of white blood cells. The latter may contribute to the increased risk of gram-negative sepsis reported in hypophosphatemic patients.[175] This is of particular concern in immunosuppressed patients receiving phosphate-poor alimentation through a central venous line.

## NEUROLOGIC MANIFESTATIONS

Manifestations at the level of the central nervous system resulting in generalized anorexia and malaise or more severe disturbances such as ataxia, seizures, and coma have been described in hypophosphatemia.[176–178] Neuromuscular abnormalities include paresthesias and weakness, the result of both myopathic changes and diminished nerve conduction.[179]

## SKELETAL ABNORMALITIES

The skeletal abnormalities associated with hypophosphatemia, particularly in vitamin D–resistant rickets, may be quite marked. In addition, bony abnormalities, including osteomalacia and pathologic fractures, have been described in antacid-induced phosphate depletion,[180, 181] as well as in hypophosphatemic patients undergoing hemodialysis who did not receive phosphate-binding gels.[182] A rheumatic syndrome resembling ankylosing spondylitis also has been reported in hypophosphatemic patients.[183]

## GASTROINTESTINAL DISTURBANCES

Gastrointestinal manifestations include anorexia, nausea, and vomiting.[177] It has been speculated that hypophosphatemia in an alcoholic patient may further impair hepatic function through hypoxic insult.

## RENAL MANIFESTATIONS

There is decreased phosphorus excretion and decreased tubular reabsorption of calcium, magnesium, bicarbonate, and glucose.[184–189] The renal conservation of phosphorus occurs early in the syndrome and is the result of a primary increase in the tubular reabsorption of the anion, as well as a decrease in GFR and consequently in the filtered load of phosphorus.[189, 190] This mechanism results in complete renal conservation of phosphorus, with net losses representing only a small fraction of total body phosphorus stores.[177] The increase in phosphorus reabsorption seen with phosphorus depletion is independent of several hormones known to influence phosphorus transport under other circumstances, including PTH, vitamin D, calcitonin, and thyroxine.[191] The possibility that serum phosphorus concentration per se (or intracellular phosphorus) may in some manner regulate its absorption along the nephron seems plausible. Hypercalciuria of enough magnitude to produce negative calcium balance is commonly seen in hypophosphatemic patients. Several factors contribute to this increase in calcium excretion, including increased calcium mobilization from bone, enhanced gastrointestinal calcium absorption, and inhibition of renal tubular calcium reabsorption.[184, 189] These effects appear to be independent of PTH activity and may be the result of a direct effect of phosphate on these transport processes.

### ACID-BASE DISTURBANCES

Renal bicarbonate wasting, diminished titratable acid excretion, and decreased ammoniagenesis have been reported in hypophosphatemia.[185, 192] However, these defects are counterbalanced to some extent by the mobilization of alkali from bone. Thus, steady-state pH may be near normal at the expense of skeletal buffers.[186]

## Differential Diagnosis of Hypophosphatemia

In general, the cause of hypophosphatemia can be determined from the medical history or from the clinical setting in which it occurs. When the cause is in doubt, measurement of the urinary phosphorus excretion level may be of help. If the urinary phosphorus concentration is less than 4 mg/dL when the serum phosphorus level is less than 2 mg/dL, renal losses can be excluded.[193] Of the three major extrarenal causes—diminished phosphorus intake, increased extrarenal losses (gastrointestinal tract), and translocation into the intracellular space—the last is the most common, especially in hospitalized patients.[146, 194] When urine phosphorus excretion is high, the differential diagnosis includes hyperparathyroidism, a primary renal tubular abnormality, or vitamin D–dependent or –resistant renal rickets. Measurements of serum calcium, PTH, and vitamin D and its metabolites, as well as urinary excretion of other solutes (glucose, amino acids, bicarbonate), usually elucidate the underlying disturbance that is responsible for the hypophosphatemia.

## Treatment of Hypophosphatemia

Several general principles apply to the treatment of patients with hypophosphatemia. As with any predominantly intracellular ion (e.g., potassium), the state of total body phosphorus stores, as well as the magnitude of phosphorus losses, cannot be readily assessed by measuring the concentration in serum. In fact, when a rapid shift of phosphorus has resulted from glucose infusion or hyperalimentation, total body stores of phosphorus may be normal, although with diminished intake and renal losses, there may be severe phosphorus depletion. Furthermore, the volume distribution of phosphorus may vary widely, reflecting in part the intensity and duration of the underlying cause.[195]

In clinical situations in which hypophosphatemia is expected (e.g., glucose infusion or hyperalimentation in alcoholic or nutritionally compromised patients during treatment of diabetic ketoacidosis), careful monitoring of the concentration of serum phosphorus is crucial. In these situations, phosphorus supplementation to prevent the development of severe hypophosphatemia may be helpful. Certainly, other contributing causes of hypophosphatemia in this setting should be identified and treated. This is especially true of the use of phosphate-binding antacids (aluminum and magnesium hydroxide) for peptic ulcer disease, which can be replaced by aluminum phosphate antacids (Phosphagel) or cimetidine (Tagamet). It is now generally recommended that hyperalimentation solutions contain a phosphorus concentration of 12 to 15 mM (37 to 46.5 mg/dL) to provide an appropriate amount of phosphorus in patients in whom renal impairment is absent.[195] Phosphorus supplementation during glucose infusion or during the treatment of ketoacidosis is usually withheld until the serum phosphorus levels decrease below 1 mg/dL. Phosphorus may be given orally to these patients and others with mild, asymptomatic hypophosphatemia in the form of skim milk, which contains 0.9 mg/mL, Nutraphos (3.3 mg/mL), or phosphorus soda (129 mg/mL). However, intestinal absorption is quite variable, and diarrhea often complicates the oral administration of phosphate-containing compounds. For these reasons, parenteral administration is usually recommended in hospitalized patients.

If oral therapy is permissible, Fleet Phospho-Soda may be given at a dose of 60 mmol daily in three doses (21 mmol/5 mL or 643 mg/5 mL). A convenient method is to provide the phosphorus together with potassium replacement in these patients. Addition of 5 mL of potassium phosphate to 1 L of intravenous fluid provides 22 mEq of potassium and 15 mmol (466 mg) of phosphorus.[195] However, because potassium losses may greatly exceed the phosphorus deficit, the repletion of potassium should not be totally linked to phosphorus therapy. In patients with severe phosphate depletion, it is difficult to determine the magnitude of the total deficit of phosphorus and to calculate a precise initial dose. It is usually prudent to proceed with caution and repair the deficit slowly. The most frequently recommended regimen is 0.08 mmol/kg body weight (2.5 mg/kg body weight) given over 6 hours for severe but uncomplicated hypophosphatemia and 0.16 mmol/kg body weight (5 mg/kg body weight) in symptomatic patients.[195] Parenteral administration should be discontinued when the serum phosphorus concentration is greater than 2 mg/dL.

Calcium administration may be needed during phosphate repletion to prevent severe hypocalcemia. Calcium must not be added to bicarbonate or phosphate-containing solutions because of the potential precipitation of calcium salts. Intravenous infusion of calcium gluconate or calcium chloride may be given until tetany abates. In addition to hypocalcemia, metastatic calcification, hypotension, hyperkalemia, and hypernatremia are potential side effects of parenteral infusion of phosphorus. These problems can be prevented by judicious use of therapy and frequent monitoring of serum electrolyte concentrations.

# HYPERPHOSPHATEMIA

Hyperphosphatemia is said to occur when serum phosphorus concentration exceeds 5 mg/dL in adults. It should be remembered that in children and adolescents, serum phosphorus levels up to 6 mg/dL may be physiologic. The most frequent cause of hyperphosphatemia is decreased excretion of phosphorus in the urine as a consequence of a fall in GFR. However, increases in serum phosphorus can also occur as a result of increased entry into the extracellular fluid due to excessive intake of phosphorus or increased release of phosphorus from tissue breakdown. The major causes of hyperphosphatemia are listed in Table 27–3.

## Causes of Hyperphosphatemia

### DECREASED EXCRETION OF PHOSPHORUS IN URINE AND DECREASED RENAL FUNCTION

In progressive renal failure, phosphorus homeostasis is maintained by a progressive increase in phosphorus excretion per nephron.[196, 197] As a consequence of this increased phosphorus excretion, it is unusual to see marked hyperphosphatemia until GFR values fall below 25 mL/min.[198] Under physiologic conditions with a GFR of 120 mL/min, a fractional excretion of 5% to 15% of the filtered load of phosphorus is adequate to maintain phosphorus homeostasis. However, as renal insufficiency progresses and the number of nephrons decreases, fractional excretion of phosphorus may increase to as high as 60% to 80% of the filtered load. In patients with renal disease, this progressive phosphaturia per nephron serves to maintain the concentration of phosphorus within normal limits in plasma. However, when the number of nephrons is greatly diminished and the dietary intake of phosphorus remains constant, phosphorus homeostasis can no longer be maintained, and hyperphosphatemia develops. This usually occurs when the GFR falls below 25 mL/min. As hyperphosphatemia develops, the filtered load of phosphorus per nephron increases, phosphorus excretion rises, and phosphorus balance is re-established, but at higher concentrations of serum phosphorus.

**TABLE 27–3.** Causes of Hyperphosphatemia

I. Decreased renal excretion of phosphate
  A. Renal insufficiency
    1. Chronic
    2. Acute
  B. Hypoparathyroidism
  C. Pseudohypoparathyroidism
    1. Type I
    2. Type II
  D. Abnormal circulating parathyroid hormone
  E. Acromegaly
  F. Tumoral calcinosis
  G. Administration of bisphosphonates
II. Increased entrance of phosphorus into the extracellular fluid
  A. Neoplastic diseases
    1. Leukemia
    2. Lymphoma
  B. Increased catabolism
  C. Respiratory acidosis
III. Administration of $PO_4$ salts or vitamin D
  A. Pharmacologic administration of vitamin D metabolites
  B. Ingestion or administration of phosphate salts
IV. Miscellaneous
  A. Cortical hyperostosis
  B. Intermittent hyperphosphatemia
  C. Artifacts

Adapted from Slatopolsky E.: Pathophysiology of calcium, magnesium, and phosphorus. In Klahr S. (ed): The Kidney and Body Fluids and Disease. New York, Plenum, 1983, p 269.

Hyperphosphatemia is a usual finding in patients with advanced renal insufficiency unless phosphorus intake has been decreased through dietary manipulations or the patient is receiving phosphate binders, such as calcium carbonate or aluminum-containing salts, that decrease the absorption of phosphate from the gastrointestinal tract.[199] In patients with acute renal failure, hyperphosphatemia is a usual finding.[200] The degree of hyperphosphatemia in patients with acute renal failure varies considerably. It is quite marked in patients with renal insufficiency secondary to severe trauma or known traumatic rhabdomyolysis, as frequently occurs in patients ingesting large amounts of alcohol or in heroin addicts.[201] The degree of hyperphosphatemia depends on the amount of phosphorus released from damaged tissue, because phosphorus intake and decreased GFR (to $<2$ mL/min) are constant across different forms of oliguric acute renal failure. In most patients with acute renal failure, hyperphosphatemia is transitory, and serum phosphorus values return toward normal as renal function improves. However, in some of these patients, infection or tissue destruction from many causes may maintain relatively high serum phosphorus values, even during the recovery phase of renal function.

### DECREASED OR ABSENT LEVELS OF CIRCULATING PARATHYROID HORMONE

Hypoparathyroidism is characterized by low or absent levels of PTH, low levels of serum calcium, and hyperphosphatemia.[202] The most common cause of hypoparathyroidism is injury to the parathyroid glands or their blood supply during thyroid, parathyroid, or radical neck surgery. Idiopathic hypoparathyroidism is a rare disease. Because PTH normally inhibits the renal reabsorption of phosphorus, its absence leads to an elevation in the Tm for phosphorus and decreased excretion of the anion in the urine. Balance is re-established when the serum phosphorus concentration rises to 6 to 8 mg/dL. At this concentration of serum phosphorus, the filtered load of phosphate is increased, exceeding the Tm for phosphorus reabsorption, and a new steady state is re-established.

Patients with hypoparathyroidism are easily diagnosed by the findings of low levels of serum calcium, hyperphosphatemia, and undetectable levels of circulating immunoreactive PTH. After several years of hypoparathyroidism, other signs may become manifest, such as cataracts and bilateral, symmetrical calcification of the basal ganglia on x-rays of the skull. The most striking symptoms in patients presenting with hypoparathyroidism are related to an increase in neuromuscular excitability resulting from a decrease in the levels of ionized calcium in serum. Some patients may not develop hypocalcemia and severe tetany, but increased neuromuscular excitability may be demonstrated by contraction of facial muscles in response to stimulus over the facial nerve (Chvostek sign) or by carpal spasm (Trousseau sign) occurring 2 or 3 minutes after inflating a blood pressure cuff around the arm above systolic blood pressure. In other patients, psychiatric disturbances, paresthesias, numbness, muscle cramps, and dysphagia may be presenting symptoms.

## PSEUDOHYPOPARATHYROIDISM

Pseudohypoparathyroidism is a relatively rare condition characterized by end-organ resistance to the action of PTH.[203] Characteristically, the kidney and skeleton do not respond appropriately to the action of PTH. Some patients with pseudohypoparathyroidism may have specific somatic characteristics such as short stature, round face, short metacarpal bones and phalanges, and some degree of mental retardation. Biochemically, these patients, like those with hypoparathyroidism, have low concentrations of serum calcium and hyperphosphatemia. However, there are two important points in the differential diagnosis. In the majority of patients with pseudohypoparathyroidism, the circulating levels of immunoreactive PTH are elevated, whereas in patients with true hypoparathyroidism, PTH levels are low or absent. Second, patients with pseudohypoparathyroidism do not respond to the administration of exogenous PTH with phosphaturia. Patients with true hypoparathyroidism demonstrate a heightened phosphaturic response to the administration of exogenous PTH.

Two major types of pseudohypoparathyroidism have been described. In type I, patients fail to increase the excretion of cAMP or phosphate in the urine in response to the administration of exogenous PTH. This abnormal response seems to be related, at least in some patients, to a defect in the guanosine triphosphate–binding protein, $G_s$, of the adenylate cyclase complex.[204, 205] In other patients, there is an increase in cAMP in response to the administration of exogenous PTH but no phosphaturic response. This condition has been termed pseudohypoparathyroidism type II.[206]

## ABNORMAL CIRCULATING PARATHYROID HORMONE

This syndrome is characterized by hyperphosphatemia, hypocalcemia, chronic tetany, and cataracts. These manifestations, as described earlier, are observed in patients with hypoparathyroidism, but these patients have normal or high serum levels of PTH. However, in contrast to patients with pseudohypoparathyroidism, they do respond to the exogenous administration of PTH with an increase in the excretion of cAMP and phosphaturia. It has been postulated that the defect in these patients relates to an abnormal form of endogenous PTH that is devoid of physiologic effects.[207] However, this hypothesis has not been substantiated by the characterization and analysis of circulating PTH in these patients.

## ACROMEGALY

Growth hormone decreases the urinary excretion of phosphorus and increases the Tm for phosphorus.[208] Hypersecretion of growth hormone may lead to the development of gigantism if the increased secretion occurs before closure of the epiphysis or to acromegaly if the excessive secretion occurs after puberty. Hyperphosphatemia has been described in patients with acromegaly. It is known that serum phosphorus concentrations are higher in children (5 to 8 mg/dL) than in adults. This may be related in part to increased levels of circulating growth hormone in children.

## TUMORAL CALCINOSIS

Although the cause of tumoral calcinosis has not been completely characterized, its pathogenesis is probably related to a primary increase in phosphorus reabsorption by the kidney.[209] This condition, which is seen more frequently in young African Americans, is characterized by hyperphosphatemia, ectopic calcification around large joints, normal levels of circulating immunoreactive PTH, and a normal response to the administration of exogenous PTH.[210, 211] The extensive calcification of soft tissues observed in patients with this condition is most likely due to an elevated phosphorus-calcium product in blood. Despite the development of hyperphosphatemia, patients with tumoral calcinosis do not develop secondary hyperparathyroidism. This may be due to the fact that circulating levels of $1,25(OH)_2D_3$ remain normal in these patients, despite hyperphosphatemia. These normal levels of $1,25(OH)_2D_3$ maintain a normal gastrointestinal absorption of calcium. This, combined with the decreased urinary calcium observed in these patients, may serve to maintain normal serum calcium values and prevent the development of secondary hyperparathyroidism.

## ADMINISTRATION OF BISPHOSPHONATES

Administration of bisphosphonates, which are used in the treatment of Paget disease and osteoporosis, may result in the development of hyperphosphatemia.[212] The mechanisms by which bisphosphonates increase serum phosphorus are not completely clear at present but may involve an alteration in phosphate distribution between different cellular compartments and a decrease in renal phosphorus excretion. It appears that both the level of circulating PTH and the urinary excretion of cAMP after administration of exogenous PTH are normal in patients receiving bisphosphonates.

## REDISTRIBUTION OF PHOSPHORUS BETWEEN INTRACELLULAR AND EXTRACELLULAR POOLS

Various syndromes of tissue breakdown may result in the development of hyperphosphatemia and subsequent hypocalcemia. Hyperphosphatemia has been described in patients with several types of lymphomas. Patients receiving treatment for lymphoblastic leukemia may develop hyperphosphatemia with a concomitant decrease in serum calcium.[213] The phosphorus load originates primarily from the destruction of lymphoblasts, which have about four times the concentration of organic and inorganic phosphorus present in mature lymphocytes.

Similar findings have been described during the treatment of Burkitt lymphoma. Cohen and colleagues reviewed the acute tumor lysis syndrome associated with the treatment of Burkitt lymphoma.[214] In 37 patients with Burkitt lymphoma, azotemia occurred in 14 patients and preceded chemotherapy in 8. Pretreatment azotemia was associated with elevated levels of lactate dehydrogenase and uric acid and sometimes with extrinsic ureteral obstruction by the tumor. Following chemotherapy, major metabolic complications related to tumor lysis were associated with large tumors and high lactate dehydrogenase levels and were manifested by hyperkalemia, hyperphosphatemia, and hyperuricemia. Elevated phosphorus levels were seen in 31% of nonazotemic patients and in all azotemic patients. Hemodialysis was required in three patients for control of azotemia, hyperuricemia, hyperphosphatemia, and/or hyperkalemia.

Tsokos and coworkers studied the renal metabolic complications of other undifferentiated lymphomas and lymphoblastic lymphomas.[215] These workers found that serum lactate dehydrogenase before chemotherapy correlated well with the stage of disease and predicted the serum levels of creatinine, uric acid, and phosphorus in the post-treatment period. Patients with lactate dehydrogenase values greater than 2000 IU were likely to develop severe hyperphosphatemia. When azotemia developed in the postchemotherapy period, it was attributed to hyperuricemia and/or hyperphosphatemia. Some of these patients had elevated serum phosphorus levels in the range of 20 to 30 mg/dL, which may contribute to the development of renal insufficiency due to calcium deposition in the kidney and other tissues.

Thus, there is a great risk of hyperphosphatemia in patients undergoing chemotherapy for rapidly growing malignant lymphomas. The best method of preventing this complication, as well as the best therapeutic intervention, has not been well defined. Initially, it appears to be useful to attempt to increase the renal excretion of phosphate during the induction of remission by chemotherapy in these patients. This requires infusion of large amounts of saline and possibly bicarbonate, which has been shown to increase renal phosphorus excretion above and beyond the mere effects of volume expansion. Acetazolamide, a potent phosphaturic agent, might also be beneficial in these individuals. The general recommendation of hemodialysis as the prime therapeutic modality for hyperphosphatemia and acute renal insufficiency resulting from tumor lysis is not based on experimental data. Although hemodialysis rapidly lowers serum phosphorus levels, it does not address the mass of phosphorus that is continually presented to the extracellular space from ongoing tissue breakdown. Thus, it is possible that combined hemodialysis and peritoneal dialysis, or even peritoneal dialysis alone, might be as beneficial, if not more so, and safer in individuals with tumor lysis syndrome.

## INCREASED CATABOLISM

Conditions characterized by increased protein breakdown (severe tissue muscle damage, severe infections) may sometimes be accompanied by hyperphosphatemia. Although the hyperphosphatemia may be related simply to translocation of phosphorus into the extracellular space, other factors seem to play a role. Hyperphosphatemia has been described in patients with ketoacidosis before treatment. After administration of intravenous fluids and insulin therapy, the entrance of glucose into the cells is usually followed by the movement of phosphorus back into the intracellular space, and some patients may develop hypophosphatemia. Thus, the combination of dehydration, acidosis, and tissue breakdown in different catabolic states may lead to hyperphosphatemia.

## RESPIRATORY ACIDOSIS

Acute respiratory acidosis may lead to a marked increase in serum phosphorus.[216] By contrast, chronic respiratory acidosis is usually not manifested by sustained elevated levels of serum phosphorus. Acute rises in $P_{CO_2}$ in experimental animals have been shown to lead to increased serum phosphorus levels. The modest degree of hyperphosphatemia seen in chronic respiratory acidosis is probably related to renal compensation and increased phosphorus excretion via the kidney to maintain phosphorus homeostasis.

## ADMINISTRATION OF PHOSPHATE SALTS OR VITAMIN D OR ITS METABOLITES

Administration of vitamin $D_3$ or its metabolites, particularly $1,25(OH)_2D_3$, may result in increases in serum phosphorus, particularly in uremic patients. These compounds likely cause hyperphosphatemia in uremic individuals by increasing phosphorus absorption from the gut and perhaps by potentiating the effect of PTH on the skeleton, with increased release of phosphorus from bone. Decreased renal function limits the compensatory mechanism of the kidney to excrete the increased load of phosphate entering the extracellular space. In addition to elevating serum phosphorus, vitamin D metabolites may result in hypercalcemia. An increase in the phosphorus-calcium product may result in tissue deposition of calcium, particularly in the kidney, leading to further deterioration in renal function.

### INGESTION OR ADMINISTRATION OF SALTS CONTAINING PHOSPHATE

Hyperphosphatemia has been observed in adults ingesting laxative-containing phosphate salts or after the administration of enemas containing large amounts of phosphate.[217, 218] Intravenous phosphate administration has been used in the treatment of hypercalcemia of malignancy. The administration of 1 to 2 g of phosphate intravenously decreases the concentration of serum calcium. Unfortunately, the severe hyperphosphatemia induced by the administration of large amounts of phosphorus intravenously may lead to calcium precipitation in important organs such as the heart and kidney, and several deaths have been reported as a consequence of this form of therapy. Hyperphosphatemia may develop in newborn infants fed cow's milk, which is higher in phosphorus content than is human milk. This may be an important factor in the genesis of neonatal tetany.

## Clinical Manifestations of Hyperphosphatemia

Most of the clinical effects of hyperphosphatemia are related to secondary changes of calcium metabolism. Hyperphosphatemia produces hypocalcemia by several mechanisms (Fig. 27–5), including decreased production of $1,25(OH)_2D_3$,[122] precipitation of calcium,[219] and decreased absorption of calcium from the gastrointestinal tract, presumably due to a direct effect of phosphorus on calcium absorption.[220] In addition to the manifestations by hypocalcemia, which are described elsewhere in this chapter, ectopic calcification is one of the important manifestations of hyperphosphatemia. The association of hyperphosphatemia and ectopic calcification has been observed in several clinical settings, including patients with chronic renal failure, hypoparathyroidism, and tumoral calcinosis. It appears that when the calcium-phosphorus product exceeds 70, the likelihood of calcium precipitation is greatly increased. In addition to the calcium-phosphorus product, local tissue factors may play an important role in calcium deposition. For example, regional changes in pH (local alkalosis) may favor calcification in tissue such as cornea and lung. In patients with severe calcification (calciphylaxis), it appears that high levels of circulating PTH may also aggravate this condition.

Hyperphosphatemia plays a key role in the development of secondary hyperparathyroidism in patients with renal insufficiency. It has been observed that

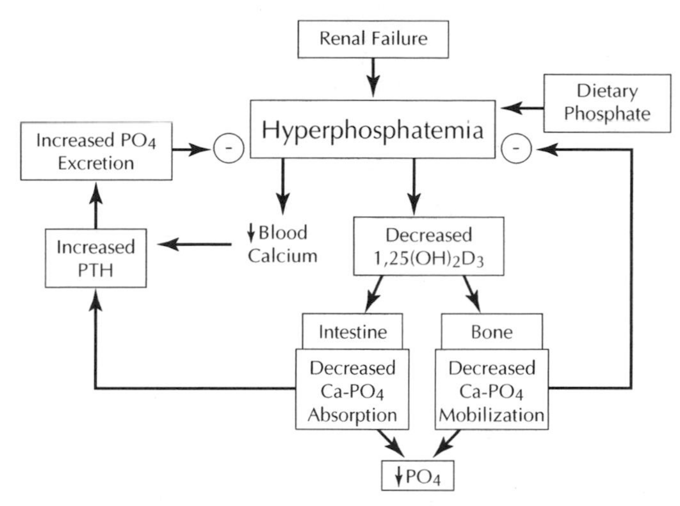


**FIGURE 27–5** ■ The relationship of hyperphosphatemia to calcium homeostasis. Hyperphosphatemia is commonly produced by decreased renal excretion associated with chronic kidney disease and normal dietary intake of phosphorus. As a result of hyperphosphatemia, there is a decrease in blood calcium and also in the production of calcitriol. Decreased calcitriol leads to a decrease in intestinal calcium phosphate absorption and a decrease in bone reabsorption, thus producing decreased phosphate mobilization. As a result, the hyperphosphatemia is ameliorated. Furthermore, the decrease in phosphate and the decrease in blood calcium increase parathyroid hormone secretion and lead to increased phosphorus excretion and further amelioration of hyperphosphatemia.

when phosphate ingestion is decreased and hyperphosphatemia is prevented in experimental animals with induced renal insufficiency, hyperparathyroidism can be prevented.[221] The mechanisms presumably relate to maintenance of serum calcium levels with prevention of hyperphosphatemia and, at the same time, continued synthesis of $1,25(OH)_2D_3$, the circulating levels of which may directly influence the secretion of PTH.[222,223] In the past decade, several investigators demonstrated that dietary phosphate markedly influences the rate of parathyroid cell proliferation and PTH synthesis and secretion, independent of changes in ionized calcium or $1,25(OH)_2D_3$.[224–227] It seems that the mechanism by which phosphorus increases PTH synthesis and secretion is post-transcriptional. Moreover, in experimental uremic rats, it has been shown that phosphate restriction suppresses parathyroid cell growth by inducing p21, a repressor of the cell cycle. Conversely, a high phosphate intake rapidly (in 3 to 5 days) induces significant parathyroid cell hyperplasia by inducing an increase in transforming growth factor-α.[228] Transforming growth factor-α, known to promote growth not only in malignant transformation but also in normal tissues,[229, 230] is enhanced in hyperplastic and adenomatous human parathyroid glands.[231]

In patients on chronic hemodialysis, the degree of hyperparathyroidism correlates well with the concentration of serum phosphorus. Patients who do not adhere to their therapeutic regimens of phosphate binders seem to develop more severe and persistent hyperphosphatemia, with marked secondary hyperparathyroidism and bone disease, than do patients who adhere carefully to dietary and therapeutic prescriptions. Vascular calcification has been observed in some patients with chronic renal insufficiency and severe calcification, hyperphosphatemia, and hyperparathyroidism, leading to necrosis and gangrene of the extremities. Slit-lamp examination may show ocular calcification, and some patients may develop acute conjunctivitis, the so-called red eye syndrome of uremia. Precipitation of calcium in the skin may be partly responsible for pruritus, a symptom that is usually seen in patients with advanced uremia. It has been reported that parathyroidectomy in such patients may alleviate the symptoms.

From the therapeutic point of view, the most efficacious way to control hyperphosphatemia is through the use of phosphate binders that decrease the absorption of phosphorus from the gastrointestinal tract. In patients with adequate renal function, expansion of the extracellular fluid with saline greatly increases phosphorus excretion in the urine and contributes to correction of the hyperphosphatemia.

In recent years, vascular calcification has become a common finding in atherosclerosis, a serious problem in diabetes, and a major cause of morbidity and mortality related to coronary artery disease in patients with end-stage renal disease on renal replacement therapy. Vascular calcification affects the media of arteries and appears to be related to the ability of extracellular inorganic phosphate levels to regulate human smooth muscle cell–related mineralization. In vitro, human smooth muscle cells cultured in high-phosphate concentrations demonstrate dose-dependent increases in mineral deposition.[38] Elevated phosphate concentrations enhance the expression of osteoblast differentiation markers in the vascular smooth muscle cells, including osteocalcin and Osf2/Cbfa-1.[38] The effects of elevated phosphate on vascular smooth muscle cells appear to be mediated by sodium-dependent phosphate transport specifically related to the type III transporter PIP 1 (Glvr-1) (Fig. 27–6). These results suggest that elevated phosphate levels cause vascular smooth muscle cells to undergo phenotypic changes that predispose to calcification. This offers a potential explanation of the phenomenon of vascular calcification under hyperphosphatemic conditions.

## Treatment of Hyperphosphatemia

Decreased absorption of phosphate from the gastrointestinal tract is a cornerstone of treatment of hyperphosphatemia. Phosphate absorption from the gastrointestinal tract can be markedly reduced either by decreasing the amount of phosphorus in the diet or by administering phosphate-binding agents capable of decreasing the absorption of phosphorus. Because protein requirements limit the amount of phosphorus restriction that can be achieved through dietary manipulation, from a practical point of view, the administration of agents that decrease phosphorus absorption from the gastrointestinal tract is the mainstay of treatment. Calcium salts have replaced aluminum salts as the traditional treatment to control hyperphospha-

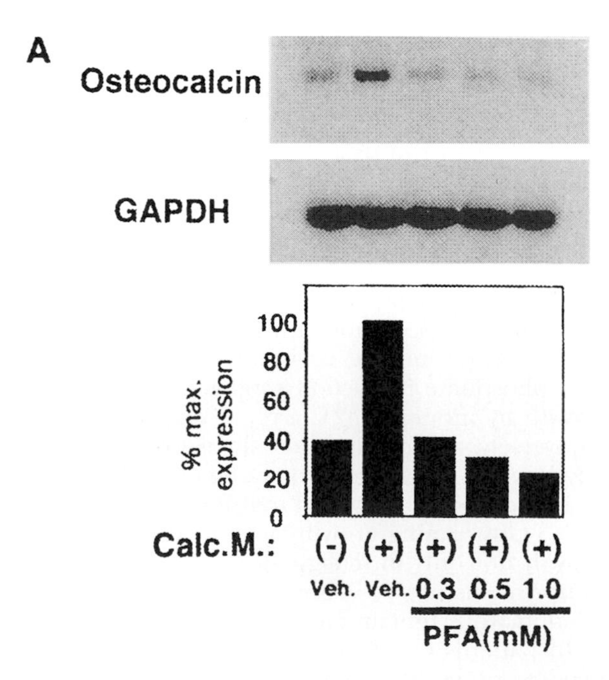


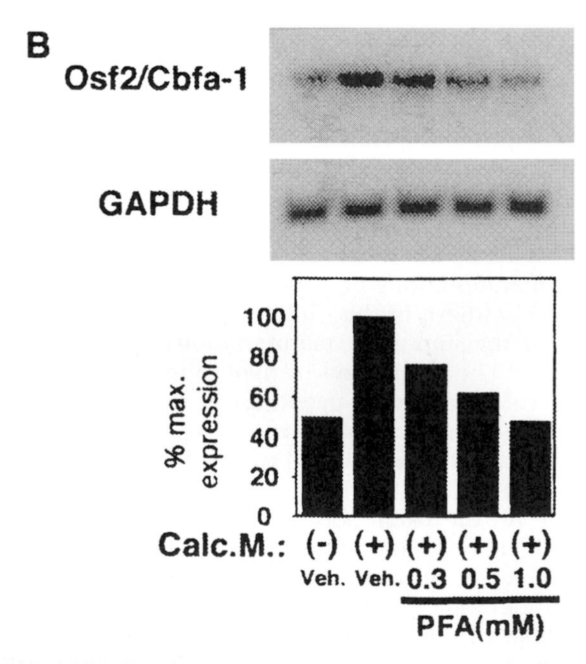


**FIGURE 27–6** ■ Regulation of vascular calcification by phosphate transport in vascular smooth muscle cells. Vascular smooth muscle cells express a type III phosphate transporter, Pit-1. As a result of hyperphosphatemia and phosphate transport, some vascular smooth muscle cells related to atherosclerotic plaques and, in the presence of diabetes or chronic kidney disease, begin to express an osteoblastic phenotype. *A,* Northern blot showing expression of osteocalcin in vascular smooth muscle cells in the presence of a medium permissive to phosphate transport (Calc.M.). The effect of the calcification medium is inhibited by phosphonoformic acid (PFA), a specific inhibitor of phosphate transport. *B,* The phosphate transport medium (Calc.M.) also induces expression of Osf2/Cbfa-1, an osteoblast-specific transcription factor. This is also blocked by PFA. Northern blot for glyceraldehyde-3-phosphate dehydrogenase (GAPDH) is a control for the Northern blot experiment demonstrating equal loading of material into each of the lanes.

temia. Most of these preparations require the administration of 2 to 4 tablets or capsules three or four times daily. If the patient develops constipation—one of the complications of such medications—magnesium salts can be incorporated into these preparations. However, if the patient has hyperphosphatemia secondary to severe renal insufficiency, magnesium should not be given because of the likelihood of producing severe hypermagnesemia, which may lead to magnesium intoxication, muscle paralysis, and death.

Aluminum toxicity, which results from prolonged administration of aluminum-containing salts as phosphate binders to patients with chronic renal insufficiency, has led to diminished use of these agents or their elimination.[232, 233] Several studies indicated that calcium carbonate is an effective agent for controlling hyperphosphatemia in chronic renal failure.[234–236] However, in the past 10 years, numerous investigators have demonstrated an increase in the number of aortic and mitral valve calcifications in dialysis patients when compared with the general population. Cardiovascular events are responsible for 40% to 60% mortality of dialysis patients.[237–240] Morbidity and mortality rates increase as the calcium-phosphorus product rises above 60. Braun and colleagues, with the use of electron beam computed tomography, demonstrated a significant deposition of calcium in the coronary arteries of dialysis patients.[241] Although coronary artery calcification gets worse with age, this abnormality has been demonstrated in young patients.[242] In fact, postmortem examination of children with renal failure demonstrated that 60% to 70% had calcification of the heart, lungs, and blood vessels.[242] Positive calcium balances of 500 to 900 mg daily were demonstrated in uremic patients receiving large doses of calcium carbonate. Thus, it is critical not only to reduce the calcium-phosphorus product to less than 60 but also to significantly decrease the calcium load that patients receive to control serum phosphorus.

To avoid these deleterious side effects, a well-tolerated, calcium-free phosphate binder was developed, sevelamer hydrochloride (Renagel). This new phosphate binder is a hydrogel of cross-linked polymer (allylamine hydrochloride) that is resistant to digestive degradation and is not absorbed from the gastrointestinal tract. Its mechanism of action relates to the presence of partially protonated amines spaced one carbon from the polymer backbone, which interact with phosphate ions by ionic and hydrogen bonding. Several short-term clinical studies in patients with end-stage renal disease have established that sevelamer hydrochloride is an effective phosphate binder without increasing the calcium load[243, 244] (see Fig. 27–5). In addition, sevelamer hydrochloride decreased low-density lipoprotein cholesterol by 30% to 40% and in long-term studies also increased high-density lipoprotein cholesterol by 20% to 30%; it did not affect triglycerides.[245] Studies in progress will provide critical information on its potential efficacy in reducing morbidity and mortality in dialysis patients.

Although decreased gastrointestinal absorption of phosphorus is an effective way to control hyperphosphatemia in patients with renal insufficiency, excretion of phosphorus through the kidney is also an important mechanism. Thus, expansion of the extracellular fluid volume may markedly increase phosphorus excretion by the kidney. This result is presumably related both to direct effects of volume expansion on the kidney, which decreases salt and water reabsorption and hence phosphorus reabsorption, and to increased PTH release, particularly as a consequence of decreased ionized calcium during volume expansion. In patients with marked renal insufficiency or with marked degrees of hyperphosphatemia due to tumor lysis or chemotherapy, peritoneal dialysis or hemodialysis may be used to remove large quantities of phosphorus from the extracellular space. Redistribution of phosphorus from the intracellular to the extracellular space can sometimes be rapidly corrected by the administration of glucose and insulin. In general, mild degrees of hyperphosphatemia can be tolerated, particularly if calcium levels are not markedly elevated. The goal in patients with chronic renal insufficiency is to keep phosphorus levels below 4.5 mg/dL to avoid in serum ionized calcium and marked development of severe hyperparathyroidism.

## REFERENCES


1. Levine BS, Kleeman CR: Hypophosphatemia and hyperphosphatemia: Clinical and pathophysiologic aspects. In Maxwell MH, Kleeman CR (eds): Clinical Disorders of Fluid and Electrolyte Metabolism. New York, McGraw-Hill, 1994, pp 1040–1045.
2. Hopkins T, Howard JE, Eisenberg H: Ultrafiltration studies on calcium and phosphorus in human serum. Bull Johns Hopkins Hosp 91:1–21, 1952.
3. Walser M: Ion association. VI. Interactions between calcium, magnesium, inorganic phosphate, citrate and protein in normal human plasma. J Clin Invest 40:723–730, 1961.
4. Fuchs R, Peterlik M: Intestinal phosphate transport. In Massry SG, Ritz E, Jahn H (eds): Phosphate and Minerals in Health and Disease. New York, Plenum Press, 1980, pp 380–385.
5. Berner W, Kinne R, Murer H: Phosphate transport into brush border membrane vesicles isolated from rat small intestine. Biochem J 160:467–474, 1976.
6. Hilfiker H, Hattenhauer O, Traebert M, et al: Characterization of a murine type II sodium-phosphate cotransporter expressed in mammalian small intestine. Proc Natl Acad Sci 95:14564–14569, 1998.
7. Matsumoto T, Fontaine O, Rasmussen H: Effect of 1,25$(OH)_2$ vitamin $D_3$ on phosphate uptake into chick intestinal brush border membrane vesicles. Biochim Biophys Acta 599:13–23, 1980.
8. Murer H, Hildmann B: Transcellular transport of calcium and inorganic phosphate in the small intestinal epithelium. Am J Physiol 240:G409–G416, 1981.
9. Norman AW: Calcium and phosphorus absorption. In Lawson DEM (ed): Vitamin D. New York, Academic Press, 1978, pp 90–93.
10. Peterlik M, Wasserman RH: Effect of vitamin D on transepithelial phosphate transport in chick intestine. Am J Physiol 234: E379–E388, 1978.
11. Kikuchi K, Ghishan FK: Phosphate transport by basolateral plasma membranes of human small intestine. Gastroenterology 93:106–113, 1987.
12. Knox FG, Osswald H, Marchand GR, et al: Phosphate transport along the nephron. Am J Physiol 233:F261–F268, 1977.
13. Pastoriza-Munoz E, Colindres RE, Lassiter WE, et al: Effect of parathyroid hormone on phosphate reabsorption in rat distal convolution. Am J Physiol 235:F321–F330, 1978.

14. Jamison RL, Arrascue JF: Calcium and phosphate reabsorption by the loop of Henle. Miner Electrolyte Metab 4:90–97, 1980.
15. Peraino RA, Suki WN: Phosphate transport by isolated rabbit cortical collecting tubule. Am J Physiol 238:F358–F362, 1980.
16. Shareghi GR, Agus ZS: Phosphate transport in the light segment of the rabbit cortical collecting tubule. Am J Physiol 242: F379–F384, 1982.
17. Chabardes D, Imbert M, Clique A, et al: PTH sensitive adenyl cyclase activity in different segments of the rabbit nephron. Pflugers Arch 354:229–239, 1975.
18. Haramati A, Haas JA, Knox FG: Adaptation of deep and superficial nephrons to changes in dietary phosphate intake. Am J Physiol 244:F265–F269, 1983.
19. Haramati A, Haas JA, Knox FG: Nephron heterogeneity of phosphate reabsorption: Effect of parathyroid hormone. Am J Physiol 246:F155–F158, 1984.
20. Hoffmann N, Thees M, Kinne R: Phosphate transport by isolated renal brush border vesicles. Pflugers Arch 362:147–156, 1976.
21. Sacktor B: Transport in membrane vesicles isolated from the mammalian kidney and intestine. In Sanadi R (ed): Current Topics in Bioenergetics. New York, Academic Press, 1977, pp 30–39.
22. Murer H, Biber J: Molecular mechanisms of renal apical Na phosphate cotransport. Annu Rev Physiol 58:607–618, 1996.
23. Werner A, Moore ML, Mantei N, et al: Cloning and expression of cDNA for a Na/Pi cotransport system of kidney cortex. Proc Natl Acad Sci U S A 88:9608–9612, 1991.
24. Kavanaugh MP, Miller DG, Zhang W, et al: Cell-surface receptors for gibbon ape leukemia virus and amphotropic murine retroviruses are inducible sodium-dependent phosphate symporters. Proc Natl Acad Sci U S A 91:7071–7075, 1994.
25. Fucentese M, Murer H, Biber J: Expression of rat renal Na/cotransport of phosphate and sulfate in Sf9 insect cells. J Am Soc Nephrol 5:860–862, 1994.
26. Tenenhouse HS, Roy S, Martel J, et al: Differential expression, abundance, and regulation of $Na^+$-phosphate cotransporter genes in murine kidney. Am J Physiol 275:F527–F534, 1998.
27. Busch AE, Schuster A, Waldegger S: Expression of a renal type I sodium/phosphate transporter (NaPi-1) induces a conductance in *Xenopus* oocytes permeable for organic and inorganic anions. Proc Natl Acad Sci U S A 93:5347–5351, 1996.
28. Verri T, Markovich D, Perego C, et al: Cloning of a rabbit renal Na-Pi cotransporter which is regulated by dietary phosphate. Am J Physiol 268:F626–F633, 1995.
29. Ritthaler T, Traebert M, Lotscher M, et al: Effects of phosphate intake on distribution of type II Na/$P_i$ cotransporter mRNA in rat kidney. Kidney Int 55:976–983, 1999.
30. Murer H, Werner A, Reshkin S, et al: Cellular mechanisms in proximal tubular reabsorption of inorganic phosphate. Am J Physiol 260:C885–C899, 1991.
31. Keusch I, Traebert M, Lotscher M, et al: Parathyroid hormone and dietary phosphate provoke a lysosomal routing of the proximal tubular Na/Pi-cotransporter type II. Kidney Int 54: 1224–1232, 1998.
32. Levi M, Kempson SA, Lotscher M, et al: Molecular regulation of renal phosphate transport. J Membr Biol 154:1–9, 1996.
33. Lotscher M, Wilson P, Nguyen S, et al: New aspects of adaptation of rat renal Na-Pi cotransporter to alterations in dietary phosphate. Kidney Int 49:1012–1018, 1996.
34. Kempson SA, Lotscher M, Kaissling B, et al: Parathyroid hormone action on phosphate transporter mRNA and protein in rat renal proximal tubules. Am J Physiol 268:F784–F791, 1995.
35. Caverzasio J, Montessuit C, Bonjour J-P: Functional role of $P_i$ transport in osteogenic cells. News Physiol Sci 11:119–125, 1996.
36. Palmer G, Guicheux J, Bonjour JP, et al: Transforming growth factor-beta stimulates inorganic phosphate transport and expresson of the type III phosphate transporter Glvr-1 in chondrogenic ATDC5 cells. Endocrinology 141:2236–2243, 2000.
37. Selz T, Caverzasio J, Bonjour JP: Regulation of Na-dependent Pi transport by parathyroid hormone in osteoblast-like cells. Am J Physiol 256:E93–E100, 1989.
38. Jono S, McKee MD, Murry CE, et al: Phosphate regulation of vascular smooth muscle cell calcification. Circ Res 87:e10–e17, 2000.
39. Schwab SJ, Hammerman MR: Mechanisms of phosphate exit across the basolateral membrane of the renal proximal tubule cell. Clin Res 32:530–535, 1984.
40. Beutner EH, Munson PL: Time course of urinary excretion of inorganic phosphate by rats after parathyroidectomy and after injection of parathyroid extract. Endocrinology 66:610–616, 1960.
41. Pullman TN, Lavender AR, Aho I, et al: Direct renal action of a purified parathyroid extract. Endocrinology 67:570–582, 1960.
42. Agus ZS, Gardner LB, Beck LH, et al: Effects of parathyroid hormone on renal tubular reabsorption of calcium, sodium and phosphate. Am J Physiol 224:1143–1148, 1973.
43. Wen SF: Micropuncture studies of phosphate transport in the proximal tubule of the dog: The relationship of sodium reabsorption. J Clin Invest 53:143–153, 1974.
44. Beck N: Effect of metabolic acidosis on renal response to parathyroid hormone in phosphorus-deprived rats. Am J Physiol 241:F23–F27, 1981.
45. Beck LH, Goldberg M: Effects of acetazolamide and parathyroidectomy on renal transport of sodium, calcium and phosphate. Am J Physiol 224:1136–1142, 1973.
46. Amiel C, Kuntziger H, Richet G: Micropuncture study of handling of phosphate by proximal and distal nephron in normal and parathyroidectomized rat: Evidence for distal reabsorption. Pflugers Arch 317:93–109, 1970.
47. Goldfarb S, Beck LH, Agus ZS, et al: Dissociation of tubular sites of action of saline, PTH and dbcAMP on renal phosphate reabsorption. Nephron 21:221–229, 1978.
48. Knox FG, Preiss J, Kim JK, et al: Mechanism of resistance to the phosphaturic effect of the parathyroid hormone in the hamster. J Clin Invest 59:675–683, 1977.
49. Le Grimellec C, Roinel N, Morel F: Simultaneous Mg, Ca, P, K and Cl analysis in rat tubular fluid. IV. During acute phosphate plasma loading. Pflugers Arch 346:189–204, 1974.
50. Evers C, Murer H, Kinne R: Effect of parathyrin on the transport properties of isolated renal brush-border vesicles. Biochem J 172:49–56, 1978.
51. Hammerman MR, Hruska KA: Cyclic AMP–dependent protein phosphorylation in canine renal brush-border membrane vesicles is associated with decreased Pi transport. J Biol Chem 257: 992–999, 1982.
52. Hayes G, Busch AE, Lang F, et al: Protein kinase C consensus sites and the regulation of renal Na/Pi-cotransport (NaPi-2) expressed in *Xenopus laevis* oocytes. Pflugers Arch 430:819–824, 1995.
53. Lotscher M, Scarpetta Y, Levi M, et al: Rapid downregulation of rat renal Na/Pi cotransporter in response to parathyroid hormone involves microtubule rearrangement. J Clin Invest 104:483–494, 1999.
54. Hoppe A, Metler M, Berndt TJ, et al: Effect of respiratory alkalosis on renal phosphate excretion. Am J Physiol 243:F471–F475, 1982.
55. Fulop M, Brazeau P: The phosphaturic effect of sodium bicarbonate and acetazolamide in dogs. J Clin Invest 47:983–991, 1968.
56. Quamme GA: Urinary alkalinization may not result in an increase in urinary phosphate excretion [abstract]. Kidney Int 25:150, 1984.
57. Mercado A, Slatopolsky E, Klahr S: On the mechanisms responsible for the phosphaturia of bicarbonate administration. J Clin Invest 56:1386–1395, 1975.
58. Puschett JB, Goldberg M: The relationship between the renal handling of phosphate and bicarbonate in man. J Lab Clin Med 73:956–969, 1969.
59. Kuntziger HE, Amiel C, Couette S, et al: Localization of parathyroid-hormone-independent sodium bicarbonate inhibition of tubular phosphate reabsorption. Kidney Int 17:749–755, 1980.
60. Cuche JL, Ott CE, Marchand GR, et al: Intrarenal calcium in phosphate handling. Am J Physiol 230:790–796, 1976.
61. Pitts RF, Alexander RS: The renal reabsorptive mechanism for inorganic phosphate in normal and acidotic dogs. Am J Physiol 142:648–662, 1944.
62. Guntupalli J, Eby B, Lau K: Mechanism for the phosphaturia of $NH_4Cl$: Dependence on acidemia but not on diet $PO_4$ or PTH. Am J Physiol 242:F552–F560, 1982.

63. Kempson SA: Effect of metabolic acidosis on renal brush border membrane adaptation to low phosphorus diet. Kidney Int 22:225–233, 1982.
64. Quamme GA, Mizgala CL, Wong NLM, et al: Effects of intraluminal pH and dietary phosphate on phosphate transport in the proximal convoluted tubule. Am J Physiol 249:F759–F768, 1985.
65. Ambuhl PM, Zajicek HK, Wang H, et al: Regulation of renal phosphate transport by acute and chronic metabolic acidosis in the rat. Kidney Int 53:1288–1298, 1998.
66. Frick A, Durasin I: Proximal tubular reabsorption of inorganic phosphate in adrenalectomized rats. Pflugers Arch 385:189–192, 1980.
67. Bonjour JP, Preston C, Fleisch H: Effect of 1,25 dihydroxyvitamin $D_3$ on renal handling of $P_i$ in thyroparathyroidectomized rats. J Clin Invest 60:1419–1428, 1977.
68. Muhlbauer RC, Bonjour J-P, Fleisch H: Tubular handling of Pi: Localization of effects of $1,25(OH)_2D_3$ and dietary Pi in TPTX rats. Am J Physiol 241:F123–F128, 1981.
69. Stoll R, Kinne R, Murer H, et al: Phosphate transport by rat renal brush border membrane vesicles: Influence of dietary phosphate, thyroparathyroidectomy, and 1,25-dihydroxyvitamin $D_3$. Pflugers Arch 380:47–52, 1979.
70. Gekle DJ, Stroder J, Rostock D: The effect of vitamin D on renal inorganic phosphate reabsorption on normal rats, parathyroidectomized rats, and rats with rickets. Pediatr Res 5: 40–45, 1971.
71. Liang CT, Barnes J, Cheng L, et al: Effects of $1,25(OH)_2D_3$ administered in vivo on phosphate uptake by isolated chick renal cells. Am J Physiol 242:C312–C318, 1982.
72. Kurnik BR, Hruska KA: Effects of 1,25-dihydroxycholecalciferol on phosphate transport in vitamin D–deprived rats. Am J Physiol 247:F177–F184, 1984.
73. Caverzasio J, Montessuit C, Bonjour J-P: Stimulatory effect of insulin-like growth factor-1 on renal Pi transport and plasma 1,25-dihydroxyvitamin $D_3$. Endocrinology 127:453–459, 1990.
74. Biber J, Murer H: Na-$P_i$ cotransport in LLC-$PK_1$ cells: Fast adaptive response to $P_i$ deprivation. Am J Physiol 249:C430–C434, 1985.
75. Brown CD, Bodmer M, Biber J, et al: Sodium-dependent phosphate transport by apical membrane vesicles from a cultured renal epithelial cell line (LLC-$PK_1$). Biochim Biophys Acta 769: 471–478, 1984.
76. Caverzasio J, Brown CD, Biber J, et al: Adaptation of phosphate transport in phosphate-deprived LLC-$PK_1$ cells. Am J Physiol 248:F122–F127, 1985.
77. Levi M, Lotscher M, Sorribas V, et al: Cellular mechanisms of acute and chronic adaptation of rat renal P(i) transporter to alterations in dietary P(i). Am J Physiol 267:F900–F908, 1994.
78. Werner A, Kempson SA, Biber J, et al: Increase of Na/$P_i$-cotransport encoding mRNA in response to low $P_i$ diet in rat kidney cortex. J Biol Chem 269:6637–6639, 1994.
79. Olsen HS, Cepeda MA, Zhang Q-Q, et al: Human stanniocalcin: A possible hormonal regulator of mineral metabolism. Proc Natl Acad Sci U S A 93:1792–1796, 1996.
80. Haas JA, Larson MV, Marchand GR, et al: Phosphaturic effect of furosemide: Role of TH and carbonic anhydrase. Am J Physiol 232:F105–F110, 1977.
81. Knochel JP: The pathophysiology and clinical characteristics of severe hyperphosphatemia. Arch Intern Med 137:203–220, 1977.
82. Kreisberg RA: Phosphorus deficiency and hypophosphatemia. Hosp Pract 12:121–128, 1977.
83. Arnaud CD, Clar OH: Primary hyperparathyroidism. In Krieger DT, Bardin CW (eds): Current Therapy in Endocrinology 1983–1984. Philadelphia and St. Louis, Decker and Mosby, 1983, pp 270–277.
84. Berson SA, Yalow RS: Parathyroid hormone in plasma in adenomatous hyperparathyroidism, uremia and bronchogenic carcinoma. Science 154:907–909, 1966.
85. Glikman RM: Malabsorption: Pathophysiology and diagnosis. In Wyngaarden JB, Smith LHJ (eds): Cecil's Textbook of Medicine. Philadelphia, WB Saunders, 1985, pp 710–719.
86. Roth KS, Foreman JW, Segal S: The Fanconi syndrome and mechanisms of tubular dysfunction. Kidney Int 20:705–716, 1981.
87. Lloyd SE, Pearce SHS, Fisher SE, et al: A common molecular basis for three inherited kidney stone diseases. Nature 379: 445–449, 1996.
88. Tieder M: Hereditary hypophosphatemic rickets with hypercalciuria. N Engl J Med 312:611–617, 1985.
89. Gazit D, Tieder M, Liberman UA, et al: Osteomalacia in hereditary hypophosphatemic rickets with hypercalciuria: A correlative clinical-histomorphometric study. J Clin Endocrinol Metab 72:229–235, 1991.
90. Scheinman SJ: X-linked hypercalciuric nephrolithiasis: Clinical syndromes and chloride channel mutations. Kidney Int 53: 3–17, 1998.
91. Gunther W, Luchow A, Cluzeaud F, et al: ClC-5, the chloride channel mutated in Dent's disease, colocalizes with the proton pump in endocytotically active kidney cells. Proc Natl Acad Sci U S A 95:8075–8080, 1998.
92. Jentsch TJ, Gunther W: Chloride channels: An emerging molecular picture. Bioessays 19:117–126, 1997.
93. Howell RR: Essential fructosuria and hereditary fructose intolerance. In Wyngaarden JB, Smith LHJ (eds): Cecil's Textbook of Medicine. Philadelphia, WB Saunders, 1985, pp 1100–1108.
94. Rosenbaum RW, Hruska KA, Korkor A, et al: Decreased phosphate reabsorption after renal transplantation: Evidence for a mechanism independent of calcium and parathyroid hormone. Kidney Int 19:568–578, 1981.
95. Falls WFJ, Stacey WK: Postobstructive diuresis: Studies in a dialyzed patient with a solitary kidney. Am J Med 54:404–412, 1973.
96. Moorhead JF, Wills MR, Ahmed KY, et al: Hypophosphatemic osteomalacia after cadaveric renal transplantation. Lancet 1: 694–697, 1974.
97. Beck LH, Goldberg M: Mechanism of the blunted phosphaturia in saline-loaded thyroparathyroidectomized dogs. Kidney Int 6:18–23, 1974.
98. Kos CH, Lemieux N, Tihy F, et al: The renal specific $Na^+$-phosphate cotransporter cDNA maps to human chromosome 5q35. J Am Soc Nephrol 4:810–816, 1993.
99. The Hyp Consortium: A gene (PEX) with homologies to endopeptidases is mutated in patients with X-linked hypophosphatemic rickets. Nat Genet 11:130–136, 1995.
100. White KE, Lorenz B, Evans WE, et al: Autosomal dominant hypophosphatemic rickets is caused by mutations in a novel gene, FGF23, that shares homology with the fibroblast growth factor family [abstract]. J Bone Miner Res 15:S153, 2000.
101. Eicher EM, Southard JL, Scriver CR, et al: Hypophosphatemia: Mouse model for human familial hypophosphatemic (vitamin D–resistant) rickets. Proc Natl Acad Sci U S A 73:4667–4671, 1976.
102. Tenenhouse HS, Scriver CR: Effect of 1,25-dihydroxyvitamin $D_3$ on phosphate homeostasis in the X-linked hypophosphatemic (Hyp) mouse. Endocrinology 109:658–660, 1981.
103. Brickman AS, Coburn JW, Kurokawa K, et al: Actions of 1,25-dihydroxycholecalciferol in patients with hypophosphatemic, vitamin D–resistant rickets. N Engl J Med 289:495–498, 1973.
104. Meyer RA Jr, Gray RW, Meyer MH: Abnormal vitamin D metabolism in the X-linked hypophosphatemic mouse. Endocrinology 107:1577–1581.
105. Beamer WG, Wilson MD, DeLuca HF: Successful treatment of genetically hypophosphatemic mice by 1-alpha-hydroxy vitamin $D_3$ but not 1,25 dihydroxy vitamin $D_3$. Endocrinology 106: 1949–1955, 1980.
106. Tenenhouse HS, Scriver CR, McInnes RR, et al: Renal handling of phosphate in vivo and in vitro by the X-linked hypophosphatemic male mouse: Evidence for a defect in the brush border membrane. Kidney Int 14:236–244, 1978.
107. Tenenhouse HS, Werner A, Biber J, et al: Renal $Na^+$-phosphate cotransport in murine X-linked hypophosphatemic rickets: Molecular characterization. J Clin Invest 93:671–676, 1994.
108. Chong SS, Kristjansson K, Zoghbi HY, et al: Molecular cloning of the cDNA encoding a human renal sodium phosphate transport protein and its assignment to chromosome 6p21.3-p23. Genomics 18:355–359, 1993.
109. Meyer RAJ, Tenenhouse HS, Meyer M, et al: The renal phosphate transport defect in normal mice parabiosed to X-linked hypophosphatemic mice persists after parathyroidectomy. J Bone Miner Res 4:523–532, 1989.

110. Nesbitt T, Coffman TM, Griffiths R, et al: Crosstransplantation of kidneys in normal and Hyp mice: Evidence that the Hyp mouse phenotype is unrelated to an intrinsic renal defect. J Clin Invest 89:1453–1459, 1992.
111. Econs MJ, Drezner MK: Tumor-induced osteomalacia: Unveiling a new hormone. N Engl J Med 330:1645–1649, 1994.
112. Rifas L, Dawson LL, Halstead LH, et al: Phosphate transport in osteoblasts from normal and X-linked hypophosphatemic mice. Calcif Tissue Int 54:505–510, 1995.
113. Ecarot B, Glorieux FH, Desbarats M, et al: Defective bone formation by Hyp mouse bone cells transplanted into normal mice: Evidence in favor of an intrinsic osteoblast defect. J Bone Miner Res 7:215–220, 1992.
114. Ecarot B, Glorieux FH, Desbarats M, et al: Effect of dietary phosphate deprivation and supplementation of recipient mice on bone formation by transplanted cells from normal and X-linked hypophosphatemic mice. J Bone Miner Res 7:523–530, 1992.
115. Hruska KA, Rifas L, Cheng S-L, et al: X-linked hypophosphatemic rickets and the murine Hyp homologue. Am J Physiol 268:F357–F362, 1995.
116. Rifas L, Avioli LV, Cheng SL: $1,25(OH)_2D_3$ corrects underphosphorylation of osteopontin in the Hyp/Y mouse osteoblast. In Bouillon R, Norman AW, Thomasset M (eds): Vitamin D, A Pluripotent Steroid Hormone: Structural Studies, Molecular Endocrinology and Clinical Applications. New York, de Gruyter, 1994, pp 700–704.
117. Cai Q, Hodgson SF, Kao PC, et al: Brief report: Inhibition of renal phosphate transport by a tumor product in a patient with oncogenic osteomalacia. N Engl J Med 330:1645–1649, 1994.
118. Glorieux FH, Marie PJ, Pettifor JM, et al: Bone response to phosphate salts, ergocalciferol, and calcitriol in hypophosphatemic vitamin D–resistant rickets. N Engl J Med 303:1023–1031, 1980.
119. Verge CF, Lam A, Simpson JM, et al: Effect of therapy in X-linked hypophosphatemic rickets. N Engl J Med 325:1875–1877, 1991.
120. Friedman NE, Lobaugh B, Drezner MK: Effects of calcitriol and phosphorus therapy on the growth of patients with X-linked hypophosphatemia. J Clin Endocrinol Metab 76:839–844, 1993.
121. Weinstein LS, Shenker A, Gejman PV, et al: Activation mutations of the stimulatory G protein in the McCune-Albright syndrome. N Engl J Med 325:1688–1695, 1991.
122. Gray RW, Wilz DR, Caldas AE, et al: The importance of phosphate in regulating plasma $1,25\text{-}(OH)_2$-vitamin D levels in humans: Studies in healthy subjects, in calcium-stone formers and in patients with primary hyperparathyroidism. J Clin Endocrinol Metab 45:299–306, 1977.
123. Frame B, Parfitt AM: Osteomalacia: current concepts. Ann Intern Med 89:966–982, 1978.
124. Eberle M, Traynor-Kaplan AE, Sklar LA, et al: Is there a relationship between phosphatidylinositol trisphosphate and F-actin polymerization in human neutrophils? J Biol Chem 265: 16725–16728, 1990.
125. Fu GK, Lin D, Zhang MY, et al: Cloning of human 25-hydroxyvitamin D 1-alpha-hydroxylase and mutations causing vitamin D–dependent rickets type 1. Mol Endocrinol 11:1961–1970, 1997.
126. Liberman UA, Eil C, Marx SJ: Resistance of 1,25-dihydroxyvitamin D: Associated with heterogeneous defects in cultured skin fibroblasts. J Clin Invest 71:192–200, 1983.
127. Feldman D, Chen T, Cone C, et al: Vitamin D resistant rickets with alopecia: Cultured skin fibroblasts exhibit defective cytoplasmic receptors and unresponsiveness to $1,25(OH)_2D_3$. J Clin Endocrinol Metab 55:1020–1022, 1982.
128. Chen TL, Hirst MA, Cone CM, et al: 1,25-Dihydroxyvitamin D resistance, rickets and alopecia: Analysis of receptors and bioresponse in cultured fibroblasts from patients and parents. J Clin Endocrinol Metab 59:383–388, 1984.
129. Malloy PJ, Hochberg Z, Pike JW, et al: Abnormal binding of vitamin D receptors to deoxyribonucleic acid in a kindred with vitamin D–dependent rickets, type II. J Clin Endocrinol Metab 68:263–269, 1989.
130. Hochberg Z, Weisman Y: Calcitriol-resistant rickets due to vitamin D receptor defects. Trends Endocrinol Metab 6:216–220, 1995.
131. Hewison M, Rut AR, Kristjansson K, et al: Tissue resistance to 1,25-dihydroxyvitamin D without a mutation of the vitamin D receptor gene. Clin Endocrinol 39:663–670, 1993.
132. Refetoff S, Weiss RE, Usala SJ: The syndromes of resistance to thyroid hormone. Endocr Rev 14:348–399, 1993.
133. McPhaul MJ, Marcelli M, Zoppi S, et al: Genetic basis of endocrine disease. 4. The spectrum of mutations in the androgen receptor gene that causes androgen resistance. J Clin Endocrinol Metab 76:17–23, 1993.
134. Smith EP, Boyd J, Frank GR, et al: Estrogen resistance caused by a mutation in the estrogen receptor gene in a man. N Engl J Med 331:1088–1089, 1994.
135. Li YC, Amling M, Pirro AE, et al: Normalization of mineral ion homeostasis by dietary means prevents hyperparathyroidism, rickets, and osteomalacia, but not alopecia in vitamin D receptor–ablated mice. Endocrinology 139:4391–4396, 1998.
136. Parker MS, Klein I, Haussler MR, et al: Tumor-induced osteomalacia: Evidence of a surgically correctable alteration in vitamin D metabolism. JAMA 245:492–493, 1981.
137. Rowe PSN, Ong ACM, Cockerill FJ, et al: Candidate 56 and 58 kDa protein(s) responsible for mediating the renal defects in oncogenic hypophosphatemic osteomalacia. Bone 18:159–169, 1996.
138. Nemere I, Norman AW: The rapid, hormonally stimulated transport of calcium (transcaltachia). J Bone Miner Res 2: 167–169, 1987.
139. Weidner N: Review and update: Oncogenic osteomalacia and rickets. Ultrastruct Pathol 15:317–333, 1991.
140. Sweet RA, Males JL, Hamstra AJ, et al: Vitamin D metabolite levels in oncogenic osteomalacia. Ann Intern Med 93:279–280, 1980.
141. Drezner MK, Feinglos MN: Osteomalacia due to 1alpha,25-dihydroxycholecalciferol deficiency: Association with a giant cell tumor of bone. J Clin Invest 60:1046–1053, 1977.
142. Ribovich ML, DeLuca HF: Effect of dietary calcium and phosphorus on intestinal calcium absorption and vitamin D metabolism. Arch Biochem Biophys 188:145–156, 1978.
143. Miyauchi A, Fukase M, Tsutsumi M, et al: Hemangiopericytoma-induced osteomalacia: Tumor transplantation in nude mice causes hypophosphatemia and tumor extracts inhibit renal 25-hydroxyvitamin D 1-hydroxylase activity. J Clin Endocrinol Metab 67:46–53, 1988.
144. Klahr S, Davis TA: Changes in renal function with chronic protein-calorie malnutrition. In Mitch WE, Klahr S (eds): Nutrition and the Kidney. Boston, Little Brown, 1988, pp 59–79.
145. Shields HM: Rapid fall of serum phosphorus secondary to antacid therapy. Gastroenterology 75:1137–1141, 1978.
146. Juan D, Elrazak MA: Hypophosphatemia in hospitalized patients. JAMA 242:163–164, 1979.
147. Larsson L, Rebel K, Sorbo B: Severe hypophosphatemia—a hospital survey. Acta Med Scand 214:221–223, 1983.
148. Betro MG, Pain RW: Hypophosphatemia and hyperphosphatemia in a hospital population. BMJ 1:273–276, 1972.
149. Ryback RS, Eckardt MJ, Pautler CP: Clinical relationships between serum phosphorus and other blood chemistry values in alcoholics. Arch Intern Med 140:673–677, 1980.
150. Seldin DW, Tarail R: The metabolism of glucose and electrolytes in diabetic acidosis. J Clin Invest 29:552–565, 1950.
151. Mostellar ME, Tuttle EPJ: Effects of alkalosis on plasma concentration and urinary excretion of urinary phosphate in man. J Clin Invest 43:138–149, 1964.
152. Aderka D, Shoenfeld Y, Santo M, et al: Life-threatening hypophosphatemia in a patient with acute myelogenous leukemia. Acta Haematol 64:117–119, 1980.
153. Matzner Y, Prococimer M, Polliack A, et al: Hypophosphatemia in a patient with lymphoma in leukemic phase. Arch Intern Med 141:805–806, 1981.
154. Zamkoff KW, Kirshner JJ: Marked hypophosphatemia associated with acute myelomonocytic leukemia: Indirect evidence of phosphorus uptake by leukemic cells. Arch Intern Med 140: 1523–1524, 1980.
155. Chesney PJ, Davis JP, Purdy WK, et al: Clinical manifestations of toxic shock syndrome. JAMA 246:741–748, 1981.

156. Lennquist S, Lindell B, Nordstrom H, et al: Hypophosphatemia in severe burns: A prospective study. Acta Chir Scand 145: 1–6, 1979.
157. Levy LA: Severe hypophosphatemia as a complication of the treatment of hypothermia. Arch Intern Med 140:128–129, 1980.
158. Silvis SE, DiBartolomeo AG, Aaker HM: Hypophosphatemia and neurologic changes secondary to oral caloric intake: A variant of hyperalimentation syndrome. Am J Gastroenterol 73: 215–222, 1980.
159. Weinsier RL, Krumdiek CL: Death resulting from overzealous total parenteral nutrition: The refeeding syndrome revisited. Am J Clin Nutr 34:393–399, 1981.
160. Kono N, Kuwajima M, Tarui S: Alteration of glycolytic intermediary metabolism in erythrocytes during diabetic ketoacidosis and its recovery phase. Diabetes 30:346–353, 1981.
161. Ditzel J: Changes in red cell oxygen release capacity in diabetes mellitus. Fed Proc 38:2484–2488, 1979.
162. Darsee JR, Nutter DO: Reversible severe congestive cardiomyopathy in three cases of hypophosphatemia. Ann Intern Med 89:867–870, 1978; retracted by Nutter DO, Glenn JF: Ann Intern Med 99:275–276, 1983.
163. Zazzo J-F, Troche G, Ruel P, et al: High incidence of hypophosphatemia in surgical intensive care patients: Efficacy of phosphorus therapy on myocardial function. Intensive Care Med 21:826–831, 1995.
164. Fuller TJ, Nichols WW, Brenner BJ, et al: Reversible depression in myocardial performance in dogs with experimental phosphorus deficiency. J Clin Invest 62:1194–1200, 1978.
165. Knochel JP, Barcenas C, Cotton JR, et al: Hypophosphatemia and rhabdomyolysis. J Clin Invest 62:1240–1246, 1978.
166. Knochel JP, Bilbrey GL, Fuller TJ: The muscle cell in chronic alcoholism: The possible role of phosphate depletion in alcoholic myopathy. Ann N Y Acad Sci 252:274–286, 1975.
167. Kretz J, Sommer G, Boland R, et al: Lack of involvement of sarcoplasmic reticulum in myopathy of acute phosphorus depletion. Klin Wochenschr 58:833–837, 1980.
168. DeFronzo RA, Lang R: Hypophosphatemia and glucose intolerance: Evidence for tissue insensitivity to insulin. N Engl J Med 303:1259–1263, 1980.
169. Bellingham AJ, Detter JC, Lenfant C: The role of hemoglobin affinity for oxygen and red cell 2,3-diphosphoglycerate in the management of diabetic ketoacidosis. Trans Assoc Am Physicians 83:113–120, 1970.
170. Lichtman MA, Miller DR, Cohen J, et al: Reduced red cell glycolysis, 2,3-diphosphoglycerate and adenosine triphosphate concentration and increased hemoglobin-oxygen affinity caused by hypophosphatemia. Ann Intern Med 74:562–568, 1971.
171. Travis SF, Sugarman HJ, Ruberg RL, et al: Alterations of red-cell glycolytic intermediates and oxygen transport as a consequence of hypophosphatemia in patients receiving intravenous hyperalimentation. N Engl J Med 285:763–768, 1971.
172. Jacob HS, Amsden T: Acute hemolytic anemia and rigid red cells in hypophosphatemia. N Engl J Med 285:1446–1450, 1971.
173. Klock JC, Williams HE, Mentzer WC: Hemolytic anemia and somatic cell dysfunction in severe hypophosphatemia. Arch Intern Med 134:360–364, 1974.
174. Craddock PR, Yawata Y, Van Santen L, et al: Acquired phagocyte dysfunction: A complication of the hypophosphatemia of parental hyperalimentation. N Engl J Med 290:1403–1407, 1974.
175. Riedler GF, Scheitlin WA: Hypophosphatemia in septicemia: Higher incidence in gram-negative than in gram-positive infections. BMJ 1:753–756, 1969.
176. Lotz M, Ney R, Bartter FC: Osteomalacia and debility resulting from phosphorus depletion. Trans Assoc Am Physicians 77: 281–295, 1964.
177. Lotz M, Zisman E, Bartter FC: Evidence for a phosphorus-depletion syndrome in man. N Engl J Med 278:409–415, 1968.
178. Prins JG, Schrijver H, Staghouwer JM: Hyperalimentation, hypophosphatemia and coma. Lancet 1:1253–1254, 1973.
179. Boelens PA, Norwood W, Kjellstrand C, et al: Hypophosphatemia with muscle weakness due to antacids and hemodialysis. Am J Dis Child 120:350–353, 1970.
180. Baker LRI, Ackrill P, Cattell WR, et al: Iatrogenic osteomalacia and myopathy due to phosphate depletion. BMJ 3:150–152, 1974.
181. Cooke N, Teitelbaum S, Avioli LV: Antacid-induced osteomalacia and nephrolithiasis. Arch Intern Med 138:1007–1009, 1978.
182. Ahmed KY, Varghese Z, Willis MR, et al: Persistent hypophosphatemia and osteomalacia in dialysis patients not on oral phosphate-binders: Response to dihydrotachysterol therapy. Lancet 1:439–442, 1976.
183. Moser CR, Fessel WJ: Rheumatic manifestations of hypophosphatemia. Arch Intern Med 134:674–678, 1974.
184. Coburn JW, Massry SG: Changes in serum and urinary calcium during phosphate depletion: Studies on mechanisms. J Clin Invest 49:1073–1087, 1970.
185. Dominguez JH, Gray RW, Lemann JJ: Dietary phosphate deprivation in women and men: Effects on mineral and acid balances, parathyroid hormone and the metabolism of 25-OH-vitamin D. J Clin Endocrinol Metab 43:1056–1068, 1976.
186. Emmett M, Goldfarb S, Agus ZS, et al: The pathophysiology of acid-base changes in chronically phosphate-depleted rats: Bone-kidney interactions. J Clin Invest 59:291–298, 1977.
187. Gold LW, Massry SG, Arieff AI, et al: Renal bicarbonate wasting during phosphate depletion: A possible cause of altered acid-base homeostasis in hyperparathyroidism. J Clin Invest 52: 2556–2561, 1973.
188. Gold LW, Massry SG, Friedler RM: Effect of phosphate depletion on renal tubular reabsorption of glucose. J Lab Clin Med 89:554–559, 1977.
189. Goldfarb S, Westby GR, Goldberg M, et al: Renal tubular effects of chronic phosphate depletion. J Clin Invest 59:770–779, 1977.
190. Muhlbauer RC, Bonjour JP, Fleisch H: Tubular localization to dietary phosphate in rats. Am J Physiol 234:E290–E294, 1978.
191. Steele TH, Stromberg BA, Larmore CA: Renal resistance to parathyroid hormone during phosphorus deprivation. J Clin Invest 58:1461–1464, 1976.
192. O'Donovan DJ, Lotspeich WD: Activation of kidney mitochondrial glutaminase by inorganic phosphate and organic acids. Nature 212:930–932, 1966.
193. Agus ZS, Goldfarb S, Wasserstein A: Disorders of calcium and phosphate balance. In Brenner BM, Rector FCJ (eds): The Kidney. Philadelphia, WB Saunders, 1981, pp 940–945.
194. Harris CA, Bauer PG, Chirito E, et al: Composition of mammalian glomerular filtrate. Am J Physiol 227:972–976, 1974.
195. Lentz RD, Brown DM, Kjellstrand CM: Treatment of severe hypophosphatemia. Ann Intern Med 89:941–944, 1978.
196. Slatopolsky E, Gradowska L, Kashemsant C: The control of phosphate excretion in uremia. J Clin Invest 45:672–677, 1966.
197. Slatopolsky E, Robson AM, Elkan I, et al: Control of phosphate excretion in uremic man. J Clin Invest 47:1865–1874, 1968.
198. Goldman R, Bassett SH: Phosphorus excretion in renal failure. J Clin Invest 33:1623, 1954.
199. Rutherford E, Mercado A, Hruska K, et al: An evaluation of a new and effective phosphate binding agent. Trans Am Soc Artif Intern Organs 19:446–449, 1973.
200. Massry SG, Arieff AI, Coburn JW, et al: Divalent ion metabolism in patients with acute renal failure: Studies on the mechanism of hypocalcemia. Kidney Int 5:437–445, 1974.
201. Koffler A, Friedler RM, Massry SG: Acute renal failure due to nontraumatic rhabdomyolysis. Ann Intern Med 85:23–28, 1976.
202. Parfitt AM: The spectrum of hypoparathyroidism. J Clin Endocrinol Metab 34:152–158, 1972.
203. Albright F, Burnett CH, Smith PH, et al: Pseudohypoparathyroidism—an example of "Seabright-Bantam syndrome." Endocrinology 30:922–932, 1942.
204. Bourne HR, Kaslow HR, Brickman AS, et al: Fibroblast defect in pseudohypoparathyroidism, type I: Reduced activity of receptor-cyclase coupling protein. J Clin Endocrinol Metab 53:636–640, 1981.
205. Farfel Z, Brickman AS, Kaslow HR, et al: Defect of receptor-cyclase coupling protein in pseudohypoparathyroidism. N Engl J Med 303:237–242, 1980.
206. Drezner M, Neelon FA, Lebovitz HE: Pseudohypoparathyroidism type II: A possible defect in the reception of the cyclic AMP signal. N Engl J Med 289:1056–1060, 1973.
207. Connors MH, Irias JJ, Golabi M: Hypo-hyperparathyroidism:

Evidence for a defective parathyroid hormone. Pediatrics 60: 343–348, 1977.
208. Lambert PP, Corvilan J: Site of action of parathyroid hormone and role of growth hormone in phosphate excretion. In Williams PC (ed): Hormones and the Kidney (Memoirs of the Society of Endocrinology, No. 13). New York, Academic Press, 1963, pp 130–139.
209. Mitnick PD, Goldbarb S, Slatopolsky E, et al: Calcium and phosphate metabolism in tumoral calcinosis. Ann Intern Med 92:482–487, 1980.
210. Lufkin EG, Wilson DM, Smith LH, et al: Phosphorus excretion in tumoral calcinosis: Response to parathyroid hormone and acetazolamide. J Clin Endocrinol Metab 50:648–653, 1980.
211. Zerwekh JE, Sanders LA, Townsend J, et al: Tumoral calcinosis: Evidence for concurrent defects in renal tubular phosphorus transport and in 1alpha,25-dihydroxycholecalciferol synthesis. Calcif Tissue Int 32:1–6, 1980.
212. Walton RJ, Russell RG, Smith R: Changes in the renal and extrarenal handling of phosphate induced by disodium etidronate (EHDP) in man. Clin Sci Mol Med 49:45–56, 1975.
213. Zusman J, Brown DM, Nesbit ME: Hyperphosphatemia, hyperphosphaturia and hypocalcemia in acute lymphoblastic leukemia. N Engl J Med 289:1335–1340, 1973.
214. Cohen LF, Balow JE, Magrath IT, et al: Acute tumor lysis syndrome: A review of 37 patients with Burkitt's lymphoma. Am J Med 68:486–491, 1980.
215. Tsokos GC, Balow JE, Spiegel RJ, et al: Renal and metabolic complications of undifferentiated and lymphoblastic lymphomas. Medicine 60:218–229, 1981.
216. Giebisch G, Berger L, Pitts RF: The extra-renal response to acute acid-base disturbances of respiratory origin. J Clin Invest 34:231–245, 1955.
217. Honig PJ, Holtzapple PG: Hypocalcemic tetany following hypertonic phosphate enemas. Clin Pediatr 14:678–679, 1975.
218. McConnell TH: Fatal hypocalcemia from phosphate absorption from laxative preparation. JAMA 216:147–148, 1971.
219. Payne JW, Walser M: Ion association. II. The effect of multivalent ions on the concentration of free calcium ions as measured by the frog heart method. Bull Johns Hopkins Hosp 105: 298–310, 1959.
220. Morgan DB: Calcium and phosphorus transport across the intestine. In Girdwood RM, Smith AW (eds): Malabsorption. Baltimore, Williams & Wilkins, 1969.
221. Slatopolsky E, Caglar S, Gradowska L, et al: On the prevention of secondary hyperparathyroidism in experimental chronic renal disease using "proportional reduction" of dietary phosphorus intake. Kidney Int 2:147–151, 1972.
222. Golden P, Mazey R, Greenwalt A, et al: Vitamin D: A direct effect on the parathyroid gland. Miner Electrolyte Metab 2: 1, 1979.
223. Slatopolsky E, Weerts C, Thielan J: Marked suppression of secondary hyperparathyroidism by intravenous administration of 1,25-dihydroxycholecalciferol in uremic patients. J Clin Invest 74:2136–2143, 1984.
224. Parfitt AM: The hyperparathyroidism of chronic renal failure: A disorder of growth. Kidney Int 52:3–9, 1997.
225. Slatopolsky E, Finch J, Denda M, et al: Phosphorus restriction prevents parathyroid gland growth: High phosphorus directly stimulates PTH secretion in vitro. J Clin Invest 97:2534–2540, 1996.
226. Silver J, Sela SB, Naveh-Man T: Regulation of parathyroid cell proliferation. Curr Opin Nephrol Hypertens 6:321–326, 1997.
227. Denda M, Finch J, Slatopolsky E: Phosphorus accelerates the development of parathyroid hyperplasia and secondary hyperparathyroidism in rats with renal failure. Am J Kidney Dis 28: 596–602, 1996.
228. Dusso AS, Lu Y, Pavlopoulos T, et al: A role of enhanced expression of transforming growth factor alpha (TGF-alpha) in the mitogenic effect of high dietary phosphorus on parathyroid cell growth in uremia [abstract]. J Am Soc Nephrol 10:617, 1999.
229. Kumar V, Bustin SA, McKay IA: Transforming growth factor alpha. Cell Biol Int 19:373–388, 1995.
230. Driman DK, Kobrin MS, Kudlow JE, et al: Transforming growth factor-alpha in normal and neoplastic human endocrinal tissues. Hum Pathol 23:1360–1365, 1992.
231. Gogusev J, Duchambon P, Stoermann-Chopard C, et al: De novo expression of transforming growth factor-alpha in parathyroid gland tissue of patients with primary or secondary uraemic hyperparathyroidism. Nephrol Dial Transplant 11: 2155–2162, 1996.
232. Berlyne GM, Ben-Ari J, Pest D, et al: Hyperaluminaemia from aluminum resins in renal failure. Lancet 2:494–496, 1970.
233. Ward MK, Feest TG, Ellis HA: Osteomalacic dialysis osteodystrophy: Evidence for a water-borne aetiological agent, probably aluminum. Lancet 1:841–845, 1978.
234. Moriniere PH, Roussel A, Tahira Y, et al: Substitution of aluminum hydroxide by high doses of calcium carbonate in patients on chronic hemodialysis: Disappearance of hyperaluminaemia and equal control of hyperparathyroidism. Proc Eur Dial Transplant Assoc 19:784–787, 1982.
235. Slatopolsky E, Weerts C, Lopez-Hilker S, et al: Calcium carbonate as a phosphate binder in patients with chronic renal failure undergoing dialysis. N Engl J Med 315:157–161, 1986.
236. Slatopolsky E, Weerts C, Norwood K, et al: Long-term effects of calcium carbonate and 2.5 mEq/liter calcium dialysate on mineral metabolism. Kidney Int 36:897–903, 1989.
237. Ribeiro S, Ramos A, Brandao A, et al: Cardiac valve calcification in hemodialysis patients: Role of calcium-phosphate metabolism. Nephrol Dial Transplant 13:2037–2040, 1988.
238. Rostand SG, Sanders C, Kirk KA, et al: Myocardial calcification and cardiac dysfunction in chronic renal failure. Am J Med 85: 651–657, 1988.
239. London GM, Dannier B, Marchais SJ, et al: Calcification of the aortic valve in the dialyzed patient. J Am Soc Nephrol 11: 778–783, 2000.
240. Guerin AP, London GM, Marchais SJ, et al: Arterial stiffening and vascular calcifications in end-stage renal disease. Nephrol Dial Transplant 13:2037–2040, 2000.
241. Braun J, Oldendorf M, Moshage W, et al: Electron beam computed tomography in the evaluation of cardiac calcification in chronic dialysis patients. Am J Kidney Dis 27:394–401, 1996.
242. Milliner DS, Zinsmeister AR, Lieberman L, et al: Soft tissue calcification in pediatric patients with end-stage renal disease. Kidney Int 38:931–936, 1990.
243. Chertow GM, Burke SK, Lazarus JM, et al: Poly[allylamine hydrochloride] (RenaGel): A noncalcemic phosphate binder for the treatment of hyperphosphatemia in chronic renal failure. Am J Kidney Dis 29:66–71, 1997.
244. Slatopolsky E, Burke SK, Dillon MA: RenaGel, a nonabsorbed calcium and aluminum-free phosphate-binder, lowers serum phosphorus and parathyroid hormone. Kidney Int 55:299–307, 1999.
245. Chertow GM, Burke SK, Dillon MA, et al: Long-term effects of sevelamer hydrochloride on the calcium × phosphate product and lipid profile of haemodialysis patients. Nephrol Dial Transplant 14:2907–2914, 1999.

CHAPTER 28

# Idiopathic Hypercalciuria and Renal Stone Disease

Charles Y. C. Pak, MD

The association of hypercalciuria with the formation of calcium-containing renal stones has been recognized for 6 decades.[1] The term *idiopathic hypercalciuria* was used to describe this condition initially because the exact cause for hypercalciuria was unknown.[2] Substantial progress has been made since then that mandates the aforementioned term be discarded.

In 1974, we suggested that hypercalciuric nephrolithiasis is heterogeneous in origin, comprised of three broad entities.[3] Named after the presumed primary disturbance, absorptive hypercalciuria is caused by an excessive intestinal absorption of calcium, renal hypercalciuria to an impaired renal tubular reabsorption of calcium, and reabsorptive hypercalciuria (primary hyperparathyroidism) to excessive bone reabsorption. All three forms have secondary disturbances that contribute to hypercalciuria. Absorptive hypercalciuria has a secondary renal leak of calcium from parathyroid suppression. In renal hypercalciuria and reabsorptive hypercalciuria of primary hyperparathyroidism, a high intestinal absorption of calcium is common from parathyroid hormone (PTH)-induced stimulation of calcitriol synthesis.

However, new questions have arisen, and controversy remains regarding hypercalciuric nephrolithiasis. This chapter reviews the current state of the field in the following order: pathogenetic importance of hypercalciuria in stone formation, pathogenesis of three forms of hypercalciuria, and diagnosis and medical management of hypercalciuric nephrolithiasis.

## PATHOGENETIC IMPORTANCE OF HYPERCALCIURIA IN STONE FORMATION

This question is considered with respect to the effect on stone formation of high calcium concentration in urine itself and the effect of high dietary intake of calcium.

### Effect of High Urinary Calcium Concentration

High urinary calcium concentration could cause crystallization of stone-forming calcium salts (i.e., calcium oxalate or phosphate) by increasing ionic activity of calcium and thus the saturation of calcium salts.[4] For the most common stone-forming salt (calcium oxalate), it was initially reported that the rise in urinary saturation plotted against the calcium concentration is not linear but reaches a plateau due to the complexation of oxalate by calcium.[5] In contrast, the saturation of calcium oxalate continued to rise with increasing oxalate concentration, reaching a much higher level. This report has led to the allegation that hyperoxaluria is more important than hypercalciuria in causing stone formation.

However, a re-examination of this study using a more reliable computer program for the calculation of urinary saturation has disclosed an equivalent effect of hypercalciuria and hyperoxaluria in raising the urinary saturation of calcium oxalate.[6] Within the range of concentrations encountered in urine, the increase in calcium concentration was equally effective as that of oxalate in enhancing urinary saturation of calcium oxalate (Fig. 28–1).

A high urinary calcium concentration could also contribute to stone formation by attenuating the inhibitor activity against the crystallization of stone-forming calcium salts.[7] Because most urinary "inhibitors" are negatively charged, calcium could bind and inactivate them.

### Effect of Dietary Calcium

The effect of dietary calcium on stone-forming propensity is complex. It depends on the physiologic state of calcium absorption, the hormonal and metabolic changes induced by absorbed calcium, and the interaction of calcium with other components in food.

**State of Calcium Absorption.** The amount of calcium excreted in urine is influenced by the state of calcium absorption. In subjects with normal intestinal calcium absorption, the absorbed calcium reaches a peak at a much lower level than in patients with absorptive hypercalciuria.[3] Thus, with increasing intake of calcium, the maximum amount of calcium excreted in urine is less than 300 mg/day in normal subjects whereas it could reach a value as high as 600 mg/day in patients with absorptive hypercalciuria. Thus, patients with absorptive hypercalciuria are at a greater risk of forming stones during a high calcium intake than are subjects with normal intestinal calcium absorption.

**Intestinal Adaptation.** Even when moderate hypercalciuria develops initially from high dietary intake of calcium, various hormonal changes normally ensue from absorbed calcium to cause a later fall in calcium

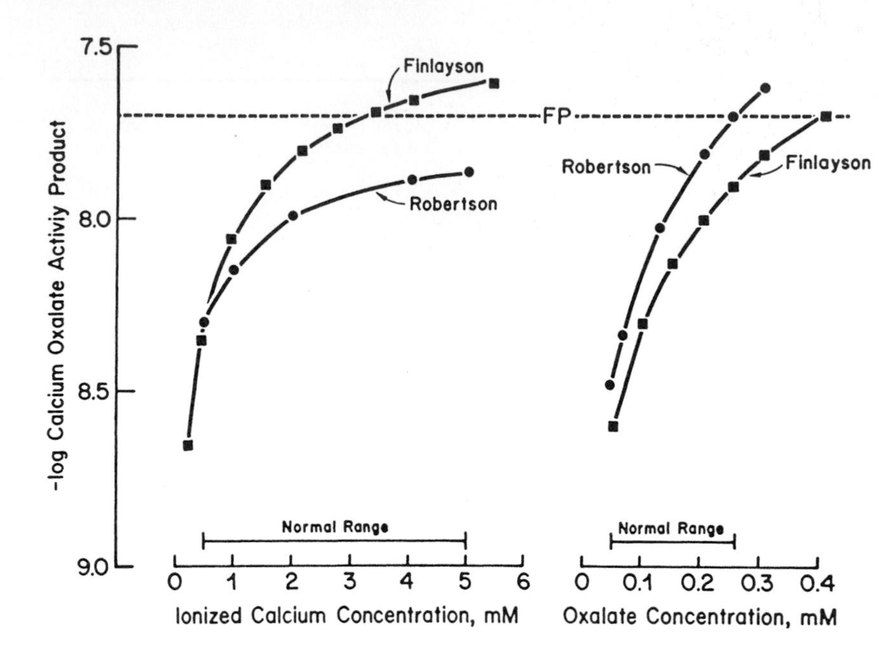


**FIGURE 28–1** ■ Effect of calcium and oxalate concentrations on the activity product of calcium oxalate in simulated urinary environment. The activity product, a measure of urinary saturation, was calculated by the method used by Robertson (used in the study by Nordin and associates, 1972) and by the more refined method used by Finlayson (1979). The formation product (FP, or limit of metastability) is shown by a *dashed horizontal line.* (From Pak CYC, Nicar M, Northcutt C: The definition of the mechanism of hypercalciuria is necessary for the treatment of recurrent stone formers. Contr Nephrol 33:136, 1982.)

excretion. Called "intestinal adaptation," this scheme implicates the suppression of parathyroid function by absorbed calcium, inhibiting calcitriol synthesis and reducing fractional (intestinal) calcium absorption[8] (Fig. 28–2). In normal subjects in whom intestinal adaptation is fully operational, urinary calcium may exceed 200 mg/day during the first week of calcium supplementation but fall below this level after 3 months of supplementation.[9] However, the intestinal adaptation may be impaired among patients with absorptive hypercalciuria, probably reflective of a primary disturbance in intestinal calcium transport. These patients generally respond to a high calcium intake by a sustained and marked increase in urinary calcium excretion[3] (Fig. 28–3). Thus, the risk of stone formation from a high calcium intake tends to be greater among patients with absorptive hypercalciuria than among normal subjects.

**Calcium-Food Interaction.** Orally administered calcium could interact with various components in food and modify urinary excretion of other risk factors. A high dietary content of calcium could lower urinary oxalate by binding oxalate in the intestinal tract.[10] Urinary phosphate excretion may also be reduced modestly by the binding of phosphate in the intestinal tract. These changes could oppose the stone-forming propensity of increased urinary calcium.

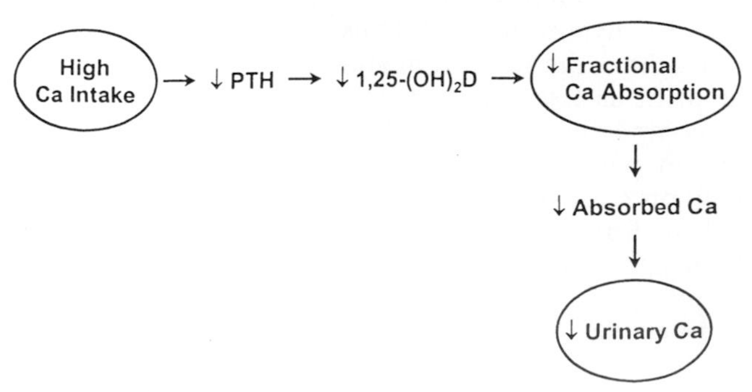


**FIGURE 28–2** ■ Intestinal adaptation following a high intake of calcium. PTH, parathyroid hormone.

The sequelae of calcium-food interaction depend on the composition of food and on the efficiency of calcium absorption. If dietary oxalate is restricted, little if any change in urinary oxalate might ensue from a higher intake of calcium. Among patients with absorptive hypercalciuria, the high calcium absorption might leave a low amount of calcium in the intestinal tract to bind oxalate.[11] Thus, relative hyperoxaluria might be found, especially during calcium restriction.

In recent epidemiologic studies, subjects in the higher quartiles of calcium intake were found to have a lower incidence of stones than in those in the lower quartiles.[12] Thus, it was inferred that a high dietary intake of calcium is protective against stone formation. However, this interpretation should be taken with caution. Subjects in the higher quartiles also took increased amounts of potential stone-protective dietary constituents, including more fluids, potassium (alkali), and magnesium.

## PATHOGENESIS OF HYPERCALCIURIA

### Absorptive Hypercalciuria

The primary abnormality in absorptive hypercalciuria is the intestinal hyperabsorption of calcium[3] (Fig. 28–4). The rise in circulating concentration of calcium from absorbed calcium enhances the renal filtered load of calcium and suppresses parathyroid function. Impaired renal tubular reabsorption of calcium from parathyroid suppression combines with increased filtered load to cause hypercalciuria.

The exact cause of the intestinal hyperabsorption of calcium is not known. Whatever theory is implicated, it must account for accompanying fasting hypercalciuria,

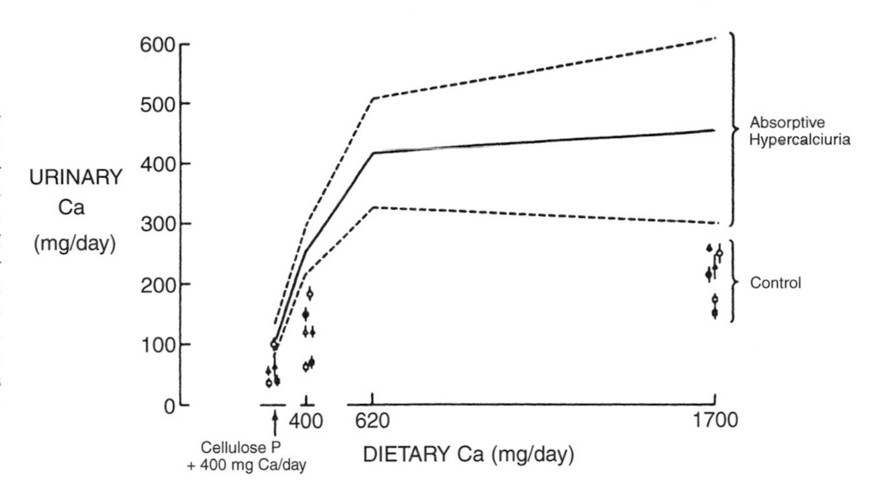


**FIGURE 28–3** ■ The dependence of urinary calcium excretion on calcium intake in patients with absorptive hypercalciuria and normal subjects. Although subjects were maintained on a metabolic diet containing 400 mg/day calcium, a lower calcium intake was produced by giving cellulose phosphate and higher intakes were produced by supplementing the diet with calcium gluconate. *Solid* and *dashed lines* indicate mean ± SD for patients with absorptive hypercalciuria. (From Pak CYC, Ohata M, Lawrence EC, et al: The hypercalciurias: causes, parathyroid functions and diagnostic criteria. J Clin Invest 54:387, 1974.)

bone loss, and familial disposition. Fasting hypercalciuria is frequently found among patients with severe absorptive hypercalciuria. It is not due to renal hypercalciuria, because parathyroid function is normal or suppressed, and inhibition of intestinal calcium absorption by sodium cellulose phosphate restores normal fasting urinary calcium without increasing serum PTH above the normal range. Moreover, the rise in fasting urinary calcium is appropriate with the decline in urinary cyclic adenosine monophosphate (AMP), indicating that the fasting hypercalciuria is acquired from parathyroid suppression.[13]

However, fasting hypercalciuria could be due in part to bone loss. Although radial shaft bone density is generally normal,[14] many patients with absorptive hypercalciuria present with low spinal bone density[15, 16] (Fig. 28–5). Thus, they may be particularly susceptible to cancellous bone loss. Few available studies of bone biopsy examination have disclosed low bone turnover.[17, 18]

Finally, approximately 50% of patients with absorptive hypercalciuria present with a positive family history of stones. The mode of inheritance appears to be autosomal dominant.[19, 20] The remaining patients, however, do not have a family history of stones. Moreover, many patients with hypercalciuria present with a history of dietary excesses, especially of animal proteins.[21] These findings suggest a possibility that absorptive hypercalciuria may occur as two major variants, genetic and acquired.

## THEORY 1. GENETIC ABSORPTIVE HYPERCALCIURIA

**Vitamin D Overproduction or Hypersensitivity.** Extensive work has been conducted on the potential etiologic role of vitamin D in absorptive hypercalciuria, because of the well-known stimulatory action of vitamin D on intestinal calcium absorption. In support of this theory, a high serum calcitriol concentration and enhanced rate of calcitriol synthesis have been reported in some patients with this condition.[22] A metabolic picture of absorptive hypercalciuria, consistent with upregulated state of calcitriol, has been reported

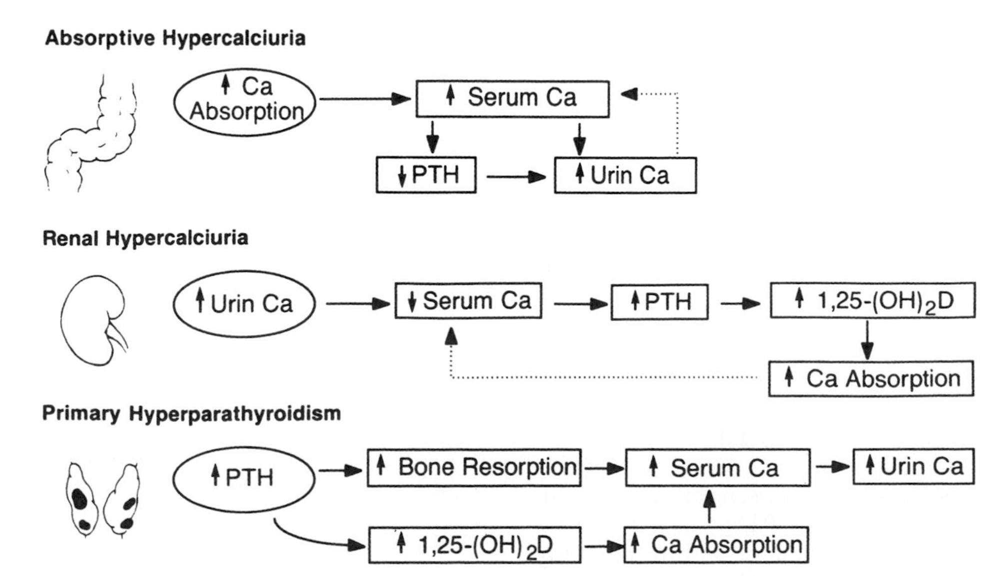


**FIGURE 28–4** ■ Pathogenetic schemes for the three main forms of hypercalciuria. (From Resnick M, Pak CYC: Urolithiasis. Philadelphia, WB Saunders, 1990, p 44.)

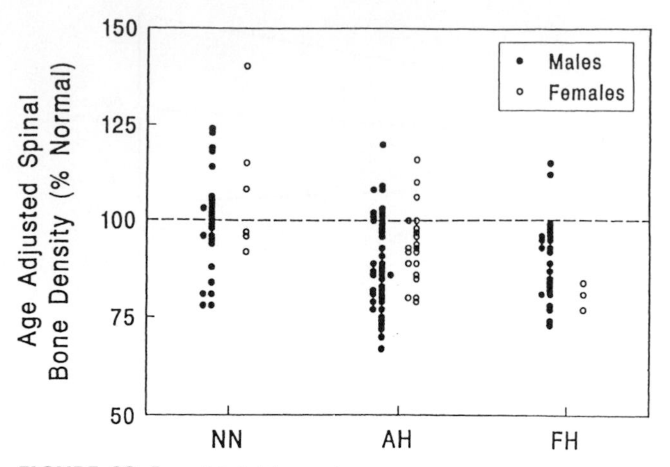


**FIGURE 28–5** ■ L2–L4 bone density in patients with absorptive hypercalciuria (AH), fasting hypercalciuria (FH), and normocalciuric nephrolithiasis (NN). Bone density is shown individually as age-adjusted values (expressed as a percentage of normal values) in men (*filled circles*) and women (*open circles*). (From Pietschmann F, Breslau NA, Pak CYC: Reduced vertebral bone density in hypercalciuric nephrolithiasis. J Bone Miner Res 7:1383–1388, 1992 with permission of the American Society for Bone and Mineral Research.)

in normal subjects after exogenous administration of 1,25-$(OH)_2$D.[23] Some workers have ascribed the vitamin D excess to hypophosphatemia from a renal phosphate leak.[24]

However, considerable evidence has accumulated that suggests that vitamin D is not involved. Serum 1,25-$(OH)_2$D concentration is not elevated in most patients,[25] and persistent hypophosphatemia is rare.[26] Treatment with steroids does not correct intestinal hyperabsorption of calcium in absorptive hypercalciuria,[27] whereas it restores normal intestinal absorption of calcium in sarcoidosis, a known state of vitamin D hypersensitivity. Thiazide does not affect calcium absorption in absorptive hypercalciuria, even though it reduces it in renal hypercalciuria, in which intestinal calcium absorption is increased from calcitriol excess of secondary hyperparathyroidism.[28] In many patients with absorptive hypercalciuria, a reduction in calcitriol synthesis by ketoconazole does not produce a reduction in calcium absorption.[29] In absorptive hypercalciuria, calcium absorption is high in the jejunum, but this is not the case in the ileum and colon.[30] In contrast, normal subjects treated with calcitriol display high calcium absorption at all three sites.[31] Finally, recent explorations using molecular biologic tools have failed to disclose any abnormality in vitamin D receptor genotype or in the cDNA sequence corresponding to the coding region of vitamin D receptor mRNA.[32]

**Unknown Gene Mutation.** Three kindreds with extensive familial history of stones were evaluated in a systematic study of autosomal genome-wide linkage analysis.[33] The probands had a metabolic picture of absorptive hypercalciuria. The phenotype was characterized by hypercalciuria, high intestinal calcium absorption, normal or low serum PTH, and low bone density. Analysis of key recombinants within the study families localized the gene to a 4.3-Mb region between markers D1S2681 (centromere) and D1S2815. Studies have revealed a mutation within a new gene mapping of this region. The functional role of the gene has not yet been elucidated.

## THEORY 2. ACQUIRED ABSORPTIVE HYPERCALCIURIA

Several schemes for the pathogenesis of absorptive hypercalciuria have been introduced. These schemes implicate abnormal phospholipid composition of cell membranes, prostaglandin excess, cytokines with bone bioactivity, increased renal mass, and acquired calcitriol excess. These schemes can be incorporated into an overall theory for acquired absorptive hypercalciuria originating from overconsumption of animal proteins (Fig. 28–6). After describing each scheme, both affirmative and negative data are reviewed.

**Abnormal Phospholipid Composition of Cell Membranes.** In patients with idiopathic calcium nephrolithiasis, the erythrocyte content of arachidonic acid was found to be high.[34] Believed to be partly due to a high animal protein diet, this disturbance was accompanied by reduced Na:K:2Cl cotransporter activity. It was suggested that the increased arachidonic acid content of cell membranes enhanced prostaglandin $E_2$ ($PGE_2$) synthesis, which in turn inhibited the cotransporter activity producing hypercalciuria. Moreover, arachidonic acid induced mRNA expression of bone resorbing cytokines (interleukin [IL]-1$\alpha$, IL-1$\beta$, as well as tumor necrosis factor [TNF]-$\alpha$) in vitro, explaining bone loss.[35]

**Prostaglandin Excess.** A diet high in animal proteins has been shown to stimulate the synthesis of $PGI_2$ and $PGE_2$.[36] The prostaglandin excess can then produce hypercalciuria by increasing the glomerular filtration rate and inhibiting Na:K:2Cl cotransporter activity. A high renal excretion of PGE has been reported in patients with idiopathic hypercalciuria.[37, 38] Intravenous infusion of $PGE_2$ enhanced urinary calcium excretion in monkeys,[39] and treatment with indomethacin or fish oil reduced calcium excretion in patients with idiopathic hypercalciuria.[34, 39–41] A high glomerular filtration rate and an enlarged renal mass have been

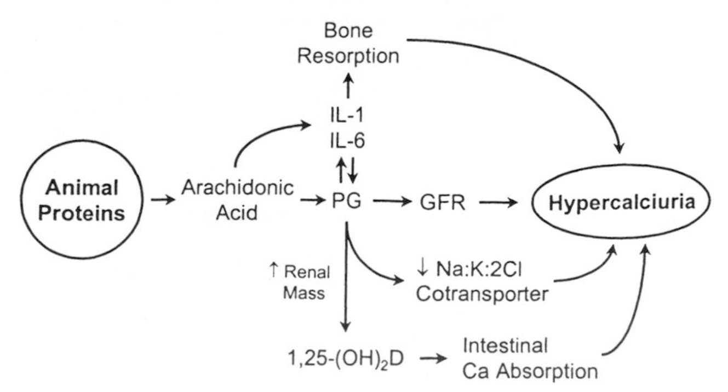


**FIGURE 28–6** ■ Pathogenetic scheme for acquired absorptive hypercalciuria.

reported among patients with idiopathic hypercalciuria.[21, 41]

Prostaglandin excess may also account for bone loss. Treatment of hypercalciuric patients with sulindac reduced urinary calcium and increased serum PTH.[42] Because this agent inhibits prostaglandin synthesis in bone but not in the kidneys, the results suggested that bone reabsorption was enhanced due to prostaglandin excess in hypercalciuric nephrolithiasis.

**Cytokines with Bone Bioactivity.** It was reported initially that IL-1 production by peripheral monocytes was enhanced in patients with fasting hypercalciuria but not in those with absorptive hypercalciuria with normal fasting urinary calcium.[16] In a later report, the monocytic synthesis of IL-1 and TNF-α was found to be high in the combined group of patients with hypercalciuric nephrolithiasis (with normal or high fasting urinary calcium).[43] The increased production of bone-reabsorbing cytokines correlated with the reduced spinal bone density.

IL-1 has been shown to stimulate $PGE_2$ synthesis.[44] Thus, cytokines may secondarily elicit the renal actions of prostaglandins enumerated earlier.

**Increased Renal Mass.** A high intake of animal proteins is common among patients with recurrent calcium nephrolithiasis. It has been suggested that such a diet could cause hyperfiltration and increased nephron mass by an unknown mechanism.[21] The latter would produce enhanced calcitriol synthesis. The ensuing intestinal hyperabsorption of calcium and increased filtered load would cause hypercalciuria. In support of this hypothesis, the glomerular filtration rate was shown to be greater than that of control subjects without stones. Moreover, serum calcitriol concentration correlated with the glomerular filtration rate.

**Enhanced Calcitriol Synthesis**. As previously discussed, the enhanced calcitriol synthesis has been ascribed to increased renal mass.[21] Moreover, $PGE_2$ has been reported to stimulate calcitriol synthesis.[45]

**Problems with the Aforementioned Schemes for Acquired Absorptive Hypercalciuria.** The aforementioned theory implicating animal protein excess requires further validation. Increased renal mass has been encountered in normocalciuric stone-formers as well as in those with hypercalciuria.[41] The scheme involving hyperfiltration is inconsistent with the reports that a progressive glomerular sclerosis develops from a long-term high-protein diet.[46] Because stone disease tends to be chronic, a reduced renal mass and impaired glomerular filtration rate would have been expected. Other groups have reported that the glomerular filtration rate does not differ between hypercalciuric and normocalciuric stone-formers.[3]

The stimulation of calcitriol synthesis by a high animal protein diet has not been directly shown. Instead, serum calcitriol concentration and intestinal calcium absorption are reduced or unaltered by an animal protein diet, compared with a vegetable protein diet.[47] If bone loss were due to the action of interleukins or TNF-α or PGE, osteoclastic reabsorption should have been increased. However, the histomorphometric analysis of biopsied bone in hypercalciuric nephrolithiasis has disclosed low bone turnover.

## Renal Hypercalciuria

The primary disturbance in renal hypercalciuria is believed to be the impairment in renal tubular reabsorption of calcium[48] (see Fig. 28–4). Some patients may display secondary stimulation of calcitriol synthesis and intestinal calcium absorption.

Although the exact cause remains elusive, the following studies support the presence of renal leak of calcium. First, some patients with hypercalciuric nephrolithiasis, albeit a minority, present with fasting hypercalciuria with secondary hyperparathyroidism. Thus, high fasting urinary calcium in the setting of normal serum calcium is accompanied by high serum PTH and/or urinary cyclic AMP and often by high serum $1,25\text{-}(OH)_2D$ and intestinal calcium absorption. The correction of fasting hypercalciuria (renal leak of calcium) by thiazide restores normal serum PTH, calcitriol, and intestinal calcium absorption.[28]

Second, patients with renal hypercalciuria show an exaggerated sodium excretion when thiazide is given to block sodium reabsorption in the distal tubule.[49] This finding, which is absent in those with absorptive hypercalciuria, indicates a defect in proximal tubular function. Third, the calciuric response to oral glucose ingestion is exaggerated in renal hypercalciuria, which is again indicative of an abnormality in proximal tubular function.[50]

## Resorptive Hypercalciuria (Primary Hyperparathyroidism)

Hypercalciuria is believed to be due primarily to an increased bone reabsorption from excessive production of PTH by abnormal parathyroid tissue (see Fig. 28–4). There is a secondary intestinal hyperabsorption of calcium from the PTH-dependent stimulation of calcitriol synthesis.

The association of calcium-containing renal stones with primary hyperparathyroidism has long been recognized. However, a much smaller percentage of patients with renal stones are diagnosed with this condition today than 4 decades ago. This trend probably reflects an earlier detection from routine analysis of serum calcium and the institution of treatment before the complication of stones develops.

Despite much progress made in the stone field, it is still unknown why some patients with primary hyperparathyroidism form stones whereas others do not. It was suggested that the biochemical presentation of stone-forming patients differs from those with bone disease. Compared with the latter group, the stone-forming group was reported to have a higher serum $1,25\text{-}(OH)_2D$, intestinal calcium absorption, and urinary calcium.[51, 52] However, this finding was not confirmed.[53] In preliminary reports, urinary inhibitors (citrate and pyrophosphate) have been shown to be lower in stone-forming patients with primary hyperparathyroidism compared with their non–stone-forming counterparts.

# DIAGNOSTIC CONSIDERATIONS

When differentiating the various forms of hypercalciuria associated with nephrolithiasis, the following tests are required or optional. Required tests are stone analysis, serum multichannel analysis, serum PTH, and 24-hour urinary calcium for a complete stone risk analysis.[54] Optional tests are fasting urinary calcium and bone densitometry.[55, 56]

**TABLE 28–1.** Diagnostic Criteria of Three Forms of Hypercalciuria

| | Absorptive Hypercalciuria | Renal Hypercalciuria | Resorptive Hypercalciuria |
|---|---|---|---|
| Serum | | | |
| Calcium | Normal | Normal | High |
| Phosphorus | Normal | Normal | Normal/low |
| PTH | Normal/low | High | High |
| Urinary | | | |
| Ca (24-hr) | High | High | High |
| Ca (fasting) | Normal/high | High | High |
| Bone density | | | |
| Radial shaft | Normal | Low | Low |
| Lumbar spine | Normal/low | Normal/low | Normal/low |

## Required Tests

**Stone Analysis.** Whenever a stone is recovered, it should be analyzed. In primary hyperparathyroidism, the calcium phosphate (hydroxyapatite) fraction constitutes a large portion of the stone. In contrast, the predominant phase is calcium oxalate in absorptive and renal hypercalciurias.

**Serum Tests.** Serum calcium concentration is invariably high in primary hyperparathyroidism but normal in absorptive and renal hypercalciurias. However, following a high calcium intake, serum calcium may be high normal or slightly elevated in absorptive hypercalciuria. Serum phosphate concentration is often low normal or low in primary hyperparathyroidism. Although serum phosphate may also be reduced in absorptive and renal hypercalciurias, this reduction tends to be transient with a spontaneous rise in serum phosphate on repeat determination.[26] Serum PTH is high in primary hyperparathyroidism and renal hypercalciuria, but it is normal or low normal in absorptive hypercalciuria.

**24-Hour Urine Tests.** Urinary calcium is greater than 250 mg/day or 4 mg/kg/day on a random diet and more than 200 mg/day on a diet restricted in calcium and sodium. In primary hyperparathyroidism, urinary pH is high normal and slightly higher than in absorptive and renal hypercalciurias. Hyperuricosuria and hypocitraturia often coexist with hypercalciuria.

## Optional Tests

**Fasting Urinary Calcium.** Fasting urinary calcium is high in primary hyperparathyroidism and renal hypercalciuria. It may also be high in severe absorptive hypercalciuria. Thus, fasting hypercalciuria alone is not sufficient to differentiate the three forms of hypercalciuria. In primary hyperparathyroidism, fasting hypercalciuria is accompanied by hypercalcemia and high serum PTH. The diagnosis of renal hypercalciuria requires the presence of high serum PTH and normocalcemia, besides fasting hypercalciuria.[57] Fasting hypercalciuria with normal serum calcium and PTH indicates severe absorptive hypercalciuria.[17]

**Bone Density.** Radial shaft bone density is often depressed in primary hyperparathyroidism and renal hypercalciuria.[14] Spinal bone density is moderately decreased in severe absorptive hypercalciuria.[15]

Diagnostic features of the different forms of hypercalciuria are compared in Table 28–1.

# MANAGEMENT OF HYPERCALCIURIC NEPHROLITHIASIS

## Conservative Management

All patients should be offered conservative measures of high fluid intake and dietary modification.

**High Fluid Intake.** A sufficient amount of fluids should be ingested to ensure a urine output of at least 2 L/day. In the absence of excessive sweating and diarrhea, this goal may be achieved by drinking about 3 L (10 glassfuls) of fluids distributed throughout the day. All types of fluids are acceptable, except for the avoidance of oxalate-rich tea and a moderate restriction of calcium-rich milk. The goal of high fluid ingestion is to dilute the urinary concentration of stone-forming constituents and thus reduce the urinary saturation of stone-forming calcium salts.[58] The value of high fluid intake in inhibiting stone formation has been shown in a placebo-controlled randomized trial.[59]

**Sodium Restriction.** A high sodium diet increases the risk of calcium stone formation, by increasing urinary calcium and reducing urinary citrate[60] (Fig. 28–7). Urinary calcium increases by about 40 to 50 mg/day for every increment in urinary sodium of 100 mEq/day. Urinary citrate decreases modestly, probably from sodium-induced bicarbonaturia. The rise in urinary sodium increases urinary saturation of sodium urate. These effects increase urinary saturation and the propensity for the crystallization of calcium salts. For these reasons, sodium restriction (100 mEq/day or 1 teaspoonful/day) is recommended.

**Avoidance of Oxalate-Rich Foods.** Oxalate-rich foods include dark greens (e.g., spinach), nuts, tea, and chocolate. Despite varying bioavailability,[61] their ingestion could increase urinary oxalate. The restriction of such foods should abrogate the mild increase in oxalate excretion occurring among patients with

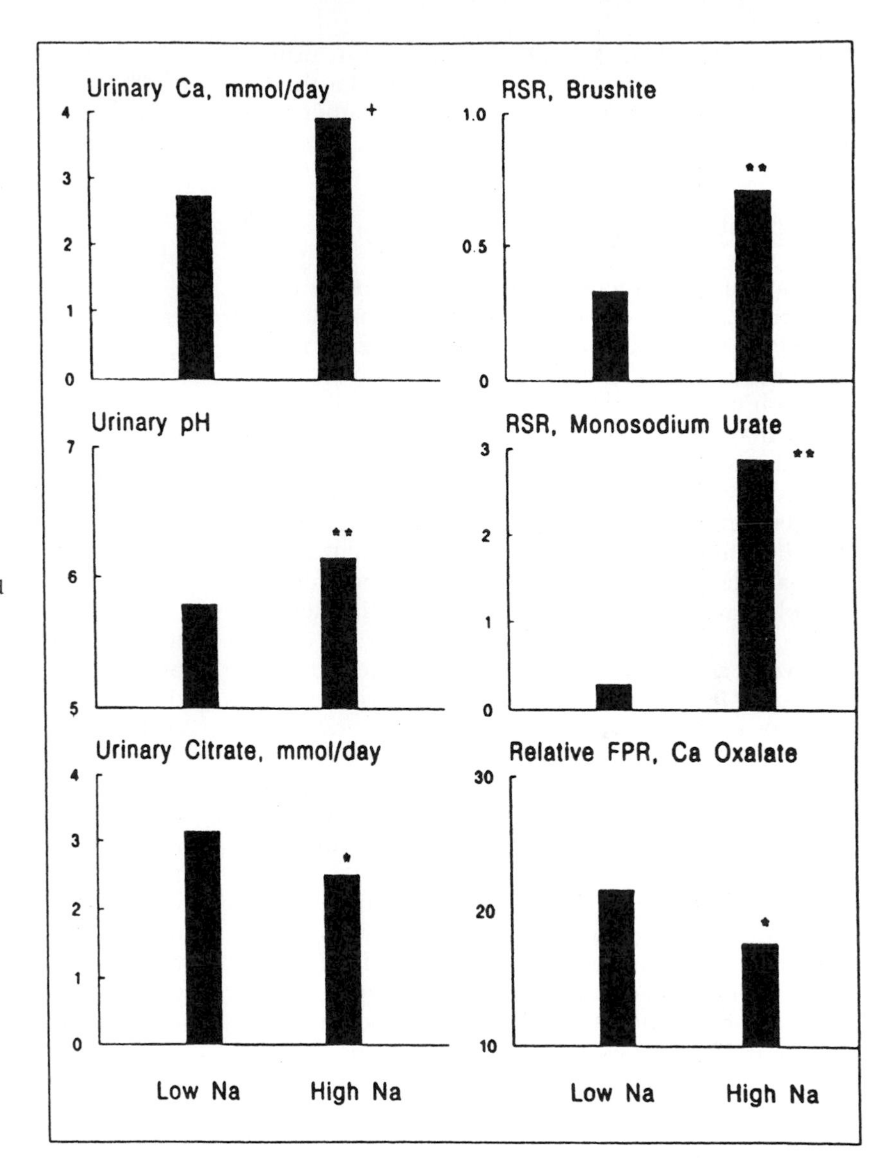


**FIGURE 28–7** ■ Effect of oral sodium load on urinary biochemistry and physicochemistry.

absorptive hypercalciuria[11] and keep urinary oxalate in the normal range.

**Increased Intake of Citrus Fruits.** The renal effects of potassium-rich citrus fruits (e.g., orange, grapefruit, and cranberry) resemble those of potassium citrate with an excess of citric acid.[62] One liter of orange juice, for example, contains 55 mEq potassium and 130 mEq of citric acid. Whereas both potassium and citrate are almost completely absorbed from the gastrointestinal tract, citrate is metabolized in vivo but potassium is not. Thus, an alkali load is delivered, resulting in an increased urinary citrate excretion. Moreover, the renal excretion of absorbed citrate that escapes oxidation in vivo adds to enhanced citrate excretion.

In contrast, potassium-poor citrus fruits (e.g., lemon and lime) do not confer an alkali load. Thus, the induced rise in urinary citrate is much less prominent than that produced by potassium-rich citrus fruits, because it occurs only by the renal excretion of a small amount of absorbed citrate that escapes oxidation.

Citrate is a known inhibitor of the crystallization of stone-forming calcium salts.[63] Thus, adequate amounts of citrus fruits, particularly as potassium-rich products, should be ingested.

**Moderate Calcium Restriction.** There has been a growing sentiment that calcium restriction may actually exaggerate stone formation and should not be undertaken among patients with recurrent formation of calcium-containing renal stones. This contention is based largely on epidemiologic studies showing that stone formation rate is inversely related to calcium intake.[13] The protective effect of calcium was ascribed to the reduction in urinary oxalate excretion from binding of oxalate by calcium in the intestinal tract. The low bone density frequently encountered in stone-forming patients was illustrated as evidence of the harmful effect of dietary calcium restriction.

The aforementioned comments may apply to stone-forming patients with normal intestinal calcium absorption and normocalciuria, but not to those with absorptive hypercalciuria. As described earlier, patients with absorptive hypercalciuria display a marked and sustained increase in urinary calcium following a high calcium intake[3] (see Fig. 28–3). The avoidance of oxalate-rich foods can largely abolish the rise in urinary oxalate from dietary calcium restriction. Lastly, low bone density may be genetic in origin rather than acquired.[33]

## Treatment with Drugs

In patients with metabolic disturbances such as hypercalciuria, conservative management alone may be insufficient to prevent a recurrence of stone formation. Thus, besides conservative management, treatment with drugs designed to correct metabolic disturbances may be required. The importance of drug treatment is shown by a superior inhibition of stone formation with drug treatment versus placebo among patients maintained on conservative management.[64] The following discussion considers drugs that are currently available for the treatment of hypercalciuric nephrolithiasis as well as those that are under development.

**Thiazide and Related Diuretics.** Thiazide diuretic is widely used for the control of hypercalciuric nephrolithiasis because of its well-known hypocalciuric action.[65] Thiazide is ideally indicated for renal hypercalciuria. By correcting renal calcium leak, it restores normal serum PTH, calcitriol, and intestinal calcium absorption.[28] Thus, it produces a sustained reduction in urinary calcium.

In absorptive hypercalciuria, thiazide is also effective in controlling hypercalciuria during the first 2 years of treatment.[66] However, beyond 2 years of treatment, urinary calcium returns to the initial hypercalciuric range in some patients. This loss of hypocalciuric action has been ascribed to the persistence of hyperabsorption of calcium owing to the failure of thiazide to reduce calcium absorption.

Some evidence exists that chlorthalidone[67] and indapamide[68] produce a sustained reduction in urinary calcium among patients with hypercalciuric nephrolithiasis, some of whom must have had absorptive hypercalciuria. The effect of these drugs on intestinal calcium absorption has not been fully investigated.

During the use of these diuretics, hypocitraturia may develop from induced hypokalemia.[69]

**Potassium Citrate.** Potassium citrate may reduce urinary calcium, probably by the calcium-sparing effect of alkali and potassium as opposed to sodium.[63] Its alkali load increases urinary pH and citrate (Fig. 28–8). The renal clearance of absorbed citrate escaping oxidation adds to the rise in urinary citrate (albeit a minor portion). The rise in urinary pH and citrate increases the amount of dissociated citrate to complex calcium, thus reducing ionic calcium concentration. This effect of potassium citrate attenuates the increase in the saturation of calcium oxalate resulting from hypercalciuria. Moreover, the rise in urinary citrate directly inhibits the crystallization of stone-forming calcium salts by retarding spontaneous nucleation, crystal agglomeration,[70] and heterogenous nucleation of calcium oxalate by sodium urate.

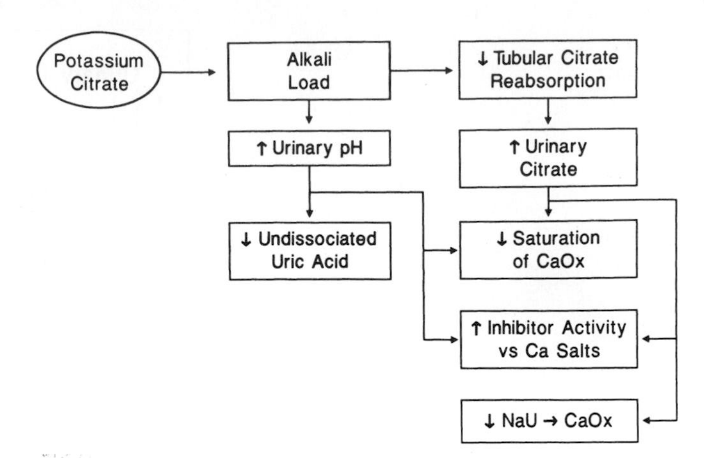


FIGURE 28–8 ■ Physiologic and physicochemical actions of potassium citrate. (From Resnick M, Pak CYC: Urolithiasis. Philadelphia, WB Saunders, 1990, p 98.)

**Allopurinol.** By reducing urinary uric acid, allopurinol was believed to retard urate-induced crystallization of calcium oxalate. This rationale formed the basis for the use of allopurinol among patients with hyperuricosuric calcium oxalate nephrolithiasis.[71] In a placebo-controlled randomized trial, allopurinol was shown to reduce stone formation in normocalciuric patients with hyperuricosuria.[72] However, the inhibitory effect was modest, with a significant difference in survival (stone-free rate) between allopurinol and placebo revealed only during the third year of treatment but not during the first 2 years. No data are available on the use of allopurinol in stone-forming subjects with hypercalciuria.

**Combined Use of Thiazide with Potassium Citrate.** When thiazide is used to treat hypercalciuric nephrolithiasis, it is advisable to co-administer potassium citrate.[73] Thiazide alone frequently causes hypokalemia, which may then reduce urinary citrate excretion by producing intracellular acidosis. Potassium chloride supplementation may avert hypokalemia and the fall in urinary citrate. However, the same amount of potassium citrate will not only prevent hypokalemia but will also increase urinary citrate to above the pretreatment value.[69]

The aforementioned drugs are compared with respect to their mode of action in Table 28–2.

**Drugs Under Development.** Slow-release neutral potassium phosphate (UroPhos-K) represents a physiologically more meaningful treatment of absorptive hypercalciuria than thiazide.[74] UroPhos-K reduces intestinal calcium absorption by inhibiting calcitriol synthesis and by binding calcium in the intestinal tract. Thus, a sustained reduction in urinary calcium is achieved in absorptive hypercalciuria with this drug, unlike with thiazide.

Moreover, this treatment reduces the urinary saturation of calcium oxalate (from reduced urinary calcium) and enhances the inhibitor activity against calcium oxalate crystallization (from increased urinary pyrophosphate and citrate).[75] However, the urinary saturation of calcium phosphate is unchanged or increased (from the more prominent increase in urinary

**TABLE 28–2.** Mode of Action of Drugs for Hypercalciuric Nephrolithiasis

| | Thiazide | Allopurinol | Potassium Citrate | Thiazide + Potassium Citrate |
|---|---|---|---|---|
| Urinary | | | | |
| Ca | Decrease | No change | Transient ↓ | Transient ↓ |
| pH | No change | No change | Increase | Increase |
| Citrate | Decrease | No change | Increase | Increase |
| Uric acid | No change | Decrease | No change | No change |
| Urinary saturation | | | | |
| Ca oxalate | Decrease | No change | Decrease | Decrease |
| Uric acid | No change | Decrease | Decrease | Decrease |
| Urate-induced Ca oxalate crystallization | No change | Decrease | Decrease | Decrease |
| Inhibitor activity against Ca oxalate | Decrease | No change | Increase | Increase |

phosphate than the decline in urinary calcium). No placebo-controlled randomized trial has been conducted to test the efficacy of UroPhos-K against recurrent stone formation.

At the same dose of potassium, potassium-magnesium citrate (Relyte) has a greater inhibitor activity against calcium oxalate crystallization compared with potassium citrate, owing to a more prominent citraturic and alkalinizing effect.[76] Moreover, Relyte increases urinary magnesium, whereas potassium citrate does not. When used in conjunction with thiazide, Relyte is effective in correcting hypokalemia and hypomagnesemia.[77] A preliminary trial indicated that Relyte alone may be effective in preventing stone formation in hypercalciuric nephrolithiasis.[78]

**Recommended Treatment.** Until UroPhos-K and Relyte become available, the first-line treatment is thiazide with potassium citrate.[56] Patients might be begun on hydrochlorothiazide 50 mg/day and potassium citrate 20 mEq twice per day (with meals). The dose of potassium citrate should be adjusted in order to maintain urinary citrate above 500 mg/day.

When thiazide is no longer effective in reducing urinary calcium, it might be substituted by indapamide 4 mg/day. When neither thiazide nor indapamide can correct hypercalciuria, potassium phosphate (currently available as a rapid release preparation) or bisphosphonate (e.g., alendronate 10 mg/day) might be considered.

## REFERENCES


1. Flocks RH: Calcium and phosphorus excretion in the urine of patients with renal or ureteral calculi. JAMA 113:1466–1471, 1939.
2. Albright F, Henneman P, Benedict PH, et al: Idiopathic hypercalciuria: A preliminary report. Proc R Soc Med 46:1077–1081, 1953.
3. Pak CYC, Ohata M, Lawrence EC, et al: The hypercalciurias: Causes, parathyroid functions and diagnostic criteria. J Clin Invest 54:387–400, 1974.
4. Pak CYC, Holt K: Nucleation and growth of brushite and calcium oxalate in urine of stone-formers. Metabolism 25:665–673, 1976.
5. Nordin BEC, Peacock M, Wilkinson R: Hypercalciuria and stone disease. In McIntyre I, Saunders WB (eds): Clinics in Endocrinology and Metabolism, vol I. Philadelphia, WB Saunders, 1972, pp 169–183.
6. Pak CYC, Nicar M, Northcutt C: The definition of the mechanism of hypercalciuria is necessary for the treatment of recurrent stone formers. In Berlyne GM, Giovannetti S, Thomas S (eds): Contributions to Nephrology, vol 33. Basel, Karger, 1982, pp 136–151.
7. Zerwekh JE, Hwang TIS, Poindexter J, et al: Modulation by calcium of inhibitor activity of naturally occurring urinary inhibitors. Kidney Int 33:1005–1008, 1988.
8. Norman DA, Fordtran JA, Brinkley LJ, et al: Jejunal and ileal adaptation to alteration in dietary calcium: Changes in calcium and magnesium absorption and pathogenetic role of parathyroid hormone and 1,25-dihydroxyvitamin D. J Clin Invest 67:1599–1603, 1981.
9. Sakhaee K, Baker S, Zerwekh J, et al: Limited risk of kidney stone formation during long-term calcium citrate supplementation in non-stone-forming subjects. J Urol 152:324–327, 1994.
10. Jaeger P, Portmann L, Jacquet A-F, et al: Influence of the calcium content of the diet on the incidence of mild hyperoxaluria in idiopathic renal stone formers. Am J Nephrol 5:40–44, 1985.
11. Hodgkinson A: Evidence for increased oxalate absorption in patients with calcium-containing renal stones. Clin Sci Mol Med 54:291–294, 1978.
12. Curhan GC, Willett WC, Rimm EB, et al: A prospective study of dietary calcium and other nutrients and the risk of symptomatic kidney stones. N Engl J Med 328:833–838, 1993.
13. Pak CYC, Galosy RA: Fasting urinary calcium and adenosine 3',5'-monophosphate: A discriminant analysis for the identification of renal and absorptive hypercalciuria. J Clin Endocrinol Metab 48:260–265, 1979.
14. Lawoyin S, Sismilich S, Browne R, et al: Bone mineral content in patients with primary hyperparathyroidism, osteoporosis, and calcium urolithiasis. Metabolism 28:1250–1254, 1979.
15. Pietschmann F, Breslau NA, Pak CYC: Reduced vertebral bone density in hypercalciuric nephrolithiasis. J Bone Miner Res 7:1383–1388, 1992.
16. Pacifici R, Rothstein M, Rifas L, et al: Increased monocyte interleukin-1 activity and decreased vertebral bone density in patients with fasting idiopathic hypercalciuria. J Clin Endocrinol Metab 71:138–145, 1990.
17. Bordier P, Ryckewart A, Gueris J, et al: On the pathogenesis of the so-called idiopathic hypercalciuria. Am J Med 63:398–409, 1977.
18. Malluche HH, Tschoepe W, Ritz E, et al: Abnormal bone histology in idiopathic hypercalciuria. J Clin Endocrinol Metab 50:654–658, 1980.
19. Coe FL, Parks JH, Moore ES: Familial idiopathic hypercalciuria. N Engl J Med 300:337–340, 1979.
20. Pak CYC, McGuire J, Peterson R, et al: Familial absorptive hypercalciuria in a large kindred. J Urol 126:717–719, 1981.
21. Hess B, Ackermann D, Essig M, et al: Renal mass and serum calcitriol in male idiopathic calcium renal stone formers: Role of protein intake. J Clin Endocrinol Metab 80:1916–1921, 1995.
22. Insogna KL, Broadus AE, Dreyer BE, et al: Elevated production rate of 1,25-dihydroxyvitamin D in patients with absorptive hypercalciuria. J Clin Endocrinol Metab 61:490–495, 1985.
23. Broadus AE, Erickson SB, Gertner JM, et al: An experimental human model of 1,25-dihydroxyvitamin D-mediated hypercalciuria. J Clin Endocrinol Metab 59:202–206, 1984.

24. Gray RW, Wilz DR, Caldas AE, et al: The importance of phosphate in regulating plasma 1,25-$(OH)_2$-vitamin D levels in humans: Studies in healthy subjects, in calcium-stone formers and in patients with primary hyperparathyroidism. J Clin Endocrinol Metab 45:299–306, 1977.
25. Kaplan RA, Haussler MR, Deftos LF, et al: The role of 1,25-dihydroxyvitamin D in the mediation of intestinal hyperabsorption of calcium in primary hyperparathyroidism and absorptive hypercalciuria. J Clin Invest 59:756–760, 1977.
26. Barilla DE, Zerwekh JE, Pak CYC: A critical evaluation of the role of phosphate in the pathogenesis of absorptive hypercalciuria. Miner Electrolyte Metab 2:302–309, 1979.
27. Zerwekh JE, Pak CYC, Kaplan RA, et al: Pathogenetic role of 1,25-dihydroxyvitamin D in sarcoidosis and absorptive hypercalciuria: Different response to prednisolone therapy. J Clin Endocrinol Metab 51:381–386, 1980.
28. Zerwekh JE, Pak CYC: Selective effect of thiazide therapy on serum 1,25-dihydroxyvitamin D and intestinal calcium absorption in renal and absorptive hypercalciurias. Metabolism 29: 13–17, 1980.
29. Breslau NA, Preminger GM, Adams BV, et al: Use of ketoconazole to probe the pathogenetic importance of 1,25-$(OH)_2D$ in absorptive hypercalciuria. J Clin Endocrinol Metab 75:1446–1452, 1992.
30. Brannan PG, Morawski S, Pak CYC: Selective jejunal hyperabsorption of calcium in absorptive hypercalciuria. Am J Med 66: 425–428, 1979.
31. Vergne-Marini P, Parker TF, Pak CYC, et al: Jejunal and ileal calcium absorption in patients with chronic renal disease: Effect of 1-hydroxycholecalciferol. J Clin Invest 57:861–866, 1976.
32. Zerwekh JE, Hughes MR, Reed BY, et al: Evidence for normal vitamin D receptor messenger ribonucleic acid and genotype in absorptive hypercalciuria. J Clin Endocrinol Metab 80:2960–2965, 1995.
33. Reed BY, Heller HJ, Gitomer WL, et al: Mapping of a common gene defect in absorptive hypercalciuria and idiopathic osteoporosis to chromosome 1q23.3-q24. J Clin Endocrinol Metab 84: 3907–3913, 1999.
34. Baggio B, Gambaro G, Zambon S, et al: Anomalous phospholipid n-6 polyunsaturated fatty acid composition in idiopathic calcium nephrolithiasis. J Am Soc Nephrol 7:613–620, 1996.
35. Priante G, Bordin L, Anglani F, et al: Arachidonic acid stimulates bone IL-1 and TNF-α mRNA expression. In Rodgers AL, Hibbert BE, Hess B, et al (eds): Urolithiasis 2000. Capetown, University of Cape Town Rodebosch, 2000, pp 259–260.
36. Kontessis P, Jones S, Dodds R, et al: Renal, metabolic and hormonal responses to ingestion of animal and vegetable proteins. Kidney Int 38:136–144, 1990.
37. Henriquez-La Roche C, Rodriguez-Iturbe B, Herrera J, et al: Increased urinary excretion of prostaglandin E in patients with idiopathic hypercalciuria. Clin Sci 75:581–587, 1988.
38. Houser M, Zimmerman B, Davidman M, et al: Idiopathic hypercalciuria associated with hyperreninemia and high urinary prostaglandin E. Kidney Int 26:176–182, 1984.
39. Buck AC, Sampson WF, Lote CJ, et al: The influence of renal prostaglandins on glomerular filtration rate (GFR) and calcium excretion in urolithiasis. J Urol 53:485–491, 1981.
40. Buck AC, Davies RL, Harrison T: The protective role of eicosapentaenoic acid (EPA) in the pathogenesis of nephrolithiasis. J Urol 146:188–194, 1991.
41. Buck AC, McLeod MA, Sampson WF: The role of renal eicosanoid metabolism in the pathogenesis of renal stone formation. In Rodgers AL, Hibbert BE, Hess B, et al (eds): Urolithiasis 2000. Capetown, University of Cape Town Rodebosch, 2000, pp 640–645.
42. Filipponi P, Mannarelli C, Pacifici R, et al: Evidence for a prostaglandin-mediated bone resorptive mechanism in subjects with fasting hypercalciuria. Calcif Tissue Int 43:61–66, 1988.
43. Weisinger JR, Alonzo E, Bellorin-Font E, et al: Possible role of cytokines on the bone mineral loss in idiopathic hypercalciuria. Kidney Int 49:244–250, 1996.
44. Dinarello CA, Cannon JG, Mier JW, et al: Multiple biological activities of human recombinant interleukin 1. J Clin Invest 77: 1734–1739, 1986.
45. Kurokawa K: Calcium-regulating hormones and the kidney. Kidney Int 32:760–771, 1987.
46. Brenner B, Meyer TE, Hostetter TH: Dietary protein intake and the progressive nature of kidney disease: The role of haemodynamically mediated glomerular injury in the pathogenesis of progressive glomerular sclerosis in aging, renal ablation and intrinsic renal disease. N Engl J Med 307:652–659, 1982.
47. Breslau NA, Brinkley L, Hill KD, et al: Relationship of animal protein-rich diet to kidney stone formation and calcium metabolism. J Clin Endocrinol Metab 66:140–146, 1988.
48. Coe FL, Canterbury JM, Firpo JJ, et al: Evidence for secondary hyperparathyroidism in idiopathic hypercalciuria. J Clin Invest 52:134–142, 1973.
49. Sakhaee K, Nicar MJ, Brater DC, et al: Exaggerated natriuretic and calciuric responses to hydrochlorothiazide in renal hypercalciuria but not in absorptive hypercalciuria. J Clin Endocrinol Metab 61:825–829, 1985.
50. Barilla DE, Townsend J, Pak CYC: An exaggerated augmentation of renal calcium excretion following oral glucose ingestion in patients with renal hypercalciuria. Invest Urol 15:486–488, 1978.
51. Broadus AE, Horst RL, Lang R, et al: The importance of circulating 1,25-dihydroxyvitamin D in the pathogenesis of hypercalciuria and renal-stone formation in primary hyperparathyroidism. N Engl J Med 302:421–426, 1980.
52. Patron P, Gardin J-P, Paillard M: Renal mass and reserve of vitamin D: Determinants of plasma 1,25$(OH)_2D_3$ in primary hyperparathyroidism. Kidney Int 31:1174–1180, 1987.
53. Pak CYC, Nicar MJ, Peterson R, et al: A lack of unique pathophysiological background for nephrolithiasis of primary hyperparathyroidism. J Clin Endocrinol Metab 53:536–542, 1981.
54. Pak CYC, Peterson R, Sakhaee K, et al: Correction of hypocitraturia and prevention of stone formation by combined thiazide and potassium citrate therapy in thiazide-unresponsive hypercalciuric nephrolithiasis. Am J Med 79:284–288, 1985.
55. Pak CYC, Griffith DP, Menon M, et al: Urolithiasis. Curr Pract Med 4:13.3–13.4, 1996.
56. Pak CYC: Medical management of nephrolithiasis: A new simplified approach for general practice. Am J Med Sci 313:215–218, 1997.
57. Pak CYC: Physiological basis for absorptive and renal hypercalciurias. Am J Physiol 237:F415–F423, 1979.
58. Pak CYC, Sakhaee K, Crowther C, et al: Evidence justifying a high fluid intake in treatment of nephrolithiasis. Ann Intern Med 93:36–39, 1980.
59. Borghi L, Meschi T, Amato F, et al: Urinary volume, water and recurrences in idiopathic calcium nephrolithiasis: A 5-year randomized prospective study. J Urol 155:839–843, 1996.
60. Sakhaee K, Harvey JA, Padalino PK, et al: Potential role of salt abuse on the risk of kidney stone formation. J Urol 150: 310–312, 1991.
61. Brinkley L, McGuire J, Gregory J, et al: Bioavailability of oxalate in foods. Urology 17:534–538, 1981.
62. Wabner CL, Pak CYC: Effect of orange juice consumption on urinary stone risk factors. J Urol 149:1405–1408, 1993.
63. Pak CYC: Citrate and renal calculi. Miner Electrolyte Metab 20: 371–377, 1994.
64. Barcelo P, Wuhl O, Servitge E, et al: Randomized double-blind study of potassium citrate in idiopathic hypocitraturic calcium nephrolithiasis. J Urol 150:1761–1764, 1993.
65. Yendt ER, Guay GF, Garcia DA: The use of thiazide in the prevention of renal calculi. Can Med Assoc J 102:614–620, 1970.
66. Preminger GM, Pak CYC: Eventual attenuation of hypocalciuric response to hydrochlorothiazide in absorptive hypercalciuria. J Urol 137:1104–1109, 1987.
67. Bushinsky DA, Favus MJ, Coe FL: Mechanism of chronic hypocalciuria with chlorthalidone: Reduced calcium absorption. Am J Physiol 247:F746–F752, 1984.
68. Borghi L, Meschi T, Guerra A, et al: Randomized prospective study of a nonthiazide diuretic, indapamide, in preventing calcium stone recurrences. J Cardiovasc Pharmacol 22:S78–S86, 1993.
69. Nicar MJ, Peterson R, Pak CYC: Use of potassium citrate as potassium supplement during thiazide therapy of calcium nephrolithiasis. J Urol 131:430–433, 1984.
70. Kok DJ, Papapoulos SE, Bijvoet OLM: Excessive crystal agglomeration with low citrate excretion. Lancet 10:1056–1058, 1986.
71. Coe FL, Raisen L: Allopurinol treatment of uric-acid disorders in calcium stone formers. Lancet 1:129–131, 1973.

72. Ettinger B, Tang A, Citron JT, et al: Randomized trial of allopurinol in the prevention of calcium oxalate calculi. N Engl J Med 315:1386–1389, 1986.
73. Pak CYC, Skurla C, Harvey J: Graphic display of urinary stone risk factors for renal stone formation. J Urol 134:867–870, 1985.
74. Heller HJ, Reza-Albarran AA, Breslau NA, et al: Sustained reduction in urinary calcium during long-term treatment with Uro-Phos-K (slow-release neutral potassium phosphate) in absorptive hypercalciuria. J Urol 159:1451–1456, 1998.
75. Breslau NA, Padalino P, Kok DJ, et al: Physicochemical effects of a new slow-release potassium phosphate preparation (Uro-Phos-K) in absorptive hypercalciuria. J Bone Miner Res 10:394–400, 1995.
76. Pak CYC, Koenig K, Khan R, et al: Physicochemical action of potassium-magnesium citrate in nephrolithiasis. J Bone Miner Res 7:281–285, 1992.
77. Wuermser LA, Reilly C, Poindexter JR, et al: Potassium magnesium citrate versus potassium chloride in thiazide-induced hypokalemia. Kidney Int 57:607–612, 1999.
78. Ettinger B, Pak CYC, Citron JT, et al: Potassium magnesium citrate is an effective prophylaxis against recurrent calcium oxalate nephrolithiasis. J Urol 158:2069–2073, 1997.

# Index

Note: Page numbers followed by the letter f refer to figures and those followed by t refer to tables.

ISBN 0-7216-8956-6